T0256073

Essentials of Spinal Cord Injury

Basic Research to Clinical Practice

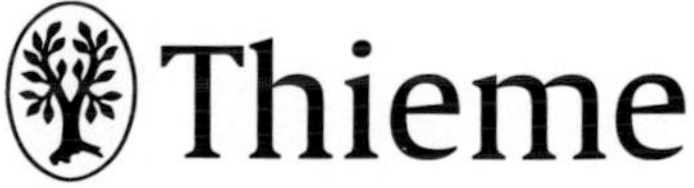

Essentials of Spinal Cord Injury

Basic Research to Clinical Practice

Michael G. Fehlings, MD, PhD, FRCSC, FACS
Professor of Neurosurgery
Gerald and Tootsie Halbert Chair in Neural Repair and Regeneration
Director, Neuroscience Program
Co-Chairman, Spinal Program
University of Toronto
Medical Director
Krembil Neuroscience Centre
Toronto Western Hospital
University Health Network
Toronto, Ontario, Canada

Maxwell Boakye, MD, MPH, FACS
Ole A., Mabel Wise, and Wilma Wise Nelson Endowed Research Chair
Associate Professor of Neurosurgery
Center for Advanced Neurosurgery
University of Louisville
Attending Neurosurgeon
Robley Rex VA Hospital
Louisville, Kentucky

John F. Ditunno Jr., MD
Professor
Department of Rehabilitation Medicine
Emeritus Director
The Regional Spinal Cord Injury Center of the Delaware Valley
Thomas Jefferson University
Philadelphia, Pennsylvania

Alexander R. Vaccaro, MD, PhD
The Everrett J. and Marion Gordon Professor of Orthopaedic Surgery
Professor of Neurosurgery
Co-Director, The Regional Spinal Cord Injury Center of the Delaware Valley
Co-Chief, Spine Surgery
Co-Director, Spine Fellowship Program
Thomas Jefferson University
The Rothman Institute
Philadelphia, Pennsylvania

Serge Rossignol, MD, PhD
Department of Physiology
Groupe de Recherche sur le Système Nerveux Central (FRSQ)
Canada Research Chair on the Spinal Cord
Université de Montréal
SensoriMotor Rehabiltation Research Team of the CIHR
Montreal, Quebec, Canada

Anthony S. Burns, MD, MSc
Associate Professor
Division of Physiatry
Department of Medicine
University of Toronto
Toronto Rehabilitation Institute
University Health Network
Toronto, Ontario, Canada

Thieme
New York · Stuttgart

Thieme Medical Publishers, Inc.
333 Seventh Ave.
New York, NY 10001

Executive Editor: Kay Conerly
Managing Editor: Judith Tomat
Editorial Director, Clinical Reference: Michael Wachinger
Production Editor: Kenneth L. Chumbley
International Production Director: Andreas Schabert
Senior Vice President, International Marketing and Sales: Cornelia Schulze
Vice President, Finance and Accounts: Sarah Vanderbilt
President: Brian D. Scanlan
Compositor: Prairie Papers Inc.
Printer: Everbest Printing Co.

Library of Congress Cataloging-in-Publication Data

Essentials of spinal cord injury : basic research to clinical practice / [edited by] Michael G. Fehlings ... [et al.].
p. ; cm.
Includes bibliographical references.
ISBN 978-1-60406-726-2 (alk. paper)—ISBN 978-1-60406-727-9 (eISBN)
I. Fehlings, Michael.
[DNLM: 1. Spinal Cord Injuries. WL 403]

617.4'82044—dc23

2012016863

Important note: Medical knowledge is ever-changing. As new research and clinical experience broaden our knowledge, changes in treatment and drug therapy may be required. The authors and editors of the material herein have consulted sources believed to be reliable in their efforts to provide information that is complete and in accord with the standards accepted at the time of publication. However, in view of the possibility of human error by the authors, editors, or publisher of the work herein or changes in medical knowledge, neither the authors, editors, nor publisher, nor any other party who has been involved in the preparation of this work, warrants that the information contained herein is in every respect accurate or complete, and they are not responsible for any errors or omissions or for the results obtained from use of such information. Readers are encouraged to confirm the information contained herein with other sources. For example, readers are advised to check the product information sheet included in the package of each drug they plan to administer to be certain that the information contained in this publication is accurate and that changes have not been made in the recommended dose or in the contraindications for administration. This recommendation is of particular importance in connection with new or infrequently used drugs.

Some of the product names, patents, and registered designs referred to in this book are in fact registered trademarks or proprietary names even though specific reference to this fact is not always made in the text. Therefore, the appearance of a name without designation as proprietary is not to be construed as a representation by the publisher that it is in the public domain.

Printed in China

5 4 3 2 1

ISBN 978-1-60406-726-2
eISBN 978-1-60406-727-9

I would like to dedicate this book to my family, colleagues, students, and patients.

Michael G. Fehlings

My greatest thanks go to all my patients whom I have met throughout the years with spinal cord injury who have educated me during their journey through treatment and rehabilitation.

Alexander R. Vaccaro

To my wife, Petrina, for her love, kindness, patience, understanding, and support, and without whom this would not have been possible. To my children, Kwame and Amie, for being fun and making this worthwhile. To my parents for all their sacrifices for me: my late father Kwaku for being the greatest dad and my hero, and my mother, Alice, for being the greatest mom with her encouragement and enduring support.

Maxwell Boakye

To my students and colleagues who have constantly renewed my interest in spinal cord research and to my family who endorsed the crazy schedule needed for this work. I acknowledge also the funding organizations, such as the Canadian Institute for Health Research (CIHR), that have unfailingly supported my research throughout these years.

Serge Rossignol

It has been and continues to be a privilege to work in such an amazing and stimulating field. We admire the many individuals whose care we have had the opportunity to participate in and are thankful to the many colleagues, teachers, and mentors whom we have had the opportunity to work with over the years.

Anthony S. Burns and John F. Ditunno Jr.

Contents

Foreword

With this textbook, *Essentials of Spinal Cord Injury: Basic Research to Clinical Practice*, the editors (Michael Fehlings, Alex Vaccaro, Max Boakye, Serge Rossignol, John Ditunno Jr., and Anthony Burns) have assembled a world-class group of contributors to produce the "Bible of Spinal Cord Injury." Their contribution to the literature deserves "Bible" status for a multitude of reasons. It is comprehensive. It covers the entire field while clearly and succinctly transmitting very detailed information. This book is an easy read, while simultaneously functioning as an incredibly easy access resource for meaningful information. Hence, it functions both as a reference and a textbook. It does both so well that the means by which this is accomplished is worthy of explanation.

First and foremost, the editors and contributors are world class—both regarding their knowledge and prior bodies of work, as well as their well-known individual and collective abilities to "tell it like it is" with clarity. Second, the field of spinal cord injury is completely covered by this textbook. This coverage ranges from epidemiology and assessment and management to the most recent breakthroughs. It covers operative and nonoperative strategies, as well as the underlying theories and principles for both. It covers the controversial and the straightforward. To use the word "comprehensive" would indeed be an understatement. Third, the layout of the chapters and the entire book is incredibly well done. To be sure, the publisher is to be given partial credit here. This last point deserves further elaboration.

Each chapter begins with *Key Points*. This provides an overview and a quick take-home message. It provides an abridged version for what is to follow and sets the tone for the perusal or indepth reading of the chapter. The illustrations are multicolored and very well done. They add substantially to the clarity and look of the book. The majority of chapters include an overview of the literature (in addition to comprehensive reference list at the end of each chapter) that provides appropriate referenced publications, study design and study information, and outcome, results, and conclusions—all in table format. This provides an invaluable "quick look" at the literature with a meaningful distillation of each publication. I found this nuance to be of particular value.

Each chapter has a *Pitfalls and Pearls* section as a summary of sorts that puts closure on the chapter. This is a very effective strategy to distill information, while once again providing the high points. The reader thus has multiple means of skimming the chapter if he or she so chooses. This begins with the *Key Points*, transitions to the overviews of the literature, and culminates with the *Pitfalls and Pearls* section. To facilitate reading even further, each section is color-coded and the chapter pages have, on opposing pages, the section title and the chapter title written on side bars. This is a very nice touch for those who would use this book as a reference source.

This book should be on the shelves of neurosurgeons, spine surgeons, nurses, intensivists, rehabilitation physicians, researchers, and students. I cannot say enough regarding the value of this book. It should be on the shelf of any clinician or scientist who harbors any interest whatsoever in the field of spinal cord injury. It is, indeed, a gem!

Edward Benzel, MD
Chairman
Department of Neurosurgery
Neurological Institute
Cleveland Clinic
Cleveland, Ohio

Preface

The management of spinal cord injury requires a solid foundation in many disciplines including neuroscience, critical care, neurophysiology, neuroimaging, surgery, and neurorehabilitation. Moreover, future advancements in spinal cord injury care will require a detailed knowledge of translational research opportunities. Mastery of these varied areas remains a challenging task that requires a breadth of knowledge, which to date has not been assembled in one text. This challenge represents the inspiration for the current text. To facilitate acquisition of expertise in spinal cord injury medicine, surgery, and translational research, we present the key concepts in one volume in an easily digestible format. Our intent is to provide practicing spinal surgeons, neurosurgeons, orthopedic surgeons, critical care physicians, rehabilitation physicians, allied health care personnel, spinal cord injury scientists, graduate students, medical students, and postdoctoral fellows with a comprehensive source of knowledge related to spinal cord injury.

The current text embraces and integrates emerging concepts in clinical medicine and surgery with neuroanatomy, neurophysiology, neuroimaging, neuroplasticity, and cellular transplantation approaches. Several challenges remain in spinal cord injury—we need better initial management of the injury, assessment of injury severity, improved prognostication, improved medical, surgical, psychosocial, rehabilitation management, and improved understanding of the art and science of spinal cord injury. It is our hope that this book will engage and attract bright, motivated students to the field and allow experts and seasoned practitioners to fine tune and broaden their knowledge. Moreover, we feel that this text will enable basic scientists with an interest in spinal cord injury to understand better the key clinical concepts underlying this challenging condition.

The overarching goal is to facilitate the acquisition of a good working knowledge of the essentials in the field. Hence, the chapters are relatively short, focused, and include keypoints, pearls, and pitfalls. The chapters are cross-referenced to enhance and highlight relationships between different areas. The book is organized into integrated sections which cover: (i) epidemiology, assessment, and clinical management; (ii) neuroanatomy, neurophysiology, and imaging; (iii) neuroplasticity, neuroprotection, and neuroregenerative approaches; (iv) controversies in management; and (v) breakthroughs of the last twenty years and emerging areas including genomics and proteomics.

This book is a culmination of the authors' attempts to learn more about spinal cord injury. The chapters have been assembled and the authors have been chosen to distill the essential knowledge into focused sections. Clinicians will learn more about exciting, varied research, and researchers will gain appreciation of evidence based management of spinal injury. Our intent is to stimulate passion for research in this field and to enable improved care and outcomes for individuals with spinal cord injury.

Contributors

Todd J. Albert, MD
Richard H Rothman Professor and Chairman
Department of Orthopaedic Surgery
Professor of Neurosurgery
Thomas Jefferson University Hospitals
President
The Rothman Institute
Philadelphia, Pennsylvania

Aileen J. Anderson, PhD
Associate Professor
Department of Physical Medicine and Rehabilitation
Department of Anatomy and Neurobiology
Sue and Bill Gross Stem Cell Center
Institute for Memory Impairments and Neurological Disorders
University of California–Irvine
Irvine, California

James W. Austin, PhD
Genetics and Development
Toronto Western Research Institute
Toronto, Ontario, Canada

Martin Baggenstos, MD
Microneurosurgical Consultants PC
Portland, Oregon

Michael S. Beattie, PhD
Professor and Director of Research
Brain and Spinal Injury Center
Department of Neurological Surgery
University of California–San Francisco
San Francisco, California

David M. Benglis Jr., MD
Associate
Department of Neuroscience
Atlanta Brain and Spine Care
Piedmont Hospital
Atlanta, Georgia

Mahmoud Benour, MD
Neurosurgery Resident
University of Calgary
Calgary, Alberta, Canada

Maxwell Boakye, MD, MPH, FACS
Ole A., Mabel Wise, and Wilma Wise Nelson Endowed Research Chair
Associate Professor of Neurosurgery
Center for Advanced Neurosurgery
University of Louisville
Attending Neurosurgeon
Robley Rex VA Hospital
Louisville, Kentucky

Kath Bogie, DPhil
Department of Orthopaedics
Case Western Reserve University
Louis Stokes Department of Veterans Affairs Medical Center
Cleveland, Ohio

Jacqueline C. Bresnahan, PhD
Professor
Brain and Spinal Injury Center
Department of Neurological Surgery
University of California–San Francisco
San Francisco, California

Keith D. Burau, PhD
Associate Professor
Division of Biostatistics
University of Texas School of Public Health
Houston, Texas

Anthony S. Burns, MD, MSc
Associate Professor
Division of Physiatry
Department of Medicine
University of Toronto
Toronto Rehabilitation Institute
University Health Network
Toronto, Ontario, Canada

Terry C. Burns, MD, PhD
Resident
Department of Neurosurgery
Stanford University
Stanford, California

David W. Cadotte, MD, MSc
Post-Doctoral Research Fellow
Neurosurgery Resident
Division of Neurosurgery
Toronto Western Hospital University Health Network
University of Toronto
Toronto, Ontario, Canada

Aleksa Cenic, MD, FRCSC, MSc
Assistant Professor
Neurosurgery
McMaster University
Hamilton, Ontario, Canada

Kevin Chao, MD
Resident
Neurosurgery
Stanford University
Stanford, California

Luis Enrique Chaparro, MD
Clinical and Research Fellow
Department of Anesthesiology and Perioperative Medicine
Queen's University
Kingston, Ontario, Canada

Yuying Chen, MD, PhD
Associate Professor
Department of Physical Medicine and Rehabilitation
University of Alabama–Birmingham
Birmingham, Alabama

B. Catharine Craven, MD, MSc, FRCPC, CCD
Assistant Professor
Department of Medicine
Toronto Rehabilitation Institute
University Health Network
University of Toronto
Toronto, Ontario, Canada

Graham H. Creasey, BSc, MB, ChB, FRCSEd
Professor of Spinal Cord Injury Medicine
Department of Neurosurgery
Stanford University
Stanford, California

Armin Curt, MD
Professor and Chairman
Spinal Cord Injury Center
University of Zurich
University Hospital Balgrist
Zurich, Switzerland

Scott D. Daffner, MD
Assistant Professor
Department of Orthopaedics
West Virginia University School of Medicine
Morgantown, West Virginia

Andrew T. Dailey, MD
Associate Professor
Departments of Neurosurgery and Orthopedics
University of Utah
Salt Lake City, Utah

Derry Dance, MD, BSc, JD
Resident
Department of Medicine
Division of Physiatry
University of Toronto
Toronto, Ontario, Canada

Michael Daubs, MD
Department of Orthopaedics
University of Utah School of Medicine
Salt Lake City, Utah

W. Dalton Dietrich, PhD
Scientific Director
The Miami Project to Cure Paralysis
University of Miami Miller School of Medicine
Miami, Florida

Volker Dietz, MD, FRCP
Professor Emeritus
Spinal Cord Injury Center
Balgrist University Hospital
Zurich, Switzerland

John F. Ditunno Jr., MD
Professor
Department of Rehabilitation Medicine
Emeritus Director
The Regional Spinal Cord Injury Center of the Delaware Valley
Thomas Jefferson University
Philadelphia, Pennsylvania

Thomas M. Dixon, PhD
Psychologist
Spinal Cord Injury Unit
Louis Stokes Department of Veterans Affairs Medical Center
Cleveland, Ohio

Doniel Drazin, MD, MA
Resident
Department of Neurosurgery
Cedars-Sinai Medical Center
Los Angeles, California

Marcel F. Dvorak, MD, FRCSC
Professor of Orthopaedics
Head
Division of Spine
Vancouver General Hospital
University of British Columbia
Vancouver, British Columbia, Canada

James M. Ecklund, MD, FACS
Medical Director
Neurosciences, Inova Health System
Chairman
Department of Neurosciences, Inova Fairfax Hospital
Professor of Surgery
Uniformed Services University
Professor of Neurosurgery
George Washington University
Professor of Neurosurgery
Virginia Commonwealth University School of Medicine–Inova
Inova Fairfax Hospital
Department of Neurosciences
Falls Church, Virginia

Peter H. Ellaway, PhD
Emeritus Professor of Physiology
Division of Experimental Medicine
Imperial College London
London, England

Stacy L. Elliott, MD
Medical Director
British Columbia Center, Sexual Medicine
Clinical Professor
Departments of Psychiatry and Urological Sciences
University of British Columbia
Principle Investigator
International Collaboration On Repair Discoveries
Vancouver, British Columbia, Canada

Aria Fallah, MD
Resident
Division of Neurosurgery
Department of Surgery
University of Toronto
Toronto, Ontario, Canada

H. Francis Farhadi, MD, PhD, FRCS(C)
Assistant Professor
Department of Neurological Surgery
Ohio State University Wexner Medical Center
Columbus, Ohio

Michael G. Fehlings, MD, PhD, FRCSC, FACS
Professor of Neurosurgery
Gerald and Tootsie Halbert Chair in Neural Repair and Regeneration
Director, Neuroscience Program
Co-Chairman, Spinal Program
University of Toronto
Medical Director
Krembil Neuroscience Centre
Toronto Western Hospital
University Health Network
Toronto, Ontario, Canada

Sharon Foster-Geeter, BSN, CWCN
SCI Wound Care Coordinator
Spinal Cord Injury Service
Louis Stokes Department of Veterans Affairs Medical Center
Cleveland, Ohio

Alyson Fournier, PhD
Associate Professor
Department of Neurology and Neurosurgery
McGill University
Montreal, Quebec, Canada

Ralph F. Frankowski, PhD
Professor
Division of Biostatistics
University of Texas Health Science Center
Houston School of Public Health
Houston, Texas

Christine C. Frick, PsyD
Clinical Psychologist
Psychology Service
VA New England Healthcare System
West Haven, Connecticut

Alain Frigon, PhD, MSc
Assistant Professor
Physiology and Biophysics
Université de Sherbrooke
Sherbrooke, Quebec, Canada

David Gendelberg, BS
Spine Research Fellow
Department of Orthopaedics
Thomas Jefferson University Hospitals
The Rothman Institute
Philadelphia, Pennsylvania

George Ghobrial, MD
Resident
Department of Neurological Surgery
Thomas Jefferson University Hospitals
Philadelphia, Pennsylania

Robert G. Grossman, MD
Chairman
Department of Neurosurgery
The Methodist Hospital
Houston, Texas

Joy D. Guingab-Cagmat, PhD
Postdoctoral Associate
Department of Psychiatry
University of Florida
Gainesville, Florida

Susan Harkema, PhD
Professor
Department of Neurological Surgery
University of Louisville
Owsley B. Frazier Chair in Neurological Rehabilitation
Rehabilitation Research Director
Kentucky Spinal Cord Injury Research Center
Research Director
Frazier Rehab Institute
Director of the NeuroRecovery Network
Frazier Rehab Institute
Louisville, Kentucky

James S. Harrop, MD
Associate Professor
Chief, Division of Spine and Peripheral Nerve Surgery
Department of Orthopedic and Neurological Surgery
Thomas Jefferson University
Philadelphia, Pennsylvania

Gregory W. J. Hawryluk, MD, PhD
Senior Resident
Division of Neurosurgery
University of Toronto
Toronto, Ontario, Canada

Jessica Hillyer, PhD
Program Director
Department of Psychology
South University
Austin, Texas

Chester Ho, MD
Associate Professor and Head
Division of Physical Medicine and Rehabilitation
Department of Clinical Neurosciences
Foothills Hospital
Calgary, Alberta, Canada

Susan P. Howley, BA
Executive Vice President Research
Christopher and Dana Reeve Foundation
Short Hills, New Jersey

R. John Hurlbert, MD, PhD, FRCSC, FACS
Associate Professor
Division of Neurosurgery
Spine Program
University of Calgary
Calgary, Alberta, Canada

Catherine E. Kang, PhD
Postdoctoral Fellow
Department of Neurology
Feinberg School of Medicine
Northwestern University
Chicago, Illinois

Rose Katz, MD
Praticien Attaché Assistant
Directrice de l'Er 6 UPMC
Physiologie et physiopathologie de la motricité chez l'Homme
Service de Médecine Physique et Rédaptation
Groupe Hospitalier Pitié-Salpêtrière
Paris, France

Paul Kennedy, DPhil
Professor of Clinical Psychology
Director, Academic and Research
Oxford Institute of Clinical Psychology Training
University of Oxford
Oxford, England

Martin J. Kilbane, PT, OCS
Supervisor of Rehabilitation Therapies
Spinal Cord Injury Center
Louis Stokes Department of Veterans Affairs Medical Center
Cleveland, Ohio

Howard Kim, PhD
Institute of Medical Science
University of Toronto
Toronto, Ontario, Canada

Firas H. Kobeissy, PhD
Assistant Research Professor
Associate Scientific Director for the Psychoproteomics Research Center
Department of Psychiatry
The Evelyn F. and William L. McKnight Brain Institute
University of Florida
Gainesville Florida

John L. Kipling Kramer, PhD
Postdoctoral Fellow
Spinal Cord Injury Center
University Hospital Balgrist
University of Zurich
Zurich, Switzerland

Andrei Krassioukov, MD, PHD, FRCPC
Professor
Department of Medicine
Division of Physical Medicine and Rehabilitation
Associate Director and Scientist
International Collaboration on Repair Discoveries
University of British Columbia
Vancouver, British Columbia, Canada

Kay Harris Kriegsman, PhD
Psychologist in Private Practice
Bethesda, Maryland

Gina L. D. Kubec, OTD
Occupational Therapist
Spinal Cord Injury and Disorders
Louis Stokes Department of Veterans Affairs Medical Center
Cleveland, Ohio

Jean-Charles Lamy, PhD
Research Associate
Université Paris Descartes
Sorbonne Paris Cité
Paris, France

Joon Y. Lee, MD
Associate Professor of Orthopaedic Surgery
Spine Division
University of Pittsburgh Medical Center
Pittsburgh, Pennsylvania

Brian Lenehan, MB, MCh, BAO, FRCS Tr. and Orth.
Consultant Orthopaedic and Spine Surgeon
Department of Trauma and Orthopaedics
Mid-Western Regional Hospitals
Limerick, Ireland

Allan D. Levi, MD, PhD, FACS
Professor of Neurosurgery
University of Miami Miller School of Medicine
Chief of Neurosurgery
University of Miami Hospital
Miami, Florida

Geoffrey Ling, MD, PhD, FAAN
Colonel, Medical Corps, United States Army
Professor and Interim Chair of Neurology
Director of Critical Care Medicine for Anesthesiology and Neurology
Uniformed Services University of the Health Sciences
Bethesda, Maryland

Daniel C. Lu, MD, PhD
Assistant Professor
Department of Neurosurgery
University of California–Los Angeles
Los Angeles, California

Angela Mailis, MD, MSc, FRCPC (Phys Med)
Director, Comprehensive Pain Program
Senior Investigator
Krembil Neuroscience Centre
Professor
Department of Medicine
University of Toronto
Toronto Western Hospital
Toronto, Ontario, Canada

Geoffrey T. Manley, MD, PhD
Professor and Vice Chairman of Neurological Surgery
University of California–San Francisco
Chief of Neurosurgery
San Francisco General Hospital
Co-Director
Brain and Spinal Injury Center
San Francisco, California

Edward M. Marchan, MD
Physician Resident
Department of Radiation Oncology
Emory University School of Medicine
Atlanta, Georgia

Catherine A. McGuinness, BSc
Consultant
Health Information
Vancouver, British Columbia, Canada

Lisa McKerracher, PhD
Adjunct Professor
Department of Neurology and Neurosurgery
McGill University
Montreal, Québec, Canada
CEO
BioAxone Biosciences Inc.
Fort Lauderdale, Florida

David J. Mikulis, MD
Professor and Director
Functional Brain Imaging Lab
Department of Medical Imaging
The University of Toronto
The University Health Network
Toronto Western Hospital
Toronto, Ontario, Canada

Steven J. Mitchell, OTR/L, ATP
Clinical Specialist, Seating/Wheeled Mobility and Assistive Technology
Spinal Cord Injury/Disorders Service
Louis Stokes Department of Veterans Affairs Medical Center
Cleveland, Ohio

Toba N. Niazi, MD
Neurological Surgery
University of Utah School of Medicine
Salt Lake City, Utah

Jens Bo Nielsen, MD, PhD
Professor
Department of Exercise and Sport Sciences
Department of Neuroscience and Pharmacology
University of Copenhagen
Copenhagen, Denmark

Vanessa K. Noonan, PhD, PT
Researcher
Department of Orthopaedics
University of British Columbia
Vancouver, British Columbia, Canada

Jeffrey B. Palmer, MD
Lawrence Cardinal Shehan Professor of Physical Medicine and Rehabilitation
Director and Physiatrist-in-Chief
Department of Physical Medicine and Rehabilitation
Johns Hopkins University School of Medicine
Baltimore, Maryland

Sara Palmer, PhD
Assistant Professor
Department of Physical Medicine and Rehabilitation
Johns Hopkins University School of Medicine
Baltimore, Maryland

Alpesh A. Patel, MD, FACS
Associate Professor
Department of Orthopaedic Surgery and Rehabilitation
Loyola University Medical Center
Chicago Illinois

Sheri L. Peterson, BS
Doctoral Candidate
Department of Anatomy and Neurobiology
Sue and Bill Gross Stem Cell Center
Institute for Memory Impairments and Neurological Disorders
University of California–Irvine
Irvine, California

Nicolas Phan, MDCM, FRCSC, FACS
Assistant Professor
Department of Surgery
Sunnybrook Health Sciences Centre
University of Toronto
Toronto, Ontario, Canada

Avraam Ploumis, MD, PhD
Assistant Professor
Orthopaedic Spine Surgeon
Department of Orthopaedics and Rehabilitation
University of Ioannina
Ioannina, Greece

Kris E. Radcliff, MD
Assistant Professor
Department of Orthopedic Surgery
Thomas Jefferson University
Philadelphia, Pennsylvania

Mary V. Ratliff, BS
OMS-III
Kentucky College of Osteopathic Medicine
University of Pikeville
Pikeville, Kentucky

Serge Rossignol, MD, PhD
Department of Physiology
Groupe de Recherche sur le Système Nerveux Central (FRSQ)
Canada Research Chair on the Spinal Cord
SensoriMotor Rehabiltation Research Team of the CIHR
Université de Montréal
Montreal, Quebec, Canada

James W. Rowland, BSc
Graduate Student
Spinal Program
University of Toronto
Toronto, Ontario, Canada

Michal Schwartz, MD
Professor
Ilze and Maurice Professorial Chair of Neuroimmunology
Department of Neurobiology
The Weizmann Institute of Science
Rehovot, Israel

J. C. Seton, MSN, RN, ACNS-BC
Louis Stokes Department of Veterans Affairs Medical Center
Cleveland, Ohio

Kimberly Sexton, MS, RD, LD
Supervisory Dietitian–Clinical Section
Home Based Primary Care and Weight Management/Health Promotion and Disease Prevention Nutrition Coordinator
Louis Stokes Department of Veterans Affairs Medical Center
Cleveland, Ohio

Mohammed Farid Shamji, MD, PhD, FRCSC
Adult Spine Surgery Fellow
Division of Neurosurgery
University of Calgary
Calgary, Alberta, Canada

Ashwini D. Sharan, MD, FACS
Associate Professor
Department of Neurosurgery
Thomas Jefferson University
Philadelphia, Pennsylvania

Ravid Shechter, PhD
Postdoctoral
Neurobiology Department
The Weizmann Institute of Science
Rehovot, Israel

Peng Shi, MD, PhD
Research Associate Professor
Department of Physiology and Functional Genomics
College of Medicine
University of Florida
Gainesville, Florida

Molly Sandra Shoichet, PhD
Professor
Department of Chemical Engineering and Applied Chemistry
Institute of Biomaterials and Biomedical Engineering, Chemistry
University of Toronto
Toronto, Ontario, Canada

Gurusukhman D. S. Sidhu, MBBS
Research Fellow
Department of Orthopedic Surgery
Thomas Jefferson University Hospitals
The Rothman Institute
Philadelphia, Pennsylvania

Harvey E. Smith, MD
Assistant Clinical Professor
Department of Orthopaedic Surgery
Tufts University School of Medicine
New England Baptist Hospital
Boston, Massachusetts

Emilie F. Smithson, MD
Buckinhamshire Hospitals
NSIC, Stoke Mandeville Hospital
Aylesbury, England

Christopher J. Sontag, BS
Doctoral Candidate
Department of Anatomy and Neurobiology
Sue and Bill Gross Stem Cell Center
Insitute for Memory Impairments and Neurological Disorders
University of California–Irvine
Irvine, California

John D. Steeves, PhD
Peter Wall Institute Distinguished Scholar in Residence
Professor of International Collaboration on Repair Discoveries
University of British Columbia
Vancouver Coastal Health
Vancouver, British Columbia, Canada

Patrick Stroman, PhD
Associate Professor
Centre for Neuroscience Studies
Queen's University
Kingston, Ontario, Canada

Ishaq Y. Syed, MS, MD
Assistant Professor
Department of Orthopaedic Surgery
Wake Forest Baptist University Medical Center
Winston-Salem, North Carolina

Violeta Talpag, MSc
Ultrasound Department
BSA Diagnostics Medical Imaging
Toronto, Ontario, Canada

Charles H. Tator, MD, PhD, FRCSC
Professor of Neurosurgery
University of Toronto
Founder, Think First Foundation
Toronto Western Hospital
Toronto, Ontario, Canada

Wolfram Tetzlaff, MD, PhD
Professor and Assoc. Director
International Collaboration on Repair Discoveries
University of British Columbia
Man in Motion Chair in Spinal Cord Injury Research
Blusson Spinal Cord Centre
Vancouver, British Columbia, Canada

Sonia Teufack, MD
Resident
Department of Neurological Surgery
Thomas Jefferson University Hospitals
Philadelphia, Pennsylvania

Aiko K. Thompson, PhD
Research Scientist
Translational Neurological Research Program
Helen Hayes Hospital and the Wadsworth Center
New York State Department of Health
West Haverstraw, New York
Associate Professor
Department of Biomedical Sciences
State University of New York–Albany
Albany, New York
Assistant Professor
Department of Neurology
Neurological Institute
Columbia University
New York, New York

Stephan Ong Tone, PhD
MD-PhD Candidate
Department of Neurology and Neurosurgery
McGill University
Montreal Neurological Institute
Montreal, Quebec, Canada

Elizabeth G. Toups, MS, RN, CCRP
Clinical Trials Manager
Department of Neurosurgery
Methodist Neurological Institute
The Methodist Hospital
Houston, Texas

Eve C. Tsai, MD, PhD, FRCS(C)
Assistant Professor
Department of Surgery
The Ottawa Hospital
Ottawa Hospital Research Institute
University of Ottawa
Ottawa, Ontario, Canada

Alexander R. Vaccaro, MD, PhD
The Everrett J. and Marion Gordon Professor of Orthopaedic Surgery
Professor of Neurosurgery
Co-Director, The Regional Spinal Cord Injury Center of the Delaware Valley
Co-Chief, Spine Surgery
Co-Director, Spine Fellowship Program
Thomas Jefferson University
The Rothman Institute
Philadelphia, Pennsylvania

Kevin K. W. Wang, PhD
Director, Center for Neuroproteomics and Biomarkers Research
Associate Director, Center for Traumatic Brain Injury Studies
Associate Professor, Psychiatry and Neuroscience
Evelyn F. and William L. McKnight Brain Institute
University of Florida
Gainesville, Florida

Michael Y. Wang, MD, FACS
Professor
Departments of Neurological Surgery and Rehabilitation Medicine
University of Miami Miller School of Medicine
Miami, Florida

Shelly Wang, MD
Resident
Department of Neurosurgery
University of Toronto
Toronto, Ontario, Canada

Monique Washington, RN, MS
Management of Information and Outcomes Coordinator
Spinal Cord Injury
Louis Stokes Department of Veterans Affairs Medical Center
Cleveland, Ohio

Jefferson R. Wilson, MD
Postdoctoral Research Fellow
Neurosurgery Resident
Division of Neurosurgery and Spinal Program
University of Toronto
Toronto, Ontario, Canada

Joshua L. White, PsyD
Psychologist, Team Leader
Veterans Addiction Recovery Center
Louis Stokes Cleveland Veterans Affairs Medical Center
Cleveland, Ohio

Jonathan R. Wolpaw, MD
Laboratory Chief and Professor
Laboratory of Neural Injury and Repair
Wadsworth Center
New York State Department of Health
State University of New York
Albany, New York

James Xie, BS
Stanford University School of Medicine
Stanford, California

Sung-Joo Yuh, MD, BSC
Neurosurgical Chief Resident
Department of Neurosurgery
University of Ottawa
The Ottawa Hospital
Ottawa, Ontario, Canada

Zhiqun Zhang, PhD
Adjunct Assistant Professor
Department of Psychiatry
Evelyn F. and William L. McKnight Brain Institute
Gainesville, Florida

Benjamin M. Zussman, BS
Medical Student
Department of Neurosurgery
Thomas Jefferson University
Philadelphia, Pennsylvania

I

Principles of Spinal Cord Injury Clinical Practice

1

Anatomy and Physiology of the Spinal Cord

Serge Rossignol

Key Points

1. The spinal cord (SC) is like all other centers of the CNS, with inputs from other brain structures, sensory information from various body parts, with processing units, and with outputs to the brain and various body parts.
2. The SC is shorter than the vertebral canal, and the correspondence between the two should be remembered when extrapolating neural symptoms based on the description of lesions, which usually can refer to vertebral segments and not spinal segments.
3. Ascending sensory tracts are generally crossed with respect to the telencephalon or diencephalon, but the crossing does not occur at the same levels. Proprioceptive/tactile inputs from one side of the body cross on the other side at the brain stem level, whereas pain/temperature inputs cross at the spinal level. This sensory dissociation is important in determining the site of spinal lesions and understanding syndromes like the Brown-Séquard syndrome (spinal hemisection).
4. Descending corticospinal fibers are mostly crossed at the level of the bulb; the red nucleus of the mesencephalon projects contralaterally; the vestibular nuclei project ipsilaterally, whereas the reticular formation projects either unilaterally or bilaterally to the cord.
5. Testing reflexes indicates the state of excitability of certain spinal pathways (motoneurons and interneurons) at different segments, and their asymmetry may help in the localization of spinal lesions.

The spinal cord (SC) is often represented in various textbooks as a longitudinal nervous structure within the vertebral canal that carries information to and from supraspinal structures via ascending sensory and descending motor pathways, respectively. The SC is also a segmented structure, and information reaching or leaving the SC flows through segmental dorsal and ventral roots, respectively. Therefore, from a purely anatomical point of view, the SC is mainly a site where long pathways course through various spinal quadrants and where various spinal segments interconnect. In spinal cord injuries (SCIs), lesions of various sizes can damage motor or sensory pathways located in dorsal, lateral, or ventral regions, and the symptoms will largely be correlated to the injured pathways and the level of injury. This is of great clinical importance after injury because the topographical distribution of sensorimotor impairments over the body will be used to categorize the impairments of the patient according to the American Spinal Injury Association (ASIA) score.

In addition, the SC, like any other structure of the central nervous system (CNS), receives and processes inputs and generates outputs. More specifically, neurons of the gray matter (motoneurons and interneurons) receive inputs from descending pathways, intersegmental propriospinal pathways, and peripheral sensory afferents through various segmental pathways. Interneurons project to other interneurons, or project their axon through ascending/descending tracts.

In the ventral horn, motoneurons integrate multiple types of inputs responsible for movement execution (i.e., they form the final common pathway). Moreover, all sensory afferents from most parts of the body converge on spinal neurons. Therefore, in reality, the SC occupies a unique and central position in the interactions between the CNS and all other structures of the body. This is why injury to the SC is so devastating; it disrupts the essential links between peripheral sensory inputs, the CNS, and the motor apparatus.

A better comprehension of the structure and physiology of the SC, a relatively old phylogenetic structure, may lead to a better understanding of the input–output processes occurring elsewhere in the CNS while also offering new avenues for treatments after SCI in humans. For instance, knowing that the SC possesses intrinsic circuits capable of generating complex movements could provide a framework for treating SCI patients, a framework in which the endogenous capacities of the SC are taken into account.[1]

Anatomy

General Disposition of the Spinal Cord

The SC is ~45 cm in length in humans and is enclosed in a multiarticulated flexible bony structure called the vertebral column. As shown in **Fig. 1.1**, the SC starts at the caudal end of the brain stem, where it exits the foramen magnum at the base of the skull. It extends to the first lumbar vertebral level (L1). The SC is more or less cylindrical (anteroposterior flattening) and follows the curvature of the vertebral column and has different thicknesses depending on the vertebral levels. For instance, at cervical level C4 to T2 and lumbosacral levels L3–S3, the SC is larger corresponding to the cervical and lumbar enlargements, respectively, where motoneurons related to muscles of the upper and lower limbs are located. **Figure 1.1** (left) shows the enlargements of the ventral horn at these two levels. The caudal end of the SC is called the conus medullaris.

It should be noted that, embryologically, the various segments of the SC are derived from the ectodermal sheet and are connected to adjacent segmental structures from the mesodermal sheet that will eventually give rise to muscles and bones. The vertebral column grows to a greater length than the SC, and to maintain established connections, the spinal roots must elongate in the thoracolumbar region and reach their target by spinal nerves exiting the vertebral column through intervertebral foramina. The result is that at lower thoracic and lumbar levels, the spinal segments are more rostral (cephalic) than the vertebral segments of the same name. As a reference, the spinous process of the fourth thoracic vertebra is located at about the level of the sixth thoracic SC segment. The spinal lumbar enlargement is aligned with the last three thoracic spinous processes. The first lumbar vertebra corresponds to the end of the cord (conus medullaris).

It is of paramount importance to understand the discrepancy between vertebral segments and spinal segments because trauma or tumors are often defined with respect to vertebral, not spinal, segments, although the latter are obviously respon-

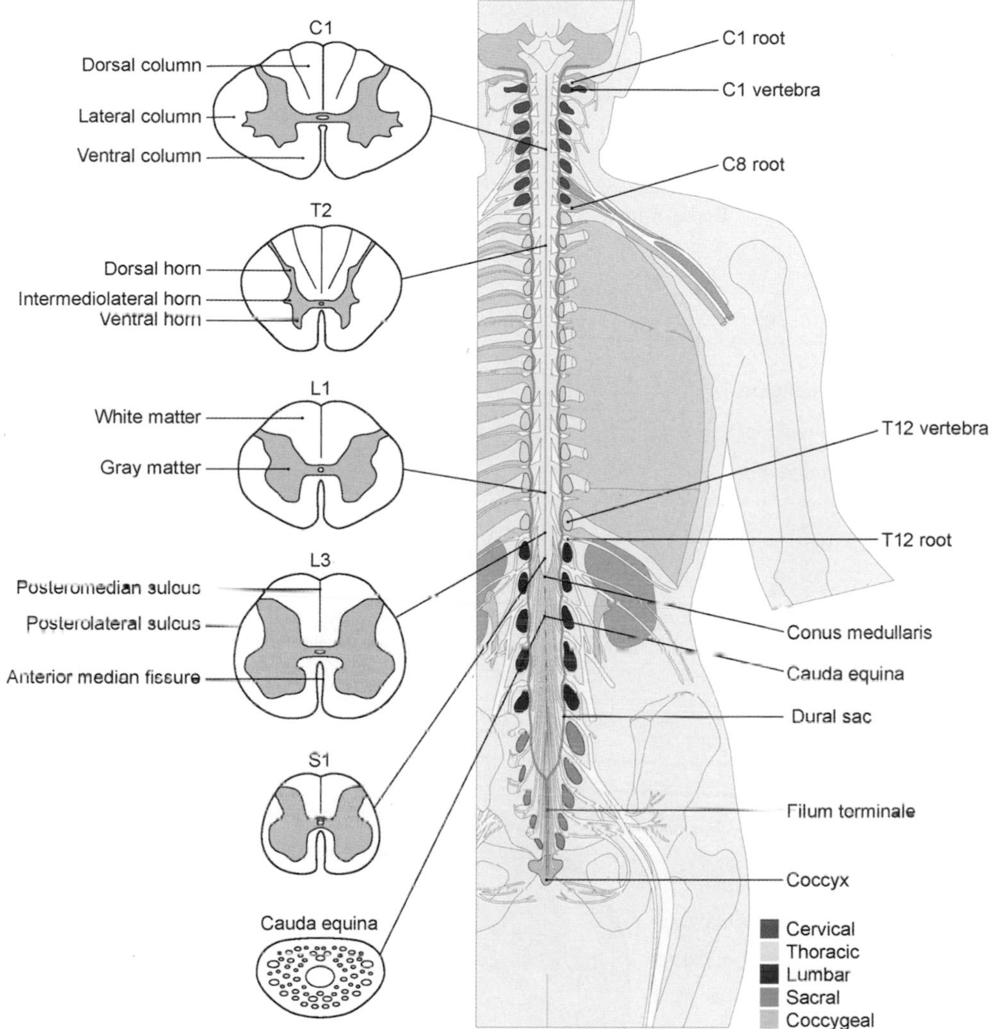

Fig. 1.1 Gross anatomy of the spinal cord showing the relationships with bony structures as well as other body parts. The axial spinal sections on the left show the distribution of the white and gray matter and are representative of each spinal level. On the right, the vertebrae are color-coded to help with identification of the various levels. (This figure is inspired by Netter,[2] Section II, plates 14 and 17.)

sible for neurological symptoms. Damage at the L1 vertebra may result in a conus medullaris syndrome, characterized by paralysis of the sphincter, bladder dysfunction, and perianal anesthesia. Lesions of the cauda equina below the L1 vertebra will produce sensorimotor deficits of the lower limbs because the cauda equina contains roots of various lumbosacral levels (see Chapter 26).

Meninges

The SC is enclosed not only by the outer bony structure of the vertebral column but also by three different meningeal layers (**Fig. 1.2**). The most external layer is thick and is called the dura mater. The dura mater does not adhere to the vertebral bone, contrary to the dura mater of the brain, which has an external periosteal layer that

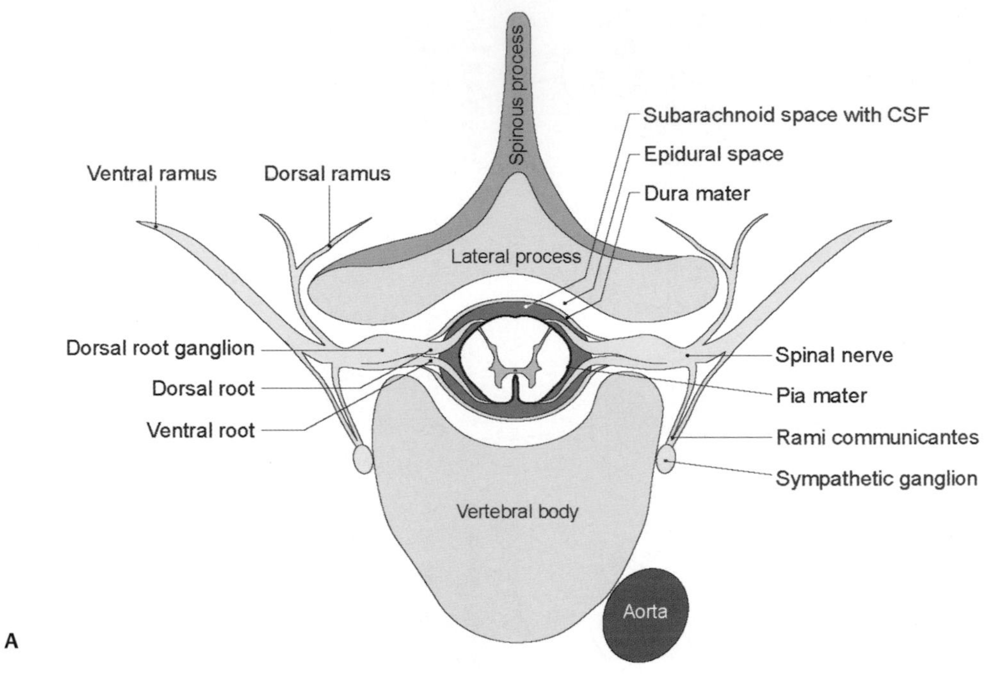

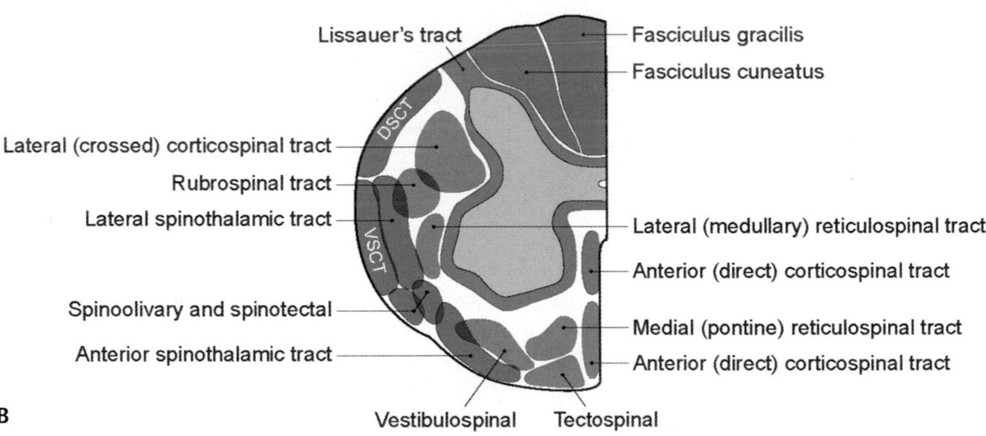

Fig. 1.2 The anatomy of a segment. **(A)** shows the principal anatomical relationships between a spinal segment, the meninges, the dorsal and ventral roots, as well as the bony structures of a typical thoracic vertebra. **(B)** represents typical ascending and descending tracts. Sensory pathways are in blue, whereas motor pathways are in red. All pathways are placed on only one side of the cord to indicate that lesions of the cord usually involve both sensory and descending motor pathways. The same fiber tracts are also on the other side of the cord, which is not represented. (This figure is inspired by Netter,[2] Section II, plate 17.)

adheres to the cranium and is separated by venous sinuses at various locations. Instead, overlying the spinal dura is the epidural space, which contains various amounts of fat and vessels, which can be prominent when visualized by magnetic resonance imaging (MRI). The epidural space is where local anesthetics are normally injected during surgery or childbirth, for example. The dura extends to sacral levels S1–2, where it forms the dural sac (**Fig. 1.1**).

Under the dura, the arachnoid space contains the cerebrospinal fluid, which is prominent in T2 MRI (**Fig. 1.3**). The arachnoid space also extends to the dural sac, and because the SC is shorter than the vertebral column, the arachnoid space at the lower lumbar level is an ideal place for lumbar puncture (L3–4 or L4–5) to retrieve cerebrospinal fluid without damaging the SC, because at this level only roots forming the cauda equina are present and will be pushed aside by the needle collecting the cerebrospinal fluid.

The third layer, the pia mater, follows the contours of the SC as well as the arteries and veins of the SC. The pia is firmly attached to the dura by a series of 22 denticulate ligaments. The pia ends as the filum terminale and, when covered by the remaining dura, forms the coccygeal ligament, which is attached to the coccyx.

Spinal Nerves and Spinal Roots

Basic Anatomy of a Segment

There are 31 pairs of spinal nerves (made of ventral and dorsal roots): eight cervical, 12 thoracic or dorsal, five lumbar, five sacral, and one coccygeal. However, at the cervical level, there are only seven vertebrae. The first cervical nerve reaches the intervertebral foramen above the vertebra, whereas the other seven cervical roots reach the foramen below the vertebral body of the same name. This naming pattern is maintained at all other levels of the vertebral canal, so that all roots emerge caudally to the vertebral body (see **Fig. 1.1**). The spinal nerves consist of ventral and dorsal roots. From the ventral gray matter, a series of filaments emerge at the level of the anterolateral sulcus and coalesce to form the ventral roots. These axons originate from motoneurons and innervate skeletal muscles. Other efferents (preganglionic sympathetic fibers) come from the intermediate gray matter in the thoracic and upper lumbar regions and innervate autonomic ganglia. These efferents leave the ventral roots through the rami communicantes to reach the ganglionic chain close to the vertebral bodies (**Fig. 1.2A**).

The dorsal roots carry sensory afferents whose unipolar cell bodies are located within dorsal root ganglia. The sensory afferents with their cell bodies and central axons are called the first-order neurons. The central axons enter the spinal cord at the level of the posterolateral sulcus, whereas the peripheral axons reach sensory receptors of different types and sensory modalities in peripheral tissues, such as the skin, muscles, and joints. The ventral and dorsal roots are ensheathed by the pia and by the arachnoid to some extent. They join laterally to form the spinal nerve and are then ensheathed by the dura as they exit the intervertebral foramina.

Each spinal segment thus contains the dorsal and ventral roots of the corresponding spinal nerve. The entry or exit of these roots defines the ventrolateral and posterolateral sulci. Moreover, deeper fissures are present on the ventral and posterior sides (posterior median sulcus and ventral sulcus) (**Fig. 1.1**). Collectively, these landmarks define the dorsal, lateral, and ventral columns where various descending and ascending tracts are located.

The familiar shape seen in a transverse section of the cord is that of the letter *H*, which results from the distribution of nerve cell bodies in the gray matter. The gray matter is in turn subdivided into dorsal, ventral, and, at some levels, intermediate horns. The SC subdivisions are often referred to as being composed of ten laminae, defined by Rexed[3] to identify the localization of particular types of neurons at various segmental levels. This numbering scheme is often used to determine the projection site of descending pathways in the gray matter.

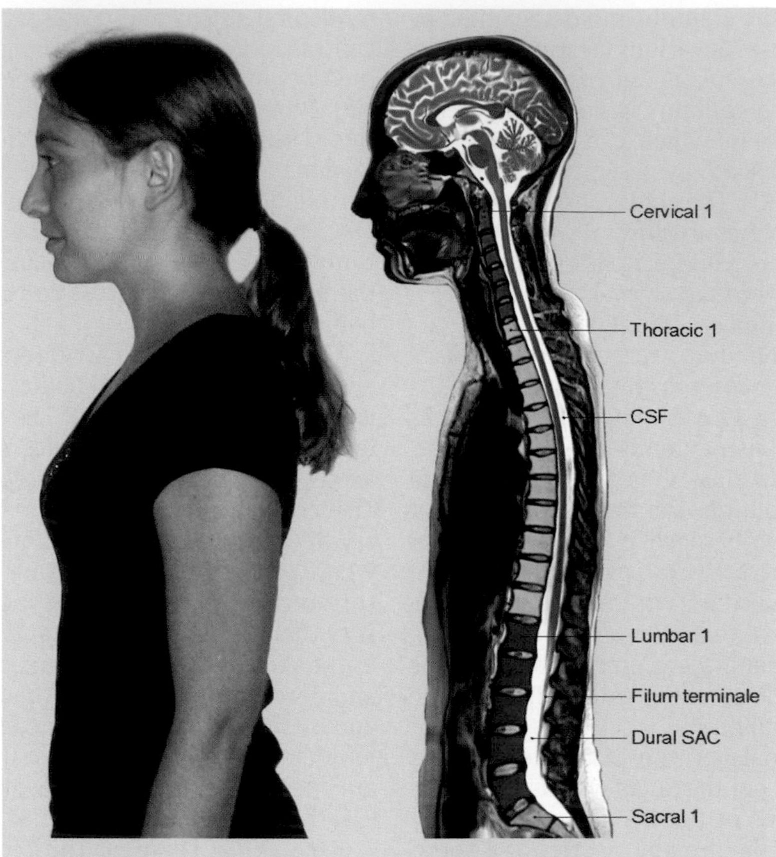

Fig. 1.3 T2 magnetic resonance imaging (MRI) scan. This figure shows a picture of a person with her corresponding MRI. The acquisition was done at 3 Tesla using a fast spin echo T2-weighted sequence (TR/TE = 3500/111ms, in-plane resolution 0.68 × 0.68 mm^2). On this anatomical MRI, one can clearly distinguish all vertebral levels: cervical (blue), thoracic (green), lumbar (red), and most of the sacral (cyan). The brain and spinal cord appear in dark gray, whereas the cerebrospinal fluid (CSF) appears in bright signal, due to differences in relaxation properties. MRI is extremely useful for defining the morphology in the spinal cord and its surrounding environment. Contrary to most schemes of the spinal cord, the relatively high ratio between the CSF and spinal cord is noticeable. (This sequence was taken by Dr. Julien Cohen-Adad at the Functional Neuroimaging Unit of the Centre de Recherche de l'Institut de Gériatrie de Montréal. We are grateful also to Claudine Gauthier, who agreed to be the subject.)

The horns of the gray matter contain different classes of functional neurons. Second-order interneurons in the dorsal horn process sensory information from the first-order (or primary) sensory afferents in the dorsal roots. They may form di-, tri-, or polysynaptic pathways, as will be seen later. Their axons may remain local within the segment or reach other segmental levels through propriospinal pathways. Ventral horns contain motoneurons of various types (α-motoneurons reaching skeletal muscle fibers and γ-motoneurons innervating extrafusal motor fibers in muscle spindles). The ventral horns are larger at the levels of the cervical and lumbar enlargements because of motoneurons innervating limb muscles. Motoneurons are also distributed spatially, so that motoneurons innervating axial or proximal muscles are located more medially than motoneurons innervating more distal muscles that control the hands or feet, which are located more laterally. The rostrocaudal distribution of motoneurons also follows the body scheme, so that more rostral segments innervate muscles of more proximal joints and vice versa for distal joints. Furthermore, motoneurons innervating muscles exerting flexion are more dorsally located than extensor motoneurons. The embryonic development of motoneuronal and interneuronal topography has been more clearly identified in recent years by the work of Jessell and Sanes[4] who have established how various genetically determined factors may dictate the fate of various types of neurons. This topography is significant in SCI because various lesions (primary or secondary) can damage specific parts of the cord and consequently affect certain functional groups of motoneurons more than others. For instance, when lesions occur dorsomedially, motoneurons that innervate proximal flexor muscles will be more affected than motoneurons that innervate distal extensors.

The lateral horn (at the thoracic and upper lumbar levels only) contains preganglionic sympathetic neurons whose axons reach the sympathetic ganglia adjacent to the vertebral bodies through white communicating rami from the ventral roots. Preganglionic parasympathetic neurons are located similarly at the S2–4 levels for visceral innervation.

Spinal White Matter

SCI may affect different portions of the SC, and it is, of course, important to have a clear idea of the distribution of long descending and ascending tracts that constitute some of the inputs and outputs of the SC. Therefore, the distribution of these tracts in a prototypic segment (**Fig. 1.2B**) is described here.

Surrounding the gray matter is the white matter, through which various myelinated (thus the name) but also unmyelinated fibers travel to interconnect segments of the cord, to carry sensory information to and from supraspinal centers. The proportion of gray and white matter differs considerably according to the spinal level (**Fig. 1.1**, left). More caudally descending tracts become smaller as more and more branches reach their targets within the SC. The opposite is true for sensory tracts, as more and more axons enter the SC, so that the tracts get larger rostrally.

Sensory Pathways

Dorsal Columns Located between the dorsal sulcus and the posterolateral sulcus where the dorsal roots enter the cord, the dorsal columns, made of the fasciculus cuneatus (upper limbs) and the fasciculus gracilis (lower limbs, below the sixth thoracic level), contain fibers mainly for fine touch discrimination and proprioceptive inputs carried by large afferents innervating muscle spindles and Golgi tendon organs of the ipsilateral side. These two tracts end in the cuneatus and gracilis nuclei of the brain stem, respectively, which then project their axons contralaterally to form part of the medial lemniscus reaching the thalamus. In the context of SCI, it is important to remember that fibers in these tracts are organized somatotopically, so that fibers originating from the lower limbs are more medial than those originating from the upper limbs.

Spinocerebellar Tracts Spinocerebellar tracts carry proprioceptive and exteroceptive information from the limbs and also from endogenous spinal processes. The *dorsal spinocerebellar tract* (DSCT) originates from cells in the Clarke column located at the base of the dorsal horn (lamina VI). These cells receive proprioceptive inputs from a limited number of muscle receptors (providing length and force feedback) and exteroceptive inputs from cutaneous receptors. The DSCT ascends ipsilaterally in the dorsal posterolateral funiculus and reaches the cerebellum through the inferior cerebellar peduncle. The cuneovestibular pathway plays the equivalent role for the upper limbs and originates from the external cuneate nucleus. The ventral *spinocerebellar tract* (VSCT) originates mainly from border cells in the ventral horn, which, contrary to the Clarke column neurons, project their axons contralaterally. This tract, and its forelimb equivalent the *rostral spinocerebellar tract*, reaches the cerebellum via the superior cerebellar peduncle. The VSCT carries information from peripheral receptors and intraspinal processes. For instance, during fictive locomotion (evoked in a decerebrate and paralyzed cat), DSCT cells may be silenced, whereas VSCT cells can continue to discharge rhythmically to provide the cerebellum with an ongoing monitor of intraspinal activity.[5,6]

Anterior and lateral *spinothalamic tracts* are located laterally and carry pain and temperature inputs from the contralateral side of the body through cross pathways passing through the anterior commissure of the SC. It should thus be realized that in the somatesthesic system, proprioceptive/tactile information is carried within the ipsilateral dorsal column and crosses to the other side in the brain stem, whereas pain/temperature information crosses to the other side at the spinal cord level itself. Consequently, following a hemisection of the SC (Brown-Séquard syndrome), there is a dissociation between proprioceptive/exteroceptive information with that of pain/temperature sensation. The proprioceptive/tactile information on the side of the hemisection will be perturbed on the side of the lesion, whereas the pain/temperature deficit will be on the other side.

Motor Pathways

It is customary to subdivide descending pathways into dorsolateral and medial groups based mainly on their control of fine motor movements of the hands and feet or postural muscles, respectively.[7,8]

The lateral corticospinal tract, after decussating at the level of the bulbar pyramids, travels through the dorsolateral funiculus along the whole cord. It is somatotopically organized so that fibers destined for cervical levels (55% of fibers) are the most medial, and those destined for the lumbar enlargement are more lateral. It should be remembered that the posterior columns are also somatotopically organized but in a reverse order. The lateral corticospinal tract contains axons originating mainly from cells of layer V in the motor cortex and the premotor cortex but the primary sensory cortex and parietal cortex also contribute ~20% of the tract. A small contingent of fibers is uncrossed and travels in a medioventral location (the anterior corticospinal tract) to reach the upper extremities only.

Besides this direct access to motoneurons and interneurons of the cord, the cortex can also reach the SC more indirectly through corticoreticular pathways and be involved in postural adjustments before or during voluntary movements. It is important to realize that corticospinal cells are involved not only in controlling muscle groups but also in regulating the excitability of various interneuronal pathways involved in sensory processing. Thus, during voluntary movement, predictable sensory information may be gated out.

The second-largest tract in the dorsolateral funiculus is the rubrospinal tract, which originates from large cells in the caudal red nucleus (magnicellular part) contralaterally. This tract is also involved in controlling distal muscles (mainly flexor muscles) and is complementary to the corticospinal tract. In humans, this tract is more rudimentary and reaches only thoracic segments.

Ventral-ventrolateral pathways include vestibular and reticular pathways. The vestibular pathway originates from the lateral vestibular nucleus, travels in the anterior part of the lateral funiculus, and projects to extensor motoneurons of the limbs and paraxial muscles to maintain equilibrium.

Reticular pathways originate from various brain stem reticular nuclei and project either ipsilaterally (from the pons) or bilaterally (from the medulla) to the ventral SC. They are involved in neck responses, interlimb coordination, and equilibrium. Because the cells of origin of these pathways receive cortical inputs, they are believed to provide a potentially more indirect access to the SC after lesion of the corticospinal tract.[9]

Propriospinal Pathways

Various spinal segments are interconnected by propriospinal pathways coursing close to the gray matter on both sides.

The tract of Lissauer is located at the entry of the dorsal roots and distributes afferent inputs to different spinal segments. Other interconnections may be established by spinal interneurons (nucleus proprius), which may project their axons to short or long pathways interconnecting more distant segments. Such pathways have become more important because it was demonstrated that, after corticospinal tract lesions, new connections could be established with the lumbosacral cord through cervical propriospinal pathways in rats.[10] In the same species, it was also shown that propriospinal pathways may be important for the expression of locomotion after partial lesions in adults,[11] or sufficient to activate the locomotor pattern in neonates.[12,13]

Autonomic Pathways

Supraspinal pathways innervating preganglionic neurons of the lateral column from T1 to L2 and S2–4 are located in the lateral column and originate from the hypothalamus via projections to the reticular formation. Depending on the level, spinal lesions may produce different symptoms, ranging from Horner syndrome, autonomic dysreflexia (see Chapter 16), bladder dysfunction, or sexual dysfunctions affecting erection or ejaculation.

Lesions of the SC will also damage pathways that carry important neuromodulators, such as serotonin and norepinephrine. The serotonergic pathway originates from subdivisions of the raphe nucleus in the brain stem while the noradrenergic pathway originates from the locus ceruleus, also in the brain stem. These projections to the SC are widespread, and neurotransmitters may be released at defined synapses or released in the SC environment by a mechanism known as volumic transmission, whereby several neurons can be influenced in a less specific way.

These pathways release their neurotransmitters at various levels of the SC, and, given the fact that receptor subtypes may be distributed differentially at various segments,[14] it can be expected that drugs acting on these receptors may affect different functions. As will be seen in Chapter 33, the use of neurotransmitter precursors or agonists, as well as antagonists, may provide important therapeutic avenues after SCI,[15] either to reactivate circuits or to diminish unwarranted activity in others.

Vascularization of the Spinal Cord

Essentially, the SC is supplied by the anterior spinal artery, two posterior spinal arteries, and several radicular arteries originating at various levels. Some knowledge of the vascular territory is important because traumatic or arteriosclerotic diseases may block arteries in specific territories, which will indiscriminately affect sensory and motor pathways as well as the gray matter.

Originating from the fusion of the two vertebral arteries, the anterior spinal artery is located in the median sulcus and gives off central branches, which irrigate the anterior two thirds of the SC. Ischemia resulting from the blockage of the anterior spinal artery or its various branches will give rise to the anterior cord syndrome, characterized initially by a flaccid paralysis due to the interruption of various descending motor tracts. Characteristically, proprioception/exteroception is preserved because the dorsal horn and the dorsal columns are spared. Posterior spinal arteries irrigate the posterior third of the cord and, consequently, ischemia of this region mainly affects dorsal column pathways. Radicular arteries vascularize the ventral and dorsal roots and also contribute to the anterior and posterior spinal arteries.

Physiology

As stated in the introduction, the SC is a bona fide neural center similar to any other central structure of the nervous system, with complex processing functions, inputs, and outputs. Here the processing functions are achieved in the gray matter through various types of interneurons. The inputs to the gray matter are not only from peripheral sensory afferents that reach the cord through the dorsal roots but also from pathways descending from the brain stem and telencephalic structures either directly or indirectly via propriospinal pathways. There is thus a very wide set of inputs from the periphery and other parts of the CNS, so that the cells in the SC gray matter have to integrate all of the inputs to produce the appropriate outputs. The outputs of the gray matter are to peripheral organs, such as skeletal muscles or ganglia of the sympathetic and parasympathetic system and to the brain stem, diencephalon, and telencephalon through various ascending pathways. Thus, damage to the SC has consequences not only for how sensory information and descending inputs are processed but also for how the SC controls peripheral organs and how it interacts with other CNS structures.

With this in mind, it is of interest to look at various sensorimotor input–output functions that may be of interest within the clinical context of SCI. Responses to peripheral or central inputs allow the assessment of the excitability level of various simple or more complex circuits or an alteration in the distribution of the evoked responses. It is thus important to know the main components of the pathways to better evaluate the nature of the changes observed. Chapters 46 and 47 deal with the evaluation of descending pathways using techniques like transcranial magnetic stimulation or electrical stimulation. The following text considers spinal pathways activated by afferent inputs from the periphery. **Figure 1.4** gives a broad overview of spinal reflex pathways that, although seemingly complex, is still very much simplified.[16]

Monosynaptic Reflex

Monosynaptic circuits are established in the SC by afferent inputs originating from sensors within primary muscle spindles that measure changes in the rate and magnitude of muscle length. The afferents from these sensors are large afferents (group Ia) that enter the cord and make monosynaptic connections with motoneurons. When the muscle is stretched, several action potentials are generated in the Ia afferent, which triggers the release of an excitatory neurotransmitter (i.e., glutamate) on the membrane of motoneurons. The motoneurons are then depolarized and, if the input is strong enough, the motoneurons will generate action potentials within the motor axon and cause a muscle contraction by liberating acetylcholine at the neuromuscular junction. The monosynaptic reflex is thus considered a simple negative-feedback system whereby muscle stretch generates a muscle contraction to oppose the stretch.

This pathway is tested in various manners, either by mechanical stretch of a given muscle (e.g., tendon tap), or by electrically stimulating the muscle nerve (see stimulation symbol on the right portion of **Fig. 1.4**), which is called the H-reflex. The state of the muscle spindles may differ in various conditions because they are innervated by γ-motoneurons whose cell bodies are also within the ventral spinal cord. These γ-motoneurons may be more or less excitable depending on the state of descending inputs. Thus the same muscle stretch can lead to muscle responses of different amplitudes depending on the state of the muscle spindles, which depends on the excitability of γ-motoneurons.[17] Therefore, the H-reflex cannot be considered identical to the stretch reflex because it bypasses the muscle spindles via direct electrical activation of the sensory axons in the muscle nerve. As such, it is not subject to fusimotor drive (γ-motoneurons), which alters the sensitivity of the muscle spindle to a given stretch.

Thus, stretch reflexes inform the clinician about the state of the muscle spindles, of the transmission from sensory afferents to the motoneurons, and of the motoneurons themselves. Alterations in the excitability at various levels will alter the amplitude of the muscle contraction in response to a tendon tap. Central conditions that alter the excitability of the α-motoneurons are of course manifested directly in the amplitude of the muscle response. After SCI, α-motoneurons may be unexcitable because of diminished or abolished excitatory inputs from de-

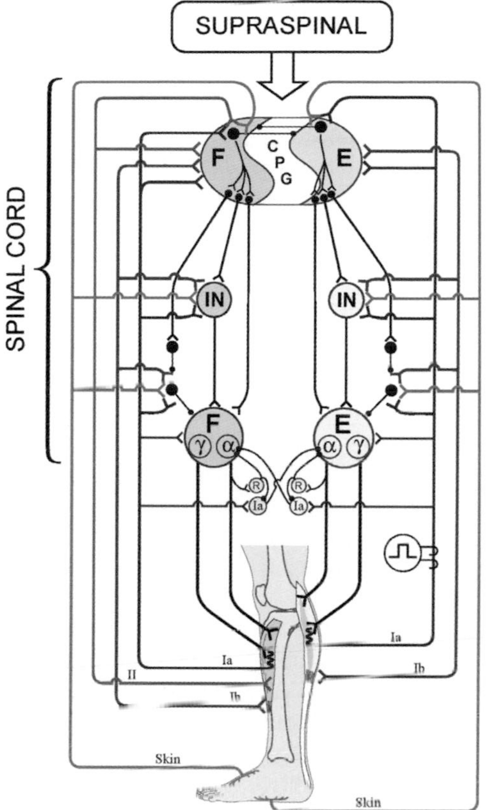

Fig. 1.4 General scheme of reflex pathways and spinal locomotor control. This figure is subdivided into three parts. The *supraspinal* levels include various descending pathways from the telencephalon and brain stem involved in activating, stopping, or modulating characteristics of the spinal central pattern generator (CPG) for locomotion. Although the supraspinal pathways are shown here to act only on the CPG, these structures also act on interneurons (IN) and motoneurons (FG and E) as well as on the excitability of transmission in reflex pathways at motoneuronal or premotoneuronal (presynaptic and/or interneuronal) levels. The *large arrow* emerging from the supraspinal level encompasses all these functions. Some of the details are discussed in the text. The *spinal cord* level includes the CPG with a generally reciprocal activity between the flexor (F) and extensor (E) sides through inhibitory interneurons. These two antagonist phases of the CPG circuitry are separated to indicate that each part may exert a function on other spinal mechanisms (represented by three output neurons emerging from each part of the CPG) as well as interact with other parts (inhibitory connections between F and E). The interneurons are represented by two large pink and blue interneurons (IN), which are interposed between afferents and motoneurons in disynaptic pathways (Ia IN) as well as other more specific inhibitory interneurons (in black) representing disynaptic inhibitory pathways (such as Ib inhibitory IN), which can also be inhibited by other interneurons in certain tasks, such as locomotion. Finally, motoneuron pools include both α-motoneurons projecting to extrafusal muscle fibers and γ-motoneurons projecting to intrafusal muscle fibers. Recurrent inhibition through Renshaw cells inhibits α-motoneurons (represented) and γ-motoneurons (not represented) and Ia interneurons responsible for reciprocal inhibition between α-motoneurons. In the periphery, one ankle flexor muscle (pink) and one extensor muscle (blue) are represented with a spindle in both. Groups Ia and II represent sensory fibers from spindles and are responsible for indicating rate and amount of muscle stretch, respectively. The stimulation symbol on the Ia fiber from the extensor illustrates direct stimulation of Ia afferents as performed during H-reflex studies. Ib fibers originate from Golgi tendon organs, which measure the force output of the muscle. Skin inputs from the dorsum or the plantar surface are indicated as projecting to flexor and extensor motoneurons. Connectivity of the various afferents is only partial and is largely based on the established literature.[17] This figure illustrates that the circuitry presents many alternatives for responses that may account for dynamic changes between responses in physiological or pathophysiological conditions.

scending pathways. Acutely, this is termed spinal shock, in which all reflexes are abolished for a while, even the monosynaptic reflex. As excitability returns, these reflexes reappear or even become exaggerated, as is the case in spasticity. Again, the state of γ-motoneuron excitability can also determine the level of responsiveness as well as the return of some membrane property (see later plateau potentials). Finally, asymmetry in monosynaptic reflexes may be used to determine asymmetrical lesions of the SC, since the inputs to the SC will then be unbalanced.

As stated, the H-reflex tests the monosynaptic pathway but bypasses changes in the excitability of muscle spindles. Changes in the amplitude of the H-reflex can thus be used to measure changes in α-motoneuron excitability but also in the excitability of presynaptic components, which can all be altered by other sensory afferents and/or descending inputs (see Chapter 48). As such, stimulating other nerves or different structures before evoking the H-reflex can be used to probe changes in presynaptic excitability, a method called conditioning. Changing presynaptic excitability will increase or decrease the H-reflex. Clinically, it is important to dissociate changes occurring at pre- (i.e., before the motoneuron) and postsynaptic (i.e., at the motoneuron) loci.

Di-, Tri-, and Multisynaptic Reflexes

Whereas the previous monosynaptic reflex may be regarded as providing a simple negative-feedback circuit to adjust muscle length, the majority of reflex pathways include one or more interneurons (**Fig. 1.4**). When one interneuron is interposed between the primary afferent and the motoneurons, it is termed a disynaptic pathway. Trisynaptic pathways have two interposed interneurons, and with more than two interneurons, the pathways are said to be polysynaptic.[18]

Such pathways offer greater versatility of responses to a particular input. For instance, a sensory afferent may project to some excitatory interneurons that will excite motoneurons and also project to inhibitory interneurons that inhibit other motoneurons. As an example, when muscle spindles are stretched, monosynaptic excitation is provided to the motoneurons from which the afferents originate (i.e., homonymous) and to close synergists (i.e., heteronymous) but the same afferents will also project to inhibitory interneurons (so-called Ia inhibitory interneurons), which project to antagonist motoneurons (**Fig. 1.4**). Thus, stretch of a muscle leads to its contraction and to the contraction of close synergists but also to inhibition of the antagonist muscle acting principally at the same joint. This is called reciprocal inhibition. These Ia interneurons in turn are controlled by Renshaw cells and by a plethora of descending inputs, so that reciprocal inhibition may be deficient after SCI, leading to more co-contraction (see Chapter 42).

One important observation in recent years has been that reflex responses to a given input may be quite different in various conditions, so that reflex responses can hardly be considered all hardwired, and alternative pathways do exist. For instance, it was shown in walking animals that the same stimulation of the skin may give rise to a flexion response in one phase of walking and to an inhibition or excitation of extensor muscles in the opposite phase of the walking cycle.[18] Another striking example of phase-dependent modulation comes from stimulation of force detectors in muscle (i.e., Golgi tendon organs). Stimulation of the Ib fibers that stem from Golgi tendon organs produce an inhibitory response in the muscle at rest but an excitatory response of the same muscle during locomotion due to the opening of locomotor-related interneuronal pathways (see **Fig. 1.4**).

Such alternative reflex pathways are also relevant in the appearance of the Babinski response, which consists of toe fanning and dorsiflexion of the big toe (corticospinal lesion) when the sole of the foot is stimulated, in contrast to the normal response of plantar flexion to the same stimulation. Alternative reflex pathways exist and, in certain conditions, the bias may favor one direction or the other. Such biases may be seen in pathological conditions, such as after SCI (see Chapter 48).

Outputs of the Gray Matter to the Periphery

There are three outputs of the gray matter to the peripheral nervous system: α-motoneurons, γ-motoneurons, and preganglionic axons.

The α-motoneurons, with cell bodies in the ventral horn, send their axons to innervate skeletal muscles. These motoneurons integrate inputs from several sources, including spinal interneurons and descending pathways. Motoneurons constitute the final output to muscles and are often considered the final common pathway. Motoneurons have several receptors with fast ionic channels that can excite [glutamate acting through *N*-methyl-D-aspartate (NMDA) receptors] or inhibit [γ-aminobutyric acid (GABA) through GABA receptors] their membrane. Motoneurons also have metabotropic receptors that produce longer-lasting changes in excitability. Indeed, motoneurons can show nonlinear characteristics, such that a given input can produce a prolonged depolarization of the membrane, which is called a persistent inward current (PIC). Of particular interest within the context of SCI is that after acute SCI, motoneurons lose the ability to generate PICs, and this is probably due in part to the lack of neuromodulators, such as noradrenaline and serotonin, which are synthesized in the brain stem and are therefore largely depleted below the injury. Using agonists of these neurotransmitters can reinstate motoneuronal excitability in acutely spinalized cats. Over the long term, there appears to be a return of PICs, and abnormal descending control of this excitability could contribute to the development of spasticity as well as other motor dysfunctions.[19]

Gamma motoneurons innervate intrafusal muscle fibers of muscle spindles, and their smaller axons also course through ventral roots. Gamma motoneurons receive a variety of supraspinal inputs and can thus indirectly set the muscle tone by altering muscle spindle sensitivity. Consequently, a large increase in excitability of γ-motoneurons may increase the sensitivity of the spindles to a point where a very small stretch can yield large muscle contractions. As a result, stretching the muscle spindle results in greater discharge of Ia afferents and a larger response in target motoneurons. A variety of conditions can change the excitability state (set) of γ-motoneurons.[20]

Finally, preganglionic neurons in the intermediolateral column send their axons through ventral roots and, through the white communicans nerves, reach the autonomic ganglia chain. These preganglionic axons also receive a variety of inputs, and their discharge will result in a greater or lesser discharge of ganglion cells, leading eventually to an increase or decrease of peripheral noradrenaline.

Complex Sensorimotor Patterns

Although the SC is traditionally described as a structure giving rise to rather simple reflexes, it is clear that it is also capable of generating, by itself, more complex movements, which are programmed through more complex genetically determined circuits.[15,21,22] For example, in the adult cat, following a complete SC transection at low thoracic levels, it is possible to elicit complex movements, such as fast paw shaking or locomotion, two rhythms with specific characteristics in terms of frequency and structure.[23] Multiple studies have shown that the basic pattern of locomotion can be evoked from the isolated SC through well-conserved mechanisms in the lamprey, a primitive vertebrate that has existed for 600 million years, as well as in large mammals.[24] Such basic pattern of rhythmic organization intrinsic to the SC has clearly been shown in rats, mice, cats, and some primates. Although many details of the circuit generating the locomotor pattern, called the central pattern generator (CPG), are not known in mammals (contrary to other species, such as the lamprey), one can question whether such circuitry also exists in humans and if it can be stimulated to express some motor functions after SCI. Some work clearly points to the existence of such spinal mechanisms in humans also.[1,25,26] Other chapters deal with the importance of these concepts for locomotor rehabilitation (Chapters 44 and 45).

Acknowledgments

The author's work has been funded continuously since 1975 by the Canadian Institute of Health Research (CIHR) through individual grants, group grants, a team grant (Multidisciplinary Team on Locomotor Rehabilitation), and a Canada Research Chair on the Spinal Cord.

Pearls

- The fact that the spinal cord is shorter than the vertebral canal allows the collection of cerebrospinal fluid from the dural sac without damaging the spinal cord itself because only spinal roots are found in the dural sac.
- The gray matter (subdivided into various horns) at the core of the spinal cord contains neurons organized in laminae, each having some role in processing information.
- The white matter, organized in columns, contains descending and ascending fiber tracts with a somatotopic organization, which explains the progressive impairments of various body parts with particular location of spinal lesions. The vascular organization is such that multiple pathways of different functions can be impaired in ischemic diseases of the spinal cord.
- There are various alternative reflex pathways, so that some peripheral inputs may yield different types of responses depending on the state of excitability of certain interneuronal pathways. Some pathological reflexes (Babinski) may represent a bias of alternative interneuronal spinal pathway due to a pathological process and not the creation of new pathways.
- The spinal cord can give rise not only to simple reflex responses but also to more complex primitive motor patterns, such as are required in basic locomotion.

Pitfalls

- The spinal cord is not just a conduit for information from the brain to the body and from the body to the brain.
- The spinal cord is like all other centers of the CNS, with inputs from other brain structures and sensory information from various body parts, with processing units, and with outputs to the brain and various body parts.
- The SC is shorter than the vertebral canal, so that the correspondence between the two should be remembered when one is extrapolating the neural symptoms based on the description of lesions, which may often refer to vertebral, not spinal, segments.
- Ascending (sensory) and descending (motor) tracts are generally crossed with respect to the telencephalon or the brain stem, but the crossing does not occur at the same levels. Proprioceptive/tactile inputs from one side of the body cross on the other side at the brain stem level, whereas pain/temperature inputs cross at the spinal level. This sensory dissociation is important in determining spinal lesions.
- Testing reflexes indicates the state of excitability of certain spinal pathways (motoneurons and interneurons), and their asymmetry may help in lesion localization.

References

1. Nadeau S, Jacquemin G, Fournier C, Lamarre Y, Rossignol S. Spontaneous motor rhythms of the back and legs in a patient with a complete spinal cord transection. Neurorehabil Neural Repair 2010;24(4):377–383
2. Netter FH. Nervous system: anatomy and physiology. In: Brass A, Dingle RV, eds. The Ciba Collection of Medical Illustrations, vol 1. 1983:1–239
3. Rexed B. The cytoarchitectonic organization of the spinal cord in the cat. J Comp Neurol 1952;96(3):414–495
4. Jessell TM, Sanes JR. Development: the decade of the developing brain. Curr Opin Neurobiol 2000;10(5):599–611
5. Arshavsky YI, Berkinblit MB, Fukson OI, Gelfand IM, Orlovsky GN. Recordings of neurones of the dorsal spinocerebellar tract during evoked locomotion. Brain Res 1972;43(1):272–275
6. Arshavsky YI, Berkinblit MB, Gelfand IM, Orlovsky GN, Fukson OI. Activity of the neurones of the ventral spino-cerebellar tract during locomotion. Biophysics (Oxf) 1972;17:926–935
7. Lawrence DG, Kuypers HGJM. The functional organization of the motor system in the monkey, II: The effects of lesions of the descending brainstem pathways. Brain 1968;91(1):15–36
8. Lawrence DG, Kuypers HGJM. The functional organization of the motor system in the monkey, I; The effects of bilateral pyramidal lesions. Brain 1968;91(1):1–14
9. Ballermann M, Fouad K. Spontaneous locomotor recovery in spinal cord injured rats is accompanied by anatomical plasticity of reticulospinal fibers. Eur J Neurosci 2006;23(8):1988–1996
10. Bareyre FM, Kerschensteiner M, Raineteau O, Mettenleiter TC, Weinmann O, Schwab ME. The injured spinal cord spontaneously forms a new intraspinal circuit in adult rats. Nat Neurosci 2004;7(3):269–277
11. Courtine G, Song B, Roy RR, et al. Recovery of supraspinal control of stepping via indirect propriospinal relay connections after spinal cord injury. Nat Med 2008;14(1):69–74
12. Cowley KC, Zaporozhets E, Schmidt BJ. Propriospinal neurons are sufficient for bulbospinal transmission of the locomotor command signal in the neonatal rat spinal cord. J Physiol 2008;586(6):1623–1635
13. Zaporozhets E, Cowley KC, Schmidt BJ. Propriospinal neurons contribute to bulbospinal transmission of the locomotor command signal in the neonatal rat spinal cord. J Physiol 2006;572(Pt 2):443–458
14. Schmidt BJ, Jordan LM. The role of serotonin in reflex modulation and locomotor rhythm production in the mammalian spinal cord. Brain Res Bull 2000;53(5):689–710
15. Rossignol S. Neural control of stereotypic limb movements. In: Rowell LB, Sheperd JT, eds. Handbook of Physiology, Section 12. Exercise: Regulation and Integration of Multiple Systems. New York: Oxford University Press; 1996:173–216
16. Frigon A, Rossignol S. Functional plasticity following spinal cord lesions. Prog Brain Res 2006; 157(16):231–260
17. Prochazka A. Proprioceptive feedback and movement regulation. In: Rowell LB, Sheperd JT, eds. Handbook of Physiology. Section 12. Exercise: Regulation and Integration of Multiple Systems. New York: American Physiological Society; 1996:89–127
18. Rossignol S, Dubuc R, Gossard JP. Dynamic sensorimotor interactions in locomotion. Physiol Rev 2006;86(1):89–154
19. Murray KC, Nakae A, Stephens MJ, et al. Recovery of motoneuron and locomotor function after spinal cord injury depends on constitutive activity in 5-HT2C receptors. Nat Med 2010;16(6): 694–700
20. Prochazka A, Hulliger M, Zangger P, Appenteng K. 'Fusimotor set': new evidence for alpha independent control of gamma motoneurones during movement in the awake cat. Brain Res 1985; 339(1):136–140
21. Sherrington CS. Flexion-reflex of the limb, crossed extension-reflex, and reflex stepping and standing. J Physiol 1910;40(1-2):28–121
22. Grillner S. Control of locomotion in bipeds, tetrapods, and fish. In: Brookhart JM, Mountcastle VB, eds. Handbook of Physiology: The Nervous System II. Bethesda, MD: American Physiological Society; 1981:1179 1236
23. Langlet C, Leblond H, Rossignol S. Mid-lumbar segments are needed for the expression of locomotion in chronic spinal cats. J Neurophysiol 2005;93(5):2474–2488
24. Grillner S, Wallén P. Cellular bases of a vertebrate locomotor system-steering, intersegmental and segmental co-ordination and sensory control. Brain Res Rev 2002;40(1-3):92–106
25. Calancie B. Spinal myoclonus after spinal cord injury. J Spinal Cord Med 2006;29(4):413–424
26. Bussel BC, Roby-Brami A, Yakovleff A, Bennis N. Evidences for the presence of a spinal stepping generator in patients with a spinal cord section. In: Amblard B, Berthoz A, Clarac F, eds. Posture and Gait: Development, Adaptation and Modulation. North Holland: Elsevier; 1988:273–278

2

Evaluation of the Patient with Spinal Cord Injury

Mahmoud Benour, Aleksa Cenic, R. John Hurlbert, and Charles Tator

Key Points

1. Initial evaluation of polytrauma patients suffering a spinal cord injury should focus on excluding immediate life-threatening systemic injuries.
2. In-depth neurological evaluation according to the ASIA score at presentation is required not only to guide immediate management but also to predict long-term recovery.
3. Functional outcomes measures, such FIM, SCIM, WISCI, and MBI, provide valuable tools in evaluating the impact of SCI on the patient's quality of life.

The worldwide annual incidence of spinal cord injury (SCI) is 15 to 40 cases per million population.[1,2] Motor vehicle crashes are the most common cause of SCI, followed by falls, sports, and violence-related injuries.[1,3] SCI commonly involves the younger age group, with the average age being 38 years.[1,3] SCI can be a devastating problem, not only for patients but also for their families (see Chapter 5 for epidemiology).

The functional outcome of SCI is dependent on the severity of the initial injury and hence is widely variable. It is well established that the initial neurological presentation is one of the most important predictors of functional outcome. This chapter explores methods of patient evaluation in the setting of acute SCI, with a view toward guiding management and predicting outcome (discussed in detail in Chapter 7).

Patient Evaluation

History

The clinical history has a special significance in SCI because it may give clues to the mechanism and severity of the injury. The history from the patient, as well as from emergency response personnel and witnesses, should be noted. Past medical history, allergies, and any surgical history should be documented. Initial presentation reported by the emergency medical response service at the scene of the injury provides pertinent information about the possible loss of neurological function.

The following clinical factors indicate a higher risk of having SCI: pain or palpation tenderness along the spinal axis, limb numbness or paresthesias, limb weakness, any loss or decrease in the level of consciousness, incontinence, and the presence of drug or alcohol intoxication.

Several mechanisms of injury that require special attention in spinal evaluation include a fall from a significant height and motor vehicle crashes involving high speed, roll-over, or ejection.

Physical Examination

The forces leading to SCI are often great enough to cause injury to other organs; thus SCI is often accompanied by multiple trauma.[4] Commonly associated injuries include long bone fractures, visceral injuries involving the chest and abdominal cavities, pelvic fractures, and head injuries. In patients with SCI, it can be difficult to diagnose long bone fractures and other injuries due to the absence of pain sensation.[5] Initial assessment of multiple trauma patients with suspected SCI includes evaluation of airway, breathing, and circulation. Following the Advanced Trauma Life Support (ATLS) guidelines will systematically reveal life- and limb-threatening injuries.[6]

Upon completing the ATLS protocol, a neurological examination may be initiated, with special attention to motor and sensory function in the upper and lower extremities. In the awake or unconscious SCI patient, thorough palpation of the axial spine (from cervical to sacral) should then be performed with documentation of any focal tenderness and physical signs of injury (e.g., bruising, lacerations, or step-off deformity).

General Physical Examination and the Systemic Effect of Spinal Cord Injury

When hypotension is present on initial presentation, it may be difficult to differentiate hypovolemic systemic shock due to significant blood loss versus hypotension as a result of neurogenic shock.[7] Hypotension, bradycardia, and warm extremities are due to cervical SCI (neurogenic shock) and not to hypovolemic shock. The latter causes hypotension, tachycardia, and cold extremities. Although septic shock can be associated with peripheral vasodilatation (warm extremities), it is accompanied by tachycardia rather than bradycardia. Septic shock is not usually part of the differential diagnosis in the trauma setting.

Spinal and Neurogenic Shock (discussed in Chapter 6)

The sympathetic and parasympathetic divisions of the autonomic nervous system maintain blood pressure and cardiac output through their regulation of the heart rate, stroke volume, and peripheral vascular resistance.

Sympathetic preganglionic fibers supplying the heart leave the spinal cord in the anterior roots of T1–5. SCI at or above these levels eliminates the descending sympathetic outflow, resulting in unopposed parasympathetic control of the heart, mediated through parasympathetic cardiac afferents that travel with the vagus nerve and thus are not affected by the SCI. A similar mechanism causes imbalance in the peripheral autonomic tone, resulting in vasodilatation also under unopposed parasympathetic control. The end-organ result is hypotension with paradoxical bradycardia and dramatically reduced cardiac output.

Massive intravenous fluid resuscitation may result in fluid overload and pulmonary edema. Blood pressure in neurogenic shock is best restored by blood transfusion to increase circulating blood volume and judicious use of vasopressors (e.g., dopamine) after volume replacement.

The term *spinal shock*, as stated by Atkinson and Atkinson, is "applied to all phenomena surrounding physiologic or anatomic spinal cord transection that result in temporary loss or depression of all or most of spinal reflex activities below the level of injury."[8] This will be discussed in more depth in Chapter 6, but is introduced here.

Spinal shock is a type of neurogenic shock and is a temporary physiological disorganization of spinal cord function that starts within minutes following injury and can last 6 weeks or longer postinjury. The most classic findings pertain to decreased tone and hyporeflexia in the setting of an upper motor neuron lesion. The exact pathophysiological mechanism is unknown but may be related to the temporary inhibition of impulse conduction in the injured cord secondary to an imbalance in ionic concentrations.[9–12] There is usually a major hemodynamic component of spinal shock, perhaps worsened by the flaccid extremity muscle tone that increases venous capacitance and contributes to a state of relative hypovolemia.

The resolution of spinal shock is marked by the return of deep tendon and other reflexes. Usually among the first to return is the bulbocavernosus reflex.[13,14] This reflex is defined as anal sphincter contraction in response to squeezing the glans penis in males. In females, the reflex may be obtained by pulling on a urethral Foley catheter or squeezing the clitoris. This reflex is of mainly historical note and plays little role in modern SCI assessment and management. Formerly, the early return of this reflex was regarded as an indication of a poor prognosis for neurological recovery.

Autonomic Dysreflexia

Autonomic dysreflexia (see also Chapter 16) is defined as "an increase in systolic blood pressure of at least 20% associated with a change in heart rate and accompanied by at least one of the following signs or symptoms: sweating, piloerection, facial flushing, headache, blurred vision, and stuffy nose."[15–17]

Autonomic dysreflexia is caused by spinal reflex mechanisms that remain intact after SCI. It is not seen in the acute (spinal shock) stage, but rather occurs once reflexes have returned and spasticity sets in. It is characterized by excessive uncontrolled sympathetic output as a result of a noxious stimulus (expected to cause pain or discomfort in a person without SCI) below the level of the lesion.[18] This response in turn results in peripheral vasoconstriction below the lesion. In lesions at T6 and above, the splanchnic vascular bed is involved, which contributes, along with peripheral vasoconstriction, to the increase in vascular tone that causes an elevation of systemic blood pressure.[16,18] Clinical manifestations vary from mild symptoms, pallor initially, followed by flushing of the face and neck and sweating in areas above the lesion and cold peripheral areas and piloerection below the spinal lesion, to acute life-threatening situations, including myocardial infarction and intracerebral hemorrhage.[16]

Neurogenic Pulmonary Edema

Neurogenic pulmonary edema results from "a protein-rich alveolar fluid leaking from the pulmonary capillaries into the interstitial tissue, most likely due to a transient severe increase in sympathetic activity associated with the injury."[19] This results in significant respiratory distress (e.g., shortness of breath) requiring mechanical ventilation to assist breathing.

The pathophysiology of neurogenic pulmonary edema in SCI is not fully understood but is believed to occur as a result of an immediate increase in blood pressure, which leads to an increase in both systemic and pulmonary vascular pressure. This increase results in a shift of blood from the high-resistance systemic circulation to the low-resistance pulmonary circulation. The increase in the pulmonary vascular pressure along with the increase in pulmonary blood volume, due to volume overload during resuscitation, contributes to the formation of pulmonary edema because of the hydrostatic effect of increased pulmonary capillary pressure. "Neurogenic pulmonary edema has been reported to occur with autonomic dysreflexia, which supports the theory that it is caused by a massive sympathetic discharge."[19,20]

Bradycardia

Heart rate and rhythm are under the control of the autonomic nervous system. The sinoatrial node is under direct influence of both the sympathetic and the parasympathetic nervous systems. Sympathetic input increases action potential production, whereas parasympathetic input decreases it.[20,21] Individuals with acute high-level SCI are more susceptible to bradyarrhythmias, including bradycardia and atrioventricular block, due to the disruption of the sympathetic input in the presence of unopposed vagal stimulation. Although bradycardia is the most common arrhythmia, supraventricular tachycardia and ventricular tachycardia have also been observed.[18] Bradycardia appears to be most common during the first 10 to 14 days after injury, and the severity correlates with the degree of SCI.[22,23] Reflex bradycardia can be triggered by procedures that increase vagal activity, such as endotracheal suctioning and laryngoscopy. Prophylactic atropine administration is recommended during such procedures.

Orthostatic Hypotension

In individuals with recent upper cervical SCI, the supine mean arterial pressure averages 57 mmHg, compared with 82 mmHg in noninjured spinal cord persons.[20] The American Autonomic Society and the American Academy of Neurology define orthostatic hypotension as a decrease in systolic blood pressure of more than 20 mmHg or a decrease in diastolic blood pressure of more than 10 mmHg with upright posture or head-up tilt to 60 degrees for at least 3 minutes.[24] Symptoms of orthostatic hypotension can include dizziness, nausea, lightheadedness, and loss of consciousness, which can be explained by cerebral hypoperfusion.[15,25–27] The probability of orthostatic hypotension increases in the presence of one or more of the following factors: (1) sympathetic nervous system dysfunction, (2) impaired baroreflex function, (3) lack of skeletal muscle pumping activity, (4) cardiovascular deconditioning due to prolonged bed rest, and (5) low plasma volume and hyponatremia.[15,25–27]

Neurological Evaluation

The most common system for assessing neurological function in SCI worldwide is the American Spinal Injury Association (ASIA) system.[12] It was formulated with the International Medical Society of Paraplegia, now renamed the International Spinal Cord Society (ISCoS). The details are discussed in Chapter 6.

Acute Spinal Cord Injury Syndromes

There are two main types of acute SCI lesions: complete and incomplete (**Table 2.1**). The distinction between complete and incomplete injury is an important first step to plan treatment and to predict functional outcome.[9,12,28]

In this chapter, cervicomedullary and reversible (transient) SCI syndromes are reviewed. More details on other syndromes are discussed in Chapter 6.

Cervicomedullary Syndrome

The cervicomedullary syndrome results from injury to the higher segments of the cervical spinal cord as well as injury to the lower segment of the brain stem—the medulla. The injury may extend to involve the area between C4 caudally, and the pons rostrally. The cervicomedullary syndrome is caused by either a traction injury associated with severe atlantoaxial dislocation or a compression injury from a burst fracture or ruptured disk of the upper cervical vertebrae. It also may occur as a result of ischemic events following a vertebral artery injury (e.g., dissection) or from a cervical spine trauma (e.g., cervical facet dislocations).[11]

The clinical features of the cervicomedullary syndrome include upper extremity weakness with minimally affected or

Table 2.1 Syndromes of Acute Spinal Cord Injury (Figs. 2.1, 2.2, 2.3, 2.4, and 2.5)

Complete spinal cord injury
Incomplete spinal cord injury • Cervicomedullary syndrome • Central cord syndrome • Anterior cord syndrome • Posterior cord syndrome • Brown-Séquard syndrome • Conus medullaris syndrome
Cauda equina syndrome
Reversible or transient syndromes

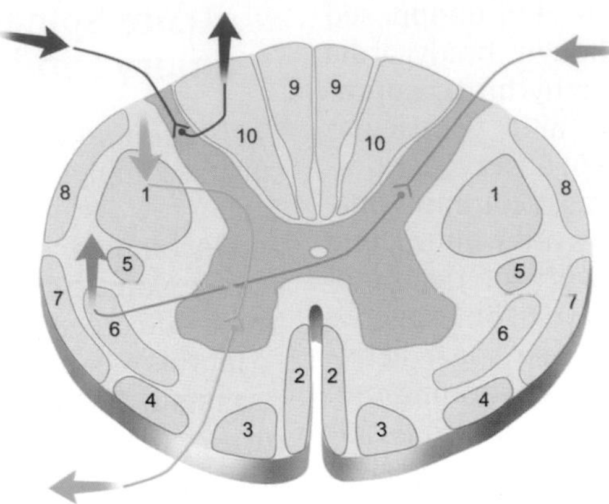

Fig. 2.1 Cross-section of the spinal cord showing the (1) lateral corticospinal tract; (2) anterior corticospinal tract; (3) medial vestibulospinal tract, reticulospinal tract, testospinal tract; (4) lateral vestibulospinal tract; (5) rubrospinal tract; (6) anterolateral spinothalamic tract; (7) ventral spinocerebellar tract; (8) dorsal spinocerebellar tract; (9) fasciculus gracilis; (10) fasciculus cuneatus.

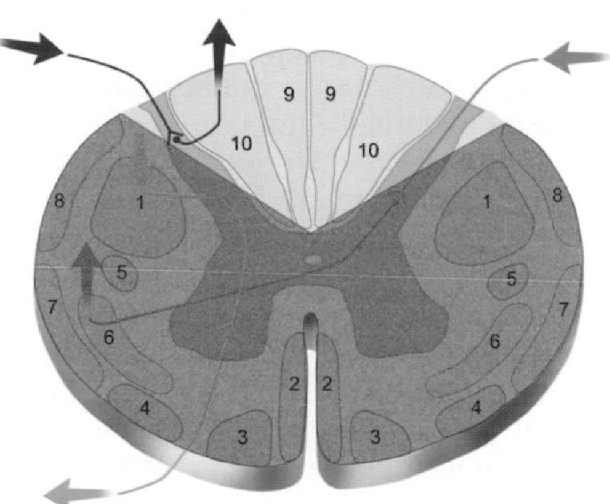

Fig. 2.2 Anterior spinal cord syndrome.

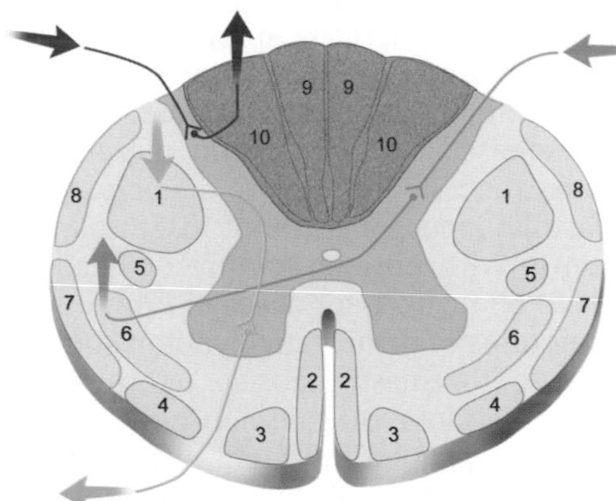

Fig. 2.3 Posterior spinal cord syndrome.

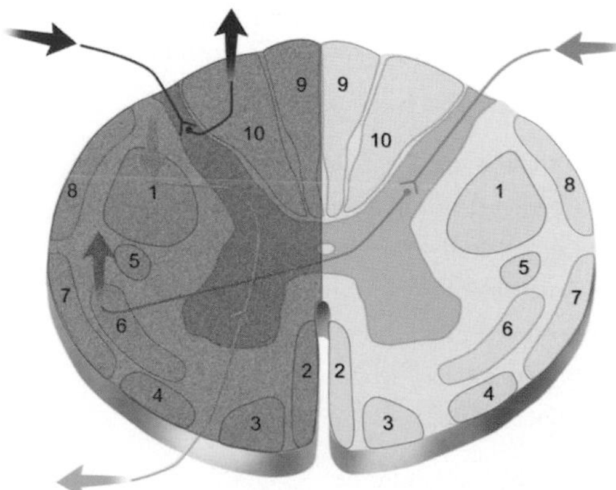

Fig. 2.4 Brown-Séquard syndrome.

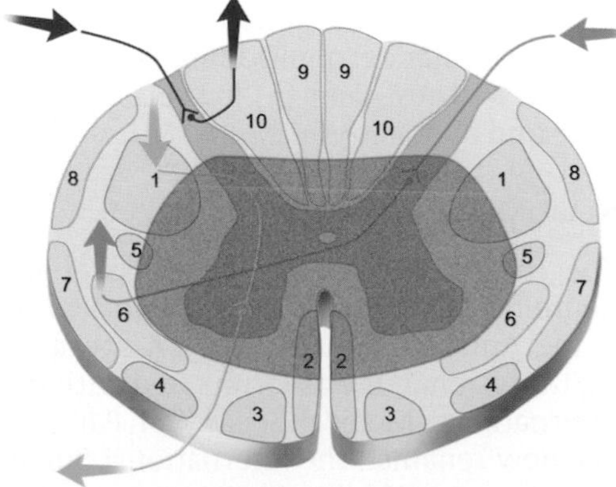

Fig. 2.5 Central cord syndrome.

spared lower extremities (mimics a central cord syndrome).[23] The most severe form presents as respiratory arrest, hypotension, motor deficit varying from tetraparesis to tetraplegia, and anesthesia from C1-4 dermatomes.[11,29]

There are three sensory nuclei for the trigeminal nerve: the main sensory nucleus, the spinal nucleus, and the mesencephalic nucleus. They form a long continuous column of cells that extend caudally from the rostral midbrain to approximately the C3 level. Involvement of the trigeminal nucleus produces facial anesthesia that exhibits the "onion skin" or Dejerine pattern in which there is sparing of the midportion of the face.[10,11,29] This Dejerine pattern results from the topographic representation of the trigeminal spinal nucleus. The most central part of the face (nose, mouth) is represented rostrally, whereas lateral facial sensation is represented caudally.[10,11,29]

Respiratory insufficiency occurs in 25% of patients and is usually mild in severity. Residual deficits are generally mild.[29]

Reversible or Transient Syndromes

The term *spinal cord concussion* was first introduced by Obersteiner in 1879: "It is a form of SCI in which complete neurological recovery occurs within 24 to 48 hours after injury."[30] The pathophysiology of spinal cord concussion is unknown. One of the theories postulated is that it is caused by a functional disturbance of the axonal membrane without disruption of its structural integrity.[31]

Burning-hands syndrome, which frequently occurs in athletes, was first described by Maroon in 1977. This syndrome is characterized by transient paresthesias and dysesthesias in the upper limbs, especially the hands. It is most commonly reported in athletes, mostly football players, and it is most likely due to a hyperextension cervical spine injury. This syndrome generally lasts up to 48 hours, typically resolving spontaneously without any significant residual deficits.[9]

Functional Outcome Assessment Scores

After SCI, the initial neurological level and completeness of injury are important predictors of neurological recovery and functional outcome. Patients with incomplete injuries have a much better chance of gaining functional independence than do those with complete injuries. After complete motor loss, patients will generally recover one motor level of function distal to the lowest motor level recorded on the initial neurological assessment. Neurological recovery after SCI usually starts early.[32,33] The majority of the neurological recovery occurs in the first year, with minimal improvement thereafter.[32,34] Neurological improvement appears to be correlated to the degree of severity of the initial presentation following SCI.[32,35]

Many functional assessment scores have been used to evaluate functional independence after SCI. The following are the more commonly used in the SCI literature.

Functional Independence Measure and Spinal Cord Independence Measure

The Functional Independence Measure (FIM) is a scoring system that uses an 18-item scale. Scoring of each item ranges from 1 to 7. A FIM score of 7 implies all tasks are performed safely without modification (complete independence). A FIM score of 1 indicates "total assistance" where less than 25% of the task is performed. Scores from 6 to 2 indicate the need of another person for assistance or supervision.[29,36,37] A more recent version of the FIM score that has been modified specifically for, and is therefore more representative of, patients with SCI is called the Spinal Cord Independence Measure (SCIM).[38] This measure includes self-care, mobility, and respiratory and sphincter management and has recently been updated and endorsed as a valid, specific measure of function for SCI.[39]

Modified Barthel Index

The Modified Barthel Index (MBI) is a five-point scoring system that assesses the patient in performing 10 items of daily living activities (e.g., personal hygiene, bathing, feeding, stair climbing). The MBI score is based on the amount of physical assistance required. There are five categories for MBI total scoring. Category 5 is the minimal dependency level, whereas category 1 is the maximal dependency.[40]

Walking Index for Spinal Cord Injury

The Walking Index for Spinal Cord Injury (WISCI) is a scoring system used to score a patient's ability to walk based on physical assistance (e.g., the need for braces and assisting devices). The lowest score, zero, is given when the patient cannot walk, and the highest score is 20 if the patient can walk with no assistance for at least 10 m. Patients with a score of 19 and below need some form of physical assistance to ambulate.[41,42]

Recovery of Neurological Function Based on the ASIA System

Results from a recent study done by Vazquez et al. showed that 35.4% of SCI patients improve from their initial neurological status, with the majority belonging to the incomplete injury group. Ninety-four percent of ASIA A patients remained as a complete injury from the time of admission to the time of discharge from the hospital, whereas a few percent showed early improvements without significant functional recovery. Of the ASIA B patients, 63% showed neurological recovery, with 33% of them becoming functional. Seventy-six percent of ASIA C patients improved neurologically and became functionally independent, whereas all ASIA D patients were functionally independent on discharge.[32] This is discussed in more detail in Chapter 7. One of the most complete analyses of recovery based on the ASIA system was reported by Fawcett et al.[43] At present, this system is the most useful for clinical trials in SCI.[44]

Conclusion

In summary, SCI remains a devastating condition affecting a young age group engaged in life-enjoying activities. Those with severe injuries usually have significant, permanent neurological and psychological deficits with which they must live for the rest of their lives. Initial examination of the SCI patient provides the most insight into prognosis and should conform with ASIA criteria. To minimize the deficits, treatment must include measures to counteract the secondary effects of SCI on other body systems, including pulmonary, cardiac, and vascular systems. Standardized outcome measures are available that measure not only neurological performance but also functional independence. It is hoped that future research in SCI will develop improved treatments.

Pearls

- Admitting ASIA score is an important measure for both the clinical management and the outcome of SCI patients.
- Awareness and early management of neurogenic shock are essential in optimizing the management of SCI and in preventing or reducing secondary injuries.

Pitfalls

- Spinal shock may last for weeks and typically ends with the development of spasticity and hyperreflexia.
- The bulbocavernosus reflex is chiefly of historical note and has little value in modern SCI assessment and management.

References

1. National Spinal Cord Injury Statistical Center (University of Alabama at Birmingham): Spinal cord injury facts and figures, April 2009
2. Sekhon LH, Fehlings MG. Epidemiology, demographics, and pathophysiology of acute spinal cord injury. Spine 2001;26(24, Suppl):S2–S12
3. Jackson AB, Dijkers M, Devivo MJ, Poczatek RB. A demographic profile of new traumatic spinal cord injuries: change and stability over 30 years. Arch Phys Med Rehabil 2004;85(11):1740–1748
4. Meguro K, Tator CH. Effect of multiple trauma on mortality and neurological recovery after spinal cord or cauda equina injury. Neurol Med Chir (Tokyo) 1988;28(1):34–41
5. Wang CM, Chen Y, DeVivo MJ, Huang CT. Epidemiology of extraspinal fractures associated with acute spinal cord injury. Spinal Cord 2001;39(11):589–594
6. Harris MB, Sethi RK. The initial assessment and management of the multiple-trauma patient with an associated spine injury. Spine 2006;31(11, Suppl):S9–S15, discussion S36
7. Kiss Z, Tator C. Neurogenic shock. In: Geller ER, ed. Shock and Resuscitation. New York: McGraw-Hill, 1993:421–440
8. Atkinson PP, Atkinson JL. Spinal shock. Mayo Clin Proc 1996;71(4):384–389
9. Tator CH. Clinical manifestations of acute spinal cord injury. In: Tator CH, Benzel EC, eds. Contemporary Management of Spinal Cord Injury: From Impact to Rehabilitation. Park Ridge, IL: American Association of Neurological Surgery; 2000:21–32
10. Green BA, Eismont FJ. Acute spinal cord injury: a systems approach. Cent Nerv Syst Trauma 1984;1(2):173–195
11. Fehlings MG, Dandie GDC, Ng WP. Clinical syndromes of spinal cord disease. In: Batjer HH, Loftus CM, eds. Textbook of Neurological Surgery, Principles and Practice. Philadelphia: Lippincott, Williams and Wilkins; 2003:1577–1583
12. Tator CH. Neurologic examination: grading scales. In: Benzel EC, ed. The Cervical Spine. 4th ed. Baltimore: Lippincott, Williams and Williams; 2000:184–195
13. Ditunno JF, Little JW, Tessler A, Burns AS. Spinal shock revisited: a four-phase model. Spinal Cord 2004;42(7):383–395
14. Ko HY, Ditunno JF Jr, Graziani V, Little JW. The pattern of reflex recovery during spinal shock. Spinal Cord 1999;37(6):402–409
15. Furlan JC, Fehlings MG. Cardiovascular complications after acute spinal cord injury: pathophysiology, diagnosis, and management. Neurosurg Focus 2008;25(5):E13
16. Teasell RW, Arnold JM, Krassioukov A, Delaney GA. Cardiovascular consequences of loss of supraspinal control of the sympathetic nervous system after spinal cord injury. Arch Phys Med Rehabil 2000;81(4):506–516
17. Krassioukov AV, Furlan JC, Fehlings MG. Autonomic dysreflexia in acute spinal cord injury: an under-recognized clinical entity. J Neurotrauma 2003;20(8):707–716
18. Blackmer J. Rehabilitation medicine, I: Autonomic dysreflexia. CMAJ 2003;169(9):931–935
19. Urdaneta F, Layon AJ. Respiratory complications in patients with traumatic cervical spine injuries: case report and review of the literature. J Clin Anesth 2003;15(5):398–405
20. Garstang SV, Miller-Smith SA. Autonomic nervous system dysfunction after spinal cord injury. Phys Med Rehabil Clin N Am 2007;18(2):275–296, vi–vii
21. Collins HL, Rodenbaugh DW, DiCarlo SE. Spinal cord injury alters cardiac electrophysiology and increases the susceptibility to ventricular arrhythmias. Prog Brain Res 2006;152:275–288
22. Piepmeier JM, Lehmann KB, Lane JG. Cardiovascular instability following acute cervical spinal cord trauma. Cent Nerv Syst Trauma 1985;2(3):153–160
23. Lehmann KG, Lane JG, Piepmeier JM, Batsford WP. Cardiovascular abnormalities accompanying acute spinal cord injury in humans: incidence, time course and severity. J Am Coll Cardiol 1987;10(1):46–52
24. The Consensus Committee of the American Autonomic Society and the American Academy of Neurology. Consensus statement on the definition of orthostatic hypotension, pure autonomic failure, and multiple system atrophy. Neurology 1996;46(5):1470
25. Sidorov EV, Townson AF, Dvorak MF, Kwon BK, Steeves J, Krassioukov A. Orthostatic hypotension in the first month following acute spinal cord injury. Spinal Cord 2008;46(1):65–69
26. Claydon VE, Steeves JD, Krassioukov A. Orthostatic hypotension following spinal cord injury: understanding clinical pathophysiology. Spinal Cord 2006;44(6):341–351
27. Shatz O, Willner D, Hasharoni A, et al. Acute spinal cord injury, I: Cardiovascular and pulmonary effects and complications. Contemp Crit Care. 2005;3:1
28. Maynard FM Jr, Bracken MB, Creasey G, et al., American Spinal Injury Association. International Standards for Neurological and Functional Classification of Spinal Cord Injury. Spinal Cord 1997;35(5):266–274
29. Dickman CA, Hadley MN, Pappas CT, Sonntag VK, Geisler FH. Cruciate paralysis: a clinical and radiographic analysis of injuries to the cervicomedullary junction. J Neurosurg 1990;73(6):850–858
30. Zwimpfer TJ, Bernstein M. Spinal cord concussion. J Neurosurg 1990;72(6):894–900
31. Schneider RC, Cherry G, Pantek H. The syndrome of acute central cervical spinal cord injury: with special reference to the mechanisms involved in hyperextension injuries of cervical spine. J Neurosurg 1954;11(6):546–577
32. Vazquez XM, Rodriguez MS, Peñaranda JM, Concheiro L, Barus JI. Determining prognosis after spinal cord injury. J Forensic Leg Med 2008;15(1):20–23
33. Cifu DX, Wehman P, McKinley WO. Determining impairment following spinal cord injury. Phys Med Rehabil Clin North Am 2001;12(3):603–612
34. Kirshblum SC, O'Connor KC. Levels of spinal cord injury and predictors for neurologic recovery. Phys Med Rehabil Clin North Am 2000;11(1):1–27
35. Tator CH. Epidemiology and general characteristics of the spinal cord-injured patient. In: Tator

CH, Benzel EC, eds. Contemporary Management of Spinal Cord Injury: From Impact to Rehabilitation. Park Ridge, IL: American Association of Neurological Surgery; 2000:15–20

36. O'Sullivan SB, Schmitz TJ. Physical Rehabilitation Assessment and Treatment. 4th ed. Philadelphia: FA Davis; 2001:1–18

37. Hall KM, Cohen ME, Wright J, Call M, Werner P. Characteristics of the Functional Independence Measure in traumatic spinal cord injury. Arch Phys Med Rehabil 1999;80(11):1471–1476

38. Catz A, Itzkovich M, Agranov E, Ring H, Tamir A. SCIM—Spinal Cord Independence Measure: a new disability scale for patients with spinal cord lesions. Spinal Cord 1997;35(12):850–856

39. Anderson K, Aito S, Atkins M, et al., Functional Recovery Outcome Measures Work Group. Functional recovery measures for spinal cord injury: an evidence-based review for clinical practice and research. J Spinal Cord Med 2008;31(2): 133–144

40. Shah S, Vanclay F, Cooper B. Improving the sensitivity of the Barthel Index for stroke rehabilitation. J Clin Epidemiol 1989;42(8):703–709

41. Morganti B, Scivoletto G, Ditunno P, Ditunno JF, Molinari M. Walking Index for Spinal Cord Injury (WISCI): criterion validation. Spinal Cord 2005;43(1):27–33

42. Ditunno JF Jr, Ditunno PL, Graziani V, et al. Walking Index for Spinal Cord Injury (WISCI): an international multicenter validity and reliability study. Spinal Cord 2000;38(4):234–243

43. Fawcett JW, Curt A, Steeves JD, et al. Guidelines for the conduct of clinical trials for spinal cord injury as developed by the ICCP panel: spontaneous recovery after spinal cord injury and statistical power needed for therapeutic clinical trials. Spinal Cord 2007;45(3):190–205

44. Tator CH. Review of treatment trials in human spinal cord injury: issues, difficulties, and recommendations. Neurosurgery 2006;59(5):957–982, discussion 982–987

3

Imaging of Acute Spinal Cord Trauma and Spinal Cord Injury

David W. Cadotte, David J. Mikulis, Patrick Stroman, and Michael G. Fehlings

Key Points

1. A systematic approach to evaluate imaging of the bony spine is presented.
2. Metrics of spinal instability are provided.
3. The use of MRI to detect ligament damage is reviewed.
4. The interpretation of MRI signal changes within the damaged spinal cord is outlined, along with measurements used to quantify compression of the spinal cord.
5. Future trends in imaging of the damaged spinal cord are discussed.

Imaging of the patient who sustains a traumatic spinal cord injury (SCI) must occur as soon as possible after life-saving measures are complete. As will be discussed in other areas of this book, hypotension and hypoxia are two factors that significantly contribute to secondary damage following SCI and should be managed appropriately before any imaging of the spine is performed.

This chapter is organized to correspond to clinical management of SCI patients with regard to imaging. Whether an emergency room physician, a community family physician, or a specialized trauma, neurosurgery, or orthopedic surgery physician, the information presented here provides a comprehensive and understandable overview of imaging issues in patients suspected of having an acute traumatic SCI. The text here avoids excessive detail regarding the biomechanics of injury and spinal fracture classification systems, which can be daunting to those not trained in this area. However, an understanding of spinal biomechanics, the importance of which cannot be overstated, allows the physician with a trained eye to anticipate injury patterns and provide a more thorough diagnosis. For example, if an anterior wedge fracture were detected in the thoracolumbar spine, a prudent clinician would understand that the integrity of the posterior longitudinal ligament may be compromised and should be investigated with magnetic resonance imaging (MRI). Several texts have been written that describe these characteristics, and clinicians who treat these fractures are referred to such texts for a comprehensive review. (Descriptions of these characteristics are beyond the scope of this chapter.)

The sections that follow outline imaging that should take place in any patient suspected of an SCI. Where appropriate, specific clinical scenarios are described in which the treating physician is faced with a decision tree. In these situations, up-to-date information is provided regarding optimal treatment strategies. The text moves on to provide an overview of different measurements that can be obtained from various imaging modalities. This information is important and can be used for several purposes, including communications with colleagues about the patient, medical record documentation, and research. The chapter concludes with a review of prospects in the field of SCI imaging. This final section highlights areas of promising research that will provide more detailed information about the state of the spinal cord after injury. This information may ultimately help to stratify patients and guide therapy.

Imaging the Spinal Cord Injury Patient

Evaluation of the Spinal Column Following Trauma

The Role of Plain Radiographs and Computed Tomographic Scans

The mechanism of injury in combination with the presenting clinical examination will determine the method of initial spinal column evaluation. The treating physician has both plain x-rays and computed tomography (CT) available to assess the bony spine and must use these tools to rule in or rule out spinal column injury. For example, a cervical spine x-ray is appropriate for minor trauma with a normal neurological examination presenting with neck pain. On the other hand, a person surviving a high-speed motor vehicle collision who has a depressed level of consciousness and is spontaneously moving the upper but not the lower extremities is more appropriately imaged with a CT scan of the spine. The goal of imaging the bony spine with radiographs is to provide a quick survey of the regional bony anatomy and to guide additional CT or MRI. This imaging information can then inform the treating spinal surgeon and is subsequently used by the surgical team for treatment planning. The following paragraphs compare the use of plain x-ray and CT as they apply to the trauma patient. Although this chapter's focus is acute imaging, it is important to consider how the patient may be followed over time, because baseline imaging studies provide valuable information over the course of treatment.

A note of caution must be conveyed when the treating physician decides to use plain x-rays as the only method of investigation. Some authors have reported fractures undetected on plain x-ray later revealed by CT scan.[1,2] The benefit of plain x-rays compared with CT is greater anatomical coverage at a lower dose of radiation. Clinical judgment must therefore be used when weighing the pretest probability of injury with the choice of imaging modality.

Although plain radiographs provide a fast means of surveying the regional anatomy in the initial evaluation of spinal trauma, especially in low-income countries where other modalities may not be readily accessible, CT scan has become the most common method of evaluation in most institutions and certainly in larger trauma centers. Some advantages of CT over plain x-ray include improved visualization of the craniocervical junction and cervicothoracic junction, improved fracture detection, and the ability to reformat images for surgical planning in three dimensions. Additionally, reformatted images enable detection of fractures that are difficult to visualize if they are in the same sectional plane as the acquired CT slices.

CT protocol should be performed with 1 mm slices enabling high-resolution reformats. Sagittal and coronal reformats are then reviewed as plain radiographs. The axial and reformatted images are then reviewed individually using both bone and soft tissue settings to assess fractures and soft tissue injury, including extradural hematoma and herniated disks.

In the cervical spine, the standard radiographic views are anteroposterior (AP), lateral, and open-mouth odontoid; a lateral swimmer's projection may also be obtained to examine the cervicothoracic junction if C7 and T1 are not adequately assessed on the true lateral projection. Dynamic flexion-extension views have a limited role in the acute setting because muscle spasm and other distracting injuries often preclude an adequate examination.[3] The dynamic study is of value during the follow-up period to assess potential ligamentous instability during recovery from injury. Both AP and lateral views are appropriate to investigate the thoracic and lumbar spine. In persons who are overweight, the image quality may be poor, and the clinician may decide to use CT as the primary imaging modality. Stability can also be assessed on flexion-extension views of the thoracic and lumbar spine.

An overview of imaging findings on plain x-rays and CT scans is presented next and is illustrated in **Fig. 3.1**, with a cervical spine plain x-ray (top) and a cervical spine CT scan (bottom), and in **Fig. 3.2**, a thoracolumbar spine CT scan reformat. These figures should be used in conjunction with the following information.

Cervical Spine

The AP radiograph of the normal spine should reveal the spinous processes positioned in the midline at each level. The vertebral bodies should be of equal height and have a smooth cortical surface. The uncovertebral joints (C3–6) should be symmetrical and vertically aligned at all levels (**Fig. 3.1**).

In evaluating the lateral radiograph, one should systematically proceed through this suggested checklist:

1. The radiograph should display the occiput through the T1 level.
2. The lines connecting the anterior and posterior margins of the vertebral bodies and the spinolaminar line (the anterior margin of the junction of the spinous process and lamina) should form a gentle convex curve with no steps or discontinuities.
3. The laminar space (the distance from the posterior aspect of the articular pillars to the spinolaminar line) should be uniform throughout the cervical spine.
4. The prevertebral soft tissues should be examined for swelling indicating possible ligamentous injury.
5. The intralaminar spaces (the space between the laminar arches) should not be widened.
6. The lateral atlantodental interval can be visualized and should not exceed 3 mm in adults.
7. The relationship between the superior and inferior articulating facets at each level should be checked for proper alignment.

The open-mouth odontoid view reveals the atlantoaxial articulation. One must examine the occipital condyles, the lateral masses of C1, the dens, and the lateral masses of C2. There should be no offsets between the occipital condyles, the lateral masses of C1, and the lateral masses of C2.

Thoracic and Lumbar Spine

When reviewing plain x-rays of the thoracic and lumbar spine, one must consider the mechanism of injury in combination with the essential assessments of alignment, bony integrity (best assessed by examining for disruptions in the cortical bone), and joint space disruption. If the mechanism of injury or neurological status warrants investigation beyond that of plain x-rays, a CT scan should be obtained. Both AP and lateral projections should be viewed together, along with a reference point for identifying the exact level, either the sacrum or the occiput. In turn, each level should be systematically approached and examined for evidence of instability. Although there are different opinions as to what constitutes instability, the following list proposed by Daffner et al.[4] offers several features to examine:

1. Displacement or translation of the vertebral body > 2 mm
    a. May indicate disruption of ligamentous support
2. Widening of the interspinous space, facet joints, or interpeduncular distance

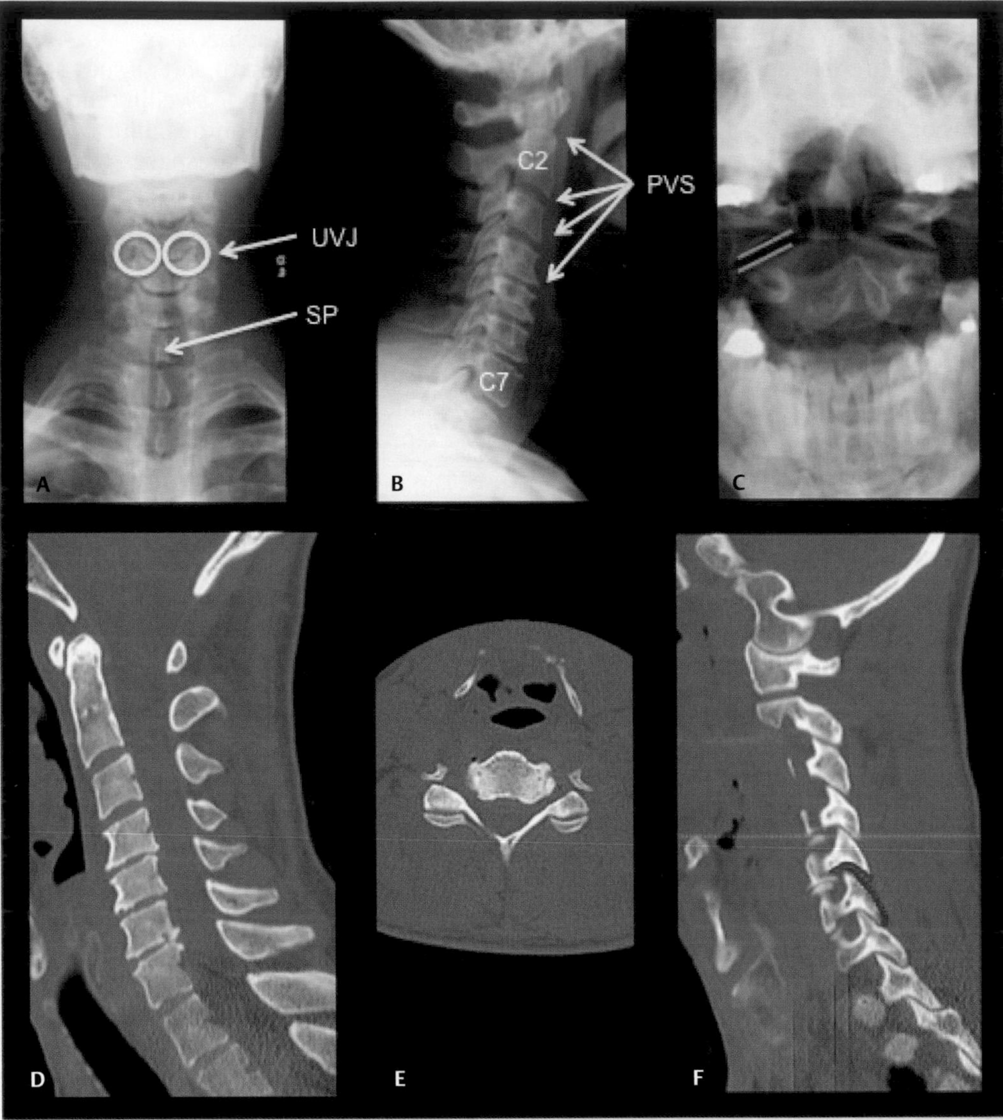

Fig. 3.1 Anteroposterior (AP) **(A)**, lateral **(B)**, and open-mouth odontoid view **(C)** plain cervical x-rays. Midsagittal computed tomography (CT) reformat **(D)**, axial CT **(E)**, corresponding to the left facets shown on the parasagittal reformat **(F)**. This case represents images obtained from a 44-year-old female who fell down a flight of stairs and presented to the hospital with neck pain. The neurological examination was normal. The T1 vertebral body could not be visualized on the lateral plain x-ray so the treating physician obtained a CT scan to ensure the absence of fracture. A prudent clinician should examine for alignment of the uncovertebral joints (UVJ) and the midline position of the spinous processes (SP) on the AP x-ray or CT reformat (not shown). The lateral x-ray (or CT) should be examined for prevertebral soft tissue swelling (PVS), good visualization from the skull base through T1, alignment of the anterior and posterior margins of the vertebral bodies, the spinolaminar line, and the lateral atlantodental interval. Either the open-mouth odontoid view (or the coronal CT reformat) should be examined for the atlantoaxial articulation (*blue lines*). The parasagittal CT reformat should be examined for alignment of the facet joints at each level (outlined in **(F)**, *red contour lines*).

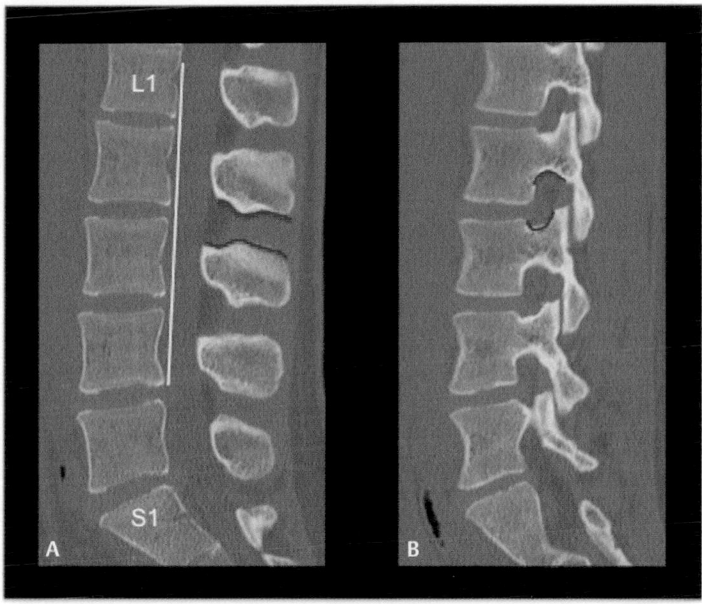

Fig. 3.2 Shown are lateral CT reformats of a 39-year-old male who was involved in a sports injury and complained of sudden onset of back pain following a moderate impact injury. The clinical examination was normal. **(A)** Midsagittal CT scan of the lumbar spine. Shown is L1-S1. **(B)** A right parasagittal image outlining the facet articulations at each level. One should examine for alignment of the vertebral bodies, the interspinous space, and the interpeduncular space (*red lines*) that may indicate ligamentous disruption and disruption of the posterior vertebral body line (*yellow line*). In addition, if a vertebral body fracture is identified, one should measure the loss of height as a percentage of normal height. See text for further description.

   a. Should be compared with levels above and below and may indicate ligamentous disruption
3. Disruption of the posterior vertebral body line
   a. Indicates disruption of either the anterior or the posterior column
4. Widening of the spinal canal on the anteroposterior view
   a. May indicate sagittally oriented trauma
5. Vertebral body height loss >50% or wedging of the vertebral body
6. Kyphosis >20 degrees across one level

Evaluation of the Spinal Cord and Surrounding Soft Tissues with MRI

While soft tissue windows on newer model multidetector CT scanners offer a reasonable glimpse into damage of soft tissues or compression of the spinal cord, nothing compares to the picture quality and diagnostic ability of modern MRI machines. Image acquisition time is longer than that required for CT scans and can range from as little as 10 minutes to more than 45 minutes depending on the extent of imaging required. The clinician should expect to gain valuable knowledge with regard to both ligamentous and neural element damage. Therefore, either of these situations must have a relatively high pretest probability before requesting a spinal MRI. Should a high degree of suspicion exist, MRI should be performed as soon as possible after the traumatic event, preferably within hours. The exception to this rule occurs when the treating physician is faced with a patient who has suffered a cervical SCI and presents with either perched or locked facets. This scenario is considered in the next paragraph. Other important aspects to consider when obtaining an MRI scan in acute SCI include identifying reversible causes of neurological deficit and interpreting signal changes within the spinal cord to gauge the extent of injury. Each of these topics is discussed here.

Special Situation: Timing of MRI in the Setting of Cervical Spinal Cord Injury with Perched or Locked Facets

One of the recent controversies in the treatment of SCI has been with regard to timing of surgical decompression. This controversy acquired momentum in recent years in favor of early surgical decompression due to a large body of animal evidence and emerging clinical evidence that suggests early decompression affords better outcome. This is supported by several recent clinical trials that seem to suggest similar findings, although not as robust. The controversy is far from being resolved, but most treating surgeons would agree on a few essential points, one of which occurs in the setting of a patient presenting with bilateral locked cervical facets. This injury causes severe cord compression and has the ability to be corrected via closed reduction. In a recent review, Fehlings and Perrin[5] outline the evidence for and against this maneuver and conclude that, in the setting of bilateral locked facets, reduction should be attempted as soon as possible in a person with an incomplete tetraplegia or in a person with deteriorating neurological function. This, of course, can only be performed in an awake, alert, and cooperative patient.

This situation outlines the set of circumstances in a rare number of cases of SCI. However, a recent question has been raised around the role of MRI in this context: should one perform an MRI scan or proceed directly on the x-ray evidence of bilateral locked facets? The arguments offered in favor of early MRI tend to be focused on other causes of spinal cord compression, such as a cervical disk herniation, that could be worsened by closed reduction. Furthermore, it is hypothesized that open surgical treatment could possibly avoid this added risk. The evidence in favor of early closed reduction without first obtaining an MRI scan is more substantial, as reviewed by Fehlings and Perrin.[5] One study specifically addressed this concern and has pointed out the safety of performing this maneuver without prior MRI.[6] Ultimately, the decision must be left up to the treating physician, given the specific circumstances of each case.

Identifying Reversible Causes of Neurological Deficit on MRI

Perhaps the greatest value of MRI in the acute setting of SCI is to identify potentially reversible causes of neurological impairment. These include extradural compressive forces, such as disk herniation or epidural hematoma that would be amenable to surgical intervention, and ligamentous instability that would result in a dynamic compression of the cord if the spinal column were not surgically stabilized.

Traumatic insults to the spinal ligaments or cervical disks are evident by hyperintensity in T2-weighted images. Although such injuries are more easily identified with MRI in comparison to x-ray or CT, one must exert some caution because the specificity is relatively low. In fact, one study identified only eight of 14 surgically proven ligamentous disruptions.[7] One must examine carefully for each of the anterior and posterior longitudinal ligaments, the interspinous ligament, the ligamentum nuchae, the ligamentum flavum, and the ligaments at the craniocervical junction: the tectorial membrane, the transverse ligament, and the alar ligaments. Any disruption should then be correlated with bony imaging on CT scan to ensure that an occult fracture was not overlooked. Furthermore, bone edema (visualized with MRI) is an indicator of a fracture, and this location should also be correlated with CT. More specific information on the interpretation of MRI signal characteristics is presented next.

Interpreting MRI Signal Changes in Acute Traumatic Injury

MRI signal abnormalities within the spinal cord can uncover reasons for acute neurological deficits and indications of prognosis. Several authors have performed postmortem analysis comparing intramedullary signal changes with gross and histopathological analysis,[8–10] associating imaging findings with hemorrhage, edema, cavitation, and transection. Although it is not within the scope of this chapter to review all the caveats of MRI signal interpretation, the reader must keep in mind the physiological process and attempt to correlate the two. Therefore, one should examine for evidence of torn ligaments, often showing up as bright signal on T2-weighted images provided that adequate fat suppression was used during image acquisition; otherwise, both fat and injured ligament have the same signal characteristics. Acute bony fracture is represented as decreased signal on T1-weighted images against the background of the high signal of marrow fat; acute bony fracture is also represented as bright signal on T2-weighted images if fat suppression is used. The spectrum of pathology in the spinal cord ranges from minimal cord edema (bright T2-weighted signal) through to cord hemorrhage (bright or dark T2-weighted signal and perhaps dark T1-weighted signal depending on the state of hemoglobin).

The standard MRI evolution of a hematoma is depicted in **Fig. 3.3**. It is often the case that hematomas in the spinal cord are not homogeneous and have signal changes in both T1- and T2-weighted images. Special iron sequences can help to confirm the presence of blood. Intramedullary signal characteristics provide valuable information to the clinician because they not only explain neurological deficits (in the absence of extramedullary compressive lesions) but also offer information with regard to prognosis whereby intraparenchymal blood is associated with a poorer prognosis (this topic will be expanded upon later in the chapter).

The use of MRI in SCI has dramatically improved our ability to accurately diagnose injury and plan optimal treatment strategies. In recent years our understanding of the signal characteristics relative to the pathophysiological process has improved our ability to visualize the nature of the damage to the spinal cord. These developments are anticipated to provide clinicians with the tools required to measure certain characteristics of the injury, such as a hematoma within the spinal cord, and provide accurate prognostic information. The role of these measurements is further discussed in the next section.

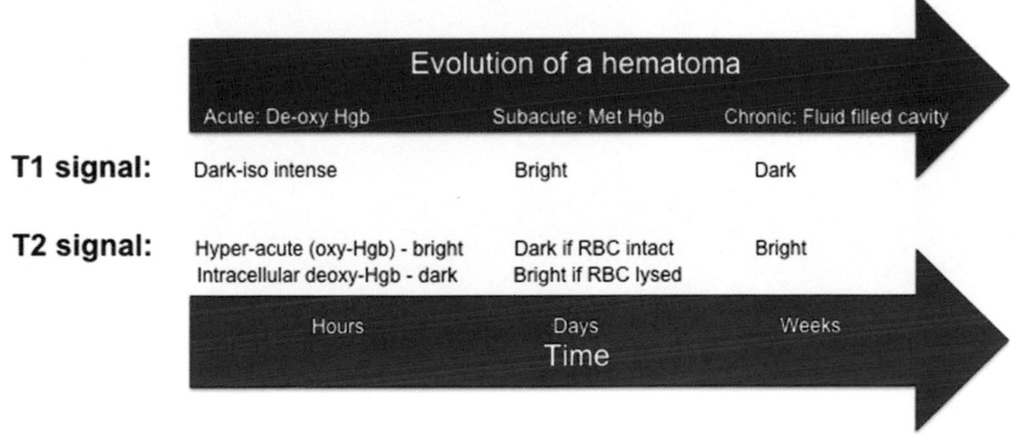

Fig. 3.3 A diagram illustrating the evolution of a hematoma (*red arrow*) over time (*blue arrow*). Shown in the middle of the two arrows are the T1- and T2-weighted signal characteristics that should be expected along the time course of blood breakdown.

MRI Measurements in the Setting of Spinal Cord Injury

The use of MRI in the setting of SCI has become commonplace at most advanced health-care centers and is considered to be standard in some. As the use of this technology increases, it is important to develop the proper measurement tools to communicate the degree of injury to other specialists. This information can be used to understand the nature and extent of injury in an individual patient and also to feed data into clinical trials. Fehlings et al.[11] have set the current standard for such measurements by outlining two important characteristics in SCI. The first is the degree of maximal canal compromise (MCC) and the second is the maximal spinal cord compression (MSCC). Each of these is depicted in **Fig. 3.4** and briefly expanded on below.

Maximal Spinal Canal Compromise

Using midsagittal CT reconstructions (or MRI scans) and the respective axial slices, one should identify the level of MCC and compare this with the normal canal diameter at the midvertebral body level above and below the lesion. This is quantified using the formula shown in **Fig. 3.4,** where D_i is the anteroposterior canal diameter at the level of maximum injury, D_a is the anteroposterior canal diameter at the nearest normal level above the level of injury, and D_b is the anteroposterior canal diameter at the nearest normal level below the level of injury.

Maximal Spinal Cord Compression

The anteroposterior cord diameter on midsagittal and axial T2 MRI scans at the level of maximum compression should be compared with the anteroposterior cord diam-

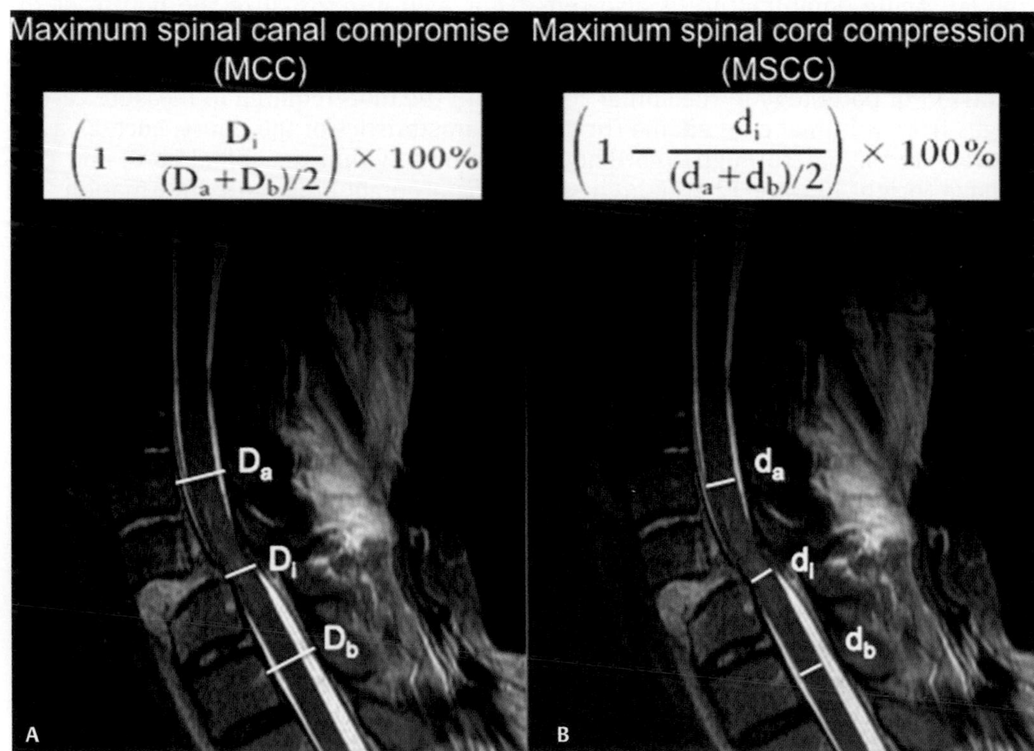

Fig. 3.4 **(A)** Midsagittal T2 magnetic resonance imaging (MRI) and equation outlining the calculation for maximal canal compromise (MCC). D_i is the anteroposterior canal diameter at the level of maximum injury, D_a is the anteroposterior canal diameter at the nearest normal level above the level of injury, and D_b is the anteroposterior canal diameter at the nearest normal level below the level of injury. **(B)** Midsagittal T2 MRI and equation outlining the calculation for the maximal spinal cord compression (MSCC), where d_i is the anteroposterior cord diameter at the level of maximum injury, d_a is the anteroposterior cord diameter at the nearest normal level above the level of injury, and d_b is the anteroposterior cord diameter at the nearest normal level below the level of injury

eter at the normal levels immediately above and below the level of injury. If cord edema is present, measurements of normal anteroposterior cord diameter should be made at midvertebral body levels just beyond the rostral and caudal extent of the cord edema at the levels where the cord appears normal. These values are quantified using the formula depicted in **Fig. 3.4**, where d_i is the anteroposterior cord diameter at the level of maximum injury, d_a is the anteroposterior cord diameter at the nearest normal level above the level of injury, and d_b is the anteroposterior cord diameter at the nearest normal level below the level of injury.

It is important to keep in mind that these measurements represent the drive to understand how the traumatic process has affected the spinal column or cord. As imaging techniques continue to evolve, such as spinal diffusion imaging, diffusion tensor imaging, and spinal functional MRI (fMRI), greater insight into the damaged tissue will be available. The next section explores some of the novel imaging techniques that are on the horizon.

Future Prospects of Imaging in Spinal Cord Injury

MRI as a Prognostic Tool Following Trauma—Current State and Future Prospects

Neurological deficit following traumatic injury to the spine occurs as a result of either direct damage to the neural elements or the secondary effects of injury, including, but not limited to, hypoxia, ischemia, or free-radical-mediated damage. The motor neurons, sensory neurons, or interneurons damaged as a result of these cascades are far from static entities, and they have the capacity to change for either better or worse. In the best-case scenario, a patient who sustains an SCI and subsequent neurological deficit will improve motor, sensory, autonomic, or sexual function to some extent. An alternative is that recovery of function will not occur or that changes in the local neuronal circuitry will result in spasticity or chronic neuropathic pain. One of the recent trends in imaging of the spinal cord has been to identify factors that are associated with prognosis. Ranging from standard MRI protocols to advanced novel pulse sequences and data analysis techniques, progress is being made toward identifying the exact nature of the traumatic event and determining prognosis.

Standard MRI

Over the course of approximately 2 decades, standard MRI protocols have provided researchers with information about the spinal cord. T1- and T2-weighted intramedullary signal characteristics quickly became a source of information that was previously unattainable. Several groups have investigated the nature of these signal characteristics and have attempted to elucidate their meaning by conducting animal experiments that correlate signal characteristics to standard histopathology techniques. The results are beyond the scope of this chapter; suffice it to say that correlations can be made between the degree of damage to the spinal cord and the observed signal changes on standard MRI sequences. A spectrum of signal characteristics exists that range from normal to complete cord transection. As one would expect, outcome at the normal end of this spectrum is more favorable. The prognostic sensitivity and specificity of standard MRI are currently being investigated. The following paragraph highlights a few of the recent studies that have been conducted in this regard.

Tewari et al.[12] demonstrate that patients with minimal cord changes on MRI are likely to improve neurologically, regardless of their initial neurological status. Increased signal in T2-weighted images alone, representing spinal cord edema, is thought to predict neurological recovery,[12–14] whereas patients with mixed changes in both T1- and T2-weighted images tend not to recover neurological function.[13] Patients with parenchymatous hemorrhage and contusion demonstrate little or no neurological recovery.[12,14,15] The rostrocaudal length of signal change was associated with the degree of recovery. For example, Shin et al.[13] report that if the signal change is two vertebral segments or less (compared with greater than two segments), the patient is more likely to recover. Similarly, Boldin et al.[16] demonstrated that if the length of the signal change within the cord is 4 mm or less, neurological recovery is more likely. Miyanji et al.[15] use a quantitative measure (as already described), MSCC, and demonstrate that the greater the compression, the less the neurological recovery. In addition, they show an association with cord swelling and hemorrhage, both of which are associated with a poor neurological recovery.

In contrast to the foregoing positive associations, one recent study demonstrated a lack of association and another was equivocal.[17,18] Tsuchiya et al.[17] obtained diffusion-weighted (DW) images along with apparent diffusion coefficient (ADC) maps in SCI patients and concluded that increased signal (i.e., reduced rate of apparent water self-diffusion) on DW images coupled with restricted diffusion may be associated with unfavorable functional prognosis, but they could not demonstrate this statistically. Miranda et al.[18] demonstrated that neither increased T2-weighted signal intensity nor the length of signal change was associated with the degree of motor deficit.

The foregoing studies demonstrate an ability of MRI to provide an indication of functional recovery following SCI. Unfortunately, the measures are crude, and the ability to predict recovery exists at the extremes of injury: those with minimal signal change are likely to improve, and those with extensive compression or hemorrhage are not.

Pearls

- The severity of cord compression, the presence of intraparenchymal hemorrhage, and the length of cord signal change are prognostic indicators of poor functional outcome after traumatic SCI.
- The presence of a spinal fracture at any level mandates a careful radiographic evaluation of the entire spine to rule out a noncontiguous fracture (which can occur in up to 15% of cases).
- The use of fat-suppressed MRI in the setting of acute trauma is essential to distinguish ligament damage from normal fat signal.

Functional Imaging of the Spinal Cord

Functional imaging of the spinal cord aims to identify regions of the spinal cord that respond with changes in neuronal activity to specific neural input. For example, application of a heat stimulus to the skin would transmit neural input through the dorsal root ganglion and synapse in the dorsal horn of the spinal cord. Neural signals are then relayed to the brain stem, and also project to local regions within the same spinal cord segment and adjacent segments via interneurons. Along with modulatory input from the brain stem, this network constitutes a degree of local processing to produce a net sensation. This activity has recently been detected with novel fMRI techniques and has the potential to more precisely delineate the nature of injury.[19–22] Therefore, fMRI of the spinal cord has the potential to supplement, and improve on, anatomical MRI with regard to prognosis. This technique also has the potential to monitor the effects of novel treatment strategies before clinical changes are observed. Lastly, spinal fMRI may be able to detect abnormal circuit reorganization following SCI that results in debilitating neuropathic pain. To date, researchers are at a loss as to the exact nature of this pain, but animal experiments seem to point in the direction of altered processing of sensory input. If this is true in human SCI, spinal fMRI may provide a specific diagnosis and open the door to novel treatment strategies.

Other spinal imaging methods on the horizon include magnetic resonance spectroscopy and diffusion-weighted imaging. These techniques are reviewed in Chapter 41 of this book.

Pitfalls

- Beware of patients with spinal trauma and ankylosing spondylitis or diffuse idiopathic skeletal hyperostosis (DISH)—these patients require careful assessment with CT and possibly MRI to rule out a nondisplaced transdiskal fracture.
- T2 signal changes on MRI in the soft tissues may represent only contusion and not actual ligamentous disruption. These signal changes should be correlated with evidence of deformity or subluxation.

References

1. Woodring JH, Lee C. Limitations of cervical radiography in the evaluation of acute cervical trauma. J Trauma 1993;34(1):32–39
2. Platzer P, Jaindl M, Thalhammer G, et al. Clearing the cervical spine in critically injured patients: a comprehensive C-spine protocol to avoid unnecessary delays in diagnosis. Eur Spine J 2006;15(12):1801–1810
3. Insko EK, Gracias VH, Gupta R, Goettler CE, Gaieski DF, Dalinka MK. Utility of flexion and extension radiographs of the cervical spine in the acute evaluation of blunt trauma. J Trauma 2002;53(3):426–429
4. Daffner RH, Deeb ZL, Goldberg AL, Kandabarow A, Rothfus WE. The radiologic assessment of post-traumatic vertebral stability. Skeletal Radiol 1990;19(2):103–108
5. Fehlings MG, Perrin RG. The timing of surgical intervention in the treatment of spinal cord injury: a systematic review of recent clinical evidence. Spine 2006;31(11, Suppl):S28–S35, discussion S36
6. Vaccaro AR, Falatyn SP, Flanders AE, Balderston RA, Northrup BE, Cotler JM. Magnetic resonance evaluation of the intervertebral disc, spinal ligaments, and spinal cord before and after closed traction reduction of cervical spine dislocations. Spine 1999;24(12):1210–1217
7. Weisskopf M, Bail H, Mack M, Stöckle U, Hoffmann R. Value of MRI in traumatic disco-ligament instability of the lower cervical spine [in German]. Unfallchirurg 1999;102(12):942–948
8. Becerra JL, Puckett WR, Hiester ED, et al. MR-pathologic comparisons of Wallerian degeneration in spinal cord injury. AJNR Am J Neuroradiol 1995;16(1):125–133
9. Quencer RM, Bunge RP, Egnor M, et al. Acute traumatic central cord syndrome: MRI-pathological correlations. Neuroradiology 1992;34(2):85–94
10. Quencer RM, Bunge RP. The injured spinal cord: imaging, histopathologic clinical correlates, and basic science approaches to enhancing neural function after spinal cord injury. Spine 1996;21(18):2064–2066
11. Fehlings MG, Rao SC, Tator CH, et al. The optimal radiologic method for assessing spinal canal compromise and cord compression in patients with cervical spinal cord injury, II: Results of a multicenter study. Spine 1999;24(6):605–613
12. Tewari MK, Gifti DS, Singh P, et al. Diagnosis and prognostication of adult spinal cord injury without radiographic abnormality using magnetic resonance imaging: analysis of 40 patients. Surg Neurol 2005;63(3):204–209, discussion 209
13. Shin JC, Kim DY, Park CI, Kim YW, Ohn SH. Neurologic recovery according to early magnetic resonance imaging findings in traumatic cervical spinal cord injuries. Yonsei Med J 2005;46(3):379–387
14. Andreoli C, Colaiacomo MC, Rojas Beccaglia M, Di Biasi C, Casciani E, Gualdi G. MRI in the acute phase of spinal cord traumatic lesions: relationship between MRI findings and neurological outcome. Radiol Med (Torino) 2005;110(5-6):636–645
15. Miyanji F, Furlan JC, Aarabi B, Arnold PM, Fehlings MG. Acute cervical traumatic spinal cord injury: MR imaging findings correlated with neurologic outcome—prospective study with 100 consecutive patients. Radiology 2007;243(3):820–827
16. Boldin C, Raith J, Fankhauser F, Haunschmid C, Schwantzer G, Schweighofer F. Predicting neurologic recovery in cervical spinal cord injury with postoperative MR imaging. Spine 2006;31(5):554–559
17. Tsuchiya K, Fujikawa A, Honya K, Tateishi H, Nitatori T. Value of diffusion-weighted MR imaging in acute cervical cord injury as a predictor of outcome. Neuroradiology 2006;48(11):803–808
18. Miranda P, Gomez P, Alday R, Kaen A, Ramos A. Brown-Sequard syndrome after blunt cervical spine trauma: clinical and radiological correlations. Eur Spine J 2007;16(8):1165–1170
19. Stroman PW. Spinal fMRI investigation of human spinal cord function over a range of innocuous thermal sensory stimuli and study-related emotional influences. Magn Reson Imaging 2009;27(10):1333–1346
20. Ghazni NF, Cahill CM, Stroman PW. Tactile sensory and pain networks in the human spinal cord and brain stem mapped by means of functional MR imaging. AJNR Am J Neuroradiol 2010;31(4):661–667
21. Kornelsen J, Stroman PW. Detection of the neuronal activity occurring caudal to the site of spinal cord injury that is elicited during lower limb movement tasks. Spinal Cord 2007;45(7):485–490
22. Stroman PW. Magnetic resonance imaging of neuronal function in the spinal cord: spinal FMRI. Clin Med Res 2005;3(3):146–156

4

Pathophysiology of Spinal Cord Injury

James W. Austin, James W. Rowland, and Michael G. Fehlings

Key Points

1. Spinal cord injury is biphasic, with the initial injury leading to a cascade of deleterious effects (the "secondary injury"), including ischemia, glutamatergic excitoxicity, inflammation, and apoptosis.
2. Early intervention to prevent the spread of the secondary damage represents a promising therapeutic opportunity.
3. A better understanding of potentially beneficial endogenous responses, such as progenitor cell proliferation, axonal sprouting, remyelination, and angiogenesis, could lead to novel therapeutic interventions.
4. The concept of translational research in SCI requires a rigorous preclinical animal-based investigative program that is coupled to a robust clinical research pathway. The concept of "forward translation" from bench to bedside should be linked to "reverse translational" investigation, where clinical observations and questions are addressed in relevant preclinical research studies.

Spinal cord injury (SCI) is biphasic in nature and represents the sum of a complex series of local and systemic secondary responses to an initial primary injury. The secondary phases of the pathophysiological processes exacerbate the initial damage while endogenous efforts to facilitate healing and regeneration struggle to succeed. Spatial and temporal dynamics of these secondary mediators are central to SCI pathophysiology and are a recurring theme throughout this chapter. Clinical observations have demonstrated that SCI is highly heterogeneous, making each patient's injury unique in cause, lesion architecture, and outcome. In line with this, there exists a need for a variety of different animal models that account for variations in human injuries, especially given that promising preclinical studies have rarely shown similar efficacy upon translation into the clinic. There are currently no effective treatment options for SCI patients. The development of a successful treatment paradigm must be based on a deep understanding of SCI pathophysiology and how the different aspects of primary and secondary injury contribute to the progression of an individual's unique injury.

Primary Injury

The spinal cord runs within the vertebral column, making it vulnerable if physical forces alter the position and structural integrity of the normally protective vertebrae. Traumatic forces, such as ones incurred from traffic accidents, diving into shallow water, or sports-related injuries, can cause the types of vertebral column complications associated with SCI and outlined in **Table 4.1**. Although the majority of SCIs are due to blunt injury, penetrating trauma due to knife or gunshot wounds occurs in a significant percentage of cases.[1] The majority of SCIs (~55%) occur at the cervical level (C1 to C7–T1), whereas 15% occur at each of the thoracic (T1–11), thoracolumbar (T11–12 to L1–2) and lumbosacral (L2–S5) regions.[2]

The spinal cord is rarely transected during injury, even in cases that result in severe neurological deficit.[2] SCI can involve shear, stretch, and more commonly contusive and compressive forces. In addition, spinal cord laceration has been observed in a small number of cases due to vertebral bone fragments or from violence with weapons.[3] Due to the heterogeneous nature of injuries, numerous animal models have been developed to mimic the human condition and shed light on the mechanisms and progression of the injury. Animal models include various weight drop devices, spinal cord compression by forceps or modified aneurysm clips, balloon compression, and hemi- or full transection injuries in mice, rats, and other small mammals (see Chapter 31). Studies in rats have demonstrated that neurological impairment increases relative to the force of trauma and the time of compression.[4] Cells, especially neurons and their axons, become permeabilized acutely following injury due to compressive and shear forces,[5,6] leading to immediate cell disability and death. The initial physical trauma also damages local vasculature, causing edema and hemorrhaging in the well-vascularized gray matter and, to a lesser extent, in the white matter. Animal studies have also demonstrated that this breach in the blood–spinal cord barrier (BSCB) leads to extravasation of markers from 730 Da in size up to red blood cell size (5 mm in diameter) 5 minutes after injury to the spinal cord.[7] Damage to the meningeal layers and spinal roots and bleeding in the subdural and subarachnoid space are also common.[8]

Acute neuroanatomical outcome includes paralysis to neurons involved in motor, sensory, and autonomic functions at the level of injury. Furthermore, axonal damage at injury level leads to miscommunication in afferent and efferent white matter tracts transmitting signals beyond

Table 4.1 Vertebral Column Injuries Associated with Spinal Cord Injury

Type of bony injury	Incidence (%)
Minor fracture (including compression)	10
Fracture dislocation	40
Dislocation only	5
Burst fracture	30
SCIWORA	5
SCIWORET (including cervical spondylosis)	10

Abbreviations: SCIWORA, spinal cord injury without obvious radiological abnormality; SCIWORET, spinal cord injury without obvious radiologic evidence of trauma.
Source: Adapted from Sekhon LH, Fehlings MG. Epidemiology, demographics, and pathophysiology of acute spinal cord injury. Spine 2001;26(24 Suppl):S2–S12.2

the injury site. Commonly, there exists a subpial rim of surviving axons traversing the lesion site in varying states of demyelination. SCI has typically been referred to as either complete or incomplete, referring to complete loss of motor and conscious sensory function below the injury site or some quantity of loss, respectively. To circumvent the ambiguity of this definition, the American Spinal Injury Association (ASIA) created a more descriptive measure called the ASIA Impairment Scale.[9]

Motor Function

Motor impairment following SCI is a result of damage to both upper and lower motor neurons. Loss of lower motor neurons in the anterior/ventral horn leads to paralysis of muscles at the level of injury. Furthermore, upper motor neuron axons passing through the level of injury, in tracts such as the corticospinal tract, are also damaged, resulting in loss of efferent input to muscles below the level of injury. Because most injuries occur at the cervical level, control of muscles of the upper limbs (in high cervical injuries), trunk, and lower limbs is commonly affected.

Sensory Function

Sensory input carrying pain and temperature information is relayed from specialized receptors in the periphery to the brain via the spinothalamic tract. These first-order neurons enter the central nervous system (CNS), ascend or descend one or two vertebral levels, and synapse on second-order sensory neurons in the dorsal/posterior horn, prior to decussating and heading rostrally toward the brain. In contrast, first-order neurons of the posterior column–medial lemniscus pathway, carrying fine touch and vibration information, enter the spinal cord and travel rostral toward the brain before decussating in the medulla. Damage to first- and second-order spinothalamic neurons/axons or first-order axons of the posterior column pathway disrupts sensory information relayed from dermatomes at and below the level of injury to the brain.

Autonomic Function

Perhaps even more devastating than the acute motor or sensory loss is the miscommunication between higher centers of the hypothalamus and limbic system and the various effector organs of the autonomic nervous system. Preganglionic cell bodies of the sympathetic system (the final neurons within the CNS that regulate sympathetic output) are found in the intermediolateral horn of the gray matter between T1 and L2. Parasympathetic preganglionic cell bodies are located in the brain stem and sacral levels of the spinal cord. The effects of injury on autonomic function depend on the anatomical level. Controls for vasoconstriction, cardiac output, and respiration are found in the T1–4 regions, whereas input to the gastrointestinal tract and associated organs as well as sexual organs is found below this level from T5 to L2. Research suggests that spinal sympathetic interneurons, which are relatively inactive in the uninjured normal spinal cord, become active following injury, resulting in impaired autonomic function commonly referred to as autonomic dysreflexia.[10] Evidence for the existence of these spinal interneurons and their role following SCI is provided by experiments that have demonstrated that sympathetic preganglionic neurons have very little spontaneous activity without excitatory input and animal transection injury models in which all sympathetic input from the brain stem is lost yet the animals still have sympathetic activity.[11] Parasympathetic branches contributing to respiration, cardiovascular control, and digestion remain intact due to their cranial nerve location (originating above the cervical spinal cord). In contrast, parasympathetic inputs to the kidneys, bladder, and sexual organs are susceptible in SCI cases due to their sacral pelvic nerve location.

Secondary Injury

The forces, severity, and location of the primary injury dictate the characteristics of secondary events, which together determine the extent of tissue and functional loss, and ultimately patient outcome. The initial trauma triggers a series of systemic, cellular, and molecular cascades that expand the lesion from the primary injury site into adjacent white and gray matter, increasing the extent of tissue loss. Concurrently, endogenous beneficial responses occur that function to limit the spread of the lesion and attempt to regenerate and reconnect damaged signaling pathways. In general, the force of injury determines the ensuing hemorrhage, which in turn dictates the extent of ischemia and secondary damage.

Overview of Secondary Injury Progression

In mammals like humans and rats, a fluid-filled cystic cavity forms at the injury epicenter and spreads radially and rostrocaudally from the injury site over time, resulting in extensive functional and morphological alteration. Infiltrating macrophages, lymphocytes, and activated microglia are present within the cavity, along with granular myelin debris and axons at various degrees of demyelination.[12] Typically, a subpial rim of tissue survives the injury and contains axons also in varying states of myelination.[13] Astrocytes proliferate and surround the cavity in an attempt to attenuate the spread of the lesion, forming a glial scar.[14] This astrogliosis also represents a physical and chemical barrier to axonal regeneration. A fibrous scar consisting of collagen and various inhibitory extracellular matrix (ECM) molecules is deposited within and surrounding the lesion. Wallerian degeneration of axons toward their cell bodies and away from the epicenter is a common fate of severed axons.[15] Severed axonal ends distal to the injury site degenerate along with disrupted myelin and are broken down, eventually being phagocytosed by macrophages. A chronic snapshot of the injury demonstrates a cystic cavity containing vascular/glial bundles,[16] regenerated nerve roots, collagenous fibers, and astrocytes. **Table 4.2** and **Fig. 4.1** summarize the spatiotemporal expression of secondary events.

The Acutely Injured Spinal Cord

Following the primary physical damage and death of neural cells, the acute secondary phase of the injury begins. Typically, the acute phase represents the first 24 to 48 hours following injury. This phase is characterized by vascular dysfunction, including ischemia, energy and ion imbalances, excitotoxicity, and early inflammatory events that lead to necrotic and, to a lesser extent, apoptotic cell death.

The immediate acute injury has often been described as the initial 2 hours postinjury.[17] Function below the injury site is immediately lost to a poorly understood phenomenon called spinal shock.[18] During this time, neurons and glia that survived but sustained mechanical damage/permeabilization from the initial injury undergo necrosis. Within minutes, edema and hemorrhaging, which correlate to injury severity,[19] result in ischemic zones at and adjacent to the injury site, causing additional necrotic cell death.[20] Microglia, responding to by-products of necrosis (DNA, ATP, K^+), become activated and secrete inflammatory cytokines that act to recruit systemic inflammatory cells. In most cases, the gross histology has not been significantly altered and may appear normal with magnetic resonance imaging.[21]

Changes in Vasculature and Blood Flow

Vasospasm and impaired autoregulation, along with the hemorrhage and loss of microcirculation observed immediately following injury, contribute to the overall ischemic pathology. Autoregulation of local spinal cord blood pressure is lost following injury, resulting in reduction of blood flow, which is further exacerbated by systemic hypotension.[22,23] Vasospasm is evident after SCI and can be caused by the injury itself or by the release of vasoactive factors such as histamine or nitric oxide (NO).[24]

Energy, Ion, and Glutamate Imbalances

Dysfunction in Na^+, K^+, Ca^{2+}, glutamate, and metabolic homeostasis is well documented and causes impairment and cell death fol-

Table 4.2 Spatiotemporal Secondary Pathophysiological Events

		Immediate (≤2 h)	Acute (≤2 d)	Subacute (≤2 w)	Intermediate (≤6 m)	Chronic (>6 m)
Epicenter	Vascular	– Rupture of blood vessels – Gray matter hemorrhage – Small white matter hemorrhages – BSCB compromise – Edema	– Hypotension – Ischemia/hypoperfusion – Hemorrhage – Maximal BSCB permeability – Edema	– Resolution of hemorrhage and edema – Angiogenesis – BSCB repair	Angiogenesis	Static
	Inflammatory	Microglial activation • cytokine secretion	Microglial activation • cytokines • NO neutrophil influx • MPO, ROS, MMP9	– Microglial activation – Macrophage infiltration • phagocytosis • trophic factor secretion – Decline in neutrophils – Lymphocyte recruitment	Activated macrophage/ microglia present	Static
	ECM	Necrotic products in ECM • DNA, ATP, K^+	– Degradation of ECM – HA	– Increase in • collagen IV, • fibronectin • laminin • CSPGs – Myelin debris • Nogo, MAG, OMgp		Static
	Chemical/ Biochemical		Glutamate • ↑ $[Ca^{2+}]i$, ROS, calpain, energy imbalances • ↓ ATP, ↑ lac/pyr ratio, loss of ion homeostasis • ↑ $[Na^+]$, $[Ca^{2+}]$, ↓ $[K^+]i$	Lipid peroxidation		Static
	Other cellular/axonal	– Axonal severing – Gray matter necrosis	– Demyelination from oligodendrocyte loss – Axonal A-β accumulation – Terminal end bulb formation in axons – Astrocyte proliferation	– Astrocyte proliferation • "Heteromorphic" at lesion borders – Myelination – Progenitor cell proliferation	– Glial scar – Axonal sprouting – Myelination	Glial and fibrous scar remain

		Immediate (≤2 h)	Acute (≤2 d)	Subacute (≤2 w)	Intermediate (≤6 m)	Chronic (>6 m)
Perilesional	Vascular			Angiogenesis	Angiogenesis	Static
	Inflammatory		Microglial activation			Static
	ECM					Static
	Biochemical			White matter glutamate excitotoxicity		
	Other cellular/axonal		– Astrocyte proliferation – Axonal swelling	– "Isomorphic astrogliosis" at remote sites –Progenitor proliferation		– Wallerian degeneration – Syrinx formation – Ligamentum flavum ossification (CSM)

With input from[8,37,98,121].

Abbreviations: BSCB, blood–spinal cord barrier; CSM, cervical spondylotic myelopathy; ECM, extracellular matrix; HA, hyaluronan; MPO, myeloperoxidase; ROS, reactive oxygen species.

Note: The time windows are largely based on preclinical studies

lowing SCI. Injury leads to increases in intracellular axonal Na^{+} and Ca^{2+} due to failure of ion pumps, inactivation of ion channels, reverse function of ion exchangers, and membrane depolarization.[25,26] Intracellular increases in astrocyte and oligodendrocyte Ca^{2+} through L-type and N-type Ca^{2+} channels and excess glutamate signaling (via metabotrophic and iontrophic glutamate receptors) may also play a role in white matter injury.[27] Impaired glutamate reuptake by astrocytes through dysfunction in glutamate transporters, cell death, and release of glutamate from neurons, axons, and glia via reversal of $Na^{(+)}$-dependent glutamate transport, all lead to increased extracellular glutamate.[28] Increased extracellular concentration of glutamate is observed within 3 hours after injury, leading to alterations in glial and axonal function and gray matter neuronal cell death.[29,30] No direct effects of glutamate on axons have been reported.

Changes in acute energy metabolism following SCI are characterized by depletion of adenosine triphosphate (ATP), an initial decrease in glucose, and increases in lactate/pyruvate ratios (indicative of hypoxia).[31,32] The resultant deficits in energy metabolism are no doubt due to hypoperfusion/ischemia–mediated decreases in oxygen and glucose availability to cells and subsequent reperfusion.

Intracellular Consequences of Acute Excessive Calcium Concentration

Excessive intracellular Ca^{2+} results in neuronal cell death and axonal degradation through activation of protein kinases and proteases and mitochondrial dysfunction. Proteases called calpains are activated acutely following SCI due to increases in intracellular Ca^{2+} and lead to the degradation of cytoskeletal proteins, such as neurofilaments and microtubules, disrupting axonal integrity and function.[33] Extreme intracellular Ca^{2+} levels are detrimental to mitochondria, causing increased reactive oxygen species (ROS) production in neurons and glia.

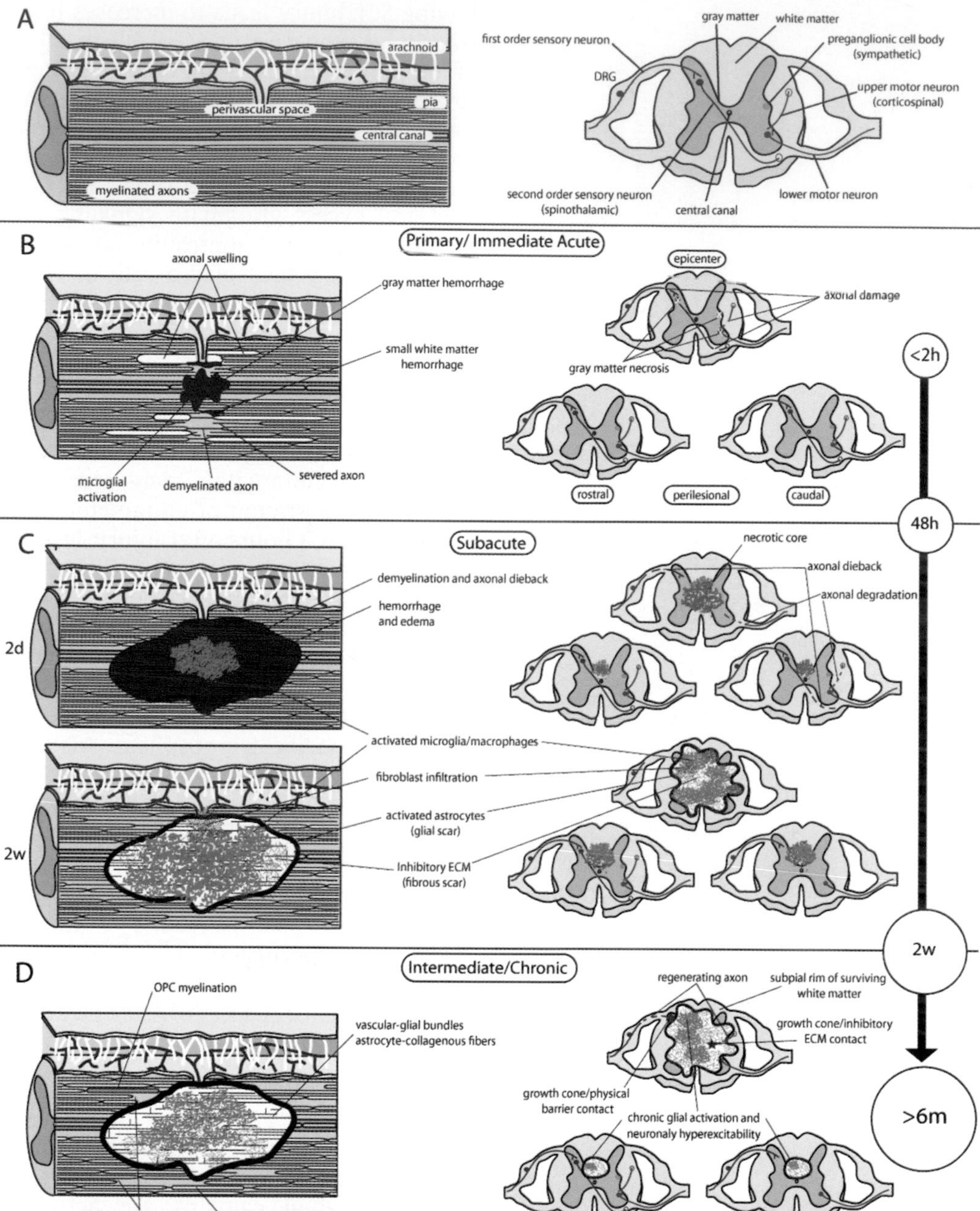

Fig. 4.1 Longitudinal and cross-sectional representation of the spinal cord at various stages following spinal cord injury. **(A)** Normal cord. **(B)** Immediate/acute injury. This phase is characterized by severing of axons at the epicenter and demyelination due to the primary injury. Gray matter hemorrhaging and small white matter hemorrhages are common. Necrosis of gray matter glia and sensory (*red*), autonomic (*green*), and motor neurons (*blue*) occurs, along with axonal swelling and accumulation of A-β protein (indicative of axonal transport failure). Microglia become activated due to necrotic by-products and secrete inflammatory cytokines and nitric oxide, further damaging tissue and recruiting systemic inflammatory cells. Necrosis of sympathetic preganglionic neurons (*green*) causes autonomic dysfunction. **(C)** Subacute injury. Hemorrhaging and edema continue, resulting in a spread of the hypoperfused/ischemic zone (*red area*). This continues the necrosis and begins apoptotic cell death. Macrophages (*green*) infiltrate, contributing to the local damage. At the epicenter, acute necrosis of lower motor neuronal cell bodies results in degradation of the leftover axons (*blue dashed line*). Severing of first-order sensory axons causes dieback toward the cell body (dorsal root ganglion, DRG). Severing of upper motor neuronal axons at the epicenter results in degradation of the distal end (*blue dashed line in caudal cross section*). *(continued on next page)*

Oxidative Stress

Increased production of ROS occurs following SCI due to metabolic imbalances and excess intracellular Ca^{2+}.[34,35] In both cases, mitochondria become dysfunctional and produce increased amounts of ROS.[36] Experimental methods for ROS detection have demonstrated that peak ROS production occurs 12 hours following injury, with levels remaining elevated until they return to basal levels within 4 to 5 weeks.[37] In addition to necrotic cell death, brief oxidative stress can cause apoptosis of oligodendrocytes[38] and neurons.[39] Mitochondrially produced ROS include superoxide (O_2^-) and hydrogen peroxide (H_2O_2). If not neutralized, O_2^- can react with NO, forming peroxynitrite (^-ONOO), one of the most reactive and detrimental free radicals known. When generation of ROS increases above the antioxidative capacities of cells, as is the case in mitochondrial dysfunction, these reactive molecules can damage proteins, DNA, and lipids. Neutrophil infiltration and associated oxidative burst have also been identified as a detrimental source of ROS in postinjured CNS tissue.[40]

Inflammation

The inflammatory response following SCI is a complex interaction of local and systemic mediators. Aspects of inflammation contribute to the secondary damage, and others, such as removal of cellular debris, aid in tissue repair. A confounding variable in SCI inflammatory research is significant differences in the inflammatory response between species[37] (even between strains[41]) of animal models, differences with each other and differences with humans.

Within hours of CNS injury, microglia are activated due to vascular compromise, loss of tissue homeostasis, and necrotic by-products (ATP, DNA, extracellular K^+). Microglia transition from ramified to amoeboid morphology upon activation and release cytokines [tumor necrosis factor-α (TNF-α), interferon-γ (IFN-γ), interleukin (IL)-6, IL-1β] and NO, which act to recruit systemic inflammatory cells and to modulate protein expression in neurons and glia, and result in neurotoxicity and myelin damage.[40–43] The first systemic immune cells to infiltrate the injured spinal cord are neutrophils. These cells arrive within several hours after injury and are found maximally within 1 to 2 days.[37,40,43] Neutrophils also release matrix metalloproteinases (MMPs) and myeloperoxidase, which is a source of ROS that can lead to lipid peroxidation. Whether the presence of neutrophils is beneficial or detrimental following SCI is undetermined.[44–46]

Blood–Spinal Cord Barrier Compromise

The BSCB remains compromised long after the initial primary mechanical damage to local vasculature due to the effects of in-

Fig. 4.1 (*Continued*) Severing of sensory fibers at the epicenter causes axonal dieback caudal to the injury site (*red dashed line in caudal section*). As the injury progresses over several weeks, hemorrhaging and edema come to an end and microglia/macrophages phagocytose cell and hemorrhagic debris. Oligodendrocytes undergo apoptotic cell death due to inflammation and white matter excitotoxicity, contributing to demyelination. Depending on the extent of damage to the meninges, fibroblasts (*orange*) proliferate and infiltrate the spinal cord, contributing to extracellular matrix remodeling. Astrocytes proliferate, acting to seal off the injury, forming a glial scar (*black outline of cavity*). Macrophages continue to infiltrate and phagocytose debris. At the level of injury, the majority of sensory and motor neurons are gone. Severed motor, sensory, and autonomic axons moving above and below the injury site have their distal ends (relative to the cell body) degraded, and the proximal ends retract. Angiogenesis also occurs (not shown). **(D)** Intermediate/chronic. The remaining debris is cleared from the lesion and microglia/macrophages remain active, contributing to neuropathic pain. Growth cones of regenerating sensory and motor neurons (*dashed lines*) meet either a physical barrier in the glial scar or an inhibitory chemical signal in the fibrous scar (due to chondroitin sulfate proteoglycans and myelin-associated proteins). Note that a subpial rim of surviving tissue exists in varying states of demyelination, representing a possible therapeutic target. In the lesion, macrophages, vascular-glial bundles, and astrocytes and collagenous fibers can be found. Remyelination is possible via either Schwann cells or oligodendrocyte precursor cells. The time windows are largely based on preclinical studies in rodent models. It has been estimated that in humans the acute injury lasts up to 2 weeks, the subacute injury extends from 2 weeks to 6 months, and the chronic injury extends beyond the period of 6 months.

flammatory mediators on endothelial cells and loss of astrocytes. Tracer studies in rats show that BSCB permeability peaks at 24 hours and remains compromised until ~2 weeks following injury.[47] The inflammatory cytokines IL-1β and TNF-α are responsible for the acute increase in vascular permeability.[48] Increased expression of ROS, NO, histamine, and matrix metalloproteinases contributes to prolonged permeability.

Apoptotic versus Necrotic Cell Death

Although there are clearly some purely necrotic causes of cell death and purely apoptotic causes, certain studies demonstrate that, depending on the intensity of the cell death insult, either necrosis or apoptosis could be the resultant cell death phenotype.[49] There is little evidence to support the idea that neurons undergo apoptosis in human SCI,[50] despite evidence of it in animal models.[51,52] Oligodendrocytes, on the other hand, undergo apoptosis following SCI,[53] and their death leads to axonal demyelination.[54] In general, acute cell death following SCI is necrotic.

The Subacutely Injured Spinal Cord

The subacute period lasts from approximately 2 days to 2 weeks following injury in animal models of SCI. In humans, it is likely that the subacute phase lasts from 2 weeks to 6 months. This phase is characterized by massive immune cell infiltration, reactive astrogliosis, remodeling of the ECM, delayed cell death, and continuing axonal demyelination/degeneration. Endogenous progenitor cell proliferation, removal of cellular debris, angiogenesis, and astrocyte containment of the injury cavity are examples of the beneficial aspects of the body's response during this period.

Inflammation

Monocytes/macrophages are recruited 2 to 3 days following injury and can remain present and activated for several weeks.[41,55–57] Once activated, macrophages are morphologically indistinguishable from resident microglia and adopt a similar cytokine expression profile. As with many aspects of inflammation, their beneficial/detrimental role in the injured spinal cord is not clear.[58–60] The possible discrepancies in these studies could be due to the timeline for prevention of infiltration. Macrophages that are activated and present within the spinal cord during the first week are potentially detrimental, whereas after that point they are essential in the recovery process. It appears that the ability of these cells to secrete growth factors and neurotrophins, as well as to phagocytose dead tissue and debris, makes them integral to wound healing and the regenerative process.[61]

T-lymphocytes enter the spinal cord maximally between 3 and 7 days following injury in response to the cytokine/chemokine signals from activated microglia and macrophages.[37,43] T-lymphocytes can regulate macrophage/microglial activity, mainly by controlling secretion of both pro- and antiinflammatory cytokines. Through cytokine signaling, CNS-specific T-cells recruit antigen-independent T-cells to the site of injury, and it is these cells that secrete various trophic factors important for regeneration and growth, such as insulin-like growth factor-1 (IGF-1) and brain-derived neurotrophic factor (BDNF).[62,63]

Subacute Cell Death and Axonal Degeneration

There are several extra- or intracellular events, including removal of trophic factors, increase in inflammatory mediators, death receptor activation, and DNA damage, that can all cause apoptosis in the subacute setting.[64] The specific components involved in the execution of apoptosis differ according to the nature of the initiator and according to cell type.

The occurrence of apoptosis in posttraumatic spinal cord tissue was recognized in humans by Emery and coworkers in 1998, through detection of terminal deoxynucleotidyl transferase dUTP nick end labeling (TUNEL) and caspase-3 activation.[50] Clinically relevant animal models of SCI have also identified apoptosis as a significant event in the injury pathophysiology, in which neurons and more so oligodendrocytes seem to be vulnerable.[65–69] Caspase-3 activation following experimental SCI has been observed as early as 4 hours and up to 8 days after injury in both neurons and oligodendrocytes at, rostral to, and caudal to the injury epicenter.[66,67,70] In addition, the presence of cytochrome c in cytoplasmic regions has been measured several hours following SCI in neurons and after several days in oligodendrocytes.[66] Delayed oligodendroglial apoptosis has been shown to occur in association with axonal degeneration, which suggests the two phenomena are linked.[67,71]

Death Receptors

The tumor necrosis factor receptor family are prototypic death receptors. Members that have been implicated in SCI include the tumor necrosis factor receptor (TNFR), Fas receptor (FasR), and the tumor necrosis factor-related apoptosis-inducing ligand (TRAIL) receptor. Deletion of the TNFR has been shown to increase damage and reduce functional recovery in experimental models of SCI. The TRAIL receptor has been associated with SCI.[72] FasR is upregulated in cases of spinal cord trauma, and blocking its activation is beneficial following injury.[67,73,74] Additionally, the p75 neurotrophin receptor can induce apoptotic cell death,[75,76] a phenomenon that has been associated with oligodendrocytes undergoing apoptosis following experimental SCI.[67] The intrinsic or extrinsic death receptor pathway can be activated following injury, and both pathways activate caspase-3. Increased intracellular Ca^{2+} can cause release of cytochrome c from mitochondria. The cleaved form of caspase-3 translocates to the nucleus, where it has the ability to further cleave over 40 different proteins. It is recognized that apoptosis may occur in the absence of caspase activation,[77] for instance, through mitochondrial release of apoptosis-inducing factor (AIF).[78]

The Mitochondria and Apoptosis

Mitochondria are key regulators of both caspase-dependent and caspase-independent apoptotic signaling. Several proapoptotic proteins in addition to cytochrome c, such as AIF, can be released from the mitochondrial intermembrane space under various circumstances. When released, AIF is translocated to the nucleus and induces cell death by triggering chromatin condensation and high molecular weight (50 KDa) fragmentation. Endonuclease activity is not inherent to AIF; thus it does not directly cleave DNA but acts to recruit or activate endonucleases.[79] There is much debate in the literature about how these proapoptotic molecules are able to escape from mitochondria, or more specifically, what causes mitochondrial outer membrane permeability (MOMP) allowing their translocation into the cytoplasm.[80] Ca^{2+} influx in surviving glial cells occurs almost immediately following injury, a phenomenon that spreads from the injury epicenter over time.[81] Mitochondrial Ca^{2+} accumulation resulting from increased intracellular Ca^{2+} concentrations has been demonstrated to cause opening of the MOMP.[82]

Demyelination

Studies in animals have demonstrated that surviving axons can be found in demyelinated states.[83] This finding has prompted numerous studies looking at stem cell transplantation with the hopes of remyelinating these axons,[84] though it is clear that stem cells can have other nonremyelinating effects, such as neurotrophic factor secretion.[85] In humans, however, studies describing SCI have not validated these findings, suggesting that demyelinated axons are not common to the human pathology.[8,86] Other studies have detected demyelinated axons in four of seven postmortem human SCI cases.[87] Technical issues or the length of time following injury that the samples were collected could explain these discrepancies.

The Glial and Fibrous Scar

Scarring in the injured spinal cord is highly dependent on the severity and type of injury. Transection injury models produce very different patterns of scarring than contusion or compression injuries.[88] Contusion/compression injuries in humans (which are the most common) can involve laceration, breaches in the dura, subarachnoid hemorrhaging, or complete obliteration of the arachnoid layers and will have very different molecular makeup and extent of scarring due to greater involvement of meningeal fibroblasts. Schwann cells have also been implicated in production of scar-related ECM molecules following human SCI.[89]

In rats and humans, astrocytes that survive the primary and acute secondary stages of injury respond by activating/proliferating and surrounding the cystic cavity in an attempt to prevent its spread. This phenomenon is typically referred to as astrogliosis or glial scarring, where astrocytes create a "heteromorphic network."[8] Although partially beneficial due to limiting the spread of the lesion, their physical presence represents a barrier to axonal regeneration whether endogenous or therapeutically initiated. Astrocytes also express and secrete chondroitin sulfate proteoglycans (CSPGs) and other inhibitory molecules, which can cause growth cone collapse and dystrophic end bulb formation in neurons.[89–92] Although astrogliosis is prevalent following SCI in rats and mice, it is not as pronounced in human SCI,[93] which may have important consequences for the development of SCI therapies that specifically target glial scarring, such as chondroitinase ABC (ChABC).[94]

Inside and around the lesion borders (fibrous scar), the ECM undergoes profound changes as a consequence of injury due to cleanup of necrotic and myelin debris, activation of glial and immune cells, and possible infiltration of fibroblasts. The hyaluronan component of the normal ECM is degraded by hyaluronidases and ROS,[95] leading to astrocyte proliferation following injury.[96] The fibrous scar consists of a collagen IV backbone, which is not inhibitory itself but is "sticky" and binds other ECM molecules.[88] Collagen IV and laminin expression are upregulated following injury and can be associated with scar formation in rats[97] and humans along with fibronectin.[89] Laminin remains upregulated into chronic time points in rats, whereas collagen IV decreases chronically, but not to basal levels. Molecules in the fibrous scar responsible for inhibition of neurite outgrowth in animal studies consist of CSPGs, such as NG2, aggrecan, neurocan, brevican, phosphacan, and versican, as well as other molecules, including tenascin and myelin inhibitory molecules, such as myelin-associated glycoprotein (MAG), oligodendrocyte myelin glycoprotein (OMgp) and Nogo A, B, and C.[91,98–102] In humans, the CSPGs NG2 and phosphacan were found in scar regions postinjury, whereas neurocan and versican were not.[103]

Astrocytes are one of the cell types responsible for producing CSPGs,[98,104,105] which are ECM molecules with membrane and secreted forms. The latter of which typically form complexes with laminin/collagen IV. CSPG expression is upregulated and typically reaches maximal expression around 1 week following SCI in animal models.[91,106,107] Other cell types responsible for the production of CSPGs include fibroblasts and immune cells such as macrophage and microglia.

How Inhibitory Molecules Prevent Regeneration

Myelin-associated inhibitory molecules bind the nogo receptor (NgR) on neurons and activate the Rho/Rock pathway leading to decreased growth cone mobility and growth cone collapse. Until recently, the receptor for CSPGs was unknown. It was found that PTPsigma, a transmembrane tyrosine phosphatase, was expressed on neurons and can act as a receptor for CPSGs.[108] CSPGs also signal through the Rho/Rock pathway. The actin cytoskeleton is the downstream target of this signaling cascade.

Angiogenesis

Endogenous angiogenesis occurs during the subacute period and is detected at 7 days postinjury in the gray matter of adult rats but diminishes as the cystic cavity spreads.[97] At more remote sites from the epicenter there is still significant angiogenesis present that has been associated with regenerating nerve fibers.[109]

Progenitor Cell Proliferation

Stem/progenitor cells have been identified in the adult mammalian spinal cord[110–112] and proliferate extensively following SCI.[113] These cells differentiate into glia because endogenous neurogenesis is generally not seen in the spinal cord. NG2 is a CSPG that is expressed on a subpopulation of progenitor cells and macrophages[91] after injury.[91,114] It has been suggested that NG2+ progenitors can differentiate into astrocytes and oligodendrocytes after trauma, with cues for progenitor differentiation coming from changes in postinjury niches.[115] In the spinal cord, cells around the central canal have been identified as a source of progenitors and proliferate following injury, generating mainly astrocytes.[116,117]

The Intermediate Phase

The intermediate period of SCI occurs from 2 weeks to 6 months postinjury. The glial and fibrous scars continue to develop, macrophages remain present and active in the lesion, severed axons continue to degenerate in perilesional areas, axonal sprouting occurs, and endogenous remyelination is observed. The severed axon portion distal to the cell body degenerates and myelin breaks down. Macrophages continue to phagocytose debris from degenerating axons/myelin breakdown globules. Regenerative axonal sprouting in corticospinal and reticulospinal tracts has been documented in rats.[118] Peripheral Schwann cells have been found to remyelinate following human SCI.[119] Oligodendrocyte precursor cells (OPCs) are also responsible for remyelination in the injured spinal cord.[110]

The Chronically Injured Spinal Cord

The chronic SCI phase is typically considered anywhere after 6 months postinjury. Wallerian degeneration of severed axons toward the cell body continues, and debilitating neuropathic pain can develop. What is left at the injury site has been described as a multilocular cystic cavity traversed by vascular-glial bundles with regenerated nerve roots.[8,120] Furthermore, astrocyte and collagenous fibers run through and surround the lesion. Within 1 to 2 years it is believed that the lesion has ceased to progress and continuing deficits are stabilized.

Posttraumatic Syringomyelia

The formation of a fluid-filled cavity (syrinx) occurs in as many as 21 to 28% of SCI patients up to 30 years following injury.[121–124] This phenomenon has been termed posttraumatic syringomyelia (PTS) and consists of syrinx or syringes with clear anatomical distinction from the central canal. Approximately one in three cases is symptomatic, with common symptoms including segmental pain due to compressive/pressure injury of spinothalamic pathways at or above the level of injury and sensory loss,[125–127] progressive asymmetrical weakness,[125,126] or increased spasticity.[121] Animal studies suggest that PTS is due to increased pressure in cerebrospinal fluid (CSF) dynamics from arachnoid lesions or cord compressions, resulting in increased inflow of CSF.[128] Indeed, in humans, PTS is associated with arachnoid scarring.[124,129]

Neuropathic Pain

The genesis of neuropathic pain is dependent on the region relative to the injury site. Typically, the divisions include "above-level," "at-level," and "below-level." Previously innocuous stimuli become noxious in SCI patients, resulting in mechanical and/or thermal allodynia. In rats, neuropathic pain is seen 4 weeks following injury and depends on injury intensity.[130] In humans, studies have shown that the number of patients exhibiting neuropathic pain is as high as 58% in some populations.[131–133] Chronic microglial and astrocyte activation produces factors that result in dorsal horn neuron hyperexcitability in remote regions from the epicenter.[134–136] Indeed, therapies that target astrocyte and microglial/macrophage activation show reduction in the incidence of neuropathic pain in animal models.[137,138]

Conclusion

The progression of SCI over time results in significant morphological and functional alteration. Inflammation, scarring, continuing axonal degeneration, and endogenous attempts at regeneration/remyelination highlight the complex interaction of local and systemic responses.

The characterization of SCI pathophysiology has come a long way in recent years;

however, there is still much to be elucidated. A greater understanding of the injured human spinal cord is needed, along with an increased variety of animal models to better mimic the heterogeneous human condition. Further defining the timeline of inflammatory and glial reactions to injury could better determine which responses should be allowed to proceed and which should be inhibited therapeutically for increased quality of life and functional recovery for patients.

Pearls

- SCI is biphasic in nature and represents a primary injury that sets off a secondary injury cascade.
- Posttraumatic ischemia will generally determine the extent of secondary tissue loss and functional impairment seen following SCI.
- Autonomic dysfunction and neuropathic pain have severe negative effects on quality of life for SCI patients. In order to reduce or prevent these, research elucidating their pathophysiological development is necessary. As such, pathophysiological research is of equal importance to that focused on improving motor function after injury.
- Only education and safety can prevent primary SCI. Early intervention to limit the spread of secondary events is paramount. Additionally, due to some drawn-out processes, subacute intervention can also be beneficial.
- The body elicits endogenous beneficial responses. Progenitor cell proliferation, axonal sprouting, remyelination, angiogenesis, and some aspects of the immune response can aid in recovery following injury. It is important to understand these processes so that interventions can harness and maximize their potential.
- Due to the complex nature of SCI, a successful treatment paradigm will target detrimental secondary processes while promoting repair processes, with or without the use of cell replacement strategies. Furthermore, temporal application of therapeutics will be a central variable.

Pitfalls

- Thus far, demyelination/remyelination in human SCI appears to be less prevalent than that observed in animal SCI studies. However, clinical trials using progenitor cells thought to be capable of remyelination, such as the one initiated (and subsequently halted for financial reasons) by Geron, may elucidate the issue further.
- To date, promising preclinical therapeutics have not enjoyed the same clinical efficacy. Considering the heterogeneous nature of human SCI, it would be beneficial if preclinical therapeutics showed effectiveness in a variety of animal models prior to initiation of clinical trials.
- Small animal models are our best source for studying the pathophysiology of SCI. However, as there are discrepancies between certain aspects of these models and humans, significant findings should be validated in nonhuman primates or studied in human postmortem tissue for an accurate representation of SCI progression in humans. Development of therapeutics and time windows for their application can then be based on clinically relevant pathophysiological events.
- Inflammatory and glial responses are both beneficial and detrimental.
  - The early astrocytic response is essential to contain the injury and minimize the spread of the secondary injury. In the chronic stage, the glial scar inhibits plasticity and regeneration.
  - Early inflammation is detrimental, whereas the later, more coordinated events, aid in tissue repair and recovery.
  - A better understanding of the nature, source, and temporal expression of the key mediators of these events will lead to identification of therapeutic targets and, more importantly, when interventions should be applied following injury

References

1. Burney RE, Maio RF, Maynard F, Karunas R. Incidence, characteristics, and outcome of spinal cord injury at trauma centers in North America. Arch Surg 1993;128(5):596–599
2. Sekhon LH, Fehlings MG. Epidemiology, demographics, and pathophysiology of acute spinal cord injury. Spine 2001;26(24, Suppl):S2–S12
3. Tator CH. Update on the pathophysiology and pathology of acute spinal cord injury. Brain Pathol 1995;5(4):407–413
4. Nyström B, Berglund JE. Spinal cord restitution following compression injuries in rats. Acta Neurol Scand 1988;78(6):467–472
5. LaPlaca MC, Simon CM, Prado GR, Cullen DK. CNS injury biomechanics and experimental models. Prog Brain Res 2007;161:13–26
6. Choo AM, Liu J, Lam CK, Dvorak M, Tetzlaff W, Oxland TR. Contusion, dislocation, and distraction: primary hemorrhage and membrane permeability in distinct mechanisms of spinal cord injury. J Neurosurg Spine 2007;6(3):255–266
7. Maikos JT, Shreiber DI. Immediate damage to the blood-spinal cord barrier due to mechanical trauma. J Neurotrauma 2007;24(3):492–507
8. Kakulas BA. Neuropathology: the foundation for new treatments in spinal cord injury. Spinal Cord 2004;42(10):549–563
9. Ditunno JF Jr, Young W, Donovan WH, Creasey G; American Spinal Injury Association. The international standards booklet for neurological and functional classification of spinal cord injury. Paraplegia 1994;32(2):70–80
10. Schramm LP. Spinal sympathetic interneurons: their identification and roles after spinal cord injury. Prog Brain Res 2006;152:27–37
11. Hong Y, Cechetto DF, Weaver LC. Spinal cord regulation of sympathetic activity in intact and spinal rats. Am J Physiol 1994;266(4 Pt 2):H1485–H1493
12. Waxman SG. Demyelination in spinal cord injury. J Neurol Sci 1989;91(1-2):1–14
13. Nashmi R, Fehlings MG. Changes in axonal physiology and morphology after chronic compressive injury of the rat thoracic spinal cord. Neuroscience 2001;104(1):235–251
14. Faulkner JR, Herrmann JE, Woo MJ, Tansey KE, Doan NB, Sofroniew MV. Reactive astrocytes protect tissue and preserve function after spinal cord injury. J Neurosci 2004;24(9):2143–2155
15. Ehlers MD. Deconstructing the axon: Wallerian degeneration and the ubiquitin-proteasome system. Trends Neurosci 2004;27(1):3–6
16. Popovich PG, Horner PJ, Mullin BB, Stokes BT. A quantitative spatial analysis of the blood-spinal cord barrier, I: Permeability changes after experimental spinal contusion injury. Exp Neurol 1996;142(2):258–275
17. Rowland JW, Hawryluk GW, Kwon B, Fehlings MG. Current status of acute spinal cord injury pathophysiology and emerging therapies: promise on the horizon. Neurosurg Focus 2008;25(5):E2
18. Ditunno JF, Little JW, Tessler A, Burns AS. Spinal shock revisited: a four-phase model. Spinal Cord 2004;42(7):383–395
19. Fehlings MG, Tator CH, Linden RD. The relationships among the severity of spinal cord injury, motor and somatosensory evoked potentials and spinal cord blood flow. Electroencephalogr Clin Neurophysiol 1989;74(4):241–259
20. Tator CH, Fehlings MG. Review of the secondary injury theory of acute spinal cord trauma with emphasis on vascular mechanisms. J Neurosurg 1991;75(1):15–26
21. Aoyama T, Hida K, Akino M, Yano S, Iwasaki Y, Saito H. Ultra-early MRI showing no abnormality in a fall victim presenting with tetraparesis. Spinal Cord 2007;45(10):695–699
22. Guha A, Tator CH, Rochon J. Spinal cord blood flow and systemic blood pressure after experimental spinal cord injury in rats. Stroke 1989;20(3):372–377
23. Guha A, Tator CH. Acute cardiovascular effects of experimental spinal cord injury. J Trauma 1988;28(4):481–490
24. Anthes DL, Theriault E, Tator CH. Ultrastructural evidence for arteriolar vasospasm after spinal cord trauma. Neurosurgery 1996;39(4):804–814
25. Stys PK, Lopachin RM. Mechanisms of calcium and sodium fluxes in anoxic myelinated central nervous system axons. Neuroscience 1998;82(1):21–32
26. Agrawal SK, Fehlings MG. Mechanisms of secondary injury to spinal cord axons in vitro: role of Na^+, $Na^{(+)}$-$K^{(+)}$-ATPase, the $Na^{(+)}$-H^+ exchanger, and the $Na^{(+)}$-Ca^{2+} exchanger. J Neurosci 1996;16(2):545–552
27. Li S, Stys PK. Mechanisms of ionotropic glutamate receptor-mediated excitotoxicity in isolated spinal cord white matter. J Neurosci 2000;20(3):1190–1198
28. Li S, Mealing GA, Morley P, Stys PK. Novel injury mechanism in anoxia and trauma of spinal cord white matter: glutamate release via reverse Na^+-dependent glutamate transport. J Neurosci 1999;19(14):RC16
29. McAdoo DJ, Xu GY, Robak G, Hughes MG. Changes in amino acid concentrations over time and space around an impact injury and their diffusion through the rat spinal cord. Exp Neurol 1999;159(2):538–544
30. Liu D, Xu GY, Pan E, McAdoo DJ. Neurotoxicity of glutamate at the concentration released upon spinal cord injury. Neuroscience 1999;93(4):1383–1389
31. Anderson DK, Means ED, Waters TR, Spears CJ. Spinal cord energy metabolism following compression trauma to the feline spinal cord. J Neurosurg 1980;53(3):375–380
32. Braughler JM, Hall ED. Effects of multi-dose methylprednisolone sodium succinate administration on injured cat spinal cord neurofilament degradation and energy metabolism. J Neurosurg 1984;61(2):290–295
33. Banik NL, Matzelle DC, Gantt-Wilford G, Osborne A, Hogan EL. Increased calpain content and progressive degradation of neurofilament protein in spinal cord injury. Brain Res 1997;752(1-2):301–306
34. Hall ED. Free radicals and CNS injury. Crit Care Clin 1989;5(4):793–805

35. Lewén A, Matz P, Chan PH. Free radical pathways in CNS injury. J Neurotrauma 2000;17(10):871–890
36. Azbill RD, Mu X, Bruce-Keller AJ, Mattson MP, Springer JE. Impaired mitochondrial function, oxidative stress and altered antioxidant enzyme activities following traumatic spinal cord injury. Brain Res 1997;765(2):283–290
37. Donnelly DJ, Popovich PG. Inflammation and its role in neuroprotection, axonal regeneration and functional recovery after spinal cord injury. Exp Neurol 2008;209(2):378–388
38. Mronga T, Stahnke T, Goldbaum O, Richter-Landsberg C. Mitochondrial pathway is involved in hydrogen-peroxide-induced apoptotic cell death of oligodendrocytes. Glia 2004;46(4):446–455
39. Bao F, Liu D. Peroxynitrite generated in the rat spinal cord induces apoptotic cell death and activates caspase-3. Neuroscience 2003;116(1):59–70
40. Carlson SL, Parrish ME, Springer JE, Doty K, Dossett L. Acute inflammatory response in spinal cord following impact injury. Exp Neurol 1998;151(1):77–88
41. Popovich PG, Wei P, Stokes BT. Cellular inflammatory response after spinal cord injury in Sprague-Dawley and Lewis rats. J Comp Neurol 1997;377(3):443–464
42. Hausmann ON. Post-traumatic inflammation following spinal cord injury. Spinal Cord 2003;41(7):369–378
43. Fleming JC, Norenberg MD, Ramsay DA, et al. The cellular inflammatory response in human spinal cords after injury. Brain 2006;129(Pt 12):3249–3269
44. Saville LR, Pospisil CH, Mawhinney LA, et al. A monoclonal antibody to CD11d reduces the inflammatory infiltrate into the injured spinal cord: a potential neuroprotective treatment. J Neuroimmunol 2004;156(1-2):42–57
45. Bao F, Chen Y, Dekaban GA, Weaver LC. An anti-CD11d integrin antibody reduces cyclooxygenase-2 expression and protein and DNA oxidation after spinal cord injury in rats. J Neurochem 2004;90(5):1194–1204
46. Stirling DP, Liu S, Kubes P, Yong VW. Depletion of Ly6G/Gr-1 leukocytes after spinal cord injury in mice alters wound healing and worsens neurological outcome. J Neurosci 2009;29(3):753–764
47. Noble LJ, Wrathall JR. Distribution and time course of protein extravasation in the rat spinal cord after contusive injury. Brain Res 1989;482(1):57–66
48. Schnell L, Fearn S, Schwab ME, Perry VH, Anthony DC. Cytokine-induced acute inflammation in the brain and spinal cord. J Neuropathol Exp Neurol 1999;58(3):245–254
49. Bonfoco E, Krainc D, Ankarcrona M, Nicotera P, Lipton SA. Apoptosis and necrosis: two distinct events induced, respectively, by mild and intense insults with N-methyl-D-aspartate or nitric oxide/superoxide in cortical cell cultures. Proc Natl Acad Sci U S A 1995;92(16):7162–7166
50. Emery E, Aldana P, Bunge MB, et al. Apoptosis after traumatic human spinal cord injury. J Neurosurg 1998;89(6):911–920
51. Lou J, Lenke LG, Ludwig FJ, O'Brien MF. Apoptosis as a mechanism of neuronal cell death following acute experimental spinal cord injury. Spinal Cord 1998;36(10):683–690
52. Yong C, Arnold PM, Zoubine MN, et al. Apoptosis in cellular compartments of rat spinal cord after severe contusion injury. J Neurotrauma 1998;15(7):459–472
53. Crowe MJ, Bresnahan JC, Shuman SL, Masters JN, Beattie MS. Apoptosis and delayed degeneration after spinal cord injury in rats and monkeys. Nat Med 1997;3(1):73–76
54. Totoiu MO, Keirstead HS. Spinal cord injury is accompanied by chronic progressive demyelination. J Comp Neurol 2005;486(4):373–383
55. Sroga JM, Jones TB, Kigerl KA, McGaughy VM, Popovich PG. Rats and mice exhibit distinct inflammatory reactions after spinal cord injury. J Comp Neurol 2003;462(2):223–240
56. Blight AR. Delayed demyelination and macrophage invasion: a candidate for secondary cell damage in spinal cord injury. Cent Nerv Syst Trauma 1985;2(4):299–315
57. Blight AR. Macrophages and inflammatory damage in spinal cord injury. J Neurotrauma 1992;9(Suppl 1):S83–S91
58. Kigerl KA, Gensel JC, Ankeny DP, Alexander JK, Donnelly DJ, Popovich PG. Identification of two distinct macrophage subsets with divergent effects causing either neurotoxicity or regeneration in the injured mouse spinal cord. J Neurosci 2009;29(43):13435–13444
59. Popovich PG, Guan Z, Wei P, Huitinga I, van Rooijen N, Stokes BT. Depletion of hematogenous macrophages promotes partial hindlimb recovery and neuroanatomical repair after experimental spinal cord injury. Exp Neurol 1999;158(2):351–365
60. Shechter R, London A, Varol C, et al. Infiltrating blood-derived macrophages are vital cells playing an anti-inflammatory role in recovery from spinal cord injury in mice. PLoS Med 2009;6(7):e1000113
61. Jones TB, McDaniel EE, Popovich PG. Inflammatory-mediated injury and repair in the traumatically injured spinal cord. Curr Pharm Des 2005;11(10):1223–1236
62. Moalem G, Gdalyahu A, Shani Y, et al. Production of neurotrophins by activated T cells: implications for neuroprotective autoimmunity. J Autoimmun 2000;15(3):331–345
63. Schwartz M, Moalem G, Leibowitz-Amit R, Cohen IR. Innate and adaptive immune responses can be beneficial for CNS repair. Trends Neurosci 1999;22(7):295–299
64. Ellis RE, Yuan JY, Horvitz HR. Mechanisms and functions of cell death. Annu Rev Cell Biol 1991;7:663–698
65. Liu XZ, Xu XM, Hu R, et al. Neuronal and glial apoptosis after traumatic spinal cord injury. J Neurosci 1997;17(14):5395–5406
66. Springer JE, Azbill RD, Knapp PE. Activation of the caspase-3 apoptotic cascade in traumatic spinal cord injury. Nat Med 1999;5(8):943–946
67. Casha S, Yu WR, Fehlings MG. Oligodendroglial apoptosis occurs along degenerating axons and is associated with FAS and p75 expression fol-

lowing spinal cord injury in the rat. Neuroscience 2001;103(1):203–218

68. Grossman SD, Rosenberg LJ, Wrathall JR. Temporal-spatial pattern of acute neuronal and glial loss after spinal cord contusion. Exp Neurol 2001;168(2):273–282
69. Abe Y, Yamamoto T, Sugiyama Y, et al. Apoptotic cells associated with Wallerian degeneration after experimental spinal cord injury: a possible mechanism of oligodendroglial death. J Neurotrauma 1999;16(10):945–952
70. McEwen ML, Springer JE. A mapping study of caspase-3 activation following acute spinal cord contusion in rats. J Histochem Cytochem 2005;53(7):809–819
71. Barres BA, Jacobson MD, Schmid R, Sendtner M, Raff MC. Does oligodendrocyte survival depend on axons? Curr Biol 1993;3(8):489–497
72. Plunkett JA, Yu CG, Easton JM, Bethea JR, Yezierski RP. Effects of interleukin-10 (IL-10) on pain behavior and gene expression following excitotoxic spinal cord injury in the rat. Exp Neurol 2001;168(1):144–154
73. Demjen D, Klussmann S, Kleber S, et al. Neutralization of CD95 ligand promotes regeneration and functional recovery after spinal cord injury. Nat Med 2004;10(4):389–395
74. Ackery A, Robins S, Fehlings MG. Inhibition of Fas-mediated apoptosis through administration of soluble Fas receptor improves functional outcome and reduces posttraumatic axonal degeneration after acute spinal cord injury. J Neurotrauma 2006;23(5):604–616
75. Frade JM, Rodríguez-Tébar A, Barde YA. Induction of cell death by endogenous nerve growth factor through its p75 receptor. Nature 1996; 383(6596):166–168
76. Casaccia-Bonnefil P, Carter BD, Dobrowsky RT, Chao MV. Death of oligodendrocytes mediated by the interaction of nerve growth factor with its receptor p75. Nature 1996;383(6602):716–719
77. Kitanaka C, Kuchino Y. Caspase-independent programmed cell death with necrotic morphology. Cell Death Differ 1999;6(6):508–515
78. Lorenzo HK, Susin SA, Penninger J, Kroemer G. Apoptosis inducing factor (AIF): a phylogenetically old, caspase-independent effector of cell death. Cell Death Differ 1999;6(6):516–524
79. Ye H, Cande C, Stephanou NC, et al. DNA binding is required for the apoptogenic action of apoptosis inducing factor. Nat Struct Biol 2002;9(9): 680–684
80. Cregan SP, Dawson VL, Slack RS. Role of AIF in caspase-dependent and caspase-independent cell death. Oncogene 2004;23(16):2785–2796
81. Mills LR, Velumian AA, Agrawal SK, Theriault E, Fehlings MG. Confocal imaging of changes in glial calcium dynamics and homeostasis after mechanical injury in rat spinal cord white matter. Neuroimage 2004;21(3):1069–1082
82. Ankarcrona M, Dypbukt JM, Bonfoco E, et al. Glutamate-induced neuronal death: a succession of necrosis or apoptosis depending on mitochondrial function. Neuron 1995;15(4): 961–973
83. Karimi-Abdolrezaee S, Eftekharpour E, Wang J, Morshead CM, Fehlings MG. Delayed transplantation of adult neural precursor cells promotes remyelination and functional neurological recovery after spinal cord injury. J Neurosci 2006;26(13):3377–3389
84. Keirstead HS, Nistor G, Bernal G, et al. Human embryonic stem cell-derived oligodendrocyte progenitor cell transplants remyelinate and restore locomotion after spinal cord injury. J Neurosci 2005;25(19):4694–4705
85. Xiao M, Klueber KM, Lu C, et al. Human adult olfactory neural progenitors rescue axotomized rodent rubrospinal neurons and promote functional recovery. Exp Neurol 2005;194(1): 12–30
86. Norenberg MD, Smith J, Marcillo A. The pathology of human spinal cord injury: defining the problems. J Neurotrauma 2004;21(4): 429–440
87. Guest JD, Hiester ED, Bunge RP. Demyelination and Schwann cell responses adjacent to injury epicenter cavities following chronic human spinal cord injury. Exp Neurol 2005;192(2): 384–393
88. Brazda N, Müller HW. Pharmacological modification of the extracellular matrix to promote regeneration of the injured brain and spinal cord. Prog Brain Res 2009;175:269–281
89. Buss A, Pech K, Kakulas BA, et al. Growth-modulating molecules are associated with invading Schwann cells and not astrocytes in human traumatic spinal cord injury. Brain 2007;130(Pt 4):940–953
90. Jones LL, Margolis RU, Tuszynski MH. The chondroitin sulfate proteoglycans neurocan, brevican, phosphacan, and versican are differentially regulated following spinal cord injury. Exp Neurol 2003;182(2):399–411
91. Jones LL, Yamaguchi Y, Stallcup WB, Tuszynski MH. NG2 is a major chondroitin sulfate proteoglycan produced after spinal cord injury and is expressed by macrophages and oligodendrocyte progenitors. J Neurosci 2002;22(7):2792–2803
92. Monnier PP, Sierra A, Schwab JM, Henke-Fahle S, Mueller BK. The Rho/ROCK pathway mediates neurite growth-inhibitory activity associated with the chondroitin sulfate proteoglycans of the CNS glial scar. Mol Cell Neurosci 2003;22(3): 319–330
93. Hagg T, Oudega M. Degenerative and spontaneous regenerative processes after spinal cord injury. J Neurotrauma 2006;23(3-4):264–280
94. Bradbury EJ, Moon LD, Popat RJ, et al. Chondroitinase ABC promotes functional recovery after spinal cord injury. Nature 2002;416(6881): 636–640
95. Noble PW. Hyaluronan and its catabolic products in tissue injury and repair. Matrix Biol 2002;21(1):25–29
96. Struve J, Maher PC, Li YQ, et al. Disruption of the hyaluronan-based extracellular matrix in spinal cord promotes astrocyte proliferation. Glia 2005;52(1):16–24
97. Loy DN, Crawford CH, Darnall JB, Burke DA, Onifer SM, Whittemore SR. Temporal progression of angiogenesis and basal lamina deposition after contusive spinal cord injury in the adult rat. J Comp Neurol 2002;445(4):308–324

98. Asher RA, Morgenstern DA, Fidler PS, et al. Neurocan is upregulated in injured brain and in cytokine-treated astrocytes. J Neurosci 2000;20(7): 2427–2438
99. Ughrin YM, Chen ZJ, Levine JM. Multiple regions of the NG2 proteoglycan inhibit neurite growth and induce growth cone collapse. J Neurosci 2003;23(1):175–186
100. McKeon RJ, Schreiber RC, Rudge JS, Silver J. Reduction of neurite outgrowth in a model of glial scarring following CNS injury is correlated with the expression of inhibitory molecules on reactive astrocytes. J Neurosci 1991;11(11):3398–3411
101. Becker CG, Becker T, Meyer RL, Schachner M. Tenascin-R inhibits the growth of optic fibers in vitro but is rapidly eliminated during nerve regeneration in the salamander *Pleurodeles waltl*. J Neurosci 1999;19(2):813–827
102. Sandvig A, Berry M, Barrett LB, Butt A, Logan A. Myelin-, reactive glia-, and scar-derived CNS axon growth inhibitors: expression, receptor signaling, and correlation with axon regeneration. Glia 2004;46(3):225–251
103. Buss A, Pech K, Kakulas BA, et al. NG2 and phosphacan are present in the astroglial scar after human traumatic spinal cord injury. BMC Neurol 2009;9:32
104. Rudge JS, Silver J. Inhibition of neurite outgrowth on astroglial scars in vitro. J Neurosci 1990;10(11):3594–3603
105. Höke A, Silver J. Proteoglycans and other repulsive molecules in glial boundaries during development and regeneration of the nervous system. Prog Brain Res 1996;108:149–163
106. Fitch MT, Silver J. Activated macrophages and the blood-brain barrier: inflammation after CNS injury leads to increases in putative inhibitory molecules. Exp Neurol 1997;148(2):587–603
107. Tang X, Davies JE, Davies SJ. Changes in distribution, cell associations, and protein expression levels of NG2, neurocan, phosphacan, brevican, versican V2, and tenascin-C during acute to chronic maturation of spinal cord scar tissue. J Neurosci Res 2003;71(3):427–444
108. Shen Y, Tenney AP, Busch SA, et al. PTPsigma is a receptor for chondroitin sulfate proteoglycan, an inhibitor of neural regeneration. Science 2009;326(5952):592–596
109. Zhang Z, Guth L. Experimental spinal cord injury: Wallerian degeneration in the dorsal column is followed by revascularization, glial proliferation, and nerve regeneration. Exp Neurol 1997;147(1):159–171
110. Horner PJ, Power AE, Kempermann G, et al. Proliferation and differentiation of progenitor cells throughout the intact adult rat spinal cord. J Neurosci 2000;20(6):2218–2228
111. Johansson CB, Momma S, Clarke DL, Risling M, Lendahl U, Frisén J. Identification of a neural stem cell in the adult mammalian central nervous system. Cell 1999;96(1):25–34
112. Weiss S, Dunne C, Hewson J, et al. Multipotent CNS stem cells are present in the adult mammalian spinal cord and ventricular neuroaxis. J Neurosci 1996;16(23):7599–7609
113. Yamamoto S, Yamamoto N, Kitamura T, Nakamura K, Nakafuku M. Proliferation of parenchymal neural progenitors in response to injury in the adult rat spinal cord. Exp Neurol 2001;172(1): 115–127
114. McTigue DM, Wei P, Stokes BT. Proliferation of NG2-positive cells and altered oligodendrocyte numbers in the contused rat spinal cord. J Neurosci 2001;21(10):3392–3400
115. Sellers DL, Maris DO, Horner PJ. Postinjury niches induce temporal shifts in progenitor fates to direct lesion repair after spinal cord injury. J Neurosci 2009;29(20):6722–6733
116. Takahashi M, Arai Y, Kurosawa H, Sueyoshi N, Shirai S. Ependymal cell reactions in spinal cord segments after compression injury in adult rat. J Neuropathol Exp Neurol 2003;62(2):185–194
117. Mothe AJ, Tator CH. Proliferation, migration, and differentiation of endogenous ependymal region stem/progenitor cells following minimal spinal cord injury in the adult rat. Neuroscience 2005;131(1):177–187
118. Hill CE, Beattie MS, Bresnahan JC. Degeneration and sprouting of identified descending supraspinal axons after contusive spinal cord injury in the rat. Exp Neurol 2001;171(1):153–169
119. Hayes KC, Kakulas BA. Neuropathology of human spinal cord injury sustained in sports-related activities. J Neurotrauma 1997;14(4):235–248
120. Kakulas BA. Pathology of spinal injuries. Cent Nerv Syst Trauma 1984;1(2):117–129
121. Backe HA, Betz RR, Mesgarzadeh M, Beck T, Clancy M. Post-traumatic spinal cord cysts evaluated by magnetic resonance imaging. Paraplegia 1991;29(9):607–612
122. Williams B. Pathogenesis of post-traumatic syringomyelia. Br J Neurosurg 1992;6(6):517–520
123. Wang D, Bodley R, Sett P, Gardner B, Frankel H. A clinical magnetic resonance imaging study of the traumatised spinal cord more than 20 years following injury. Paraplegia 1996;34(2):65–81
124. Klekamp J, Batzdorf U, Samii M, Bothe HW. Treatment of syringomyelia associated with arachnoid scarring caused by arachnoiditis or trauma. J Neurosurg 1997;86(2):233–240
125. Edgar R, Quail P. Progressive post-traumatic cystic and non-cystic myelopathy. Br J Neurosurg 1994;8(1):7–22
126. Rossier AB, Foo D, Shillito J, Dyro FM. Posttraumatic cervical syringomyelia. Incidence, clinical presentation, electrophysiological studies, syrinx protein and results of conservative and operative treatment. Brain 1985;108(Pt 2):439–461
127. Schurch B, Wichmann W, Rossier AB. Post-traumatic syringomyelia (cystic myelopathy): a prospective study of 449 patients with spinal cord injury. J Neurol Neurosurg Psychiatry 1996;60(1):61–67
128. Stoodley MA. Pathophysiology of syringomyelia. J Neurosurg 2000;92(6):1069–1070; author reply 1071–1073
129. Schwartz ED, Falcone SF, Quencer RM, Green BA. Posttraumatic syringomyelia: pathogenesis, imaging, and treatment. AJR Am J Roentgenol 1999;173(2):487–492

130. Bruce JC, Oatway MA, Weaver LC. Chronic pain after clip-compression injury of the rat spinal cord. Exp Neurol 2002;178(1):33–48

131. Siddall PJ, Taylor DA, McClelland JM, Rutkowski SB, Cousins MJ. Pain report and the relationship of pain to physical factors in the first 6 months following spinal cord injury. Pain 1999;81(1-2):187–197

132. Finnerup NB, Johannesen IL, Sindrup SH, Bach FW, Jensen TS. Pain and dysesthesia in patients with spinal cord injury: a postal survey. Spinal Cord 2001;39(5):256–262

133. Werhagen L, Budh CN, Hultling C, Molander C. Neuropathic pain after traumatic spinal cord injury—relations to gender, spinal level, completeness, and age at the time of injury. Spinal Cord 2004;42(12):665–673

134. Hulsebosch CE, Hains BC, Crown ED, Carlton SM. Mechanisms of chronic central neuropathic pain after spinal cord injury. Brain Res Brain Res Rev 2009;60(1):202–213

135. Detloff MR, Fisher LC, McGaughy V, Longbrake EE, Popovich PG, Basso DM. Remote activation of microglia and pro-inflammatory cytokines predict the onset and severity of below-level neuropathic pain after spinal cord injury in rats. Exp Neurol 2008;212(2):337–347

136. Gwak YS, Hulsebosch CE. Remote astrocytic and microglial activation modulates neuronal hyperexcitability and below-level neuropathic pain after spinal injury in rat. Neuroscience 2009;161(3):895–903

137. Bao F, Chen Y, Schneider KA, Weaver LC. An integrin inhibiting molecule decreases oxidative damage and improves neurological function after spinal cord injury. Exp Neurol 2008;214(2):160–167

138. Gwak YS, Crown ED, Unabia GC, Hulsebosch CE. Propentofylline attenuates allodynia, glial activation and modulates GABAergic tone after spinal cord injury in the rat. Pain 2008;138(2):410–422

5

Epidemiology of Traumatic Spinal Cord Injury

Yuying Chen

Key Points

1. The epidemiological statistics relating to spinal cord injury (SCI) are bittersweet: relatively low incidence, young age of most victims, typically with lifelong disability, high costs of health care, yet mostly preventable.
2. This chapter reviews the basic facts and figures about SCI, including incidence, prevalence, life expectancy, etiologic risk factors, neurological deficits, associated injuries, and trends over time in the United States.
3. It is hoped that the prevention and control of SCI as well as the planning and coordination of SCI care and services over a patient's lifetime will be significantly improved through a better understanding of SCI epidemiology.

Spinal cord injury (SCI), typically defined as an acute traumatic lesion of the spinal cord resulting in any degree of sensory/motor deficit or bladder/bowel dysfunction temporarily or permanently,[1] accounts for only a small proportion of all injuries; but the associated disabilities and life changes render SCI one of the most catastrophic injuries. Because disabilities are typically permanent, yet many SCIs are potentially preventable, understanding the epidemiological profile of SCI is essential for injury prevention and control and also for strategic planning of clinical and supportive SCI services throughout the region and country. This chapter uses data from the statewide population-based surveillance systems in the United States, the National SCI Statistical Center (NSCISC), and several population-based studies to summarize the quantitative and qualitative features of SCI.

Incidence

To better estimate the impact of SCI, beginning in the early 1980s, many US states established a population-based surveillance system and mandated by law the reporting of new cases of SCI to state health departments.[1] Hospitals were the primary sources of information, but some states also required reporting from public/private health and social agencies, physicians, emergency medical services staff, and chief medical examiners. Based on reports published by the state SCI registries[2–13] and previous incidence studies at the regional[14–17] and national levels,[18–20] the annual incidence of SCI in the United States varies from 25 new cases per million population in West Virginia from 1985 to 1988[2] to 83 new cases per million population in Alaska from 1991 to 1993.[13] Taking all estimates together, excluding those who die at the scene of the accident, the average is ~40 new SCI cases per million population per year. Given the current size of the US population, this totals ~12,000 new SCIs each year. The incidence of prehospital SCI deaths has been estimated by several studies,[11,12,16,17] ranging from four cases per million in Utah from 1989 to 1991 to 21 cases per million in Northern California from 1970 to 1971.

Risk Factors for Spinal Cord Injury

The incidence of SCI is typically reported to be lowest for the pediatric group and highest for persons in their late teens and twenties and declines consistently thereafter; this is supported by virtually all previous incidence studies. SCI occurs predominantly among men across all age groups. The male to female incidence rate ratio is about 4:1 and varies by age.[2,8,10–12] The incidence rates are higher for blacks than for whites, especially among men and for violence-related SCI. The whites to blacks incidence rate ratio is 1.4:2.0 overall[8,10,11,14,17,18] but is 6.3:17.8 for SCI with violence-related etiology.[5,8,10,11] Using the state of Mississippi as an example, the relative incidence of SCI between male and female, between blacks and whites, and across age groups is depicted in **Fig. 5.1**.[11]

Approximately 22 to 50% of new SCI cases report alcohol use or test positive for blood alcohol at the time of injury.[2,8,10–14,20,21] The association with alcohol consumption is particularly common among Native Americans, with injuries occurring between 10 pm and 4 am, pedestrian injuries, and cervical injuries.[10,13,21] SCI occurs most frequently on weekends, accounting for ~55% of total injuries.[8,22] The incidence of SCI also increases during the warm weather months, with 38 to 44% of total injuries occurring during May through August,[8,22] which is largely attributable to higher frequencies of diving and other recreational sport mishaps in summer.

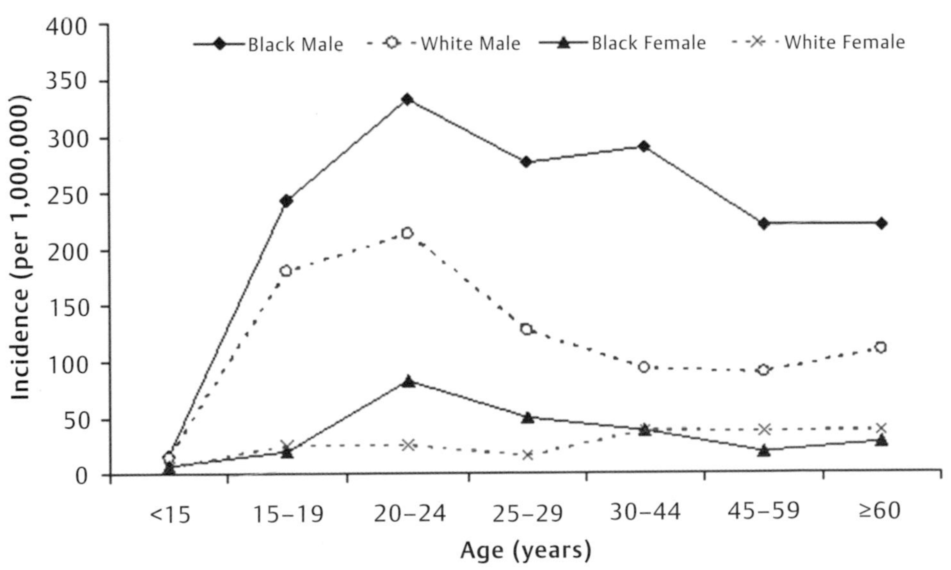

Fig. 5.1 Annual incidence rate (per million population) of spinal cord injury in Mississippi, United States 1992–1994.[11]

External Causes of Injury

External causes of SCI are often grouped into five categories: motor vehicle crashes, violence, sports/recreational activities, falls, and all other causes. Vehicular crashes, predominantly automobile crashes, are the leading cause of SCI in all US states and across sexes and racial groups except blacks, for whom violence is also a common cause. For example, in the state of Oklahoma, the annual incidence of SCI from violence is the same as that from vehicular crashes in the black population—21 new cases per million. Approximately 74% of violence-related SCIs are due to gunshot wounds.[10] Falls are typically the next leading cause of injury, followed by sports/recreational activities. Approximately 72% of falls are attributable to falls from a height, whereas diving mishaps account for ~46 to 75% of SCIs due to recreational sports.[8,10,22] Acts of violence are usually reported as the fourth leading grouped etiology of SCI among whites.

The injury etiology also varies by age groups.[8,10,23] The recreational sport mishaps are common among persons younger than 15 years of age, whereas falls rank first among persons older than age 65 years. The activity that has a high frequency as a cause of injury may suggest being risky to a specific group, but also could be attributable to a relatively high participation rate of such an activity among this specific group.

International Variation

Work in understanding the global epidemiology of SCI has been prolific. Foremost in this work is the recent establishment of a living data repository structure by the International Spinal Cord Society to allow documentation and mapping of SCI statistics around the world[24] (http://www.iscos.org.uk/page.php?content=57). For example, the incidence rate is noted to be more than twice as high in North America than in Australia (15 per million) and western Europe (16 per million). The external cause of injury also varies by countries and regions (**Fig. 5.2**). The international variation could be explained, to a large extent,

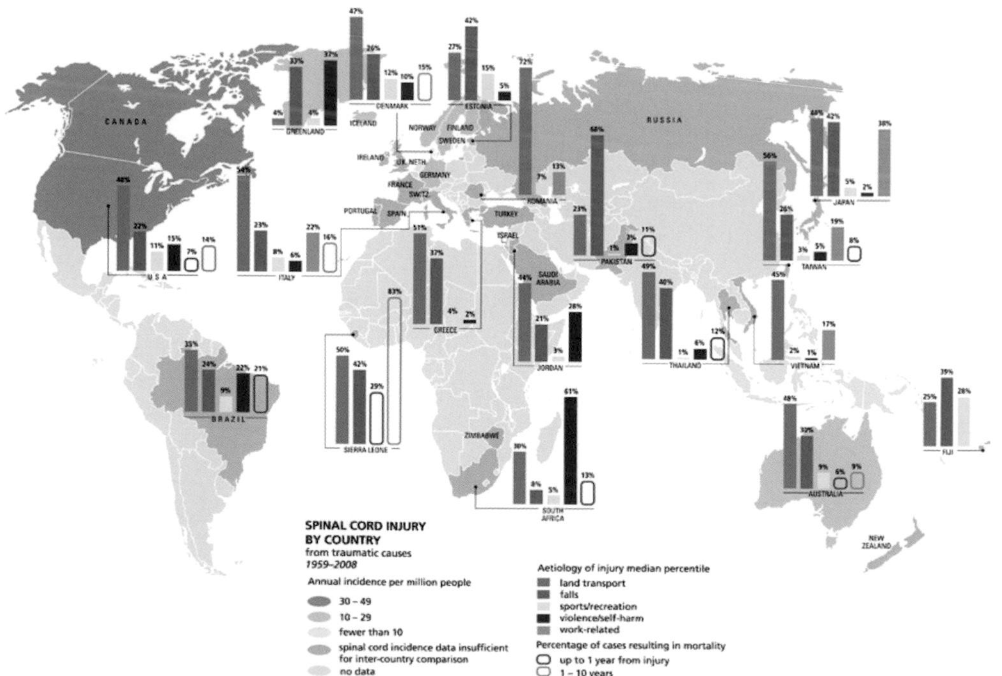

Fig. 5.2 Global mapping of spinal cord injury from traumatic causes by country 1959–2008. (From Cripps RA, Lee BB, Wing P, Weerts E, Mackay J, Brown D. A global map for traumatic spinal cord injury epidemiology: towards a living data repository for injury prevention. Spinal Cord 2011;49:493–501. Reprinted with permission.)

by the differences in underlying population characteristics (age, race, sex) and external factors (urbanization, road condition, policy measures, such as implementation of seat-belt restraint laws, etc.). It can also be attributable to the differences in reporting procedures, case definition, and completeness of case ascertainment.

Trends

There have not been any population-based incidence studies of SCI in the United States since the early 1990s. It is not clear whether the incidence has changed in recent years. Data from the SCI Model System, however, provide insight into the relative contribution of each factor to the occurrence of SCI over time. The regional SCI Model System program was established in the early 1970s with funding from what is now the National Institute on Disability and Rehabilitation Research. All Model System centers are required to collect and submit data on their patients to a national database managed by the NSCISC.[24] As of April 2009, this database contains data from 26 SCI Model System centers on 37,489 patients injured between 1973 and 2009.

Analyzing data from the NSCISC database, we observed a steady increase in age at injury over time, from an average of 28.9 years in 1973 to 1979 to 38.1 in 2000 to 2009 (**Table 5.1**). The percentage of individuals who are age 65 or older has also increased from 3.1% to 8.8% during the same period. The male to female ratio changed from 4.5 in 1973 to 1979 to 3.7 in 2000 to 2009. Moreover, a substantial trend has

Table 5.1 Demographic and Injury Profile of New Injuries: Trends over 35 Years

	Year of injury			
Characteristics	**1973–1979**	**1980–1989**	**1990–1999**	**2000–2009**
Total SCI cases	4563	10,271	12,585	10,070
Age at injury				
Mean (years)	28.9	31.5	35.3	38.1
% ≥ 65 years	3.1	4.9	7.8	8.8
Sex: % female	18.2	17.6	19.8	21.2
Race/ethnicity (%)				
Non-Hispanic Whites	76.8	68.2	59.8	64.7
Non-Hispanic Blacks	14.2	20.4	24.3	20.0
Hispanic origin	6.0	8.4	12.3	11.9
Other	3.0	3.0	3.6	3.4
Grouped etiology (%)				
Vehicular crashes	46.9	44.4	40.8	46.5
Falls	16.5	18.5	20.6	24.0
Violence	13.3	16.9	21.8	12.2
Sports	14.3	12.3	8.5	9.5
Other	9.0	7.9	8.3	7.8
Neurological impairment (%)				
Tetraplegia, complete	25.6	21.8	24.6	22.2
Tetraplegia, incomplete	28.5	32.8	29.5	35.6
Paraplegia, complete	28.1	25.0	26.8	24.6
Paraplegia, incomplete	17.8	20.4	19.1	17.6

also been observed in the racial/ethnic distribution of persons enrolled in the NSCISC database over time, the percentage of persons of Hispanic origin increasing from 6.0% to 11.9% over the last 3 decades.

The observed trend in the demographic profile of new SCI cases seems to reflect the changes in the general US population (i.e., advancing age and increasing racial/ethnic diversity), but could also be attributable to periodic changes in the identities and locations of participating SCI Model System centers, changes in referral patterns to Model System centers, and changes in eligibility criteria for inclusion in the NSCISC database. The increase or decrease of underlying age-, sex-, and race-specific incidence rates over the last few decades is also possible.

Vehicular crashes have consistently been the leading cause of injury among persons who are enrolled in the NSCISC database (**Table 5.1**). The percentage of SCIs from falls has increased steadily over time, from 16.5% during 1973 to 1979 to 24.0% in 2000 to 2009. The percentage of violent etiology increased substantially between 1973 and 1999, but significantly dropped in 2000 and after. Sporting injuries continuously declined for ~25 years and were steady over the past 10 years. The proportional nature of these statistics can only reflect the relative importance of the contribution of these external factors to the causation of SCI but cannot present the underlying changes in the cause-specific incidence over time. Population-based studies are needed to further understand these trends in external causes of injury and also in the demographic profile of SCI.

Level and Completeness of Injury

The level of SCI as classified by the International Standards for Neurological Classification of Spinal Cord Injury,[25] is mostly at the cervical level among persons in the NSCISC database (53.2%), followed by thoracic (35.6%) and lumbosacral levels (11.2%). The most common segment is C5 (15.4%) and C4 (14.4%), followed by C6 (10.9%), T12 (6.7%), C7 (5.4%), and L1 (5.1%).[26] At the time of discharge from inpatient rehabilitation, 47.5% of persons have neurologically complete injuries according to the American Spinal Injury Association (ASIA) Impairment Scale (AIS A), 10.7% have incomplete injuries with sensory sparing (AIS B), 12.0% have incomplete injuries with nonfunctional motor capabilities below the lesion level (AIS C), 29.1% had incomplete injuries with functional motor capabilities below the lesion level (AIS D), and 0.7% had essentially complete neurological recovery (AIS E).[26]

External causes of injury play a meaningful role in determining the preserved neurological function.[8,23,26] Approximately three quarters of violence-related SCIs result in paraplegia, with 1.5 times more complete injuries than incomplete injuries (42.5% vs 25.6%).[23] In contrast, up to 88.0% of recreational sports-related SCIs result in tetraplegia with an almost identical frequency of complete and incomplete injuries (43.5% vs 44.5%). Vehicular crashes and falls usually result in tetraplegia, 54.9% and 57.7%, respectively, and incomplete tetraplegia is slightly more common in falls than in vehicular crashes (37.2% vs 32.3%).[23]

There seems to be a trend toward increased likelihood of an incomplete cervical injury over the last 3 decades (**Table 5.1**). As the frequency of violence-related SCI decreases, the percentage of paraplegia seems to decrease over the past 20 years.

Life Expectancy

Life expectancy of persons with SCI has improved significantly during the past few decades but remains below normal.[27] The NSCISC data show that the overall mortality is ~4.5% during the first year of injury, 2.1% at postinjury year 2, and 1.3 to 2.5% per year thereafter.[26] The median life expectancy is ~33 years after injury but varies considerably by level and completeness of injury, status of ventilator use, age, sex, and other factors.[27,28] The recent estimates of life expectancy from the NSCISC databases are depicted by age at injury, ventilator dependency, and level and completeness of injury in **Table 5.2**.

Prevalence

Prevalence reflects the number of persons with an SCI who are currently alive, which is primarily a function of incidence (number of new cases each year) and mortality (number of deceased cases each year). The prevalence of SCI has been estimated by studies that were based on the mathematical relationship of incidence, survival, and prevalence[29,30]; extrapolated data from a regional disability survey[31]; data from the National Health Interview Survey[32]; and involved a nationwide probability sample of small geographic areas and institutions.[33] The reported prevalence ranges from 525 cases per million population in 1975 to 1124 cases per million population in 1981. Utilizing a complex mathematical model including age-sex-specific incidence, survival, and baseline prevalence, a recent study estimated ~250,000 persons living with SCI in 2004 in the United States and projects an increase to 270,000 persons in 2014 due to improved life expectancy.[34]

Demographic Profile of Prevalent Cases

The average age of all persons living with SCI using this calculation, including new and existing cases, in the United States has been estimated to be 41 years in 1988, which is ~10 years older than the average age among new cases in the NSCISC database during the same period. In the report published by Berkowitz et al. in 1988, 5.4% of those with SCIs were below age 25, 54.2% were aged between age 25 and 44, 27.8% between age 45 and 64, and 12% were aged 65 or older.[35] Because women usually have a longer life expectancy than men, the male to female prevalence ratio is typically lower than that observed among new SCI cases (2.6 vs 4.0). The white to nonwhite ratio among persons with SCI who were alive in 1988 was 1.5, similar to the ratio among new cases.[35]

Table 5.2 Life Expectancy (Years) for Persons with Spinal Cord Injury

		Life expectancy (years)				
		Non–ventilator dependent				Ventilator dependent
		AIS D	AIS A, B, or C			
Age at injury (years)	2004 US population	Any level	Paraplegia	C5–8	C1–4	Any level
10	68.5	62.2	54.2	48.9	44.2	25.2
20	58.8	52.6	44.8	39.8	35.3	18.1
30	49.3	43.3	36.1	31.4	27.5	13.3
40	39.9	34.1	27.3	23.1	19.6	8.0
50	30.9	25.5	19.5	15.9	13.0	4.2
60	22.5	17.7	12.7	9.8	7.6	1.8
70	15.1	11.2	7.3	5.3	3.8	0.3
80	9.1	6.0	3.4	2.2	1.3	<0.1

Among those surviving the first 24 hours of injury.
Abbreviations: AIS, American Spinal Injury Association Impairment Scale.

Associated Injuries

SCI is often accompanied by other injuries that significantly impact clinical management decision making and treatment outcomes.[36] The following severe injuries that occur at the same time as SCI are recommended by the International SCI Standards and Data Sets to be documented in any clinical and research database: (1) moderate to severe traumatic brain injury (TBI; Glasgow Coma Scale ≤ 12), (2) extraspinal fractures requiring surgery, (3) severe facial injuries affecting sense organs, (4) major chest injury requiring chest tube or mechanical ventilation, (5) traumatic amputations of an arm or leg (or injuries severe enough to require surgical amputation), (6) severe hemorrhage, and (7) damage to any internal organ requiring surgery.[37] Among persons enrolled in the NSCISC database between 2006 and 2009, 42.7% had one or more of the aforementioned injuries at the same time as SCI. The presence of these injuries was particularly common among persons injured from violence (61.8%) and motor vehicle crashes (50.8%). Conversely, among persons injured in recreational sports mishaps and falls, 26.6% and 29.1%, respectively, had one or more of these injuries associated with SCI.

There have been detailed investigations of the incidence and risk factors of extraspinal fractures and TBI associated with acute SCI.[38–40] Overall, extraspinal fractures occurred in 28% of all new SCIs, with rib/sternum fractures most common, followed by upper extremity, lower extremity, and skull fractures. These extraspinal fractures were most common among SCIs caused by motor vehicle crashes and among persons with thoracic and lumbosacral injuries. In a hospital-based sample of 198 persons with SCI, 60% had a co-occurring TBI (34% mild, 10% mild complicated, 6% moderate, and 10% severe). The presence of TBI was most common among SCIs from motor vehicle crashes and falls and among persons with cervical injuries.

Conclusion

Taking all previously reported statistics together, the overall annual incidence of SCI is ~40 cases per million population in the United States or ~12,000 new cases each year. The number of people in the United States who are alive and have SCI is estimated to be ~250,000 in 2004 and 270,000 in 2014. Life expectancy of persons with SCI has improved significantly during the past few decades but remains below normal.

The risk of SCI is generally higher for persons of age 15 to 24 years, males, and blacks. The external cause of SCI varies by age groups, race/ethnicity, and sex. Overall, motor vehicle crashes are the leading cause of injury. Violent etiology is also common among black males. Falls rank first among persons older than age 65 years, whereas recreational sport mishaps are more common among individuals of age 15 years or younger.

External causes of injury have a major effect on the level and extent of the preserved neurological function and also the presence of other severe injuries. With knowledge of the epidemiology of SCI, spinal injuries can potentially be prevented through strategic planning and policy measures. The clinical and other lifelong supportive services of persons with SCI can also be better organized and coordinated.

Pearls

- The prevention of SCI must be multifaceted, accounting for the variation in causes associated with age, race, and sex. For example, in the United States, prevention programs targeting blacks must address violence issues, whereas those targeting Native Americans should focus on issues related to alcohol and vehicular crashes. Prevention programs for older adolescents and young adults should target motor vehicle crashes and risk-taking behaviors such as diving, whereas prevention programs for older adults should target falls.
- The latest trends in the demographic profile of new injuries reveal an increase in age at injury, percentage of individuals of Hispanic origin, and percentage of women, which strongly suggest the needs for clinical staff diversification and cultural competency training and also expertise in gerontology, geriatrics, and women's health.

Pitfalls

- There have not been any population-based incidence studies of SCI in the United States since the 1990s. As a result, it is not known whether the number of new injuries every year has increased, decreased, or remained the same in recent years.
- It is challenging to compare the facts and figures of SCI among studies, particularly across different countries, because of the variation in case definition, categorization of etiologic factors, and other methodological parameters. As a result, artificial differences may be observed or real differences missed.

References

1. Harrison CL, Dijkers M. Spinal cord injury surveillance in the United States: an overview. Paraplegia 1991;29(4):233–246
2. Woodruff BA, Baron RC. A description of nonfatal spinal cord injury using a hospital-based registry. Am J Prev Med 1994;10(1):10–14
3. Colorado Department of Public Health and Environment, Disease Control and Environmental Epidemiology Division. 1996 Annual Report of the Traumatic Spinal Cord Injury Early Notification System. Denver: Colorado Department of Transportation Printing Office; 1997
4. Relethford JH, Standfast SJ, Morse DL; Centers for Disease Control (CDC). Trends in traumatic spinal cord injury—New York, 1982-1988. MMWR Morb Mortal Wkly Rep 1991;40(31):535–537, 543
5. Bayakly AR, Lawrence DW. Spinal Cord Injury in Louisiana 1991 Annual Report. New Orleans: Louisiana Office of Public Health; 1992
6. Virginia Department of Rehabilitation Services. Spinal Cord Injury in Virginia: A Statistical Fact Sheet. Fishersville: Virginia Spinal Cord Injury System; 1993
7. Johnson SC. Georgia Central Registry: Spinal Cord Disabilities and Traumatic Brain Injury. Warm Springs, GA: Roosevelt Warm Springs Institute for Rehabilitation; 1992
8. Acton PA, Farley T, Freni LW, Ilegbodu VA, Sniezek JE, Wohlleb JC. Traumatic spinal cord injury in Arkansas, 1980 to 1989. Arch Phys Med Rehabil 1993;74(10):1035–1040
9. Buechner JS, Speare MC, Fontes J. Hospitalizations for spinal cord injuries, 1994-1998. Med Health R I 2000;83(3):92–93
10. Price C, Makintubee S, Herndon W, Istre GR. Epidemiology of traumatic spinal cord injury and acute hospitalization and rehabilitation charges for spinal cord injuries in Oklahoma, 1988-1990. Am J Epidemiol 1994;139(1):37–47
11. Surkin J, Gilbert BJ, Harkey HL III, Sniezek J, Currier M. Spinal cord injury in Mississippi. Findings and evaluation, 1992-1994. Spine 2000;25(6):716–721
12. Thurman DJ, Burnett CL, Jeppson L, Beaudoin DE, Sniezek JE. Surveillance of spinal cord injuries in Utah, USA. Paraplegia 1994;32(10):665–669
13. Warren S, Moore M, Johnson MS. Traumatic head and spinal cord injuries in Alaska (1991-1993). Alaska Med 1995;37(1):11–19
14. Burke DA, Linden RD, Zhang YP, Maiste AC, Shields CB. Incidence rates and populations at risk for spinal cord injury: a regional study. Spinal Cord 2001;39(5):274–278
15. Clifton GL. Spinal cord injury in the Houston-Galveston area. Tex Med 1983;79(9):55–57
16. Griffin MR, Opitz JL, Kurland LT, Ebersold MJ, O'Fallon WM. Traumatic spinal cord injury in Olmsted County, Minnesota, 1935-1981. Am J Epidemiol 1985;121(6):884–895
17. Kraus JF, Franti CE, Riggins RS, Richards D, Borhani NO. Incidence of traumatic spinal cord lesions. J Chronic Dis 1975;28(9):471–492

18. Bracken MB, Freeman DH Jr, Hellenbrand K. Incidence of acute traumatic hospitalized spinal cord injury in the United States, 1970-1977. Am J Epidemiol 1981;113(6):615–622
19. Kalsbeek WD, McLaurin RL, Harris BS III, Miller JD. The National Head and Spinal Cord Injury Survey: major findings. J Neurosurg 1980;(Suppl): S19–S31
20. Vitale MG, Goss JM, Matsumoto H, Roye DP Jr. Epidemiology of pediatric spinal cord injury in the United States: years 1997 and 2000. J Pediatr Orthop 2006;26(6):745–749
21. Garrison A, Clifford K, Gleason SF, Tun CG, Brown R, Garshick E. Alcohol use associated with cervical spinal cord injury. J Spinal Cord Med 2004; 27(2):111–115
22. Nobunaga AI, Go BK, Karunas RB. Recent demographic and injury trends in people served by the Model Spinal Cord Injury Care Systems. Arch Phys Med Rehabil 1999;80(11):1372–1382
23. Jackson AB, Dijkers M, Devivo MJ, Poczatek RB. A demographic profile of new traumatic spinal cord injuries: change and stability over 30 years. Arch Phys Med Rehabil 2004;85(11):1740–1748
24. Stover SL, DeVivo MJ, Go BK. History, implementation, and current status of the National Spinal Cord Injury Database. Arch Phys Med Rehabil 1999;80(11):1365–1371
25. Marino RJ, Barros T, Biering-Sorensen F, et al; ASIA Neurological Standards Committee 2002. International standards for neurological classification of spinal cord injury. J Spinal Cord Med 2003;26(Suppl 1):S50–S56
26. National Spinal Cord Injury Statistical Center. 2008 Annual Report for the Spinal Cord Injury Model Systems. Birmingham, AL: National Spinal Cord Injury Statistical Center; 2009
27. DeVivo MJ, Krause JS, Lammertse DP. Recent trends in mortality and causes of death among persons with spinal cord injury. Arch Phys Med Rehabil 1999;80(11):1411–1419
28. Krause JS, Devivo MJ, Jackson AB. Health status, community integration, and economic risk factors for mortality after spinal cord injury. Arch Phys Med Rehabil 2004;85(11):1764–1773
29. DeVivo MJ, Fine PR, Maetz HM, Stover SL. Prevalence of spinal cord injury: a reestimation employing life table techniques. Arch Neurol 1980; 37(11):707–708
30. Kurtzke JF. Epidemiology of spinal cord injury. Exp Neurol 1975;48(3 pt. 2):163–236
31. Ergas Z. Spinal cord injury in the United States: a statistical update. Cent Nerv Syst Trauma 1985;2(1):19–32
32. Collins JG. Types of injuries and impairments due to injuries. Vital Health Stat 10 1986;(159): 87–1587
33. Harvey C, Rothschild BB, Asmann AJ, Stripling T. New estimates of traumatic SCI prevalence: a survey-based approach. Paraplegia 1990;28(9): 537–544
34. Lasfargues JE, Custis D, Morrone F, Carswell J, Nguyen T. A model for estimating spinal cord injury prevalence in the United States. Paraplegia 1995;33(2):62–68
35. Berkowitz M, Harvey C, Greene C, Wilson SE. The Economic Consequences of Traumatic Spinal Cord Injury. New York, NY: Demos; 1992
36. Fine PR, Stover SL, DeVivo MJ. A methodology for predicting lengths of stay for spinal cord injury patients. Inquiry 1987;24(2):147–156
37. DeVivo M, Biering-Sørensen F, Charlifue S, et al; Executive Committee for the International SCI Data Sets Committees. International Spinal Cord Injury Core Data Set. Spinal Cord 2006;44(9): 535–540
38. Chen Y, DeVivo MJ. Epidemiology of extraspinal fractures in acute spinal cord injury: data from the model spinal cord injury care systems 1973–1999. Top Spinal Cord Inj Rehabil 2005; 11:18–29
39. Macciocchi S, Seel RT, Thompson N, Byams R, Bowman B. Spinal cord injury and co-occurring traumatic brain injury: assessment and incidence. Arch Phys Med Rehabil 2008;89(7): 1350–1357
40. Wang CM, Chen Y, DeVivo MJ, Huang CT. Epidemiology of extraspinal fractures associated with acute spinal cord injury. Spinal Cord 2001; 39(11):589–594

6

Spinal Cord Injury Classification

Sonia Teufack, James S. Harrop, and Ashwini D. Sharan

Key Points

1. The outcome of SCI greatly correlates with the extent of neurological injury and initial functional impairment.
2. The simplest and most useful method of classification of acute SCI is into complete and incomplete injuries. The ASIA classification is the most widely used international system to document sensory and motor impairment following SCI.
3. The ZPP applies to complete SCI or ASIA A and refers to all segments below the neurological level of injury with some preservation of motor or sensory function. Over time, some patients may spontaneously recover functional motor strength within the ZPP.

Spinal cord injuries (SCIs) constitute a major source of social and economic burden to our society. Every year, more than 12,000 Americans suffer an SCI as a direct result of trauma.[1] Over the past decades, significant progress has been made in the evaluation and management of patients with SCI; furthermore, most SCI clinicians and researchers maintain an investigative mindset that continuously fuels further improvement of SCI assessment and treatment.

The initial neurological evaluation of SCI patients is critical because it dictates the acute management and determines the long-term prognosis. It is crucial to identify the level as well as the completeness of an SCI. Based on the American Spinal Injury Association/International Medical Society of Paraplegia (ASIA/IMSOP) standards, the level of injury is defined as the most caudal level of normal motor and sensory function.[2] The simplest and most useful method of classification of acute SCI is into complete and incomplete injuries.

Because the outcome for SCI patients greatly correlates with the extent of neurological injury and initial functional impairment, it is important to have a reliable and reproducible method of classification of SCI. Several grading systems have been produced over the years.

History of Spinal Cord Injury Classification

First Classification System: Frankel Grade

Clinicians have used various scales to grade neurological deficits following SCI. In 1969, Frankel and colleagues[3] published the first classification system for acute SCI based on a study conducted in Stoke Mandeville Hospital over a period of 10 years. They retrospectively evaluated 682 SCI patients and designed a five-grade system based on the neurological function of these patients. Grade A designated patients with complete loss of motor and sensory function below the level of injury, including loss of sacral function. Grade B was for patients with complete loss of motor function but sensory preservation including sacral sparing. Grades C and D described patients who had retained some motor function; however, this motor function was judged useless in grade C as opposed to useful in grade D. Patients assigned to grade E had full neurological function. Following its publication, the Frankel scale was widely used; it was easily applicable and was uniquely based on gross motor and sensory evaluation of patients. However, it had significant limitations; for instance, it did not clearly segregate patients in groups C and D. The Frankel scale was also not sensitive enough to reflect significant motor function improvement of a patient into a better Frankel grade.[4,5] Several modifications of the Frankel scale were published in the following years, but they all lacked sensitivity.[6–9]

Evolution of Classification Systems

Since the establishment of the Frankel classification system, several others have followed. Bracken et al.[10] designed a grading system in 1978, based on a prospective study of 133 SCI patients at the Yale University School of Medicine. They segregated motor and sensory neurological deficits into a five-scale and a seven-scale system, respectively. The motor scale included the following categories: (1) antigravity movement in all myotomes, (2) and (3) trace contraction in some muscles of a myotome, (4) absence of contraction at or below the iliopsoas, (5) absent contraction in the first palmar interosseus or higher. The sensory scale was based on pinprick evaluation and listed seven categories: (1) normal, (2) some segments decreased, (3) some segments absent, (4) paraparesis, (5) quadriparesis, (6) paraplegia, and (7) quadriplegia. This scale demonstrated a strong correlation between changes in motor and sensory scores and patients' outcome at discharge. However, it had a significant flaw in that cross-classification of the motor and sensory scales showed a discrepancy. This system fell out of favor because it was difficult to memorize and perform at the bedside. It also failed to integrate motor and sensory exams and did not account for sacral function.

Lucas and Ducker[11] at the Maryland Institute for Emergency Medical Services also published a motor classification system in the late 1970s. They conducted a review of 436 SCI patients with a single-level vertebral trauma and proposed a classification based on the motor index initial (MIi). The MIi was defined as the sum of motor function for each muscle group tested, divided by the number of motor groups tested (up to 14). Motor function was graded 0 to 5, with 5 normal, 4 functional, 3 fair, 2 poor, 1 trace, and 0 absent. In their series, MIi was directly related to recovery rate. This classification system was never widely used, but it introduced a standardized method of motor examination that inspired subsequent grading scales.[8]

Several other classification systems were introduced in the early 1980s. Klose and colleagues[12] published the University of Miami Neuro-spinal Index (UMNI), which combined both sensory and motor scales. Motor function was recorded by testing 44 muscle groups. A score of 0 was given for no function, 1 for flicker of contraction, 2 for movement without gravity, 3 for movement against gravity, 4 for movement overcome by resistance, and 5 for normal power, for a total of 0 to 220 points. The sensory function was tested by evaluating pinprick and vibration on the right and left sides of the body at all 30 segments of the spinal cord. A score of 0 was given for absent sensation, 1 for present but abnormal, 2 for normal, for a total of 0 to 240 points. This classification was found useful because it had good interrater reliability and could be used to closely monitor patients' progression. However, it was cumbersome to perform and compute and did not evaluate sacral function.

In 1981, Chehrazi and colleagues[13] developed a classification scale also known as the Yale Scale. This scale was a composite of numerical motor and sensory scales and assessed the severity of SCI and prognosis for recovery. The motor scale was computed by averaging the strength of muscle groups below the injury level, graded 0 to 5 as described by the Royal Medical Research Council of Great Britain (**Table 6.1**). The sensory scale was the average of pinprick, position, and deep pain senses. Pinprick and position were graded 0 to 2 in dermatomes below the level of injury. Deep pain was assessed by compression of the Achilles tendon or toe, with 1 given for correct localization and 0 for no localization. A total of 0 to 10 points could be achieved, with 0 indicating complete absence of motor and sensory function and 10 intact motor and sensory function. This classification system had good reliability and was easily memorized and performed at the patient's bedside. However, like most previous scales, it failed to evaluate sacral function.

Table 6.1 Muscle Strength Grading Scale in Accordance with the British Medical Research Council System

Grade	Muscle strength
0	Complete paralysis
1	Flicker
2	Movement with gravity eliminated
3	Movement against gravity but no resistance
4	Movement against gravity and resistance
5	Full strength

American Spinal Injury Association/International Medical Society of Paraplegia Standards

In 1984, ASIA held a conference in Chicago to define standards for the neurological classification of SCI patients. The neurological assessment focused on the examination of 10 muscle groups, five in the upper extremities and five in the lower extremities, graded 0 to 5 points. Sensory evaluation was only recorded as the most cephalad level of normal sensation, and the Frankel classification was used to grade the functional status of patients. In 1989, the ASIA standards were revised to provide better sensory examination,[5] with the assessment of light touch and pinprick sensation. In 1991, Priebe and Waring[14] evaluated the interobserver reliability of the 1984 and 1989 ASIA grading systems. They found that the 1989 ASIA standards had greater accuracy, but they still had a less than optimal coefficient of reliability (k = 0.67).

In 1992, ASIA standards for the neurological classification of SCI patients were revised for a second time, in association with the IMSOP[15] (**Fig. 6.1** and **Table 6.2**).

Table 6.2 American Spinal Injury Association Impairment Scale

A	Complete: no motor or sensory function, including in sacral segments
B	Incomplete: Sensory but no motor function is preserved below the level of injury, including in sacral segments
C	Incomplete: motor function is preserved below the level of injury, and the majority of key muscles below the level of injury have a muscle grade <3/5
D	Incomplete: motor function is preserved below the level of injury, and the majority of key muscles below the level of injury have a muscle grade ≥3/5
E	Normal: motor and sensory functions are normal

Source: The American Spinal Injury Association: International Standards for Neurological Classification of Spinal Cord Injury, Reprint 2008. Chicago, IL. Reprinted with permission.

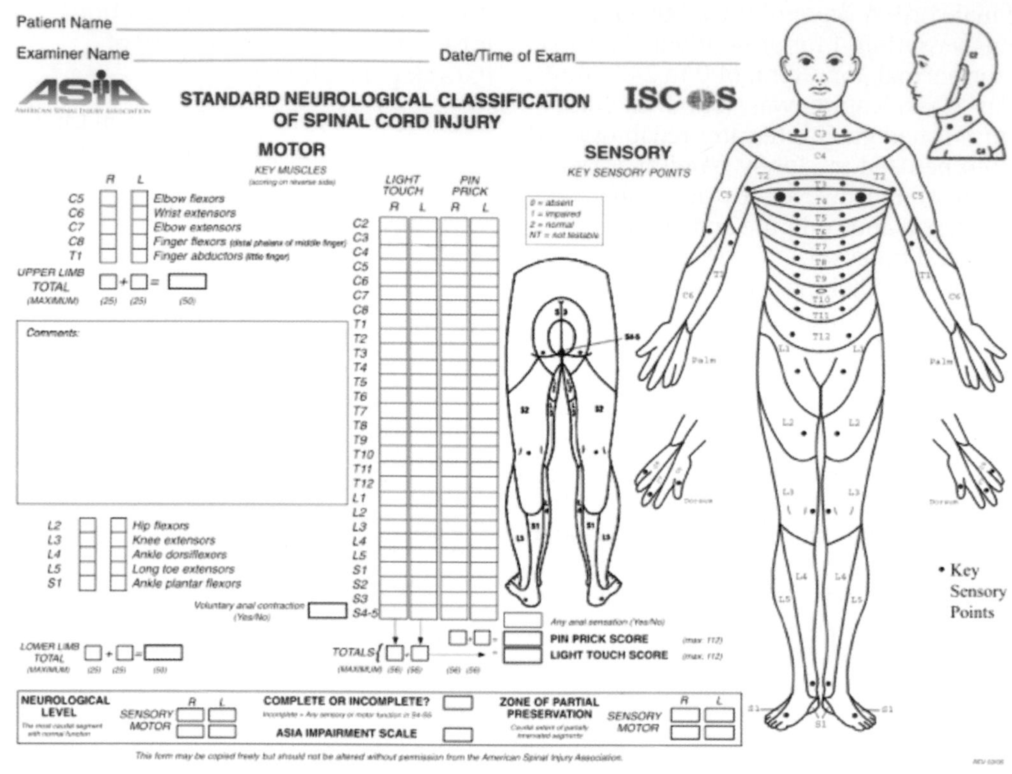

Patient Name ____________________

Examiner Name ____________________ Date/Time of Exam ____________________

ASIA — AMERICAN SPINAL INJURY ASSOCIATION

STANDARD NEUROLOGICAL CLASSIFICATION OF SPINAL CORD INJURY

ISCoS

MOTOR

KEY MUSCLES (scoring on reverse side)

	R	L	
C5			Elbow flexors
C6			Wrist extensors
C7			Elbow extensors
C8			Finger flexors (distal phalanx of middle finger)
T1			Finger abductors (little finger)
UPPER LIMB TOTAL (MAXIMUM)	(25)	(25)	= (50)

Comments:

	R	L	
L2			Hip flexors
L3			Knee extensors
L4			Ankle dorsiflexors
L5			Long toe extensors
S1			Ankle plantar flexors
LOWER LIMB TOTAL (MAXIMUM)	(25)	(25)	= (50)

Voluntary anal contraction (Yes/No)

	LIGHT TOUCH R	LIGHT TOUCH L	PIN PRICK R	PIN PRICK L
C2				
C3				
C4				
C5				
C6				
C7				
C8				
T1				
T2				
T3				
T4				
T5				
T6				
T7				
T8				
T9				
T10				
T11				
T12				
L1				
L2				
L3				
L4				
L5				
S1				
S2				
S3				
S4-5				
TOTALS (MAXIMUM)	(56)	(56)	(56)	(56)

SENSORY

KEY SENSORY POINTS

0 = absent
1 = impaired
2 = normal
NT = not testable

Any anal sensation (Yes/No)

PIN PRICK SCORE (max: 112)

LIGHT TOUCH SCORE (max: 112)

NEUROLOGICAL LEVEL — The most caudal segment with normal function — SENSORY R L — MOTOR R L

COMPLETE OR INCOMPLETE? — Incomplete = Any sensory or motor function in S4-S5

ASIA IMPAIRMENT SCALE

ZONE OF PARTIAL PRESERVATION — Caudal extent of partially innervated segments — SENSORY R L — MOTOR R L

This form may be copied freely but should not be altered without permission from the American Spinal Injury Association.

Fig. 6.1 American Spinal Injury Association Standard Neurological Classification of Spinal Cord Injury

In addition to the previous assessments of motor function, sensory level, and Frankel functional impairment, the new standards incorporated the Functional Independence Measure (FIM). The FIM was developed in an effort to provide a uniform appraisal of disability for SCI patients.[7,16] It evaluates patients' functional status based on their ability to perform activities of daily living, including self-care, control of bowel and bladder function, ambulation, as well as social interaction. The advantage of using the FIM over time is that it records socioeconomically meaningful improvements in the neurological function of SCI patients. Subsequent studies of the ASIA/IMSOP scale found that it provided a good discrimination in severity of SCI and predictability of outcome.[17,18] However, it was found to have weak interobserver reliability, principally for the grading of incomplete SCI.[19,20] Additional updates were made to the ASIA/IMSOP standards in 1996, with inclusion of the ASIA Impairment Scale, the ASIA Motor Index Score, the ASIA Sensory Scale, and the FIM. These updates further refined the assessment and classification of acute SCI and are widely recognized and used.

Functional and Anatomical Classification of Spinal Cord Injury

Level of Injury: Skeletal versus Neurological

The relationship and numbering or labeling of the osseous spinal column and the spinal cord parenchyma can be confusing. As humans develop from infancy to adulthood, the spinal column undergoes greater rostrocaudal growth than the spinal cord. This results in the distal spinal cord being stretched from the sacrum to approximately L1 osseous spinal column level. The spinal cord parenchymal level (neurologic level) then is displaced from its original osseous level. This can result in a patient having an osseous injury but a different neurologic level of injury. In the upper cervical area, spinal cord segments overlay the same number of vertebral bodies; however, as one progresses caudally to the thoracic area, spinal cord segments overlay vertebral bodies of one then two levels below. Ultimately, the T11 vertebral body corresponds to the L1 spinal cord segment, and the conus medullaris is located between L1 and L2 vertebral bodies. For example, a T11 burst fracture often results in a patient having a neurologic injury level of L1.

The skeletal level of injury refers to the level of maximal vertebral column damage on the radiograph. The neurological level of injury is the most caudal level at which motor and sensory functions are intact. Depending on the location of the injury, the skeletal level may correspond to the neurological level; however, it may also correspond to the neurological level one to two segments below. In the assessment of acute SCI, it is important to record a sensory level, which is the most caudal dermatome with 2/2 score for light touch and pinprick, as well as a motor level, which is the most caudal key muscle with a strength of 3 or above while the segment above is normal or 5/5, for the left and right side of the body independently.

Complete Spinal Cord Injury (ASIA A)

Patients suffering from a complete SCI have no preservation of motor and sensory function below the level of injury, including in the sacral segments. These patients are defined as ASIA A. Complete SCI above the C3 level can result in death from respiratory failure without immediate intervention with cardiopulmonary resuscitation (CPR). Patients with complete SCI can also develop loss of autonomic function and spinal shock. In addition, they can have bowel and bladder dysfunction with incontinence in the acute posttraumatic phase. At a later time they become hyperreflexic, and unlike incomplete SCI, very few patients with complete SCI will recover meaningful neurological function.[21,22]

Zone of Partial Preservation

The zone of partial preservation (ZPP) applies to complete SCI or ASIA A and refers to all segments below the neurological level of injury with some preservation of motor or sensory function. Most patients with complete SCI will have a ZPP of varying size a few segments below the neurological level. Over the period of time following the injury, some patients may spontaneously recover functional motor strength within the ZPP.

This concept becomes crucial in the evaluation of efficacy of treatment modalities for SCI patients, because a clear distinction should be made between spontaneous recovery within the ZPP and further neurological function improvement from medical interventions.[23]

Incomplete Spinal Cord Injury (ASIA B, C, D)

SCIs with any residual motor or sensory function more than three segments below the level of injury are considered incomplete. Signs of preserved long-tract function include sensation or voluntary movement in the lower extremities, sacral sparing with preserved perianal sensation, and voluntary rectal sphincter contraction. Patients with incomplete SCI can be classified in syndromes based on correlation of spinal cord anatomy and presenting symptoms.

Central Cord Syndrome

Central cord syndrome (CCS) is the most common type of incomplete SCI syndrome. Its occurrence is bimodal; in younger patients it may occur following severe high-energy, high-velocity spinal column trauma, as opposed to a more common incidence in the elderly after a forward fall or other minor hyperextension injuries.[24,25] CCS may occur whether or not the injury results in spinal column fracture or dislocation.[26,27] In elderly patients, this is often seen in patients with cervical stenosis secondary to cervical spondylosis resulting in reduced spinal canal diameter.

The pathognomonic physical finding of CCS is a disproportionate loss of motor function in the upper extremities compared with the lower extremities. More loss of distal extremity function is typically noted compared with proximal musculature strength because CCS in the cervical region usually results in severe hand paresis. Sensory deficits are variable; one of the early manifestations of CCS can be loss of pain and temperature sensation in a capelike pattern at the level of injury. This results from the damage of crossing spinothalamic fibers. Tactile sensation remains intact because posterior column fibers are preserved. In some cases, patients develop an acute or delayed hyperesthesia or allodynia in the proximal upper extremities.

There is no neuroanatomical evidence to explain the physical finding of disproportionate upper extremity weakness in CCS. Several theories have been hypothesized, one of which is that the centermost region of the spinal cord is more susceptible to injury from cord compression and edema,[28] and long tract fibers are arranged somatotopically, with upper extremity fibers central to lower extremity fibers. Evaluation of patients with CCS should include cervical spine x-ray and computed tomography (CT) to evaluate for canal stenosis, spondylosis, and fractures; cervical spine magnetic resonance imaging (MRI) to look for traumatic disk herniation, ligamentous injury, and cord edema or hematoma. Several studies have shown a correlation between the length of rostrocaudal edema and neurological deficit, as well as a gradual improvement of function with decreased cord edema over time.[29,30] The presence of spinal cord hematoma is associated with a worse prognosis.[31]

The best treatment method for CCS remains controversial. Current practice options published by the AANS and CNS include blood pressure augmentation for cord perfusion, early reduction of fracture dislocation injuries, and surgical decompression for persistent cord compression and deterioration of function.[32] Almost all patients with CCS will have some degree of neurological recovery. It usually starts in the lower extremities, followed by the bladder, proximal upper extremities, and finally fine hand movement which are most limited or absent.[33] Younger patients have a significantly higher recovery rate than older patients; 97% versus 41% recovery of ambulation, respectively.[25]

Brown-Séquard Syndrome

Brown-Séquard syndrome refers to spinal cord hemisection injury. The most common mechanism of literal cord hemisection is penetrating trauma by a missile or a knife wound. Other mechanisms of functional cord hemisection include radiation myelopathy and hemicord compression from a large herniated disc,[34,35] epidural hematoma/collection, tumor, or arteriovenous malformation.

The classical clinical presentation is ipsilateral motor paralysis from the injury to the descending corticospinal tract, and dissociated sensory loss with ipsilateral loss of proprioception and vibratory sense from injury to the ascending posterior column as well as contralateral loss of pain and temperature sensation one to two levels below the level of injury from damage to the crossing spinothalamic fibers. In addition, ipsilateral compromise of lateral columns can result in autonomic dysregulation with cutaneous hyperemia and anhydrosis. Over time, injury to the ipsilateral descending corticospinal fibers can result in spastic paralysis below the level of injury as well as hyperreflexia and Babinski response, with contralateral sparing. Lesions that cause Brown-Séquard syndrome can also injure anterior horn cells and associated nerve roots; in these instances, patients can develop flaccid paralysis, hyporeflexia, and muscle atrophy as well as anesthesia and analgesia in the corresponding segments.

Of all incomplete SCIs, Brown-Séquard syndrome has the best prognosis.[36] Approximately 90% of patients will recover functional motor strength and will be able to ambulate independently.[37]

Anterior Cord Syndrome

Anterior cord syndrome (ACS) is also known as anterior spinal artery syndrome and is thought to result from spinal cord ischemia in the territory supplied by the anterior spinal artery. ACS is the second most common type of incomplete SCI. The mechanisms of injury are thought to be anterior spinal artery occlusion versus direct anterior cord compression from a traumatic herniated disk[38] or dislodged bone fragments in cervical flexion and extension injuries.

The clinical presentation is paraplegia or tetraplegia for injuries higher than C7, from damage to the descending corticospinal, rubrospinal, and vestibulospinal tracts. Sensory deficits are dissociated, with bilateral loss of pain and temperature sensations from injury to the spinothalamic fibers but preservation of proprioception and vibratory senses from intact posterior column below the level of injury.

During the evaluation of ACS, it is essential to determine whether it results from anterior spinal artery occlusion or direct anterior cord compression because the latter may require surgical decompression. Patients should be promptly evaluated with x-ray, CT, MRI, or myelography as needed. Patients with ACS have the worst prognosis for recovery of neurological function and require longer periods of rehabilitation.[36]

Posterior Cord Syndrome

Posterior cord syndrome (PCS) is a rare type of incomplete SCI; in its pure form it is characterized by selective injury to the posterior column. Traumatic PCS could be attributed to an expanding extradural lesion overlying the posterior cervical canal or the ligamentum flavum buckling in the setting of cervical spondylosis. However, during the initial evaluation of pure PCS, the differential diagnosis should also include tabes dorsalis and demyelinating diseases, such as multiple sclerosis.

Patients present with characteristic loss of proprioception and vibratory sense distal to the level of injury, sometimes accompanied by pain and burning paresthesias. Often, patients will develop sensory ataxia and loss of balance during a Romberg maneuver that will increase with eye closure.

Conus Medullaris Syndrome

The spinal cord terminates into a tapered end, the conus medullaris, most commonly at the L1 vertebral body or L1-2 disk interspace level in adults.[39] This section of the spinal cord contains the lumbar and sacral nerve root segments and is prone to injury because it is located at the transition point between the relatively fixed thoracic spine and the more flexible lumbar spine.[40]

Injuries to the conus medullaris from disk herniation or fracture usually result in a symmetrical pattern of upper and lower motor neuron dysfunction. In the acute phase, symptoms can include bilateral flaccid lower extremity paralysis, saddle anesthesia, loss of rectal tone and volition, and urinary retention. Over time, patients may develop muscular atrophy or spasticity, positive Babinski response and hyperreflexia. Overall, patients with conus medullaris syndrome have a relatively poor prognosis for recovery of bowel and bladder function.

Cauda Equina Syndrome

Cauda equina syndrome (CES) results from an injury to the nerve roots emanating from the conus medullaris, at the level of L2 and below. This is not a type of SCI. Common etiologies are large herniated disk, burst fractures, epidural hematomas, compressive tumors, and ankylosing spondylitis. Unlike conus medullaris syndrome, CES tends to be asymmetrical and display only lower motor neuron symptoms.

In the setting of an acute CES, patients may present with radicular pain, patchy paralysis, saddle anesthesia, and arreflexia involving more than one nerve root. During initial evaluation, it is critical to evaluate patients for sphincter disturbances, particularly urinary retention as well as urinary and fecal incontinence.[41] Presence of urinary retention at any time during evaluation of a patient has 90% sensitivity for the diagnosis of CES. Timing of surgical decompression in CES remains controversial; some studies showed no benefit with early surgical intervention.[42,43] However, surgical decompression within 48 hours of onset of symptoms is recommended to improve the potential for recovery of bowel and bladder function.[44]

Spinal Shock

Spinal shock (see also Chapter 2) has been used to describe two very different phenomena following SCI. For instance, the term has been used inaccurately to describe neurogenic shock resulting from loss of sympathetic tone and bradycardia and hypotension in the trauma patient. Neurogenic shock is different from hypovolemic shock and should always be distinctly identified in an SCI patient with evidence of internal or external bleeding. Treatment includes judicious use of fluid resuscitation, pressors, and elevation of the patient's legs.

True spinal shock refers to the temporary loss or depression of all or most spinal reflex activity below the level of the injury. In patients with complete SCI, spinal shock will precede a period of gradual progression to hypertonia, hyperreflexia, and spasticity. Ditunno et al.[45] proposed a four-phase model describing the evolution of spinal shock over time. Phase 1, which occurs during the first 24 hours, is characterized by complete loss or depression of all reflexes below the level of injury. This phenomenon is thought to result from disruption of signaling between cerebral and spinal cord neurons. Phase 2 occurs from 24 to 72 hours postinjury and is marked by the return of polysynaptic reflexes, such as the bulbocavernosus reflex. This reflex can be monitored by performing a rectal examination and either pinching the glans penis or tugging on the Foley to observe involuntary contraction of the rectal sphincter. The later phases 3 and 4 are the hallmark of interneuron and lower motor neuron sprouting. Phase 3 may occur within 4 weeks and is mediated by axon-supported synaptic growth, whereas phase 4 occurs in the following weeks to month with soma-supported synaptic growth. These phases are characterized by a progression to hyperreflexia and spasticity.

Conclusion

Over the years, a variety of classification systems have been created for the evaluation of SCIs. The ASIA classification system is currently the most widely used. It takes into account the patient's neurological exam in terms of motor, sensory, and sacral function; it also evaluates the patient's functional status. The ASIA system has a good interrater validity and reliability and is a good predictive tool of functional outcomes of SCI patients.

Pearls

- The initial neurological evaluation of SCI patients is critical because it dictates the acute management and determines the long-term prognosis.
- ASIA/IMSOP standards are described in **Fig. 6.1** and are commonly used to describe SCI.
- Some common forms of incomplete SCI syndromes are described in the chapter and include central cord syndrome, Brown-Séquard syndrome, anterior and posterior cord syndrome, conus syndrome, and cauda equina syndrome.

Pitfalls

- Spinal cord injury is a devastating event for which we have yet to find a cure. Several treatment methods have been introduced over the years to minimize subsequent nerve damage and improve functional recovery. However, there are not yet methods to reverse injury or replace damaged neurons.
- SCI requires a lifelong commitment to rehabilitation and adaptation to acquired disabilities.
- SCIs constitute a major source of social and economic burden to our society because they generally affect a younger population and may lead to lifetime disability.

References

1. National Spinal Cord Injury Statistical Center. Spinal cord injury: facts and figures at a glance. J Spinal Cord Med 2005;28(4):379–380
2. American Spinal Injury Association, International Spinal Cord Society. International Standards for Neurological Classification of Spinal Cord Injury. 6th ed. Chicago, IL: American Spinal Injury Association; International Spinal Cord Society; 2006
3. Frankel HL, Hancock DO, Hyslop G, et al. The value of postural reduction in the initial management of closed injuries of the spine with paraplegia and tetraplegia, I: Paraplegia 1969;7(3):179–192
4. American Spinal Injury Association. Standards for Neurological Classification of Spinal Injury Patients. Chicago, IL: American Spinal Injury Association; 1984
5. American Spinal Injury Association. Standards for Neurological Classification of Spinal Injury Patients. Chicago, IL: American Spinal Injury Association; 1989
6. Benzel EC, Larson SJ. Functional recovery after decompressive spine operation for cervical spine fractures. Neurosurgery 1987;20(5):742–746
7. Ditunno JF Jr. New spinal cord injury standards, 1992. Paraplegia 1992;30(2):90–91
8. Maynard FM Jr, Bracken MB, Creasey G, et al; American Spinal Injury Association. International standards for neurological and functional classification of spinal cord injury. American Spinal Injury Association. Spinal Cord 1997;35(5):266–274
9. Wells JD, Nicosia S. Scoring acute spinal cord injury: a study of the utility and limitations of five different grading systems. J Spinal Cord Med 1995;18(1):33–41
10. Bracken MB, Webb SB Jr, Wagner FC. Classification of the severity of acute spinal cord injury: implications for management. Paraplegia 1978;15(4):319–326
11. Lucas JT, Ducker TB. Motor classification of spinal cord injuries with mobility, morbidity and recovery indices. Am Surg 1979;45(3):151–158
12. Klose KJ, Green BA, Smith RS, Adkins RH, MacDonald AM. University of Miami Neuro-Spinal Index (UMNI): a quantitative method for determining spinal cord function. Paraplegia 1980;18(5):331–336
13. Chehrazi B, Wagner FC Jr, Collins WF Jr, Freeman DH Jr. A scale for evaluation of spinal cord injury. J Neurosurg 1981;54(3):310–315
14. Priebe MM, Waring WP. The interobserver reliability of the revised American Spinal Injury Association standards for neurological classification of spinal injury patients. Am J Phys Med Rehabil 1991;70(5):268–270
15. American Spinal Injury Association, International Medical Society of Paraplegia. Standards for Neurological and Functional Classification of Spinal Cord Injury Patients. Chicago, IL: American Spinal Injury Association and International Medical Society of Paraplegia; 1992
16. Keith RA, Granger CV, Hamilton BB, Sherwin FS. The functional independence measure: a new tool for rehabilitation. Adv Clin Rehabil 1987;1:6–18
17. Bednarczyk JH, Sanderson DJ. Comparison of functional and medical assessment in the classification of persons with spinal cord injury. J Rehabil Res Dev 1993;30(4):405–411
18. Waters RL, Adkins R, Yakura J, Vigil D. Prediction of ambulatory performance based on motor scores derived from standards of the American Spinal Injury Association. Arch Phys Med Rehabil 1994;75(7):756–760
19. Cohen ME, Ditunno JF Jr, Donovan WH, Maynard FM Jr. A test of the 1992 international standards for neurological and functional classification of spinal cord injury. Spinal Cord 1998;36(8):554–560
20. Jonsson M, Tollbäck A, Gonzales H, Borg J. Inter-rater reliability of the 1992 international standards for neurological and functional classification of incomplete spinal cord injury. Spinal Cord 2000;38(11):675–679
21. La Rosa G, Conti A, Cardali S, Cacciola F, Tomasello F. Does early decompression improve neurological outcome of spinal cord injured patients? Appraisal of the literature using a meta-analytical approach. Spinal Cord 2004;42(9):503–512
22. Sapkas GS, Papadakis SA. Neurological outcome following early versus delayed lower cervical spine surgery. J Orthop Surg (Hong Kong) 2007;15(2):183–186
23. Fawcett JW, Curt A, Steeves JD, et al. Guidelines for the conduct of clinical trials for spinal cord injury as developed by the ICCP panel: spontaneous recovery after spinal cord injury and statistical power needed for therapeutic clinical trials. Spinal Cord 2007;45(3):190–205
24. Ishida Y, Tominaga T. Predictors of neurologic recovery in acute central cervical cord injury with only upper extremity impairment. Spine 2002;27(15):1652–1658, discussion 1658
25. Penrod LE, Hegde SK, Ditunno JF Jr. Age effect on prognosis for functional recovery in acute, traumatic central cord syndrome. Arch Phys Med Rehabil 1990;71(12):963–968
26. Epstein N, Epstein JA, Benjamin V, Ransohoff J. Traumatic myelopathy in patients with cervical spinal stenosis without fracture or dislocation: methods of diagnosis, management, and prognosis. Spine 1980;5(6):489–496
27. Miranda P, Gomez P, Alday R. Acute traumatic central cord syndrome: analysis of clinical and radiological correlations. J Neurosurg Sci 2008;52(4):107–112, discussion 112
28. Turnbull IM. Chapter 5. Blood supply of the spinal cord: normal and pathological considerations. Clin Neurosurg 1973;20:56–84
29. Selden NR, Quint DJ, Patel N, d'Arcy HS, Papadopoulos SM. Emergency magnetic resonance imaging of cervical spinal cord injuries: clinical correlation and prognosis. Neurosurgery 1999;44(4):785–792, discussion 792–793
30. Schaefer DM, Flanders A, Northrup BE, Doan HT, Osterholm JL. Magnetic resonance imaging of acute cervical spine trauma. Correlation with severity of neurologic injury. Spine 1989;14(10):1090–1095
31. Flanders AE, Spettell CM, Tartaglino LM, Friedman DP, Herbison GJ. Forecasting motor recovery

after cervical spinal cord injury: value of MR imaging. Radiology 1996;201(3):649–655

32. Management of acute central cervical spinal cord injuries. Neurosurgery 2002;50(3, Suppl): S166–S172

33. Harrop JS, Sharan A, Ratliff J. Central cord injury: pathophysiology, management, and outcomes. Spine J 2006;6(6, Suppl):198S–206S

34. Sayer FT, Vitali AM, Low HL, Paquette S, Honey CR. Brown-Sèquard syndrome produced by C3-C4 cervical disc herniation: a case report and review of the literature. Spine 2008;33(9):E279–E282

35. Groen RJ, Middel B, Meilof JF, et al. Operative treatment of anterior thoracic spinal cord herniation: three new cases and an individual patient data meta-analysis of 126 case reports. Neurosurgery 2009;64(3, Suppl):145–159, discussion 159–160

36. McKinley W, Santos K, Meade M, Brooke K. Incidence and outcomes of spinal cord injury clinical syndromes. J Spinal Cord Med 2007;30(3): 215–224

37. Roth EJ, Park T, Pang T, Yarkony GM, Lee MY. Traumatic cervical Brown-Sequard and Brown-Sequard-plus syndromes: the spectrum of presentations and outcomes. Paraplegia 1991;29(9): 582–589

38. Schaefer DM, Flanders AE, Osterholm JL, Northrup BE. Prognostic significance of magnetic resonance imaging in the acute phase of cervical spine injury. J Neurosurg 1992;76(2): 218–223

39. Malas MA, Salbacak A, Büyükmumcu M, Seker M, Köylüoğlu B, Karabulut AK. An investigation of the conus medullaris termination level during the period of fetal development to adulthood. Kaibogaku Zasshi 2001;76(5):453–459

40. Gray H, ed. Anatomy, Descriptive and Surgical. New York: Bounty Books; 1977. Pick T. P. and Howden R., eds.

41. Shapiro S. Cauda equina syndrome secondary to lumbar disc herniation. Neurosurgery 1993; 32(5):743–746, discussion 746–747

42. O'Laoire SA, Crockard HA, Thomas DG. Prognosis for sphincter recovery after operation for cauda equina compression owing to lumbar disc prolapse. Br Med J (Clin Res Ed) 1981; 282(6279):1852–1854

43. Kostuik JP, Harrington I, Alexander D, Rand W, Evans D. Cauda equina syndrome and lumbar disc herniation. J Bone Joint Surg Am 1986;68(3): 386–391

44. Ahn UM, Ahn NU, Buchowski JM, Garrett ES, Sieber AN, Kostuik JP. Cauda equina syndrome secondary to lumbar disc herniation: a meta-analysis of surgical outcomes. Spine 2000;25(12): 1515–1522

45. Ditunno JF, Little JW, Tessler A, Burns AS. Spinal shock revisited: a four-phase model. Spinal Cord 2004;42(7):383–395

7

Spontaneous Recovery Patterns and Prognoses after Spinal Cord Injury

Doniel Drazin and Maxwell Boakye

Key Points

1. Performing the neurological examination at 72 hours following the injury provides a more accurate assessment and may be important with respect to therapeutic interventions and trials.
2. The greatest gains in motor skills occur in the first 3 months, with most recovery complete by 9 months; additional recovery, however, can also occur up to 12 to 18 months post-SCI.
3. The ASIA Impairment Scale (AIS) and ASIA motor scores are considered to be the best predictors of spontaneous recovery.

Physicians and patients alike seek new and accurate information regarding the prognosis for recovery following a spinal cord injury (SCI). Having an awareness of the patterns of spontaneous recovery can help physicians in weighing risks and benefits and making treatment decisions regarding their patients with SCI. Accurate determination of injury severity and prognosis is important for proper planning of rehabilitation and allocation of appropriate resources. Recent studies reveal that a significant number of patients will spontaneously recover from SCI with no medical treatment at all.[1] The American Spinal Injury Association (ASIA) Impairment Scale (AIS) and ASIA motor scores (see Chapter 6, this volume, for more discussion) are considered to be the best predictors of spontaneous recovery.[2,3] Patterns of spontaneous recovery following SCI have become evident through analysis of the ASIA scores of control groups from recent SCI clinical trials.[1] Additional information has been available from numerous databases, including the Model Spinal Cord Injury System (MSCIS) database and retrospective cohort studies. Ditunno, Waters, and Kirshblum have written a great deal regarding prediction of neurological recovery after SCI, and their work should be reviewed for more comprehensive examination of this topic.[2,4–16]

Neurological Level of Injury

The neurological level of injury (NLI) is defined as the lowest level of the spinal cord that shows normal bilateral sensory and motor function. It is recognized that segments with normal function may vary by modality (motor function vs sensory) and body side (right vs left). Therefore, the four different segments can be classified as right-motor, right-sensory, left-motor, and left-sensory. Often, however, a patient's NLI is designated by a single motor level and a single sensory level. The zone of partial preservation refers to segments below the level of injury in patients with complete injuries, where there is partial preservation of motor or sensory function.

Timing of Exam

It is often difficult to perform an accurate neurological examination immediately following an injury because the patient has suffered "spinal shock" and may be sedated, in addition to various other reasons. It is generally agreed that performing the neurological examination at 72 hours following the injury provides a more accurate assessment and may be important with respect to therapeutic interventions and trials.[11] Many of the early studies used either 72 hours to 1 week or 30 days for the initial examination.[11,12]The timing of the exam is important because differences in motor and sensory scores from sequential neurological examinations are a predictor of the patient's expected recovery (or deterioration).

General Aspects of Motor Recovery

Various retrospective cohort studies have revealed key factors that predict spontaneous motor recovery. Of utmost importance is whether the injury was complete versus incomplete, the level of injury, initial strength of muscles in the first caudal level below the injury, and presence of pinprick sensation in the sacral segments. Empirical findings are discussed in this chapter as they relate to patients with complete tetraplegia, complete paraplegia, incomplete tetraplegia, and incomplete paraplegia. Additional predictors of spontaneous outcome after SCI, including motor-evoked potentials, somatosensory-evoked potentials, and conventional and diffusion tensor magnetic resonance imaging, have been discussed in detail in other chapters (see Chapters 43 and 46) and will not be discussed here.

The greatest gains in motor skills occur in the first 3 months, with most recovery complete by 9 months; additional recovery, however, can also occur up to 12 to 18 months post-SCI.[1] Patients with higher initial ASIA impairment scores (indicating a less severe injury) experience greater degrees and faster rates of motor recovery. The majority of motor recovery occurs within the first level below the ASIA motor level. Little or no recovery occurs at more than two spinal levels below the initial ASIA level.[1,12] Studies show that recovery is faster and more complete in muscles that have retained a degree of voluntary function. The prognosis for muscles in the zone of partial preservation with no function is poor.

Kirshblum et al. reviewed 5-year data on 987 patients from the 16 MSCIS locations and showed that, after 5 years postinjury, 94.4% with ASIA A scores initially remained ASIA A.[3] Additionally, it was noted that 3.5% improved from ASIA A to ASIA B, 1.05% improved each from ASIA A to C and to D[3] (**Table 7.1**).

Data show that only 20% of patients who received initial ASIA A scores (complete

Table 7.1 Predictors of Good Motor Recovery

Incomplete injury
Presence of pinprick sensation at the level of injury, in the zone of partial preservation, or at sacral segments
Antigravity strength in the first caudal level below injury level
Presence of some recovery in the first month after injury
Rapid rate of recovery in the first week to month
Brown-Séquard and central cord syndromes have better prognosis than anterior cord syndromes

SCI) experience some level of spontaneous recovery within the first year.[1] Between 15 and 40% of patients with initial ASIA B scores converted to ASIA C status, up to 40% of patients with initial ASIA B scores converted to ASIA D status, and 60 to 80% of patients with initial ASIA C scores converted to ASIA D status[1] (**Fig. 7.1A, B, C**). Patients with initial ASIA A scores recovered ~5 points during the first year, whereas patients with initial ASIA B scores gained ~31 points.[1]

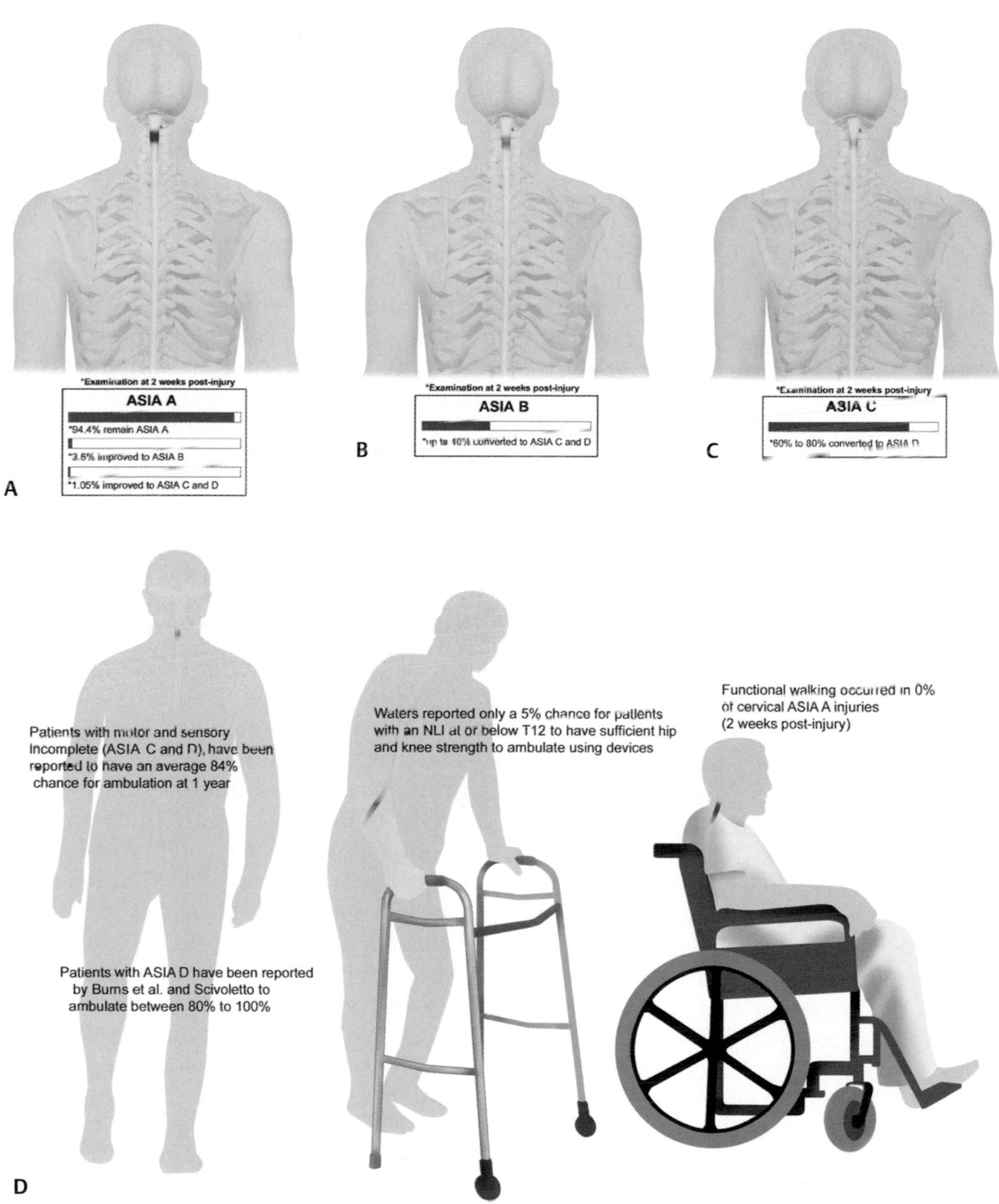

Fig. 7.1 **(A–C)** Spontaneous neurological rates based on 2 weeks postinjury ASIA scores. About 20% of ASIA A (complete SCI) patients experience some level of spontaneous recovery within the first year. Between 15 and 40% of patients with initial ASIA B scores converted to ASIA C or D status, and 60 to 80% of patients with initial ASIA C scores converted to ASIA D status.[14] **(D)** Impact of injury severity and level on ambulatory function. Cervical ASIA A injuries have worst prognosis with regard to likelihood of ambition. Patients with injury levels at or below T12 had 5% chance of ambulation with devices.[4,5,11,22,29,35]

Recovery in Complete Tetraplegia

Most complete tetraplegia patients (66 to 90%) spontaneously regain one root level of function.[4] C4-level injuries appear to have a lower rate of recovery in C5 biceps muscles compared with recovery of the next caudal neurological level in patients with C5 injuries. In one study, 33% of complete tetraplegia patients with a C4 injury with 0/5 biceps strength regained antigravity strength (3/5) at 6 months, 38% at 1 year, and 53% at 2 years.[4] In comparison, 40% of complete tetraplegia patients with a C5 injury with 0/5 strength in wrist extensors regained antigravity strength at 6 months, 51% at 1 year, and 64% at 2 years.[4] It is important to test the C5 muscles rather than C6 muscles when assessing recovery at the next caudal level in C4 tetraplegics in order not to underestimate the extent of recovery.[2]

The initial strength of the muscles is another important predictor of likelihood of achieving antigravity strength. Complete tetraplegics with no strength (0/5) at the next caudal level at 1 month follow-up were able to recover 27% of the time to antigravity strength, while patients with some strength (1 to 2/5) initially were able to recover 97% of the time to regain antigravity strength at the next caudal level at 1-year follow-up.[2] In addition, the faster a muscle with no initial strength (0/5) recovers some strength (>0/5), the better the prognosis is for recovery.[15] Wu et al. noted that patients who developed certain milestones (1/5 at 1 month and 2/5 by 2 months) had a greater chance (86%) for recovery to antigravity or more by 1 year.[15]

Over all, Waters et al. found that motor score improvement averaged 8.6 ± 4.7 points in patients with a complete injury between C4 and C7, whereas the control group ASIA A patients (from the National Acute Spinal Cord Injury Study [NASCIS] II database) gained 4.6 points after 1 year.[1,12]

Recovery in Complete Paraplegia

The extent of recovery of lower extremity (LE) functioning in patients with complete paraplegia on admission appears to be related to the level of injury. In one study (N = 148), patients with an NLI above T9 did not regain any LE function 1 year postinjury, whereas 38% of patients with an NLI below T9 regained some LE functioning.[9] Of patients who had complete paraplegia upon admission, only 4% rehabilitated to incomplete status, with half of these patients (2%) recovering bowel and bladder control.[9]

Recovery in Incomplete Tetraplegia

Incomplete injuries are associated with a wider range of neurologic recovery.[7] Although patients with complete lesions may improve one and sometimes two levels, individuals with incomplete lesions often have recovery at multiple levels below the neurological level of injury. Those with incomplete injuries will achieve a plateau of recovery to the next level more rapidly than complete lesions in 9 to 12 months. In comparison to complete injuries, patients with motor incomplete injuries had an average increase in motor score improvement of 10.6 ± 6.9.[10] In the NASCIS II control group, patients with initial ASIA B, C/D injuries improved 31.3 and 12.9 points, respectively.[1] The improvement in motor scoring, however, is limited by the "ceiling effect," because the ASIA D patients can only recover a few points to normal strength. This "ceiling effect" has been described in the literature and is important to consider when trying to assess various therapies or to design clinical trials for patients with incomplete tetraplegia.[8]

The appearance of some motor function early (within 1 month) has been suggested as a predictor of better functional outcome. Waters et al. reported recovery from 1 month to antigravity at 1 year to be 20% for an initial 0/5 score, 73% for 1/5, and 100% for a 2/5 score.[10] Ditunno et al. reported that recovery to at least grade 3/5 in the elbow flexors and extensors and the wrist extensors was more likely if the patient had exhibited voluntary movement in those muscles 1 week following injury.[4] The presence of a muscle flicker in the lower extremities has been found to be a high predictor (86%) of recovery.[17] Ditunno et al. also reported that the initial strength of a patient's elbow flexors could predict a recovery of the individual's wrist extensors.[7]

Within the category of incomplete tetraplegia, there are three separate incomplete syndromes: central cord syndrome, Brown-Séquard syndrome. and anterior cord syndrome, each with distinguishing motor and sensory loss patterns. Central cord syndrome is often seen in older individuals due to hyperextension of the neck. In central cord syndrome, motor loss is more severe in the upper extremities than in the lower extremities. These patients often have motor recovery comparable to other incomplete tetraplegics, although a relatively lower percentage of these patients achieve ambulatory ability.[2,18] In one study,[19] ASIA motor scores improved from a mean of 58.7 at injury to a mean of 92.3 at long-term follow-up (mean = 70 hours). Despite the large improvement in motor scores, significant disability and loss of functionality remained. The persistence of weakness in the upper extremities may compromise the patients' ability to use ambulatory assistive devices.[2]

Brown-Séquard syndrome results from an ipsilateral hemisection SCI leading to ipsilateral hemiplegia and proprioceptive loss and contralateral hemianalgesia. These patients usually have a favorable prognosis, with 75% of patients achieving ambulatory capacity, with a 30 point increase in ASIA motor score in one study at long-term follow-up.[2,20]

Anterior cord syndrome involves a loss of motor function and pinprick sensation with preservation of light touch sensation and joint position sense.[3] Anterior cord syndrome has a poorer prognosis than the other incomplete syndromes. Only 10 to 20% of patients experience motor recovery.[2] In one study,[21] patients with anterior cord syndrome recovered 22 motor points (final motor score, 38); those with a central cord syndrome gained 29 motor points (final motor score, 76); and those with Brown-Séquard syndrome gained 30 motor points (final motor score, 73).

Recovery in Incomplete Paraplegia

According to Waters et al., patients with incomplete paraplegia showed a spontaneous average gain of 12 lower extremity motor score points 1 year after injury. Further, of the 54 patients with incomplete paraplegia they evaluated, 76% were able to ambulate 1 year postinjury.[22]

Sensory Recovery

Sensory functioning for the ASIA scale is graded on a range from 0 to 2, with 0 being absent and 2 being normal. Studies show an association between sensory and motor recovery.[14] In fact, motor recovery can be predicted by the maintenance of pinprick sensation post-SCI.[23] Sensory and motor gains tend to occur within the same time frame. The extent of sensory recovery may be unrelated to motor recovery, in part due to the reliance upon the patient's subjective assessment of sensory perception (as opposed to the more objective motor assessments).[1] Usually, however, spontaneous recovery of sensation follows a time course pattern similar to that of spontaneous recovery of motor function.

For ASIA A patients (sensory complete, motor complete), the presence of some sensation at the level of injury increases the chances of recovery.[24] Specifically, the presence of bilateral pinprick sparing has been noted to be a favorable predictor of motor recovery. Patients who are ASIA B (sensory incomplete, motor complete) who were noted to have intact bilateral sacral pinprick sensation had a good likelihood (37%) of regaining lower extremity antigravity strength in at least one muscle.[17,25]The correlation between spontaneous recovery and pinprick was also demonstrated by Poynton et al.[26] in that muscles with 0/5 strength but pinprick preservation at the same level were associated with 92% recovery to antigravity for incomplete injuries, and 77% for complete injuries at 1 year. Conversely, if there was no pinprick preservation, recovery to antigravity or greater was 1.3% for complete and 3.9% for incomplete injuries at 1 year. In terms of specific motor recovery related to sensation, Browne et al. found that five of six patients who recovered to antigravity from 0/5 strength initially at C6 had C5 pinprick sensation, whereas only two of nine without C5 pinprick sensation recovered to antigravity.[24] Over all, the presence of intact pinprick sensation at C5 was highly predictive of antigravity or greater motor recover at C6.

The Sygen study (GM-1 ganglioside or Sygen) results showed that patients with sacral pinprick sensation were more likely (results not statistically significant) to recover ambulatory function.[1,27]

The fact that pinprick preservation is a more important predictor of motor recovery than light touch is due to the anatomical proximity of pinprick fibers to the motor fibers in the spinal cord.[2] The lateral spinothalamic tracts containing pinprick fibers are located just ventral to the lateral corticospinal tracts that contain the motor fibers. Preservation of pinprick would suggest an injury that probably spares the lateral spinothalamic tract and therefore likely spares the lateral corticospinal tract.

Ambulation

Recovery of ambulation is an important goal for patients with SCI and is a significant milestone in rehabilitation. Some researchers have defined the motor requirements for ambulation to be antigravity (ASIA score > 3/5) in both the hip flexors on one side and the quadriceps on the contralateral side. Functional walking occurred in 0% of cervical ASIA A injuries and 8.5% of thoracic and lumbar ASIA A injuries.[28,29] Waters reported only a 5% chance for patients with an NLI at or below T12 to have sufficient hip and knee strength to ambulate using devices.[30] None of the complete tetraplegics achieved ambulatory ability.[28,29] Of complete paraplegics, only 5% were able to ambulate at the community level at 1- and 2-year follow-up. All patients who recovered the ability to ambulate had an NLI at or below T12.[9] Ambulation was reported from 0 to 89% in patients with ASIA B, depending largely on preservation of pinprick sensation.[25] As already mentioned, pinprick sensation preservation predicts a more favorable prognosis. In patients with ASIA B, Crozier et al. found an 11% rate of ambulation, whereas Waters et al. reported 0%.[25,31] However, ambulation ranged from 33 to 89% in those with pinprick preservation.[25,31]

With respect to patients with motor and sensory incomplete SCI (ASIA C and D), the field has proven that spontaneous recovery of walking function occurs for a majority of patients.[20,25,31–33] Specifically, Crozier et al. and Maynard et al. reported these patients to have an average 84% chance for ambulation at 1 year.[25,33] However, practitioners should consider that age, timing of motor recovery, and lower/upper extremity strength are factors that influence the chance of ambulation in these patients. For example, in ASIA C patients older than 50, Scivoletto and Di Donna found that 25% and Burns et al. found that 42% had a chance of ambulation, whereas those younger than 50 had a 71% and 91% chance of ambulation, respectively.[29,32] Scivoletto and Di Donna and Burns et al. reported ambulation between 80 and 100% in patients with ASIA D at discharge from inpatient rehab.[29,32] Early recovery of a minimum of antigravity quadriceps strength in at least one quadriceps by 2 months was shown to be an excellent predictor of ambulatory recovery.[34]

Recently, predictive factors for ambulation were determined by Zörner and colleagues.[35] Among predictors like age, gender, sensation, motor scores, and somatosensory evoked potentials, lower extremity motor score (LEMS) was identified as the single best predictor for walking. In combination with LEMS, somatosensory evoked potentials and ASIA scale scores increased the prediction of ambulatory outcome in tetraparetic subjects to 92% and 100%, respectively. This model, however, was less successful at predicting ambulatory outcome in paraparetic patients.[35]

The importance of the LEMS in predicting ambulation was also confirmed in previous studies.[10] In incomplete tetraplegics, an initial LEMS of 20 or greater was associated with attainment of community ambulation at 1 year postinjury. Overall, patients with incomplete tetraplegia had a 46% chance of community ambulation at 1 year; patients with LEMS between 10 and 19 had a 63% chance of ambulation and patients with LEMS greater than or equal to 20 achieved a 100% rate of community ambulation.[10] Ambulatory success depended on upper extremity motor score, with mean score of 16.1 in nonambulators versus 30.3 for community ambulators. In contrast, only 21% of patients with LEMS between 1 and 9 achieved community ambulation. In incomplete paraplegics, all patients with a 1 month LEMS of > 10 points ambulated at 1 year follow-up and 70% with LEMS between 1 and 9 ambulated at 1 year follow-up[22] (**Table 7.2**).

Demographic Factors That May Affect Recovery

Gender

A few studies have examined the role of gender and SCI. Sipski et al. reviewed data from 14,433 patients from the MSCIS and found that women had greater changes in ASIA motor scores after 1 year than men.[30] A functional outcome comparison, however, yielded higher functional independence measure (FIM) motor scores for men with ASIA A or B injuries, except for those with C1–4 and C-6 neurological levels. It should be noted that at the time of admission, men had more severe injuries (i.e., more likely to have complete SCI) than women. Interestingly, in this study, except for an increased risk for men to develop pulmonary embolus, there were no other gender effects on the development of other medical complications. Similarly, Furlan et al. found no gender differences in inpatient mortality associated with acute traumatic SCI.[36]

Table 7.2 Favorable Predictors of Ambulation

Age < 50
Injury level below T9
Preservation of pinprick sensation
American Spinal Injury Association grade ≥ C
Antigravity strength in at least one quadriceps by 2 months
Lower extremity motor score > 10 at 1 month
Initial lower extremity motor score of 30 or greater (community ambulation)

Age

Several studies have examined the relationship between age and outcome after SCI. Scivoletto et al. reviewed 284 SCI subjects more than 50 years old and found that the younger individuals had better recovery in terms of their ASIA impairment levels and increased ASIA motor scores.[37] Older individuals had more medical complications but also had shorter lengths of stay and performed better on a few activities of daily living (ADL). Younger individuals tended to have more favorable outcomes with walking and bladder/bowel independence. In another study by Fisher et al. that looked at 70 ASIA A patients, there was a trend toward better neurological recovery for patients under 24 years old.[38] Van Hedel and Curt reviewed the records of 98 ASIA A/B subjects and found that functional outcomes, as measured by a spinal cord independence measure, decreased significantly with increasing age.[39] It is hypothesized that older patients will have greater morbidity and mortality rates. Boakye et al., using the national inpatient sample, found that patients more than 45 years of age had a higher risk of in-hospital mortality following acute SCI.[40]

Comorbidities

Comorbidities affect morbidity and mortality after injury and hence may directly or indirectly influence recovery. Boakye et al. found that patients who had three or more medical comorbidities had a 1.8 times higher risk of mortality and were 1.45 times as likely to be discharged to an institution other than home than those with no comorbidities.[40] In a retrospective cohort study (N = 297) of patients with acute traumatic SCI, Furlan et al. found that comorbidities confounded the age-related differences in mortality during initial hospitalization following an acute traumatic SCI.[36] In addition, this study demonstrated that the Charlson Comorbidity Index (CCI) is a reliable and valid way to measure comorbidities for the purpose of predicting in-hospital mortality for patients with acute traumatic SCI after controlling for age. Thus, a measure of comorbidities (using the CCI) appears to be an important factor when one is drawing conclusions about mortality rates following SCI.

Conclusion

It is important for health-care professionals to be knowledgeable about the patterns of spontaneous recovery in patients with SCI, as well as the factors that affect recovery after treatments for SCI. This information will assist physicians in properly informing patients of their likely prognoses, explaining the risks and benefits of interventions, and, most importantly, making treatment decisions.

Pearls

- Patients without initial motor or sensory function below the injury may still achieve excellent recovery.
- The most important factors are the completeness of injury, the initial strength of muscles at the first caudal level, and the level of neurological injury.
- The rate and extent of recovery are greatest within the first 6 months after injury, but recovery can continue for many months thereafter for up to 2 years.
- Preservation of pinprick sensation at the level of injury in the zone of partial preservation or in the sacral segments are favorable predictors of motor recovery and future ambulation.

Pitfalls

- Avoid using the 24-hour ASIA exam as a predictor of outcome. Use the 72-hour exam.
- Frequently, the C5 exam can be confused with the C6 in patients who have C4 injury levels.
- Failure to diagnose an incomplete injury (preservation of sensation in a sacral segment) results in inaccurate assessment of prognosis.

References

1. Fawcett JW, Curt A, Steeves JD, et al. Guidelines for the conduct of clinical trials for spinal cord injury as developed by the ICCP panel: spontaneous recovery after spinal cord injury and statistical power needed for therapeutic clinical trials. Spinal Cord 2007;45(3):190–205
2. Kirshblum SC, O'Connor KC. Predicting neurologic recovery in traumatic cervical spinal cord injury. Arch Phys Med Rehabil 1998;79(11): 1456–1466
3. Maynard FM Jr, Bracken MB, Creasey G, et al; American Spinal Injury Association. International Standards for Neurological and Functional Classification of Spinal Cord Injury. Spinal Cord 1997;35(5):266–274
4. Ditunno JF Jr, Stover SL, Freed MM, Ahn JH. Motor recovery of the upper extremities in traumatic quadriplegia: a multicenter study. Arch Phys Med Rehabil 1992;73(5):431–436
5. Ditunno JF Jr, Formal CS. Chronic spinal cord injury. N Engl J Med 1994;330(8):550–556
6. Ditunno JF Jr, Cohen ME, Hauck WW, Jackson AB, Sipski ML. Recovery of upper-extremity strength in complete and incomplete tetraplegia: a multicenter study. Arch Phys Med Rehabil 2000;81(4):389–393
7. Ditunno JF Jr, Sipski ML, Posuniak EA, Chen YT, Staas WE Jr, Herbison GJ. Wrist extensor recovery in traumatic quadriplegia. Arch Phys Med Rehabil 1987;68(5 Pt 1):287–290
8. Kirshblum SC, O'Connor KC. Levels of spinal cord injury and predictors of neurologic recovery. Phys Med Rehabil Clin N Am 2000;11(1):1–27, vii
9. Waters RL, Yakura JS, Adkins RH, Sie I. Recovery following complete paraplegia. Arch Phys Med Rehabil 1992;73(9):784–789

10. Waters RL, Adkins RH, Yakura JS, Sie I. Motor and sensory recovery following incomplete tetraplegia. Arch Phys Med Rehabil 1994;75(3):306–311
11. Brown PJ, Marino RJ, Herbison GJ, Ditunno JF Jr. The 72-hour examination as a predictor of recovery in motor complete quadriplegia. Arch Phys Med Rehabil 1991;72(8):546–548
12. Waters RL, Adkins RH, Yakura JS, Sie I. Motor and sensory recovery following complete tetraplegia. Arch Phys Med Rehabil 1993;74(3):242–247
13. Kirshblum S, Millis S, McKinley W, Tulsky D. Late neurologic recovery after traumatic spinal cord injury. Arch Phys Med Rehabil 2004;85(11):1811–1817
14. Stauffer ES, Ditunno JF Jr, Waters RL, Kirshbaum S. Neurologic recovery following injuries to the cervical spinal cord and nerve roots. Spine 1984;9(5):532–534
15. Wu L, Marino RJ, Herbison GJ, Ditunno JF Jr. Recovery of zero-grade muscles in the zone of partial preservation in motor complete quadriplegia. Arch Phys Med Rehabil 1992;73(1):40–43
16. Ditunno JF, Cohen ME, Fomral C, Whiteneck G. Functional outcomes. In: Stover SL, Delisa JA, Whiteneck GG, eds. Spinal Cord Injury. Clinical Outcomes from the Model Systems. Gaithersburg, MD: Aspen; 1995:170–184
17. Folman Y, el Masri W. Spinal cord injury: prognostic indicators. Injury 1989;20(2):92–93
18. Waters RL, Adkins RH, Sie III, Yakura JS. Motor recovery following spinal cord injury associated with cervical spondylosis: a collaborative study. Spinal Cord 1996;34(12):711–715
19. Dvorak MF, Fisher CG, Hoekema J, et al. Factors predicting motor recovery and functional outcome after traumatic central cord syndrome: a long-term follow-up. Spine 2005;30(20):2303–2311
20. McKinley W, Santos K, Meade M, Brooke K. Incidence and outcomes of spinal cord injury clinical syndromes. J Spinal Cord Med 2007;30(3):215–224
21. Pollard ME, Apple DF. Factors associated with improved neurologic outcomes in patients with incomplete tetraplegia. Spine 2003;28(1):33–39
22. Waters RL, Adkins RH, Yakura JS, Sie I. Motor and sensory recovery following incomplete paraplegia. Arch Phys Med Rehabil 1994;75(1):67–72
23. Oleson CV, Burns AS, Ditunno JF, Geisler FH, Coleman WP. Prognostic value of pinprick preservation in motor complete, sensory incomplete spinal cord injury. Arch Phys Med Rehabil 2005;86(5):988–992
24. Browne BJ, Jacobs SR, Herbison GJ, Ditunno JF Jr. Pin sensation as a predictor of extensor carpi radialis recovery in spinal cord injury. Arch Phys Med Rehabil 1993;74(1):14–18
25. Crozier KS, Graziani V, Ditunno JF Jr, Herbison GJ. Spinal cord injury: prognosis for ambulation based on sensory examination in patients who are initially motor complete. Arch Phys Med Rehabil 1991;72(2):119–121
26. Poynton AR, O'Farrell DA, Shannon F, Murray P, McManus F, Walsh MG. Sparing of sensation to pin prick predicts recovery of a motor segment after injury to the spinal cord. J Bone Joint Surg Br 1997;79(6):952–954
27. Geisler FH, Dorsey FC, Coleman WP. Recovery of motor function after spinal-cord injury—a randomized, placebo-controlled trial with GM-1 ganglioside. N Engl J Med 1991;324(26):1829–1838
28. Ditunno JF, Scivoletto G, Patrick M, Biering-Sorensen F, Abel R, Marino R. Validation of the walking index for spinal cord injury in a US and European clinical population. Spinal Cord 2008;46(3):181–188
29. Scivoletto G, Di Donna V. Prediction of walking recovery after spinal cord injury. Brain Res Bull 2009;78(1):43–51
30. Sipski ML, Jackson AB, Gómez-Marín O, Estores I, Stein A. Effects of gender on neurologic and functional recovery after spinal cord injury. Arch Phys Med Rehabil 2004;85(11):1826–1836
31. Waters RL, Adkins R, Yakura J, Vigil D. Prediction of ambulatory performance based on motor scores derived from standards of the American Spinal Injury Association. Arch Phys Med Rehabil 1994;75(7):756–760
32. Burns SP, Golding DG, Rolle WA Jr, Graziani V, Ditunno JF Jr. Recovery of ambulation in motor-incomplete tetraplegia. Arch Phys Med Rehabil 1997;78(11):1169–1172
33. Maynard FM, Reynolds GG, Fountain S, Wilmot C, Hamilton R. Neurological prognosis after traumatic quadriplegia. Three-year experience of California Regional Spinal Cord Injury Care System. J Neurosurg 1979;50(5):611–616
34. Crozier KS, Cheng LL, Graziani V, Zorn G, Herbison G, Ditunno JF Jr. Spinal cord injury: prognosis for ambulation based on quadriceps recovery. Paraplegia 1992;30(11):762–767
35. Zörner B, Blanckenhorn WU, Dietz V, Curt A; EM-SCI Study Group. Clinical algorithm for improved prediction of ambulation and patient stratification after incomplete spinal cord injury. J Neurotrauma 2010;27(1):241–252
36. Furlan JC, Kattail D, Fehlings MG. The impact of co-morbidities on age-related differences in mortality after acute traumatic spinal cord injury. J Neurotrauma 2009;26(8):1361–1367
37. Scivoletto G, Morganti B, Ditunno P, Ditunno JF, Molinari M. Effects on age on spinal cord lesion patients' rehabilitation. Spinal Cord 2003;41(8):457–464
38. Fisher CG, Noonan VK, Smith DE, Wing PC, Dvorak MF, Kwon BK. Motor recovery, functional status, and health-related quality of life in patients with complete spinal cord injuries. Spine 2005;30(19):2200–2207
39. van Hedel HJ, Curt A. Fighting for each segment: estimating the clinical value of cervical and thoracic segments in SCI. J Neurotrauma 2006;23(11):1621–1631
40. Boakye M, Patil CG, Santarelli J, Ho C, Tian W, Lad SP. Laminectomy and fusion after spinal cord injury: national inpatient complications and outcomes. J Neurotrauma 2008;25(3):173–183

8

Management of Spinal Cord Injury in the Intensive Care Unit

Nicolas Phan

Key Points

1. Clinical management of SCI in the ICU is centered on the identification, prevention, and treatment of secondary insults, with a specific emphasis on maintaining adequate perfusion and oxygenation of injured nervous tissue.
2. Hemodynamic instability and ventilatory failure are common after SCI, especially in cervical and high thoracic injuries, and can occur in a delayed fashion.
3. The ICU provides the optimal environment for early detection and treatment of cardiovascular instability and respiratory failure in patients with SCI and can potentially reduce complications and improve outcome after SCI.

The treatment of spinal cord injury (SCI) has evolved significantly over the past decades. Treatment of acute SCI in the intensive care unit (ICU) (**Fig. 8.1**) can provide several benefits, such as monitoring and management of cardiopulmonary dysfunction. Although some centers have created units dedicated solely to the treatment of patients with SCI,[1–4] this type of specialized care has not been universally accepted, and there is still a wide range of management strategies within regions and even within specific institutions. Specifically, the question of whether patients with acute SCI benefit from care in the ICU has not been fully answered. This chapter describes the scientific rationale behind ICU management of SCI and the main issues specific to SCI that can be addressed in an intensive care setting.

Rationale for Spinal Cord Injury Management in the ICU

The pathophysiology of SCI is generally separated into primary and secondary injury mechanisms. Primary injury occurs at the time of trauma, and common mechanisms include mechanical compression, laceration, shear, and penetrating injury. Although these processes are heterogeneous, they all result from external mechanical forces transferred to the spinal cord tissue. The primary injury event initiates a cascade of secondary injury mecha-

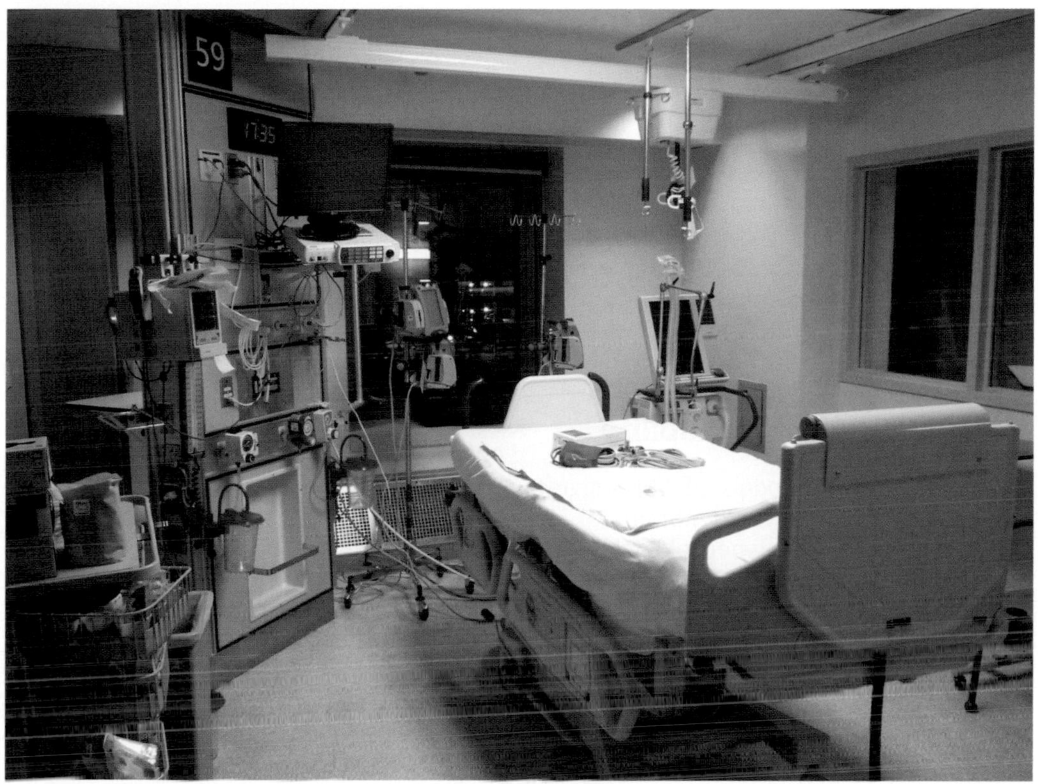

Fig. 8.1 Typical intensive care unit room set up with multimodal monitoring at Sunnybrook Health Sciences Centre, Toronto, Canada.

nisms, including (1) vascular injury and compromise that can lead to loss of autoregulation, vasospasm, thrombosis, and hemorrhage; (2) electrolyte imbalances, cellular integrity loss, energy metabolism failure, and edema; (3) neurotransmitter accumulation and toxicity, free radical buildup, and lipid peroxidation; and (4) delayed cell death or apoptosis.[5–7]

The molecular mechanisms involved in this secondary injury cascade are similar to those involved in other types of neurological injury, such as traumatic brain injury (TBI) and acute ischemic stroke. These various pathways of cellular injury have been the focus of extensive preclinical work on neuroprotection for SCI. However, at present, clinical trials targeting secondary injuries have shown only limited benefit in patients.

An additional critical aspect of secondary injury after SCI is avoidance of *secondary insults*. Secondary insults are clinical events that would otherwise be well tolerated but exacerbate damage to vulnerable tissue that has been "primed" by the initial injury. Examples of secondary insults frequently encountered early in SCI that can be identified and managed in an intensive care setting are hypotension, hypoxia, fever, and hyperglycemia. Hypotension and hypoxia result in decreased substrate delivery of oxygen and glucose to the injured cord, whereas pyrexia may further increase metabolic demand, and hyperglycemia may exacerbate ongoing injury mechanisms.

The absolute primacy of the "ABCs" of trauma patients with confirmed or suspected SCI cannot be overemphasized. Adequate perfusion and oxygenation of injured nervous tissue are essential to optimize recovery. Even brief periods of hypoperfusion and hypoxia can trigger secondary injury cascades, which increase morbidity and mortality and decrease chances of neurological recovery.[7]

Current clinical approaches to the management of SCI in the ICU are centered on these concepts of primary and secondary SCI. Likewise, the identification, prevention, and treatment of secondary insults are the principal focus of neurointensive care management for patients with acute SCI.

Hemodynamic Instability

Studies in animal models of SCI suggest ischemia is a common denominator or end-result of continuing neurological compromise following the primary injury.[8] At the spinal cord level, direct injury to the microcirculation results in vasospasm and loss of autoregulation, leading to alteration in spinal cord blood flow.[6] At the systemic level, acute SCI is often associated with hemodynamic instability. This is particularly more common and pronounced in cervical and complete SCI. Hypotension in the setting of SCI and trauma can have multiple etiologies: (1) Loss of sympathetic vasomotor tone results in a decrease in systemic vascular resistance and pooling of blood in the peripheral vasculature. (2) Interruption of sympathetic input to the thoracic region results in unopposed parasympathetic outflow to the cardiac fibers, which leads to arrhythmias. The most commonly seen arrhythmia is bradycardia, although supraventricular and ventricular tachycardia can also occur.[9] Arrhythmias tend to be more common in the first 2 weeks following injury and more pronounced in more severe injuries.[9] (3) Since a significant proportion of SCI patients also have multisystem injuries, hypovolemia from internal bleeding can be a significant contributor to hypotension. Typically, hypotension related to hypovolemia is associated with tachycardia, whereas hypotension seen with severe SCI is often coupled with bradycardia.

Systemic hypotension in the setting of SCI, with coincidental loss of autoregulatory function in the microcirculation, further compromises local spinal cord perfusion and blood flow and exacerbates spinal cord ischemia.[6,8] The first line of treatment is volume resuscitation using 1 to 2 L of crystalloids. Volume expansion alone may not be sufficient to restore normotension if the increase of venous return is not matched by an accompanying increase in cardiac output; the addition of vasopressor pharmacological agents may be required. The choice of vasopressor should be an agent that has both α- and β-adrenergic actions, such as dopamine or norepinephrine. Dobutamine can help increase the cardiac output but also causes a decrease in systemic vascular resistance, which can compound the hemodynamic effect of SCI and is therefore less useful. Phenylephrine has a purely α-adrenergic effect and should be used with caution because the increase in cardiac afterload and lack of β-adrenergic response, especially in cervical SCI, can result in reflex bradycardia.[10,11]

Restoration of normal hemodynamic parameters is the primary goal and can be demonstrated by adequate urine output, resolution of systemic acidosis, and return of normal mentation in conscious patients. The absolute values for blood pressure and cardiac output that are required to achieve this will vary between patients. The appropriate end point necessary to achieve adequate spinal cord perfusion and blood flow is more difficult to define. There is good evidence from animal studies that hypotension contributes to spinal cord ischemia after injury and can worsen the initial insult and reduce the potential for neurological recovery.[12] Similar evidence is lacking in human SCI. The effect of hypotension in human TBI has been studied comprehensively and inference from the TBI literature seems appropriate.[13] Prospectively collected data from the Traumatic Coma Data Bank demonstrated that hypotension, defined as systolic blood pressure of less than 90 mmHg and hypoxia, defined as PaO_2 below 60 mmHg, were independently associated with a significant increase in morbidity and mortality after severe TBI.[13] A single episode of hypotension was associated with a 50% increase in mortality.

Despite the lack of similar human studies in SCI, therapeutic interventions aimed at correcting hypotension and maintaining threshold levels of mean arterial pressure (MAP) to improve spinal cord perfusion have promising potential. Several reports of case series suggest that treatment of hypotension and resuscitation to maintain MAP at high-normal levels, 85 to 90 mmHg, may enhance neurological outcome after acute traumatic SCI.[1–4,14,15]

Vale et al.,[3] in 1997, reported their experience with a nonrandomized, prospective pilot study in the assessment of aggressive medical resuscitation and blood pressure management in 77 consecutive ASCI patients. All patients were managed in the ICU with invasive monitoring, including pulmonary artery catheters and arterial lines, while blood pressure was optimized to maintain MAP above 85 mmHg for 7 days after injury. The average admission MAP for complete cervical SCI patients was 66 mmHg. Nine of 10 (90%) patients with complete cervical SCI required vasopressors after volume replacement, compared with 13 of 25 (52%) with incomplete cervical injuries, and 9 of 29 (31%) with thoracic injuries. At 1 year follow-up, three of 10 complete cervical SCI patients regained ambulatory capacity, and two patients regained bladder function. Incomplete cervical SCI patients fared better. Twenty-three regained ambulatory function at 12-month follow-up, only four of whom had initial examination scores consistent with walking. Twenty-two of 25 (88%) patients regained bladder control. Thirty-one of 35 (89%) cervical SCI patients and 27 of 29 (93%) thoracic level SCI patients were treated surgically. The results were independent of neurological function at admission and timing of surgery. The authors concluded that the enhanced neurological outcome identified in their series after acute SCI was the result of early and aggressive volume resuscitation and blood pressure augmentation and was cumulative to and/or distinct from any potential benefit provided by surgery.

The results of this study and five other case series[1,2,4,14,15] showing similar trends have led to the establishment of blood pressure treatment guidelines, with the understanding that class I evidence from randomized controlled trials on the subject are unlikely to be obtained in the future for acute SCI.[10] Correction of hypotension (systolic BP <90 mmHg) is offered as a strong treatment option,[10] whereas class III evidence from the literature suggests that maintenance of MAP at 85 to 90 mmHg after ASCI for 7 days is safe and may improve spinal cord perfusion and, ultimately, neurological outcome.[3,10]

Respiratory System and Complications

Respiratory complications are a major cause of mortality and morbidity in patients with SCI.[16] Respiratory failure is common in SCI patients and occurs more often in cervical and complete SCI.[17] The two phases of respiration, inspiration and expiration, are both affected after SCI. The process of inspiration requires the contraction of the diaphragm and the internal intercostals, which allows chest expansion. Accessory muscles can be recruited for increased respiratory activity. The C3-5 spinal cord segments and corresponding nerve roots innervate the diaphragm, and injuries above the C3 level result in apnea and the need for immediate ventilatory support. In the acute phase, flaccid paralysis of the intercostals leads to an overall decrease in size of the thoracic cavity when the diaphragm contracts. This results in a significantly diminished forced vital capacity to ~70% of normal.[18] Expiration is principally a passive process but can be augmented by contraction of the abdominal musculature. The loss of abdominal wall function in SCI leads to a similar decrease in expiratory force with accompanying impairment in the ability to cough and clear secretions.[18] With time, the respiratory musculature becomes more spastic and the chest wall more rigid, with a resulting improvement in ventilatory function. Most of this improvement is seen during inspiration, with a return of forced vital capacity and maximal inspiratory force to ~60% of baseline.[18] The loss of sympathetic tone in the acute phase also results in increased bronchial tone from unopposed cholinergic bronchoconstriction.[18] In addition, mucus production is increased while ciliary muscle activity is decreased.

All of these respiratory changes can lead to relative hypoxemia and exacerbate spinal cord ischemia after acute SCI. It is therefore paramount to identify patients at risk for respiratory failure and complications. The altered mechanics of respiration lead to a pattern of shallow breaths, which can be initially compensated by an increase in respiratory rate. However, rapid shallow breathing does not adequately move the air out of the dead space zones, which do not participate in gas exchange, and also promotes atelectasis. The overall result is a higher work of breathing and decreased gas exchange, superimposed on diminished inspiratory force. Approximately one third of patients with cervical SCI will require endotracheal intubation and ventilatory support.[19] Careful monitoring and some degree of judgment are necessary to identify patients before respiratory decompensation occurs. A decrease in vital capacity <1 L as well as rising respiratory rate and arterial PCO_2 are good indicators of impending respiratory failure. It is best to use a proactive approach of early intubation under controlled circumstances before the patient's condition becomes an emergency to avoid devastating consequences, such as prolonged hypoxia, which can exacerbate secondary injury to the spinal cord. In the setting of a cervical spine injury, orotracheal intubation can be performed safely by experienced practitioners using manual in-line traction.[20] In their retrospective review of 186 patients with low cervical SCI (C5-T1), Hassid et al. reported 58% complete SCI, with an overall intubation rate of 68%, tracheostomy rate of 69%, and mortality rate of 15%. Patients with incomplete SCI required intubation less frequently, at 38%, but still had a high proportion of tracheostomy (50%) for intractable pulmonary failure.[16] Their data emphasize the need for rapid and comprehensive assessment of respiratory status in all patients with SCI, especially in cervical levels. Lu et al. reported eight cases of mid-low cervical SCI who developed delayed apnea with catastrophic consequences.[17] Associated findings included the presence of diffuse, extensive cord lesions, respiratory distress, and bradycardia with or without associated hypotension, even when transient and self-limited. Sleep was also found to be an at-risk period of time in five of the eight cases. Evidence from animal models has attributed this type of delayed clinical deterioration and respiratory failure to progressively expanding cord lesion.[6] In summary, patients with cervical SCI often present initially without any evidence of respiratory compromise but have a high risk of developing respiratory failure during the initial course of their clinical progression.

Patients with thoracic SCI are also more at risk for respiratory complications than patients with lower injuries. Cotton et al. reviewed 11,080 patients with thoracic and lumbar spinal injuries, with 596 having a thoracic SCI. Respiratory complication rates were higher in high thoracic SCI (T1-6, 51%), than in lower thoracic injuries (T7-12, 34.5%) and thoracic fractures without SCI (27.5%).[21] The need for intubation, risk of pneumonia, and mortality were all more prevalent in the higher thoracic SCI group. Aside from altered breathing mechanics associated with denervation of the upper thoracic segments, a potential explanation for the increased risk of respiratory complications in this group is the higher Injury Severity Score (ISS). A greater amount of force is usually required to produce significant damage to the thoracic spine because of the increased stiffness provided by the supporting rib cage and costotransverse articulations and ligaments. This is associated with greater risk of injury to the thoracic cavity, such as flail chest wall segments, pulmonary contusions, pneumo-/hemothoraces, and cardiac injuries.

A significant proportion of respiratory morbidity and mortality in SCI is attributable to pneumonia. Ventilator-associated pneumonia (VAP) is a direct consequence of intubation and prolonged ventilation.

The risk of developing VAP increases by 1 to 3% per day of intubation.[22] *Streptococcus pneumoniae* and *Haemophilus influenzae* are the pathognomonic organisms in the early period (< 4 days), whereas gram-negative species and *Staphylococcus aureus* are the usual causative agents in later periods. Overall mortality of VAP has been reported as 27%, and as high as 43% when due to *Pseudomonas aeruginosa*.[23] Diagnosis of VAP is challenging because many associated radiographic findings are nonspecific, and laboratory abnormalities are common in critically ill patients. Increasing amounts of secretions may be an indicator of early pneumonia, but many patients have copious secretions without an associated infection. Empirical treatment without clear evidence of actual infection can lead to the selection of antibiotic-resistant organisms, whereas delayed treatment can have serious consequences. Recommendations from the American College of Chest Physicians for the diagnosis of VAP include temperature > 38°C or < 36°C, leukocytosis or leukopenia, purulent secretions, and hypoxemia. These criteria, in combination with an abnormal chest radiograph showing air bronchograms or alveolar infiltrates, warrant starting antibiotic therapy tailored to organisms grown from tracheal aspirates.[11]

Respiratory mechanics improve steadily after the acute period, allowing weaning from ventilatory support, especially if the level of injury is at C4 or below.[24] The average period of ventilator dependence is strongly related to the level of injury: 65 days for patients with C1-4 levels, 22 days in patients with C5-8 levels, and 12 days for patients with thoracic injuries.[25] Parameters that suggest a patient is ready for weaning include rise in forced vital capacity, FIO_2 requirement < 50%, minute ventilation < 10 L, and resolution of any respiratory complications, such as pneumonia.[11] The majority of patients take 2 weeks or more before they are ready for weaning.[19] Early mobilization helps the process of weaning in most patients. However, it has been shown that quadriplegic patients have better ventilatory mechanics in the supine position than in the upright position.[26] Flaccid abdominal musculature allows the abdominal contents to descend in the upright position, which overdistends the diaphragm and decreases its contraction efficiency. This may be helped with the use of abdominal binders.[27] Changes in ventilation mode can also assist the weaning process; they include T-piece trials, continuous positive airway support, and pressure support mode.[28] Each method has specific advantages, and, although it is not clear which is superior, pressure support ventilation has become increasingly prevalent because it allows for slow titration of the amount of ventilatory support.[28] The use of tracheostomy offers clear advantages in patients with SCI who require prolonged ventilation: (1) The amount of dead space and resistance across the smaller airway is decreased. (2) It permits easier suctioning of secretions (pulmonary toileting). (3) It allows for periods of spontaneous breathing to alternate with mechanical support without manipulating the airway. (4) It is more comfortable for the patient. (5) It may decrease the incidence of pneumonia. For patients who require an anterior cervical surgical stabilization, it is generally recommended to wait 1 to 2 weeks between the two procedures to avoid contamination of the surgical wound by respiratory secretions. Cameron et al. recently reported their experience before and after implementation of an interdisciplinary tracheostomy team supervising SCI patients with tracheostomies.[29] They found a significant decrease in median length of stay, decrease in median duration of cannulation, increase in the use of speaking valve, and decrease in time to valve trial, and no tracheostomy-related emergency, compared with two events in the preimplementation period.

Spine Clearance in the Unconscious Patient

The incidence of cervical spine injury in polytrauma patients is relatively small, ~ 1 to 3%. Even so, the potential for devastating consequences from neurological compromise related to a missed diagnosis requires that all trauma victims be managed with the expectation that a spinal injury is present. This implies that the cervical, thoracic, and lumbar spines have to be "cleared" during the hospital stay. Prolonged supine immobilization has significant morbidity, including pressure sores, raised intracranial pressure (ICP), airway and respiratory complications, difficulty with central venous access, gastric reflux and aspiration, and limitations in physiotherapy care. Most of these complications can occur quickly after admission and can progress rapidly after 48 to 72 hours. Furthermore, there is some evidence that rigid collars do not restrict the displacement of unstable cervical injuries.[30]

The presence of severe TBI is associated with an increased risk of cervical spine injury. A Glasgow Coma Scale score of < 8 has been shown to be associated with a 50% increase in incidence of cervical spine injury.[31] Moreover, the management of many polytrauma patients requires sedation for other reasons such as ventilatory care or the need for repeat/multiple surgeries, and clinical assessment may therefore be impossible for prolonged periods. In the unconscious or unexaminable patient, imaging modalities occupy a central role in clearing the spine. The overall complications related to prolonged immobilization and rigid cervical collar are not insignificant and have to be balanced against the small risk of an undetected or unstable ligamentous injury missed by radiological modalities. There is currently no standardized approach in the clearance of the cervical spine in unconscious and intubated patients,[31] which reflects the difficulty this problem poses in the ICU.

Several imaging modalities have been used to clear the cervical spine. Cross-table lateral plain radiographs require the visualization of the entire cervical spine, including the craniocervical junction and the cervicothoracic junction. When these images are anatomically and technically adequate, their radiographic sensitivity in detecting cervical injuries is ~80%.[31] It is estimated that a single lateral plain radiograph will miss ~15% of injuries, and typically 50% of these films are inadequate.[31] The addition of an open-mouth view for odontoid visualization and an anteroposterior view to better asses the facet joints and rotation abnormalities increases the sensitivity to ~90%. The odontoid view is often obscured in unconscious patients by artifact from endotracheal and gastric tubes and cervical collars, and ~25 to 50% of films are inadequate for proper interpretation.

Computed tomography (CT) has evolved rapidly in recent years, and it is difficult to interpret older studies of its efficacy in spinal injury detection. Improvements like thinner axial slice acquisition (1.5 to 2 mm), sagittal and coronal reconstructions, and digital viewing may all have helped in bringing CT to the forefront of imaging modalities for spinal clearance. Directed CT scanning involves scanning of only the nonvisualized or suspicious areas identified on plain films. Most studies show that the addition of directed CT detects an additional 10% of injuries not seen on plain films.[31] CT scanning of the entire cervical spine detects significantly more injuries than plain films or directed scanning. Studies have shown a sensitivity approaching 100% for entire spine CT and improvement in detection of 10%.[31]

Magnetic resonance imaging (MRI) is the investigation of choice for spinal cord evaluation in SCI. However, its role in spinal clearance is less clear. MRI has a theoretical advantage over CT in detecting ligamentous injuries. MRI is extremely sensitive for soft tissue injuries, but the significance of many detected abnormalities is unknown. Most abnormalities severe enough to require surgical fusion can be detected by CT.[32]

Dynamic fluoroscopy involves passively manipulating the cervical spine under real-time imaging and has the advantage of demonstrating actual instability under stress. The main limitation of this method is the inability to obtain an anatomically adequate study, particularly at the cervicothoracic junction, which is missed in ~40% of cases. There are also legitimate concerns regarding cervical manipulation in unconscious patients. In their comprehensive review of cervical spinal clearance, Morris and McCoy found 10 separate studies on dynamic fluoroscopy.[31] Of a total of 887 patients, only 10 (0.9%) cervical injuries were detected by dynamic fluoroscopy, five (0.6%) of which required surgery, with an overall number of 177 that needed treatment.[31] None of the studies included high-resolution CT of the entire cervical spine as part of their investigation. Spiteri et al. did a retrospective review of their clearance protocol over 10 years and found 87 patients with unstable injuries, 85 of which were identified by CT, with a sensitivity of 97.7% and a specificity of 100%.[33] Of the two cases that were missed, dynamic screening detected one (sensitivity 98.8%, specificity 100%), and missed the other. Review of the second case confirmed that the abnormality, an atlantooccipital dislocation, was identifiable on CT. The authors concluded that high-resolution CT alone could be reliably used to clear the cervical spine and indicated that dynamic screening was removed from their routine clearance protocol.

Role of the ICU in the Management of Spinal Cord Injury

Patients with acute SCI frequently experience hypotension, arrhythmias, hypoxemia, airway compromise, and pulmonary dysfunction.[3,16,17,28,34] Hemodynamic instability and ventilatory failure can occur in a delayed fashion in patients who appear stable early during their postinjury course. The general consensus that secondary insults in the form of hypotension and hypoxia can further compromise the injured cord, combined with the high incidence of associated multisystem injuries, provide a sound basis for admitting, monitoring, and treating SCI patients in an intensive care setting in the acute phase.

A few clinical series have tried to determine whether patients with acute SCI benefit from care in the ICU. In 1984, Tator et al. reported their experience in the care of 144 patients treated in the Acute Spinal Cord Injury Clinic at Sunnybrook Medical Centre between 1974 and 1979 and compared their results to a previously published cohort of patients treated in the same area from 1948 and 1973.[2] Some of their core principles included early referrals, rapid transfer time, and early admission to their specialized unit, as well as aggressive treatment of hypotension and respiratory failure. The median interval time from injury to admission was 4.9 hours, compared with 12 hours in the previous period. Neurological status was assessed in 95 patients, of whom 41 (43%) had neurological improvement, 52 (55%) did not change, and only two had neurological deterioration. Mortality rates were significantly lower, at 6.9%, compared with 14.0% in the earlier group, and the authors attributed this mainly to improved respiratory care. Length of stay in the ICU was also reduced by ~50% for both complete and incomplete injuries.

Levi et al. treated 50 patients with acute cervical SCI according to an aggressive protocol that included invasive hemodynamic monitoring with arterial lines and pulmonary artery catheters, and treatment with volume and vasopressors to maintain adequate cardiac output and MAP > 90 mmHg.[1] Eight patients presented with SBP < 90 mmHg at admission, and 82% of patients required vasopressor support in addition to volume replacement to achieve the target MAP. Patients with complete injuries had 5.5 times the rate of vasopressor requirement compared with incomplete injuries. The authors reported improvement in neurological function in 40% of patients, whereas 42% remained unchanged, and the overall mortality was 18%. There was minimal morbidity with invasive hemodynamic monitoring. The authors concluded that hemodynamic monitoring in the intensive care setting allows early recognition of cardiac dysfunction and hemodynamic instability with a potential to reduce morbidity and mortality after SCI.

The study from Vale et al.[3] is described in an earlier section. Their group also reported a high incidence of vasopressor requirement in SCI patients, and improved neurological outcomes with invasive monitoring in the ICU and aggressive blood pressure treatment compared with previously published studies. The authors chose the high-normal target for MAP of 85 mmHg arbitrarily based on their previous experience with TBI patients, and a length of treatment of 7 days based on data from experimental SCI studies showing a period for maximal spinal cord edema lasting between 3 and 5 days. There were no complications related to the invasive hemodynamic monitoring.

Casha and Christie recently did a comprehensive literature review of cardiopulmonary management after SCI.[35] Their findings confirm that (1) the incidence of cardiorespiratory complications after acute SCI is high and warrants care in specialized monitoring units; (2) the period of greatest risk for hemodynamic instability ranges between 1 and 2 weeks, whereas respiratory failure requiring mechanical ventilation can last weeks; (3) a target MAP >85 mmHg in the first week after acute SCI is recommended, although the evidence is weak; (4) high cervical and complete SCI are the strongest predictive risk factors for cardiopulmonary complications; and (5) atelectasis and copious secretions are frequent obstacles to ventilatory weaning, and there is weak evidence to support that chest physiotherapy and aggressive suctioning are useful in the prevention of further respiratory complications.

Multimodal Monitoring for Spinal Cord Injury

The difficulty in finding objective, absolute targets and treatment thresholds for hemodynamic, respiratory, and metabolic parameters to optimize neurological recovery and prevent secondary injuries represents a unique challenge in SCI. In the treatment of TBI, new technologies have been applied with success to complement standard monitoring modalities in the ICU. These techniques allow for the measurement of cerebral physiological and metabolic parameters related to oxygen delivery, cerebral blood flow, and metabolism with the goal of improving the detection and management of secondary brain injury. They include jugular venous bulb oximetry, parenchymal brain tissue oxygen tension monitoring, cerebral microdialysis, and intraparenchymal cerebral blood flow (CBF) monitoring. Initial observational data suggest that these monitoring tools provide unique information that may help to individualize management in severe TBI.[36] Multimodality neuromonitoring in TBI is generally achieved with the placement of intraparenchymal probes. This type of monitoring is not desirable in SCI; intraparenchymal probe placement in injured cord tissue, or even in nearby normal areas, carries too great a risk for further injury. Noninvasive techniques, such as imaging, or less invasive extramedullary and extradural or surface monitors could provide alternatives to this problem.

We know little about the physiological changes that occur within the spinal cord in the early at-risk period after human SCI. A better understanding of these variables would help significantly, especially in the ICU, where rapid changes in clinical condition or shifts in therapeutic approach could be tailored based on the prevention of secondary injury. Concepts taken from the TBI field can be extrapolated to SCI.

Intraspinal Pressure

ICP monitoring is central to the management of patients with severe head injury. Elevated ICP is associated with increased mortality and worsened outcome.[37] Despite the lack of large randomized trials examining the effect of ICP monitoring on outcome, ICP treatment remains a core component of the guidelines for severe head injury management. Direct intraparenchymal spinal cord pressure monitoring is not feasible in humans. In TBI, ventricular catheters provide a cheap, reliable way of monitoring ICP and have the added benefit of allowing cerebrospinal fluid drainage to treat rises in ICP. A similar technique can be applied for SCI. Lumbar subarachnoid catheters can be inserted and give a reading of the intrathecal pressure, which is closely related to local tissue pressure.[38] Lumbar catheters are routinely used in neurosurgery and spinal surgery for the treatment of cerebrospinal fluid (CSF) leaks with minimal morbidity. Pressure readings can be obtained using standard transducers and will vary with the position of the catheter and patient. Readings could also be limited in the event that spinal cord swelling obstructs the normal flow of CSF along the neuraxis. In theory, spinal pressure monitoring could be useful in determining whether monitoring and CSF drainage help in neurological recovery or if changes occur after surgical spinal decompression.

Spinal Perfusion Pressure and Blood Flow

Through autoregulation, the normal cerebral vasculature maintains an adequate blood flow across a wide range of mean arterial blood pressure. The spinal cord and intracranial microcirculations are similar, including their ability for pressure autoregulation. Local vascular alterations and systemic hypotension following SCI can potentiate the ischemic injury. Similarly, induced systemic hypertension may increase the amount of hemorrhagic necrosis. Therefore, the relationship between systemic blood pressure and spinal cord blood flow is of vital importance for the management of patients with SCI.

CBF optimization is a foundation of TBI treatment.[37] Unfortunately, bedside measurement of CBF is not easily or widely obtainable. The concept of cerebral perfusion pressure (CPP) has been used as a more easily applicable alternative and is defined as the difference between the MAP and the ICP: CPP = MAP – ICP. It is the driving force for CBF through the cerebral vascular resistance. Because episodes of hypotension and raised ICP are both associated with worsened outcome in TBI, it is not surprising to find that episodes of low CPP are also associated with poorer outcome.[39] The concept of spinal perfusion has also been used in a similar fashion. The pressure conducted through the spinal cord microcirculation is the gradient between the spinal arterial inflow and the venous outflow pressures. The inflow pressure is directly dependent on the MAP. The venous outflow is more difficult to determine. However, as in the cerebral compartment, the venous pressure can be approximated to be close to, or slightly higher than, the surrounding intrathecal pressure to prevent collapse of the venous system.[38] Again in this situation, a lumbar catheter would allow direct measurement of the CSF pressure and approximation of the venous outflow pressure. Spinal cord perfusion pressure could be calculated as MAP–intrathecal pressure.

Therapies aimed at augmenting spinal cord perfusion pressure and blood flow can be applied in the ICU if appropriate measurements can be obtained. In TBI, it was initially postulated that induced hypertension to target CPP > 70 mmHg with volume expansion and vasopressor agents would improve outcome. There is now a growing body of evidence to suggest that routinely artificially maintaining CPP above such high levels may not be beneficial and carries a risk of severe extracerebral complications, such as acute respiratory distress syndrome (ARDS). Thus the guideline-recommended CPP threshold is to target a CPP between 60 and 70 mmHg and avoid levels below 50 mmHg.[37] Such guidelines do not exit for SCI, mainly because normal and pathological parameters have not yet been established. The current recommended treatment option of maintaining MAP at 85 mmHg for 7 days is based on a single uncontrolled pilot study.[3,10] In pathological states where pressure autoregulation is altered, treatment based solely on perfusion pressure can potentially lead to perfusion breakthrough and secondary injury in the form of hemorrhage and edema.

Knowledge of local spinal cord blood flow and vascular resistance can facilitate treatment decisions by determining if pressure autoregulation is intact or impaired. Hypothetically, patients with intact pressure autoregulation could benefit from higher MAP parameters, whereas more cautious settings could be applied to those with impaired autoregulation. Finally, it is possible that augmenting spinal cord perfusion pressure by lowering intrathecal pressure instead of increasing MAP has a more substantial effect in improving spinal cord blood flow. The concept of CSF drainage to prevent spinal cord ischemia is well established in thoracoabdominal aneurysm repair, where segmental arterial feeders and aortic cross-clamping can put the spinal cord at risk of infarction.[40] The mechanism involved is not completely understood but may be related to a relative decrease in venous pressure with CSF drainage, leading to an increased arteriovenous pressure gradient (perfusion pressure) beyond the control of autoregulatory mechanisms. The spinal cord venous pressure itself also appears to be important in spinal cord perfusion. It is closely related to the central venous pressure because the cerebrospinal venous system is valveless. Etz et al. recently reported a retrospective analysis of 20 cases of paraplegia after thoracoabdominal aortic aneurysm repair and found significantly higher mean central venous pressures in the early postoperative period compared with a control group.[41] The same is true in TBI, where elevations in central venous pressure are often accompanied by rises in ICP. Knowledge of the venous outflow pressure, which could be approximated by measuring intrathecal pressure, and local spinal cord blood flow would be essential in individualizing and optimizing treatment in SCI. Spinal cord blood flow measurement has been obtained in the past in animal models with invasive techniques. Magnetic resonance technology using arterial spin labeling has recently been used successfully to image local blood flow in the mouse spinal cord with relatively good spatial resolution.[42] Evolution of this technique to human SCI should be feasible and would yield new insight in microcirculatory changes after SCI and could potentially guide treatment. The ICU provides the ideal environment for this type of multimodal monitoring and blood-flow-targeted therapies.

Brain tissue oxygen tension ($P_{bt}O_2$) monitoring is now routinely used in specialized neurocritical care centers for the treatment of TBI. An intraparenchymal oxygen electrode measures $P_{bt}O_2$ when placed in the white matter. Despite the growing clinical use of this new technology, the specific determinants of low $P_{bt}O_2$ following severe TBI remain poorly defined. There is some indication that $P_{bt}O_2$ is more closely related to CBF and arteriovenous oxygen tension difference than oxygen delivery and metabolism.[43] Normal $P_{bt}O_2$ is > 20 mmHg; duration and depth of $P_{bt}O_2$ below 15 mmHg are associated with worsened outcome.[44] Noninvasive tissue oxygen monitoring techniques do not currently exist. Near-infrared spectroscopy has been used to measure brain tissue oxygen saturation, but this technique has not been applied to SCI. It is also unclear whether tissue oxygen tension and saturation monitoring detect the same physiological and pathophysiological changes in CNS injury.

Conclusion

Patients with SCI are at increased risk of hemodynamic, respiratory, and systemic deterioration, which can be life threatening and may potentiate secondary injury mechanisms. Several small, uncontrolled studies indicate that invasive monitoring and aggressive treatment of secondary insults in the ICU are associated with decreased mortality, improved neurological recovery, reduced length of hospital stay, and lower complication rates. Strict avoidance and rapid treatment of hypotension and hypoxia are essential in optimizing neurological recovery after SCI. Specialized neurocritical care units provide the ideal environment for the treatment and monitoring of SCI patients. Guideline-based standardized protocols using multimodal monitoring offer a potential novel approach to the management of SCI and may be implemented successfully with the help of new technologies and dedicated treatment facilities.

Pearls

- The core principle of ICU management of SCI is the prevention of secondary injury mechanisms and insults.
- It is recommended that patients be treated with vasopressors to keep an SBP >85 mmHg for a duration of 1 week after injury.
- A proactive approach of early intubation under controlled circumstances is recommended to avoid hypoxia and secondary SCI.
- CT scanning of the entire cervical spine using thin axial cuts and sagittal and coronal reconstructions is highly sensitive in detecting injuries and is the study of choice for cervical spine clearance in the unconscious patient.
- Monitoring in an intensive care setting with early detection and treatment of cardiovascular instability and respiratory failure can potentially reduce complications and improve outcome after SCI.
- (**Table 8.1**)

Pitfalls

- Patients with SCI are at increased risk for hemodynamic instability and respiratory compromise.
- Cervical and complete injuries are most commonly associated with hemodynamic instability and respiratory complications.
- Hemodynamic instability after acute SCI is common, with an incidence as high as 90% in complete cervical injuries.
- Respiratory complications are a major cause of morbidity and mortality after SCI.
- Approximately one third of patients with cervical SCI will require endotracheal intubation and ventilatory support.
- Careful monitoring and some degree of judgment are necessary to identify patients before respiratory decompensation occurs. A decrease in vital capacity to <1 L, rising respiratory rate, and elevated arterial PCO_2 are good indicators of impending respiratory failure
- Cervical spine clearance in unconscious and sedated patients in the ICU is challenging.
- (**Table 8.2**)

Table 8.1 Spinal Cord Injury in the ICU: Pearls

1. Key role of intensive care unit in spinal cord injury (SCI) treatment is prevention of secondary injury
2. Guidelines suggest treating SCI patients with vasopressors to keep an SBP >85 mmHg for 1 week after injury
3. Patients at risk of respiratory failure should be intubated early
4. Computed tomographic scanning of the entire cervical spine is the tool of choice for cervical spine clearance in the unconscious patient
5. Admission to specialized care centers with invasive monitoring and treatment of hemodynamic instability and respiratory failure can reduce complications and improve outcome after SCI

Table 8.2 Spinal Cord Injury in the ICU: Pitfalls

1. Patients with spinal cord injury (SCI) are at increased risks for hemodynamic instability and respiratory compromise
2. Cervical and complete SCIs are most commonly associated with hemodynamic instability and respiratory complications
3. Hemodynamic instability after acute SCI is common, as high as 90% in complete cervical injuries
4. Respiratory complications are a major cause of morbidity and mortality after SCI
5. One third of patients with cervical SCI will require intubation and ventilatory support
6. Patients at risk for respiratory decompensation need to be identified early; indicators of impending failure include vital capacity <1 L, rising respiratory rate, and elevated arterial PCO_2
7. Cervical spine clearance in unconscious and sedated patients in the intensive care unit is challenging

References

1. Levi L, Wolf A, Belzberg H. Hemodynamic parameters in patients with acute cervical cord trauma: description, intervention, and prediction of outcome. Neurosurgery 1993;33(6):1007–1016, discussion 1016–1017
2. Tator CH, Rowed DW, Schwartz ML, et al. Management of acute spinal cord injuries. Can J Surg 1984;27(3):289–293, 296
3. Vale FL, Burns J, Jackson AB, Hadley MN. Combined medical and surgical treatment after acute spinal cord injury: results of a prospective pilot study to assess the merits of aggressive medical resuscitation and blood pressure management. J Neurosurg 1997;87(2):239–246
4. Wolf A, Levi L, Mirvis S, et al. Operative management of bilateral facet dislocation. J Neurosurg 1991;75(6):883–890
5. Hall ED, Wolf DL. A pharmacological analysis of the pathophysiological mechanisms of posttraumatic spinal cord ischemia. J Neurosurg 1986;64(6):951–961
6. Tator CH, Fehlings MG. Review of the secondary injury theory of acute spinal cord trauma with emphasis on vascular mechanisms. J Neurosurg 1991;75(1):15–26
7. Fehlings MG, Phan N. Spinal cord and related injuries. In: Brinker MR, ed. Orthopaedic Trauma. Philadelphia: Saunders; 2001
8. Tator CH. Experimental and clinical studies of the pathophysiology and management of acute spinal cord injury. J Spinal Cord Med 1996;19(4): 206–214
9. Lehmann KG, Lane JG, Piepmeier JM, Batsford WP. Cardiovascular abnormalities accompanying acute spinal cord injury in humans: incidence, time course and severity. J Am Coll Cardiol 1987;10(1):46–52
10. Hadley MN. Blood pressure management after acute spinal cord injury. Neurosurgery 2002; 50(3, Suppl):S58–S62
11. Ball PA. Critical care of spinal cord injury. Spine 2001;26(24, Suppl):S27–S30
12. Guha A, Tator CH, Rochon J. Spinal cord blood flow and systemic blood pressure after experimental spinal cord injury in rats. Stroke 1989;20(3): 372–377
13. Chesnut RM, Marshall LF, Klauber MR, et al. The role of secondary brain injury in determining outcome from severe head injury. J Trauma 1993;34(2):216–222
14. Levi L, Wolf A, Rigamonti D, Ragheb J, Mirvis S, Robinson WL. Anterior decompression in cervical spine trauma: does the timing of surgery affect the outcome? Neurosurgery 1991;29(2): 216–222
15. Zäch GA, Seiler W, Dollfus P. Treatment results of spinal cord injuries in the Swiss Paraplegic Centre of Basle. Paraplegia 1976;14(1):58–65
16. Hassid VJ, Schinco MA, Tepas JJ, et al. Definitive establishment of airway control is critical for optimal outcome in lower cervical spinal cord injury. J Trauma 2008;65(6):1328–1332
17. Lu K, Lee TC, Liang CL, Chen HJ. Delayed apnea in patients with mid- to lower cervical spinal cord injury. Spine 2000;25(11):1332–1338
18. McMichan JC, Michel L, Westbrook PR. Pulmonary dysfunction following traumatic quadriplegia: recognition, prevention, and treatment. JAMA 1980;243(6):528–531
19. Gardner BP, Watt JW, Krishnan KR. The artificial ventilation of acute spinal cord damaged patients: a retrospective study of forty-four patients. Paraplegia 1986;24(4):208–220
20. Shatney CH, Brunner RD, Nguyen TQ. The safety of orotracheal intubation in patients with unstable cervical spine fracture or high spinal cord injury. Am J Surg 1995;170(6):676–679, discussion 679–680
21. Cotton BA, Pryor JP, Chinwalla I, Wiebe DJ, Reilly PM, Schwab CW. Respiratory complications and mortality risk associated with thoracic spine injury. J Trauma 2005;59(6):1400–1407, discussion 1407–1409
22. Craven DE. Epidemiology of ventilator-associated pneumonia. Chest 2000;117(4, Suppl 2): 186S–187S
23. Fagon JY, Chastre J, Hance AJ, Montravers P, Novara A, Gibert C. Nosocomial pneumonia in ventilated patients: a cohort study evaluating attributable mortality and hospital stay. Am J Med 1993;94(3):281–288
24. Wicks AB, Menter RR. Long-term outlook in quadriplegic patients with initial ventilator dependency. Chest 1986;90(3):406–410
25. Jackson AB, Groomes TE. Incidence of respiratory complications following spinal cord injury. Arch Phys Med Rehabil 1994;75(3):270–275
26. Estenne M, De Troyer A. Mechanism of the postural dependence of vital capacity in tetraplegic subjects. Am Rev Respir Dis 1987;135(2): 367–371
27. Goldman JM, Rose LS, Williams SJ, Silver JR, Denison DM. Effect of abdominal binders on breathing in tetraplegic patients. Thorax 1986;41(12): 940–945
28. Mansel JK, Norman JR. Respiratory complications and management of spinal cord injuries. Chest 1990;97(6):1446–1452
29. Cameron TS, McKinstry A, Burt SK, et al. Outcomes of patients with spinal cord injury before and after introduction of an interdisciplinary tracheostomy team. Crit Care Resusc 2009;11(1): 14–19
30. Hughes SJ. How effective is the Newport/Aspen collar? A prospective radiographic evaluation in healthy adult volunteers. J Trauma 1998; 45(2):374–378
31. Morris CG, McCoy E. Clearing the cervical spine in unconscious polytrauma victims, balancing risks and effective screening. Anaesthesia 2004; 59(5):464–482
32. Benzel EC, Hart BL, Ball PA, Baldwin NG, Orrison WW, Espinosa MC. Magnetic resonance imaging for the evaluation of patients with occult cervical spine injury. J Neurosurg 1996;85(5): 824–829
33. Spiteri V, Kotnis R, Singh P, et al. Cervical dynamic screening in spinal clearance: now redundant. J Trauma 2006;61(5):1171–1177, discussion 1177
34. Hadley MN. Management of acute spinal cord injuries in an intensive care unit or other moni-

tored setting. Neurosurgery 2002;50(3, Suppl): S51–S57
35. Casha S, Christie S. A systematic review of intensive cardiopulmonary management after spinal cord injury. J Neurotrauma 2011;28(8): 1479–1495
36. Rosenthal G, Hemphill JC, Sorani M, et al. The role of lung function in brain tissue oxygenation following traumatic brain injury. J Neurosurg 2008;108(1):59–65
37. Brain Trauma Foundation AAoNSA. Congress of Neurological Surgeons (CNS), AANS/CNS Joint Section on Neurotrauma and Critical Care Guidelines for the management of severe traumatic brain injury. J Neurotrauma 2007;24(Suppl 1):S1–S106
38. Greitz D. Unraveling the riddle of syringomyelia. Neurosurg Rev 2006;29(4):251–263, discussion 264
39. Andrews PJ, Sleeman DH, Statham PF, et al. Predicting recovery in patients suffering from traumatic brain injury by using admission variables and physiological data: a comparison between decision tree analysis and logistic regression. J Neurosurg 2002;97(2):326–336
40. Coselli JS, Lemaire SA, Köksoy C, Schmittling ZC, Curling PE. Cerebrospinal fluid drainage reduces paraplegia after thoracoabdominal aortic aneurysm repair: results of a randomized clinical trial. J Vasc Surg 2002;35(4):631–639
41. Etz CD, Luehr M, Kari FA, et al. Paraplegia after extensive thoracic and thoracoabdominal aortic aneurysm repair: does critical spinal cord ischemia occur postoperatively? J Thorac Cardiovasc Surg 2008;135(2):324–330
42. Duhamel G, Callot V, Decherchi P, et al. Mouse lumbar and cervical spinal cord blood flow measurements by arterial spin labeling: sensitivity optimization and first application. Magn Reson Med 2009;62(2):430–439
43. Rosenthal G, Hemphill JC III, Sorani M, et al. Brain tissue oxygen tension is more indicative of oxygen diffusion than oxygen delivery and metabolism in patients with traumatic brain injury. Crit Care Med 2008;36(6):1917–1924
44. Valadka AB, Gopinath SP, Contant CF, Uzura M, Robertson CS. Relationship of brain tissue PO_2 to outcome after severe head injury. Crit Care Med 1998;26(9):1576–1581

9

Concomitant Traumatic Brain Injury and Spinal Cord Injury

Daniel C. Lu, Nicolas Phan, Michael S. Beattie, and Geoffrey T. Manley

Key Points

1. Many cases of SCI, especially cervical cord injury, are accompanied by concomitant brain injury.
2. Individuals with SCI who also incurred mild or moderate TBI may be expected to have less functional recovery than those with SCI alone.
3. Concurrent SCI and TBI remain underdiagnosed and understudied. More attention to this complication of SCI is needed to improve both acute treatment and rehabilitation.

Traumatic spinal cord injury (SCI), and especially cervical SCI, is often accompanied by traumatic brain injury (TBI), although the reported coincidence varies widely between studies. A recent report of TBI complications in military personnel in Iraq reported a significant incidence of SCI (9.8%) along with other multiple traumas.[1] According to the Spinal Cord Model Systems dataset, 28.2% of SCI patients have at least a mild brain injury with loss of consciousness, whereas 11.5% have a TBI severe enough to demonstrate cognitive or behavioral changes.[2] The complications associated with this "dual-diagnosis" are well known in the rehabilitation setting[3] but may be underdiagnosed.[4] A recent study by Macciocchi et al.[5] estimated that 60% of SCI patients had at least mild TBI, and a prior retrospective study from this same center showed a substantial loss of recovery associated with dual diagnosis versus SCI alone.[6]

Identification of potential injury to the spine is critical in the evaluation of patients with blunt traumatic multisystem injuries. Depending on the mechanism of injury, the majority of patients with the dual diagnosis of TBI and SCI have injury to the cervical spine. However, assessment of the cervical spine in trauma victims presents specific challenges. Injuries in other systems can mask cervical column pain or discomfort, and obtundation from closed head injury or sedation limits the ability to perform an adequate clinical exam. Failure to recognize cervical injuries can have disastrous consequences. Few conditions are as devastating as cervical SCI and quadriplegia. Early diagnosis and acute management of identified or potential cervical spinal column injury and SCI are therefore essential in the treatment of the trauma patient.

The epidemiology of SCI has been studied in more detail than that of spinal column injuries. Cervical spine injury occurs in ~2 to 3% of patients with blunt trauma who undergo imaging studies.[7] The incidence of SCI in the United States is estimated to be between 40 and 50 cases per million people per year, giving rise to 12,000 new cases per year.[8] The global incidence of SCI has not been precisely studied, but estimates range from 10 to 83 cases per million population annually.[9] Cervical SCI is more frequent than thoracic and lumbar injuries. Furthermore, there has been a small relative increase in the proportion of cervical SCIs, from 54.5% between 1973 and 1979 to 56.5% between 2000 and 2003.[10]

Individuals with SCI who also incurred mild or moderate TBI will have less functional recovery than those with SCI alone. This hypothesis is based upon both clinical consensus and limited practice-based and epidemiological evidence. Specifically, individuals who sustained a documented or undocumented mild to moderate TBI in addition to an SCI would evidence impaired cognitive function at admission, achieve smaller functional gains during rehabilitation, and require longer periods of rehabilitation than peers who sustained only an SCI. The cognitive and emotional sequelae of TBI hold the potential to adversely affect learning and skills acquisition and should, therefore, be assessed in relation to impact on the rehabilitation process. A retrospective, single-institution study[6] has established that patients with SCI and comorbid TBI evidence smaller functional gains with rehabilitation. These results point to the importance of accurate and timely diagnosis and treatment of SCI in the setting of TBI. This chapter reviews the phenomenon of dual diagnosis, focusing on the cervical spinal cord, and discusses the challenges in diagnosis and management.

Dual Injury Definition

TBI is defined as damage to brain tissue caused by an external mechanical force as evidenced by medically documented loss of consciousness or posttraumatic amnesia (PTA) due to brain trauma or by objective neurological findings that can be reasonably attributed to TBI on physical examination or mental status examination. Within TBI, there is a broad spectrum of processes that account for brain injury (i.e., concussion, epidural hematoma, subdural hematoma, parenchymal contusion, diffuse axonal injury, etc.).

Similarly, SCI is defined as damage to the spinal cord caused by an external force. This injury would manifest itself in loss of motor or sensory function attributable to the level of SCI. The initial acute injury sustained during the inciting event can cause cord contusion, hematoma formation, or continued compression of the spinal cord. Various mechanisms can lead to such injury and have been well described by various groups, such as the AO Fracture Classification System (www.aofoundation.org).

A patient is defined as having a dual injury diagnosis if he suffers from both of the foregoing injuries. In looking at the world's largest database of SCI and TBI (the Spinal Cord Injury Model Systems of Care and the Traumatic Brain Injury Model Systems of Care, www.nscisc.uab.edu) there are common themes within these two patient populations: both have average ages in the 30s, the majority are male, and motor vehicle accidents and falls are the top causes of injuries. In the SCI population, the majority of patients have cervical injuries (50.7%), followed by thoracic (35.1%) and lumbosacral injuries (11%). **Figures 9.1** and **9.2** illustrate two representative clinical cases of concomitant TBI and SCI.

Clinical Assessment

A complete and detailed initial physical exam in a patient with dual diagnosis is crucial because further progression or improvement of neurological deficits can determine the management course (i.e., surgical vs conservative) as well as the prognosis. In patients with suspected head injury, an admission computed tomographic (CT) scan of the head to evaluate for surgical lesions is important. While

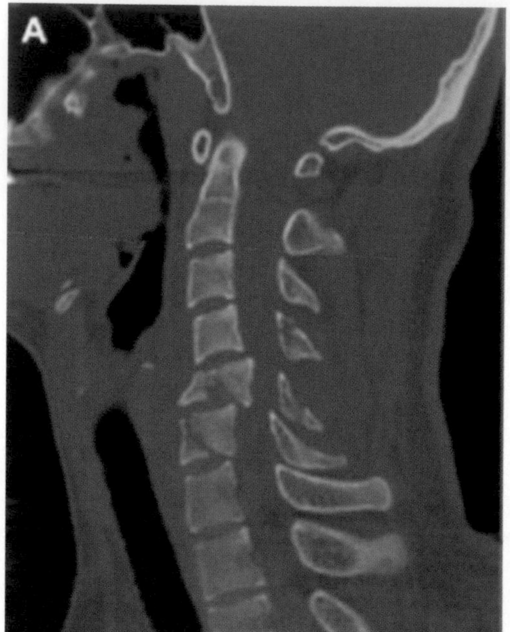

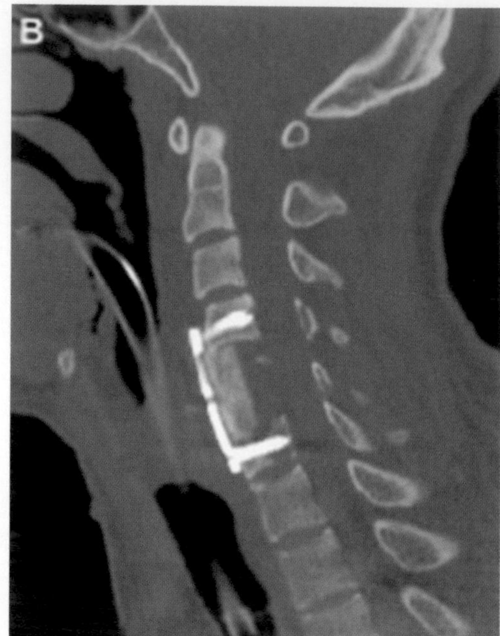

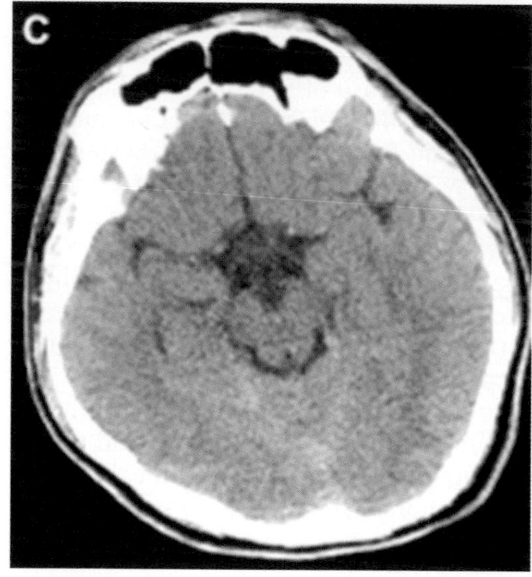

Fig. 9.1 This 22-year-old male was walking in the street during a windstorm. A billboard fell on the back of his head, resulting in loss of consciousness and hyperflexion of his cervical spine. He was intubated at the scene. His level of consciousness improved after resuscitation, but he was found to have a complete spinal cord injury with C5 level. **(A)** Admission midsagittal computed tomographic (CT) scan showing fractured C5 and C6 vertebral bodies and posterior elements. The posterior part of the C5 vertebral body is dislocated posteriorly within the spinal canal. **(B)** Postoperative midsagittal CT scan showing reduction and fusion of fracture deformity, done 48 hours after admission. **(C)** Admission brain CT scan at the level of the basal cisterns. The brain CT scan did not show any abnormality, consistent with severe concussion.

there is a tendency to focus on injuries to the head, injuries to the spinal cord should not be overlooked. In these patients, cervical spine injury must be assumed, and adequate radiographic images of the cervical spine should be obtained. Imaging should show all levels from the occiput to T1. If this cannot be achieved with plain radiographs, a CT scan with sagittal and coronal reconstructions should be obtained. Although this can exclude fractures or dislocation, magnetic resonance imaging (MRI) or dynamic fluoroscopy is required to rule out ligamentous injury. In awake patients, motor, sensory, reflex, and autonomic components should be thoroughly evaluated and the deficit levels noted. The spine should be palpated at each level, noting any tenderness, “step-off” deformities, or swellings.

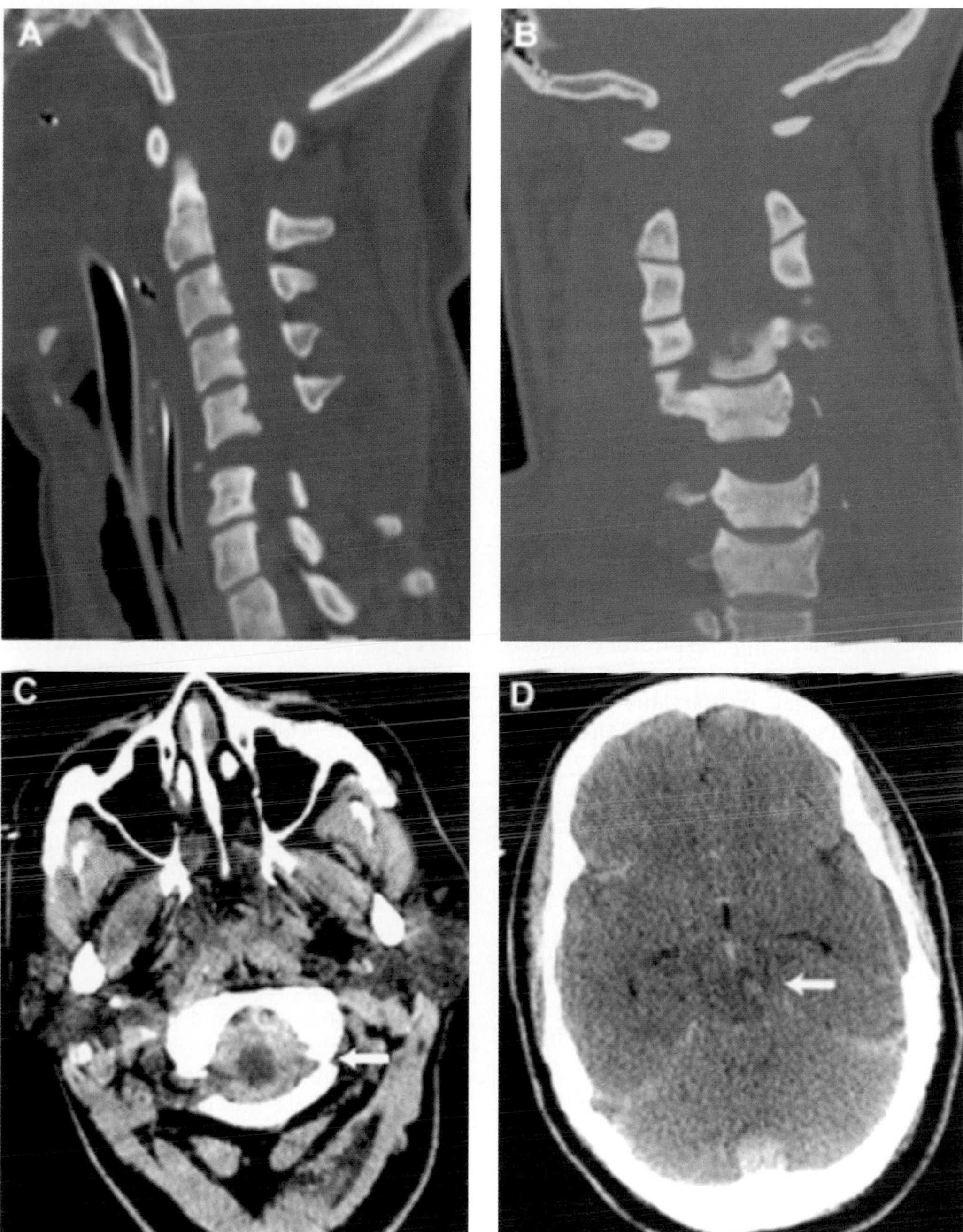

Fig. 9.2 This 42-year-old female was a pedestrian hit by an SUV at high speed. The Glasgow Coma Scale score at the scene was 3, and she had absent vital signs. Bystanders at the scene and emergency medical service revived her. She did not regain any neurological function after resuscitation and required inotropic support for neurogenic shock. **(A,B)** Sagittal and coronal computed tomographic (CT) scan of the cervical spine showing severe fracture dislocation and distraction at C5-6. **(C)** CT scan of the brain showing thick subarachnoid hemorrhage (SAH) at the craniocervical junction (*arrow*). **(D)** CT scan of the brain showing tight basal cisterns and hemorrhage within the brain stem (*arrow*). Because of the patient's poor neurological status and evidence of brain stem injury, aggressive management was not instigated. After discussion with the family, life support was withdrawn.

Complete versus Incomplete Spinal Cord Injury

SCI can result in complete or incomplete neurological deficits. In complete SCI, both motor and sensory components are absent below the level of injury, down to the lowermost sacral segments (S4 and S5). Sensations are absent, with paralysis and flaccid muscle tone. However, there may be partial motor or sensation present at the level just caudal to the injury with complete neurological deficit below this level. Reflexes are absent acutely but may become hyperactive with time. Patients can present with urinary retention with absent rectal tone, and males can present with priapism. The loss of sympathetic tone may result in neurogenic shock, which is more common in SCIs above the T6 level. Complete injury above the C3-5 level may also result in phrenic nerve paralysis and respiratory failure. In incomplete injury, motor or sensory components may be partially preserved below the level of injury. Incomplete SCI has better prognosis for recovery of function, whereas only 1 to 2% of patients with complete SCI recover significant distal cord function.

Spinal Shock

Spinal shock refers to the loss of somatic motor, sensory, and sympathetic autonomic function after SCI. Although the mechanism is unclear, it is thought to be due to loss of nerve conduction from deranged levels of electrolytes and neurotransmitters. The presence of spinal shock can cause significant confusion in the initial neurological assessment. The low blood pressure, if not treated aggressively, can also lead to secondary brain injury in patients with a dual diagnosis. The effect of spinal shock in regard to autonomic dysfunction, such as the bulbocavernosus reflex, and reflex dysfunctions may persists for days to weeks after SCI. However, the clinician should assume that its effects on the somatic motor and sensory examination have resolved by 1 hour after the initial injury.

ASIA/IMSOP Clinical Assessment Scale

Numerous clinical assessment scales have been developed to evaluate SCI patients. All of these scales assess either neurological or functional capacities of SCI patients to gauge loss or gain of function over time with consistent interrater reliability. Although it is routine to obtain and record the Glasgow Coma Scale (GCS) score for TBI patients, standardized assessment of SCI is not consistently performed. The most commonly used scale is the one developed by the American Spinal Injury Association (ASIA) in conjunction with the International Medical Society of Paraplegia (IMSOP). This scale divides patients into five grades of neurological deficits. Grade A denotes complete injury with no motor or sensory function. Grades B through D denote incomplete injuries below the anatomical level of the insult. Grade B denotes preserved sensory but no motor function, Grade C denotes preserved motor function with muscle strength grade less than 3, and Grade D denotes preserved motor function with muscle strength grade 3 or greater. Grade E denotes normal motor and sensory function. Furthermore, functional assessment tools have been developed, such as the Functional Independence Measure (FIM).[11] The FIM scores the patient's ability to perform activities of daily living, such as eating, grooming, and toileting. Thus, recovery over time can be measured in both neurological and functional components by incorporating the ASIA/IMSOP scale with the FIM. This combination of assessment tools not only measures the patient's neurological improvements over time but also incorporates improvements in functional capacities that may occur in the absence of neurological improvement.

Management

Acute Interventions

Every trauma patient subjected to significant mechanisms of injury is suspected to have a spinal injury until proven otherwise. Patients with cervical injuries are particularly vulnerable during transfer procedures due to the higher mobility of the cervical spine and the relative importance of the cervical spinal cord at risk. The absolute primacy of the "ABCs" cannot be overemphasized, especially in the setting of a TBI and an SCI. Adequate perfusion and oxygenation of injured brain and spinal cord are essential to optimize recovery. Even brief periods of hypoperfusion and hypoxia can trigger secondary injury mechanisms, which increase morbidity and mortality and decrease chances of neurological recovery.[12] Complete immobilization of the entire spine from the onset is necessary to prevent further injury to an already damaged spinal column or cord. If endotracheal intubation is required, the cervical spine is maintained in a neutral position without extension by applying gentle in-line traction. These important measures, which are implemented guidelines in the Advanced Trauma Life Support (ATLS) protocols, have contributed to a reduction in the ratio of quadriparesis to paraparesis in patients with multisystem trauma.[13]

The restoration of systemic hypotension to normotension is now a recognized principle of the emergency management in SCI based on the recognition that there is vascular compromise of the injured cord by local microcirculatory events. Initial resuscitation consists of volume replacement with crystalloids and blood products if persistent bleeding is suspected. Hypotension from neurogenic shock is much less common than hypovolemia in trauma patients, even in those with SCI, and is considered only after adequate volume replacement has been achieved and potential sources of ongoing bleeding have been ruled out. Treatment of hypotension in this case involves vasopressor agents.

Furthermore, prevention of hypoperfusion and hypotension is particularly important during surgical intervention, especially for other nonneurological injuries, such as orthopedic injuries, where intraoperative blood loss can be pronounced. We therefore recommend that nonurgent surgeries be postponed during the first week of the acute injury period to reduce the chance of secondary brain and spinal cord injuries. If urgent surgical intervention is necessary, specific instructions are to keep the mean arterial blood pressure above 80 mmHg or the cerebral perfusion pressure between 60 mmHg and 70 mmHg if an intracranial pressure monitor is present. The hemoglobin is also maintained at 10 g/dL to ensure adequate oxygen delivery.

It is recommended that all TBI patients with an admission GCS score of less than 8 be subjected to intracranial pressure monitoring. We attempt to place ventriculostomy catheters in most patients so that the cerebrospinal fluid (CSF) can be evacuated to relieve intracranial pressure. Even if the patient is taken to surgery, such CSF diversion can be a temporizing measure before surgical decompression is completed. Additionally, such monitoring may serve as a way to assess intracranial pressure during nonintracranial surgical intervention (spine, orthopedic, vascular, etc.).

The use of osmotic agents has demonstrated efficacy in TBI patients with intracranial hypertension.[14] However, the use of mannitol or hypertonic saline in treatment of SCI has not been demonstrated. Current use of osmotic agents in addressing SCI has been anecdotal and limited to published case reports with limited outcome data. However, recent data from a rat model of cervical SCI showed that 5% hypertonic saline given periodically over the 8 hours following injury reduced MRI indices of hemorrhage and edema.[15] Because hypertonic saline has been indicated for TBI,[16] this treatment may be an example of one that would be useful for combined SCI/TBI. Currently, we recommend that osmotic agents be used to treat intracranial hypertension if needed and not be used solely for SCI because there is no measureable end point for cord-specific treatment. Thus, although preclinical studies suggest a potential role for hypertonic saline in the treatment of SCI, more clinical studies are needed.

Intravenous corticosteroid therapy is the only pharmacological therapy currently used in the acute treatment of SCI. Two randomized, controlled trials, NASCIS

II and NASCIS III, published in 1990 and 1997, respectively, have shown benefits in patients treated with methylprednisolone in the acute setting.[17,18] A bolus of 30 mg/kg of methylprednisolone is given to patients seen within 8 hours of their injury. If the initial bolus is given within 3 hours, the treatment is continued with a continuous infusion of 5.4 mg/kg/h of methylprednisolone for 24 hours, whereas patients who received the initial bolus between 3 and 8 hours receive an infusion for 48 hours. The use of corticosteroids in the treatment of SCI has come under criticism since its inception.[19] Some critics have suggested that the benefits claimed in the original studies were not clinically significant and are outweighed by the risks and complications of the high-dose corticosteroid treatment. However, expert panels have maintained their support of this treatment as a recommendation but not a guideline in the treatment of SCI.[20] Patients with cervical SCI can benefit the most from gaining functional levels or be significantly more impaired by losing only one level. For example, maintenance or acquisition of C6 musculature provides a major increment in the functional status of quadriplegic patients, allowing them to transfer from bed, propel a wheelchair, and live independently. A gain or loss of level(s) in the setting of a mid- to lower-thoracic SCI is less likely to affect the final functional recovery and may therefore not warrant steroid treatment, especially in higher-risk patients.

The use of steroids for SCI in the dual diagnosis patient is particularly problematic given the recent results of the CRASH trial.[21] This mega trial demonstrated that patients receiving methylprednisolone for the treatment of TBI did worse. The TBI patients in this trial had severe TBI, defined as a GCS score of 8 or less. The study did not address the effect on patients with mild and moderate TBI. This raises the question of whether to treat a trauma patient with both SCI and TBI with steroids. Given the complexity and heterogeneity of these injuries in humans, small- and large-animal models of combined injury treated with steroids will likely provide information to guide future clinical trails.

Role and Timing of Surgical Intervention

The timing of surgery for intracranial pathology is relatively straightforward in comparison to a spinal pathology. For an intracranial space-occupying lesion, such as a hematoma, surgical decompression is performed when the size of the lesion or CT characteristics meet the criteria for surgical intervention or medical therapy fails to address the rise in intracranial pressure. During cranial surgery, it is important to note the possibility of cervical or spinal injury and to keep the head in a neutral position in a cervical collar with spinal precautions. In patients with known spine fractures and instability, a fluoroscope can be helpful to evaluate the patient before, during, and after positioning.

Likewise, if the patient is taken to the operating theater to address a spinal pathology, it is important note the intracranial pressure during surgery. If there is any concern regarding the intracranial pressure during surgery due to an intracranial lesion, an intracranial pressure monitor should be placed and measures taken to decrease the pressure (elevation of the head, osmotic therapy, hyperventilation, etc.) if it is indeed elevated during surgery. For cervical injuries, surgical fusion is required when injuries to the cervical spine result in instability. Classification systems like the SLIC system can be used to determine the need for fusion.[22] With the SLIC system, injuries with a score of 5 or more are all treated surgically, whereas those with a score of 3 or less are treated nonsurgically. A score of 4 is considered equivocal. There are two types of surgical approaches to the spine, anterior and posterior. Anterior approaches are best suited in the setting of mechanical failure of the anterior two columns, such as in vertebral body burst fracture, or when the spinal cord is compressed by elements located anteriorly, such as disrupted herniated disks. Posterior approaches can be used when no compressive elements are present anteriorly, when the posterior elements are severely disrupted, or when reduction from an anterior approach is not feasible or has failed. Severe injuries, such as in translation/

rotation injuries, or when the three columns are disrupted, sometimes warrant both anterior and posterior procedures, referred to as 360 degree procedures.

Thoracolumbar injuries follow a similar treatment algorithm. Classification with the TLICS can be used to determine the need for surgical stabilization.[23] TLICS and the Magerl/AO classification were demonstrated to have good correlation for surgical management prediction.[24] With the TLICS system, injuries with a score of 5 or more are treated surgically, whereas those with a score of 3 or less are treated nonsurgically. A score of 4 is equivocal. The surgical procedure is determined by the following general principles: (1) incomplete neurological injury requires an anterior procedure if compression from anterior spinal elements is present; (2) posterior ligamentous complex disruption requires a posterior procedure; and (3) combined incomplete neurological injury and posterior ligamentous complex disruption generally require a circumferential stabilization procedure.

The role and timing of surgical decompression in the setting of an SCI remain among the most controversial topics in spinal surgery, due to the lack of well-executed randomized, controlled trials.[25] Early decompression and stabilization of spinal column fractures allow early mobilization to prevent complications, such as pulmonary and urinary infections, decubitus ulcers, and deep vein thrombosis. Neurological worsening associated with persistent spinal cord compression by disk, bone fragments, or dislocated elements is a widely accepted indication for early surgery. Although it seems intuitive that early decompression after SCI may improve neurological recovery, the question remains for the most part unanswered. It has been thought in the past that early spinal surgery increases morbidity and mortality in patients with SCI.[26] However, modern techniques of spine surgery as well as advances in neurocritical care and neuroanesthesia have allowed these patients to undergo early surgery without a significant increase in complications.[27] Animal and radiological studies have shown that mechanical factors, such as persistent compression, are important in the pathogenesis and recovery from SCI.[28,29] Moreover, several prospective series suggest that early decompression can be performed safely and may improve outcome.[27,30,31] A meta-analysis of published clinical studies up to the year 2000 suggested that early decompression within 24 hours resulted in better outcomes compared with delayed decompression and conservative management.[32] Based on the foregoing assumptions, early decompression and stabilization may provide patients with SCI an optimal window neurological recovery, early mobilization, and rehabilitation.

Subacute Interventions

The most commonly used antiepileptic drug, phenytoin, is given routinely for seizure prevention during recovery from TBI.[33] This drug has been shown to be neuroprotective, in addition to (or in part because of) reduction of seizures and hyperexcitability. Previous studies have demonstrated the lack of efficacy in preventing long-term seizures with phenytoin use.[34] Additionally, the side effects of antiepileptics, including motor and cognitive dysfunction, could potentially retard recovery and rehabilitation. Therefore, short-term use of phenytoin is advised. However, the issue is complicated by the presence of preclinical data suggesting that agents like phenytoin that reduce Na^+-channel permeability may have a neuroprotective effect in both SCI[35] and TBI.

Neuropathic pain is often a side effect of SCI. In a recent animal study, a commonly used pain medication, morphine, was shown to impair recovery of locomotion in a rat thoracic SCI model.[36] It is important to note that drugs used to reduce neuropathic pain after injury, such as gabapentin and opiates, may retard recovery and the cognitive and plasticity processes needed for rehabilitation after dual injuries and should be used only as necessary. And yet these drugs may also be neuroprotective. This points out the need for good animal models of SCI plus TBI to address some of these issues. Such models are conspicuously lacking.

Conclusion

The dual diagnosis of concomitant brain injury and SCI has only recently been recognized as a distinct diagnostic entity despite its high prevalence in the traumatic setting. Thorough clinical and radiographic evaluation of the spine, particularly the cervical spine, is essential following blunt head trauma. In the setting of SCI, early diagnosis and treatment are necessary to prevent neurological deterioration. This may not always be possible in the dually diagnosed patient with a severe TBI and active neurocritical care issues, such as elevated ICP. Although questions remain regarding optimal timing of surgical treatment and medical management of SCI, it is likely that the evolving multidisciplinary approach will lead to improved treatment, recovery, and outcome for patients with concomitant TBI and SCI.

Pearls

- Every trauma patient subjected to significant mechanisms of injury is suspected to have a spinal injury until proven otherwise.
- Early spinal decompression (<24 hours) may provide SCI patients an optimal window of neurological recovery, early mobilization, and rehabilitation.
- Surgical parameters in concomitant injury are mean arterial pressure >80 mmHg, cerebral perfusion pressure 60 to 70 mmHg, hemoglobin >10 g/dL.

Pitfalls

- Full spine survey is essential in a comatose patient because contiguous and noncontiguous spine injuries are present in up to 20% of patients.
- Manipulation of the cervical spine during head positioning for cranial decompression could further exacerbate spinal injuries.
- Intracranial pathology (hematoma, edema) could progress during spinal surgery. It is therefore essential to perform intracranial pressure monitoring in patients with intracranial pathology undergoing spinal surgery.

References

1. Bell RS, Vo AH, Neal CJ, et al. Military traumatic brain and spinal column injury: a 5-year study of the impact blast and other military grade weaponry on the central nervous system. J Trauma 2009;66(4, Suppl):S104–S111
2. Lin VW, Cardenas DD. Spinal Cord Medicine: Principles and Practice. NY, New York: Demos; 2002
3. Sommer JL, Witkiewicz PM. The therapeutic challenges of dual diagnosis: TBI/SCI. Brain Inj 2004;18(12):1297–1308
4. Tolonen A, Turkka J, Salonen O, Ahoniemi E, Alaranta H. Traumatic brain injury is under-diagnosed in patients with spinal cord injury. J Rehabil Med 2007;39(8):622–626
5. Macciocchi S, Seel RT, Thompson N, Byams R, Bowman B. Spinal cord injury and co-occurring traumatic brain injury: assessment and incidence. Arch Phys Med Rehabil 2008;89(7):1350–1357
6. Macciocchi SN, Bowman B, Coker J, Apple D, Leslie D. Effect of co-morbid traumatic brain injury on functional outcome of persons with spinal cord injuries. Am J Phys Med Rehabil 2004;83(1):22–26
7. Hoffman JR, Schriger DL, Mower W, Luo JS, Zucker M. Low-risk criteria for cervical-spine radiography in blunt trauma: a prospective study. Ann Emerg Med 1992;21(12):1454–1460
8. McDonald JW, Sadowsky C. Spinal-cord injury. Lancet 2002;359(9304):417–425
9. Wyndaele M, Wyndaele JJ. Incidence, prevalence and epidemiology of spinal cord injury: what learns a worldwide literature survey? Spinal Cord 2006;44(9):523–529
10. National Spinal Cord Injury Statistical Center. Spinal cord injury. Facts and figures at a glance. J Spinal Cord Med 2005;28(4):379–380
11. Ditunno JF Jr. Functional assessment measures in CNS trauma. J Neurotrauma 1992;9(Suppl 1):S301–S305
12. Tator CH, Fehlings MG. Review of the secondary injury theory of acute spinal cord trauma with emphasis on vascular mechanisms. J Neurosurg 1991;75(1):15–26
13. Vale FL, Burns J, Jackson AB, Hadley MN. Combined medical and surgical treatment after acute spinal cord injury: results of a prospective pilot study to assess the merits of aggressive medical resuscitation and blood pressure management. J Neurosurg 1997;87(2):239–246
14. Sorani MD, Manley GT. Dose-response relationship of mannitol and intracranial pressure: a metaanalysis. J Neurosurg 2008;108(1):80–87
15. Nout YS, Mihai G, Tovar CA, Schmalbrock P, Bresnahan JC, Beattie MS. Hypertonic saline attenu-

ates cord swelling and edema in experimental spinal cord injury: a study utilizing magnetic resonance imaging. Crit Care Med 2009;37(7): 2160–2166
16. Ware ML, Nemani VM, Meeker M, Lee C, Morabito DJ, Manley GT. Effects of 23.4% sodium chloride solution in reducing intracranial pressure in patients with traumatic brain injury: a preliminary study. Neurosurgery 2005;57(4):727–736, discussion 727–736
17. Bracken MB, Shepard MJ, Collins WF, et al. A randomized, controlled trial of methylprednisolone or naloxone in the treatment of acute spinal-cord injury. Results of the Second National Acute Spinal Cord Injury Study. N Engl J Med 1990;322(20):1405–1411
18. Bracken MB, Shepard MJ, Holford TR, et al. Administration of methylprednisolone for 24 or 48 hours or tirilazad mesylate for 48 hours in the treatment of acute spinal cord injury. Results of the Third National Acute Spinal Cord Injury Randomized Controlled Trial. National Acute Spinal Cord Injury Study. JAMA 1997;277(20): 1597–1604
19. Hurlbert RJ. The role of steroids in acute spinal cord injury: an evidence-based analysis. Spine 2001;26(24, Suppl):S39–S46
20. Fehlings MG. Editorial: recommendations regarding the use of methylprednisolone in acute spinal cord injury: making sense out of the controversy. Spine 2001;26(24, Suppl):S56–S57
21. Edwards P, Arango M, Balica L, et al; CRASH trial collaborators. Final results of MRC CRASH, a randomised placebo-controlled trial of intravenous corticosteroid in adults with head injury-outcomes at 6 months. Lancet 2005;365(9475): 1957–1959
22. Vaccaro AR, Hulbert RJ, Patel AA, et al; Spine Trauma Study Group. The subaxial cervical spine injury classification system: a novel approach to recognize the importance of morphology, neurology, and integrity of the disco-ligamentous complex. Spine 2007;32(21):2365–2374
23. Vaccaro AR, Lehman RA Jr, Hurlbert RJ, et al. A new classification of thoracolumbar injuries: the importance of injury morphology, the integrity of the posterior ligamentous complex, and neurologic status. Spine 2005;30(20):2325–2333
24. Joaquim AF, Fernandes YB, Cavalcante RA, Fragoso RM, Honorato DC, Patel AA. Evaluation of the thoracolumbar injury classification system in thoracic and lumbar spinal trauma. Spine 2011;36(1):33–36
25. Fehlings MG, Tator CH. An evidence-based review of decompressive surgery in acute spinal cord injury: rationale, indications, and timing based on experimental and clinical studies. J Neurosurg 1999;91(1, Suppl):1–11
26. Marshall LF, Knowlton S, Garfin SR, et al. Deterioration following spinal cord injury: a multicenter study. J Neurosurg 1987;66(3):400–404
27. Fehlings MG, Perrin RG. The role and timing of early decompression for cervical spinal cord injury: update with a review of recent clinical evidence. Injury 2005;36(Suppl 2):B13–B26
28. Guha A, Tator CH, Endrenyi L, Piper I. Decompression of the spinal cord improves recovery after acute experimental spinal cord compression injury. Paraplegia 1987;25(4):324–339
29. Delamarter RB, Sherman J, Carr JB. Pathophysiology of spinal cord injury. Recovery after immediate and delayed decompression. J Bone Joint Surg Am 1995;77(7):1042–1049
30. Tator CH, Duncan EG, Edmonds VE, Lapczak LI, Andrews DF. Comparison of surgical and conservative management in 208 patients with acute spinal cord injury. Can J Neurol Sci 1987;14(1): 60–69
31. Waters RL, Adkins RH, Yakura JS, Sie I. Effect of surgery on motor recovery following traumatic spinal cord injury. Spinal Cord 1996;34(4): 188–192
32. La Rosa G, Conti A, Cardali S, Cacciola F, Tomasello F. Does early decompression improve neurological outcome of spinal cord injured patients? Appraisal of the literature using a meta-analytical approach. Spinal Cord 2004;42(9): 503–512
33. Temkin NR, Dikmen SS, Wilensky AJ, Keihm J, Chabal S, Winn HR. A randomized, double-blind study of phenytoin for the prevention of post-traumatic seizures. N Engl J Med 1990;323(8): 497–502
34. Temkin NR. Antiepileptogenesis and seizure prevention trials with antiepileptic drugs: meta-analysis of controlled trials. Epilepsia 2001;42(4):515–524
35. Schwartz G, Fehlings MG. Evaluation of the neuroprotective effects of sodium channel blockers after spinal cord injury: improved behavioral and neuroanatomical recovery with riluzole. J Neurosurg 2001;94(2, Suppl):245–256
36. Hook MA, Moreno G, Woller S, et al. Intrathecal morphine attenuates recovery of function after a spinal cord injury. J Neurotrauma 2009;26(5):741–752

10

Pharmacotherapy in Acute Spinal Cord Injury: Focus on Steroids

Edward M. Marchan, George Ghobrial, Benjamin M. Zussman, James S. Harrop, and Alpesh A. Patel

Key Points

1. High-dose steroids are commonly used in the treatment of acute spinal cord injury.
2. Significant limitations exist in both the animal and the clinical literature supporting the use of steroids in acute spinal cord injury.
3. Potential complications exist that are associated with high-dose steroids in patients with acute spinal cord injury.
4. Given the risks and benefits, high-dose steroids should be used cautiously and with careful observation in patients with acute spinal cord injury.

Incidence of Acute Spinal Cord Injury

Advances in the understanding of basic physiology and neurobiology in spinal cord injury (SCI) and the development of therapeutic strategies have progressed at a frustratingly slow rate. This is in spite of the estimated incidence of traumatic SCI in the United States of 15 to 40 new cases per million population, or 12,000 cases annually.[1–3] Although the figures for incidence are high due to the impact on the younger population, the estimates of prevalence vary from ~ 183,000 to 230,000 cases in the United States, or the equivalent of 700 to 900 cases per million. The direct cost of SCI is estimated to be in excess of $7 billion annually[1,2] and bears the greater cost of loss of life, productivity, emotional suffering, and diminished quality of life for patients and families.[1–3]

Historical Pharmacological Treatment

During the last 2 decades, new hope emerged for patients with SCI in the form of several promising therapies heading toward clinical trial. These proposed therapies included tirilizad mesylate, GM-1 ganglioside, thryotropin-releasing hormone (TRH), gacyclidine, naloxone, and nimodipine. Unfortunately, these therapies were unable to demonstrate efficacy for neurological improvement and thus were not accepted by the medical community.[4–6]

The only therapeutic intervention for acute SCI that has been widely utilized has been the use of high-dose intravenous methylprednisolone (MPSS). Despite initial enthusiasm and continued clinical use, the role of MPSS remains controversial. The potential benefits of MPSS have been brought into question as the complications associated with the administration of high-dose MPSS have been clarified. This chapter reviews pharmacological treatment strategies for acute SCI with a focus on the basic and clinical science data supporting and refuting the use of high-dose MPSS.

Basic Science

Pharmacology of Corticosteroids

Acute SCI is believed to involve a two-step mechanism.[2] The primary mechanism involves the initial, traumatic mechanical injury due to local deformation and energy transformation directly on the spinal cord parenchymal tissue. The secondary mechanism encompasses a cascade of biochemical and cellular processes that are initiated by the primary process, often leading to further cellular damage and potentiating cell death (**Fig. 10.1**).[2] The secondary mechanism of acute SCI was first postulated by Allen[7] in 1911 after he described an improvement in neurological function with the removal of posttraumatic hematomyelia in dogs after a traumatically induced acute SCI. The effects of free radicals, as advocated by Demopoulos et al.,[8] were thought to be crucial to the injury process. The focus of research has shifted to the role of calcium, opiate receptors, and lipid peroxidation. Recently, research has implicated apoptosis, intracellular protein synthesis inhibition, and glutaminergic mechanisms, among a myriad of pathophysiological pathways that mediate secondary injury mechanisms (**Fig. 10.1**).

There is considerable evidence that the primary mechanical injury initiates a plethora of secondary injury mechanisms, including the following: (1) vascular changes, including ischemia, impaired autoregulation, and microcirculatory derangements[9]; (2) ionic derangements[10]; (3) neurotransmitter accumulation, including serotonin or catecholamines and extracellular glutamate, the latter causing excitotoxic cell injury (**Fig. 10.1**)[11]; (4) arachidonic acid release and free radical production[11] and lipid peroxidation[12]; (5) endogenous opioids; (6) inflammation; (7) loss of adenosine triphosphate–dependent cellular processes; and (8) programmed cell death or apoptosis.[2]

Methylprednisolone has been proposed to act by reducing secondary injury, in part by the scavenging of lipid peroxyl radicals.[13] Consequently, MPSS is thought to inhibit the lipid peroxidation (LP) cascade and, hence, preserve neurons, axons, myelin, and intracellular organelles, including the mitochondria and nucleus, by preventing free radical injury. However, more recent studies have suggested that methylprednisolone acts preferentially on glial cells with a diminished effect on neurons.

MPSS has also been shown to inhibit oligodendrocyte death via activation of the glucocorticoid receptor (GR) (**Fig. 10.1**), which binds to the STAT5 receptor resulting in the upregulation of the expression of the *blc-X$_l$* gene.[13] In monocytes, macrophages, and T lymphocytes, the response to the activation of the GR is opposite, resulting in apoptosis. It is postulated that the antiapoptotic effects are due to the increased expression of the neuroprotective cytokine erythropoietin, which is seen in oligodendrocytes.

Dosing Strategies

Increasing knowledge of the posttraumatic LP mechanism in the 1970s and early 1980s prompted the search for a neuroprotective pharmacological strategy aimed at antagonizing oxygen radical-induced LP in a safe and effective manner. Attention was focused on the possibility that glucocorticoid steroids might be effective inhibitors based upon their high lipid solubility as well as their ability to intercalate into artificial membranes be-

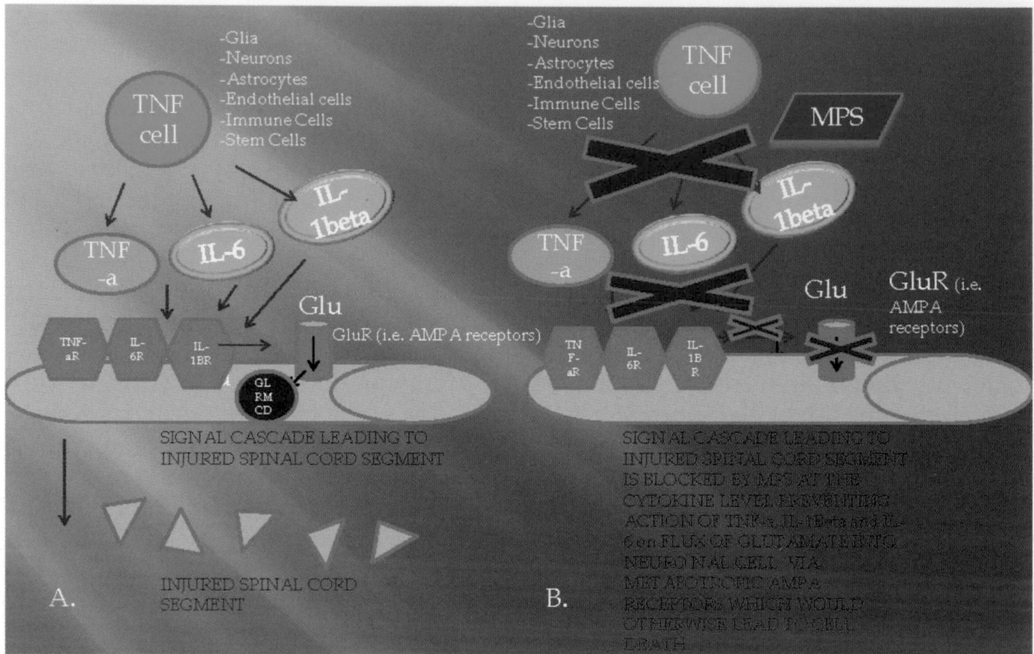

Fig. 10.1 Mechanistic diagram describing the potential action of methylprednisolone (MPS) on cytokine [tumor necrosis factor-α, (TNF- α), interleukin (IL)-6, IL-1β] formation and release by TNF-producing cells (i.e., glia, neurons, astrocytes, endothelial cells, immune cells) in the extracellular milieu of the injured spinal cord tissue. **(A)** In the acute spinal cord injury setting, release of TNF-α, IL-6, IL-1β by a TNF cell leads to binding of these cytokines to each of their respective receptors (TNF-αR, IL-6R, IL-1βR) in the neuronal cell membrane. Subsequently, a signal is sent for opening of the metabotropic glutamate receptor (GluR) (i.e., AMPA receptor) leading to an extracellular to intracellular flux of glutamate (Glu) into the cell, which facilitates glutamate receptor–mediated cell death (GLRMCD). **(B)** Administration of MPS in the first 8 hours of injury (preferably during the first 4 hours) leads to an inhibition of cytokine formation in the extracellular milieu, consequently blocking the process of GLRMCD.

tween the hydrophobic polyunsaturated fatty acids of the membrane phospholipids, thereby limiting the propagation of LP chain reactions.[13]

Hall and Braughler[14] investigated the effects of high-dose MPSS (15 to 90 mg/kg IV) on spinal cord electrophysiology. In an initial set of experiments in cats, it was observed that the administration of an intravenous bolus of MPSS could indeed inhibit posttraumatic LP in spinal cord tissue, but that the doses required for this effect were much higher (30 mg/kg) than previously hypothesized or than those empirically employed in the clinical treatment of acute central nervous system (CNS) injury. Further experimental studies, also conducted in cat SCI models, showed that the 30 mg/kg dose of MPSS not only prevented LP but, in parallel, also inhibited posttraumatic spinal cord ischemia. Braughler and Hall[14] found that a 30 mg/kg dose of MPSS followed at 2 hours by a 15 mg/kg dose provides significantly better protection against injury-induced ischemia and Ca^{2+}-dependent neurofilament degradation than a single 30 mg/kg dose. With many of these therapeutic parameters (LP, secondary ischemia, aerobic energy metabolism), the dose–response for MPSS followed a sharp U-shaped pattern. The neuro- and vasoprotective effect is partial with a dose of 15 mg/kg, optimal at 30 mg/kg, and diminishes at higher doses (60 mg/kg).

The antioxidant neuroprotective action of MPSS is closely linked to the drug's tissue pharmacokinetics.[14] For instance, when MPSS tissue levels are at their peak following administration of a 30 mg/kg intravenous dose, lactate levels in the injured cord are inhibited. The subsequent administration of a second dose (15 mg/kg IV), at the time at which the levels after the first dose have declined by 50%, acts to maintain the peak suppression of lactate and more effectively maintains adenosine triphosphate (ATP) generation and energy charge.[15,16] These findings suggested that prolonged MPSS therapy might better suppress the secondary injury process and lead to better outcomes compared with the effects of a single large intravenous dose. Indeed, subsequent experiments in a cat spinal injury model demonstrated that animals treated with MPSS using a 48-hour antioxidant dosing regimen had improved recovery of motor function over a 4-week period.[13]

Animal Spinal Cord Injury Data

Glucocorticoids have been repeatedly shown to inhibit axonal sprouting and synaptogenesis in various CNS regions.[17,18] Although it is not known whether these actions occur concomitantly with the acute antioxidant neuroprotective effects, the potential of steroids to attenuate posttraumatic plasticity mechanisms is a serious concern. Thus the potential for steroid side effects, inhibition of plasticity mechanisms, and even neurotoxic actions underscores the fact that glucocorticoids like MPSS are a far-from-ideal approach to dealing with the posttraumatic oxidative stress and LP-related damage and consequent need for antioxidant dosing that continues beyond the first 24 to 48 hours.

Despite concerns about the potential inhibitory and neurotoxic effects of MPSS, it is encouraging that high doses of MPSS have actually been reported to diminish axonal dieback of vestibulospinal fibers and to promote their terminal sprouting in transected rat spinal cords.[19] Thus the question of whether high-dose MPSS is neuroprotective or neurotoxic may depend on dose selection, timing, and duration of administration and the particular neuronal population in question.

Clinical Studies

Randomized, Controlled Trials

NASCIS I

Three landmark National Acute Spinal Cord Injury studies examined the use of MPSS for acute traumatic SCI. The first NASCIS study, published in 1984 and 1985,[20] compared a high-dose with a low-dose cohort of methylprednisolone (level of evidence: III). The investigated groups included a high-dose methylprednisolone treatment (1000 mg bolus/d) versus the standard dose (100 mg bolus/d) in 330 patients for 10 days after SCI. A placebo was judged unethical because of an assumed benefit from steroid administration and was therefore excluded.[21] Motor scores were determined based on the Bracken scale, from the examination of seven muscle groups on each side of the body scored on a 6-point scale. The authors reported the motor and sensory scores from the right side of the body only.

No difference in neurological recovery of motor function or pinprick and light touch sensation was observed between the two treatment groups at 6 weeks and at 6 months after injury (p = 0.63 at 6 weeks, and p = 0.59 at 6 months). The lack of a treatment effect was independent of the severity of the initial lesion or the time from injury to starting treatment.

To the contrary, significant complications were reported in both treatments, more often in the high-dose MPSS group. Early mortality was statistically greater in the high-dose protocol (relative risk of 3.1 and 1.9, ≤14 and 15 to 28 days after injury, respectively). Wound infections were also more prevalent in the high-dose regimen (relative risk of 3.6). Subsequent animal studies completed after NASCIS I suggested that higher doses were required for neuroprotection than were included in the NASCIS I study,[15,22] influencing development of the NASCIS II trial.[23]

NASCIS II

The NASCIS II study was designed as a prospective, randomized, controlled clinical trial (level of evidence: II). The study examined intravenous high-dose MPSS (30 mg/kg bolus with 5.4 mg/kg/h for 23 hours); the opioid antagonist naloxone, a proposed neuroprotective drug; and placebo. Intervention was initiated within 24 hours of injury. In the initial analysis of all patients randomized within 24 hours, there was no neurological benefit in either the MPSS-treated group or the naloxone group compared with placebo at 1 year follow-up of 487 enrolled patients. Though not reaching statistical significance, greater complication rates, including wound infection and pulmonary embolism, were found in the steroid group compared with both naloxone and placebo.

A post hoc analysis was performed and demonstrated significant differences in patients receiving steroids within 8 hours of injury. Motor and sensory improvements were reported at 6 months, though only motor improvements were found at 1-year follow-up. No benefits were found for administering MPSS in acute nonpenetrating SCI more than 8 hours after injury. Though vigorously defended, no evidence has been presented to support use of the 8-hour stratification, making it an otherwise arbitrary time point found to be significant in the post hoc analysis. Additionally, the calculated motor score differences (16.0 vs 11.2) do not translate into functionally significant improvements.

One of the major critiques of this study is that all primary outcome measures of NASCIS II were negative. It is interesting to see that no table or graph exists where data are displayed as a function of time and subjected to mathematical algorithms to establish a correlation. With the multiple post hoc comparisons required to discover these differences, it remains quite possible that the observations reflect random chance alone.[21]

The NASCIS II has also been widely criticized for its failure to include outcomes important to the patient. This was criticized sharply by Hurlbert,[21] raising questions concerning the clinical importance of reported neurological recovery among patients treated within 8 hours. To correct this oversight, the NASCIS III protocol included the American Spinal Injury Association (ASIA) Functional Independence Measure (FIM) assessment. Furthermore, Bracken and Holford[24] also published a retrospective estimate of functional recovery in NASCIS II from results modeled in the NASCIS III study. In that report, the authors claimed that the MPSS therapy-related motor function recovery observed in NASCIS II predicted a clinically important recovery in the FIM.[24] However, there was a lack of robustness in statistical modeling, limiting the value of this retrospective evaluation.

NASCIS III

The NASCIS III trial compared the 24-hour infusion of MPSS used in NASCIS II to a 48-hour high-dose MPSS infusion as well as a treatment group that received tirilizad mesylate, a 21-aminosteroid and antioxidant without the negative perceived glucocorticoid effects.[23–25] All patients had their treatment initiated within 8 hours of SCI. No placebo group was included because it was again deemed ethically inappropriate to withhold at least the initial large bolus of MPSS. This trial demonstrated no sustained benefit to high-dose MPSS with respect to motor and sensory scores among the 499 randomized patients at 1-year follow-up. Again, a post hoc analysis noted that patients receiving the MPSS bolus between 3 to 8 hours after injury demonstrated improved neurological function at 6 weeks and 6 months, but not at 1 year, when they were given MPSS for 48 hours rather than 24 hours. Patients treated within 3 hours after SCI demonstrated no differences between 24- and 48-hour infusions.

Timing of Administration

Bracken et al., as a result of NASCIS III, recommended that, within 3 hours of injury, patients receive a 24-hour infusion, whereas for those treated between 3 and 8 hours postinjury, a 48-hour MPSS regimen was better than the 24-hour regimen of the NASCIS II protocol.[25] Due to the post hoc analysis in the NASCIS II trial, attention was placed on the particular issue of drug delivery within 8 hours and MPSS physiology.

Hurlbert[21] demonstrated that a physiological rationale does not exist for the selection of 8 hours as a determinant of steroid efficacy. This author stated that the 8-hour window is strictly arbitrary and represents a post hoc finding that is inherently flawed, making this time window questionable.

Complications with the Use of MPSS

The NASCIS II and III studies reported potential complications due to high-dose steroid administration that may have serious negative ramifications for patients. In the NASCIS II trial there was a 1.5-fold higher incidence of gastrointestinal hemorrhage, twofold higher incidence of wound infection, and threefold higher incidence of pulmonary embolism in the MP group as compared with controls. Similarly, in NASCIS III, the 48-hour regimen was associated with a twofold higher rate of severe pneumonia, a fourfold higher rate of severe sepsis, and a sixfold higher incidence of death than in the 24-hour group.[21]

Although the differences did not reach statistical significance, the trend is concerning because the impact of these complications can be catastrophic. Further, it is important to note that a priori sample size calculations, based on NASCIS II data, indicate over 1400 patients (sample size for binomial proportion, b = 0.8) would be required to prove statistically that no differences in the rate of wound infection exist between both groups.[21]

Of more concern is the observation in NASCIS III of a sixfold higher incidence of death due to respiratory complications in the 48-hour MP group than in the 24-hour MP group ($p = 0.056$), suggesting a higher mortality rate associated with a 48-hour protocol.[21] However, the potential for complications associated with 48-hour high-dose MPSS must be balanced against the results of NASCIS III wherein the extension of dosing to 48 hours produces a significantly better neurological outcome compared with the 24-hour regimen in patients treated after 3 hours.

CRASH Study

The foregoing NASCIS III morbidities are akin to the worrisome complications discovered in the recent CRASH trial, which studied steroids in head injury. In this study, head-injured patients with a Glasgow Coma Scale score of 14 or less received either a loading dose of 2 g of methylprednisolone followed by a 0.4 g/h infusion for 48 hours or matching placebo within 8 hours of injury. This randomized, controlled trial was stopped early when it was discovered at interim analysis that steroid-treated patients had significantly higher all-cause 2-week mortality (21.1% vs 17.9%, $p = 0.0001$).[26] Subsequent follow-up demonstrated that 6-month mortality was also higher in steroid-treated patients (25.7% vs 22.3%, $p = 0.0001$.[28] Interestingly, complications, such as seizures, gastrointestinal bleeding, and infection, were similar in both groups. The authors noted that they were unsure of the mechanism of increased mortality with steroids. The lack of an identifiable etiology, however, does not diminish the validity or importance of the results.[26]

Penetrating Trauma Indications

At the present time, none of the data from the three NASCIS studies support the use of methylprednisolone for penetrating trauma. These authors concluded that patients who sustain an SCI secondary to a gunshot wound or other penetrating injury to the spine should not be treated with steroids until the efficacy of such treatment is proven in a controlled study.[27]

Medicolegal Aspects of Corticosteroid Use

The utility of high-dose methylprednisolone infusion for acute SCI has not been clearly defined in the medical literature. Methylprednisolone is presently being used off label in the United States for SCI because there is no US Food and Drug Administration (FDA)-approved indication for this use.[28] Despite the fact that subsequent clinical studies and critical reviews have challenged the validity of the recommendations that followed the NASCIS studies, failure to administer steroids in acute SCI has been cited in litigation against physicians due to the potential "neuroprotective effect."[28] There is certainly an inherent conflict for clinicians when questioning the potential therapeutic benefit versus complications, given the medicolegal ramifications.

Critical Appraisal of Data—Evidence-Based Medicine

Randomized trials of MPSS for the treatment of acute SCI have shown that significant improvements in motor function recovery may exist after treatment with the high-dose regimen within 8 hours of injury. However, this improvement effect appears modest, if present at all, and does not appear to result in significant functional clinical recovery. Nonetheless, even small changes in motor recovery, typically assessed in the MPSS trials on one side of the body, do have the potential to be amplified into meaningful improvements in quality of life.[29]

The NASCIS II trial results did provide some evidence for the safety of high-dose MPSS.[23] However, this is counteracted by evidence in NASCIS III of a rise in mortality due to pneumonia, respiratory distress syndrome, or respiratory failure (grouped together) in the 48-hour methylprednisolone group.[24,25] This result was based on six deaths in the 48-hour group and one in the 24-hour group (RR = 6.0; 95% CI 0.73 to 49.3).

Conclusion

At present, high-dose MP therapy, although not FDA approved in the United States for acute SCI treatment, continues to be an option for initial medical treatment. Evidence-based medicine has evaluated the potential harmful effects of MPSS versus any modest neurological benefits.

Bracken[29] has addressed various criticisms and misunderstandings in the form of a recent meta-analysis of the NASCIS and non-NASCIS trials of MPSS in acute SCI. The conclusion was that "high-dose MPSS given within 8 hrs of acute SCI is a safe and modestly effective therapy that may result in important clinical recovery for some patients, although further trials are needed to identify superior pharmacological therapies and to test drugs that may sequentially influence the post-injury cascade."[29] In 2001, the Spine Focus Panel[30,31] reported that, although methylprednisolone is only modestly neuroprotective, it is clearly indicated in acute SCI because of its favorable risk/benefit profile and the lack of alternative therapies. However, a significant minority of respondents were of the opinion that the evidence supporting the use of steroids in SCI was weak and did not justify the use of this medication. The Spine Focus Panel agreed that, given the devastating impact of SCI and the modest efficacy of MP, clinical trials of other therapeutic interventions are urgently needed.

Although it is clear that substantial criticisms have emerged and are valid in regard to the administration of MPSS, the lack of available alternatives makes one reconsider whether to eliminate MPSS from the list of available options. It can be concluded, as a Class II recommendation, that in nonpenetrating trauma, MPSS used within 3 hours of injury at a 30 mg/kg loading dose followed by 5.4 mg/kg/h is not an unreasonable selection for SCI.[31] In scenarios where between 3 and 8 hours have elapsed, MPSS used at the dose given earlier for 48 hours becomes a viable option only after the family and the patient are aware of the complications that can occur with long-term administration. Any use of the drug for nonpenetrating trauma more than 8 hours after injury should be avoided.

Nevertheless, other groups, such as the AANS/CNS, have been less hopeful on the potential of MPSS to become a standard treatment even in specific settings. Guidelines were published in 2002 by this joint section emphasizing that the available medical evidence does not support a significant clinical benefit from the administration of MPSS in the treatment of patients after SCI for a duration of either 24 or 48 hours.[32] They state that "the neurological recovery benefit of methylprednisolone when administered within 8 hours of ASCI has been suggested but not convincingly proven."[32] Furthermore, the accepted position on methylprednisolone in the treatment of acute human SCI is that it should be prescribed knowing that the evidence suggesting harm is more consistent than the evidence for the benefit.[32]

Another aspect of this controversy that may have dispelled many of these conflicts is based on the fact that MPSS has not gone through the FDA approval process. It is necessary to ask why it has not been presented to the FDA. If the evidence is not strong enough to be presented to the FDA, then is it strong enough that methylprednisolone should be the treatment of choice for acute SCI?[28]

At the least, the experience with high-dose MPSS can shape the future of SCI research. Hopefully, we, as a community of scientists and physicians, have learned enough from this 20-year-old debate to perform better research so that as new compounds are developed, we can subject them to studies that have fewer methodological flaws.

Pearls

- There remains little clinical evidence for high-dose steroids in acute SCI.
- Judicious use of high dose steroids in acute SCI can reduce associated complications.
- Patients and families should be educated as to the evidence-based risks and benefits of high-dose steroids in acute SCI.

Pitfalls

- High-dose steroids are likely overutilized in acute SCI.
- Patients on a high-dose steroid protocol must be carefully managed to avoid complications.
- Data are insufficient to support extended (>24 h) use of high-dose steroids for acute SCI.

References

1. DeVivo MJ. Causes and costs of spinal cord injury in the United States. Spinal Cord 1997;35(12):809–813
2. Sekhon LH, Fehlings MG. Epidemiology, demographics, and pathophysiology of acute spinal cord injury. Spine 2001;26(24, Suppl):S2–S12
3. Kraus JF, Silberman TA, McArthur DL. Epidemiology of spinal cord injury. In: Benzel EC, Cahill DW, McCormack P. Principles of Spine Surgery. New York, NY: McGraw-Hill; 1996:41–58
4. Baptiste DC, Fehlings MG. Pharmacological approaches to repair the injured spinal cord. J Neurotrauma 2006;23(3-4):318–334
5. Kwon BK, Tetzlaff W, Grauer JN, Beiner J, Vaccaro AR. Pathophysiology and pharmacologic treatment of acute spinal cord injury. Spine J 2004;4(4):451–464
6. Lammertse DP. Update on pharmaceutical trials in acute spinal cord injury. J Spinal Cord Med 2004;27(4):319–325
7. Allen AR. Surgery of experimental lesions of spinal cord equivalent to crush injury of fracture dislocation of spinal column. A preliminary report. J Am Med Assoc 1911;57:878–880
8. Demopoulos HB, Flamm ES, Pietronigro DD, Seligman ML. The free radical pathology and the microcirculation in the major central nervous system disorders. Acta Physiol Scand Suppl 1980;492:91–119
9. Tator CH. Update on the pathophysiology and pathology of acute spinal cord injury. Brain Pathol 1995;5(4):407–413
10. Young W, Koreh I. Potassium and calcium changes in injured spinal cords. Brain Res 1986;365(1):42–53
11. Faden AI, Simon RP. A potential role for excitotoxins in the pathophysiology of spinal cord injury. Ann Neurol 1988;23(6):623–626
12. Hall ED, Yonkers PA, Horan KL, Braughler JM. Correlation between attenuation of posttraumatic spinal cord ischemia and preservation of tissue vitamin E by the 21-aminosteroid U74006F: evidence for an in vivo antioxidant mechanism. J Neurotrauma 1989;6(3):169–176
13. Xu J, Chen S, Chen H, et al. STAT5 mediates antiapoptotic effects of methylprednisolone on

oligodendrocytes. J Neurosci 2009;29(7):2022–2026

14. Hall ED, Braughler JM. Acute effects of intravenous glucocorticoid pretreatment on the in vitro peroxidation of cat spinal cord tissue. Exp Neurol 1981;73(1):321–324
15. Braughler JM, Hall ED. Effects of multi-dose methylprednisolone sodium succinate administration on injured cat spinal cord neurofilament degradation and energy metabolism. J Neurosurg 1984;61(2):290–295
16. Braughler JM, Hall ED. Lactate and pyruvate metabolism in injured cat spinal cord before and after a single large intravenous dose of methylprednisolone. J Neurosurg 1983;59(2):256–261
17. Scheff SW, Benardo LS, Cotman CW. Hydrocortison administration retards axon sprouting in the rat dentate gyrus. Exp Neurol 1980;68(1):195–201
18. Scheff SW, Cotman CW. Chronic glucocorticoid therapy alters axon sprouting in the hippocampal dentate gyrus. Exp Neurol 1982;76(3):644–654
19. Oudega M, Vargas CG, Weber AB, Kleitman N, Bunge MB. Long-term effects of methylprednisolone following transection of adult rat spinal cord. Eur J Neurosci 1999;11(7):2453–2464
20. Bracken MB, Shepard MJ, Hellenbrand KG, et al. Methylprednisolone and neurological function 1 year after spinal cord injury. Results of the National Acute Spinal Cord Injury Study. J Neurosurg 1985;63(5):704–713
21. Hurlbert RJ. Methylprednisolone for acute spinal cord injury: an inappropriate standard of care. J Neurosurg 2000;93(1, Suppl):1–7
22. Hall ED, Braughler JM. Glucocorticoid mechanisms in acute spinal cord injury: a review and therapeutic rationale. Surg Neurol 1982;18(5):320–327
23. Bracken MB, Shepard MJ, Collins WF, et al. A randomized, controlled trial of methylprednisolone or naloxone in the treatment of acute spinal-cord injury. Results of the Second National Acute Spinal Cord Injury Study. N Engl J Med 1990;322(20):1405–1411
24. Bracken MB, Holford TR. Neurological and functional status 1 year after acute spinal cord injury: estimates of functional recovery in National Acute Spinal Cord Injury Study II from results modeled in National Acute Spinal Cord Injury Study III. J Neurosurg 2002;96(3, Suppl):259–266
25. Bracken MB, Shepard MJ, Holford TR, et al. Administration of methylprednisolone for 24 or 48 hours or tirilazad mesylate for 48 hours in the treatment of acute spinal cord injury. Results of the Third National Acute Spinal Cord Injury Randomized Controlled Trial. National Acute Spinal Cord Injury Study. JAMA 1997;277(20):1597–1604
26. Roberts I, Yates D, Sandercock P, et al; CRASH trial collaborators. Effect of intravenous corticosteroids on death within 14 days in 10008 adults with clinically significant head injury (MRC CRASH trial): randomised placebo-controlled trial. Lancet 2004;364(9442):1321–1328
27. Heary RF, Vaccaro AR, Mesa JJ, et al. Steroids and gunshot wounds to the spine. Neurosurgery 1997;41(3):576–583, discussion 583–584
28. Coleman WP, Benzel D, Cahill DW, et al. A critical appraisal of the reporting of the National Acute Spinal Cord Injury Studies (II and III) of methylprednisolone in acute spinal cord injury. J Spinal Disord 2000;13(3):185–199
29. Bracken MB. Methylprednisolone and acute spinal cord injury: an update of the randomized evidence. Spine 2001;26(24, Suppl):S47–S54
30. Fehlings MG; Spine Focus Panel. Summary statement: the use of methylprednisolone in acute spinal cord injury. Spine 2001;26(24, Suppl):S55
31. Fehlings MG. Editorial: recommendations regarding the use of methylprednisolone in acute spinal cord injury: making sense out of the controversy. Spine 2001;26(24, Suppl):S56–S57
32. Pharmacological therapy after acute cervical spinal cord injury. Neurosurgery 2002;50(3, Suppl):S63–S72

11

Halo Application and Closed Skeletal Reduction of Cervical Dislocations

Scott D. Daffner

Key Points

1. Closed traction reduction is indicated in the setting of cervical fracture, subluxation, or dislocation that causes malalignment and canal compromise in an awake patient capable of giving a reliable neurological exam throughout the process. It is contraindicated in obtunded patients or any patients who have a distracting injury, or patients with skull fractures that preclude placement of tongs or a halo.

2. Stainless steel Gardner-Wells tongs should be utilized for high-weight reductions; reduction using a halo ring should only be performed when low weights will be required.

3. The initial traction weight should be only 5 lb to evaluate for unrecognized atlantooccipital dissociation. Weight is then increased by 10 lb increments added about every 10 minutes (to allow for ligamentotaxis). Serial lateral radiographs and neurological exams are performed after every increase in weight.

4. Once reduced, the cervical spine should be stabilized with either continued traction of ~ 20 lb or application of a halo vest until definitive surgical fixation is performed.

Cervical facet dislocations result from a flexion-distraction mechanism applied to the spine and are due to traumatic failure of the posterior ligamentous construct (facet capsules, interspinous ligament, supraspinous ligament) under tension. Injuries may be purely ligamentous in nature or may be associated with fractures of the articular processes. Bilateral injuries result from a pure flexion-distraction force, whereas unilateral injuries involve flexion-distraction with an accompanying rotational force. Radiographically, unilateral dislocation can be distinguished from bilateral dislocation by an offset of the spinous processes from midline on the anteroposterior cervical radiograph. On the lateral film, the relative rotation of the facet joints above and below the level of injury manifests as the so-called bow tie sign, in which both the right and left facets at a given level can be seen distinctly, as compared with nonrotated levels where the facets are superimposed. Typically, anterolisthesis at the level of injury is less than 25% of the vertebral body anteroposterior diameter. Bilateral facet dislocations, on the other hand, typically result in at least 50% anterior translation. Bilateral perched facets (not fully dislocated) demonstrate relatively large posterior distraction and focal kyphosis of the vertebral endplates. On axial computed tomographic (CT) scans, dislocated facets have a characteristic appearance, with reversal of the normal alignment of the facet joints such that the rounded portions of the articular processes are opposed, rather than the flat articular surfaces ("reverse hamburger bun sign"). Perched facets may manifest on axial CT images as the so-called naked facet sign, in which one articular surface is visualized by itself without its associated counterpart.

Cervical facet dislocations frequently present with complete or incomplete spinal cord injuries and represent a situation that requires urgent or emergent decompression. In most cases, once the dislocation is reduced, the local spinal cord compression is alleviated. Whether this emergent reduction is performed via closed or open technique, pre– or post–magnetic resonance imaging (MRI), is still a matter of great debate.[1–4] What follows is a technical description of the procedure for closed traction reduction of cervical facet dislocations.

Closed reduction can be safely and expeditiously performed in most situations. It requires the application of either Gardner-Wells tongs or a halo ring to the patient's skull and the use of sequentially increasing traction to distract the dislocated segments and gradually unlock them, allowing reduction of the dislocation. Although weights of up to 140 lb may be safely applied to Gardner-Wells tongs, most manufacturers suggest no more than 35 to 40 lb of traction be applied through a halo ring.[5] One of the reasons for this has to do with the pin design and placement. The cranial pins of Gardner-Wells tongs are angled slightly superiorly, which allows them to insert into the skull in a manner allowing greater resistance to longitudinally applied forces. Halo rings, on the other hand, are designed to provide stability in axial, sagittal, and coronal planes but are not designed to resist significant longitudinally applied forces. The angle of insertion of halo cranial pins is perpendicular to the surface of the skull; thus they have decreased pullout strength. In addition, most modern halo devices utilize a carbon fiber ring and titanium pins, which have decreased resistance to pullout compared with stainless steel. Recently, carbon fiber Gardner-Wells tongs have become available that are MRI compatible. Unfortunately, the carbon fiber tongs combined with titanium pins have a certain amount of flexibility or plastic deformity, much more so than stainless steel tongs, and can therefore tolerate lower weights before the stress causes the tongs to bend and the pins to partially disengage, potentially ripping through the patient's scalp.[6] Carbon fiber tongs with titanium can support only ~50–70 lb of force. Any application of a halo ring or carbon fiber tongs requires review the manufacturer's guidelines for weight tolerance.

After reduction, the cervical spine must be stabilized until there is definitive surgical fixation. If surgical fixation is to be performed shortly after reduction, the patient may remain in light traction until surgery. If surgery is to be delayed, or if further studies (e.g., MRI) are to be performed, the patient may be stabilized in a halo orthosis in the interim. For injuries that are amenable to reduction under lighter traction (facet fracture-dislocations, perched facets) it is easiest to apply the halo ring initially and utilize it for the reduction. It may then be locked into the vest. In other cases, such as pure facet dislocations, the need for greater traction will require the use of tongs. In these situations, the halo ring and vest may be applied after reduction is achieved.

Closed traction reduction is indicated in the setting of cervical fracture, subluxation, or dislocation that causes malalignment and canal compromise.[5,7] Application of a halo ring or Gardner-Wells tongs is contraindicated in patients with skull fractures. In addition, closed reduction may only be performed in an awake patient capable of giving a reliable neurological exam throughout the process. Therefore it is contraindicated in obtunded patients or any patients who have a distracting injury.

Application of a Halo Ring

The technique for applying the halo ring is no different in the setting of cervical dislocation than when it is applied for other purposes. All materials should be gathered at the bedside before starting. This includes material for skin preparation (razor, Betadine, etc.), local anesthetic, all parts of the halo (ring, vest, posts, connectors), and the torque wrenches required for assembly. Several sizes of ring and vest should be available because an ill-fitting vest provides little stability. The patient should be placed on a firm mattress (RotoRest bed, KCI, San Antonio, TX, or a Jackson table, Mizuho OSI, Union City, CA). The patient is carefully logrolled, maintaining cervical precautions, and the posterior half of the vest, with vertical bars attached, is placed behind the patient. During a reduction, placement of a rolled towel between the patient's shoulder blades, posterior to the vest, can aid in allowing cervical extension if needed. The approximate locations for pin placement are identified, shaved, and prepped.

The ring is positioned just inferior to the equator of the skull, leaving at least 1 to 1.5 cm of clearance above the ears. Most halo devices include plastic or rubber pads, which can be placed through screw holes in the ring to aid in positioning. The anterior pin location is over the lateral eyebrow, avoiding the more medially located supraorbital and supratrochlear nerves and the temporal artery laterally (**Fig. 11.1**).[7] Posterior pin placement should be just posterior to the ear, avoiding the mastoid. The underlying skin and subcutaneous tissue are infiltrated with local anesthetic. This is most easily performed by placing the needle through the selected pin hole in the ring. The underlying periosteum should also be anesthetized. The pins are inserted through the selected holes and advanced through the skin until fingertight. A small stab incision at the pin site may be helpful in patients with unusually tough skin or if blunt-tipped pins are utilized. Next, the pins are sequentially tightened to the required torque. This is best accomplished by tightening opposite corners at the same time (e.g., anterior right and posterior left, then switching). Required torque varies based on the manufacturer

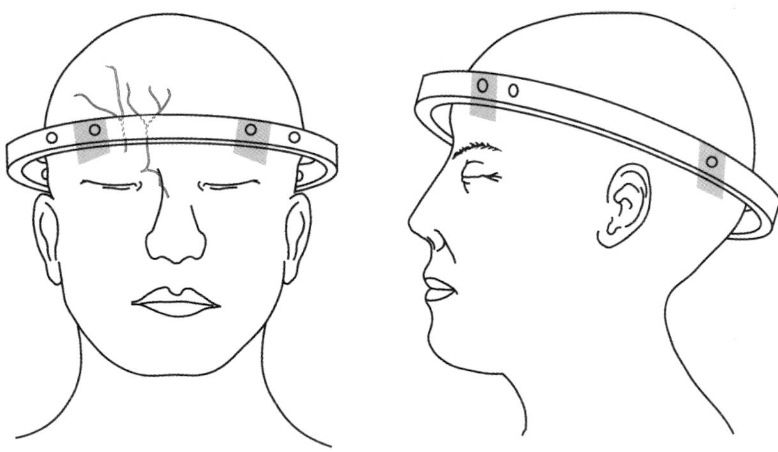

Fig. 11.1 Placement of the halo ring is just inferior to the equator of the skull, leaving ~ 1 to 1.5 cm above the ears. Anterior pins are placed over the lateral eyebrow, avoiding the supraorbital and supratrochlear nerves medially. Posterior pins are placed just posterior to the ear, avoiding the mastoid.

but is usually 6 or 8 inch-pounds. When the anterior pins are being placed, it is imperative that patients tightly close their eyes or that the surgeon pulls the eyelids down. Failure to do so may allow soft tissue to be trapped by the pin such that the eyelid may be unable to fully close.

If a closed reduction is to be performed, most halo systems include a traction bale, which is either integrated with the ring or may be attached to it. The traction rope is hooked to the bale, and the reduction is performed (yet to be described). Following reduction, with mild traction still applied, the posterior posts may be attached to the ring. The anterior half of the vest is applied, the anterior posts connected, and all attachments tightened. All pin sites and connections must be retorqued ~24 hours after placement.

Placement of a halo on a child is accomplished in much the same manner. The only major difference is that more pins are placed under less torque. This is due to the increased risk of pin penetration in the relatively thin cortices of the cranium. Typically 6 to 10 pins are used with a maximum of 2 inch-pounds of torque.

Application of Gardner-Wells Tongs

In preparation for a closed reduction, the patient should be positioned supine on a firm mattress (RotoRest bed or a Jackson table). The area above the ears is sterilely prepped. The pins are placed just below the equator of the skull ~1 cm above the ear. For neutral alignment, the pins should be parallel to the tragus. To create more of an extension vector, the pins may be placed more anteriorly. For a flexion vector (more frequently required for reduction of a facet dislocation), the pins may be placed slightly posteriorly. Care must be taken to align the pins identically on each side; failure to do so will result in an unequal traction vector. One pin has an "indicator" button that pops out when appropriate torque is reached.

As mentioned previously, reduction of facet dislocations typically requires high-weight traction (over 100 lb). Therefore, stainless steel tongs are preferred because the MRI-compatible graphite tongs can fail at high weight.[6] Frequently utilized tongs should undergo regular recalibration or replacement to prevent pullout or failure at low weights.[8]

High-Weight Closed Skeletal Reduction

The indications and contraindications for closed skeletal reduction of cervical facet dislocations have been described previously. When performing this procedure, it is imperative to understand your facility's supplies and limitations. At a minimum, a firm mattress and dedicated portable radiography or fluoroscopy are essential. The author's preference is to perform reductions with the patient placed in a RotoRest bed fitted with an overhead traction frame. This allows easy adjustment of the traction vector as needed during the procedure (**Fig. 11.2**). Alternatives include performing the procedure on a Jackson radiolucent table. Depending on space availability, one may perform the procedure in the emergency department, radiology suite, or operating room.

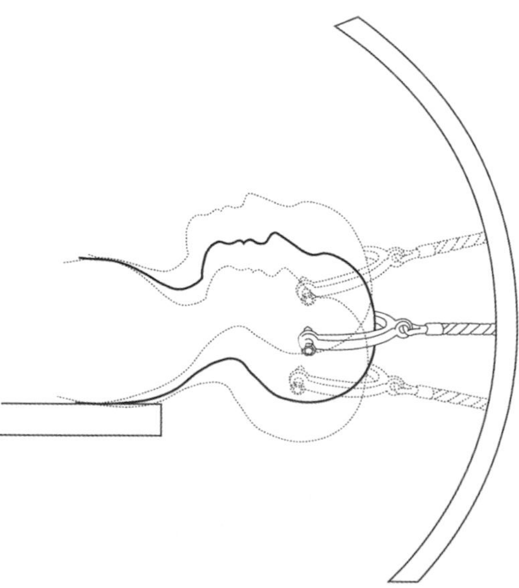

Fig. 11.2 The patient is placed supine with a bump between the shoulders. The traction frame allows adjustment of the traction vector. Initial traction is longitudinal with some flexion to unlock the facets. Once the facets are perched or reduced, the vector is switched to slight extension, and the weight can be reduced.

Prior to the procedure, informed consent should be obtained from the patient. Given the possibility that the procedure may need to be aborted secondary to neurological deterioration and an emergent open reduction performed, the consent should also include possible open reduction and stabilization. The procedure may only be safely performed on an awake patient without distracting injuries who can provide reliable serial neurological exams. Use of light sedation, muscle relaxants, and/or analgesia may allow the patient to be more relaxed, aiding in the reduction; however, care must be taken not to overmedicate the patient to the point that the person cannot provide feedback or be examined.

The patient is positioned supine on the RotoRest bed, and a small bump may be placed vertically between the patient's shoulder blades to allow mild neck extension after the completion of the reduction. The bed is placed in 10 to 15 degrees of reverse Trendelenburg position to resist the pull of traction. The shoulder pads of the RotoRest bed are placed down to act as countertraction as well as to aid in radiographic visualization of the cervical spine. Alternatively, soft restraints around the ankle may provide some countertraction.

Traction is set up to pull in neutral or slight flexion. Initially, 5 lb of traction is applied. A lateral radiograph is taken to evaluate for any potential atlantooccipital dissociation. If this is apparent, the closed reduction is stopped immediately. After the initial film, weights are added in 10 lb increments approximately every 10 minutes. After each weight is added, the patient is asked about any pain or paresthesias, and a complete motor and sensory exam is performed. Lateral cervical radiographs are taken after each weight is added (**Fig. 11.3**). Weight is added un-

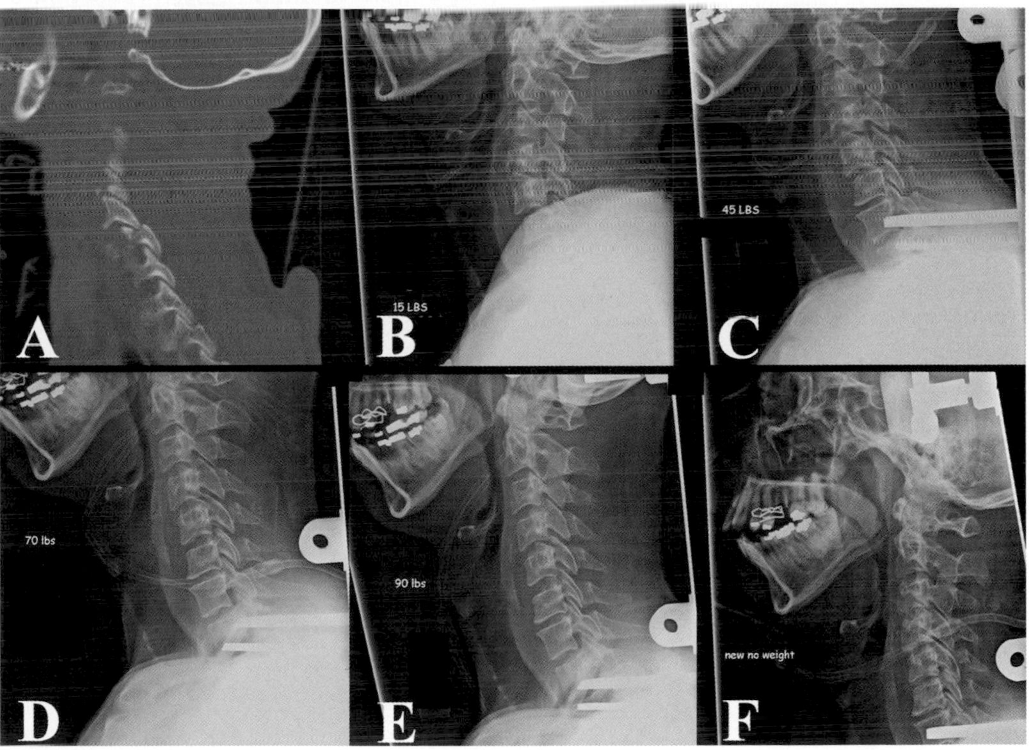

Fig. 11.3 **(A)** A 48-year-old man presented with a right C5–C6 unilateral facet fracture dislocation. **(B–E)** Selected images from high-weight traction reduction with Gardner-Wells tongs demonstrate increasing distraction of the joints with sequentially increasing weights until the C5–C6 facets were perched. **(F)** After reduction was achieved, the traction vector was shifted into slight extension and weight reduced. The patient remained in slight traction overnight and underwent posterior cervical fusion the following day.

til the facets appear perched. The inferior articular process of the cranial level must be clear of the superior articular process of the caudal vertebra. At this point, the traction vector may be redirected to slight extension, and the weight is reduced. Radiographs should confirm that the facet has slid back into proper alignment. The spine may then be stabilized by retaining 20 lb of traction via the Gardner-Wells tongs. Alternatively, the patient may then be placed into a halo orthosis for immobilization until definitive surgical fixation is performed.

True facet dislocations may require weights up to 140 lb to reduce. Fracture-dislocations (particularly if the superior articular facet is fractured) typically require less weight to reduce but are more unstable once reduced. If any change in neurological status is noted during the reduction, the procedure is immediately halted, the weight partially released, and the cervical spine immobilized. An emergent MRI scan is performed and the patient should be taken to the operating room for open reduction.[9] Failure of a reduction to progress may indicate entrapment of a disk fragment, fracture fragment, or other soft tissue. This necessitates an MRI scan and possible open reduction.

Conclusion

Closed traction reduction can successfully alleviate spinal cord compression caused by cervical facet dislocations. In patients capable of providing a reliable examination and without any distracting injuries, it should be performed expeditiously. An important factor for performing a successful reduction is knowing your individual institution's resources, particularly the type of bed, equipment (halo or Gardner-Wells tongs, stainless steel or carbon fiber), and imaging (portable x-ray or C-arm) that are available. The reduction may be maintained either by applying a halo vest orthosis or by maintaining light traction with tongs; the latter option may be preferable if the patient will have surgical stabilization within 24 hours. Primary open reduction and stabilization may be indicated for obtunded patients, incomplete spinal cord injuries, or patients otherwise unable to tolerate closed reduction. Failure to obtain closed reduction or development of a new neurological deficit during the reduction maneuver necessitates an emergent MRI scan and consideration for open reduction and stabilization. Because of the potential need for emergent operative treatment, closed reduction of cervical facet dislocations should ideally be performed only at an institution capable of performing any needed surgery.

Pearls

- The use of light sedation, muscle relaxants, and/or analgesia may facilitate easier closed reduction; care must be taken, however, to avoid oversedating patients such that they can no longer provide a reliable neurological exam or feedback.
- If halo immobilization is planned following closed reduction, the posterior portion of the halo vest should be placed under the patient prior to performing the reduction. This helps facilitate placement of the vest and posts while minimizing the need to move the patient, thereby reducing the risk of re-dislocation due to patient manipulation.
- When a halo ring is being applied to the skull, the patient's eyes should be tightly closed or the surgeon should hold the eyelids shut. Otherwise, the pins may "tack" the skin to the skull in such a way that the eyelids cannot completely shut, resulting in dry eyes and other associated problems.
- Halo pins should be retorqued 24 hours after application, and again at 10 to 14 days after application.

Pitfalls

- Graphite (radiolucent) Gardner-Wells tongs with titanium skull pins may deform and disengage when high weights are used. Therefore, stainless steel tongs and pins should be utilized whenever possible.
- Patients must be carefully examined prior to placing tongs or halo to exclude skull fractures. Tong or halo placement is contraindicated in such patients.
- The initial weight for reduction should not exceed 10 lb; after placing the initial weight, a lateral radiograph must be carefully scrutinized to evaluate for atlantooccipital dissociation. If present, the traction should be removed immediately and the patient prepared for open reduction and stabilization.
- Patients must be examined after each weight has been added. They should never be left alone during the reduction process because neurological symptoms may take several minutes to evolve.
- If a closed reduction fails to progress, or if neurological deterioration occurs, the patient should be prepared for surgery for open reduction and stabilization. An MRI scan should be performed prior to surgery to evaluate for any mechanical blockage of the reduction or any compressive lesions explaining neurological symptoms.

References

1. Grauer JN, Vaccaro AR, Lee JY, et al. The timing and influence of MRI on the management of patients with cervical facet dislocations remains highly variable: a survey of members of the Spine Trauma Study Group. J Spinal Disord Tech 2009; 22(2):96–99
2. Star AM, Jones AA, Cotler JM, Balderston RA, Sinha R. Immediate closed reduction of cervical spine dislocations using traction. Spine 1990;15(10):1068–1072
3. Eismont FJ, Arena MJ, Green BA. Extrusion of an intervertebral disc associated with traumatic subluxation or dislocation of cervical facets. Case report. J Bone Joint Surg Am 1991;73(10): 1555–1560
4. Payer M. Immediate open anterior reduction and antero-posterior fixation/fusion for bilateral cervical locked facets. Acta Neurochir (Wien) 2005; 147(5):509–513, discussion 513–514
5. Cotler JM, Herbison GJ, Nasuti JF, Ditunno JF Jr, An H, Wolff BE. Closed reduction of traumatic cervical spine dislocation using traction weights up to 140 pounds. Spine 1993;18(3):386–390
6. Blumberg KD, Catalano JB, Cotler JM, Balderston RA. The pullout strength of titanium alloy MRI-compatible and stainless steel MRI-incompatible Gardner-Wells tongs. Spine 1993;18(13): 1895–1896
7. Bransford RJ, Stevens DW, Uyeji S, Bellabarba C, Chapman JR. Halo vest treatment of cervical spine injuries: a success and survivorship analysis. Spine 2009;34(15):1561–1566
8. Lerman JA, Haynes RJ, Koeneman EJ, Koeneman JB, Wong WB. A biomechanical comparison of Gardner-Wells tongs and halo device used for cervical spine traction. Spine 1994;19(21):2403–2406
9. Wimberley DW, Vaccaro AR, Goyal N, et al. Acute quadriplegia following closed traction reduction of a cervical facet dislocation in the setting of ossification of the posterior longitudinal ligament: case report. Spine 2005;30(15):E433–E438

12

Principles of Surgical Management of Spinal Trauma Associated with Spinal Cord Injury

Toba N. Niazi, Michael Daubs, and Andrew T. Dailey

Key Points

1. The goals of surgical intervention are multifactorial and include decompression of the neural elements, establishing a stable spine to prevent painful deformity or neurological decline and to allow for early mobilization of the patient.
2. Unique classification systems exist for each different region of the spine and provide a mechanism for communication between clinicians.
3. Decompression alone of the injured spinal cord is often contraindicated and must be supplemented with a stabilizing or fusion procedure.
4. Evidence is accumulating that early decompression (defined as within 24 hours of the injury) and stabilization of a patient with spinal cord injury may lead to improved neurological outcomes.

The earliest reports of spinal column injury with neurological deficits, referred to as spinal cord injury (SCI), date back to 2500 BC in the Edwin Smith Surgical papyrus.[1] The view at that time that a SCI was "an ailment not to be treated" remained the attitude of physicians for centuries. In 1262, Theodoric of Bologna wrote a surgical text, *Chiurgica de Theodoric*,[1] in which he discussed the surgical treatment of spinal column disorders. This text stressed the importance of the reestablishment of proper alignment by reduction and stabilization to heal these injuries. Contemporary spine surgeons uphold the philosophy of stabilization and decompression.

Despite early recognition, SCI remains a significant cause of morbidity and mortality, with ~10,000 to 12,000 cases occurring annually in the United States,[2–4] primarily in younger adults.[4] The financial and social costs associated with SCI are enormous; medical costs alone are in excess of US$7 billion a year.[3] Such large figures clearly indicate the need to establish which injuries require surgical intervention and when such a procedure should be performed. With innovations in neuroanesthesia, the advent of antibiotics, and advances in surgical techniques and instrumentation, contemporary spine surgeons can be more confident in the ability to manage spinal trauma in an operative fashion than were their predecessors. Because of the wide array of injuries that can afflict the spinal column, the role of surgery is hard to define globally, and the decision to proceed operatively must instead be made on a case-by-case basis. Specific surgical goals in the management of all SCI should include (1) the establishment of a balanced and stable spine, (2) the preservation or improvement in neurological function, and (3) the quick return of the patient to an optimal level of functional capacity.[5] In each case, the surgeon must evaluate whether the surgical risks outweigh potential benefits and judge whether surgery can achieve the aforementioned goals more effectively than nonoperative treatment.

Historically, many physicians took the stance that spine surgery for acute SCI is warranted in only those patients who have progressive neurological deterioration or in those with gross spinal instability. Prior to the 1970s, the only operative treatment available was laminectomy without instrumentation, and this was avoided because of the higher incidence of neurological complications and worse clinical outcomes.[6,7] Guttman[8] advocated the use of postural techniques combined with bed rest to achieve reduction and spontaneous fusion of the spine. Dall,[9] Harris et al.,[10] and Bedbrook[7] all indicated that neither spinal surgery nor anatomical alignment of the spinal column improved the neurological outcome in patients with acute SCI, with the exception of bilateral locked facets. Although many studies agreed in their findings about nonoperative treatment, these reports were retrospective case series and provided only Class III data. In addition, nonoperative treatment is not without risks: Up to 10% of patients with incomplete cervical SCI have neurological deterioration while being treated in an exclusively nonoperative manner.[11]

With improved surgical care, outcomes after surgical treatment of spinal trauma patients have improved and made the surgical treatment of SCI a viable option. Several factors weigh in favor of a surgical approach in many cases. For example, with modern techniques, surgery can accelerate the rehabilitation process by reducing the complications associated with prolonged immobilization, decreasing morbidity for the patient and indirectly decreasing the medical costs. Similarly, stabilizing the spine through instrumentation and fusion should prevent spinal deformity, which may manifest at a later time as progressive pain, loss of function, and neurological deterioration. The decreased length of hospitalization, quicker rehabilitation, and earlier return to society are all clear advantages to surgical intervention.[12,13] In addition, operative intervention can decrease the cascade of secondary injury associated with SCI by decreasing the degree of neural compression.[14,15]

Primary and Secondary Mechanisms of Spinal Cord Injury

Acute SCI results from a combination of primary and secondary injury mechanisms. The primary injury is the initial insult that transmits direct mechanical trauma to the spinal cord and may involve a contusion, laceration, blast injury, ischemic event, or direct shearing of spinal cord axons. It often results in fragments of the vertebral body or disk material directly causing neural compression.[14–16] This leads to a cascade of biochemical events known as the secondary injury mechanism, leading to ischemia, neurogenic shock, hemorrhage, vasospasm, edema, ionic derangements, neurotransmitter accumulation, production of free radicals, inflammation, and apoptosis. It is this secondary injury cascade that damages the neural elements in the hours after injury.[14–16] Rabinowitz et al.[17] demonstrated in canine studies that the severity of the pathological changes and degree of recovery were directly related to the duration of acute compression. In essence, persistent compression of the spinal cord is a potentially reversible form of secondary injury. Pharmacological treatment, closed fracture reduction, and surgical decompression are employed to reduce the zone of injury attributed to the secondary cascade.[14–16]

Class III studies have shown a benefit of surgical treatment at various time points.

In their evaluation of early decompression, Wagner and Chehrazi[18] found no difference in recovery but cited a study by Hamel et al. who retrospectively evaluated the role of surgical intervention on neurological outcome after acute SCI in the cervical spine. Those authors found that 53% of patients treated with surgical decompression and fusion retained the ability to walk, whereas only 23% of those patients treated conservatively retained this function. Surgery also appears to benefit patients with long-standing compression of the spinal cord, regardless of the duration of time from injury. Bohlman and Anderson[19] described a series in which 58 patients who had remote cervical spine trauma with incomplete injuries underwent anterior decompressive and fusion procedures. Half of the patients demonstrated a marked improvement in their functional status. Fehlings et al. have presented the initial results of a large multicenter observational study (STASCIS) looking at 6- and 12-month outcomes following surgery and decompression for cervical SCI. Acute decompression, defined as decompression within 24 hours of the injury, led to a significant improvement in American Spinal Injury Association (ASIA) motor classification at 6 and 12 months. When completed, this study will provide strong level II evidence that early decompression is beneficial for long-term outcome in motor function.[20]

Spinal Stability

White and Punjabi[21] defined stability as the "ability of the spine under physiologic loads to limit patterns of displacement so as not to damage or irritate the spinal cord or nerve roots and in addition to prevent incapacitating deformity or pain due to structural changes." Any traumatic spinal injury that disrupts the biomechanical stability of the spine contributes not only to neurological injury but also to musculoskeletal injury that in turn will affect the functional status of the patient. Surgery helps to reestablish the alignment of the spine and subsequently stabilize the spinal column to prevent further neurological injury, deformity, and pain.[22]

Several classification systems have been developed that attempt to predict the degree of instability after spinal trauma. None of these systems has been universally adopted, and none has prospectively analyzed the ability to predict instability.[23] What is inherent in all classification systems is that both osseous and ligamentous structures contribute to the stability of the spine and are not independent of one another, although instability in either alone can cause neurological deterioration.[23] Kostuik[24] demonstrated that disruption of the ligamentous structures in the cervical, thoracic, or lumbar regions without osseous injury predisposed to spinal deformity with associated neurological deterioration. This is most devastating in cases of occipitocervical dislocation, bilateral facet disruption, and transverse ligamentous disruption.[25]

Nonoperative management of spinal instability in the setting of trauma has not always been successful. Anderson and Bohlman[26] prospectively studied a series of patients with cervical spinal injuries that were treated with halo vests and immobilization. In these patients, imaging in both the supine and the upright positions demonstrated intervertebral motion. The authors also noted that changes in body posture translated into either a compressive or a distractive force at the injury level while the patient was in a halo orthotic device. Because of the length of the spinal column and the different function of each region, unique biomechanical properties exist at each level of the spinal column. Thus we will consider the role of surgical intervention at each level separately.

Cervical Spine

The degree of motion from the cervical spine is due to this region's unique ligamentous and osseous anatomy. This unique anatomy, however, predisposes it to the risk of major injury and subsequent catastrophic neurological injury. Within the cervical spine, it is imperative in the setting of trauma to adequately visualize the cervicothoracic junction because this region accounts for 17% of all cervical spine fractures.[27]

The cervical spine is often viewed as two distinct regions, the upper cervical spine (occiput to C2) and the subaxial or lower cervical spine (C3–7). The upper cervical spine deals with flexion and extension between the occiput and the atlas and allows rotation of the head through the atlantoaxial junction. The ligamentous structures in this region are of critical importance because they provide most of the stability in this region. Many of the injuries of the upper cervical spine are not associated with SCI because of the generous canal size and the relatively small osseous volume at C1 and C2. This chapter concentrates on injuries of this region with a relatively higher incidence of SCI. The unique anatomy of the occipitocervical junction and the difficulty of approaching the upper cervical spine from an anterior approach make posterior stabilization and fusion the preferred choice for most injuries in this region. Occipitocervical dislocations are uncommon ligamentous injuries that result from hyperflexion and distraction during high-impact blunt trauma.[28] These are unstable and frequently fatal injuries that cause neurological injury from stretching, compression, and distortion of the spinal cord, brain stem, and cranial nerves.[29] Vertebral artery injury also accounts for significant morbidity and mortality in this region. Occipitocervical junction injuries were often recognized in a delayed fashion on routine cervical radiographs, but the use of routine computed tomographic (CT) scans in the polytrauma patient has led to more timely recognition of this injury.[30] Initial management of these injuries focuses on immobilization to limit further injury, with or without a halo orthosis, and never with traction. Nonoperative management of these injuries does not provide definitive treatment because of the significant ligamentous disruption that cannot heal even with prolonged external immobilization. Operative stabilization involves an occipitocervical arthrodesis with rigid internal fixation after restoration of alignment.

Transverse ligamentous injuries are unstable injuries that may result in SCI. Occasionally, these are isolated injuries, but often they are associated with C1 or C2 fractures. Integrity of this ligament is the key to stability of the C1–2 region.[31] These injuries can be diagnosed by recognizing a widened atlantodental interval on lateral radiographs or displacement of the C1 lateral masses on an open-mouth odontoid view or coronal CT reconstruction. Transverse ligamentous injuries are classified into two categories based on their radiographic appearance.[31] Type I injuries involve disruption of the midportion (Ia) or periosteal (Ib) insertion laterally. Type II injuries involve fractures that disconnect the C1 lateral mass tubercle from the transverse ligament through either a comminuted fracture (IIa) or an avulsion fracture (IIb). Type I fractures are purely ligamentous injuries that often do not heal by immobilization alone, so posterior C1–2 arthrodesis is indicated. Type II injuries have a 74% chance of healing with halo immobilization, so that may be tried before surgical intervention if the patient prefers.[31] Isolated axis and odontoid fractures rarely cause significant compromise of the spinal canal or neurological injury and will not be discussed here.

In the subaxial cervical spine (C3–7), the osseous and ligamentous structures play an equal role in stability. The spinal canal in this region is smaller than that in the upper cervical spine, which predisposes to SCI with any compressive or translational forces. As a result, those patients with congenitally narrowed cervical spinal canals are more at risk for devastating neurological injury with trauma. In 1982, Allen and colleagues[32] described a mechanistic classification of subaxial cervical spine trauma. This classification divides mid- and low-cervical fractures into six groups based on force vector and incremental tissue failure. Abnormal sagittal alignment between adjacent vertebrae implies ligamentous failure, suggesting a shear force mechanism because ligaments do not fail with compression. The three most common injury types are compressive flexion, compressive extension, and distractive flexion. Vertical compression injuries occur with intermediate frequency, distractive extension and lateral flexion injuries occur the least. Neurological injury within all six subgroups is common.[32]

Compressive flexion injuries are caused by a ventral and axially directed load of increasing intensity. Compressive fractures without subluxation and facet injury are more stable injuries, whereas injuries with increased ventral osseous and dorsal ligamentous injury tend to be unstable. If the spine can be aligned in the sagittal plane, surgical intervention through an anterior approach with corpectomy and instrumented fusion with a structural graft is sufficient. If alignment requires direct reduction of the facet joint or there is significant posterior facet damage, a dorsal approach with stabilization is often warranted.

Compressive extension injuries range from unilateral vertebral arch fractures to bilateral laminar fractures and finally to vertebral arch fractures with full ventral displacement of the vertebral body. The general surgical objective involves a dorsal approach with reduction and stabilization followed by adjunctive ventral reconstruction if there is significant vertebral body comminution and displacement.

Distractive flexion injuries, also known as fracture dislocation injuries, are often devastating injuries (**Fig. 12.1**) and are caused by flexion and distraction forces with or without an element of rotation. These injuries include perched, jumped, and locked facets and have the potential for progressive neurological deterioration. Failure of all posterior ligamentous structures (ligamentum flavum, facet capsule, interspinous ligament) has been demonstrated in patients with both unilateral and bilateral facet dislocation.[33] Most injuries within this spectrum are unstable and require surgical stabilization after reduction and decompression.[32,33] Magnetic resonance imaging (MRI) is useful to identify a herniated disk fragment prior to open or closed reduction procedures, especially if

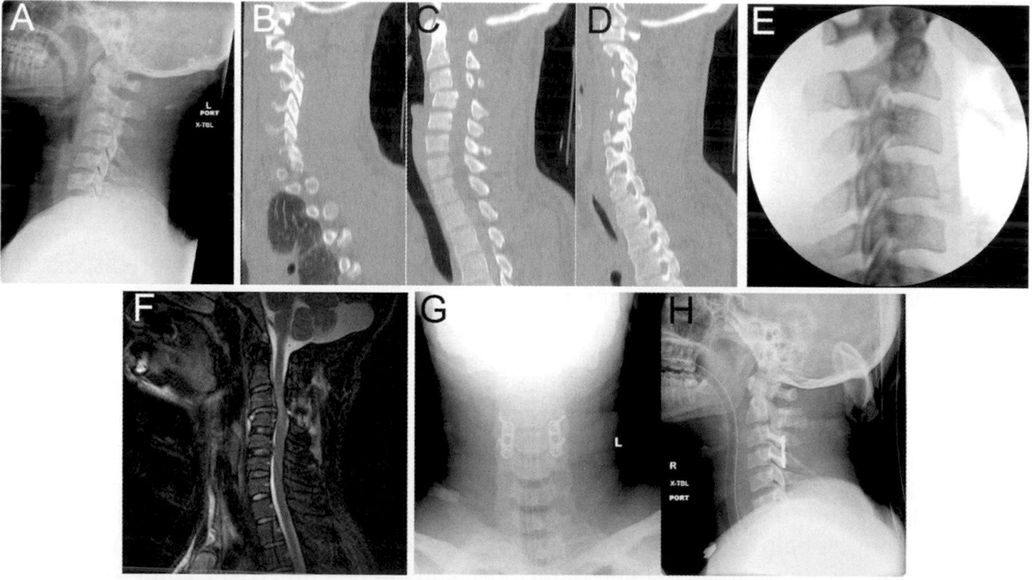

Fig. 12.1 **(A)** Lateral x-ray of the cervical spine showing C3-4 fracture dislocation in a 22-year-old man. The patient had an American Spinal Injury Association motor score of 0 with some sensory sparing initially. **(B–D)** Computed tomographic scans of the cervical spine showing associated perched facets. **(E)** Despite the application of 80 lb of traction, the fracture could not be reduced, and the patient developed respiratory difficulty. **(F)** Sagittal short tau inversion recovery sequence magnetic resonance imaging showing significant posterior ligamentous injury with cord signal change and cord compression. The patient underwent posterior spinal fusion. Postoperatively, he recovered to 4/5 strength in his deltoids, but his sensory examination remained unchanged. **(G)** Anteroposterior and **(H)** lateral x-rays showing C3-4 posterior spinal fusion.

the patient is unconscious and unable to be examined.[33] Definitive management of facet injuries (unilateral, bilateral) begins with closed reduction through skull traction to restore proper alignment. If proper alignment is obtained, then a ventral decompression and stabilization is the preferred surgical approach; if proper alignment is not attainable, a dorsal decompression and stabilization is needed.

Vertical compression injuries describe cervical burst fractures due to axial loading. This type of injury involves more osseous injury than ligamentous injury. Those patients who have incomplete neurological injuries should be ventrally decompressed with stabilization. Our bias is that most of these injuries should be surgically stabilized to prevent kyphosis and chronic pain, although external immobilization may also be employed.

Distractive extension injuries are generally found in older patients who experience a fall and a blow to the head causing avulsion of the anterior longitudinal ligament and the ventral disk space widening.[33] These patients typically present with a central cord syndrome due to underlying canal stenosis with weakness of the upper extremities and more than the lower extremities. Spontaneous recovery of the central cord syndrome is common if stability is preserved.[32] This represents a very dangerous injury in patients with ankylosing spondylitis or those with diffuse idiopathic skeletal hyperostosis who have two rigid moment arms adjacent to a fracture.[32] Unstable injuries are treated with a ventral reconstructive and plating procedure restoring the ventral or anterior tension band. Lateral flexion injuries are the least common, typically do not produce neurological deficits, and are generally stable and do not require surgical intervention.[32]

Thoracic Spine and Thoracolumbar Junction

The thoracic spine differs from the cervical spine in that it articulates with the rib cage and sternum and is more rigid; it also has coronally oriented facet joints, a kyphotic alignment, and a smaller spinal canal to spinal cord ratio. Because of the stability of the thoracic spine, high-velocity trauma is needed to destabilize this region. However, the small spinal canal leads to a high incidence of SCI when there is a dislocation in the thoracic spine. The thoracolumbar junction (T10–L2) marks the transition from a rigid thoracic spine to a mobile lumbar spine. In this region, there is a gradual change in facet orientation to a sagittal angle, and the facet joints support a third of the axial load at this level. For these reasons, the thoracolumbar junction is vulnerable to injury and accounts for ~50% of all vertebral body fractures and 40% of all SCI.[34] Burst fractures are the most common type of injury, followed by seat belt or Chance-type fractures.[34,35] Petitjean and colleagues[35] also noted a strong correlation between abdominal visceral injuries and thoracolumbar fractures.

Several factors must be considered when assessing thoracic fractures. The first is the anatomical stability of the surrounding structures, such as the ribs and sternum. The degree of normal kyphosis versus traumatic kyphosis due to ligamentous injury needs to be assessed because older patients tend to have a greater degree of kyphosis than their younger counterparts.[36] It is important to assess the degree of spinal canal compromise and the extent of neurological injury because these factors can determine the surgical approach. In the absence of neurological injury or canal compromise, these fractures may be managed conservatively.

Several classification systems have been proposed for thoracic and lumbar trauma, although none has gained universal acceptance. These systems are based on either morphological or mechanistic classification of the injury pattern. The Denis classification system[37] was a single-center experience based on the morphological description of 412 thoracic and thoracolumbar fractures. This system divides the spine into three columns: the anterior column (anterior longitudinal ligament and anterior two thirds of the vertebral body), the middle column (posterior longitudinal ligament and posterior one third of the vertebral body), and the posterior column (the facet joints, neural arch, and posterior ligaments).[37] In this classification scheme, anterior column injury is a stable compression fracture. Burst fractures are defined as failure of the anterior and middle columns and are attributed to axial loading. Flexion distraction injuries, such as those caused by a seat belt, are due to failure of the middle and posterior columns and are unstable injuries. Fracture dislocations in the Denis classification scheme are considered failure of all three columns with significant instability and neurological compromise. Denis[37] reported that up to 20% of patients with severe burst fractures and retropulsion of osseous fragments into the spinal canal or posterior column injuries treated conservatively with an external orthotic brace had subsequent neurological compromise.

An alternative classification system proposed by Magerl et al. was based on the mechanism of injury and has been termed the AO classification.[38] Three major groups of injuries were proposed, with progressive incidence of SCI, and are noted as types A, B, or C. Type A injuries have axial load or compression, Type B injuries have a distraction mechanism, and Type C injuries have multidirectional forces or rotational instability. Each fracture pattern is divided into three subtypes, each subtype has two to three subgroups, and each subgroup may have several subdivisions, for a total of 53 fracture patterns or classifications. The complexity of the system has led to confusion during attempts to define injuries past the level of subtype and has shown low to moderate intra- and interobserver reliability.[39] This led to a recent attempt at classification termed the Thoracolumbar Injury Classification System (TLICS).[40–42] Three characteristics of the injury are assessed and rated using a point system. The injury mechanism is inferred from radiographic studies, with compression injuries receiving 1 point, burst fractures 2 points, translational or rotational injuries 3 points, and distraction injuries 4 points. The integrity of the posterior ligamentous complex is also inferred from radiological studies, with intact ligaments receiving 0 points, clearly disrupted ligaments 3 points, and injuries in which the condition of the ligament is ambiguous 2 points. Finally, the system directly assesses neurological injury. Patients with an intact neurological examination receive 0 points, those with a nerve root injury or complete SCI receive 2 points, and those with incomplete SCI or a cauda equina injury receive 3 points. The sum of the severity score can then be used as a guide to determine whether the patient is better served by operative or nonoperative intervention. Patients with 3 or fewer points are candidates for nonoperative treatment, those with 5 or more points are operative candidates, and those with 4 points have treatment guided by surgeon preference.

There has been no universally accepted treatment algorithm for thoracolumbar spine injuries despite the myriad of classification schemes. Universally accepted indications for surgical intervention in the thoracic spine include incomplete neurological injury, greater than 50% loss of height of the vertebral body with posterior ligamentous disruption, fracture dislocations, or any three-column injury (**Fig. 12.2**).[43] Patients with an incomplete neurological injury who underwent operative decompression and stabilization procedures have been shown to have an enhanced neurological recovery compared with nonoperatively treated patients.[44] Surgical decompression in patients with complete neurological deficits has not demonstrated true benefit in terms of neurological improvement, although it can restore sagittal and coronal alignment and reduce pain and periods of immobilization.[45,46] Furthermore, in patients in whom the spinal deformity is not corrected, persistent extradural osseous compression with resultant cerebrospinal fluid obstruction poses an additional risk of posttraumatic syrinx, which is a well-recognized cause of delayed neurological deterioration above the level of the original injury in patients with SCI.[47]

Ventral or dorsolateral approaches in addition to instrumentation may be em-

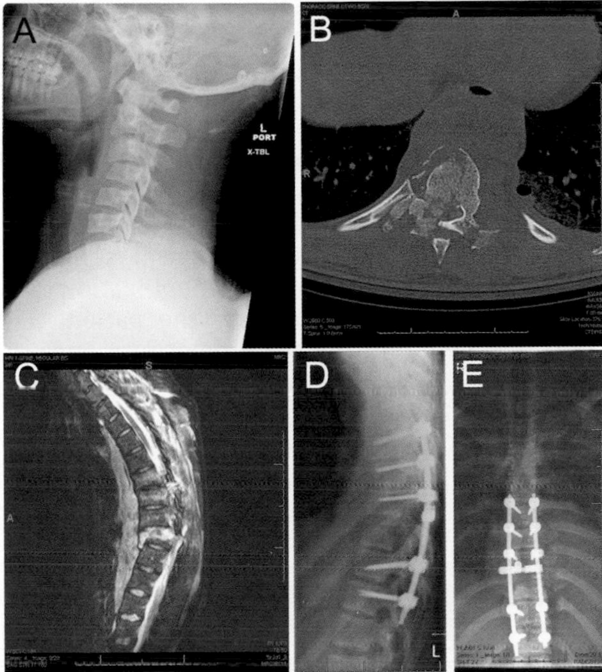

Fig. 12.2 A 35-year-old man presented with T9 fracture dislocation. **(A,B)** Sagittal and axial computed tomographic (CT) scans demonstrating T9 burst fracture dislocation and complete canal compromise. At presentation, he was without motor or sensory function below the level of the fracture. **(C)** Sagittal short tau inversion recovery magnetic resonance imaging showing significant anterior and posterior ligamentous injury with transection of the spinal cord. He underwent posterior spinal fusion with instrumentation from T6 to T11. After surgery his neurological condition remained compromised. **(D)** Anteroposterior and **(E)** lateral x-rays of the thoracic spine demonstrating T6-11 posterior spinal fusion with instrumentation.

ployed to decompress the neural elements and stabilize the spine. Dorsal decompression without instrumentation should not be performed as an isolated treatment strategy because this technique removes the posterior ligamentous complex where the integrity of the anterior and middle columns is already damaged.[6,7] Removal of the posterior tension band promotes kyphosis and may result in further neurological injury due to draping of the neural elements over the traumatic kyphotic deformity.[6,7] The ventral approach allows direct decompression of the spinal cord. The major limitation of the ventral approach is the risk of injury to the viscera and major vascular structures. However, either standalone ventral decompression and fusion or staged reconstruction of the vertebral body using a graft or expandable cage after posterior stabilization provides better biomechanical stability than posterior short segment instrumentation alone.

Burst fractures with retropulsed fragments and loss of vertebral body height require application of distractive forces to realign the spinal column and restore the spinal canal. Dorsal distraction techniques using ligamentotaxis in patients with an intact posterior tension band reduce the retropulsed bone fragments ventrally out of the spinal canal. Overdistraction, however, can incur further neurological deterioration, so careful ligamentotaxis under fluoroscopic guidance is imperative. After posterior reduction, the integrity of the anterior and middle columns should be carefully assessed because posterior reconstruction alone may have a high failure rate.[48,49]

Lower Lumbar Spine

The lower lumbar spine (L3-5) accounts for only 4% of all spinal fractures because of the large size, extensive muscular attachments, and stability of obliquely angled facets of the vertebrae.[50] The spinal cord typically ends at the L1–2 level, leading to a lower incidence of neurological injury in lower lumbar fractures. Because of the inherent stability conferred by the pelvis and the iliolumbar ligaments, fractures in this region without neurological deficit have been successfully treated by bracing alone.[51,52] Patients with fracture dislocations and burst fractures associated with a neurological deficit have generally been candidates for surgical intervention. The advent of segmental transpedicular fixation allows decompression and stabilization in this region from a posterior approach. These systems allow surgeons to restore lumbar lordosis and minimize the number of segments that need to be fused.[51] However, severe compression with comminution and destruction of the vertebral body can effectively be treated from an anterior approach.[53] This approach is typically reserved for patients with persistent canal stenosis, continuing neurological deficits, and significant biomechanical stressors.

The rationale for surgical intervention in patients with incomplete neurological injury is fairly robust, but surgical intervention in patients with complete nerve root injuries from lumbar fracture typically does not improve neurological outcome. Despite the lack of evidence for neurological improvement, we believe that surgical decompression and stabilization are important because they can result in a shorter intensive care stay; decreased morbidity associated with a recumbent position; and decreased pain, progressive deformity, and potential for neurological deterioration in the future.[53]

Conclusion

In summary, advances in surgical technique and instrumentation have made surgery in the setting of SCI an effective option. The ability to decompress the canal may result in neurological improvement if done expeditiously after the injury. Furthermore, surgical stabilization can lead to early mobilization and faster reintegration for the patient. Finally, preventing late deformity and associated complications, such as pain and syringomyelia, needs to be considered in the treatment of young patients with SCI.

Pearls and Pitfalls

- Decompression of an SCI through a laminectomy alone is generally *not* indicated.
- Early decompression and stabilization for SCI can be done safely, and evidence is accumulating that it may improve neurological outcome.
- Both mechanistic and morphological classification systems have been devised for description of spinal column trauma. Although no system is universally accepted, these aid the clinician in description of injury pattern and prediction of stability in SCI.

References

1. Deshaies EM, DiRisio D, Popp AJ. Medieval management of spinal injuries: parallels between Theodoric of Bologna and contemporary spine surgeons. Neurosurg Focus 2004;16(1):E3
2. Kraus JF, Franti CE, Riggins RS, Richards D, Borhani NO. Incidence of traumatic spinal cord lesions. J Chronic Dis 1975;28(9):471–492 PubMed
3. DeVivo MJ. Causes and costs of spinal cord injury in the United States. Spinal Cord 1997;35(12):809–813
4. Sekhon LH, Fehlings MG. Epidemiology, demographics, and pathophysiology of acute spinal cord injury. Spine 2001;26(24, Suppl):S2–S12
5. Waters RL, Meyer PR Jr, Adkins RH, Felton D. Emergency, acute, and surgical management of spine trauma. Arch Phys Med Rehabil 1999;80(11):1383–1390
6. Bedbrook GM. Spinal injuries with tetraplegia and paraplegia. J Bone Joint Surg Br 1979;61-B(3):267–284
7. Bedbrook GM. Treatment of thoracolumbar dislocation and fractures with paraplegia. Clin Orthop Relat Res 1975;(112):27–43
8. Guttmann L. Surgical aspects of the treatment of traumatic paraplegia. J Bone Joint Surg Br 1949;31B(3):399–403
9. Dall DM. Injuries of the cervical spine, II: Does anatomical reduction of the bony injuries improve the prognosis for spinal cord recovery? S Afr Med J 1972;46(31):1083–1090
10. Harris P, Karmi MZ, McClemont E, Matlhoko D, Paul KS. The prognosis of patients sustaining severe cervical spine injury (C2-C7 inclusive). Paraplegia 1980;18(5):324–330
11. Katoh S, el Masry WS, Jaffray D, et al. Neurologic outcome in conservatively treated patients with

incomplete closed traumatic cervical spinal cord injuries. Spine 1996;21(20):2345–2351

12. Duh MS, Shepard MJ, Wilberger JE, Bracken MB. The effectiveness of surgery on the treatment of acute spinal cord injury and its relation to pharmacological treatment. Neurosurgery 1994;35(2): 240–248, discussion 248–249

13. McKinley W, Meade MA, Kirshblum S, Barnard B. Outcomes of early surgical management versus late or no surgical intervention after acute spinal cord injury. Arch Phys Med Rehabil 2004; 85(11):1818–1825

14. Bunge RP, Puckett WR, Becerra JL, Marcillo A, Quencer RM. Observations on the pathology of human spinal cord injury: a review and classification of 22 new cases with details from a case of chronic cord compression with extensive focal demyelination. Adv Neurol 1993;59:75–89

15. Kakulas BA. Pathology of spinal injuries. Cent Nerv Syst Trauma 1984;1(2):117–129

16. Dolan EJ, Tator CH, Endrenyi L. The value of decompression for acute experimental spinal cord compression injury. J Neurosurg 1980;53(6): 749–755

17. Rabinowitz RS, Eck JC, Harper CM Jr, et al. Urgent surgical decompression compared to methylprednisolone for the treatment of acute spinal cord injury: a randomized prospective study in beagle dogs. Spine 2008;33(21):2260–2268

18. Wagner FC Jr, Chehrazi B. Early decompression and neurological outcome in acute cervical spinal cord injuries. J Neurosurg 1982;56(5): 699–705

19. Bohlman HH, Anderson PA. Anterior decompression and arthrodesis of the cervical spine: long-term motor improvement, I: Improvement in incomplete traumatic quadriparesis. J Bone Joint Surg Am 1992;74(5):671–682

20. Fehlings MG, Vaccaro AR, Aarabi B, et al. One year outcomes of the STASCIS study: a prospective multicenter trial to evaluate the role and timing of decompression in patients with cervical spinal cord injury. J Neurosurg 2009;110(5):A1044

21. White AA, Panjabi MM. Kinematics of the spine. In: Clinical Biomechanics of the Spine. Philadelphia, PA: JB Lippincott; 1990:92–97

22. Mirza SK, Krengel WF III, Chapman JR, et al. Early versus delayed surgery for acute cervical spinal cord injury. Clin Orthop Relat Res 1999; (359):104–114

23. Sethi MK, Schoenfeld AJ, Bono CM, Harris MB. The evolution of thoracolumbar injury classification systems. Spine J 2009;9(9):780–788

24. Kostuik JP. Dysfunction of the spinal stability system and its restabilization. In: Holtzman R, McCormick PC, Farcy JC, eds. Spinal Instability. New York, NY: Springer-Verlag; 1993:39–44

25. Levine A, Eismont F, Garfin S, Zigler J. Spine Trauma. Philadelphia: WB Saunders; 1998

26. Anderson PA, Bohlman HH. Anterior decompression and arthrodesis of the cervical spine: long-term motor improvement, II: Improvement in complete traumatic quadriplegia. J Bone Joint Surg Am 1992;74(5):683–692

27. Kwon BK, Vaccaro AR, Grauer JN, Fisher CG, Dvorak MF. Subaxial cervical spine trauma. J Am Acad Orthop Surg 2006;14(2):78–89

28. Alker G. Computed Tomography with and without Myelography. Philadelphia, PA: JB Lippincott; 1989

29. Bucholz RW, Burkhead WZ. The pathological anatomy of fatal atlanto-occipital dislocations. J Bone Joint Surg Am 1979;61(2):248–250

30. Bellabarba C, Mirza SK, West GA, et al. Diagnosis and treatment of craniocervical dislocation in a series of 17 consecutive survivors during an 8-year period. J Neurosurg Spine 2006;4(6):429–440

31. Dickman CA, Greene KA, Sonntag VK. Injuries involving the transverse atlantal ligament: classification and treatment guidelines based upon experience with 39 injuries. Neurosurgery 1996; 38(1):44–50

32. Allen BL Jr, Ferguson RL, Lehmann TR, O'Brien RP. A mechanistic classification of closed, indirect fractures and dislocations of the lower cervical spine. Spine 1982;7(1):1–27

33. Vaccaro AR, Madigan L, Schweitzer ME, Flanders AE, Hilibrand AS, Albert TJ. Magnetic resonance imaging analysis of soft tissue disruption after flexion-distraction injuries of the subaxial cervical spine. Spine 2001;26(17):1866–1872

34. Singh K, Erdos J, Sah A, Vaccaro AR, McLain RF. The value of surgical intervention in spinal trauma. In: Benzel EC, ed. Spine Surgery: Techniques, Complication Avoidance, and Management. Vol 2. Elsevier, Churchill, Livingstone; 1999:1367–1378

35. Petitjean ME, Mousselard H, Pointillart V, Lassie P, Senegas J, Dabadie P. Thoracic spinal trauma and associated injuries: should early spinal decompression be considered? J Trauma 1995; 39(2):368–372

36. Panjabi MM, Takata K, Goel V, et al. Thoracic human vertebrae: quantitative three-dimensional anatomy. Spine 1991;16(8):888–901

37. Denis F. The three column spine and its significance in the classification of acute thoracolumbar spinal injuries. Spine 1983;8(8):817–831

38. Magerl F, Aebi M, Gertzbein SD, Harms J, Nazarian S. A comprehensive classification of thoracic and lumbar injuries. Eur Spine J 1994;3(4): 184–201

39. Wood KB, Khanna G, Vaccaro AR, Arnold PM, Harris MB, Mehbod AA. Assessment of two thoracolumbar fracture classification systems as used by multiple surgeons. J Bone Joint Surg Am 2005;87(7):1423–1429

40. Vaccaro AR, Lehman RA Jr, Hurlbert RJ, et al. A new classification of thoracolumbar injuries: the importance of injury morphology, the integrity of the posterior ligamentous complex, and neurologic status. Spine 2005;30(20):2325–2333

41. Vaccaro AR, Zeiller SC, Hulbert RJ, et al. The thoracolumbar injury severity score: a proposed treatment algorithm. J Spinal Disord Tech 2005;18(3):209–215

42. Harrop JS, Vaccaro AR, Hurlbert RJ, et al; Spine Trauma Study Group. Intrarater and interrater reliability and validity in the assessment of the mechanism of injury and integrity of the posterior ligamentous complex: a novel injury severity scoring system for thoracolumbar injuries. Invited submission from the Joint Section Meeting On Disorders of the Spine and Peripheral Nerves, March 2005. J Neurosurg Spine 2006;4(2):118–122

43. Cantor JB, Lebwohl NH, Garvey T, Eismont FJ. Nonoperative management of stable thoracolumbar burst fractures with early ambulation and bracing. Spine 1993;18(8):971–976
44. Mumford J, Weinstein JN, Spratt KF, Goel VK. Thoracolumbar burst fractures: the clinical efficacy and outcome of nonoperative management. Spine 1993;18(8):955–970
45. Fehlings MG, Perrin RG. The role and timing of early decompression for cervical spinal cord injury: update with a review of recent clinical evidence. Injury 2005;36(Suppl 2):B13–B26
46. Fehlings MG, Tator CH. An evidence-based review of decompressive surgery in acute spinal cord injury: rationale, indications, and timing based on experimental and clinical studies. J Neurosurg 1999;91(1, Suppl):1–11
47. Holly LT, Johnson JP, Masciopinto JE, Batzdorf U. Treatment of posttraumatic syringomyelia with extradural decompressive surgery. Neurosurg Focus 2000;8(3):E8
48. McLain RF, Sparling E, Benson DR. Early failure of short-segment pedicle instrumentation for thoracolumbar fractures: a preliminary report. J Bone Joint Surg Am 1993;75(2):162–167
49. Sasso RC, Renkens K, Hanson D, Reilly T, McGuire RA Jr, Best NM. Unstable thoracolumbar burst fractures: anterior-only versus short-segment posterior fixation. J Spinal Disord Tech 2006; 19(4):242–248
50. Calenoff L, Chessare JW, Rogers LF, Toerge J, Rosen JS. Multiple level spinal injuries: importance of early recognition. AJR Am J Roentgenol 1978;130(4):665–669
51. Seybold EA, Sweeney CA, Fredrickson BE, Warhold LG, Bernini PM. Functional outcome of low lumbar burst fractures: a multicenter review of operative and nonoperative treatment of L3-L5. Spine 1999;24(20):2154–2161
52. An HS, Simpson JM, Ebraheim NA, Jackson WT, Moore J, O'Malley NP. Low lumbar burst fractures: comparison between conservative and surgical treatments. Orthopedics 1992;15(3): 367–373
53. Dai LD. Low lumbar spinal fractures: management options. Injury 2002;33(7):579–582

13

Venous Thromboembolism Prophylaxis

Avraam Ploumis

Key Points

1. Venous thromboembolism has a serious impact on patients with spinal cord injury.
2. Diagnosis and treatment of thromboembolism are analyzed.
3. Various forms of venous thromboprophylaxis are discussed extensively.

Venous thromboembolism (VTE), consisting of both deep venous thrombosis (DVT) and pulmonary embolism (PE), is a leading cause of mortality and morbidity following acute spinal cord injury (SCI) and offer considerable discomfort and delay in rehabilitation for the patients who suffer from it.[1,2]

SCI has a major global health impact, with a reported annual incidence of 15 to 40 cases per million, and the majority of these injuries occur in young adults from 16 to 30 years of age.[3] The frequency of DVT and PE in untreated spinal trauma (spinal fracture with or without SCI) patients has been reported to be between 67% and 100%.[4–8] Pulmonary embolism is the third most common cause of death in those patients who survive longer than 24 hours after injury.[9,10]

The American College of Chest Physicians and the Consortium of Spinal Cord Medicine have recommended specific thromboprophylaxis guidelines for SCI patients.[1,11–14] However, routine utilization of thromboprophylaxis measures has great variability due to case-specific risk factors,[14,15] low compliance in hospitals,[16] questionable efficacy,[17] potential complications, and a dearth of high-quality (level I) evidence-based recommendations. In the Spinal Cord Injury Risk Assessment for Thromboembolism (SPIRATE) study, there was a recommendation for more vigorous prophylaxis in SCI patients who are older, obese, and have flaccid paralysis or cancer.[18] Moreover, there is uncertainty regarding the length of thromboembolic prophylaxis in the setting of SCI due to questions regarding the role of screening tests for DVT.[19]

Risk Factors for Venous Thromboembolism in Spinal Cord Injury Patients

The level of thromboembolic risk is determined by numerous variables. Trauma greatly increases the risk of DVT and PE by causing immobility as well as a hypercoagulable state.[11] The risk for VTE appears to be the greatest during the first 12 weeks after injury, when flaccidity, paralysis, and immobilization of the extremities predominate. The pathophysiology of VTE in SCI involves stasis, hypercoagulability, and vessel intimal injury (the Virchow triad)[20,21] on the basis of abnormal platelet function and altered fibrinolytic activity in patients with SCI.[22,23]

Technical factors may also affect the risk of thromboembolic events following surgery.[24–26] The method of surgical approach can increase the risk of DVT and PE. Incidence rates are highest for surgeries at lumbar levels and surgeries that require an anterior approach. Moreover, the combination of these two factors increases the risk even further, most likely because an anterior approach to the lumbar spine often requires retraction of the common iliac veins and the venae cavae.[24–26] An anterior approach also has an increased risk of pelvic clot formation.[24] Other surgical factors that can increase the risk of DVT and PE include length of the procedure, prolonged postoperative immobilization, and prone positioning.[25–27]

Patient demographics can also contribute to thromboembolic risk. Increased age, male gender, smoking habits, obesity, lower limb fractures, and disease states, such as hypertension, heart failure, diabetes, and cancer, all increase the risk of DVT and PE in patients.[1,25–27] Even though spasticity has been suggested to reduce the incidence of thromboembolism, this has not been proven adequately.[28] Finally, there exists an association between the occurrence of DVT and heterotopic ossification following traumatic SCI.[29]

Natural History of DVT/PE in the Absence/Presence of Thromboprophylaxis

Without prophylaxis, clinical studies using venography as a diagnostic tool for DVT have shown high rates of calf DVT (40 to 80%) in patients suffering from major trauma and SCI.[5,27,30,31] Specifically for spinal injuries without prophylaxis, the incidence of DVT reached up to 62%, with SCI and surgery as independent risk factors.[5] Proximal embolization has been detected in 50% of established DVT without treatment.[32] Death attributed to PE has been found to reach up to 35% of patients with SCI without prophylaxis for thromboembolism.[33] The majority of VTE incidents occur in the acute rehabilitation phase of SCI, whereas in chronic SCI, the incidence of DVT/PE is 1.1%/0.3%, respectively.[1,34]

On the contrary, the incidence of DVT is at least 9.4% in patients with acute SCI who undergo thromboprophylaxis with low-molecular-weight heparin during the acute stage,[19] with a mortality rate of 9.7% among SCI patients with DVT/PE.[19]

Postthrombotic syndrome can lead to prolongation of rehabilitation in 12% of SCI patients with DVT who were followed for 3 years.[35] Recurrent leg edema, skin breakdown, pain, relapsing DVT and pulmonary complications appear generally in conjunction with postthrombotic syndrome.[33]

Diagnosis of Venous Thromboembolism

The gold standard for DVT diagnosis is venography.[19] However, due to the invasive character and side effects of this procedure, duplex ultrasonography has replaced venography in diagnosis of DVT.[19] Of course, clinical suspicion, together with history/clinical examination (edema of the leg, increase of calf diameter, and localized tenderness along the deep venous system) (**Fig. 13.1**) and risk factor assessment, are critical to reach the correct diagnosis.[36] In mild clinical suspicion of DVT or in cases of technically inadequate ultrasonography, D-dimer measurements within normal limits can exclude DVT.[36] Computed tomography (CT) or magnetic resonance imaging (MRI) venography could overcome the technical limitations of ultrasonographic diagnosis of DVT, but further clinical studies are needed to ensure its accuracy.[37] However, routine screening for DVT in adults with acute traumatic SCI under thromboprophylaxis is not recommended.[19]

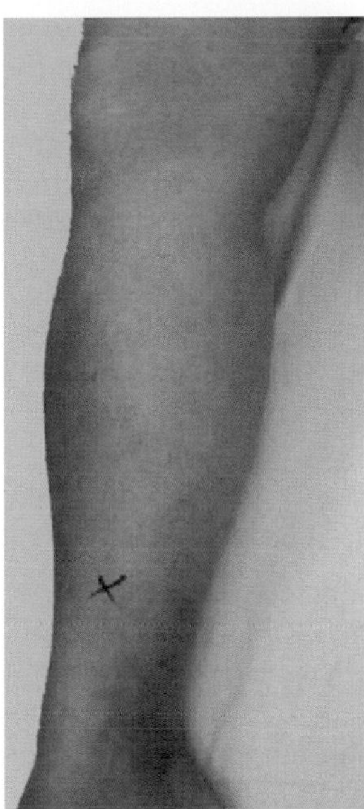

Fig. 13.1 Clinical photograph of calf edema suspicious for deep venous thrombosis.

Similar to DVT, diagnosis of PE can be made by combining history, clinical findings, and diagnostic tests (electrocardiogram, blood gas values, troponin levels, D-dimer values, chest radiography).[38] However, objective diagnostic tests for diagnosis of PE include CT pulmonary angiography (CTPA), ventilation perfusion (V/Q) scan, or true pulmonary angiography, with CTPA being the superior of all three.[38]

Start of Thromboprophylaxis in Spinal Cord Injury Patients

Hypercoagulability has been shown to start within a few hours after SCI and persists for at least 2 to 3 weeks.[8] Prophylactic pharmacological treatment for thrombosis should, therefore, be initiated as soon as possible after injury,[39] and ideally within 72 hours.[1] In cases involving intracranial bleeding, hemothorax, intraabdominal bleeding, or other active hemorrhage, pharmacological prophylaxis is contraindicated until the patient is hemodynamically and neurologically stabilized.[11] Mechanical forms of prophylaxis, however, may be initiated as soon as possible.[1,11]

Duration of Thromboprophylaxis in Spinal Cord Injury Patients

The risk for VTE appears to be the greatest during the first 12 weeks after injury, when flaccidity, paralysis, and immobilization of the extremities predominate.[40] The higher incidence of DVT episodes is within the first 2 weeks post-SCI and decreases thereafter.[30]

Most thromboembolic events occur within 2 to 3 months of injury.[41–43] In a retrospective cohort study of 16,240 SCI patients, almost all (88%) thromboembolic events occurred in the first 3 months following SCI.[44] Only a few studies have shown occurrence of VTE within the rehabilitation phase or later than 3 months postinjury.[45–47] Recent studies report the utilization of thromboprophylaxis for up to 3 months.[39,48–50] In a recent meta-analysis,[51] the recommended duration of thromboprophylaxis was at least 3 months from the time of SCI or for as long the inpatient rehabilitation period lasts.[1] Very few studies suggest the use of thromboprophylaxis beyond 3 months, irrespective of muscle tone state,[52] and many support discontinuing pharmacological prophylaxis when lower extremity mobility is purposeful.[1,6] In patients with a history of previous DVT or PE, thromboprophylaxis with oral anticoagulants should be extended from 6 months to 1 year depending on the presence of other risk factors.[43]

Modes of Thromboprophylaxis in Spinal Cord Injury Patients and Comparisons among Different Modes

Methods of thromboprophylaxis include mechanical methods, pharmaceutical agents, or a combination of the above. Electrical stimulation as a means of VTE prophylaxis has not proven to be efficient.[30] Although mechanical prophylaxis with intermittent pneumatic compression devices is a commonly employed method of VTE prevention in SCI patients, its effectiveness has also been questioned.[53,54] Pharmacological options include unfractionated heparin (UFH) and low-molecular-weight heparin (LMWH). Mechanical and pharmacological modalities may offer more effective prophylaxis in combination than when used alone; however, this has not been well-established, and a combined approach also raises compliance and cost-related issues.[30,55–64]

Comparison of Mechanical Alone versus Combined Mechanical and Chemical Thromboprophylaxis Methods in Spinal Cord Injury Patients

Several studies support the beneficial effect of mechanical prophylaxis alone even in the presence of risk factors (**Table 13.1**).[54,65] The results of a meta-analysis showed no statistically significant reduction in incidence of VTE with the addition of pharmacological prophylaxis.[51] Mechanical methods alone provided a quantifiable reduction in VTE,[65] and their use is recommended early after injury for at least the first 2 weeks in all patients.[1,11] The value of additional pharmacological prophylaxis should be weighed in terms of risks versus benefits specific to each patient.

Table 13.1 Risk Factors for Venous Thromboembolism in Spinal Cord Injury Patients

Patient	Age (>70 years)
	Gender (male)
	Medical comorbidities (cancer, diabetes, obesity, cardiopulmonary diseases)
	History of deep vein thrombosis and/or pulmonary embolism
	Smoking status
Injury	Completeness of SCI (motor complete vs motor incomplete)
	Other traumatic injuries (head, thoracoabdominal, extremity fracture)
	Severity of trauma
Operative procedure	Operative approach (anterior vs posterior)
	Spinal canal decompression (decompression vs fusion)
	Number of spinal levels fused (three or more)
	Level of injury (cervical vs thoracolumbar)

Comparison of UFH versus LMWH in Acute Spinal Cord Injury Patients

A meta-analysis of studies with SCI patients showed that the use of LMWHs was associated with statistically significant fewer episodes of DVT compared with UFH.[51] Furthermore, no statistical difference was detected between LWMH and UFH for the prevention of PE.[51] This is consistent with a similar meta-analysis in general orthopedic surgery patients.[66] Comparisons of LMWH formulations revealed no difference in efficacy between enoxaparin and dalteparin, whereas fondaparinux was more efficacious than enoxaparin.[49,65]

Inferior Vena Cava Filter Insertion in Spine Trauma

The use of inferior vena cava (IVC) filters has expanded in trauma patients, including those with SCI. However, objective criteria for their use in SCI patients have yet to be clearly defined. A review of the literature by Johns et al.[67] found that IVC filter placement in SCI patients is effective in preventing pulmonary emboli and has a low complication rate. Indications for filter placement include patients who have had pulmonary emboli despite adequate anticoagulation, patients with documented pulmonary embolus who have a contraindication to anticoagulation, patients with concomitant long bone fractures, or patients with free-floating iliofemoral thrombus.[67,68] Additionally, filters may be useful in patients with high cervical injuries, poor cardiopulmonary reserve, or IVC thrombus formation despite adequate anticoagulation.[67] Only

20% of survey respondents stated that they recommend IVC filters for their SCI patients despite this supporting evidence.[69]

Complications of Pharmacological Prophylaxis in Spinal Cord Injury Patients

Bleeding has been found to range between 0.9 to 11% in two previous meta-analyses comparing LMWH and standard heparin in general and orthopedic surgery.[66,70] However, the definition of bleeding was heterogeneous across the studies. There is conflicting evidence on the safety of LMWH and standard heparin in studies with SCI patients.

In a recent meta-analysis, bleeding was found to be significantly more likely when UFH was used; however, other heparin-related complications were minimal and not statistically different between LMWH and UFH.[51]

Compliance and Cost-Related Issues of Thromboprophylaxis

Even though thromboprophylaxis with adjusted-dose UFH produces a cost savings over LMWH,[71] the increased bleeding complications associated with UFH and the need for regular monitoring of activated partial thromboplastin time (aPTT) values have led to the use of LMWH in almost all SCI patients according to guidelines of chest physicians, of the American Association of Neurological Surgeons/Congress of Neurological Surgeons (AANS/CNS), and of the Consortium for Spinal Cord Medicine.[1,11,13] In addition, there is only moderate compliance with the published evidence-based guidelines on thromboprophylaxis among health care professionals and patients, which needs to be improved.[16,72]

The cost of thromboembolism in patients with SCI has a major impact on the already high annual cost to the national economy (annual cost to the US economy for SCI patients is $7.2 billion, added cost for thromboembolism $178 million, 1995 data).[73] This translates to 1 to 2 weeks' extension of acute care hospitalization and an increase of costs by 35%.[74]

Treatment of Venous Thromboembolism

Once venous thromboembolism (DVT or PE) diagnosis is established, as soon as possible, intravenous unfractionated or subcutaneous low-molecular heparin treatment should be initiated unless there is a serious bleeding risk. This should be replaced solely by oral warfarin when the international normalized ratio (INR) is within the therapeutic range (2 to 3) and should be continued for 6 weeks to 6 months, depending on the potential benefits and risks for each patient.[19]

Conclusion

The latest guidelines of the American College of Chest Physicians and the Consortium for Spinal Cord Medicine for thromboprophylaxis in acute spinal trauma, together with recent meta-analyses on the same subject,[1,11–13,51] offer the following evidence-based conclusions/recommendations (**Table 13.2**):

1. Mechanical prophylaxis in both legs should be used for at least the first 2 weeks following acute SCI (level I evidence).
2. Adjuvant pharmacological thromboprophylaxis agents should be initiated within 72 hours of injury if no active bleeding or coagulopathy exists.
3. LMWH is more effective than UFH in DVT prevention in patients with acute SCI; however, PE prevention is equivalent (level I evidence).
4. Fewer bleeding complications were noted when comparing LMWH to UFH in patients with acute SCI (level I evidence).

5. Duration of thromboprophylaxis in patients with complete motor paralysis or in patients with incomplete motor paralysis but with additional VTE risk factors should last for at least 3 months after their injury or for as long their rehabilitation period lasts.
6. IVC filters are only rarely used in SCI patients who have contraindications to receiving anticoagulation or when anticoagulation is not effective.

Table 13.2 Guidelines for Thromboprophylaxis in Spinal Cord Injury Patients

Duplex ultrasonography of the deep vein system and a clinical examination are critical for correct diagnosis of deep vein thrombosis
Mechanical prophylaxis (at least anti-embolism compression stockings) in both legs should be used for at least the first 2 weeks following acute spinal cord injury
Adjuvant pharmacological thromboprophylaxis agents should be initiated within 72 hours of injury if no active bleeding or coagulopathy exists
Low-molecular-weight heparin is more effective and safer than unfractionated heparin in deep vein thrombosis prevention in patients with acute spinal cord injury
Duration of thromboprophylaxis in patients with complete motor paralysis or in patients with incomplete motor paralysis but with additional VTE risk factors should last for at least 3 months

Pearls

- D-dimer measurement within normal limits can exclude DVT.
- Mechanical prophylaxis for DVT of the lower extremities is the essential first measure in all patients with acute SCI.
- LMWH is more effective as DVT prophylaxis than UFH for SCI patients.

Pitfalls

- Increased muscle tone in the lower extremities does not protect from venous thromboembolism in patients with SCI.
- Thromboprophylaxis should not be terminated before 3 months from initiation of traumatic SCI.

References

1. Consortium for Spinal Cord Medicine. Prevention of thromboembolism in spinal cord injury. J Spinal Cord Med 1997;20(3):259–283
2. Green D, Hull RD, Mammen EF, Merli GJ, Weingarden SI, Yao JS. Deep vein thrombosis in spinal cord injury: summary and recommendations. Chest 1992;102(6, Suppl):633S–635S
3. Sekhon LH, Fehlings MG. Epidemiology, demographics, and pathophysiology of acute spinal cord injury. Spine 2001;26(24, Suppl):S2–S12
4. Brach BB, Moser KM, Cedar L, Minteer M, Convery R. Venous thrombosis in acute spinal cord paralysis. J Trauma 1977;17(4):289–292
5. Geerts WH, Code KI, Jay RM, Chen E, Szalai JP. A prospective study of venous thromboembolism after major trauma. N Engl J Med 1994; 331(24):1601–1606
6. Myllynen P, Kammonen M, Rokkanen P, Böstman O, Lalla M, Laasonen E. Deep venous thrombosis and pulmonary embolism in patients with acute spinal cord injury: a comparison with nonparalyzed patients immobilized due to spinal fractures. J Trauma 1985;25(6):541–543
7. Petäjä J, Myllynen P, Rokkanen P, Nokelainen M. Fibrinolysis and spinal injury. Relationship to post-traumatic deep vein thrombosis. Acta Chir Scand 1989;155(4-5):241–246
8. Rossi EC, Green D, Rosen JS, Spies SM, Jao JS. Sequential changes in factor VIII and platelets preceding deep vein thrombosis in patients with spinal cord injury. Br J Haematol 1980;45(1): 143–151
9. DeVivo MJ, Krause JS, Lammertse DP. Recent trends in mortality and causes of death among persons with spinal cord injury. Arch Phys Med Rehabil 1999;80(11):1411–1419
10. Waring WP, Karunas RS. Acute spinal cord injuries and the incidence of clinically occurring thromboembolic disease. Paraplegia 1991;29(1): 8–16
11. Geerts WH, Pineo GF, Heit JA, et al. Prevention of venous thromboembolism: the Seventh ACCP Conference on Antithrombotic and Thrombolytic Therapy. Chest 2004;126(3, Suppl):338S–400S
12. Geerts WH, Bergqvist D, Pineo GF, et al; American College of Chest Physicians. Prevention of venous thromboembolism: American College of Chest Physicians Evidence-Based Clinical Prac-

tice Guidelines (8th Edition). Chest 2008;133(6, Suppl):381S–453S
13. Early acute management of adults with acute spinal cord injury: a clinical practice guideline for health-care professionals. J Spinal Cord Med 2008;31(4):408–479
14. Colwell CW Jr; Annenberg Center for Health Sciences and Quadrant Medical Education. Thromboprophylaxis in orthopedic surgery. Am J Orthop 2006;(Suppl):1–9, quiz 10–11
15. Colwell CW. Evidence-based guidelines for venous thromboembolism prophylaxis in orthopedic surgery. Orthopedics 2007;30(2):129–135, quiz 136–137
16. Yu HT, Dylan ML, Lin J, Dubois RW. Hospitals' compliance with prophylaxis guidelines for venous thromboembolism. Am J Health Syst Pharm 2007;64(1):69–76
17. Steier KJ, Singh G, Ullah A, Maneja J, Ha RS, Khan F. Venous thromboembolism: application and effectiveness of the American College of Chest Physicians 2001 guidelines for prophylaxis. J Am Osteopath Assoc 2006;106(7):388–395
18. Green D, Hartwig D, Chen D, Soltysik RC, Yarnold PR. Spinal Cord Injury Risk Assessment for Thromboembolism (SPIRATE Study). Am J Phys Med Rehabil 2003;82(12):950–956
19. Furlan JC, Fehlings MG. Role of screening tests for deep venous thrombosis in asymptomatic adults with acute spinal cord injury: an evidence-based analysis. Spine 2007;32(17):1908–1916
20. Merli GJ, Crabbe S, Paluzzi RC, Fritz D. Etiology, incidence, and prevention of deep vein thrombosis in acute spinal cord injury. Arch Phys Med Rehabil 1993;74(11):1199–1205
21. Anderson FA Jr, Spencer FA. Risk factors for venous thromboembolism. Circulation 2003;107(23, Suppl 1):I9–I16
22. Furlan JC, Fehlings MG. Cardiovascular complications after acute spinal cord injury: pathophysiology, diagnosis, and management. Neurosurg Focus 2008;25(5):E13
23. Winther K, Gleerup G, Snorrason K, Biering-Sørensen F. Platelet function and fibrinolytic activity in cervical spinal cord injured patients. Thromb Res 1992;65(3):469–474
24. Dearborn JT, Hu SS, Tribus CB, Bradford DS. Thromboembolic complications after major thoracolumbar spine surgery. Spine 1999;24(14): 1471–1476
25. Oda T, Fuji T, Kato Y, Fujita S, Kanemitsu N. Deep venous thrombosis after posterior spinal surgery. Spine 2000;25(22):2962–2967
26. Platzer P, Thalhammer G, Jaindl M, et al. Thromboembolic complications after spinal surgery in trauma patients. Acta Orthop 2006;77(5):755–760
27. Brambilla S, Ruosi C, La Maida GA, Caserta S. Prevention of venous thromboembolism in spinal surgery. Eur Spine J 2004;13(1):1–8
28. Iversen PO, Groot PD, Hjeltnes N, Andersen TO, Mowinckel MC, Sandset PM. Impaired circadian variations of haemostatic and fibrinolytic parameters in tetraplegia. Br J Haematol 2002;119(4): 1011–1016
29. Colachis SC III, Clinchot DM. The association between deep venous thrombosis and heterotopic ossification in patients with acute traumatic spinal cord injury. Paraplegia 1993;31(8): 507–512
30. Merli GJ, Herbison GJ, Ditunno JF, et al. Deep vein thrombosis: prophylaxis in acute spinal cord injured patients. Arch Phys Med Rehabil 1988;69(9):661–664
31. Clagett GP, Anderson FA Jr, Heit J, Levine MN, Wheeler HB. Prevention of venous thromboembolism. Chest 1995;108(4, Suppl):312S–334S
32. Carabasi RA III, Moritz MJ, Jarrell BE. Complications encountered with the use of the Greenfield filter. Am J Surg 1987;154(2):163–168
33. Davies GC, Salzman EW. The pathogenesis of deep vein thrombosis. In: Joist JH, Sherman LA, eds. Venous and Arterial Thrombosis: Pathogenesis, Diagnosis, Prevention, and Therapy. New York, NY: Grune and Stratton; 1979:1–22
34. Kim SW, Charallel JT, Park KW, et al. Prevalence of deep venous thrombosis in patients with chronic spinal cord injury. Arch Phys Med Rehabil 1994;75(9):965–968
35. Monreal M, Martorell A, Callejas JM, et al. Venographic assessment of deep vein thrombosis and risk of developing post-thrombotic syndrome: a prospective study. J Intern Med 1993; 233(3):233–238
36. Zierler BK. Ultrasonography and diagnosis of venous thromboembolism. Circulation 2004; 109(12, Suppl 1):I9–I14
37. Orbell JH, Smith A, Burnand KG, Waltham M. Imaging of deep vein thrombosis. Br J Surg 2008;95(2):137–146
38. Tapson VF. Acute pulmonary embolism. N Engl J Med 2008;358(10):1037–1052
39. Silver JR. The prophylactic use of anticoagulant therapy in the prevention of pulmonary emboli in one hundred consecutive spinal injury patients. Paraplegia 1974;12(3):188–196
40. Watson N. Anticoagulant therapy in the treatment of venous thrombosis and pulmonary embolism in acute spinal injury. Paraplegia 1974;12(3):197–201
41. El Masri WS, Silver JR. Prophylactic anticoagulant therapy in patients with spinal cord injury. Paraplegia 1981;19(6):334–342
42. Naso F. Pulmonary embolism in acute spinal cord injury. Arch Phys Med Rehabil 1974;55(6): 275–278
43. Perkash A. Experience with the management of deep vein thrombosis in patients with spinal cord injury, II: A critical evaluation of the anticoagulant therapy. Paraplegia 1980;18(1): 2–14
44. Jones T, Ugalde V, Franks P, Zhou H, White RH. Venous thromboembolism after spinal cord injury: incidence, time course, and associated risk factors in 16,240 adults and children. Arch Phys Med Rehabil 2005;86(12):2240–2247
45. Investigators SCIT; Spinal Cord Injury Thromboprophylaxis Investigators. Prevention of venous thromboembolism in the rehabilitation phase after spinal cord injury: prophylaxis with low-dose heparin or enoxaparin. J Trauma 2003; 54(6):1111–1115
46. Perkash A, Prakash V, Perkash I. Experience with the management of thromboembolism in patients with spinal cord injury, I: Incidence, diagnosis and role of some risk factors. Paraplegia 1978;16(3):322–331
47. Perkash A, Sullivan G, Toth L, Bradleigh LH, Linder SH, Perkash I. Persistent hypercoagulation associ-

ated with heterotopic ossification in patients with spinal cord injury long after injury has occurred. Paraplegia 1993;31(10):653–659

48. Investigators SCIT; Spinal Cord Injury Thromboprophylaxis Investigators. Prevention of venous thromboembolism in the acute treatment phase after spinal cord injury: a randomized, multicenter trial comparing low-dose heparin plus intermittent pneumatic compression with enoxaparin. J Trauma 2003;54(6):1116–1124, discussion 1125–1126

49. Chiou-Tan FY, Garza H, Chan KT, et al. Comparison of dalteparin and enoxaparin for deep venous thrombosis prophylaxis in patients with spinal cord injury. Am J Phys Med Rehabil 2003;82(9):678–685

50. Lohmann U, Gläser E, Braun BE, Bötel U. Prevention of thromboembolism in spinal fractures with spinal cord injuries. Standard heparin versus low-molecular-weight heparin in acute paraplegia [in German]. Zentralbl Chir 2001;126(5): 385–390

51. Ploumis A, Ponnappan RK, Maltenfort MG, et al. Thromboprophylaxis in patients with acute spinal injuries: an evidence-based analysis. J Bone Joint Surg Am 2009;91(11):2568–2576

52. Gaber TA. Significant reduction of the risk of venous thromboembolism in all long-term immobile patients a few months after the onset of immobility. Med Hypotheses 2005;64(6): 1173–1176

53. Comerota AJ, Katz ML, White JV. Why does prophylaxis with external pneumatic compression for deep vein thrombosis fail? Am J Surg 1992;164(3):265–268

54. Green D, Rossi EC, Yao JS, Flinn WR, Spies SM. Deep vein thrombosis in spinal cord injury: effect of prophylaxis with calf compression, aspirin, and dipyridamole. Paraplegia 1982;20(4):227–234

55. Agnelli G, Piovella F, Buoncristiani P, et al. Enoxaparin plus compression stockings compared with compression stockings alone in the prevention of venous thromboembolism after elective neurosurgery. N Engl J Med 1998;339(2):80–85

56. Agu O, Hamilton G, Baker D. Graduated compression stockings in the prevention of venous thromboembolism. Br J Surg 1999;86(8): 992–1004

57. Amaragiri SV, Lees TA. Elastic compression stockings for prevention of deep vein thrombosis. Cochrane Database Syst Rev 2000; (3):CD001484

58. Lassen MR, Borris LC, Christiansen HM, et al. Prevention of thromboembolism in 190 hip arthroplasties: comparison of LMW heparin and placebo. Acta Orthop Scand 1991;62(1):33–38

59. Merli GJ, Crabbe S, Doyle L, Ditunno JF, Herbision GJ. Mechanical plus pharmacological prophylaxis for deep vein thrombosis in acute spinal cord injury. Paraplegia 1992;30(8):558–562

60. Nurmohamed MT, van Riel AM, Henkens CM, et al. Low molecular weight heparin and compression stockings in the prevention of venous thromboembolism in neurosurgery. Thromb Haemost 1996;75(2):233–238

61. Ramos R, Salem BI, De Pawlikowski MP, Coordes C, Eisenberg S, Leidenfrost R. The efficacy of pneumatic compression stockings in the prevention of pulmonary embolism after cardiac surgery. Chest 1996;109(1):82–85

62. Törngren S. Low dose heparin and compression stockings in the prevention of postoperative deep venous thrombosis. Br J Surg 1980;67(7): 482–484

63. Wille-Jørgensen P, Hauch O, Dimo B, Christensen SW, Jensen R, Hansen B. Prophylaxis of deep venous thrombosis after acute abdominal operation. Surg Gynecol Obstet 1991;172(1):44–48

64. Wille-Jørgensen P, Thorup J, Fischer A, Holst-Christensen J, Flamsholt R. Heparin with and without graded compression stockings in the prevention of thromboembolic complications of major abdominal surgery: a randomized trial. Br J Surg 1985;72(7):579–581

65. Turpie AG, Bauer KA, Eriksson BI, Lassen MR. Fondaparinux vs enoxaparin for the prevention of venous thromboembolism in major orthopedic surgery: a meta-analysis of 4 randomized double-blind studies. Arch Intern Med 2002; 162(16):1833–1840

66. Nurmohamed MT, Rosendaal FR, Büller HR, et al. Low-molecular-weight heparin versus standard heparin in general and orthopaedic surgery: a meta-analysis. Lancet 1992;340(8812):152–156

67. Johns JS, Nguyen C, Sing RF. Vena cava filters in spinal cord injuries: evolving technology. J Spinal Cord Med 2006;29(3):183–190

68. Maxwell RA, Chavarria-Aguilar M, Cockerham WT, et al. Routine prophylactic vena cava filtration is not indicated after acute spinal cord injury. J Trauma 2002;52(5):902–906

69. Ploumis APR, Ponnappan RK, Sarbello J, et al. Thromboprophylaxis in traumatic and elective spinal surgery: analysis of questionnaire response and current practice of spine trauma surgeons. Spine 2010;35(3):323–329

70. Eriksson BI, Kälebo P, Anthymyr BA, Wadenvik H, Tengborn L, Risberg B. Prevention of deep-vein thrombosis and pulmonary embolism after total hip replacement. Comparison of low-molecular-weight heparin and unfractionated heparin. J Bone Joint Surg Am 1991;73(4):484–493

71. Wade WE, Chisholm MA. Venous thrombosis after acute spinal cord injury: cost analysis of prophylaxis guidelines. Am J Phys Med Rehabil 2000;79(6):504–508

72. Burns SP, Nelson AL, Bosshart HT, et al. Implementation of clinical practice guidelines for prevention of thromboembolism in spinal cord injury. J Spinal Cord Med 2005;28(1):33–42

73. DeVivo MJ, Whiteneck GG, Charles ED Jr. The economic impact of spinal cord injury. In: Stover SL, DeLisa JA, Whiteneck GG, eds. Spinal Cord Injury: Clinical Outcomes from the Model Systems. Gaithersburg, MD: Aspen; 1995:234–271

74. Tator CH, Duncan EG, Edmonds VE, Lapczak LI, Andrews DF. Complications and costs of management of acute spinal cord injury. Paraplegia 1993;31(11):700–714

14

Sexuality and Fertility after Spinal Cord Injury

Stacy L. Elliott

Key Points

1. Sexuality is a high priority for men and women with SCI.
2. Level and completeness of injury will determine the capacity for psychogenic/reflexogenic genital arousal and the ability to ejaculate.
3. Orgasm is possible in ~ 40 to 50% of men and women after SCI.
4. Pregnancy and labor, but not fertility, are affected in women with SCI: fertility is affected in men due to erection and ejaculation difficulties as well as altered semen quality post-SCI.
5. Therapeutic effectiveness is maximized by using a comprehensive Sexual Rehabilitative Framework.

Sex after spinal cord injury (SCI) matters—a lot. Those of us working in the field of SCI rehabilitation for years have understood the importance of sexual and fertility rehabilitation to men and women with SCI. Sexuality is even recognized as an activity of daily living by the American Occupational Therapy Association, thereby rendering it a rehabilitation priority. Its significance is exemplified in a recent survey by Anderson[1] on what gain of function was most important to quality of life in 681 persons with SCI (of 681 participants, 25% were female, 65% were male, and 10% chose to participate anonymously): the majority of individuals with paraplegia felt regaining sexual function was their highest priority, and for individuals with quadriplegia, it was the second-highest priority (preceded only by regaining hand and arm function), placing sexual function above the return of sensation, walking, and bladder and bowel function. Furthermore, the vast majority of individuals with SCI felt their injury has altered their sexual sense of self and that improving their sexual function would improve their quality of life.[2,3]

Health care professionals are often either too intimidated to discuss the topic of sexuality with their patients with SCI, or they feel they do not have the skills or knowledge to handle the questions raised.

Understanding how changes to sexuality occur following SCI and how they can be assessed and therapeutically managed in a comprehensive way will serve to promote long-term gains rather than short-term solutions. Utilization of a Sexual Rehabilitative Framework is a practical method for addressing the complexities of sexuality as it relates to the various psychological, physical, medical, and relationship changes that occur with SCI.

The Mind–Body Interaction

Sexuality is much more than the performance of sexual acts. Sexual response is a feedback loop or circuit that is dependent on the emotional context, physical reactions, and influence of moment-to-moment, reinforcing triggers or negative distracters.[4] The vast majority of men and women with SCI find it difficult to become physically aroused, and more women (74.7%) than men (48.7%) have difficulty becoming psychologically aroused.[2,3] Furthermore, loss of sensory or motor ability or both forces an appreciation of the power of "brain or cerebral sex." Focusing on cerebrally initiated sexual response can, despite lost abilities, result in an adapted but very satisfying sexual experience. Those areas that remain sensate take on a sexually arousing role (i.e., neck and ear stimulation has led to "eargasms" after quadriplegia), even if such body areas were not in the sexual repertoire prior to injury. In other words, the brain is always adapting its "software" despite the "hardware" being altered after SCI. This form of sexual neuroplasticity is a new science and Vancouver (BC, Canada) researchers have begun testing early "sexual sensory substitution" methods on subjects to try and regain sexual perception below the level of injury.[5]

Neurophysiology of the Sexual Response

Arousal is triggered by many inputs into the cerebral cortex: all the five senses to the brain, afferent sensory, and hormonal influences are assessed to generate a neuronal signal coordinated in the limbic system, hypothalamus, and other midbrain structures. Brain descending pathways are both excitatory and inhibitory: in a nonsexual situation, a strong inhibitory tone exists. When a peripheral or central sexual stimulation reaches a sufficient level, then increasing excitatory and reduced inhibitory signals activate the spinal centers to trigger genital arousal and ejaculation. In other words, the efferent outflow of signals from the brain down the spinal cord is impeded until our brain "allows" these messages to pass: when the healthy brain "feels safe," the inhibition is removed and the spinal reflexes are released.

In able-bodied individuals, sexual arousal involves coordinated participation of all three nervous systems: (1) sacral parasympathetic (pelvic nerve), (2) thoracolumbar sympathetic (hypogastric and lumbar sympathetic chain), and (3) somatic (pudendal) nerves.[6] After leaving the spinal cord, these nerves travel jointly through the pelvic plexus and cavernous nerve to the genitalia (**Fig. 14.1**). The genital structures of both men and women respond with increased vasocongestion and neuromuscular tension and become engorged with blood (tumescent) via smooth muscle relaxation in the erectile tissues. Nitric oxide (NO) is the primary neurotransmitter responsible for smooth muscle relaxation in both sexes. While neuronal NO (nNO) is of major significance in the sexual response, NO is also generated from healthy endothelium (eNO). Genital arousal consists of penile erection in men. In women, there is vulvar swelling, clitoral engorgement, and vaginal lubrication and accommodation. In men, a stocking-like elastic structure (tunica albuginea) surrounds the erectile corporeal bodies (corpora cavernosa) and veins pierce through it to drain the cavernosa. When the tunica is stretched by the expanding corporeal bodies, venous outflow is stopped by kinking of the veins, allowing for increased intracavernosal pressure to build and penile erection to occur (veno-occlusive mechanism). Penile rigidity is enhanced by pelvic floor contraction. Women

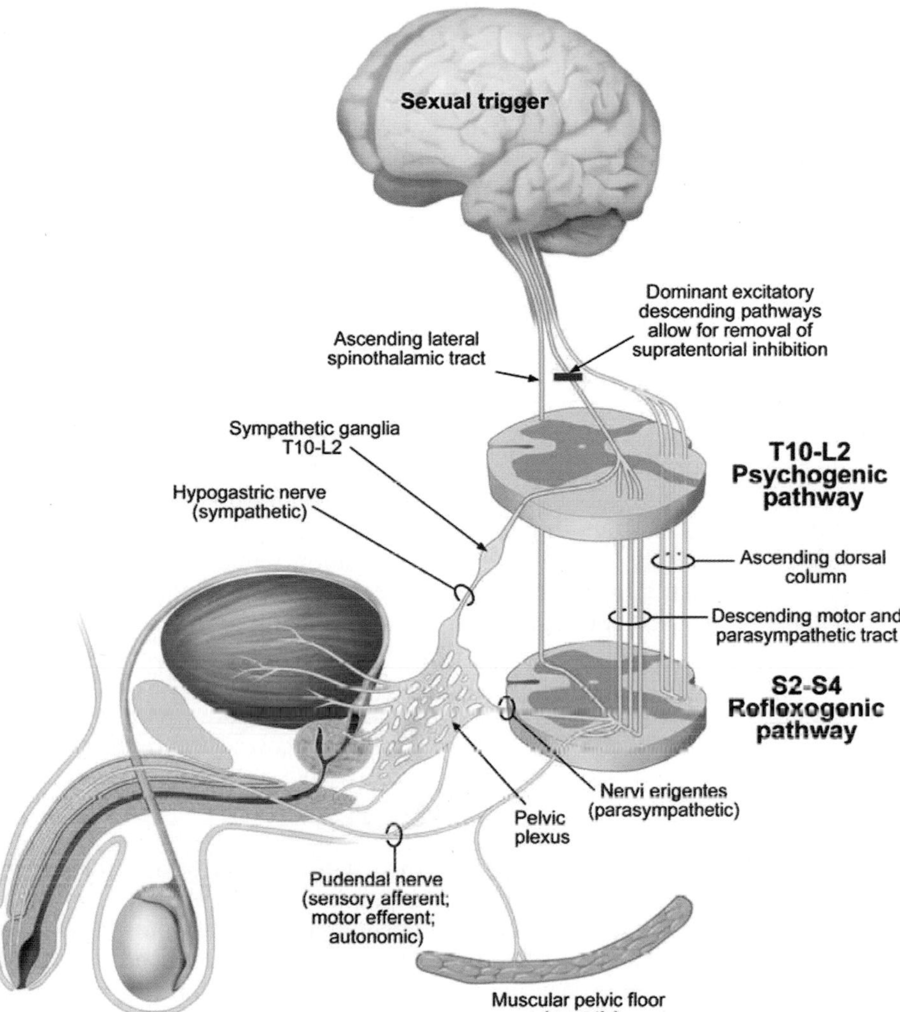

Fig. 14.1 Although both excitatory and inhibitory descending signals from the brain are possible, an excitatory signal must dominate in order to remove the supratentorial inhibition that exists on spinal sexual reflexes. Such signals are transmitted to the genitalia through two pathways: the "psychogenic pathway," rising from the sympathetic spinal cord center at T10–L2, and the "reflexogenic pathway," starting from the intermediolateral nuclei from S2–S4 and exiting as the nervi erigentes. Both sympathetic (hypogastric nerve and plexus) and parasympathetic nerves unite in the pelvic plexus. The pelvic plexus contains parasympathetic, sympathetic, and afferent somatic fibers, and in men, the cavernous nerve is the largest nerve exiting the pelvic plexus. For erection, parasympathetic dominance must prevail at the penile tissue level to promote smooth muscle relaxation via nitric oxide release: after spinal cord injury (SCI) the reflexogenic pathway provides the parasympathetic innervation if the psychogenic pathway is damaged. Sympathetic fibers from the psychogenic center (via hypogastric nerve), which normally signal smooth muscle contraction (primarily via noradrenalin), also carries pro-erectile fibers as evidenced in the SCI population who have damaged their sacral cord yet are still able to retain some erectile potential. Interneurons in the spinal cord connect the psychogenic and reflexogenic pathways in a reinforcing way: interneuronal spinal cord damage can also affect erectile quality even if both pathways remain intact. The pudendal nerves from S2–S4 comprise both motor efferent (neuronal cell bodies in Onuf's nucleus) and sensory afferent fibers. The reflex component of the reflexogenic pathway consists of an afferent sensory component from the genitalia entering the sacral cord via the pudendal nerve, and an efferent component comprised of parasympathetic signals (nervi erigentes), and somatic signals (pudendal nerve), the latter of which is responsible for the contraction of the striated pelvic-perineal muscles, including the ischiocavernosus and bulbospongiosus.

have a much thinner tunical structure around the clitoral bodies.

Local genital arousal and vasocongestion is primarily under parasympathetic dominance; sympathetic stimulation will cause detumescence of genital structures. With higher arousal levels, orgasmic release (often accompanied by ejaculation in men) can be experienced if the physiological orgasmic threshold is crossed.[6] The ejaculation reflex, primarily a sympathetic phenomenon, consists of seminal emission and propulsatile ejaculation, and propels sperm and seminal fluid (semen) distally out the urethral opening. Orgasm is the pleasurable peak feeling of sexual release and may be initiated from genital stimulation (genital orgasm) or from erogenous zones outside the genitals, including the brain (nongenital orgasm). However, a satisfying sexual experience is not dependent on orgasmic ability.

Sexual Function after Spinal Cord Injury

Genital arousal is controlled by two distinct pathways: the *psychogenic* pathway located between T10 and L2 in the spinal cord, and the *reflex* pathway, located in the sacral (S2–4) cord. There is also some evidence that the vagus nerve may be involved in orgasm in women with SCI.[7] Studies have shown the neurological ability to achieve psychogenic arousal after SCI can be predicted in both men and women by the combined degree of preservation of surface sensation to pinprick and light touch in the T11–L2 dermatomes.[8] The natural ability of men with SCI (without using medication or assistive devices) to have an erection from either psychogenic or reflexogenic sources will depend on the level and completeness of the lesion. This ability is reported to be 62%, but about two thirds of men with SCI find their erections either to be unreliable or to be of short duration.[9] Because of this, at least 60% report the use of some form of erection enhancement.[9]

Ejaculation potential depends, like erection, on the level and completeness of the lesion, but it is more likely in men who have preserved bladder and bowel control, spasticity, the ability to achieve a psychogenic erection, the ability to retain an erection, and when there is direct penile manipulation versus vaginal intercourse.[6,10] Unless significant increases in blood pressure (BP) occur with sexual stimulation, ejaculation is unlikely to happen.[10] The chance of either reaching ejaculation or experiencing orgasm after SCI appears to be modestly enhanced by the utilization of oral erection medications[11] or sympathomimetic drugs such as mididrone.[10]

Approximately 40 to 50% of men and women after SCI are able to reach either self-defined or laboratory-recorded orgasmic release, although the length and intensity of stimulation required to reach orgasm may exceed preinjury requirements.[8] In both sexes, having a complete versus incomplete injury (regardless of level of injury), having an intact sacral reflex arc, and having genital sensation are more predictive of orgasm.[6,8] For men, orgasm is more likely when ejaculation is possible, although some men are orgasmic without ejaculation after SCI.[8] Newer studies are finding that, for some men with SCI, the pleasurable or orgasmic experience at ejaculation is related to the phenomenon of autonomic dysreflexia (AD). AD, a potentially dangerous condition of episodic hypertension triggered by noxious and nonnoxious afferent stimuli below the level of the SCI lesion that is well known in the SCI population,[6] can also result in such unpleasant symptoms (severe headache, nausea, sweating, etc.) that sex is not enjoyable or is even avoided. That said, researchers have found that few orgasmic sensations are reported when AD is not produced with sexual stimulation, pleasurable climactic sensations are reported when mild to moderate AD occurs, and unpleasant or painful sensations are reported with severe AD.[12] While studies have not yet been completed on women with SCI, the data from men with SCI, which encourage sexual rehabilitation emphasizing self-ejaculation, self-exploration, and cognitive reframing to maximize the perception of sexual sensations and climax, may well apply to women with SCI.

Changes to Fertility after Spinal Cord Injury

Fertility Issues in Men Following Spinal Cord Injury

Compared with women with SCI, men's fertility is significantly affected because erectile function, ejaculatory ability, and semen quality are all compromised secondary to the neurological changes following SCI. In fact, at least 90% of men with SCI do not have the ability to father a child through the act of sexual intercourse[13,14] given that anejaculation (lack of seminal emission or propulsatile ejaculation) is common. Other ejaculatory dysfunctions (e.g., retrograde ejaculation, etc.) can also occur after SCI.[14]

Methods of Sperm Retrieval

Methods of sperm retrieval have been devised for men with SCI. Ejaculation can be provoked either by the use of powerful vibrators, which provide strong afferent stimulus to the spinal cord to trigger the efferent ejaculatory reflex (penile vibratory stimulation [PVS]), or by "jump starting" the efferent component of the ejaculatory reflex by the use of periprostatic electrical stimulation via an anal probe (electroejaculation [EEJ]). Cumulative success rates of ejaculation of ~86% have been reported using either PVS or EEJ in men with SCI,[15] but they have more recently been found to be up to 100% when all sperm retrieval methods, including surgical aspiration, are utilized.[10] Finger massage of the prostate and seminal vesicles can also mechanically express stored sperm that can then be used for insemination when PVS or EEJ is not available, but it is not clear whether this is yet indicated in men with SCI.[16] Surgical sperm retrieval methods (where sperm are surgically retrieved from the internal accessory glands) are also possible, but the use of this in men with SCI when other less invasive and costly methods are available, is controversial.[16]

PVS is the first-line treatment for anejaculation for men with SCI and is most successful in men with SCI above T10 (88% success rate) where the sacral reflex is preserved as compared with men with a level of injury at T11 or below (15% success rate).[17] Since there is an art and a science to PVS, the more experienced clinicians or clients have better ejaculatory success; however, the vibrator itself seems to be the critical element. Low amplitude, low frequency vibrators (obtained commercially) are not as successful as a vibrator of high amplitude (i.e., 2.5 mm excursions of the vibrating head) and frequency (i.e., speed of 90 to 100 Hz) such as the Ferticare (Multicept APS, Denmark). The vibrator is placed on the frenulum or "signature spots" found on the glans penis to trigger ejaculation, usually within minutes.[6] If PVS is initially unsuccessful, additional stimulus can be tried to facilitate ejaculation, such as the application of two vibrators ("sandwich technique"), use of abdominal electrical stimulation (AES) in addition to PVS,[17] or the use of phosphodiesterase V inhibitors (PDE5i) that may encourage ejaculation after SCI.[11] The use of mididrone, a sympathomimetic drug, with or without PVS, is also helpful to induce ejaculation in some men but should be utilized with caution in men who experience AD because it can increase AD severity.[10]

Those individuals who do not respond to PVS or other efforts should then be referred for EEJ. An electrical current, delivered through an anal probe with the man in a lateral decubitus or supine position, stimulates seminal emission. The Seager Electroejaculator (Dalzell Medical Systems, The Plains, VA) remains the only approved device for this procedure.[14] The ejaculate is then milked through the urethra and collected and utilized for insemination techniques. Men with incomplete or lower injuries will require anesthetic for EEJ, whereas others may tolerate the procedure in an outpatient setting. It is imperative to note that, during both PVS and EEJ, men must be monitored for AD, especially if the lesion is T6 or above.[6] Any man with SCI who wishes to pursue ejaculation utilizing a sympathomimetic medication or PVS at home for either fertility or pleasure reasons should first be evaluated for AD risk management with ejaculation in a clinic capable of continuous hemodynamic monitoring. AD can produce not only severe hypertension (and its concomitant cardiovascular risks, such as stroke)[6] but cardiac arrhythmias as well.[18] The use of prophylactic medication should also be considered prior to ejaculation attempts in those men prone to AD.[14,19]

Changes in Semen Quality and Insemination Options

Men with SCI have, from ~2 weeks postinjury,[16] permanent changes in their semen quality, with abnormal sperm motility and viability, although sperm count per se remains normal.[16]Abnormal accessory gland function, possibly from dissinnervation of the prostate gland and seminal vesicles, may be the cause of abnormalities in the seminal plasma. It does not appear that elevated scrotal temperature, infrequency of ejaculation, duration of injury, or methods of bladder management account for the lowered sperm motility, but rather that immune regulatory dysfunction and numerous abnormalities in the seminal fluid, including various toxic biochemical substances and abnormal levels of white blood cells (leukocytospermia), appear to be the culprits.[16] A treatment utilizing monoclonal antibodies to interfere with the action of damaging levels of cytokines in the seminal plasma of men with SCI may represent a future intervention to assist with poor semen quality after SCI.[20]

Where possible, if the semen can be safely obtained and it is of adequate quality, the least invasive reproductive technology during well-timed ovulatory cycles should be utilized, that is, the use of home intravaginal insemination (IVI) via syringe transfer to the vagina, or by intrauterine insemination (IUI) where the semen is specially prepared and placed directly into the uterus. Factors such as very poor semen quality or advancing age or fertility issues of the female partner encourage the expedited use of higher technology, such as in vitro fertilization (IVF), where the sperm and oocyte are placed together to fertilize in a petri dish, and the ensuing embryo(s) are placed into the uterus or cryopreserved for a later cycle. Intracytoplasmic sperm injection (ICSI), where a single sperm is injected directly into the egg, can be utilized to force fertilization. Such high-level interventions (i.e., using ejaculated or fresh testicular sperm in an ICSI cycle), may result in better conception rates per cycle.[21] However, decisions regarding method of retrieval and insemination must also include a cost–benefit ratio.[14] A review of pooled fertility data revealed a pregnancy rate of 51% and live birth rate of 40% in partners of men with SCI.[15] It appears that pregnancy outcomes (utilizing IUI, ICF, or ICSI) using sperm from men with SCI seem to be similar to those using sperm from non-SCI men with male-factor infertility: the reader is directed to an excellent review of sperm retrieval, semen quality, and pregnancy rates in partners of men with SCI.[16]

Contraception, Fertility, and Pregnancy in Women Following Spinal Cord Injury

Female fertility is usually not affected by SCI. Transient hypothalamic pituitary hypogonadism with associated amenorrhea (lasting an average of 6 months) occurs in ~40% of women and is not associated with the extent of the neurological deficit.[22] However, menstruation almost always resumes, and somewhere between 14 and 20% of women with SCI subsequently have at least one pregnancy.[22,23]

Few accessible examination beds have resulted in women with SCI, in general, receiving less gynecological care, including fewer mammograms and PAP smears.[24] Birth control is more of an issue than fertility for women after SCI. For example, barrier methods (diaphragms and condoms) may not be practical for women with compromised hand function or self-care potential. The use of birth control pills (BCPs) is generally not favored in women with SCI due to the thrombotic risk secondary to estrogen, but they are used in selected women with SCI who are at lower risk (more mobile, etc.). Women with SCI who have concomitant brain injury and/or memory issues would not be appropriate candidates for the daily BCP. Progesterone-only methods of birth control can result in unpredictable bleeding or spotting, and there is some speculation about the use of depot-medroxyprogesterone (DMPA) and skeletal health, particularly in women with SCI, who are already at risk for osteoporosis.[25] Perforation or expulsion of intrauterine devices (IUDs) may go unnoticed in women with SCI or may only present symptomatically as spasm or AD. Unfortunately, inadequate information about birth control and pregnancy is common among young women with SCI (only 10% receive adequate information during rehabilitation), and about half of women with SCI in their childbearing years do not desire pregnancy.[26] It has also been reported in a study of 128 women with SCI that of those who became pregnant, 40% chose to terminate.[22]

During pregnancy, chronic bacteriuria and recurrent urinary tract infections are common, and preventative strategies are not well delineated.[27] Bowel emptying is delayed, and perineal hygiene becomes more difficult. Transferring difficulties increase due to alterations in the center of balance, increased spasticity, and weight gain. There is an increased risk of skin breakdown and pedal edema, thrombophlebitis, and deep vein thrombosis. Postpartum depression is also more common in women with SCI.[26]

Since the uterus is innervated from T10 through L1, preterm delivery is a risk in about one third of women with SCI, and about one fourth of women with SCI are not able to feel preterm labor.[26] Premature cervical dilation, premature labor, and small-for-date infants (etiology unknown) are more common in women with SCI than in women without SCI, but the risk of spontaneous abortion is the same in both populations.[27,28] Autonomic dysreflexia is a serious complication in 85% of women with complete or incomplete lesions at or above the T5-6 level. During labor, AD can result in uteroplacental vasoconstriction with secondary fetal hypoxia and bradycardia, as well as put the mother at risk for stroke and other hypertensive complications.[6,26] Because of this, labor requires a multidisciplinary team approach, with the capacity for hemodynamic monitoring to distinguish preeclampsia from AD, anesthetic capacity, and the ability to reposition the woman every few hours during labor to prevent skin breakdown. Although most women with SCI deliver vaginally, there is a higher risk of cesarean section, and vacuum and forceps extraction, especially if there is AD or fetal distress.[26] Breast feeding may be a problem in women with injury above T4 due to loss of suckling afferent pathways to facilitate letdown reflex, and lactation may cease after 3 months or so because of inadequate response to nipple stimulation.[28]

The Comprehensive Approach to Sexuality after Spinal Cord Injury

Although sexual satisfaction is reportedly lower in both men and women after SCI, three fourths of persons after SCI are satisfied with life circumstances: predictors include having a good relationship with a partner, having some mobility, having fewer SCI consequences (i.e., fewer bladder, bowel, skin, and AD complications) and experiencing mental well-being.[3,6] The multidisciplinary utilization of a Sexual Rehabilitation Framework is very helpful to look at medical or psychological factors that impede or improve sexual and reproductive function, and may serve to prevent the development of unnecessary sexual and fertility anxieties. Regardless of the health care discipline of the clinician, the framework provides the opportunity to outline appropriate therapeutic options in line with the client's priorities: particular aspects of the sexual or reproductive concerns can then be addressed according to the clinician's expertise and the others referred.

Components of the framework and potential therapeutic suggestions are noted in the following paragraphs.

Sexual Drive or Sexual Interest

Sexual drive (libido) has a *biological* (urge to seek out sexual activity) and *motivational* component (physical or emotional sexual payoff). Managing biological or medical factors, such as replacement of hormones, treating depression, addressing incontinence or fatigue, or altering medications that interfere with sexual function, can greatly improve sexual motivation and payoff. Psychological and relationship issues affecting sexual motivation also need to be addressed. Once the main source of dissatisfaction is identified, addressing its etiology can direct therapy to the appropriate resource.

Sexual Functioning Abilities

The following areas should be assessed: (1) genital arousal (erection capacity in men and awareness of pelvic fullness or vaginal lubrication in women), (2) ejaculation ability in men, (3) orgasmic potential in both sexes, and (4) pain with sexual acts. Treatments for genital arousal difficulties include the use of PDE5i that are reliant on the availability of both nNO and eNO sources in the genital area. Most men with SCI (> 80%) will respond well to the choices of PDE5i, which include sildenafil (Viagra, Pfizer, Inc., New York, NY) as needed and vardenafil (Levitra and Staxyn, Bayer Pharmaceuticals Corp., Pittsburgh, PA), whose maximal effect is from 1 to 4 hours after it is taken, or the longer-acting (24 to 48 hour in SCI) tadalafil (Cialis, Lilly USA, Indianapolis, IN) as needed or Cialis Once-a-Day. Men with reduced nNO (lower cord injuries) or eNO (smokers, men with hyperlipidemia) will not respond as well to the PDE5i. Other choices for erection enhancement include the use of a vacuum device (VED). The VED consists of a cylinder (placed over the flaccid penis) and a pump that generates a vacuum, drawing blood into the penile tissues to create an erection that is maintained by a penile ring placed at the penile base. If an erection can be attained but not maintained, the use of penile rings alone can be tried. In both cases the ring should not be left on for more than 45 minutes: this can be a potential hazard in men who cannot feel their penis. Intracavernosal (penile) injections of single or mixed medications (prostaglandin E1, papaverine, and phentolamine) that directly relax the cavernosal smooth muscle are very effective but run the risk of priapism, so appropriate technique training and dosing instructions are necessary. Surgical penile prostheses destroy the cavernosal tissue so are only utilized when reversible methods prove unsatisfactory or there are other bladder management issues where a prosthesis for erection may be helpful.

For women with SCI, fewer options exist, and studies are sparse. Small but significant improvements in subjective arousal in women with SCI have been seen with sildenafil, especially when accompanied with manual and visual stimulation.[29] EROS-CT (Clitoral Therapy Device, Urometrics Inc., St. Paul, MN), a small, battery-powered vacuum device designed to enhance clitoral engorgement by increasing blood flow to the clitoris, is the only US Food and Drug Administration cleared-to-market device available by prescription to treat female sexual dysfunction.[30] Theoretically, for some women with SCI, there may be some benefit in clitoral responsiveness, and there may be an additional training effect from EROS-CT on the pelvic floor in those women who have retained a bulbocavernosus reflex, which in turn may reinforce remaining sacral reflexes.

Ejaculation disorders are treated by various methods noted under fertility. Orgasmic potential in both sexes can be improved by several techniques that increase genital stimulation, improve awareness of sensate areas, or allow for cerebral inputs to be appreciated at a higher level. Men and women should be encouraged to learn new body maps of erogenous areas, and to learn and practice mindfulness techniques around sexual inputs. While the use of relaxation, meditation, fantasy, recalling positive sexual experiences, breathing, and "going with the flow" can improve orgasmic potential, being with a trusted and long-term partner is the most predictive factor in orgasmic attainment after SCI.[31] Vibrators are commonly used externally on the clitoris or internally on the cervix, but can also provoke AD in susceptible women.

Persistence with physical stimulation in the context of security and intimacy can lead to reinforcement of new neural pathways and contribute to neuroplasticity. Neuroplasticity depends on focused repetition of a new task, attention to signals occurring in the moment, and an openness and positivity in their interpretation. Health care professionals can assist men and women with SCI in this process by actively intervening with therapeutic suggestions to reduce medical interferences, such as pain, spasticity, AD, and incontinence; this will reduce the distractions and allow the freedom to focus. A full description of the pros and cons of therapies for sexual dysfunction in men and women with SCI is available in other readings.[9,19,32]

Fertility and Contraception Concerns

Assessment is needed regarding questions and expectations around fertility and contraception. Some women with SCI feel they are less fertile than they were preinjury or that they are not capable of pregnancy, labor, or parenthood. During pregnancy, multidisciplinary attention to the consequences of SCI noted earlier is essential. Men need to be assessed for ejaculatory capacity and sperm quality, whether the purpose be for fertility or contraception. It is important to preserve the client's parenting rights while addressing the realistic issues of physical accessibility and emotional energy parenting requires.

The Medical Consequences of Spinal Cord Injury

Many medical issues specific to having a SCI can impede sexual function. Therapies should be directed at reducing the interferences, with various disciplines involved in such management.

Depression

This may be transient or chronic, but it is common enough for appropriate assessment and treatment to be done routinely. Depression will negatively affect all aspects of sexual functioning, as can treatment for depression (e.g., selective serotonin re-uptake inhibitor medication).

Spasticity

Spasm can be necessary for mobility or transferring, but it can also impede sexual activities. Spasticity is noted to occur 26 to 38% of the time that a person with SCI is engaged in sexual activity.[3] Although the use of antispasmodic medication can improve quality of life, it can also interfere with the sexual spinal cord reflexes: alternately, some men use ejaculation as a means to reduce spasm for several hours.[33]

Autonomic Dysreflexia

Careful questioning around symptoms of AD should be done with the knowledge that a significant portion of AD is silent but not benign.[34] Unless a proper clinical assessment is done, both the client and the medical professional can be falsely reassured that an asymptomatic client does not experience significant AD (hypertension or bradycardia). The use of a portable inflatable blood pressure (BP) cuff during daily activities can provide valuable information regarding BP changes, including those during private sexual activity. AD interfered with the motivation to be sexual in 28% of women and 16% of men in a recent survey.[2,9] AD can be triggered with arousal as well as orgasm, and the occurrence of AD during typical bladder or bowel care was a significant variable predicting the occurrence and distress of AD during sexual activity.[3] Preventative medication for AD (prazocin, nifedipine, etc.) can improve the motivation to be sexual or pursue fertility.[6]

Pain Management

Pain is counterintuitive to relaxation and sexual arousal. Medication should be taken at a time to maximize its effectiveness prior to sexual activity. During physical therapy rehabilitation, bed positioning can be explored to see whether specific support cushioning may prove helpful for reduction of pain or spasm during private sexual activity.

Medications

Several medications can affect sexual function.[35] Notably in the SCI population, antidepressants (which can suppress libido and interfere with arousal and orgasmic capacity), anticholinergics for bladder function, and drugs that reduce testosterone levels (cimetidine, spironolactone, etc.) can affect sexual function potential. Antispasmodics, such as intrathecal baclofen, have been noted to interfere with erection and ejaculation in men (and possibly interfere with orgasm in women), and cardiac medications can interfere with already compromised autonomic functions.[6] The timing, reduction, or substitution of medications that affect sexual function should be attempted.[35]

Motor and Sensory Influences

Sensory and motor potential is critical in the assessment of sexual function. The ability to caress, hold, or position a partner depends on muscle strength and core balancing abilities. Transferring or turning independently in a bed needs to be assessed and assistive devices recommended by therapists as needed. Positioning cushions are now on the market. Sensory mapping (body mapping) needs to be done by the client (and/or partner) to understand what areas are insensate, what have some (or even high) arousal potential (i.e., often a zone around the area of injury), and what areas are to be avoided due to hypersensitivity. This body mapping is a critical learning stage in sexual rehabilitation. The use of sexual aids such as feathers, massage oils, vibrators for genital and nongenital use, and the use of fantasy are all part of remapping the brain to recognize new or different stimuli as "sexual," even if they had not been tried pre-injury. This exploration assists with acceptance of and positive feelings about the "new" post-SCI sexual body. A helpful free manual for "hands-on" types of options for persons with disability is called PleasurAble, and is downloadable from the Disability Health Resource Network (www.dhrn.ca) under Disability Resources.

Bowel and Bladder Issues

One the most often reported and distressing issues around sexuality post-SCI is that of bladder and bowel incontinence, or the fear of such, during sexual activity. Although a survey noted that concerns around bladder and bowel during sexual activity were not strong enough to deter the majority of the population from engaging in sexual activity, in the subset of individuals who were concerned about bladder or bowel incontinence during sexual activity this was a highly significant issue.[3] If the difficulties are significant enough, or the management issues are too cumbersome, delay in or withdrawal from sexual activity can occur. Assertive attempts to manage urinary incontinence issues by medications, intermittent catheterization, or even the consideration of bladder augmentation or continent urinary diversions may need to be examined. Diligence in reduction of urinary tract infections (UTIs) is also important for sexuality and fertility. Bowel management issues can delay or interfere with sexual enjoyment as well; bowel routines and reliable continence are paramount for the promotion of sexual activity.

Sexual Self-View and Self-Esteem

Dealing with SCI sequelae (altered body image, diminished independence, continence, hygiene, etc.) can alter one's sense of sex appeal and sense of masculinity or femininity. Loss of confidence or former abilities at work or athletics, role reversal among partners, and the lack of support or loyalty of friends, family, and employers can further drain self-esteem. These specific issues need to be addressed to turn negatives into positives, and persistence with self-sexual exploration can realign the feeling of sexual wholeness, albeit in a new body.

Partnership Issues

The context in which sexual activity is occurring (or not occurring) is critical in the evaluation of partnership potential. Clinicians need to initiate these discussions around partnership and peer counseling because they can be extremely useful in sexual adjustment.[24]

Constructing a chart for the Sexual Rehabilitation Framework is a practical method to assess sexuality and fertility in persons with an SCI or any disability or chronic illness (**Table 14.1**).

For example, a 36-year-old married man with C6 complete quadriplegia of 3 years duration may have an assessment that looks like the example in **Table 14.2**. The same chart could be done for a 22-year-old single woman with incomplete paraplegia in a wheelchair: her issues may be about her potential to become genitally aroused and to achieve orgasm, continence issues around sexual activity, mobility to social events and meeting partners, safe birth control options, and whether she could conceive and carry a normal pregnancy to term and vaginally deliver.

Future Expectations

A large-scale cross-sectional questionnaire inclusive of 350 respondents over four European countries identified sexual activity as the area of greatest unmet need for persons with SCI.[36] Based on these stated priorities, the need for sexual and fertility rehabilitation is high, but the available studies addressing these issues are relatively low. Treatment of sexual disorders in men and women with SCI is most successful when clients and clinicians follow three principles of sexual rehabilitation[4]:

- *Maximize* the remaining capacities of the total body before relying on medications or aids (learning new body maps, breathing, visualization methods, mindfulness exercises, etc.).
- *Adapt* to residual limitations by utilizing specialized therapies (use of vibrators, training aids, PDE5i, vacuum device aids, etc.).
- *Stay open* to rehabilitative efforts and new forms of sexual stimulation, with a positive and optimistic outlook.

Although the physiology of sexual response has been relatively well mapped out by laboratory studies, the many facets involved in the interpretation of arousal and pleasure are not. Unlike motor and sensory recovery, sexuality after SCI has the potential to continue evolving long after the physical body has reached its maximum "somatic" recovery: this "sexual neuroplasticity" is best demonstrated by the stories provided by men and women with SCI and other neurological disabilities. Because it is well documented that improvement in quality of sexual health will lead to improvement

Table 14.1 Chart for the Sexual Rehabilitation Framework

Sexual area	Spinal cord injury effect	Action plan and/or referral
Sexual drive/interest		
Sexual functioning abilities		
Fertility and contraception		
Medical consequences of spinal cord injury		
Motor and sensory influences		
Bladder and bowel influences		
Sexual self-view and self-esteem		
Partnership issues (± parenting)		

Table 14.2 Example of a Chart for the Sexual Rehabilitation Framework of a 36-Year-Old Married Man with C6 Complete Quadriplegia of 3 Years Duration

Sexual area	Spinal cord injury effect	Action plan and/or referral
Sexual drive/interest	Returned to preinjury level	No action
Sexual functioning abilities	Problems with maintenance of reflex erection Anorgasmia	First-line erectile dysfunction therapies: try PDE5i daily or as needed for patient preference; consider ring or injection if PDE5i failure Attempt ejaculation first Encourage cerebral arousal techniques
Fertility and contraception	Anejaculation Not an issue at present	Trial of PVS by local expert. EEJ if PVS + AES failure. Maybe in future if ejaculating at home?
Medical consequences of spinal cord injury	Baclofen user History of autonomic dysreflexia Bladder health History of pressure sores	Consider lower dose prior to sperm retrieval Prior to sperm retrieval, consider utilization of antihypertensives Reduce UTIs prior to fertility attempts Instruction in sexual positioning to avoid this by PT, OT, rehabilitative nursing
Motor and sensory influences	Spasm can interfere with sexual activity Poor hand function Lack of sexual feeling below injury, but painful hyperesthesia at injury line	Have PT assess sexual positioning potential Have OT design assistive aids for ICI or ring placement if needed Learn body mapping to incorporate appropriate sensate/arousal areas
Bladder influences and bowel influences	Wants to have different bladder management around sexual issues Managed well around sexual activity	Urology consult Use of condoms to prevent dripping Catheterization prior possible? No action
Sexual self-view and self-esteem	Feels physically "adjusted" but less masculine	Not wishing to pursue at the present time
Partnership issues (parenting)	Some insecurity around relationship Wife in role of caregiver and intimate partner	Psychology consult with wife regarding interpersonal relationships and fertility goals Boundaries around two issues need to be defined

Abbreviations: AES, abdominal electrical stimulation; EEJ, electroejaculation; ICI, intracavernosal injection; OT, occupational therapist; PT, physical therapist; PVS, penile vibratory stimulation; UTI, urinary tract infection.

in quality of life,[3] and since dedicated men and women with SCI are excellent physiological models to answer our future questions about sexual potential, research efforts around sexual rehabilitation in this population must continue to be supported. Fortunately, there are newer resources addressing the area of sexuality and SCI, such as Spinal Cord Injury Rehabilitation Evidence (SCIRE) (www.icord.org/scire) and the Consortium for Spinal Cord Medicine Clinical Practice Guidelines on Sexuality and Reproductive Health in Adults with Spinal Cord Injury that has been recently published by the Paralyzed Veterans of America (www.pva.org). Even more difficult issues, such as supporting sexual health and intimacy in care facilities, are available as guidelines for viewing.[37]

Much more research in the area of sexual and fertility rehabilitation is needed. With the new International Standards to Document Remaining Autonomic Function after SCI,[38] including those of Sexual and Reproductive Function,[39] it is hoped the role of visceral, cardiovascular, and other autonomic contributions to sexual function and pleasure will be better delineated in the future. Furthermore, to adequately assess the complex issue of sexual health, it is recommended that future sexual health outcome measures include both quantitative and qualitative data as well as address several key issues identified by the men and women with SCI.[24] The future improved quality of life for men and women with SCI will depend upon high-quality research in the area of sexual and fertility rehabilitation by dedicated professionals.

Pearls

- The use of the Sexual Rehabilitative Framework serves to demystify the area of sexual issues related to SCI into manageable options that fit into the context of that person's life. It also demonstrates the multidisciplinary nature of the sexual health/fertility rehabilitative team.
- The issues of pleasure should be considered as legitimate as those of sexual function and fertility. Encouragement utilizing the sexual rehabilitation principles will result in more gratifying experiences for men and women with SCI than an approach oriented toward a more medical solution.
- Fertility is not affected in women with SCI as it is in men, but issues around pregnancy and delivery require special expertise to prevent unnecessary complications. Fertility options for men include successful sperm retrieval and assistive reproductive technology, allowing most men with SCI to become biological fathers.

Pitfalls

- Genitocentric views of sexual functioning will be detrimental to men and women with SCI because sexuality must be dealt with in the context of the whole person.
- Because approximately half of men and women with either incomplete or complete SCI are able to achieve orgasm, those that do not within the first few years of injury should be encouraged to continue to pursue a form of pleasurable orgasmic attainment. Until the neurology is better understood, the chance of orgasm (genital or nongenital) should not be dismissed, because orgasmic potential is not solely tied to somatic limitations (albeit those with injuries to their sacral cord or pudendal nerve are less likely to achieve orgasm than those with higher levels of injury), and neuroplasticity may play a substantial role.
- There are fewer therapeutic modalities for sexual problems in women with SCI than for men, but treatments are being investigated. Clinicians should still encourage women with SCI to experiment, including the use of PDE5i (where indicated), vibrostimulation, or other enhancers. Women with SCI should be respectfully encouraged to act as research subjects in this area.

References

1. Anderson KD. Targeting recovery: priorities of the spinal cord-injured population. J Neurotrauma 2004;21(10):1371–1383
2. Anderson KD, Borisoff JF, Johnson RD, Stiens SA, Elliott SL. Spinal cord injury influences psychogenic as well as physical components of female sexual ability. Spinal Cord 2007;45(5):349–359
3. Anderson KD, Borisoff JF, Johnson RD, Stiens SA, Elliott SL. The impact of spinal cord injury on sexual function: concerns of the general population. Spinal Cord 2007;45(5):328–337
4. Stevenson R, Elliott S. Sexual disorders with comorbid psychiatric and physical illness. In: Clinical Manual of Sexual Disorders. Washington, DC: American Psychiatric Publishing; 2009:59–94
5. Borisoff JF, Elliott SL, Hocaloski S, Birch GE. The development of a sensory substitution system for the sexual rehabilitation of men with chronic spinal cord injury. J Sex Med 2010;7(11): 3647–3658
6. Elliott S. Sexuality after spinal cord injury. In: Spinal Cord Injury Rehabilitation. Philadelphia, PA: Davis; 2009:513–529
7. Komisaruk BR, Whipple B, Crawford A, Liu WC, Kalnin A, Mosier K. Brain activation during vaginocervical self-stimulation and orgasm in women with complete spinal cord injury: fMRI evidence of mediation by the vagus nerves. Brain Res 2004;1024(1-2):77–88
8. Alexander M, Rosen RC. Spinal cord injuries and orgasm: a review. J Sex Marital Ther 2008; 34(4):308–324
9. Anderson KD, Borisoff JF, Johnson RD, Stiens SA, Elliott SL. Long-term effects of spinal cord injury on sexual function in men: implications for neuroplasticity. Spinal Cord 2007;45(5):338–348
10. Courtois F, Charvier K, Leriche A, Vézina JG, Jacqemin G. Sexual and climactic responses in men with traumatic spinal injury: a model for rehabilitation. Sexologies 2009;18:79–82
11. Giuliano F, Rubio-Aurioles E, Kennelly M, et al; Vardenafil Study Group. Vardenafil improves ejaculation success rates and self-confidence in men with erectile dysfunction due to spinal cord injury. Spine 2008;33(7):709–715
12. Courtois F, Charvier K, Leriche A, et al. Perceived physiological and orgasmic sensations at ejaculation in spinal cord injured men. J Sex Med 2008; 5(10):2419–2430
13. Kolettis PN, Lambert MC, Hammond KR, Kretzer PA, Steinkampf MP, Lloyd LK. Fertility outcomes after electroejaculation in men with spinal cord injury. Fertil Steril 2002;78(2):429–431
14. Ohl DA, Quallich SA, Sønksen J, Brackett NL, Lynne CM. Anejaculation: an electrifying approach. Semin Reprod Med 2009;27(2):179–185
15. DeForge D, Blackmer J, Garritty C, et al. Fertility following spinal cord injury: a systematic review. Spinal Cord 2005;43(12):693–703
16. Brackett NL, Ibrahim E. Fertility after spinal cord injury. In: Spinal Cord Injury Rehabilitation. Philadelphia, PA: Davis; 2009:531–547
17. Kafetsoulis A, Brackett NL, Ibrahim E, Attia GR, Lynne CM. Current trends in the treatment of infertility in men with spinal cord injury. Fertil Steril 2006;86(4):781–789
18. Claydon VE, Elliott SL, Sheel AW, Krassioukov A. Cardiovascular responses to vibrostimulation for sperm retrieval in men with spinal cord injury. J Spinal Cord Med 2006;29(3):207–216
19. Elliott S, Bono CM, Cardenas DD, Frost FS, Hammond MC, et al. Sexual dysfunction and infertility in men with spinal cord disorders In: Spinal Cord Medicine: Principles and Practice. 2nd ed. New York, NY: Demos Medical; 2010:409–428
20. Ibrahim E, Brackett NL, Aballa TC, Lynne CM. Safety of a novel treatment to improve sperm motility in men with spinal cord injury. Fertil Steril 2009; 91(4, Suppl):1411–1413
21. Kanto S, Uto H, Toya M, Ohnuma T, Arai Y, Kyono K. Fresh testicular sperm retrieved from men with spinal cord injury retains equal fecundity to that from men with obstructive azoospermia via intracytoplasmic sperm injection. Fertil Steril 2009;92(4):1333–1336
22. Bughi S, Shaw SJ, Mahmood G, Atkins RH, Szlachcic Y. Amenorrhea, pregnancy, and pregnancy outcomes in women following spinal cord injury: a retrospective cross-sectional study. Endocr Pract 2008;14(4):437–441
23. Jackson AB, Wadley V. A multicenter study of women's self-reported reproductive health after spinal cord injury. Arch Phys Med Rehabil 1999; 80(11):1420–1428
24. Abramson CE, McBride KE, Konnyu KJ, Elliott SL; SCIRE Research Team. Sexual health outcome measures for individuals with a spinal cord injury: a systematic review. Spinal Cord 2008; 46(5):320–324
25. Guilbert ER, Brown JP, Kaunitz AM, et al. The use of depot-medroxyprogesterone acetate in contraception and its potential impact on skeletal health. Contraception 2009;79(3):167–177
26. Ghidini A, Healey A, Andreani M, Simonson MR. Pregnancy and women with spinal cord injuries. Acta Obstet Gynecol Scand 2008;87(10): 1006–1010
27. Salomon J, Schnitzler A, Ville Y, et al. Prevention of urinary tract infection in six spinal cord-injured pregnant women who gave birth to seven children under a weekly oral cyclic antibiotic program. Int J Infect Dis 2009;13(3):399–402
28. Sipski ML. The impact of spinal cord injury on female sexuality, menstruation and pregnancy: a review of the literature. J Am Paraplegia Soc 1991;14(3):122–126
29. Sipski ML, Rosen RC, Alexander CJ, Hamer RM. Sildenafil effects on sexual and cardiovascular responses in women with spinal cord injury. Urology 2000;55(6):812–815
30. Billups KL. The role of mechanical devices in treating female sexual dysfunction and enhancing the female sexual response. World J Urol 2002;20(2):137–141
31. Tepper MS, Whipple B, Richards E, Komisaruk BR. Women with complete spinal cord injury: a phenomenological study of sexual experiences. J Sex Marital Ther 2001;27(5):615–623
32. Elliott S. Sexual functioning in women with spinal cord disorders. In: Lin VW, ed. Spinal Cord

Medicine: Principles and Practice. 2nd ed. New York, NY: Demos Medical; 2010:In Press

33. Laessøe L, Nielsen JB, Biering-Sørensen F, Sønksen J. Antispastic effect of penile vibration in men with spinal cord lesion. Arch Phys Med Rehabil 2004;85(6):919–924

34. Ekland MB, Krassioukov AV, McBride KE, Elliott SL. Incidence of autonomic dysreflexia and silent autonomic dysreflexia in men with spinal cord injury undergoing sperm retrieval: implications for clinical practice. J Spinal Cord Med 2008; 31(1):33–39

35. Balon R. Medications and sexual function and dysfunction. In: Balon R, Seagraves RT, eds. Clinical Manual of Sexual Disorders. Washington, DC: American Psychiatric Publishing; 2009:95–118

36. Kennedy P, Lude P, Taylor N. Quality of life, social participation, appraisals and coping post spinal cord injury: a review of four community samples. Spinal Cord 2006;44(2):95–105

37. Supporting Sexual Health and Intimacy in Care Facilities: Guidelines for Supporting Adults Living in Long-Term Care Facilities and Group Homes in British Columbia, Vancouver Coastal Health Authority July 15, 2009, Canada. http://www.vch.ca/media/FacilitiesLicensing_SupportingSexualHealthandIntimacyinCareFacilities2.pdf

38. Alexander MS, Biering-Sorensen F, Bodner D, et al. International standards to document remaining autonomic function after spinal cord injury. Spinal Cord 2009;47(1):36–43

39. Alexander MS, Bodner D, Brackett NL, Elliott S, Jackson AB, Sønksen J; Ad Hoc Committee American Spinal Injury Association. Development of international standards to document sexual and reproductive functions after spinal cord injury: preliminary report. J Rehabil Res Dev 2007; 44(1):83–90

15

Interdisciplinary Essentials in Pressure Ulcer Management

Kath Bogie, Chester Ho, Monique Washington, Sharon Foster-Geeter, J. C. Seton, Steven J. Mitchell, Martin J. Kilbane, Gina L. D. Kubec, Kimberly Sexton, Thomas M. Dixon, Christine C. Frick, and Joshua L. White

Key Points

1. Effective pressure ulcer (PU) management requires consideration of multiple intrinsic and extrinsic factors.
2. A comprehensive multidisciplinary approach is essential to achieve successful PU management outcomes. Individual members of the multidisciplinary team contribute their own expertise while collaborating and communicating with other team members about risk modification.
3. Many pressure ulcers are preventable with the use of appropriate, currently available interventions. The clinician's focus is on modification of as many medical risk factors as possible. The nursing process facilitates assessment and evaluation of PU status and assists in determining new strategies. Physical, occupational, and other rehabilitation therapists develop individualized, comprehensive plans for pressure management based on patient and family education together with assessment and selection of support surfaces and positioning devices for effective pressure relief. Nutrition, psychosocial status, and patient education are all critical factors in PU prevention and management.
4. Biomedical engineering enables technological advances in PU prevention and assessment.

To successfully prevent pressure ulcer (PU) formation, it is essential to understand the fundamental concept that there are multiple intrinsic and extrinsic factors leading to the development of PUs. Having a PU not only greatly impacts a person's quality of life, it also places a heavy burden on the health care system in treatment costs.[1] Recent trends in health care delivery suggest a comprehensive multidisciplinary approach to achieve successful wound management outcomes.[2] The team typically includes physicians, nurses, physical therapists, occupational therapists, dietitians, and psychologists, together with some input from biomedical engineers (**Fig. 15.1**). This chapter addresses the essentials of PU management from the perspectives of a multidisciplinary PU management team.

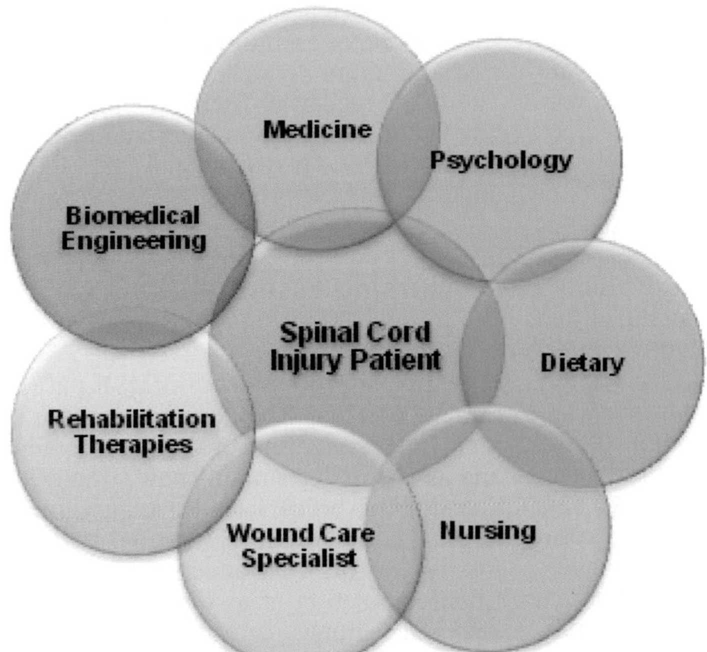

Fig. 15.1 Multidisciplinary wound care model: spinal cord injury patient at risk/with a pressure ulcer.

Medical Essentials in Pressure Ulcer Management

The clinician must address as many medical risk factors as possible while realizing that some may be rather difficult to correct or eliminate. These factors can be arbitrarily divided into intrinsic and extrinsic risk factors. Intrinsic factors refer to the internal medical factors of the individual. These include motor paralysis, muscular atrophy, mobility impairment, sensory impairment, nutritional impairment, anemia, and vascular compromise due to large-vessel disease or microvascular disease. Many medical conditions and lifestyle choices may lead to increased intrinsic PU risk factors, such as diabetes mellitus or any medical condition that results in anemia and impaired nutrition; neuromuscular diseases, such as poliomyelitis, amyotrophic lateral sclerosis, or critical illness polyneuropathy; and any acquired condition, such as spinal cord injury (SCI), stroke, or traumatic brain injury, that leads to impaired mobility and/or sensory loss. Lifestyle choices like smoking[3] and alcoholism are also associated with an increased risk of PU development (see the Psychology section). Some intrinsic risk factors may be more easily corrected than others. For instance, smoking may be more reversible than muscular atrophy secondary to a neuromuscular disease.

Extrinsic factors are environmental in nature and include the local environment of the skin (e.g., moisture level, which may be affected by sweating and bowel/bladder incontinence), interface pressure and shear force between the skin and the support surface (while seated or in bed), friction,[4] and psychosocial support. Many extrinsic factors interact with the intrinsic factors. For instance, mobility impairment may lead to bowel and bladder incontinence, which in turn will affect the local skin microenvironment by creating excessive skin moisture, hence increasing the risk of PU development. Another example is nutritional impairment, which may lead to muscular atrophy, hence negatively impacting on the interface pressure between the weight-bearing skin areas of the body and the supporting surface. Some extrinsic factors are more easily addressed than others. For instance, providing the appropriate support surfaces may reduce the interface pressure fairly easily, but lack of psychosocial support may be much more difficult to address.

Medical Approaches to Pressure Ulcer Prevention

It is clear that intrinsic and extrinsic PU risk factors are often interdependent and complex, requiring a comprehensive interdisciplinary team approach to successfully prevent PU development. The primary approach involves the identification of significant risk factors by the various team members, each focusing on their own area of expertise while collaborating and communicating with the other team members about risk modification.[5] This often necessitates the establishment of a multidisciplinary skin care team. All members are specialists in PU prevention and treatment, with one taking the leadership role. For example, a patient with a history of poorly controlled diabetes mellitus, peripheral vascular disease, and smoking has been admitted to the inpatient rehabilitation unit following a stroke that has resulted in left hemiplegia, bladder incontinence, and dysphagia. This individual has multiple intrinsic and extrinsic risk factors for PU development, and a suitable team management approach is shown in **Table 15.1**. The specific role of each discipline will be discussed in more detail later in this chapter. The team regularly discusses progress in risk factor modification and monitors skin status closely. This is a highly interactive and collaborative process.

Nursing Essentials in Pressure Ulcer Management

The nursing process is an integral part of nursing practice that allows for the assessment and evaluation of PU management and assists in determining new strategies.[6] The nursing process for PU management begins with nurses, assessing patients for risk factors that affect nursing care.[6] Upon completion of a comprehensive assessment, nurses create client-specific care plans determined by an individual's risk factors and based on clinical practice guidelines (CPGs). Nurses also plan for the implementation of the individualized care plan, apply nursing interventions accordingly, evaluate current wound care practices and modalities in use, and determine if specific expected outcomes have been met.[6] Documentation is a key communication tool that captures the established basis for initial and revised care plan development.

Table 15.1 Multidisciplinary Team Management of At-Risk Patient

Specialty	Role
Physician	Provide optimal management of underlying clinical conditions, e.g., diabetes and peripheral vascular disease
Nurse	• Complete nursing pressure ulcer risk assessment score • Ensure appropriate positioning and pressure relief while in bed • Perform appropriate management of bladder incontinence
Dietitian	Aggressively address nutritional issues arising with diabetes and dysphagia
Physical and occupational therapists	Address seating and positioning issues
Psychologist	• Address potential cognitive issues that may impair the patient's understanding of pressure ulcer prevention • Provide smoking cessation counseling

Risk Assessment Scales

Screening tools like risk assessment scales are designed to help clinicians identify high-risk patients.[7] The importance of completing comprehensive patient evaluations cannot be overstated. These include determining available support systems (such as home care resources), the patient's PU risk factors, and any existing PUs. There are a variety of PU risk assessment tools or scales available. It is important to validate assessment scales as reliable in use within their intended population.[8] For example, the Salzberg scale focuses on PU risk assessment factors specifically for persons with SCI. These factors include restricted activity level, degree of immobility, level of injury, urinary incontinence, autonomic dysreflexia, advanced age, the presence of comorbidities, as well as residence and nutrition (hypoalbuminemia or anemia).[9] However, there is much controversy regarding whether this specific scale is the best predictor. Studies to determine initial PU development prediction and recurrence using the Salzberg scale are favorable but must be considered preliminary at this time.[10] Other PU risk assessment scales include the Norton, Waterlow, Gosnell, Knoll, and Braden.[11] The Braden scale is currently most used in the United States and has been found to have the best predictive value in a review of seven risk assessment scales used with individuals with SCI.[8] Other multicenter prospective studies have published replicated findings that have strongly suggested the Braden scale to be a valid and reliable tool.[11,12] The Braden scale consists of six subscales: sensory perception, moisture, activity, mobility, nutrition, and friction/shear,[7] each with a numerical range of scores. The friction/shear subscale ranges from 1 to 3; the other subscales range from 1 to 4 (1 = lowest possible score). Lower scores indicate higher risk for PU development.[7] Nurses and other health care professionals can use the Braden scale as an outline for risk assessment and care plan development.

Clinical Practice Guidelines

The National Pressure Ulcer Advisory Panel (NPUAP), in collaboration with the Agency for Healthcare Research and Quality (AHRQ), encourages prevention as the first line of defense against PUs.[13] Prevention is much less costly than treatment, and the AHRQ CPG v3 suggests the need to increase education and quality improvement methods.[14] Forward-thinking tactics such as these foster the development of prevention initiatives useful for high-risk areas of care. The AHRQ CPG 3 advises that patients be assessed for risk on admission and periodically as determined by the unit or facility (e.g., daily or weekly).[15] The NPAUP CPG further advises the need for reassessment at regular intervals based on changes in patient condition, acuity levels and current care settings.[16] There are a variety of CPGs in addition to those from AHRQ and NPUAP, including the National Guideline Clearinghouse created by the American Medical Directors Association (AMDA),[17] Quality Improvement Organization (QIO) guidelines,[18] Wound, Ostomy and Continence Nurses Society (WOCN) best practice guidelines,[19] National Institutes for Health and Clinical Excellence (NICE) guidelines,[20] and Consortium for Spinal Cord Medicine Clinical Practice Guidelines.[21] Each guideline contains similar recommendations regarding risk assessment, prevention, PU assessment, measurement, treatment, and documentation; however, they also contain significant differences. The best CPG for an individual facility can thus vary based on overall facility policy. It is important to follow updated published guidelines and best practice methods that focus on prevention and treatment central to good patient care.[22]

Nursing Care Planning

Current practices in PU prevention and management support the nursing process in addition to comprehensive collaborative efforts.[23] The patient-specific nursing care plan should be based on education relating to self-care deficits and assistive education relating to PU prevention, moisture assessment, and bowel and bladder management.[24] Nurses must determine the patient's readiness to learn and the patient's current level of relevant knowledge.

Education-based PU prevention protocols targeted at specific risk factors may reduce future PU development.[25] Structured education protocols can increase a patient's knowledge base, correcting misguided beliefs and improving understanding of personal risk.[26] Teaching strategies should focus on identifying both internal and external factors, which the patient may have some control over. For at-risk individuals with no current PU, the care plan should include preventative education focused on daily skin inspection and keeping bed linens dry, clean, and wrinkle free.[24] Individuals and their families should be involved in the planning and implementation process as well. Patients' involvement in their own care will increase autonomy and may be beneficial for implementation.

Bowel and Bladder Management

Loss of bowel and bladder control is one of many complications consequent to SCI. In the SCI population it is important to focus on the strategies relating to moisture, nutrition, friction, and shear.[27,28] Nurses must be aware of the impairments and difficulties bowel and bladder management may present. In addition to medications and dietary recommendations, nurses must create care plans based on guidelines for avoiding high-risk behaviors and conditions that can lead to impaired skin integrity.[29]

When applying facility CPG recommendations to the Braden subscale relating to moisture, nurses create a care plan based on nursing assessment and diagnosis of individuals with SCI found to be at risk for impaired skin integrity relating to moisture.[30] The goal is removal of excess moisture, especially for those who perspire heavily and experience fecal and urinary incontinence, without drying out the client's skin.[7] Protective barriers, such as creams, drying powders, or moisture-absorbing pads, should be applied as appropriate. Nurses should also teach and assist patients to become active participants in the care and maintenance of external or internal urinary devices (external catheters, indwelling catheters, or intermittent catheterization devices) to ensure proper elimination and decrease moisture exposure.[31] Regularly scheduled bowel care is also important. Encouraging patients to be active in daily skin inspections and providing information and assistance with methods and devices reinforce effective bowel and bladder management.

Documentation and Home-Care Management

In addition to minimizing modifiable risks for their patients, nurses help to maximize independence. Planning and implementation of a nursing care plan should be based on measurable goals. Standardized documentation of care plan development, implementation, evaluation, and actual outcomes is important. Documentation is also invaluable for continuous evaluation and improvement of the nursing process and current care. Education and instruction can increase self-care compliance in anticipation of required needs at home.[24] When teaching new behaviors or tasks, an immediate demonstration of the activity should be used to assess a patient's understanding. Nurses must also ensure the behavior is being performed consistently over a determined time frame.[26] For example, daily skin inspections should be completed consistently for 5 days, and three to five reasons for adherence to bowel and bladder management plans should be verbalized. Follow-up evaluations can determine if patients are achieving expected outcomes This aspect of nursing care planning enables review of the nursing process and records the appropriate cost-effective services provided as well as information provided to clients and families.

Current Nursing Practices in Pressure Ulcer Treatment

Many PUs are preventable with the use of appropriate interventions,[32] and appropriate pressure relief must always be provided. Although 2-hour turn schedules are commonly used in nursing practice, the rationale for this time interval is not well established.[23] It has been suggested that regular turn schedules combined with low-air-loss support surfaces are required to maximize benefit.[32]

Pressure Ulcer Assessment

Pressure Ulcer Staging

To make the best decision for PU treatment, the wound must be assessed and its stage or grade determined. Wound characteristics of importance include size, location, and wound bed appearance. The NPUAP has been instrumental in developing a standard approach to wound staging to accurately communicate the degree of tissue damage.[33] In 2007, a category of suspected deep tissue injury (DTI) was added to the overall classification.[34] Other PUs are categorized in four stages or as unstageable (**Table 15.2**). Stage II through IV PUs may exhibit a yellow, tan, gray, or brown substance called slough. Tissue surrounding the wound should also be assessed to determine local skin health.

It is also important to note that the initial staging of a PU dictates the permanent description of the wound, even when it has healed. For example a stage IV ulcer that is now healed will be a "healed stage IV." Its stage will never be reversed to a stage I or zero.

Pressure Ulcer Measurement

Currently, wound measurements are obtained by measuring wound edge to wound edge and recording first the length, then the width, and then the depth. Advances in technology are needed (see the Biomedical Engineering section). Irregularly shaped wounds can make measurement more difficult. Wound measurement is al-

Table 15.2 NPAUAP Classification of Pressure Ulcers

Pressure ulcer type	Characteristics
Suspected Deep Tissue Injury	Localized area of intact skin with dark discoloration beyond that of an individual's normal skin color
Stage I	Detectable nonblanchable areas of intact skin with the appearance of persistent redness in lightly pigmented skin. Patients with darker skin may present with darker tones in skin color, such as a deepened red, blue, or purple hue.
Stage II	Shallow or superficial wound, such as an abrasion or crater that involves partial-thickness skin loss. Partial-thickness skin loss could involve the epidermis, dermis or both.
Stage III	Full-thickness skin loss. Presents clinically as a deep crater most often involving damage to subcutaneous fat. May extend down to underlying fascia, although bone, tendon, and muscle are not visible.
Stage IV	Full-thickness skin loss extending beyond underlying fascia with evidence of tissue destruction, necrosis, and/or the damage of muscle, bone, and supporting structures
Unstageable	Full-thickness skin loss with wound bed covered in slough or eschar. True depth cannot be determined until the wound is chemically debrided, removed by sharp debridement, or allowed to fall off naturally.

ways based on the face of a clock, although orientation of the clock face varies with wound location. Specifically, wounds on the feet will use the heel as the 12 o'clock landmark and the toes as the 6 o'clock landmark. Wounds anywhere else on the body use the client's head as 12 o'clock with the toes at 6 o'clock. Head to toe is always used for length and side to side for width.[33] Measurements are typically taken using a cotton tip applicator and a disposable ruler. Wound depth is measured with the applicator in the deepest area of the wound bed, grasping the applicator with the thumb and forefinger and maintaining the finger placement upon withdrawal and ruler measurement. In addition to wound area irregularities, tunnels, epiboly (premature closure of the wound edges), sinus tracts, and areas of undermining may be present as well. It is important to use the clock system to describe the location and direction of PU irregularities, always taking precautions not to lose the applicator in tunneled areas of the wound.

Wound Bed Assessment in Pressure Ulcers

Wound bed assessment includes tissue type and characteristics, exudate, and environment.[35] Tissue destruction is either partial or full thickness; however, the descriptions of tissue characteristics vary.

Tissue color within the wound bed is an important characteristic. In general, reddish pink to red indicates healthy tissue with a good blood flow. Granulation tissue is living viable tissue with a puffy, bubbled, reddish pink appearance. Poor blood flow results in tissues that appear pale pink. In wounds that extend beyond the superficial layers, the epithelial tissue may be pearly pink. In superficial wounds, epithelial tissue may develop in islands. Necrotic (dead) tissues come in a variety of colors: necrotic (dark/black), necrotic slough (yellow/green/gray/tan), or necrotic eschar (dark or black, thick hard crust). Yellow and green usually indicate infection. Overhydrated moist tissues appear white and macerated.

Wound exudate colors also communicate vital information. Clear or serous fluids and sanguineous (bloody) drainage are normal in the acute inflammatory phases of wound healing. Increases in the amount of drainage could be troublesome. Colors indicative of necrosis and infection in the wound bed are also indicative of infection if found in drainage (purulence) as well.

Temperature, moisture, and the presence of bacteria all influence wound management. Wound healing occurs at normal body temperatures.[36] Temperature decreases are related to loss of moisture from the wound. Moisture vapor within tissue is lost with every dressing change, and it can take the body hours to return to adequate body temperature. Even a 2°C decrease can delay wound healing.[35]

Nutrient-rich moisture within a wound bed indicative of good blood supply is desirable. A dry wound bed slows healing and increases the likelihood of scar formation.[37] Nurse education of patients includes the need to prevent the wound from drying out.[38] However, copious amounts of odoriferous fluid are undesirable. Wounds should be cleaned prior to assessment to avoid confusion with the odor of a treatment option.

Bacteria inhibit wound healing by competing for nutrients and oxygen, Necrosis or bacteria within a wound cause odors that can be described as pungent, foul, strong, fecal, or musty. Bacteria-ridden wounds can also smell sour or sweet. Documentation of wound bed assessments relays vital information to several disciplines and assists in determining a selection among treatment options.

Selection of Pressure Ulcer Dressings: Treatment Options

Treatments and dressing choices should be based on clinical intention, wound location and type, product availability, and cost. Preventative treatments, such as protective dressings applied directly to the skin, protect against initial skin breakdown. Adhesive dressings provide a protective environmental barrier. Nonadhesive moisture control barriers, such as creams, ointments, gels, pastes, and skin sealants, can also protect against breakdown. Product selection for wound treatment should focus on wound characteristics and appearance and provide improved wound healing.

Cleansing of the wound bed is an important component of PU care, thus it is important to select the optimal cleansing solution prior to dressing placement.[39] Although common in home use, tap water cleansing is not clinically recommended due to variable quality. Normal saline is currently most used in practice and is a cost-effective isotonic solution that will not cause tissue damage. Commercial cleansers are usually recommended to facilitate removal of wound bed debris, which could lead to infection. These solutions should be used carefully; they may harm healthy tissue if they are not applied as directed. It is important to pat surrounding skin dry after irrigation and before the application of a clean dressing to prevent maceration or damage of viable tissue due to cleansing or debriding solutions.

Selection of an appropriate debriding agent is also important. Debriding products include solutions, ointments, and creams containing enzymes that digest necrotic nonviable tissue and promote epithelialization. Wound dressings range from gauze to hydrocolloids, impregnated matrixes to foams, and more. Dressings for open wounds with depth can absorb drainage, add moisture, reduce bacteria, combat infection, and control odor. One should choose a dressing that facilitates a moist environment conducive of wound healing (**Table 15.3**).

Rehabilitation Therapist Essentials in Pressure Ulcer Management

Physical, occupational, and other rehabilitation therapists in the SCI interdisciplinary team play a critical role in PU prevention and management. Therapists develop individualized, comprehensive plans for pressure management based on patient and family education, together with assessment and selection of support surfaces and positioning devices.

Pressure Ulcer Education

There are two main goals in PU education; the first is to have patients and caregivers understand who is at risk, the barriers to remaining ulcer free, their specific risk factors, and how modifications in habits, actions, and environment can prevent skin breakdown. The second is that prevention will begin as a therapist-directed activity but will gradually shift to an entirely patient-initiated practice in all areas of life and at all times. Gibson suggested that, though patients were knowledgeable about PUs and motivated to look after their health, they tended to rely too heavily on the SCI unit rather than be independent with their care.[40] King et al. found that, although patients may believe they are at risk and that prevention is important, they do not follow through with corresponding preventative actions.[41]

Effective education must be initiated early, provided on an individualized basis, and approached in a hands-on manner.[42] It has been shown that individualized education and structured monthly follow-up can effectively reduce the frequency, or delay recurrence, of PUs.[43] Education should be an ongoing process provided to anyone at risk, including patients with acute injuries and individuals aging with an SCI, even though they may have successfully avoided a PU thus far.

There are many barriers to remaining PU free. The most preventable barrier is that patients are unaware of their risk. SCI often occurs due to a traumatic accident with multiple complications; prevention of something that *may* happen is low on the priority list, and therefore education never occurs. If patients are made aware of their elevated risk, they are frequently not told the consequences of having a PU, nor where or what to look for. Without the sensation of pain, a PU can quickly form and go unnoticed until a host of secondary complications have arisen. Therefore, it is imperative to the health and well-being of the patient that education begins early in the rehabilitation process and continues throughout the life span.

Table 15.3 Categories of Wound Dressings

Category	Stage	Drainage	Description
Alginates	II III IV	Moderate–heavy	Alginates are derived from brown seaweed. This dressing forms a gel when it comes in contact with exudates within the wound bed. Alginate has the ability to absorb excessive drainage. Can remain in place for 24–48 hours.
Antimicrobial	II III IV	N/A	Antimicrobials are used to reduce the microbial load when signs and symptoms of infection are present in the wound bed. There are many products in this category supplied in a variety of consistencies—gels, ointments, impregnated gauze, pads.
Collagen	III IV	Light–heavy	Collagen dressings derived from cowhides encourage the formation of newly formed collagen and granulation tissue.
Composites	I II III IV	Light–heavy	Composite dressings combine multiple dressings to perform a variety of functions, such as a bacterial barrier, absorption, and adhesion. Can serve as a primary or secondary dressing.
Enzymatic debrider	III IV Unstageable with slough or necrosis	No depth Minimal drainage	Enzymatic debriders loosen necrotic tissue from the wound bed by digestion of collagen from necrotic tissue.
Foams	II III IV	Light–heavy	Polyurethane dressings with small pores to absorb drainage. Nonadherent and have a waterproof outer layer. Foam dressings provide a moist wound environment and can be helpful when hypergranulation tissue is present in a wound bed.
Hydrocolloids	II III	Light–moderate	Hydrocolloids are composed of gelatin, pectin, or carboxymethylcellulose. These occlusive dressings prevent oxygen, bacteria, or fluids from contacting the wound bed, and they also provide autolysis.
Hydrogels	II III IV	Light–moderate	Hydrogels contain up to 90% water, thus facilitating moisture in the wound bed. They have a cooling effect for painful wounds.
Impregnated gauze dressings	II III IV	Light–heavy	Impregnated gauze is impregnated with a variety of products, e.g., hydrogel, iodine, petrolatum or xeroform, and sodium chloride. Wicks away exudates and maintains a moist wound environment.
Negative pressure wound vacuum (NPWT)	III IV	Light–heavy	Used when fast wound healing is indicated. Healing occurs by pulling the edges together and filling the wound bed with granulation tissue. Can be used on chronic or acute wounds. Can be used in combination with other treatment modalities.
Protective barriers	I II	None–moderate	Protective barriers are implemented to protect the intact skin or partial-thickness wounds from exposure to urine, stool, or any other body fluids.
Skin equivalents	III IV	Light–heavy	Skin equivalents are bioengineered tissues that promote the proliferation of key cells in wound healing by forming a collagen-based matrix.
Wound fillers	III IV	Light–heavy	Wound fillers manage and maintain moisture in a wound bed. Require a secondary dressing for containment.

Patients need to be made aware of the risk factors that lead to increased incidence of PUs.[44] Schubart et al. analyzed the educational needs of adults with SCI and found that awareness of lifelong risk for PU development, including the ability to self-assess risk factors and how risk changes over time, was one of the most important needs of this population.[44] Nonmodifiable risk factors include required medications, genetics, body type, comorbidities like diabetes, level of injury, and the individual's cognition. Age is another risk factor due to decreased flexibility, lack of functional mobility, and reduced financial resources as well as increased body mass and escalating caregiver burden. Modifiable risk factors include nutrition, body weight, skin care, and pressure management. Individuals who maintain a normal weight, return to meaningful roles in life, and do not have a history of tobacco use, suicidal behaviors, self-reported incarcerations, alcohol abuse, or drug abuse are less like to develop a PU.[45] Rehabilitation therapists tend to focus on modifiable risk factors to teach individualized prevention strategies for different activities.

Skin Inspection

Skin care education is important for individuals with SCI and encompasses several components.[44] Patients must control skin contact with moisture, including a bowel and bladder continence program and managing sweat. One of the most frequently taught preventive behaviors is daily visual and tactile skin checks. This can be facilitated through a flexible mirror that can be held at various angles in order for the patient to check all common PU locations. Alternative techniques or inspection by a caregiver may be necessary for individuals with restricted mobility. Individuals should learn the most frequently affected body locations, what skin changes to be aware of, and the importance of reporting any skin changes to their doctor in a timely manner.[46]

Pressure Management for Pressure Ulcer Prevention

Pressure management is a modifiable risk factor that therapists should address through a 24-hour plan of care for all at-risk patients. This includes selection of appropriate pressure relief technique(s), wheelchair, wheelchair cushion, mattress, and positioning while in bed. The goal of effective pressure management is to ensure skin integrity while maximizing independence with activities of daily living.

Establishment of an Individualized Pressure Management Program

It is important to realize that those with new injuries are unlikely to realize they are at any risk of PUs due to lack of protective sensation and the ironic fact that the primary behavior associated with PU development is inactivity rather than behavior.[9] Until the individual acquires the necessary insight and skills, performance of a pressure management regimen will initially be the responsibility of members of the interdisciplinary team. As the individual achieves an understanding of the risks and consequences of PUs and becomes able to perform these techniques, responsibility for pressure management is shifted to the individual.

Techniques to Shift Weight and Redistribute Pressure

To establish a regimen of pressure management that will be effective for a given individual, the rehabilitation therapist must identify which pressure relief techniques are most effective, provide the individual with various forms of feedback to demonstrate their effectiveness, and reinforce the need to perform these techniques with the appropriate frequency and duration. Although the term *pressure relief* is frequently used to describe weight shifts, in reality these techniques are used to shift pressure from one location to another or redistribute it across a greater surface area. Numerous studies have been performed on the effectiveness of weight shifts in preventing PU development; however, there is currently no consensus on which technique is most effective. Similarly, there has been no definitive research to indicate the optimum frequency and duration of performing pressure relief. This lack of consensus is due to differences in methodology and measurement variables. Some studies have been based on the measurement of interface pressures with the support surface, whereas others have looked at tissue oxygen perfusion.[47–49] There is, however, universal consensus that weight shifts are essential to preventing PUs. The CPGs currently recommend that therapists help the individual establish a specific pressure relief regimen within the individual's capability and that this regimen be performed every 15 to 30 minutes.[46]

For individuals with sufficient upper extremity function and sitting balance, the full push-up, side or lateral lean, and forward lean are the three most commonly used techniques. While the wheelchair push-up can eliminate pressure over the ischial tuberosities, studies of tissue oxygen perfusion suggest that tissue must be unloaded for well over 60 seconds to return to baseline levels. This may be impractical for many individuals with SCI and over time may subject the joints of the upper extremities to excessive stress. For these reasons, techniques that involve leaning may increasingly be gaining favor.

For individuals who lack the physical ability to effectively perform weight shifts, prescription of a mechanical tilt or recline system is recommended. Coggrave and Rose found that at least 65 degrees of tilt was required to recover oxygen perfusion in unloaded tissue.[47] Other studies have found a combination of a 45 degree tilt and a 120 degree recline provided the greatest reduction of interface seating pressure.[50] These authors and others have found that, although individuals frequently accessed their power tilt function, very few tilted further than 45 degrees.[50,51]

Pressure Mapping

Interface pressure mapping can be an effective tool for providing feedback regarding the pressure-reducing properties of a wheelchair cushion, specialty mattresses, and other support surfaces. To utilize this technology therapeutically, however, it is important to understand system capabilities. Most clinically available pressure mapping systems include sensors that measure vertical pressure only and cannot detect shear forces, friction, or the effects of any contour provided by the seating system. Unless routinely recalibrated, the sensitivity of sensor mats will change over time. Thus, caution should be exercised when one is comparing current versus historical results. This is especially true in the absence of frequent recalibration.

Pressure mapping can be used to assess the effectiveness of different types of cushions, identify uneven pressure distribution due to asymmetry, and optimize overall pressure distribution of a seating system through changes in its configuration. Perhaps its most effective use, however, is its ability to demonstrate the effectiveness of weight shifts and other pressure management strategies.

Support Surface Selection

Rehabilitation therapists play a primary role in support surface selection. When assessing pressure-reducing properties of support surfaces, such as wheelchair cushions and specialty mattresses, therapists must consider both the pressure being exerted by the support surface and the forces exerted by the support surface due to shear, friction, moisture, and other factors. No single clinical tool or standard can definitively determine which support surface will be best for an individual. Therefore, therapists must rely on a combination of their clinical judgment and objective findings, such as pressure mapping, to select appropriate support surfaces.

Specialty Mattress Selection

When choosing a mattress, it is important to consider comfort, individual risk factors, and the caregiver's capabilities. Mattresses are divided into static (low-tech) and dynamic (high-tech) categories. Static mattresses and overlays consist of foam, static air, water, or gel. Dynamic mattresses use alternating pressure, low-air loss, or air-fluidized surfaces to provide therapeutic pressure management. A systematic review of support surfaces concluded that, when compared with standard hospital mattresses, both static and dynamic surfaces can reduce PU incidence.[52] These authors also found that research on the relative efficacy of static and dynamic surfaces is currently inconclusive. Current clinical recommendations are that at-risk individuals should use a static mattress and those with a history of PU should utilize a dynamic surface.

Wheelchair Seating Selection

Cushion selection is a key part of pressure management for an individual following SCI. Clinicians must be knowledgeable about the properties of the various types of cushions to select the best cushion for each individual. Cushions usually use the properties of air, fluid, various densities of foam, or a combination. Air- and fluid-based cushions use the principle of providing immersion of bony prominences to maximize the amount of surface area, thus decreasing pressure. Foam cushions provide less immersion but provide better stability, which can reduce shear or redistribute pressure away from bony prominences onto areas that can tolerate additional pressure.

Rehabilitation therapists who specialize in providing seating/wheeled mobility also incorporate pressure management and reduction of shear into every aspect of an individual's wheelchair and seating system. Scoliosis, pelvic obliquities, and other postural deformities are frequently complications of SCI, and the resulting asymmetry can result in uneven pressure distribution over bony prominences. Lateral trunk support utilizing contoured backs and other devices can help prevent deformity progression and redistribute pressure away from the affected area.

Positioning

Following selection of an appropriate support surface, positioning must be considered. CPGs recommend that cushions and positioning aids should be used to decrease pressure on high-risk areas or areas with current PUs. It has been shown that optimal side-lying is achieved when cushions are used to position the patient at a 30 degree angle to bed surface, with 30 degrees of hip flexion and 35 degrees of knee flexion, making sure the lower leg is below the midpoint of the body.[53,54] Common practice is to turn the patient every 2 hours (see the nursing discussion above), but there is insufficient evidence to establish a protocol in this area. It is also recommended that the head of the bed be kept at or below 45 degrees unless medical complications preclude this.[55] The duration of head elevation should also be minimized. Head elevation leads to increased sacral region pressure and shearing forces as gravity pulls the patient down the length of the bed.

Transfers

Therapists train and educate patients on all aspects of transfers, such as when transferring from bed to wheelchair. To ensure skin protection during transfers, it is important to educate patients on avoiding excessive shearing forces and friction. Therapists train patients on performance of appropriate transfer techniques for their functional level during the acute rehabilitation. Transfers can be broken down into four categories: independent self-transfer in short or long sitting; self-technique with adaptive equipment, such as a transfer board, caregiver-assisted technique with or without adaptive equipment; or the totally dependent transfer with adaptive equipment, such as a lift device. Regardless of the transfer utilized, therapists must educate the patient and caregiver on the proper technique to reduce risk of skin breakdown. Patients are trained to ensure adequate buttock clearance to prevent excessive shearing forces. Inadequate buttock clearance during lateral transfers causes excessive shearing and repetitive skin microtrauma. Assessment of transfers does not end following acute rehabilitation, and periodic assessments of transfer technique may be required. For example, as patients age, they may experience a decline in their level of function and lose the ability to properly transfer independently. Retraining on transfers with assistance may be required to reduce the risk of skin breakdown.

Spasticity

Therapists provide patient and caregiver education and training on the importance of maintaining adequate lower-extremity range of motion for positioning in a wheelchair and lying in bed. This is extremely important to prevent limb contractures, which can cause excessive pressure points on bony prominences. Most patients with fully preserved upper-extremity strength can be instructed on performing self–range-of-motion (ROM) exercises independently. When patients are unable to perform self–ROM independently, they are educated on how to instruct caregivers on providing proper lower-extremity ROM exercises.[56]

Adjuvant Treatment Modalities

Rehabilitation therapists are involved with PU adjunctive care utilizing therapeutic modalities or biophysical agents. Biophysical agents include hydrotherapy, ultrasound, electrical stimulation, radio frequency, electromagnetism, phototherapy, and negative pressure. Current research has not substantially demonstrated a superior adjunctive therapy modality or biophysical agent utilized in PU management, and more research is needed.[57–59]

Postsurgical Flap Procedure for Wound Closure Management

Following a surgical flap procedure for wound closure, patients are usually placed on bed rest for approximately 6 weeks, usually determined by the individual surgeon. During this time, therapists provide essential education of the patient, caregivers, and fellow medical staff members on proper bed positioning to ensure pressure relief for optimal healing of the postsurgical site. Therapists provide bedside upper extremity strengthening to improve strength in preparation for transfer training. At 6 weeks, therapists initiate lower-extremity ROM exercise, including achieving 90 degree hip flexion, in preparation for wheelchair sitting. Following remobilization, therapists will evaluate transfers, wheelchair positioning, and cushioning to ensure optimal pressure relief is maintained. Prior to discharge, overall sitting time is usually increased gradually over 2 to 3 weeks up to a total of 5 hours of sitting daily.[46]

Nutritional Essentials in Pressure Ulcer Management

Nutrition is integral to the effective medical management of individuals with SCI. In the acute phase, individuals are hypermetabolic, and nutritional needs are increased. Chronically, energy expenditure is less than that for able-bodied individuals. Individuals with SCI are at increased risk for obesity, diabetes, metabolic syndrome, and cardiovascular disease.[60]

The Metropolitan Life Insurance tables have been used as a guide to determine the target body weight for SCI individuals; however, they require adjustment to correct for loss of body mass due to paralysis. Neither body mass index (BMI) nor skinfold measurement should be used to measure body composition in individuals with SCI.[60] There are two methods for adjusting the tables.[60,61]

1. Paraplegia (a) 5 to 10% lower than table weight or (b) 10 to 15 lb lower than table weight
2. Quadriplegia, (a) 10 to 15% lower than table weight or (b) 15 to 20 lb lower than table weight

Energy expenditure is decreased in individuals with SCI, more so with quadriplegia than with paraplegia, due to denervated muscle.[62] As a measure of nutrition in SCI, 24-hour urine urea nitrogen has been shown to be unreliable.[46] Indirect calorimetry is the preferred method for determining energy needs in critically ill patients.[60] The Harris-Benedict equation is used to estimate the daily calorie requirements using basal metabolic rate (BMR). Specifically;

- Male: BMR = 66 + (13.7 × weight in kg) + (5 × height in cm) – (6.76 × age in years)

- Female: BMR = 655 + (9.6 × weight in kg) + (1.8 × height in cm) – (4.7 × age in years)

In people with SCI, the Harris-Benedict equation may be used acutely based on admission weight with an injury factor of 1.2 and a stress factor of 1.1, if indirect calorimetry is not available.[60] During rehabilitation, energy needs may be determined using 22.7 kcal/kg for individuals with quadriplegia and 27.9 kcal/kg for individuals with paraplegia.[60,62]

Daily protein needs during acute SCI should be calculated using 2.0 g protein/kg actual body weight. During rehabilitation, protein needs should be calculated using 0.8 g to 1.0 g protein/kg of body weight for maintenance of adequate protein stores in patients without PUs or infection.[60]

Essential Nutrients for Pressure Ulcer Prevention

A registered dietitian should assess all individuals with SCI for risk factors associated with PU development. Nutritional assessment includes evaluation of biochemical parameters together with other factors, such as daily food/fluid intake, changes in weight status, diagnosis, lifestyle, and medications. The maintenance of nutrition-related parameters is associated with a reduced risk of PU development.[60]

Nutritional Assessment for Pressure Ulcer Healing

Nutritional assessment for PU healing includes all factors assessed for PU prevention. When a PU is present, visceral protein may be lost. Historically, serum albumin levels have been used as an indicator of visceral protein status. However, albumin has a half-life of 12 to 21 days and may be influenced by nonnutritional factors, such as infection, acute stress, surgery, and hydration status. Although prealbumin may also be influenced by stress and inflammation, it has been proven to be a more useful indicator in assessing the effectiveness of nutritional intervention due to its shorter half-life of 2 to 3 days.[63,64] Prealbumin is a negative acute phase reactant and will transiently decrease in the presence of inflammation and stress (e.g., immediately postsurgery).[64] Concurrent assessment of C-reactive protein can differentiate whether prealbumin is being affected by stress and inflammation. Prealbumin levels may also be maintained during states of malnutrition.[1,60]

Essential Nutrients for Wound Healing

Energy/calories promote anabolism, synthesis of collagen and nitrogen, and healing. Energy needs for individuals with SCI and PUs may be estimated using predictive equations if indirect calorimetry is not available, using either 30 to 40 kcal/kg body weight daily or the Harris-Benedict value times stress factor (1.2 for stage II PU, 1.5 for stage III and IV PU).[60]

Protein is essential for collagen synthesis. Protein losses occur through wound exudates, leading to deficiencies that delay wound healing.[65] Daily protein loss has been shown to increase from 2 to 1.5 g/kg body weight with a stage II PU to 1.5 to 2.0 g/kg for stage III and IV PUs.[60,65] High protein levels (>2 g/kg) have been found to contribute to dehydration in the elderly.[65] Thus protein needs should be individualized because higher protein intakes may be contraindicated in individuals with concomitant renal or hepatic impairment.

Fluid Needs for Individuals with Spinal Cord Injury and Pressure Ulcers

Current recommendations for fluids are based on guidelines for the non-SCI population. The normal daily fluid requirement is 30 to 40 mL/kg. Additional fluids (10 to 15 mL/kg) may be required when using air fluidized beds set at temperatures more than 31 to 34°C (88 to 93°F).[60]

Vitamins and Minerals

Adequate vitamin and mineral intake is best achieved through the consumption of a balanced diet. Optimal micronutrient intakes to promote PU healing are not currently known due to insufficient research.

Deficiencies of specific nutrients have been associated with impaired or delayed wound healing. Supplements should be offered when deficiencies are confirmed or suspected or when dietary intake is poor.[65] Individuals with SCI and a PU should consider taking a daily multivitamin and mineral supplement.[60] Caution should be used with administration of individual supplements of micronutrients. Intakes of vitamins and minerals should not exceed 100% RDA. Only when a true deficiency exists should a single micronutrient supplement be provided. Appropriateness of supplement administration should be reviewed by a registered dietitian every 7 to 10 days.[60]

Ascorbic acid is essential for collagen synthesis. Deficiency of ascorbic acid has been associated with delayed tissue repair and impaired immune function. Ascorbic acid supplements have been shown to promote wound healing only in patients with an ascorbic acid deficiency. Individuals at risk for ascorbic acid deficiency include the elderly, smokers, those who abuse drugs, and those who are medically stressed.[65] Current recommendations for daily vitamin C supplementation in individuals with deficiency are 100 to 200 mg for those with stage I and II PU and 1000 to 2000 mg for those with stage III and IV PU.[60,65] Individuals with renal failure are at increased risk of developing oxalate stones, and ascorbic acid supplementation should not exceed 60 to 100 mg daily.[65]

Zinc is necessary for cell replication and growth and is important for protein and collagen synthesis. Zinc deficiencies are common in individuals with diarrhea, malabsorption, or hypermetabolic stress.[65] If zinc supplementation is indicated, it should be administered in divided doses at no more than 40 mg of elemental zinc per day for no more than 2 to 3 weeks.[1,65] Zinc supplementation offers no benefit for those who are not deficient. High serum zinc levels may inhibit healing by impairing phagocytosis and interfering with copper metabolism.[1,60,65] Supplementation with zinc is contraindicated in individuals with stomach or duodenal ulcers. Zinc toxicity symptoms include nausea, vomiting, loss of appetite, abdominal cramps, diarrhea, and headache.[66]

Nutritional Needs and Neurogenic Bowel

To promote optimal stool consistency, a daily minimum of 1.5 L fluid is required for individuals with SCI and neurogenic bowel.[60] Fluid needs are estimated as either 1 mL/kcal estimated energy needs plus 500 mL, or 40 mL per kg body weight plus 500 mL.[60] Fiber intake should be initiated at 15 g/d then gradually increased to no more than 30 g/d.[60] Fiber intakes more than 20 g/d may result in undesirable prolonged intestinal transit time.[60]

Biomedical Engineering Essentials in Pressure Ulcer Management: Biomedical Approaches to Risk Assessment

Technical Developments in Pressure Mapping: Accuracy of Measurement and Improved Data Analysis

Interface pressure (IP) mapping is the most widely used technique for objective evaluation of individuals at risk for PU development. As discussed elsewhere in this chapter, direct applied pressure at the skin surface is by no means the only cause of ischemia leading to tissue breakdown. Interface pressure measurement should always be considered as one of several components in overall patient evaluation when assessing PU risk status. With that caveat, interface pressure mapping can provide much critically valuable information.

To provide accurate information about loading conditions at the interface between a patient and the support surface, be it a cushion or a mattress, the sensor used should not disrupt the interface conditions by its presence. Thus sensors must be thin, flexible, and accurate. For clinical use, assessment systems should also be reliable, be easy to set up and calibrate, and have clear output data. Over the past decade, technological advances in sensor design and image processing software have greatly improved both the accuracy and the usability of commercially available interface pressure mapping systems. This has led to the potential for increased clinical use in seating evaluations. For example, one leading company, Tekscan Inc. (South Boston, MA), has seen sales of clinical pressure mapping systems more than double for the past 5 years, compared with a decade ago.

The primary uses of interface pressure mapping are to provide information on the postural effects of seating system configuration and on the pressure distributive effects of various cushion options. However, interface pressure mapping also has the potential to be an important educational and monitoring tool for both patients and clinicians.

Real-time pressure maps provide biofeedback so that the patient can immediately see the effects of weight shifting and other pressure relief maneuvers. For example, it has been found that, although paraplegics are generally taught to relieve pressure intermittently using lifts, the majority cannot perform a lift that totally relieves pressure under the ischial regions. However, individuals with some trunk control are able to effectively decrease regional interface pressures by leaning either side to side or forward.[47] They can also maintain this posture for a sustained period, which allows regional blood flow to increase gradually, relieving localized ischemia.

Advances in IP sensors and hardware have been accompanied by research into analytical approaches. Currently commercially available systems include software that provides the clinician with average and peak pressures, either for the total contact area or for user-selected regions of interest (ROI), such as the ischial or sacral areas. Selection of ROI is very user intensive and cannot reliably quantify significant changes between assessments. It has been suggested that health care professionals use pressure maps qualitatively rather than quantitatively (i.e., by visual impression rather than mean or maximum pressures). Human visual perception is more sensitive to spatial changes that occur with movement rather than changes in color alone.[67] When considering interface pressure maps, this corresponds to peaks of high pressure as opposed to regions of evenly distributed pressure. Thus, subjective rankings of pressure maps obtained from very different surfaces may agree well with peak pressures but not mean pressures.[68]

Just as advanced image processing techniques are increasing the amount of information obtained from techniques like computed tomography (CT) and magnetic resonance imaging (MRI), so sophisticated data analysis methods provide an opportunity to get more out of the massive amounts of data obtained from interface pressure mapping assessments. For the most part, these developments arise from research studies where the goal is to examine similarities between study participants For example, Brienza et al. employed a data reduction approach known as singular value decomposition (SVD) to compare pressure and shape contour maps for seated subjects.[69] Eitzen[70] used a frequency analysis method to determine how often all observed pressure values occurred over an extended assessment period. This approach makes greater use of available data obtained over an extended assessment. Comparison of output distribution graphs can also visually represent differences between assessments. However, Eitzen felt it was too technically challenging to show real-time changes in frequency distribution during an assessment.

Our group has developed an automated analytic tool that determines changes between all regions of the contact area without any requirement for user selection of ROI. The Longitudinal Analysis with Self-Registration (LASR) statistical algorithm was therefore developed to compare multiple datasets obtained over time or under different conditions. Because the whole contact area is analyzed, significant differences across the entire spatial contact area can be determined for both static and dynamic assessments. This can include repeated short-term assessments, such as assessing several different seating cushions for a patient or evaluating the effect of changing the configuration of a patient's wheelchair (e.g., tilt-in-space or with footrest adjustment). Individuals with SCI are also often seen repeatedly over several years, and many factors related to PU risk will change over time. It is important to be able to make valid comparisons between pressure maps obtained over long time intervals. It is also most efficient in clinical settings for pressure maps to be analyzed in a real-time, or near-real-time, manner to aid clinical interpretation and decision making.

Pressure mapping produces large-volume datasets, which generally require extended processing times, thus limiting the ability to provide real-time analysis. LASR employs efficient data-mining techniques to allow rapid maximum information recovery from the large volume of data obtained for each subject assessed. In our current research, LASR has been used to show that gluteal electrical stimulation is effective in changing seating interface pressures in a manner that may indicate improved tissue health.[71] The LASR tool is available at our Web site (stat.case.edu/lasr).

Blood Flow Measurement: Tissue Oxygen and Blood Flow

Blood carries nutrients, including oxygen, to the tissues. Blood flow is thus essential for maintenance of tissue viability (i.e., prevention of PUs). Several noninvasive techniques are available, including transcutaneous blood gas measurement, laser Doppler flowmetry, and photoplethysmography. Animal studies have also used contrast-enhanced MRI to monitor changes indicative of deep tissue injury.[72]

In vascular disease management, peripheral blood flow measurement has a long history of use in determining the level of lower limb amputation.[73,74] In the field of PU management, blood flow monitoring has largely been limited to research applications.[75–78] However, Coggrave and Rose showed that transcutaneous blood oxygen measurement can readily be incorporated into clinical seating evaluations and can provide valuable insights for improving PU prevention practice.[47]

Biomedical Technology Advances in Pressure Ulcer Measurement

Changes in wound size are a major component of monitoring wound healing. Accurate wound measurement is challenging in clinical practice. Almost all PUs are irregular in shape and often have indistinct margins, and it may be difficult to position the patient reproducibly for repeated measurements. Standard clinical techniques often use manual linear measurement of maximum wound length, width, and depth (see the nursing discussion above). Digital imaging is becoming increasingly common in clinical practice as new technology becomes available.[79] Our group performed a pilot study to compare the reliability of the standard clinical measurement tool, linear measurement, with two electronic devices, specifically the Visitrak automated digitizing table (Smith and Nephew, Largo, FL), and the VeVMD digital image analysis software (Vistamedical, Winnipeg, MB, CA).[80] Forty two-dimensional (2-D) "wound" templates of varying sizes were created and mounted on a contrasting background to maximize ease of margin delineation. Wound size was measured using all three techniques by clinical personnel blinded to the actual wound size and experienced in wound evaluation. It was found that intraobserver variability was not significant for any technique. However, interobserver variation was significant ($p < 0.01$) for linear measures at all wound sizes and for electronic measures with larger wounds only. These findings indicate that the standard clinical technique of linear wound measurement is neither reliable nor accurate, even when employed by experienced clinicians. The Visitrak and VeVMD systems showed improved measurement accuracy with some dependence on the size of the wound.

Wound depth was not considered in our pilot study, but it is recognized to be a significant factor in successful wound healing. Further research is still needed to determine accurate methods for wound depth measurement. One promising approach is the use of stereophotogrammetry to construct three-dimensional (3-D) images from stereotactic 2-D images. Two images of an object viewed from slightly different angles can be combined to give an image with a perception of depth. The technique was first applied to wound measurement over 20 years ago.[81] Although patient assessment was quick and noninvasive, image processing was slow at that time and required extensive observer training. Advances in digital technology and image analysis have recently led to the development of more clinically useful systems. The LifeViz™ 3-D system (Quantificare Inc., Santa Clara, CA) is a cost-effective stereophotogrammetry system that was initially developed, tested, and validated by a team of imaging experts at the University of Glamorgan, Wales. The LifeViz™ system uses the same principles as the human visual system to achieve depth perception. A specialized lens combined with conventional digital camera equipment obtains two views of the wound from slightly different angles. Images can be readily analyzed to determine several variables, including wound area, length, width, circumference, and volume. Both digital images and quantified outcome measures can be included in the patient's record. It should be noted that, although 3-D imaging provides more accurate information than linear measurement, caution is still required when assessing PUs that exhibit significant undermining or tunneling.

Psychological Essentials in Pressure Ulcer Management

There is evidence that substance abuse, cigarette smoking, and depression are risk factors for PU development for individuals with SCI. Since the 1970s, research has examined several psychosocial variables that may either increase vulnerability to PU development or serve as buffers against them. The role of psychology on the interdisciplinary wound care team involves identifying and treating contributory mental health conditions and fostering adaptive behavior. Psychosocial factors should be considered in all cases when assessing for patients' risk for developing a PU or when treating wounds that have already occurred. Many of these psychosocial factors can be modified to improve outcomes and need to be considered as part of an interdisciplinary care plan. Possible protective influences include knowledge of and adherence to behavioral prevention strategies (see Rehabilitation Therapists), strong social support, problem-solving skills, and employment. Although the research evidence for psychosocial variables is sometimes mixed, understanding behavioral mechanisms in PU development remains important for individualized treatment

SCI clinicians place a great deal of weight on psychosocial variables in PU prevention and management. A survey of SCI specialty physicians and nurses found that 97% agreed with the following statement: "In the vast majority of cases, when patients are compliant with prevention measures, pressure ulcers can be avoided." Ninety-one percent also agreed that "patient lack of responsibility is an important risk factor for developing pressure ulcers," and over 75% endorsed that a history of mental health problems and active substance abuse represent important issues to consider in hospital admission and discharge decisions.[82] The clinicians in the survey considered that, regardless of injury level, individuals with strong social support were less likely to be admitted for a PU and required less wound healing for discharge.

Physiological Vulnerabilities to Pressure Ulcers

Substance Abuse

The SCI population has a higher base rate of alcohol and substance use than the general population.[83,84] Some studies suggest a link between alcohol/drug abuse and PU development.[45,85] By definition, substance abuse involves impairment in an individual's ability to perform daily functions.[86] Therefore, it is reasonable to be concerned that substance abuse among individuals with SCI may interfere with their consistent performance of PU preventative behaviors.[83] Postinjury use of illicit drugs and misuse of prescription drugs increase the likelihood of PUs. The effects of alcohol use/abuse are less clear, with several studies failing to find a significant association.[3,87,88] Heinemann and Hawkins suggest that a history of preinjury problem drinking or substance abuse may point to an impairment in coping skills and predispose people to PUs even in the absence of current use.[89]

Cigarette Smoking

Nicotine constricts blood vessels and decreases blood flow, especially to the extremities.[90] Decreased blood flow increases the risk of tissue breakdown and can hinder the healing process of an existing wound. Accordingly, cigarette smoking has been targeted as a behavioral risk factor for PU management. The evidence for the relationship between smoking and PU risk is clear-cut. Smith et al. showed that smoking significantly increased the odds of PU development.[88] Other studies have suggested that a history of past smoking, such as the lifetime number of cigarettes smoked, also relates to PU incidence.[3,45] The implementation of smoking cessation interventions among SCI patients represents a critical area for risk reduction

Depression

Although most individuals who sustain an SCI do not become depressed, having an SCI does increase the risk of depression. Up to 30% of individuals with an SCI will experience a depressive disorder.[91] Depression may interfere with an individual's energy level, motivation, and ability to concentrate and problem solve, thereby affecting the ability to engage in PU prevention tasks.

Investigations of the link between PUs and depressive symptoms have shown mixed results. Some studies have supported the association between PU development and depressive symptoms,[3,45,88] whereas others demonstrate no correlation.[89,92] Although the relationship remains inconclusive, the high incidence of depression in SCI requires careful assessment for depressive symptoms in all patients, so that those who need it have access to treatment.

Physiological Buffers from Pressure Ulcers

Several demographic and lifestyle factors have been identified as protective against PUs. Variables with empirical support include having a college education, being married, being employed, living an overall healthy lifestyle (specifically exercise and healthy diet were found to be protective), having an internal locus of control, and possessing good problem solving skills.[3,45,85,93] It is interesting to note that individuals with SCI who are employed have a lower incidence of PUs. One might speculate that employment would increase sitting time and distract from preventative behaviors, potentially increasing the odds of developing a PU. In contrast, research clearly shows that employment is a protective factor that correlates with positive health outcomes.

Patient Education/Preventative Behaviors

Educating patients with SCI regarding PU prevention should be central to the initial rehabilitation process (see Rehabilitation Therapists). Knowledge of and adherence to these strategies are widely believed to be strong buffers against developing PUs. The evidence that following self-care recommendations reduces PU incidence is currently inconclusive.[3,45,94,95] These findings should not detract from the importance of patient education but rather indicate the multifaceted nature of PU prevention. Most individuals with SCI possess both psychosocial vulnerabilities and buffers to PU development.[85] PU development is likely when risk factors outweigh protective factors, and the relationship among variables may be complex. For example, a previous history of PUs may be considered a risk factor for one person, but for another it may produce increased vigilance and act as a buffer.[85]

Intervention

Psychologists on SCI treatment teams can assist in PU prevention and management by identifying psychosocial risk and protective factors and providing intervention accordingly. Depression can be successfully treated among individuals who have an SCI with the use of antidepressant medication or psychotherapy or both.[96]

Smoking cessation and substance abuse treatment can also be addressed. It can be difficult for individuals with SCI to attend substance abuse group treatment sessions while hospitalized, especially if they are on bed rest. However, patients on bed rest are also unable to engage in tobacco or substance use. This period of abstinence provides an opportunity to help patients examine their use and potentially enhance motivation for behavioral change. Motivational interviewing is an effective counseling approach for these types of behavioral changes.[97,98] Nicotine replacement therapy can also aid patients willing to pursue smoking cessation. Although there are several behavioral interventions that can help individuals stop smoking, there is evidence that many individuals interested in smoking cessation are never offered such treatment.[99] It is recommended that patients' readiness to stop smoking be assessed and interventions be tailored accordingly.[99]

Prior to PU treatment it is important to have a discussion with the patient about the expectations of a wound care plan, such as bed rest and smoking cessation. If patients are aware of and agree to a treatment plan ahead of time, the likelihood that they will be adherent to treatment expectations may increase.

Pearls

- Pressure ulcer management must address the whole patient, not just the wound(s).
- Pressure ulcer management by an interdisciplinary team is integral to successful outcomes.
- Nutritional and psychological evaluation must be included in pressure ulcer management.

Pitfalls

- A "one-size-fits-all" approach cannot succeed.
- Pressure ulcer risk is variable; patients should be assessed regularly.
- Pressure ulcer education is a continuing process for both patients and clinicians.

References

1. Dorner B, Posthauer ME, Thomas D. The role of nutrition in pressure ulcer prevention and treatment. National Pressure Ulcer Advisory Panel White Paper. http://www.npuap.org/Nutrition%20White%20Paper%20Website%20Version.pdf Accessed September 12, 2009
2. Ho CH, Bogie KM. Integrating wound care research into clinical practice. Ostomy Wound Manage 2007;53(10):18–25
3. Krause JS, Broderick L. Patterns of recurrent pressure ulcers after spinal cord injury: identification of risk and protective factors 5 or more years after onset. Arch Phys Med Rehabil 2004; 85(8):1257–1264
4. Edlich RF, Winters KL, Woodard CR, et al. Pressure ulcer prevention. J Long Term Eff Med Implants 2004;14(4):285–304
5. Bergstrom N, Braden B, Kemp M, Champagne M, Ruby E. Multi-site study of incidence of pressure ulcers and the relationship between risk level, demographic characteristics, diagnoses, and prescription of preventive interventions. J Am Geriatr Soc 1996;44(1):22–30
6. Bååth C, Hall-Lord ML, Idvall E, Wiberg-Hedman K, Wilde Larsson B. Interrater reliability using Modified Norton Scale, Pressure Ulcer Card, Short Form-Mini Nutritional Assessment by registered and enrolled nurses in clinical practice. J Clin Nurs 2008;17(5):618–626
7. Ayello EA, Braden B. Why is pressure ulcer risk assessment so important? Nursing 2001; 31(11):75–79
8. Mortenson WB, Miller WC; SCIRE Research Team. A review of scales for assessing the risk of developing a pressure ulcer in individuals with SCI. Spinal Cord 2008;46(3):168–175
9. Salzberg CA, Byrne DW, Cayten CG, van Niewerburgh P, Murphy JG, Viehbeck M. A new pressure ulcer risk assessment scale for individuals with spinal cord injury. Am J Phys Med Rehabil 1996;75(2):96–104
10. Guihan M, Garber SL, Bombardier CH, Goldstein B, Holmes SA, Cao L. Predictors of pressure ulcer recurrence in veterans with spinal cord injury. J Spinal Cord Med 2008;31(5):551–559
11. Anthony D, Parboteeah S, Saleh M, Papanikolaou P. Norton, Waterlow and Braden scores: a review of the literature and a comparison between

the scores and clinical judgement. J Clin Nurs 2008;17(5):646–653
12. Braden BJ, Bergstrom N. Clinical utility of the Braden scale for predicting pressure sore risk. Decubitus 1989;2(3):44–46, 50–51
13. Catania K, Huang C, James P, Madison M, Moran M, Ohr M. Wound wise: PUPPI: the Pressure Ulcer Prevention Protocol Interventions. Am J Nurs 2007;107(4):44–52, quiz 53
14. Pressure Ulcers in Adults: Prediction and Prevention: Clinical Practice Guideline No. 3. AHCPR Pub. No. 92–0047. The Agency for Healthcare Research and Quality (AHRQ); 1992. http://www.ahrq.gov. Accessed June, 5, 2009
15. Treatment of Pressure Ulcers: Clinical Guideline No. 15. AHCPR Publication No. 95–0652. The Agency for Healthcare Research and Quality (AHRQ). 1994. http://www.ahrq.gov. Accessed June, 15, 2009
16. National Pressure Ulcer Advisory Panel. Pressure ulcers in America: prevalence, incidence, and implications for the future. An executive summary of the National Pressure Ulcer Advisory Panel monograph. Adv Skin Wound Care 2001;14(4):208–215 Erratum in: Adv Skin Wound Care 2002;15(6):E1–E3; author reply E3
17. National Guideline Clearinghouse. Pressure ulcers. American Medical Directors Association: Professional Association. 1996. http:// www.cpgnews.org/PU?index.cmf. Accessed June, 5, 2009
18. The Quality Improvement Organization. Medicare Quality Improvement Community Initiatives. http://www.medqic.org. Accessed June, 5, 2009
19. The Wound, Ostomy, and Continence Nurses Society (WOCN). http://www.wocn.org. Accessed May 1, 2012
20. National Institute for Health and Clinical Excellence. The Prevention and Treatment of Pressure Ulcers. Quick Reference Guide. 2005, http://www.nice.org.uk/nicemedia/pdf/CG029quickrefguide.pdf. Accessed May 1, 2012
21. Consortium for Spinal Cord Medicine Clinical Practice Guidelines. Pressure ulcer prevention and treatment following spinal cord injury: a clinical practice guideline for health-care professionals. J Spinal Cord Med 2001;24(Suppl 1):S40–S101
22. Benbow M. Guidelines for the prevention and treatment of pressure ulcers. Nurs Stand 2006; 20(52):42–44
23. Bluestein D, Javaheri A. Pressure ulcers: prevention, evaluation, and management. Am Fam Physician 2008;78(10):1186–1194
24. Iowa Intervention Project. Nursing Interventions Classification (NIC). 3rd ed. St. Louis, MO: Mosby; 2000
25. Horn SD, Bender SA, Ferguson ML, et al. The National Pressure Ulcer Long-Term Care Study: pressure ulcer development in long-term care residents. J Am Geriatr Soc 2004;52(3):359–367
26. Garber SL, Rintala DH, Holmes SA, Rodriguez GP, Friedman J. A structured educational model to improve pressure ulcer prevention knowledge in veterans with spinal cord dysfunction. J Rehabil Res Dev 2002;39(5):575–588 Erratum in: J Rehabil Res Dev 2002;39(6):71
27. Consortium for Spinal Cord Medicine. Bladder management for adults with spinal cord injury: a clinical practice guideline for health-care providers. J Spinal Cord Med 2006;29(5):527–573
28. Francis K. Physiology and management of bladder and bowel continence following spinal cord injury. Ostomy Wound Manage 2007;53(12): 18–27
29. Iowa Outcomes Project. Nursing Outcomes Classification (NOC). 2nd ed. St. Louis: Mosby; 2000
30. Ralph SS, Craft-Rosenberg M, Herdman TH, Lavin MA. North American Nursing Diagnosis Association: Nursing Diagnosis Definitions and Classifications 2003–2004. Philadelphia, PA: NANDA International; 2003
31. Barber DB, Woodard FL, Rogers SJ, Able AC. The efficacy of nursing education as an intervention in the treatment of recurrent urinary tract infections in individuals with spinal cord injury. SCI Nurs 1999;16(2):54–56
32. Benbow M. Pressure ulcer prevention and pressure-relieving surfaces. Br J Nurs 2008; 17(13):830–835
33. Sardina D, Morgan N. Skin and Resource Manual. Lake Geneva, WI: Wound Care Education Institute; 2006
34. Updated Staging System, National Pressure Ulcer Advisory Panel, 2007. http://www.npuap.org/pr2.htm. Accessed May 1, 2012.
35. Cannon BC, Cannon JP. Management of pressure ulcers. Am J Health Syst Pharm 2004;61(18): 1895–1905, quiz 1906–1907
36. Kramer JD, Kearney M. Patient, wound, and treatment characteristics associated with healing in pressure ulcers. Adv Skin Wound Care 2000;13(1):17–24
37. Sibbald RG, Williamson D, Orsted HL, et al. Preparing the wound bed—debridement, bacterial balance, and moisture balance. Ostomy Wound Manage 2000;46(11):14–22, 24–28, 30–35, quiz 36–37
38. Pieper B, Sieggreen M, Nordstrom CK, et al. Discharge knowledge and concerns of patients going home with a wound. J Wound Ostomy Continence Nurs 2007;34(3):245–253, quiz 254–255
39. Moore ZEH, Cowman S. Wound cleansing for pressure ulcers. Cochrane Database Syst Rev 2005; 4(4):CD004983 10.1002/14651858.CD004983.pub2
40. Gibson L. Perceptions of pressure ulcers among young men with a spinal injury. Br J Community Nurs 2002;7(9):451–460
41. King RB, Porter SL, Vertiz KB. Preventive skin care beliefs of people with spinal cord injury. Rehabil Nurs 2008;33(4):154–162
42. May L, Day R, Warren S. Evaluation of patient education in spinal cord injury rehabilitation: knowledge, problem-solving and perceived importance. Disabil Rehabil 2006;28(7):405–413
43. Rintala DH, Garber SL, Friedman JD, Holmes SA. Preventing recurrent pressure ulcers in veterans with spinal cord injury: impact of a structured education and follow-up intervention. Arch Phys Med Rehabil 2008;89(8):1429–1441
44. Schubart JR, Hilgart M, Lyder C. Pressure ulcer prevention and management in spinal cord-injured adults: analysis of educational needs. Adv Skin Wound Care 2008;21(7):322–329

45. Krause JS, Vines CL, Farley TL, Sniezek J, Coker J. An exploratory study of pressure ulcers after spinal cord injury: relationship to protective behaviors and risk factors. Arch Phys Med Rehabil 2001;82(1):107–113
46. Consortium for Spinal Cord Medicine Clinical Practice Guidelines. Pressure ulcer prevention and treatment following spinal cord injury: a clinical practice guideline for health-care professionals. J Spinal Cord Med 2001;24(Suppl 1):S40–S101
47. Coggrave MJ, Rose LS. A specialist seating assessment clinic: changing pressure relief practice. Spinal Cord 2003;41(12):692–695
48. Hobson DA. Comparative effects of posture on pressure and shear at the body-seat interface. J Rehabil Res Dev 1992;29(4):21–31
49. Makhsous M, Priebe M, Bankard J, et al. Measuring tissue perfusion during pressure relief maneuvers: insights into preventing pressure ulcers. J Spinal Cord Med 2007;30(5):497–507
50. Ding D, Leister E, Cooper RA, et al. Usage of tilt-in-space, recline, and elevation seating functions in natural environment of wheelchair users. J Rehabil Res Dev 2008;45(7):973–983
51. Sonenblum SE, Sprigle S, Maurer C. Monitoring power upright and tilt-in-space wheelchair use. Paper presented at: RESNA Annual Meeting; June 21–26, 2006; Atlanta, GA. www.mobilityrerc.gatech.edu/publications/MonitoringPowerUpright.pdf. Accessed August 10, 2009
52. McInnes E, Bell Syer SE, Dumville JC, Legood R, Cullum NA. Support surfaces for pressure ulcer prevention. Cochrane Database Syst Rev 2008;(4):CD001735
53. Colin D, Abraham P, Preault L, Bregeon C, Saumet JL. Comparison of 90 degrees and 30 degrees laterally inclined positions in the prevention of pressure ulcers using transcutaneous oxygen and carbon dioxide pressures. Adv Wound Care 1996;9(3):35–38
54. Garber SL, Campion LJ, Krouskop TA. Trochanteric pressure in spinal cord injury. Arch Phys Med Rehabil 1982;63(11):549–552
55. Goetz LL, Brown GS, Priebe MM. Interface pressure characteristics of alternating air cell mattresses in persons with spinal cord injury. J Spinal Cord Med 2002;25(3):167–173
56. Atiyeh BS, Hayek SN. Pressure sores with associated spasticity: a clinical challenge. Int Wound J 2005;2(1):77–80
57. American Physical Therapy Association. W. M. S. I. G. The guide for integumentary/wound management content in professional physical therapist education. 2008. www.aptasce-wm.org/documents/guidelines/SCEWMWoundRecs.pdf. Accessed August 15, 2009
58. Reddy M, Gill SS, Kalkar SR, Wu W, Anderson PJ, Rochon PA. Treatment of pressure ulcers: a systematic review. JAMA 2008;300(22):2647–2662
59. Sussman C, Bates-Jensen B. Wound Care: A Collaborative Practice Manual. 3rd ed. Philadelphia, PA: Lippincott Williams & Wilkins; 2007
60. American Dietetic Association. Spinal Cord Injury (SCI) Evidence-Based Nutrition Practice Guideline. 2009, June. http://www.adaevidencelibrary.com/topic.cfm?cat=3485. Accessed September 12, 2009
61. Blissitt PA. Nutrition in acute spinal cord injury. Crit Care Nurs Clin North Am 1990;2(3):375–384
62. Rodriguez DJ, Benzel EC, Clevenger FW. The metabolic response to spinal cord injury. Spinal Cord 1997;35(9):599–604
63. Bernstein LH, Leukhardt-Fairfield CJ, Pleban W, Rudolph R. Usefulness of data on albumin and prealbumin concentrations in determining effectiveness of nutritional support. Clin Chem 1989;35(2):271–274
64. Beck FK, Rosenthal TC. Prealbumin: a marker for nutritional evaluation. Am Fam Physician 2002;65(8):1575–1578 Erratum in: Am Fam Physician 2002;66(12):2208
65. Stechmiller JK. Nutrition support for wound healing. Support Line 2009;31(4):2–8
66. Office of Dietary Supplements, National Institutes of Health. Dietary supplement fact sheet: zinc. 2009, June 30. http://ods.od.nih.gov/FactSheets/Zinc.asp. Accessed September 14, 2009
67. Stoppel CM, Boehler CN, Sabelhaus C, Heinze HJ, Hopf JM, Schoenfeld MA. Neural mechanisms of spatial- and feature-based attention: a quantitative analysis. Brain Res 2007;1181:51–60
68. Stinson MD, Porter-Armstrong AP, Eakin PA. Pressure mapping systems: reliability of pressure map interpretation. Clin Rehabil 2003;17(5):504–511
69. Brienza DM, Lin CT, Karg PE. A method for custom-contoured cushion design using interface pressure measurements. IEEE Trans Rehabil Eng 1999;7(1):99–108
70. Eitzen I. Pressure mapping in seating: a frequency analysis approach. Arch Phys Med Rehabil 2004;85(7):1136–1140
71. Bogie K, Wang X, Fei B, Sun J. New technique for real-time interface pressure analysis: getting more out of large image data sets. J Rehabil Res Dev 2008;45(4):523–535, 10, 535
72. Stekelenburg A, Strijkers GJ, Parusel H, Bader DL, Nicolay K, Oomens CW. Role of ischemia and deformation in the onset of compression-induced deep tissue injury: MRI-based studies in a rat model. J Appl Physiol 2007;102(5):2002–2011
73. Cheng EY. Lower extremity amputation level: selection using noninvasive hemodynamic methods of evaluation. Arch Phys Med Rehabil 1982;63(10):475–479
74. Poredos P, Rakovec S, Guzic-Salobir B. Determination of amputation level in ischaemic limbs using $tcPO_2$ measurement. Vasa 2005;34(2):108–112
75. Mayrovitz HN, Smith JR. Adaptive skin blood flow increases during hip-down lying in elderly women. Adv Wound Care 1999;12(6):295–301
76. Knight SL, Taylor RP, Polliack AA, Bader DL. Establishing predictive indicators for the status of loaded soft tissues. J Appl Physiol 2001;90(6):2231–2237
77. Sachse RE, Fink SA, Klitzman B. Multimodality evaluation of pressure relief surfaces. Plast Reconstr Surg 1998;102(7):2381–2387

78. Bergstrand S, Lindberg LG, Ek AC, Lindén M, Lindgren M. Blood flow measurements at different depths using photoplethysmography and laser Doppler techniques. Skin Res Technol 2009; 15(2):139–147
79. Fischetti LF, Paguio EC, Alt-White AC. Digitized images of wounds: a nursing practice innovation. Nurs Clin North Am 2000;35(2): 541–550
80. Haghpanah S, Bogie K, Wang X, Banks PG, Ho CH. Reliability of electronic versus manual wound measurement techniques. Arch Phys Med Rehabil 2006;87(10):1396–1402
81. Bulstrode CJ, Goode AW, Scott PJ. Stereophotogrammetry for measuring rates of cutaneous healing: a comparison with conventional techniques. Clin Sci (Lond) 1986;71(4):437–443
82. Guihan M, Goldstein B, Smith BM, Schwartz A, Manheim LM. SCI health care provider attitudes about pressure ulcer management. J Spinal Cord Med 2003;26(2):129–134
83. Tate DG, Forchheimer MB, Krause JS, Meade MA, Bombardier CH. Patterns of alcohol and substance use and abuse in persons with spinal cord injury: risk factors and correlates. Arch Phys Med Rehabil 2004;85(11):1837–1847
84. Heinemann AW, Keen M, Donohue R, Schnoll S. Alcohol use by persons with recent spinal cord injury. Arch Phys Med Rehabil 1988;69(8): 619–624
85. Clark FA, Jackson JM, Scott MD, et al. Data-based models of how pressure ulcers develop in daily-living contexts of adults with spinal cord injury. Arch Phys Med Rehabil 2006;87(11): 1516–1525
86. American Psychiatric Association. Diagnostic and Statistical Manual of Mental Disorders. 4th ed., text revision. Washington, DC: American Psychiatric Association; 2000
87. Hawkins DA, Heinemann AW. Substance abuse and medical complications following spinal cord injuries. Rehabil Psychol 1998;43(3):219–231
88. Smith BM, Guihan M, LaVela SL, Garber SL. Factors predicting pressure ulcers in veterans with spinal cord injuries. Am J Phys Med Rehabil 2008;87(9):750–757
89. Heinemann AW, Hawkins D. Substance abuse and medical complications following spinal cord injury. Rehabil Psychol 1995;40(2):125–140
90. Ting M. Wound healing and peripheral vascular disease. Crit Care Nurs Clin North Am 1991; 3(3):515–523
91. Craig A, Tran Y, Middleton J. Psychological morbidity and spinal cord injury: a systematic review. Spinal Cord 2009;47(2):108–114
92. Fuhrer MJ, Rintala DH, Hart KA, Clearman R, Young ME. Depressive symptomatology in persons with spinal cord injury who reside in the community. Arch Phys Med Rehabil 1993;74(3):255–260
93. Herrick S, Elliott T, Crow F. Self-appraised problem-solving skills and the prediction of secondary complications among persons with spinal cord injuries. J Clin Psychol Med Settings 1994;1(3):269–283
94. Garber SL, Rintala DH, Rossi CD, Hart KA, Fuhrer MJ. Reported pressure ulcer prevention and management techniques by persons with spinal cord injury. Arch Phys Med Rehabil 1996;77(8):744–749
95. Regan MA, Teasell RW, Wolfe DL, Keast D, Mortenson WB, Aubut JA; Spinal Cord Injury Rehabilitation Evidence Research Team. A systematic review of therapeutic interventions for pressure ulcers after spinal cord injury. Arch Phys Med Rehabil 2009;90(2):213–231
96. Kemp BJ, Kahan JS, Krause JS, Adkins RH, Nava G. Treatment of major depression in individuals with spinal cord injury. J Spinal Cord Med 2004;27(1):22–28
97. Miller BR, Rollnick S. Motivational Interviewing: Preparing People for Change. 2nd ed. New York, NY: Guilford Press; 2002
98. Rollnick S, Miller BR, Butler CC. Motivational Interviewing in Health Care: Helping Patients Change Behavior. New York, NY: Guilford Press; 2008
99. Weaver FM, Miskevics S, Clemmons N, Janke EA, LaVela SL, Spring B. Smoking behavior and readiness to change in male veterans with spinal cord injuries. Rehabil Psychol 2007;52(3):304–310

16

Autonomic Dysreflexia and Cardiovascular Complications of Spinal Cord Injury

Andrei Krassioukov

Key Points

1. In addition to motor and sensory deficits, individuals with spinal cord injury (SCI) face lifelong abnormalities in blood pressure control.
2. The acute period of cervical and upper thoracic SCI commonly presents with hypotension and bradycardia, a condition known as neurogenic shock.
3. As neurogenic shock resolves, unpredictable episodes of life-threatening hypertension, known as autonomic dysreflexia, could occur and will require prompt management.
4. In general, individuals with SCI have low resting arterial blood pressure. They also experience episodes of extremely low blood pressure when they are transferred to a wheelchair or attempt to stand up, a condition known as orthostatic hypotension.
5. Individuals with SCI at or above the sixth thoracic segment are at greater risk for abnormal cardiovascular control and the development of autonomic dysreflexia.

Paralysis and loss of sensation are the most recognized consequences that occur following spinal cord injury (SCI). Young and healthy individuals are the most common victims of this devastating condition. Injury to the fragile neuronal structures in the spinal cord results not only in devastating paralysis in these individuals but also in significant functional alterations of the autonomic nervous system (ANS).[1] Although the injury itself generally affects only a few segments of the spinal cord, the effect of this local disruption can commonly be seen in all autonomic functions below the level of injury, including bladder, bowel, respiration, temperature regulation, sexual function, and, most crucially for initial survival, cardiovascular control. From the moment of the injury, on a daily basis, individuals with SCI even following completion of rehabilitation face the challenge of their unstable blood pressure, which frequently results in persistent hypotension or episodes of uncontrolled hypertension.[2] Immediately following injury there is hypotension with bradycardia, a typical manifestation of neurogenic shock.[2] This condition is usually more pronounced with cervical injuries, lasts up to 6 weeks, and requires monitoring and management within the intensive care unit setting. With initial mobilization of subjects with SCI, orthostatic hypotension commonly becomes a significant issue.[3] With reconditioning, the symptoms of orthostatic hypotension will subside in many subjects; however, some patients will have lifelong orthostatic intolerance. Opposite to orthostatic hypotension, individuals with injuries above six thoracic segments could experience significant episodes of hypertension known as autonomic dysreflexia.[4] These episodes of unpredictable hypertension could initially occur in early stages following SCI and, if not managed promptly, could be life threatening.

These cardiovascular abnormalities have been well documented in human studies, as well as in animal models. The recognition and management of these cardiovascular dysfunctions following SCI represent challenging clinical issues.[5] Moreover, the latest clinical observations suggest that cardiovascular disorders are among the most common causes of morbidity and mortality in individuals with SCI.[6] Until recently, the majority of basic science and clinical investigations were focused on finding a cure for paralysis and reestablishing motor function. Unfortunately, little attention has been paid to the function of the ANS following SCI. This chapter focuses on the range of clinical issues associated with abnormal cardiovascular control following SCI.

Neural Control of the Cardiovascular System

Cardiovascular functions depend on coordinated neural control from the sympathetic and parasympathetic components of the ANS. Peripheral blood vessels receive predominantly sympathetic innervations, whereas the heart has dual sympathetic and parasympathetic innervations (**Table 16.1**). Supraspinal neurons within the rotroventralateral medulla (RVLM) and the sympathetic preganglionic neurons (SPNs) within the spinal cord are responsible for the tonic sympathetic control of the vessels and the heart. Cell bodies of SPNs are located within the lateral horns of the spinal gray matter of the thoracic and upper lumbar spinal segments (T1–L2, **Fig. 16.1**). These neurons receive supraspinal tonic and inhibitory nervous system control via spinal autonomic pathways—pathways that are commonly disrupted following SCI.[7] Conversely, vagal (CN X) parasympa-

Table 16.1 Autonomic Innervations of the Cardiovascular System

Target organ	Sympathetic (adrenergic)	Parasympathetic (cholinergic)
Heart		
Cardiac muscle	β1 and β2: increase in contractility	M2: decrease in contractility
Sinoatrial (SA) node	β1 and β2: increase in heart rate	M2: decrease in heart rate
Atrioventricular (AV) node	β1: increase in conduction	M2: decrease in conduction
Blood vessels		
Smooth muscles of blood vessel (arteries/veins)	α1: vessel contraction	M3: vessel dilation *arteries of the cavernous tissue (erectile tissue) also have parasympathetic innervations

*Indicates aberration or exception to the rule.

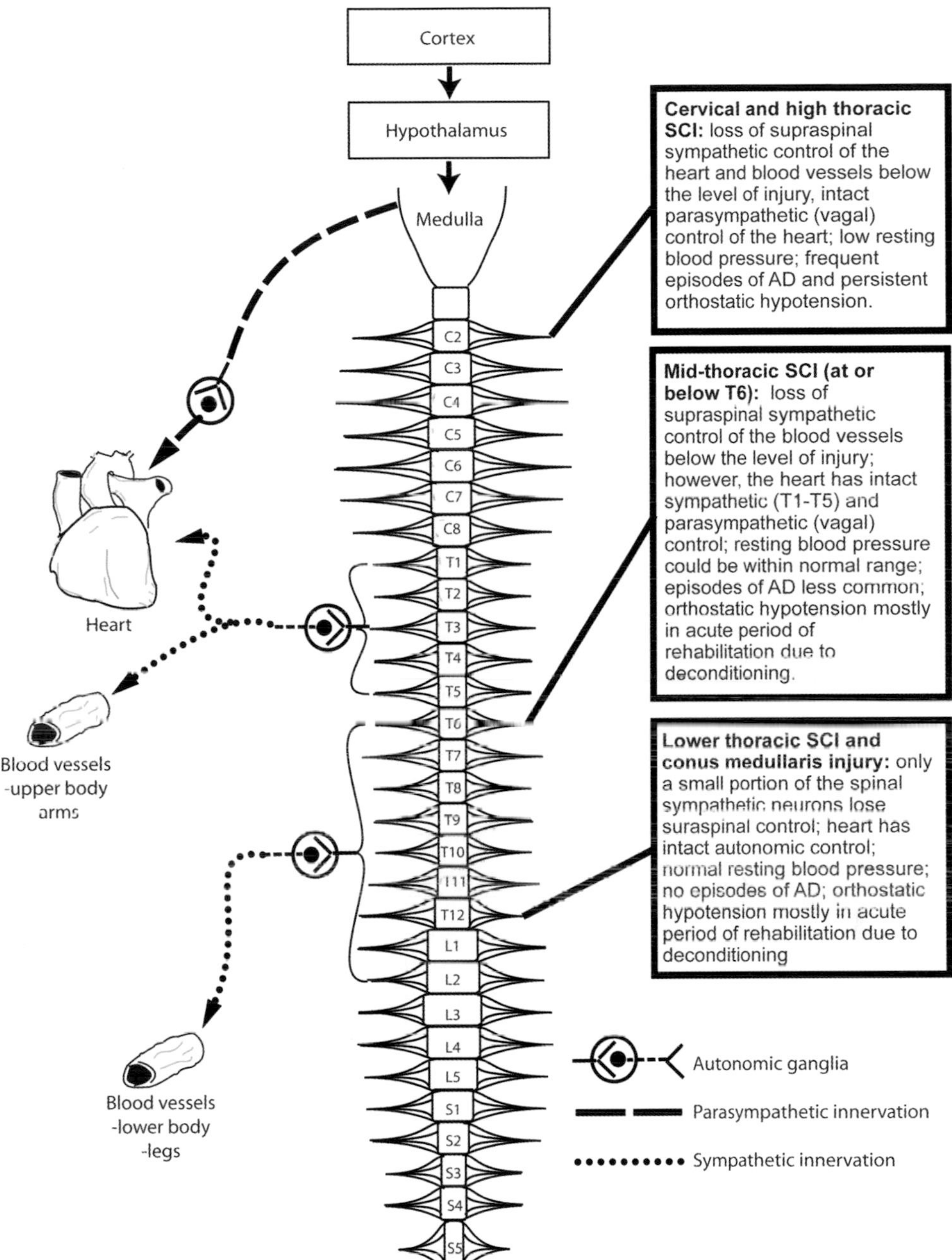

Fig. 16.1 Schematic diagram of autonomic control of cardiovascular systems and possible cardiovascular outcomes following spinal cord injury. The cerebral cortex and hypothalamus provide excitatory and inhibitory inputs to the various nuclei within the medulla oblongata involved in cardiovascular control. The parasympathetic control of the heart exits at the level of the brain stem via the vagus nerve (CN X). The preganglionic fibers of the vagus nerve then synapse with postganglionic parasympathetic neurons in ganglia on or near the target organ. Descending sympathetic input from the rostroventralateral medulla (RVLM) provide tonic control to spinal sympathetic preganglionic neurons (SPNs) involved in cardiovascular control. SPNs are found within the lateral horn of the spinal cord in segments T1–L2 and exit the spinal cord via the ventral root. They then synapse with postganglionic neurons located in the sympathetic chain (paravertebral ganglia). Finally, the sympathetic postganglionic neurons synapse with the target organs (heart and blood vessels). Afferent feedback for cardiovascular control from the central and peripheral baroreceptors is not shown.

thetic pathways, which exit supraspinally, are generally intact in individuals with SCI. As a result of the anatomical structure of the ANS, the level of SCI has important consequences for the autonomic dysfunctions observed after injury. Cardiac function, for example, is under dual control of sympathetic (SPNs from T1–5 levels) and parasympathetic (vagus, CN X) nervous systems (**Fig. 16.1**). Following high cervical SCI, parasympathetic (vagal) control will remain intact, whereas the sympathetic nervous system will lose its tonic autonomic control. On the other hand, in individuals with injury below the sixth thoracic segment, both the sympathetic and parasympathetic control of the heart are intact. As a result of injury level, individuals with tetraplegia versus those with paraplegia will have very different cardiovascular responses to injury.[3,8] It is important to appreciate that similar relationships can exist between the level of SCI and function of organs that are under autonomic control (lungs, urinary bladder, bowel, sweat glands, etc.).

Acute Postinjury Period and Neurogenic Shock

In the acute period, especially with injury at the cervical level, patients present clinically with severe hypotension and persistent bradycardia. This phenomenon is known as neurogenic shock.[1] Clinical observations strongly suggest that the extent to which prolonged and severe hypotension requiring vasopressive therapy correlates well with the severity of the SCI, with cervical or high thoracic injury, and can last up to 5 weeks after injury.[9] In one study, Glenn and Bergman reported that severe hypotension was present in all 31 tetraplegic subjects assessed with severe SCI, half of whom required pressor therapy to maintain arterial blood pressure.[10] In addition to this pronounced hypotension, many patients with acute SCI experience severe abnormalities in heart rate. In the acute postinjury stage, bradycardia has been reported in between 64 and 77% of patients with cervical SCI, with the most severe and frequent episodes within the first 5 weeks.[11] Bradycardia is a less severe problem when the injury is in the upper thoracic spinal cord because cardiac sympathetic neurons remain under brain stem control, leaving vagal and sympathetic influences more in balance. Both the level and the completeness of injury are important determinants of bradycardia severity. Indeed, we have also shown that the initial hypotension and bradycardia observed after injury persisted in the individuals with more severe injury of the descending cardiovascular autonomic pathways.[7] Moreover, all individuals in this group required vasopressor therapy to maintain systolic arterial blood pressure above 90 mmHg.[12] In contrast, individuals with less severe injury to the descending cardiovascular pathways tended to have higher blood pressure and heart rate, although minor and short-term hypotension and low heart rates were occasionally observed.

In addition to neurogenic shock, the acute phase of SCI is also associated with "spinal shock."[13] Although some authors use these terms interchangeably, it is important to recognize that they are two clinically important and distinct conditions. Neurogenic shock is characterized by changes in autonomic blood pressure control following SCI, whereas spinal shock is characterized by a marked reduction or abolition of sensory, motor, and reflex function of the spinal cord below the level of injury.[13] Clinically, spinal shock is characterized by flaccid paralysis and areflexia.

Autonomic Dysreflexia

Following the recovery from the neurogenic shock, resting hypotension is common among the majority of individuals with high thoracic and cervical SCI. However, the majority of these individuals could also experience episodes of pronounced hypertension (systolic blood pressure up to 300 mmHg), known as autonomic dysreflexia (AD) (**Fig. 16.2**). These episodes are triggered by painful or nonpainful sensory

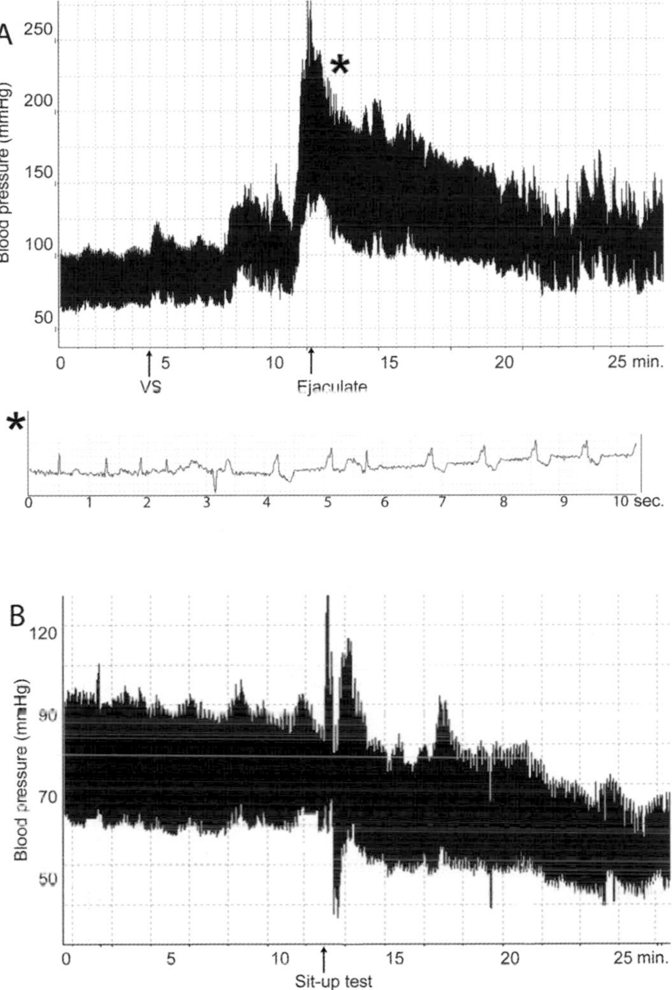

Fig. 16.2 Cardiovascular responses to vibrostimulation in a male with spinal cord injury (SCI). **(A)** Case of autonomic dysreflexia in a male with cervical SCI (C7 AIS B according to the American Spinal Injury Association Impairment Scale, motor complete, sensory incomplete) during the vibrostimulation (VS) procedure for sperm retrieval. Blood pressure (BP), obtained via finger cuff, and three-lead electrocardiography (ECG) were recorded continuously during the procedure. BP (*top diagram*) during the procedure and a 10 second sample of ECG recorded at the time of ejaculation (*bottom diagram*) are shown. Prior to VS there was relative hypotension (100/65 mmHg) with a regular heart rate of 78 bpm. With initiation of VS there was a gradual increase in arterial blood pressure suggestive of a typical episode of AD. Finally, at the time of ejaculation arterial BP surged to 280/150 mmHg, accompanied by bradycardia (38 bpm) and a short run of premature ventricular contractions (PVCs, indicated by the *asterisk* on the blood pressure recording) was observed 3 minutes following ejaculation (ECG recording at the bottom). At 15 minutes following ejaculation, arterial BP was still slightly elevated (130 mmHg, heart rate 66 bpm). During the next 30 to 35 minutes, arterial BP and heart rate gradually returned to resting values. This episode of AD was accompanied by significant spasms in the upper and lower extremities, profuse sweating on the forehead and neck, and piloerection on the forearms. Interestingly, during this episode of AD, the patient reported only a mild headache (personal observations). **(B)** Case of orthostatic hypotension in an individual with cervical C8 AIS A SCI during the orthostatic testing (sit-up test). Instrumentation for BP and ECG was conducted using the same settings as in **(A)**. Supine resting arterial BP was measured as 95/65 mmHg, with heart rate of 74 bpm. Following passive sit-up (*arrow*) the arterial BP decreased and at 3 minutes of seating was measured at 70/55 mmHg with heart rate of 90 bpm. The patient also complained of slight dizziness. During the next 10 minutes of monitoring, arterial BP continued to be low, and the test was stopped due to increased dizziness and light-headedness (personal observations).

stimulation below the level of SCI, such as a full bladder or bowel. This condition is reported to occur in 50 to 90% of people with cervical and high thoracic SCI[14] and generally occurs in individuals with SCI at or above T6, below which the main sympathetic outflow exits the spinal cord. We have found that AD can occur in the acute phase of SCI as early as 4 days after severe cervical injury.[15] Although this possibility should always be considered in the clinical setting, it remains the case that AD typically develops over time after SCI. Cardiovascular dysfunction, including AD, increases with the level and severity of injury.[16] Even among complete tetraplegics, the clinical presentation of AD is variable and ranges from uncomfortable symptoms to life-threatening crises.[17,18] In a recent survey of people with SCI, the elimination of AD was identified by both paraplegics and tetraplegics as a high priority in improving their quality of life.[19] Despite the clinical significance of abnormal cardiovascular control and AD following SCI, the factors that underlie this condition are still under discussion among clinical and basic scientists. SCI research has focused heavily on paralysis, and cardiovascular control and autonomic dysfunction have been generally neglected by both the clinical and research communities.

The majority of episodes of AD are self-limited or even asymptomatic (or "silent") for individuals with chronic SCI.[20,21] Most episodes of AD are easily managed by the individual with SCI or by a caregiver, by eliminating the inciting stimulus (i.e., via bladder emptying, bowel evacuation, change in position, or other measures[4]). However, it is also common that episodes of AD require pharmacological interventions or urgent hospitalization due to malignant presentation.[22] A major concern with the repetitive and significant blood pressure elevation in AD (which distinguishes these hypertensive episodes in individuals with SCI from hypertension in able-bodied individuals) is a possible shear injury to the blood vessel endothelium that could predispose these individuals to cardiovascular complications in the future.[23]

The mechanisms underlying the development of AD are still poorly understood. However, there are some experimental animal and clinical data suggesting that autonomic instability is a main contributing factor in the development of this condition. As described earlier in this chapter, changes occurring within the spinal autonomic circuits in both the acute and chronic stages following SCI have been identified among the possible causes of the AD.[14]

It is important to note, however, that, although AD occurs more often in the chronic stage of SCI at or above the sixth thoracic segment, there is clinical evidence of early episodes of AD in the first days and weeks after the injury.[15,24] In fact, it seems likely that AD is underrecognized in the acute phase of SCI.[15] It is also worth mentioning that despite the fact that AD is unpleasant[22] and a life-threatening emergency,[17] some wheelchair athletes with SCI voluntarily induce it before the competition to enhance their performance.[25] Self-induced AD is commonly referred to as "boosting," and it is considered unethical and illegal by the International Paralympics Committee Medical Commissions. Therefore, Paralympians are subject to medical examination before the competitions.

Orthostatic Hypotension

In addition to dramatic elevations in blood pressure due to episodes of AD, many individuals with SCI also experience episodes of extremely low blood pressure when they are transferred to a wheelchair or attempt to stand up. This is referred to as orthostatic hypotension (OH), and it is particularly common in the acute phase of injury.[26] The Consensus Committee of the American Autonomic Society and the American Academy of Neurology define OH as a decrease in systolic blood pressure of 20 mmHg or more, or in diastolic blood pressure of 10 mmHg or more, upon the assumption of an upright posture from a supine position, regardless of whether symptoms occur.[27] The symptoms of OH in individuals with SCI are similar to those in able-bodied individuals[28] and include fatigue or weakness, light-headedness, dizziness, blurred vision, dyspnea, and restlessness.[29,30] However, OH can also be asymptomatic; Illman and colleagues reported that 41.1% of cord-injured individuals who developed OH were asymptomatic, despite significant blood pressure falls.[31] In a recent study from our laboratory, we also found that OH could persist asymptomatically in the chronic stage of SCI, despite a marked decrease in arterial blood pressure.[32] In this study, blood pressure decreases indicative of OH were observed in 7/14 (50%) of cervical SCI subjects, and 2/11 (18%) of thoracic SCI subjects. Symptomatic OH was present in five (36%) cervical SCI subjects and two (18%) thoracic SCI subjects and required early termination of the test in two cervical SCI subjects.[32] Asymptomatic OH is also reported in other able-bodied populations with autonomic disturbances and is likely a result of protective alterations in cerebral autoregulation despite cerebral hypoperfusion.[33–35]

Concerning the incidence and prevalence of OH in this population, orthostatic maneuvers performed during physiotherapy and mobilization are reported to induce blood pressure changes, diagnostic of OH, in 74% of cord-injured individuals, suggesting that OH is a common phenomenon among the cord-injured population.[31]

Several mechanisms have been proposed for the development of OH in the SCI population. Interruption of sympathoexcitatory efferent pathways from the brain stem to the spinal SPNs involved in vasoconstriction causes failure of short-term-reflex blood pressure regulation.[36] This leads to pooling of blood in the viscera and dependent vasculature below the level of injury. Resting catecholamine levels are also lower in individuals with cervical SCI compared with those with paraplegia and able-bodied individuals, and there is no significant increase in epinephrine or norepinephrine levels when quadriplegic individuals undergo a head-up tilt.[3] Individuals with SCI are also reported to have impaired baroreflex function,[37] smaller plasma volumes due to hyponatremia,[30] and possible cardiovascular deconditioning, at least in the early period following SCI, due to prolonged periods of bed rest.[38] Any combination of these factors can further increase the likelihood and severity of OH. On the other hand, there are several changes that occur after SCI that can mitigate the severity of OH, including the recovery of spinal sympathetic reflexes, development of spasticity and increased muscle tone, and changes in the renin-angiotensin system. While these changes have the potential to reduce the severity of OH, the reality is that OH remains a significant problem for the majority of the SCI population.

Deconditioning and Cardiovascular Control Following Spinal Cord Injury

A possible contributor to the high cardiovascular morbidity and mortality among individuals with SCI is a decreased ability to exercise and the resulting deconditioning.[39,40] There is strong evidence from the able-bodied population that physical inactivity is associated with cardiovascular morbidity and mortality.[41] The age-adjusted 2-year incidence of heart disease in the Canadian population is less than 1% for moderately active people and 2.3% for their sedentary counterparts. There is also evidence from the able-bodied population of an inverse relationship between the weekly amount of physical activity and both incidence of and mortality due to all cardiovascular disease.[42] Although exercise, including passive movement of the paralyzed limbs, is routinely used in clinical practice, there are few data to describe how exercise affects the cardiovascular outcome of SCI. Our own clinical data indicate that locomotor training (i.e., weight-supported movement on a treadmill) ameliorates cardiovascular control in SCI.[43]

Both short-term inactivity due to bed rest[44] and long-term inactivity due to paralysis following SCI[45,46] result in vascular adaptations in the inactive and paralyzed muscles, including reduced vessel diameter, decreased blood flow, increased shear stress, increased peripheral resistance, and decreased arterial compliance. In able-bodied populations, decreased central arterial compliance is associated with the incidence and progression of cardiovascular diseases.[47] However, it is important to recognize that even structural alterations due to inactivity can be ameliorated with regular physical activity both in able-bodied individuals and in individuals with SCI.[48,49] For example, regular endurance exercise improves endothelial function and arterial compliance in able-bodied individuals.[50] Both animal data[51] and recent clinical evidence[52] suggest that vascular adaptations occur within days or weeks of the onset of training. There are only a few studies examining whether the vascular changes following SCI are reversible by training, and what the time course of these training-induced vascular adaptations might be.[53,54] Our recent study evaluated compliance in large and small arteries before and after a 2-week training program using functional electrical stimulation leg cycle ergometry (FES-LCE).[54] It appears that FES-LCE is effective in improving small-artery compliance in females with SCI.

Evaluation of Autonomic Functions Following Spinal Cord Injury

Until recently, the impact of an SCI on a person's neurological function was evaluated through the use of only motor and sensory assessment that is a part of the International Standards for the Neurological Classification of Spinal Cord Injury. This assessment does not examine the status of autonomic dysfunctions in persons with SCI. Recently, the American Spinal Injury Association (ASIA) and the International Spinal Cord Society (ISCoS) proposed the strategy to document remaining autonomic neurological function following SCI.[55] It has to be recognized that the complexity of organization of the ANS and its involvement in the control of almost every bodily system make it difficult to select appropriate clinical tests for individuals with SCI. The proposed autonomic classification system includes four components: general autonomic, bladder, bowel, and sexual functions (**Fig. 16.3**). The general autonomic component of the classification chart includes evaluation of cardiovascular dysfunction in individuals with SCI.

Conclusion

In addition to motor and sensory deficits, individuals with SCI face lifelong abnormalities in blood pressure control.[14,56] The severity of these cardiovascular dysfunctions is affected by both the level and the completeness of injury to spinal autonomic pathways. Clinical evidence suggests that individuals with SCI on a daily basis can experience severe episodes of hypertension (known as AD)[4] and, conversely, marked falls in blood pressure during positional change (OH).[36] The long-term impact of dramatic blood pressure oscillations on vascular structure in the SCI population is unknown. However, one recent study indicates that carotid intima-media thickness is increased in individuals with SCI.[57] Hypertensive crises can be life threatening and can result in seizures,[58] myocardial ischemia,[59] cerebral vascular accident,[18] and death.[17] Furthermore, individuals with SCI have an increased risk of developing heart disease and stroke, and cardiovascular dysfunction is one of the leading causes of death for people with SCI.[6] Both AD and OH are known to prevent and delay rehabilitation and significantly impair the overall quality of life of individuals with SCI.[22,31] Therefore, early recognition and timely management of cardiovascular dysfunctions in this population are crucial.

Autonomic Standards Assessment Form

Patient Name:______________________ Anatomic Diagnosis: Supraconal □, Conal □, Cauda Equina □

General Autonomic Function

System/Organ	*Findings*	*Abnormal conditions*	*Check mark*
Autonomic control of the heart	Normal		
	Abnormal	Bradycardia	
		Tachycardia	
		Other dysrhythmias	
	Unknown		
	Unable to assess		
Autonomic control of blood pressure	Normal		
	Abnormal	Resting systolic blood pressure below 90 mmHg	
		Orthostatic hypotension	
		Autonomic dysreflexia	
	Unknown		
	Unable to assess		
Sweating control	Normal		
	Abnormal	Hyperhidrosis above lesion	
		Hyperhidrosis below lesion	
		Hypohidrosis below lesion	
	Unknown		
	Unable to assess		
Temperature regulation	Normal		
	Abnormal	Hyperthermia	
		Hypothermia	
	Unknown		
	Unable to assess		

p. 1

Fig. 16.3 Autonomic Standards Assessment Form. *(Continued on page 190)*

Fig. 16.3 (*Continued*)

Broncho-pulmonary control	Normal		
	Abnormal	Unable to voluntarily breathe requiring full ventilatory support	
		Impaired voluntary breathing requiring partial vent support	
		Voluntary respiration impaired does not require vent support	
	Unknown		

Lower Urinary Tract, Bowel and Sexual Function

System/Organ	*Findings*	*Score*
Lower Urinary Tract		
Awareness of the need to empty the bladder		
Ability to prevent leakage (continence)		
Bladder emptying method		
Bowel		
Sensation of need for a bowel movement		
Continence of stool		
Voluntary sphincter contraction		
Sexual Function		
Psychogenic genital arousal		
Reflex genital arousal		
Orgasm		
Ejaculation (male only)		
Menses (female only)		

2=Normal function, 1=Reduced or Altered Neurological Function

0=Complete loss of control NA=Unable to assess due to preexisting or concomitant problems

Fig. 16.3 (*Continued*)

Detailed Urodynamic Classification

System/Organ	*Findings*	*Check mark*
Sensation during filling	Normal	
	Increased	
	Reduced	
	Absent	
	Non-specific	
Detrusor Activity	Normal	
	Overactive	
	Underactive	
	Acontractile	
Sphincter	Normal urethral closure mechanism	
	Normal urethral function during voiding	
	Incompetent	
	Detrusor sphincter dyssynergia	
	Non-relaxing sphincter	

Date of Injury ____________ Date of Assessment: ____________ Examiner: ____________

This form may be freely copied and reproduced but not modified (Sp Cord, 2009, 47, 36-43)

This assessment should use the terminology found in the International SCI Data Set

(ASIA and ISCoS - http://www.asia-spinalinjury.org/bulletinBoard/dataset.php)

p. 3

Fig. 16.3 Autonomic Standards Assessment Form. These standards were reviewed and approved by the American Spinal Injury Association (ASIA) and the International Spinal Cord Society (ISCoS), and four components of the autonomic classification are proposed: general autonomic, bladder, bowel, and sexual functions.[55] A general anatomical component is utilized to document the overall impact of spinal cord injury (SCI) on autonomic function. A classification chart is provided for the autonomic control of cardiovascular, bronchopulmonary, and sudomotor function, including thermoregulation. A chart is provided for the examiner to describe and grade the neurological control of lower urinary tract, bowel, and sexual responses. Finally, a chart is provided detailing a urodynamic evaluation that should be completed on all patients. This information is recorded in a document for each person with SCI. Documentation of the cardiovascular dysfunctions following SCI is included in the General Autonomic Function component of the chart and should be made via checks in the appropriate boxes. The information is determined based on a combination of neurological examination and clinical history. The recognition and assessment of cardiac dysrhythmias, abnormal resting arterial blood pressure, and episodes of autonomic dysreflexia or orthostatic hypotension should be documented.

Conclusion

Cardiovascular dysfunctions are common in individuals with SCI. Injury level and severity directly correlate with the magnitude of these dysfunctions. Following high cervical SCI, parasympathetic (vagal) control will remain intact, whereas the sympathetic nervous system will lose its tonic autonomic control to the spinal circuits. On the other hand, in individuals with injury below the sixth thoracic segment, both the sympathetic and the parasympathetic control of the heart are intact. As a result of injury level, individuals with tetraplegia versus those with paraplegia will have very different cardiovascular responses to injury. It is important to appreciate that similar relationships can exist between the level of SCI and function of organs that are under autonomic control (bladder, bowel, sweat gland, etc.). Plastic changes within the central and peripheral autonomic circuits are possibly responsible for the abnormal autonomic control following SCI: disruption of the descending autonomic pathways, alterations in the morphology of spinal autonomic neurons, sprouting of aberrant dorsal root afferents, formation of inappropriate synaptic connections, plastic changes within the peripheral ganglia, and changes within the peripheral neurovascular responsiveness.

Pearls

- Spinal cord injury (SCI) is a condition that results not only in devastating paralysis but also in significant alterations of the autonomic nervous system affecting various organs and systems: cardiovascular, urinary, gastrointestinal, sexual, thermoregulatory, and others.
- Restoration of sexual and other autonomic-related functions (including blood pressure control) are among the most important functional priorities for individuals with SCI.
- Unstable blood pressure control, including autonomic dysreflexia and orthostatic hypotension, is commonly seen in individuals with injuries at the sixth thoracic spinal cord segment and above.

Pitfalls

- Unstable autonomic control following SCI could be responsible for the increased risk of heart disease and stroke among these individuals.
- If untreated, an episode of autonomic dysreflexia could result in seizures, intracranial hemorrhage, myocardial infarction, or death.
- If autonomic evaluation is not performed in conjunction with motor and sensory examination as a part of SCI assessment, it could result in underappreciation of the complexity of this devastating injury.

References

1. Krassioukov AV, Karlsson AK, Wecht JM, Wuermser LA, Mathias CJ, Marino RJ; Joint Committee of American Spinal Injury Association and International Spinal Cord Society. Assessment of autonomic dysfunction following spinal cord injury: rationale for additions to International Standards for Neurological Assessment. J Rehabil Res Dev 2007;44(1):103–112
2. Krassioukov A, Claydon VE. The clinical problems in cardiovascular control following spinal cord injury: an overview. Prog Brain Res 2006;152: 223–229
3. Claydon VE, Krassioukov AV. Orthostatic hypotension and autonomic pathways after spinal cord injury. J Neurotrauma 2006;23(12):1713–1725
4. Krassioukov A, Warburton DE, Teasell R, Eng JJ; Spinal Cord Injury Rehabilitation Evidence Research Team. A systematic review of the management of autonomic dysreflexia after spinal cord injury. Arch Phys Med Rehabil 2009;90(4):682–695
5. Krassioukov A. Autonomic function following cervical spinal cord injury. Respir Physiol Neurobiol 2009;169(2):157–164
6. Garshick E, Kelley A, Cohen SA, et al. A prospective assessment of mortality in chronic spinal cord injury. Spinal Cord 2005;43(7):408–416
7. Furlan JC, Fehlings MG, Shannon P, Norenberg MD, Krassioukov AV. Descending vasomotor pathways in humans: correlation between axonal preservation and cardiovascular dysfunction after spinal cord injury. J Neurotrauma 2003;20(12): 1351–1363

8. Wecht JM, Weir JP, Bauman WA. Blunted heart rate response to vagal withdrawal in persons with tetraplegia. Clin Auton Res 2006;16(6): 378–383
9. Hadley M. Blood pressure management after acute spinal cord injury. Neurosurgery 2002;50(3, Suppl):S58–S62
10. Glenn MB, Bergman SB. Cardiovascular changes following spinal cord injury. Top Spinal Cord Inj Rehabil 1997;2(4):47–53
11. Winslow EB, Lesch M, Talano JV, Meyer PR Jr. Spinal cord injuries associated with cardiopulmonary complications. Spine 1986;11(8):809–812
12. Hadley MN, Walters BC, Grabb PA, et al. Guidelines for the management of acute cervical spine and spinal cord injuries. Neurosurgery 2002; 50:S1–S199
13. Ditunno JF, Little JW, Tessler A, Burns AS. Spinal shock revisited: a four-phase model. Spinal Cord 2004;42(7):383–395
14. Mathias CJ, Frankel HL. Autonomic disturbances in spinal cord lesions. In: Bannister R, Mathias CJ, eds. Autonomic Failure, A Textbook of Clinical Disorders of the Autonomic Nervous System. 4th ed. Oxford: Oxford Medical Publications; 2002;839–881
15. Krassioukov AV, Furlan JC, Fehlings MG. Autonomic dysreflexia in acute spinal cord injury: an under-recognized clinical entity. J Neurotrauma 2003;20(8):707–716
16. Helkowski WM, Ditunno JF Jr, Boninger M. Autonomic dysreflexia: incidence in persons with neurologically complete and incomplete tetraplegia. J Spinal Cord Med 2003;26(3):244–247
17. Eltorai I, Kim R, Vulpe M, Kasravi H, Ho W. Fatal cerebral hemorrhage due to autonomic dysreflexia in a tetraplegic patient: case report and review. Paraplegia 1992;30(5):355–360
18. Pan SL, Wang YH, Lin HL, Chang CW, Wu TY, Hsieh ET. Intracerebral hemorrhage secondary to autonomic dysreflexia in a young person with incomplete C8 tetraplegia: a case report. Arch Phys Med Rehabil 2005;86(3):591–593
19. Anderson KD. Targeting recovery: priorities of the spinal cord-injured population. J Neurotrauma 2004;21(10):1371–1383
20. Ekland MB, Krassioukov AV, McBride KE, Elliott SL. Incidence of autonomic dysreflexia and silent autonomic dysreflexia in men with spinal cord injury undergoing sperm retrieval: implications for clinical practice. J Spinal Cord Med 2008;31(1): 33–39
21. Kirshblum SC, House JG, O'Connor KC. Silent autonomic dysreflexia during a routine bowel program in persons with traumatic spinal cord injury: a preliminary study. Arch Phys Med Rehabil 2002; 83(12):1774–1776
22. Elliott S, Krassioukov A. Malignant autonomic dysreflexia in spinal cord injured men. Spinal Cord 2006;44(6):386–392
23. Steins SA, Johnson MC, Lyman PJ. Cardiac rehabilitation in patients with spinal cord injuries. Phys Med Rehabil Clin N Am 1995;6(2):263–296
24. Silver JR. Early autonomic dysreflexia. Spinal Cord 2000;38(4):229–233
25. Harris P. Self-induced autonomic dysreflexia ('boosting') practised by some tetraplegic athletes to enhance their athletic performance. Paraplegia 1994;32(5):289–291
26. Sidorov EV, Townson AF, Dvorak MF, Kwon BK, Steeves J, Krassioukov A. Orthostatic hypotension in the first month following acute spinal cord injury. Spinal Cord 2008;46(1):65–69
27. Consensus statement on the definition of orthostatic hypotension, pure autonomic failure, and multiple system atrophy. The Consensus Committee of the American Autonomic Society and the American Academy of Neurology. Neurol (Tokyo) 1996;46:1470
28. Cleophas TJM, Kauw FHW, Bijl C, Meijers J, Stapper G. Effects of beta adrenergic receptor agonists and antagonists in diabetics with symptoms of postural hypotension: a double-blind, placebo-controlled study. Angiology 1986;37(11):855–862
29. Sclater A, Alagiakrishnan K. Orthostatic hypotension: a primary care primer for assessment and treatment. Geriatrics 2004;59(8):22–27
30. Frisbie JH, Steele DJR. Postural hypotension and abnormalities of salt and water metabolism in myelopathy patients. Spinal Cord 1997; 35(5):303–307
31. Illman A, Stiller K, Williams M. The prevalence of orthostatic hypotension during physiotherapy treatment in patients with an acute spinal cord injury. Spinal Cord 2000;38(12):741–747
32. Claydon VE, Krassioukov AV. Orthostatic hypotension and autonomic pathways after spinal cord injury. J Neurotrauma 2006;23(12): 1713–1725
33. Mathias CJ, Mallipeddi R, Bleasdale-Barr K. Symptoms associated with orthostatic hypotension in pure autonomic failure and multiple system atrophy. J Neurol 1999;246(10):893–898
34. Houtman S, Colier WN, Oeseburg B, Hopman MT. Systemic circulation and cerebral oxygenation during head-up tilt in spinal cord injured individuals. Spinal Cord 2000;38(3):158–163
35. Gonzalez F, Chang JY, Banovac K, Messina D, Martinez-Arizala A, Kelley RE. Autoregulation of cerebral blood flow in patients with orthostatic hypotension after spinal cord injury. Paraplegia 1991;29(1):1–7
36. Krassioukov A, Eng JJ, Warburton DE, Teasell R; Spinal Cord Injury Rehabilitation Evidence Research Team. A systematic review of the management of orthostatic hypotension after spinal cord injury. Arch Phys Med Rehabil 2009;90(5): 876–885
37. Wecht JM, De Meersman RE, Weir JP, Spungen AM, Bauman WA. Cardiac autonomic responses to progressive head-up tilt in individuals with paraplegia. Clin Auton Res 2003;13(6):433–438
38. Vaziri ND. Nitric oxide in microgravity-induced orthostatic intolerance: relevance to spinal cord injury. J Spinal Cord Med 2003;26(1):5–11
39. Phillips WT, Kiratli BJ, Sarkarati M, et al. Effect of spinal cord injury on the heart and cardiovascular fitness. Curr Probl Cardiol 1998;23(11):641–716
40. Banerjea R, Sambamoorthi U, Weaver F, Maney M, Pogach LM, Findley T. Risk of stroke, heart attack, and diabetes complications among veterans with spinal cord injury. Arch Phys Med Rehabil 2008;89(8):1448–1453

41. Wannamethee SG, Shaper AG. Physical activity in the prevention of cardiovascular disease: an epidemiological perspective. Sports Med 2001; 31(2):101–114
42. Lee IM, Paffenbarger RS Jr. Associations of light, moderate, and vigorous intensity physical activity with longevity. The Harvard Alumni Health Study. Am J Epidemiol 2000;151(3):293–299
43. Harkema SJ, Ferreira CK, van den Brand RJ, Krassioukov AV. Improvements in orthostatic instability with stand locomotor training in individuals with spinal cord injury. J Neurotrauma 2008;25(12):1467–1475
44. Bleeker MW, De Groot PC, Rongen GA, et al. Vascular adaptation to deconditioning and the effect of an exercise countermeasure: results of the Berlin Bed Rest study. J Appl Physiol 2005;99(4): 1293–1300
45. de Groot PC, Bleeker MW, Hopman MT. Magnitude and time course of arterial vascular adaptations to inactivity in humans. Exerc Sport Sci Rev 2006;34(2):65–71
46. de Groot PC, Bleeker MW, van Kuppevelt DH, van der Woude LH, Hopman MT. Rapid and extensive arterial adaptations after spinal cord injury. Arch Phys Med Rehabil 2006;87(5):688–696
47. Celermajer DS, Sorensen KE, Gooch VM, et al. Non-invasive detection of endothelial dysfunction in children and adults at risk of atherosclerosis. Lancet 1992;340(8828):1111–1115
48. Schmidt-Trucksäss A, Schmid A, Brunner C, et al. Arterial properties of the carotid and femoral artery in endurance-trained and paraplegic subjects. J Appl Physiol 2000;89(5):1956–1963
49. Schmidt-Trucksäss AS, Grathwohl D, Frey I, et al. Relation of leisure-time physical activity to structural and functional arterial properties of the common carotid artery in male subjects. Atherosclerosis 1999;145(1):107–114
50. Clarkson P, Montgomery HE, Mullen MJ, et al. Exercise training enhances endothelial function in young men. J Am Coll Cardiol 1999;33(5): 1379–1385
51. McAllister RM, Laughlin MH. Short-term exercise training alters responses of porcine femoral and brachial arteries. J Appl Physiol 1997;82(5): 1438–1444
52. Allen JD, Geaghan JP, Greenway F, Welsch MA. Time course of improved flow-mediated dilation after short-term exercise training. Med Sci Sports Exerc 2003;35(5):847–853
53. de Groot P, Crozier J, Rakobowchuk M, Hopman M, MacDonald M. Electrical stimulation alters FMD and arterial compliance in extremely inactive legs. Med Sci Sports Exerc 2005;37(8):1356–1364
54. Zbogar D, Eng JJ, Krassioukov AV, Scott JM, Esch BT, Warburton DE. The effects of functional electrical stimulation leg cycle ergometry training on arterial compliance in individuals with spinal cord injury. Spinal Cord 2008;46(11):722–726
55. Alexander MS, Biering-Sorensen F, Bodner D, et al. International standards to document remaining autonomic function after spinal cord injury. Spinal Cord 2009;47(1):36–43
56. Claydon VE, Hol AT, Eng JJ, Krassioukov AV. Cardiovascular responses and postexercise hypotension after arm cycling exercise in subjects with spinal cord injury. Arch Phys Med Rehabil 2006;87(8):1106–1114
57. Matos-Souza JR, Pithon KR, Ozahata TM, Gemignani T, Cliquet A Jr, Nadruz W Jr. Carotid intima-media thickness is increased in patients with spinal cord injury independent of traditional cardiovascular risk factors. Atherosclerosis 2009;202(1):29–31
58. Yarkony GM, Katz RT, Wu YC. Seizures secondary to autonomic dysreflexia. Arch Phys Med Rehabil 1986;67(11):834–835
59. Ho CP, Krassioukov AV. Autonomic dysreflexia and myocardial ischemia. Spinal Cord 2010;48(9):714–715

17

Pain after Spinal Cord Injury

Angela Mailis and Luis Enrique Chaparro

Key Points

1. Pain after traumatic or other forms of injury to the spinal cord is very common (estimated to affect 25 to 96% of patients). However, estimates of prevalence, severity, and duration of pain are highly variable in the published literature due to methodological and other differences between the studies.

2. SCI-associated pain can be nociceptive somatic (with musculoskeletal pain common in both the acute and the chronic stage of SCI), nociceptive visceral (originating from bladder, bowel, and kidney problems), neuropathic (above, at, and below level), or a combination.

3. SCI-related pain can be treated with medications, physical and occupational therapies, psychologically based treatments, and surgery. Generally, the treatment should be multimodal.

Spinal cord lesions are usually traumatic, but spinal cord damage can also be the result of multiple other causes (iatrogenic, inflammatory, neoplastic, vascular or skeletal pathology, or congenital). Persisting pain is one of the commonest and most debilitating consequences of spinal cord injury (SCI).[1] Following the inability to walk and bowel or bladder dysfunction, a significant number of individuals with SCI consider chronic pain as a very disabling complication.[2] There is a strong association between pain and psychological factors or social disability. Indeed, psychological factors have a stronger association with pain than the medical condition per se in patients with SCI pain.[3,4] In addition, the pain intensity is strongly correlated with concomitant sleep disorders,[2] while pain, fatigue, and weakness are major contributors to social disability.[5]

Epidemiology

Estimates of the prevalence, severity, and duration of pain after SCI are highly variable in the published literature. The variability is due to differences among the studies in regard to pain definitions, terminology, classification, inclusion criteria, and reporting methods, as well as etiological and demographic factors. An earlier evidence report,[6] which reviewed 132 studies, found serious methodological limitations in most. Nevertheless, the report concluded that the prevalence of chronic pain after SCI varied from 40 to 75%, whereas pain was reported as moderate to severe in 25 to 60% of those with pain, was often associated with psychological and psychiatric comorbidity and was severe enough to impair daily function. A very recent review[7] of the literature that used different inclusion criteria identified 42 studies, with reported prevalence ranging between 26 and 96%, unaffected by sex/gender, complete/incomplete SCI, or paraplegia/tetraplegia. A 5-year follow-up study[8] reported prevalence of persistent severe pain up to 58%, which was, however, not associated with either the level or the type of injury. In a community survey of 384 patients with SCI, 79% of respondents reported current pain, which was significantly more common in persons with less education, unemployed, or not at school. Most common locations of current pain were the back (61%), hips and buttocks (61%), and legs and feet (58%). Upper extremity pain was experienced by 76% after the injury and by 69% of patients at the time of the survey. Those with tetraplegia were significantly more likely to have neck and shoulder pain than patients with paraplegia. On average, respondents reported a high level of pain intensity and a moderate level of pain interference with activities, and they rated treatments received for pain as being only somewhat helpful.[9]

Clinical Manifestations

A comprehensive taxonomy has been proposed by the International Association for the Study of Pain Task Force on pain after SCI,[10] which has been helpful in subsequent studies. The taxonomy details mechanism of pain and the system as well as specific structure involved and classifies the pain as follows: nociceptive musculoskeletal or visceral and neuropathic above level, at level, and below level.

Nociceptive musculoskeletal pain is common in both the acute and the chronic stage of SCI. Most of the time, upper extremity pain is attributed to overuse. Musculoskeletal spinal pain is due to fractures, surgical fixations, osteoporosis, or muscle spasms and tends to be more common after thoracic spinal injury and surgical procedures within 2 weeks after the lesion.[11] Nociceptive visceral pain originating from bladder, bowel, and kidney problems is manifested by cramps and dull pain and is associated with nausea, autonomic reflex abnormalities, and dysautonomia. Autonomic dysreflexia is frequently associated with injuries above T6 and is manifested by episodic headaches, sudden increases in blood pressure, and cerebral hemorrhage.[12]

SCI neuropathic pain, like other neuropathic pain syndromes, can be idiosyncratic (i.e., not all patients will develop such pain[13]). Particularly the below-level pain (central pain) is caused by lesions of the primary somatosensory pathway passing through the ventrocaudal nucleus of the thalamus, especially the spinothalamic tract.[14] The causative lesion may be massive or, to the contrary, minimal; sensory loss varies from minimal to complete anesthesia; pain onset can be immediate or delayed and can be ongoing, paroxysmal, or stimulus evoked; and different pain characteristics may have different underlying mechanisms. Above-level neuropathic pain is frequently related to compressive neuropathies (e.g., carpal tunnel syndrome), whereas below-level neuropathic pain is considered central pain secondary to the original injury. At-level neuropathic pain is related to nerve root or spinal cord compression or damage.[15] Above- or at-level neuropathic pain is more frequently observed after cervical spinal injuries or central cord syndromes, and below-level neuropathic pain is more often associated with anterior cord lesions.[16] Siddall and colleagues[10,17] showed a prevalence of 41% at-level neuropathic pain, 34% below-level neuropathic pain, and 5% visceral pain in a 5-year follow-up study of patients with SCI. One of the main characteristics of at-level pain is its early onset, primarily within the first 3 months after the injury. The prevalence increases with high pain intensity and early onset. Two cardinal symptoms in at-level neuropathic pain are allodynia and pain of severe intensity. Examples of neuropathic pain are shown in **Fig. 17.1**.

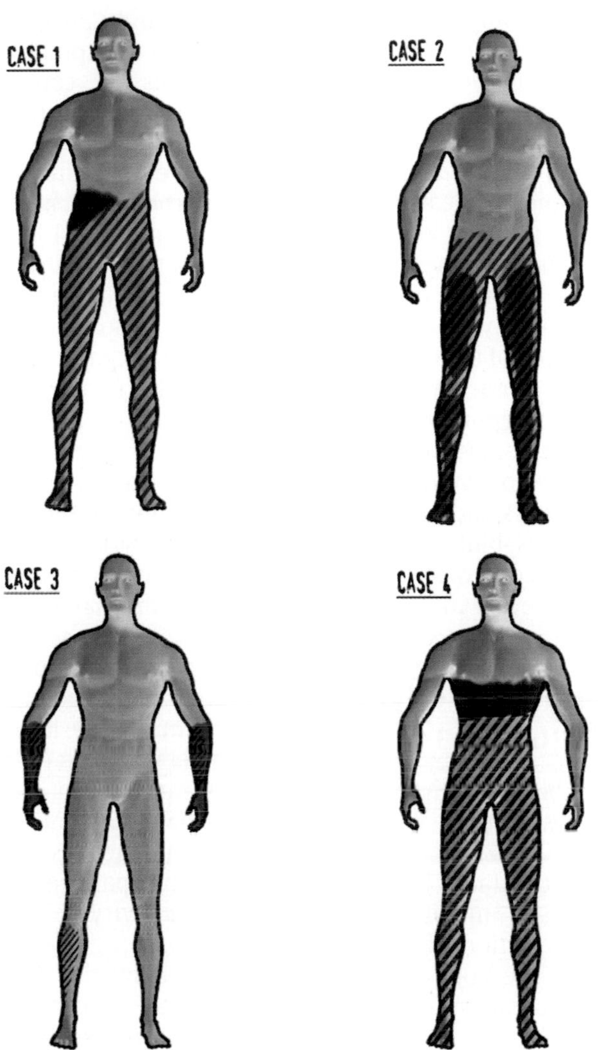

Fig. 17.1 Case 1: Complete anesthesia and paralysis below the T6 level. Pain is reported in the right flank (below-level). Case 2: Partial sensory and motor loss after T9-10 fracture with severe complaints of bilateral leg pain (below-level). Case 3: Incomplete SCI after C6-7 fracture/dislocation. Patient presents with generalized hypereflexia, minor weakness in the right arm and leg, and hypoesthesia in medial forearms and right leg, while pain involves both forearms (below-level). Case 4: T4 fracture with severe hyperalgesia, allodynia, and pain in the transitional zone (at-level) associated with complete anesthesia and paralysis below. Pain is shown in the dark-shaded areas whereas sensory loss is shown by the lined areas.

Tasker et al. reviewed the essential features of 127 personal cases.[18] Nearly two thirds of the injuries were traumatic in origin; three quarters of the patients were male; more than half of the patients were younger than 40 years of age; 42% of the lesions were cervical, followed by thoracolumbar lesions (37%). The authors pointed out that "it was curious that some patients with no detectable neurological deficit (4% of their series) had similar pain syndromes with some patients with complete cord transection." In another series,[19] onset of pain was reported immediately after the injury in 17% of the patients, less than a month in 13%, 1 to 6 months in 19%, 6 to 12 months in 8%, 1 to 5 years in 13%, and after more than 5 years in 2%.

Pain in syringomyelia (idiopathic, associated with Chiari malformation or after traumatic SCI) deserves a brief mention. Spinal cord lesions of any type can lead to syringomyelia. Unusually long latencies between the injury and the development of pain should raise suspicion of cavitation. In one series,[18] 12.6% of patients with spinal cord lesions subsequently developed a syrinx characterized by delayed onset of pain a year or more than a year after the spinal cord lesion. A survey of the Canadian Syringomyelia Network participants during their 1996 convention reported a 97.5% prevalence of pain.[20] The same study reported that pain was the sole symptom at onset in 59% of the patients and was cited as the primary cause of disability in 69% of the sufferers, and was rated as moderate in 70% of the patients, and severe in 11%.

Pain Mechanisms Underlying Spinal Cord Injury Pain

Several reviews have been published regarding the pathophysiological changes that occur after SCI.[1,15,21–23] Early on, Levitt and Levitt[24] studied central SCI pain in monkeys. Autotomy (as a manifestation of pain) appeared after section of the anterolateral quadrant of the cord or after hemisection with preservation of some sensation in ipsilateral nociceptive pathways, whereas pain never seemed to appear after posterior quadrant or funicular section. After further manipulations of the cord, the researchers concluded that the appearance of pain could not be related to any lesion of specific cord pathways. In humans, one of the earliest studies was conducted by Lenz et al.[25] in a patient with SCI during deep brain stimulation. He reported missing receptive fields from the denervated area, increased numbers of thalamic neurons without a receptive field, expansion into the thalamic region of the deafferented part of neurons with receptive fields in the border zone of the deafferented area, mismatch between receptive and projected fields from stimulation, and spontaneous spikes from cells within the deafferented area. Pagni and Canavero[26] reported a patient with a T9 spinal cyst whose single photon emission computed tomography (SPECT) showed diminished perfusion of the contralateral thalamus. Cyst resection resulted in elimination of pain and normalization of the SPECT, an effect that was also transiently produced by IV administration of propofol prior to surgery, suggesting that the responsible mechanisms are not necessarily always due to structural changes.

In summary, in central pain after spinal cord or brain damage, the lesion could be anywhere in the neuraxis from the dorsal horn to the cerebral cortex, and most commonly is associated with interruption of the spinothalamocortical nociceptive pathways. In SCI, loss of balance between different sensory channels, loss of spinal inhibitory mechanisms, and/or pattern generators within the injured cord have been proposed as possible mechanisms. Canavero[27] proposed that "irrespective of the location of the lesion, central pain is generated by disturbance in the normal oscillatory mechanisms between the cortex and the thalamus." Increased burst activity may be related to loss of inhibitory drive on *N*-methyl-D-aspartate (NMDA) receptors or increased activity at NMDA receptor sites. The presence of glutamatergic hypertonus is suggested by the relief of central pain by ketamine,[28,29] propofol,[30] and barbiturates.[31] Indeed, excitatory neurotransmitters across the dorsal horns play a special role in the development of at-level neuropathic pain.[22] Such pain can subsequently progress to below-level neuropathic pain; therefore common mechanisms may be involved.[32] Below-level neuropathic pain seems to be related to central mechanisms of pain,[23] as discussed earlier. This type of pain is severe, can be evoked or spontaneous, and has a tendency to appear in later stages of the injury (> 2 years).[15,17] This later onset indicates a slow neuronal degeneration process and subsequent hyperactivity secondary to deafferentation.[17] Human studies have shown that below-level pain is quite frequent in partial lesions (more often in anterior lesions) and has been reported to occur in 50% of tetraplegics.[17,33]

Therapeutic Approaches to Spinal Cord Injury Pain

Pharmacological Management

We conducted a systematic literature review through PubMed using the MeSH terms "Spinal Cord Injuries" AND "Pain" limited to clinical trials. In **Table 17.1**, we present 25 clinical trials, ten of which included parenteral administration of drugs; therefore, their results are not clinically applicable. A qualitative assessment of the included studies shows that SCI barely responds to pharmacological approaches. Probably, some of the pharmacological strategies have failed to demonstrate a significant benefit due to small sample size (underpower studies). In our clinical perspective, we would recommend pregabalin for patients with concomitant anxiety, and antidepressants (we would opt for duloxetine) in patients with concomitant depression. Additionally, we would recommend, as a second line of treatment, the use of opioids under direct supervision by clinicians who are familiar with the aforementioned drugs. Ketamine could be used only for inpatients and always accompanied by concomitant treatment with a benzodiazepine to avoid potential hallucinatory effects. For curious clinicians, we recommend a simple but cleverly developed tool at PubMed called "Clinical Queries" (search by "Clinical Study Category": spinal cord injury pain).

Physical and Occupational Therapies

The goal of physical therapies in general in SCI is to try to maintain, and if possible increase, strength, range of movement, balance, and coordination. Occupational therapies aim to increase functionality through performance of simple and complex real-life activities. However, few such therapies aim directly at pain of neuropathic origin. Desensitization (a procedure that brings hyperesthetic and allodynic skin into gradual contact with different textures, such as cotton, wool, etc.) aims to desensitize the skin, as in the areas of transitional zone pain and hyperpathia. In our experience, the effect is usually quite unsatisfactory. Oral medications seem to have a better but still limited chance of addressing skin hyperesthesia. Given anecdotal reports of the effect of acupuncture in some SCI pain, a study is currently in process as a multicenter randomized, controlled trial in Canada (clinical trials government identifier: NCT00523016) to test electroacupuncture versus sham acupuncture in SCI patients with burning pain.

Psychological Approaches

Chronic pain after SCI significantly interferes with activities of daily living, such as sleep, household chores, exercise, and work, and is reflected in negative coping, lower quality of life, and a significant incidence of depression. Rudy et al.[34] found that psychological factors, such as self-efficacy perception, movement-related pain, fear, and cognitive coping, are strongly correlated with physical performance. Other factors, such as age, sex, and pain duration, were not associated with the magnitude of the physical performance. The main goals of treatment in general relate to improvement of the quality of life and early social reintegration and require some training in pain-coping skills and cognitive behavioral therapy, as well as adaptation to social, sexual, and communication skills.

Invasive Treatments

Considerations for surgical treatment should be given when the cord lesion creates disabling pain that fails to respond to conservative measures. The surgical options should be thoroughly discussed after consideration of efficacy, risk, and complexity of the procedure, as well as the nature of pain (because SCI pain has more than one component). The procedures are mentioned only briefly here because extensive review is beyond the scope of this chapter. The types of pain that require surgical consideration[13] are ongoing (steady) burning, dysesthetic pain and intermittent paroxysmal shooting pains (neuralgic pains), below the level of the injury (central pains). A summary[13] of invasive procedures follows: rhizotomy, preferably percutaneous, may help with "single root pain," particularly to relieve allodynia in a single root distribution. Cor-

Table 17.1 Drug Trials and Outcome

Trial	Medication: dosing	Design	Outcome	NNT
Antidepressants				
1. Cardenas et al.[38]	Amitriptyline: 10–125 mg/day	Parallel	Amitriptyline = placebo	NA
2. Rintala et al.[39]	Amitriptyline (150 mg/day) vs gabapentin 3600 mg/day	Crossover	Amitriptyline > gabapentin = placebo	NA
3. Vranken et al.[40]	Duloxetine: 60–120 mg/day	Parallel	Duloxetine = placebo	NA
4. Davidoff et al.[41]	Trazodone: 150 mg/day	Parallel	Trazodone = placebo	9 (1.8–∞)
Anticonvulsants				
5. Levendoglu et al.[42]	Gabapentin: 3600 mg/day	Crossover	Gabapentin > placebo	NA
6. Tai et al.[43]	Gabapentin: 1800 mg/day	Crossover	Gabapentin = placebo	∞
7. Finnerup et al.[44]	Lamotrigine: 400 mg/day	Crossover	Lamotrigine = placebo	∞
8. Finnerup et al.[45]	Levetiracetam: 500–1500 mg/day	Crossover	Levetiracetam = placebo	NA
9. Siddall et al.[46]	Pregabalin: 600 mg/day	Parallel	Pregabalin > placebo	NA
10. Vranken et al.[47]	Pregabalin: 150–600 mg/day	Parallel	Pregabalin > placebo	NA
11. Harden et al.[37]	Topiramate: 25–800 mg/day	Parallel	Topiramate = placebo	NA
12. Drewes et al.[48]	Valproate: 2400 mg/day	Crossover	Valproate = placebo	10 (2.7–∞)
13. Herman et al.[49]*	Baclofen (spinal): 50 µg (single bolus)	Crossover	Baclofen > placebo	NA
Local anesthetics				
14. Finnerup et al.[50]*	Lidocaine (single IV bolus): 5 mg/kg	Parallel	Lidocaine > placebo	4 (1.8–∞)
15. Attal et al.[51]*	Lidocaine (single IV bolus): 5 mg/kg	Crossover	Lidocaine > placebo	5 (1.6–∞)
16. Chiou-Tan et al.[52]	Mexiletine: 450 mg/day	Crossover	Mexiletine = placebo	NA

Intravenous anesthetics				
17. Kvarnström et al.[29]*	Ketamine (intravenous): 0.4 mg/kg	Crossover	Ketamine > placebo = lidocaine	2 (1.36–∞)
18. Eide et al.[28]*	Ketamine (intravenous): 60 μg/kg + 6 μg/kg/min vs alfentanil	Crossover	Ketamine = alfentanil > placebo	NA
19. Amr[53]	Ketamine (intravenous): 80 mg/day + gabapentin (900 mg/day) for one week vs gabapentin alone	Parallel	Combination = gabapentin alone	NA
20. Canavero et al.[30]*	Propofol (intravenous): 0.2 mg/kg	Crossover	Propofol > placebo	NA
21. Mailis-Gagnon et al.[31]*	Sodium amobarbital: 4–7 mg/kg vs lidocaine	Parallel	Sodium amobarbital > lidocaine	NA
Opioids				
22. Attal et al.[54]	Morphine (intravenous): 9–30 mg	Crossover	Morphine = placebo	3 (1.6–40)
23. Norrbrink et al.[55]	Tramadol: 50 mg TID to 400 mg/day	Parallel	Tramadol > placebo	NA
24. Siddall et al.[56]*	Morphine 0.2–1 mg (spinal) vs clonidine 50–100 mcg (spinal) vs combination	Crossover	Combination > morphine = clonidine > placebo	7.5 (2.1–∞)
Cannabinoids				
25. Rintala et al.[57]	Dronabinol (5–25 mg) vs diphenhydramine (25–75 mg)	Crossover	Dronabinol = diphenhydramine	NA

Abbreviations: NA, not available; NNT, number needed to treat.
*Parenteral administration.

dotomy may work better in radicular or paroxysmal pain (but not steady ongoing pain), but the effect may decrease with time. In one series, pain returned in 6/25 cases[13] anytime between 1 and 21 years after the procedure. Cordectomy relates to two procedures: removing a segment of the spinal cord, or cord transection above the level of the SCI. Such procedures seem to work better for lesions below the T10 level and may affect both steady, ongoing pain and paroxysmal pains. Dorsal root entry zone (DREZ) lesion is a rather popular procedure for at-level pain, though it has also been reported in some patients to ameliorate below-level ongoing dysesthetic pains.

However, below-level central ongoing dysesthetic pains seem to better respond to neuroaugmentative procedures, primarily dorsal column stimulation (DCS), applicable only in incomplete SCI, and deep brain stimulation (DBS). Peripheral nerve stimulation does not have a place in the management of SCI pain. Successful DCS must generate paresthesias in the area of pain by electrode insertion in the epidural space at appropriate levels above the injury level. However, in SCI this may be difficult, as previous procedures or the trauma itself may have altered the epidural space, or cord lesions often damage the dorsal columns. The literature[13] shows long-term relief with DCS in some patients with ongoing pain and incomplete SCI, whereas the results were poor for paroxysmal pain. DCS, in general, is considered to have a low success rate in SCI. DBS is worth considering when DCS is technically impossible. In an older literature review of six series,[35] DBS was reported to have variable success, ranging from 0 to 59% (for ongoing pain), and resulted in some serious complications, including intracerebral hematomas, superficial infections, and so forth, while almost one in two patients experienced technical problems, such as lead migration, requiring revisions. In case of pain associated with syringomyelia, drainage of the cyst and decompression may relieve somewhat the paroxysmal pains, but not the steady ones, and the results are at best partial. Milhorat et al.[36] reported that 41% of 37 operated patients either did not improve or actually worsened after surgical decompression.

Pearls

- SCI pain arises from multiple mechanisms (above, at, and below the level of the lesion). It is a significant problem for SCI patients, affecting anywhere between one to three of every four patients.
- Treatment must be multimodal, including combination of medications, physical modalities, psychological treatments, and interventional treatments.
- SCI patients may require polypharmacy, including opioids and neuropathic adjuvants (though only pregabalin has demonstrated a positive effect in clinical studies).
- Certain rules must be observed when instituting pharmacotherapy (e.g., medications should be introduced in a sequence and not simultaneously), whereas each trial must be time- and dose-contingent. Treatment effectiveness must be documented in regard to pain and function.

Pitfalls

- Not all pains are the same in SCI. The underlying pathophysiology (central or peripheral, neuropathic or nociceptive) affects application of treatment modalities.
- The effect of psychological factors, cognition, and coping mechanisms in SCI pain and related disability should not be underestimated.
- Because SCI-related pain may be difficult to treat, it is unrealistic to expect pain elimination.

References

1. Siddall PJ, Loeser JD. Pain following spinal cord injury. Spinal Cord 2001;39(2):63–73
2. Widerström-Noga EG, Felipe-Cuervo E, Yezierski RP. Chronic pain after spinal injury: interference with sleep and daily activities. Arch Phys Med Rehabil 2001;82(11):1571–1577
3. Störmer S, Gerner HJ, Grüninger W, et al. Chronic pain/dysaesthesiae in spinal cord injury patients: results of a multicentre study. Spinal Cord 1997; 35(7):446–455
4. Summers JD, Rapoff MA, Varghese G, Porter K, Palmer RE. Psychosocial factors in chronic spinal cord injury pain. Pain 1991;47(2):183–189
5. Jensen MP, Kuehn CM, Amtmann D, Cardenas DD. Symptom burden in persons with spinal cord injury. Arch Phys Med Rehabil 2007;88(5):638–645
6. Jadad A, O'Brien MA, Wingerchuk D, et al. Management of chronic central neuropathic pain following traumatic spinal cord injury. Evid Rep Technol Assess (Summ) 2001;1(45):1–5
7. Dijkers M, Bryce T, Zanca J. Prevalence of chronic pain after traumatic spinal cord injury: a systematic review. J Rehabil Res Dev 2009;46(1): 13–29
8. Siddall PJ. Management of neuropathic pain following spinal cord injury: now and in the future. Spinal Cord 2009;47(5):352–359
9. Turner JA, Cardenas DD, Warms CA, McClellan CB. Chronic pain associated with spinal cord injuries: a community survey. Arch Phys Med Rehabil 2001;82(4):501–509
10. Siddall PJ, Yezierski RP, Loeser JD. Taxonomy and epidemiology of spinal cord injury pain. In: Yezierski RP, Burchiel KJ, eds. Spinal Cord Injury Pain: Assessment, Mechanisms, Management. Progress in Pain Research and Management, Vol 23. Seattle, WA: IASP Press; 2002:9–24
11. Berić A. Post-spinal cord injury pain states. Pain 1997;72(3):295–298
12. Karlsson AK. Autonomic dysreflexia. Spinal Cord 1999;37(6):383–391
13. Tasker R. Spinal cord injury and central pain. In: Aronoff GM, ed. Evaluation and Treatment of Chronic Pain. Baltimore, MD: Lippincott Williams & Wilkins; 1998:131–146
14. Leijon G, Boivie J, Johansson I. Central post-stroke pain—neurological symptoms and pain characteristics. Pain 1989;36(1):13–25
15. Finnerup NB, Jensen TS. Spinal cord injury pain—mechanisms and treatment. Eur J Neurol 2004;11(2):73–82
16. Que JC, Siddall PJ, Cousins MJ. Pain management in a patient with intractable spinal cord injury pain: a case report and literature review. Anesth Analg 2007;105(5):1462–1473
17. Siddall PJ, McClelland JM, Rutkowski SB, Cousins MJ. A longitudinal study of the prevalence and characteristics of pain in the first 5 years following spinal cord injury. Pain 2003;103(3): 249–257
18. Tasker RR, DeCarvalho GT, Dolan EJ. Intractable pain of spinal cord origin: clinical features and implications for surgery. J Neurosurg 1992; 77(3):373–378
19. Tasker RR. Pain resulting from central nervous system pathology (central pain), In: Bonica JJ, ed. The Management of Pain. Philadelphia, PA: Lea & Febiger; 1990:264–280
20. Cohodaveric T, Mailis-Gagnon A, Montanera W. Syringomyelia: pain, sensory abnormalities, and neuroimaging. J Pain 2000;1:54–66
21. Eide PK. Pathophysiological mechanisms of central neuropathic pain after spinal cord injury. Spinal Cord 1998;36(9):601–612
22. Yezierski RP. Spinal cord injury: a model of central neuropathic pain. Neurosignals 2005;14(4): 182–193
23. Finnerup NB, Johannesen IL, Fuglsang-Frederiksen A, Bach FW, Jensen TS. Sensory function in spinal cord injury patients with and without central pain. Brain 2003;126(Pt 1):57–70
24. Levitt M, Levitt JH. The deafferentation syndrome in monkeys: dysesthesias of spinal origin. Pain 1981;10(2):129–147
25. Lenz FA, Tasker RR, Dostrovsky JO, et al. Abnormal single-unit activity recorded in the somatosensory thalamus of a quadriplegic patient with central pain. Pain 1987;31(2):225–236
26. Pagni CA, Canavero S. Functional thalamic depression in a case of reversible central pain due to a spinal intramedullary cyst. Case report. J Neurosurg 1995;83(1):163–165
27. Canavero S. Dynamic reverberation: a unified mechanism for central and phantom pain. Med Hypotheses 1994;42(3):203–207
28. Eide PK, Stubhaug A, Stenehjem AE. Central dysesthesia pain after traumatic spinal cord injury is dependent on N-methyl-D-aspartate receptor activation. Neurosurgery 1995;37(6):1080–1087
29. Kvarnström A, Karlsten R, Quiding H, Gordh T. The analgesic effect of intravenous ketamine and lidocaine on pain after spinal cord injury. Acta Anaesthesiol Scand 2004;48(4):498–506
30. Canavero S, Bonicalzi V, Pagni CA, et al. Propofol analgesia in central pain: preliminary clinical observations. J Neurol 1995;242(9):561–567
31. Mailis-Gagnon A, Yegneswaran B, Bharatwal B, Krassioukov AV. Effects of intravenous sodium amobarbital vs lidocaine on pain and sensory abnormalities in patients with spinal cord injury. J Spinal Cord Med 2009;32(1):49–53
32. Burchiel KJ, Hsu FP. Pain and spasticity after spinal cord injury: mechanisms and treatment. Spine 2001;26(24, Suppl):S146–S160
33. Berić A, Dimitrijević MR, Lindblom U. Central dysesthesia syndrome in spinal cord injury patients. Pain 1988;34(2):109–116
34. Rudy TE, Lieber SJ, Boston JR, Gourley LM, Baysal E. Psychosocial predictors of physical performance in disabled individuals with chronic pain. Clin J Pain 2003;19(1):18–30
35. Tasker RR, Vilela Filho O. Deep brain stimulation for the control of intractable pain. In: Youmans JR, ed. Neurological Surgery. 3rd ed. Philadelphia: WB Saunders; 1996:3512–3527
36. Milhorat TH, Kotzen RM, Mu HT, Capocelli AL Jr, Milhorat RH. Dysesthetic pain in patients with syringomyelia. Neurosurgery 1996;38(5):940–946, discussion 946–947

37. Harden RN, Brenman E, Saltz S, Houle T. Topiramate in the management of spinal cord injury pain: a double-blind, randomized, placebo-controlled pilot study. In: Yezierski R, Burchiel K, eds. Spinal Cord Injury Pain: Assessment, Mechanisms, Management. 1st ed. Seattle, WA: IASP Press; 2002:393–408
38. Cardenas DD, Warms CA, Turner JA, Marshall H, Brooke MM, Loeser JD. Efficacy of amitriptyline for relief of pain in spinal cord injury: results of a randomized controlled trial. Pain 2002;96(3): 365–373
39. Rintala DH, Holmes SA, Courtade D, Fiess RN, Tastard LV, Loubser PG. Comparison of the effectiveness of amitriptyline and gabapentin on chronic neuropathic pain in persons with spinal cord injury. Arch Phys Med Rehabil 2007;88(12): 1547–1560
40. Vranken JH, Hollmann MW, van der Vegt MH, Kruis MR, Heesen M, Vos K, Pijl AJ, Dijkgraaf MG. Duloxetine in patients with central neuropathic pain caused by spinal cord injury or stroke: a randomized, double-blind, placebo-controlled trial. Pain 2011;152(2):267–273
41. Davidoff G, Guarracini M, Roth E, Sliwa J, Yarkony G. Trazodone hydrochloride in the treatment of dysesthetic pain in traumatic myelopathy: a randomized, double-blind, placebo-controlled study. Pain 1987;29(2):151–161
42. Levendoglu F, Ogun CO, Ozerbil O, Ogun TC, Ugurlu H. Gabapentin is a first line drug for the treatment of neuropathic pain in spinal cord injury. Spine (Phila Pa 1976) 2004;29(7):743–751
43. Tai Q, Kirshblum S, Chen B, Millis S, Johnston M, DeLisa JA. Gabapentin in the treatment of neuropathic pain after spinal cord injury: a prospective, randomized, double-blind, crossover trial. J Spinal Cord Med 2002;25(2):100–105
44. Finnerup NB, Sindrup SH, Bach FW, Johannesen IL, Jensen TS. Lamotrigine in spinal cord injury pain: a randomized controlled trial. Pain 2002;96(3):375–383
45. Finnerup NB, Grydehoj J, Bing J, Johannesen IL, Biering-Sorensen F, Sindrup SH, Jensen TS. Levetiracetam in spinal cord injury pain: a randomized controlled trial. Spinal Cord 2009;47(12):861–867
46. Siddall PJ, Cousins MJ, Otte A, Griesing T, Chambers R, Murphy TK. Pregabalin in central neuropathic pain associated with spinal cord injury: a placebo-controlled trial. Neurology 2006; 67(10):1792–1800
47. Vranken JH, Dijkgraaf MG, Kruis MR, van der Vegt MH, Hollmann MW, Heesen M. Pregabalin in patients with central neuropathic pain: a randomized, double-blind, placebo-controlled trial of a flexible-dose regimen. Pain 2008;136(1–2): 150–157
48. Drewes AM, Andreasen A, Poulsen LH. Valproate for treatment of chronic central pain after spinal cord injury. A double-blind cross-over study. Paraplegia 1994;32(8):565–569
49. Herman RM, D'Luzansky SC, Ippolito R. Intrathecal baclofen suppresses central pain in patients with spinal lesions. A pilot study. Clin J Pain 1992;8(4):338–345
50. Finnerup NB, Biering-Sorensen F, Johannesen IL, Terkelsen AJ, Juhl GI, Kristensen AD, Sindrup SH, Bach FW, Jensen TS. Intravenous lidocaine relieves spinal cord injury pain: a randomized controlled trial. Anesthesiology 2005;102(5):1023–1030
51. Attal N, Gaude V, Brasseur L, Dupuy M, Guirimand F, Parker F, Bouhassira D. Intravenous lidocaine in central pain: a double-blind, placebo-controlled, psychophysical study. Neurology 2000;54(3):564–574
52. Chiou-Tan FY, Tuel SM, Johnson JC, Priebe MM, Hirsh DD, Strayer JR. Effect of mexiletine on spinal cord injury dysesthetic pain. Am J Phys Med Rehabil 1996;75(2):84–87
53. Amr YM. Multi-day low dose ketamine infusion as adjuvant to oral gabapentin in spinal cord injury related chronic pain: a prospective, randomized, double blind trial. Pain Physician 2010;13(3):245–249
54. Attal N, Guirimand F, Brasseur L, Gaude V, Chauvin M, Bouhassira D. Effects of IV morphine in central pain: a randomized placebo-controlled study. Neurology 2002;58(4):554–563
55. Norrbrink C, Lundeberg T. Tramadol in neuropathic pain after spinal cord injury: a randomized, double-blind, placebo-controlled trial. Clin J Pain 2009;25(3):177–184
56. Siddall PJ, Molloy AR, Walker S, Mather LE, Rutkowski SB, Cousins MJ. The efficacy of intrathecal morphine and clonidine in the treatment of pain after spinal cord injury. Anesth Analg 2000;91(6):1493–1498
57. Rintala DH, Fiess RN, Tan G, Holmes SA, Bruel BM. Effect of dronabinol on central neuropathic pain after spinal cord injury: a pilot study. Am J Phys Med Rehabil 2010;89(10):840–848

18

Essentials of Spinal Cord Injury: Psychosocial Aspects of Spinal Cord Injury

Paul Kennedy and Emilie F. Smithson

Key Points

1. Depression is neither universal nor inevitable following SCI.
2. However, approximately one third of patients experience significant mood disorder postinjury.
3. Chronic neuropathic pain is common and complicates adjustment.
4. Coping Effectiveness Training reduces anxiety and depression postinjury.

Sustaining a spinal cord injury (SCI) leads to major changes in an individual's everyday life. The individual must adjust not only to a potential reduction in physical ability but also to changes in occupational status, in leisure activities, and in social and intimate relationships. The limited privacy of the hospital setting during rehabilitation and the increased reliance on nursing staff for intimate needs can intensify emotional reactions, and, faced with multiple stressors like these, it is not surprising that people with SCI can experience clinical anxiety, depression, and posttraumatic stress disorder (PTSD). The critical psychological issues over time are described in **Table 18.1**.

Depression

In a study by Migliorini and colleagues,[1] 37% of a community sample of individuals with SCI experienced depression, 30% anxiety, and 25% stress, and 8.4% met the diagnostic criteria for PTSD. A review by Craig and colleagues[2] estimated the frequency of depression during rehabilitation to be ~30%. Pollard and Kennedy[3] reported the longitudinal results of a study of emotional impact in people with SCI and found that rates of depression remained relatively stable after 10 years; 38% of the sample reached clinical cutoff scores on the Beck Depression Inventory at 12 weeks and 35% at 10 years postinjury.

Table 18.1 Key Psychological Issues
Acute phase
Screen for cognitive impairment
Check preinjury psychological/psychiatric status
Screen for posttraumatic stress disorder and acute stress disorder
Normalize emotional responses and convey safety
Provide support to family
Rehabilitation phase
Assess mood
Identify appraisals and coping strategies
Decatastrophize and challenge negative predictions
Provide access to effective role models
Provide individual psychological therapy for adjustment disorders
Provide group coping effectiveness training
Assess needs and arrange goal planning
Provide psychoeducation and peer counseling
Foster engagement in social activity and vocational planning
Predischarge phase
Promote self-management
Coordinate community visits
Finalize vocational goals
Engage in pain management
Provide psychosexual counseling
Arrange for community psychological support

However, contrary to the historical assumptions of Siller[4] regarding the psychological distress of patients following SCI, research has found it is neither universal nor necessary for individuals to experience depression during the process of adjustment to SCI, and that the majority of people sustaining an SCI go on to lead satisfying and rewarding lives. Furthermore, research has found that the presence of psychosocial adjustment problems following SCI is related more to emotional responses and coping than to injury or impairment variables,[5] and it has been suggested that psychopathology arises not as a direct result of the spinal injury itself but from the social, environmental, and health problems related to the injury.

Although suicide rates in SCI populations have been estimated to be up to six times higher than in the general population, the reliability of these estimations has been questioned by researchers due to the inclusion of people sustaining spinal injury following a suicide attempt[6]; thus their SCI would likely be due to preinjury psychological difficulties. A retrospective review of mortality in individuals sustaining an SCI following deliberate self-harm found that 24% of deaths were a result of suicide; however, over 60% of deaths could be attributed to medical complications, such as bladder infections.[6] In the SCI population, indirect forms of self-harm, such as self-neglect, are more prevalent than actual suicide attempts, which in turn can lead to potentially fatal medical complications, such as bladder infections and pressure ulcers (**Table 18.1**).

Concurrent Traumatic Brain Injury

The majority of individuals sustain SCIs due to traumatic circumstances, such as falls, traffic accidents, and sporting accidents,[7] and as a consequence it is not unusual for rehabilitation to be complicated by comorbid traumatic brain injury (TBI). Estimates of TBI in the SCI population range from 16 to 59%. However, Macciocchi and colleagues[8] argue that identification and classification of TBI are varied and at times unreliable. In a prospective study of 198 admissions to a traumatic SCI rehabilitation center, the research group used stringent diagnostic classification measures and found evidence that 60% of patients had also sustained a TBI. Cognitive impairments in attentional processes, memory, and problem solving have been estimated to be present in up to 50% of individuals with SCI.[9] The findings highlight the importance of performing early neuropsychological assessment to ensure that additional support is provided and patients' functional outcomes are maximized in rehabilitation. A review of the complications arising from brain injury highlights how cognitive deficits can interfere with the SCI patient's capacity to learn new compensatory skills and achieve optimum independence.[10] In addition to the complications arising from traumatic injury and factors like cerebral hypoxia and anoxia, cognitive functions and subsequent rehabilitation outcomes are also affected by preinjury substance or alcohol misuse.

Alcohol and Substance Abuse

Intoxication at time of injury has been implicated in 39 to 50% of SCI cases,[11,12] and preinjury alcohol use patterns are found to be strongly related to consumption following injury. Continued alcohol and substance misuse can have a detrimental effect on the individual's rehabilitation, leading to longer stays in the hospital and an increased likelihood of depression, pressure ulcers, and urinary tract infections.[13] Elliot and colleagues[14] found 23% of inpatients had significant alcohol problems and that these individuals not only scored higher on measures of depressive behavior but were over two and a half times more likely to develop a pressure sore in the 3 years following injury. Such variations in outcomes may be understood in terms of the coping strategies employed by people with substance misuse problems, which have been found to differ from those who do not abuse alcohol. Research has found substance misuse to be linked to greater use of avoidance coping strategies and less acceptance of injury,[15] which in turn has been associated with poorer adjustment and increased likelihood of psychological difficulties. Initial screening of patients to assess alcohol and substance misuse is beneficial when providing the enhanced care packages and support that such individuals require during rehabilitation.

In addition to the negative impact on rehabilitation and adjustment, people with alcohol problems report greater pain interference and intensity of pain following injury. Tate and colleagues[13] conducted a retrospective analysis of 3041 people with SCI and found that the 14% of participants classified as having alcohol abuse problems reported significantly worse pain outcomes and lower life satisfaction scores.

Chronic Pain

Prevalence estimates of chronic pain in SCI vary widely, with estimates ranging from 25 to 45%[16] up to 96%.[17] Pain interference is associated with lower scores on ratings of life satisfaction[18] and quality of life measures.[19] The presence of neuropathic pain has been related to lower scores on measures of physical health status[20] and has also been found to have a negative effect on occupational status after injury.[21] Higher ratings of pain have also been linked to affectivity and psychopathology, such as expressed anger and negative cognitions,[22] and higher pain severity has been linked to lower scores on measures of acceptance of injury[23] and greater catastrophizing.[24] A study of 190 individuals with SCI by Widerström-Noga and colleagues[25] found that a small group of individuals reported a low psychosocial impact of pain despite experiencing moderately high pain severity. When the characteristics of these individuals were explored, analysis revealed higher levels of positive interpersonal support from significant others compared with people with moderately high pain severity and high psychosocial impact. These findings reinforce the importance of social support to many aspects of rehabilitation and adjustment for people with SCI.

Role of Social Supports

Social support has been found to be related to psychological outcomes and adjustment after SCI,[26] has been identified as a predictor of early mortality,[27] and has been associated with low hopelessness and depression scores.[28] Qualitative research provides additional evidence for the importance of social support to the individual learning to live with spinal injury. Both family and peer support have been reported as facilitating the adjustment process, and patient feedback underscores the benefit of services providing informal support and advice to people with SCI throughout rehabilitation.

Following discharge from the hospital, family members often assume the role of primary caregivers, assisting with daily activities, such as feeding, dressing, and transfers, and with personal care, such as bladder and bowel management. Many family members adopt this new role with little or no education and support, and as a result encounter problems with overload, financial strain, impaired quality of life, and health and emotional problems.[29,30]

Contrary to early assumptions that assumed parental SCI to have a negative impact on children's adjustment, research has found children of fathers with SCI to be well adjusted, emotionally stable, and not affected in terms of body image, recreational interests, and personal relationships.[31] Alexander et al.[32] found no significant differences between children of mothers with SCI and children of able-bodied mothers on measures of personality. Ghidini and colleagues[33] investigated the impact of pregnancy and childbearing in women with SCI and found that 96% reported motherhood increased their quality of life and that they would consider having more children in the future. However, although the information available on pregnancy and childbearing during rehabilitation had not influenced the women's decisions to start families, only 11% of women asked felt that the information they received was adequate.

Sexuality Following Spinal Cord Injury

Following SCI, neurological changes frequently result in sexual dysfunction. Such difficulties can lead to emotional distress for individuals with SCI and have a negative impact on their quality of life. In addition to the changes in sexual function arising as a direct result of spinal trauma, patient concerns about bowel and bladder accidents, their altered body image, autonomic dysreflexia, pain interference, and spasticity have all been reported as factors that discourage the pursuit of physical relationships.[34] Using the responses to an Internet-based survey, Anderson and colleagues[34] found that the majority of respondents reported that SCI altered their sexual sense of self and that improvements in sexual function would improve their quality of life. Similarly, Phelps and colleagues[35] studied married/cohabiting men with SCI living in the community and found that 42% of respondents were dissatisfied with their sex lives and 50% experienced feelings of sexual inadequacy. In the first 18 months following discharge from hospital, sexual activity was reported as one of the areas with which people were most dissatisfied and was clearly an area in which rehabilitation services could be improved by the provision of further support and information.[36]

Determinants of Quality of Life and Postinjury Adjustment

When comparing ratings on quality of life measures, scores obtained from SCI populations are generally lower than those obtained from the general population.[5] However, in-depth analysis of these findings has revealed that ratings are linked to secondary complications, activity limitations, and barriers to participation,[37,38] rather than factors relating to the injury itself or degrees of physical ability[39,40]; the majority of people with SCI report themselves to be happy and satisfied with life.[41] Research has found scores on measures of life satisfaction to be directly related to involvement in productive activities, such as employment, and leisure pursuits.[42] Qualitative research into quality of life confirms quantitative findings that have highlighted the importance of meaningful relationships, responsibility, sense of control over one's own life, and engagement in meaningful activity in increasing the individual's quality of life.[43] Psychosocial issues, such as relationships, families, and peer group support,[44] and psychological factors, such as negative appraisals of disability,[45] are found to have a greater impact on functional outcomes than the neurological level of injury or impairment severity. A comprehensive review by Chevalier and colleagues[46] highlighted the important contributory role of appraisals and coping strategies in the long-term adjustment to spinal injury. Negative coping strategies, such as disengagement or avoidance, have been linked to increased levels of depression and emotional distress in persons with SCI,[47] and decreased levels of life satisfaction and participation.[48] A paper by Kennedy et al.[49] examined the relationships between initial appraisals of injury and subsequent coping responses. The study found that people who initially interpret the injury as a challenge are more likely to use adaptive coping strategies, such as acceptance. At 1 year, follow-up scores on measures of quality of life, anxiety, and depression were considerably better for individuals who viewed their injury as a challenge compared with those who initially interpreted their injury as a loss or a threat. The vast amount of literature and research into the relationship of appraisals, coping, and adjustment has led to the development of appraisal and coping measures specific to people with SCI—the Appraisals of Disability: Primary and Secondary Scale[50] and the Spinal Cord Lesion-Related Coping Strategies Questionnaire.[51] Not only can these measures be used to further our understanding of the adjustment process in people with SCI, but also they can assist in tailoring cognitive behavioral therapies to suit the specific appraisal and coping patterns of the individual.

Cognitive Behavioral Therapy and Other Psychological Interventions

As is the case in other psychological services, cognitive-behavioral approaches are the most commonly used therapeutic intervention in the SCI population due to the strong evidence base for positive outcomes. Cognitive behavioral therapy (CBT) may be used to challenge negative cognitions about disability, support patients during the acute phase of injury, or continue with ongoing care for those with a preexisting history of psychological problems. Craig and colleagues[52] found that patients receiving CBT during hospital admission were less likely to be readmitted 2 years after injury, less likely to use prescription or illegal drugs, and more likely to report themselves as having adjusted to living with SCI compared with a control group receiving care as usual.

The association between appraisals and coping strategies and scores on measures of anxiety and depression[47,49] has led to the development of psychoeducational intervention programs specifically tailored for use in the SCI population. Coping Effectiveness Training (CET)[15] aims to equip patients with the knowledge and the confidence to apply adaptive coping strategies to managing the changes arising from a spinal injury. A study by Kennedy and colleagues[15] compared patients completing the CET program with those receiving standard care and found significantly reduced anxiety and depression scores in the intervention group compared with controls. In addition to the psychological benefits, qualitative data obtained from patients participating in CET highlighted the importance of group discussion to the newly injured person and the benefit of information sharing with peers, thus reiterating the need for services that provide patients with the opportunity for informal peer support during rehabilitation.

Norrbrink Budh et al.[53] developed a comprehensive cognitive, behavioral, and educational program specifically for individuals with SCI and neuropathic pain. Although no significant changes in pain intensity were found following the intervention, results from a 12-month follow-up revealed decreased levels of anxiety and depression compared with baseline measures, suggesting the intervention enabled patients to cope effectively with their pain and to minimize the psychological impact.

Goal Planning

The overarching aim of SCI rehabilitation is to provide the individual with the necessary skills and the confidence to manage the changes and challenges arising from injury. This has been implemented in clinical care with the Needs Assessment and Goal Planning Program, which is integrated into patient care at the National Spinal Injuries Centre (NSIC) at Stoke Mandeville Hospital, Aylesbury, England. Goal setting theory has endorsed the individual's involvement in the process as essential to its success and maintenance of change. In SCI, the patient may have to relearn basic skills and also acquire new techniques to maintain health in addition to receiving large amounts of information and advice on aspects of their injury. The Needs Assessment Checklist (NAC)[54] functions to identify areas of need through standardized assessment of knowledge and ability across rehabilitation domains. What differentiates this measure from most outcome measures, and makes it particularly suitable to the SCI population, is the acknowledgment of both physical and verbal independence. From the NAC, key areas of need are identified, and the multidisciplinary team works with the patient in a goal-planning meeting to set clear, identifiable, and achievable goals to work toward during rehabilitation. Following the introduction of the program at the NSIC, patients spent more time participating in therapy and involved in rehabilitation activities, thus demonstrating goal planning to be an effective way of reducing patient disengagement and of increasing their activity levels and involvement in therapy.

Conclusion

SCI is much more than an injury to the spinal cord. It leads to profound changes in everyday life—leisure, activity, employment, and relationships—and has a substantial impact on psychological health and personality. Most people with SCI leave the hospital to return to satisfying and fulfilling lives, enjoy strong and rewarding relationships with family and friends, and participate in a variety of leisure activities. However, for some, the impact on their lives is such that they experience enduring adjustment difficulties that can lead to significant psychological problems. The issues discussed here have highlighted the need for comprehensive, person-centered rehabilitation services incorporating theoretical models of appraisals, coping, and adjustment into therapeutic care.

Pearls

- Up to one third of people with SCI have treatable depression.
- There is a high prevalence of chronic pain that complicates adjustment.

Pitfalls

- Traumatic brain injury is underdiagnosed.
- Failure to address psychological and adjustment issues will limit functional outcomes.

References

1. Migliorini C, Tonge B, Taleporos G. Spinal cord injury and mental health. Aust N Z J Psychiatry 2008;42(4):309–314
2. Craig A, Tran Y, Middleton J. Psychological morbidity and spinal cord injury: a systematic review. Spinal Cord 2009;47(2):108–114
3. Pollard C, Kennedy P. A longitudinal analysis of emotional impact, coping strategies and post-traumatic psychological growth following spinal cord injury: a 10-year review. Br J Health Psychol 2007;12(Pt 3):347–362
4. Siller J. Psychological situation of the disabled with spinal cord injuries. Rehabil Lit 1969; 30(10):290–296
5. Martz E, Livneh H, Priebe M, Wuermser LA, Ottomanelli L. Predictors of psychosocial adaptation among people with spinal cord injury or disorder. Arch Phys Med Rehabil 2005;86(6): 1182–1192
6. Kennedy P, Rogers B, Speer S, Frankel H. Spinal cord injuries and attempted suicide: a retrospective review. Spinal Cord 1999;37(12):847–852
7. Spinal Cord Injury Information Network. Spinal Cord Injury Facts and Statistics at a Glance. April 2009. http://images.main.aub.edu/spinalcord/pdffiles/factsApr09.pdf. Accessed August 2009
8. Macciocchi S, Seel RT, Thompson N, Byams R, Bowman B. Spinal cord injury and co-occurring traumatic brain injury: assessment and incidence. Arch Phys Med Rehabil 2008;89(7): 1350–1357
9. Davidoff GN, Roth EJ, Richards JS. Cognitive deficits in spinal cord injury: epidemiology and outcome. Arch Phys Med Rehabil 1992;73(3):275–284
10. Arzaga D, Shaw V, Vasile AT. Dual diagnoses: the person with a spinal cord injury and a concomitant brain injury. SCI Nurs 2003;20(2): 86–92
11. Heinemann AW, Keen M, Donohue R, Schnoll S. Alcohol use by persons with recent spinal cord injury. Arch Phys Med Rehabil 1988;69(8): 619–624
12. Burke DA, Linden RD, Zhang YP, Maiste AC, Shields CB. Incidence rates and populations at risk for spinal cord injury: A regional study. Spinal Cord 2001;39(5):274–278
13. Tate DG, Forchheimer MB, Krause JS, Meade MA, Bombardier CH. Patterns of alcohol and substance use and abuse in persons with spinal cord injury: risk factors and correlates. Arch Phys Med Rehabil 2004;85(11):1837–1847
14. Elliot TR, Kurylo M, Chen Y, Hicken B. Alcohol abuse history and adjustment following spinal cord injury. Rehabil Psychol 2002;47:278–290
15. Kennedy P, Duff J, Evans M, Beedie A. Coping effectiveness training reduces depression and anxiety following traumatic spinal cord injuries. Br J Clin Psychol 2003;42(Pt 1):41–52
16. Richards JS. Chronic pain and spinal cord injury: review and comment. Clin J Pain 1992;8(2): 119–122
17. Dijkers M, Bryce T, Zanca J. Prevalence of chronic pain after traumatic spinal cord injury: a systematic review. J Rehabil Res Dev 2009;46(1): 13–29
18. Budh CN, Osteråker AL. Life satisfaction in individuals with a spinal cord injury and pain. Clin Rehabil 2007;21(1):89–96
19. Putzke JD, Richards JS, Hicken BL, DeVivo MJ. Interference due to pain following spinal cord injury: important predictors and impact on quality of life. Pain 2002;100(3):231–242
20. Noonan VK, Kopec JA, Zhang H, Dvorak MF. Impact of associated conditions resulting from spinal cord injury on health status and quality of life in people with traumatic central cord syndrome. Arch Phys Med Rehabil 2008;89(6):1074–1082
21. Meade MA, Barrett K, Ellenbogen PS, Jackson MN. Work intensity and variations in health and personal characteristics of individuals with spinal cord injury (SCI). J Vocat Rehabil 2006;25:13–19
22. Summers JD, Rapoff MA, Varghese G, Porter K, Palmer RE. Psychosocial factors in chronic spinal cord injury pain. Pain 1991;47(2):183–189
23. Wade JB, Price DD, Hamer RM, Schwartz SM, Hart RP. An emotional component analysis of chronic pain. Pain 1990;40(3):303–310
24. Turner JA, Jensen MP, Warms CA, Cardenas DD. Catastrophizing is associated with pain intensity, psychological distress, and pain-related disability among individuals with chronic pain after spinal cord injury. Pain 2002;98(1-2):127–134
25. Widerström-Noga EG, Felix ER, Cruz-Almeida Y, Turk DC. Psychosocial subgroups in persons with spinal cord injuries and chronic pain. Arch Phys Med Rehabil 2007;88(12):1628–1635
26. North NT. The psychological effects of spinal cord injury: a review. Spinal Cord 1999;37(10): 671–679
27. Krause JS, Carter RE. Risk of mortality after spinal cord injury: relationship with social support, education, and income. Spinal Cord 2009;47(8): 592–596
28. Beedie A, Kennedy P. Quality of social support predicts hopelessness and depression post spinal cord injury. J Clin Psychol Med Settings 2002;9:227–234
29. Vitaliano PP, Zhang J, Scanlan JM. Is caregiving hazardous to one's physical health? A meta-analysis. Psychol Bull 2003;129(6):946–972
30. Post MWM, Bloemen J, de Witte LP. Burden of support for partners of persons with spinal cord injuries. Spinal Cord 2005;43(5):311–319
31. Buck FM, Hohmann GW. Personality, behavior, values, and family relations of children of fathers with spinal cord injury. Arch Phys Med Rehabil 1981;62(9):432–438
32. Alexander CJ, Hwang K, Sipski ML. Mothers with spinal cord injuries: impact on marital, family, and children's adjustment. Arch Phys Med Rehabil 2002;83(1):24–30
33. Ghidini A, Healey A, Andreani M, Simonson MR. Pregnancy and women with spinal cord injuries. Obstet Gynecol Surv 2009;64:141–142
34. Anderson KD, Borisoff JF, Johnson RD, Stiens SA, Elliott SL. The impact of spinal cord injury on sexual function: concerns of the general population. Spinal Cord 2007;45(5):328–337
35. Phelps J, Albo M, Dunn K, Joseph A. Spinal cord injury and sexuality in married or partnered men: activities, function, needs, and predictors of

sexual adjustment. Arch Sex Behav 2001;30(6): 591–602
36. Kennedy P, Sherlock O, McClelland M, Short D, Royle J, Wilson C. A multi-centre study of the community needs of people with spinal cord injuries: the first 18 months. Spinal Cord 2010;48(1): 15–20
37. Barker RN, Kendall MD, Amsters DI, Pershouse KJ, Haines TP, Kuipers P. The relationship between quality of life and disability across the lifespan for people with spinal cord injury. Spinal Cord 2009;47(2):149–155
38. Lund ML, Nordlund A, Bernspång B, Lexell J. Perceived participation and problems in participation are determinants of life satisfaction in people with spinal cord injury. Disabil Rehabil 2007;29(18):1417–1422
39. Westgren N, Levi R. Quality of life and traumatic spinal cord injury. Arch Phys Med Rehabil 1998;79(11):1433–1439
40. Manns PJ, Chad KE. Determining the relation between quality of life, handicap, fitness, and physical activity for persons with spinal cord injury. Arch Phys Med Rehabil 1999;80(12):1566–1571
41. Carpenter C, Forwell SJ, Jongbloed LE, Backman CL. Community participation after spinal cord injury. Arch Phys Med Rehabil 2007;88(4): 427–433
42. Schönherr MC, Groothoff JW, Mulder GA, Eisma WH. Participation and satisfaction after spinal cord injury: results of a vocational and leisure outcome study. Spinal Cord 2005;43(4):241–248
43. Whalley Hammell K. Quality of life after spinal cord injury: a meta-synthesis of qualitative findings. Spinal Cord 2007;45(2):124–139
44. Holicky R, Charlifue S. Ageing with spinal cord injury: the impact of spousal support. Disabil Rehabil 1999;21(5-6):250–257
45. Kennedy P, Smithson E, McClelland M, Short D, Royle J, Wilson C. Life satisfaction, appraisals and functional outcomes in spinal cord-injured people living in the community. Spinal Cord 2010; 48(2):144–148
46. Chevalier Z, Kennedy P, Sherlock O. Spinal cord injury, coping and psychological adjustment: a literature review. Spinal Cord 2009;47(11): 778–782
47. Kennedy P, Marsh N, Lowe R, Grey N, Short E, Rogers B. A longitudinal analysis of psychological impact and coping strategies following spinal cord injury. Br J Health Psychol 2000;5:157–172
48. Hansen N, Tate D. Avoidance coping, perceived handicap, and coping strategies of persons with spinal cord injury. SCI Psychosocial Processes 1994;7:195
49. Kennedy P, Lude P, Elfström ML, Smithson E. Cognitive appraisals, coping and quality of life outcomes: a multi-centre study of spinal cord injury rehabilitation. Spinal Cord 2010;48(10):762–769
50. Dean RE, Kennedy P. Measuring appraisals following acquired spinal cord injury: a preliminary psychometric analysis of the appraisals of disability. Rehabil Psychol 2009;54(2):222–231
51. Elfström ML, Rydén A, Kreuter M, Persson LO, Sullivan M. Linkages between coping and psychological outcome in the spinal cord lesioned: development of SCL-related measures. Spinal Cord 2002;40(1):23–29
52. Craig A, Hancock K, Dickson H. Improving the long-term adjustment of spinal cord injured persons. Spinal Cord 1999;37(5):345–350
53. Norrbrink Budh C, Kowalski J, Lundeberg T. A comprehensive pain management programme comprising educational, cognitive and behavioural interventions for neuropathic pain following spinal cord injury. J Rehabil Med 2006; 38(3):172–180
54. Kennedy P, Hamilton LR. The needs assessment checklist: a clinical approach to measuring outcome. Spinal Cord 1999;37(2):136–139

19

Posttraumatic Kyphotic Deformity of the Cervical Spine

Kris E. Radcliff, David Gendelberg, Gurusukhman D. S. Sidhu, and Alexander R. Vaccaro

Key Points

1. The absolute indication for surgery for posttraumatic kyphotic deformity is progressive neurological deficit. Isolated progression of kyphosis more than 5 degrees is considered by some authors to be a relative indication for reconstruction for impending instability.
2. Anterior release and reconstruction facilitate mobilization of the spine and direct decompression of the neural elements. Posterior reconstruction enhances stability and restoration of lordosis.
3. The reported complication rate of circumferential reconstruction is 33% in the literature, with a 5% permanent complication rate usually related to anterior structures. Preoperative patient counseling is essential.

Kyphosis is a common deformity after a variety of cervical spine traumatic injuries.[1] The pathogenesis of kyphosis is an alteration of the biomechanics of the cervical spine. The normal cervical spine sagittal alignment is 40 degrees of lordosis, with the result that the weight-bearing axis of the spine lies in the posterior vertebral body and posterior elements.[2,3] Kyphosis may lead to progressive kyphotic deformity, compromise of the adjacent spinal motion segments, and potentially even neurological symptoms. Kyphosis shifts the weight-bearing axis of the spine anteriorly, increasing the axial load on the vertebral bodies and disks. As kyphosis increases, so does the flexion movement, thereby increasing the likelihood of adjacent segment changes and progressive deformity. Cervical kyphosis may also result in compression of the anterior spinal cord against the posterior aspect of the vertebral body at the apex of the deformity (**Fig. 19.1**). This shift leads to increased mechanical stress on the anterior aspect of the spinal cord and possible ischemia.[4,5,6,7]

Clinically, a consequence of loss of bony ligamentous competence is often a loss of alignment. Kyphosis may develop after any injury morphology, including compression, distraction, or translation.[8] Compressive injuries may result in insufficiency of the vertebral bodies to manage axial load. Distractive injuries may result in kyphosis, either gradually due to posterior ligamentous laxity, disk injury with resultant disk

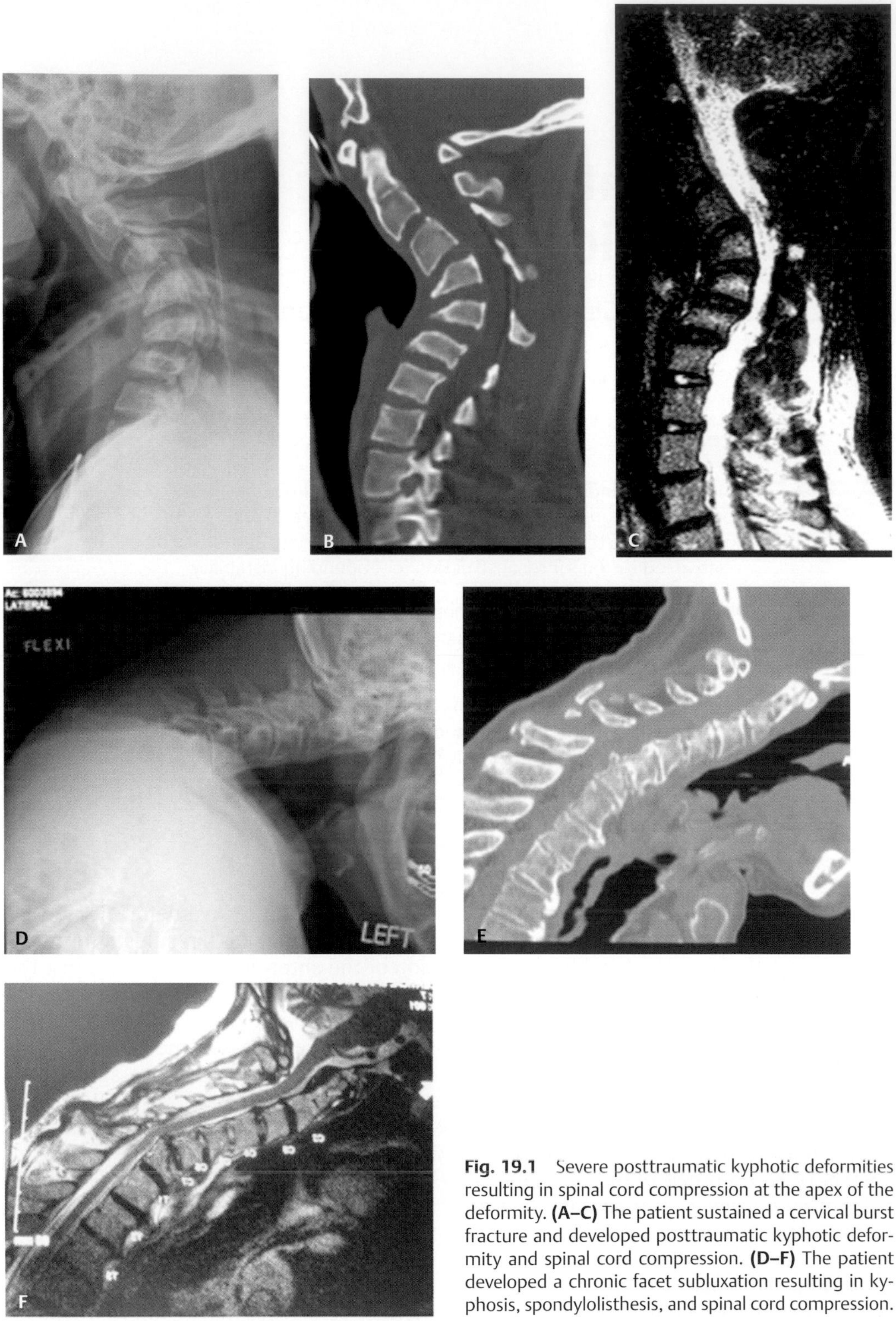

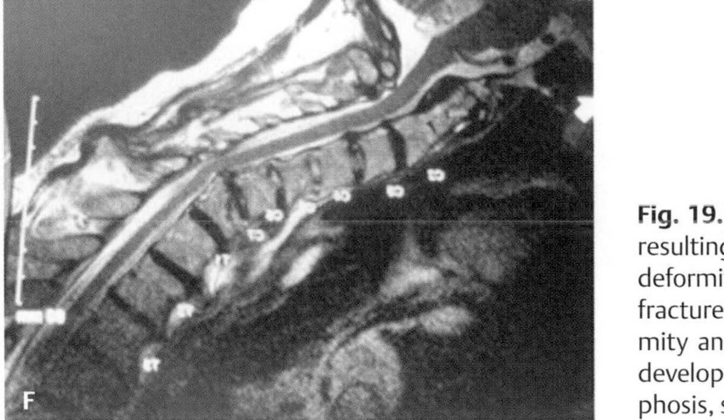

Fig. 19.1 Severe posttraumatic kyphotic deformities resulting in spinal cord compression at the apex of the deformity. **(A–C)** The patient sustained a cervical burst fracture and developed posttraumatic kyphotic deformity and spinal cord compression. **(D–F)** The patient developed a chronic facet subluxation resulting in kyphosis, spondylolisthesis, and spinal cord compression.

desiccation, and spondylosis, or acutely due to late dislocation and instability. Translation may result from flexion compression or flexion distraction injuries. Spondylolisthesis results in relative kyphosis of the motion segment.

The precise incidence of posttraumatic kyphosis is variable depending upon the injury and its treatment. The rate of kyphotic deformity appears to be highest after conservative treatment of cervical compressive injuries. Koivikko et al. reported on the radiographic outcome of conservative and operative treatment of cervical burst fractures.[9] Mean kyphosis in the conservatively treated patients (12.6 ± 10 degrees) was greater than that in the anterior cervical decompression and fusion (ACDF)-plating group (–2.2 ± 13.9 degrees) ($p = 0.00003$). Furthermore, kyphotic deformity progressed late in 8/34 patients in the conservative treatment group and in 4/35 surgically treated patients. There were no neurological deficits reported with progression of kyphosis. Fisher et al. studied patients with flexion teardrop (compression) injuries and found increased mean kyphosis of 11.4 degrees (range, 0 to 35 degrees) in the halo-thoracic vest (HTV) group compared with the anterior cervical plating group (3.5 degrees, 0 to 14°).[10] Furthermore, five patients in the HTV group were classified as failures, with average kyphosis of 4 degrees.

Distraction injuries, conservatively or operatively managed, may result in loss of cervical lordosis. Lifeso and Colucci retrospectively reviewed the outcomes of 29 patients with cervical flexion distraction injuries and reported that, following posterior fusion, there was a 27% failure rate (3/11) related to late kyphosis.[11] Of the 18 patients treated with an ACDF, there was no late collapse, pseudarthrosis, or persistent radiculopathy. Woodworth et al. report that 1 of 17 (5.8%) patients with posterior ligamentous injury treated with ACDF went on to a progressive kyphotic deformity.[12] The patient remained neurologically intact and fused in a kyphotic position and required no further treatment. In a retrospective review of patients who underwent treatment for flexion distraction injuries, Johnson et al. identify a 13% incidence of radiographic failures after ACDF-plating associated with end plate fracture and facet fracture. Of the 11 patients who developed radiographic failure, nine had a pseudarthrosis and significant pain and two had a solid fusion and no pain. There were no neurological deficits associated with progression of radiographic deformity.[13]

Posttraumatic kyphotic deformity may develop as a result of iatrogenic removal of the posterior tension band (i.e., laminectomy). The development of postlaminectomy kyphosis secondary to multilevel cervical laminectomies has been well described in both the pediatric and adult populations, with frequencies as high as 50% and 14%, respectively.[14,15,16,17]

Clinical signs of posttraumatic cervical kyphotic deformity may include neurological deficit, neck pain, or change in posture. Any changes in neurological status or pain in a patient who has previously sustained cervical spine trauma should prompt aggressive clinical evaluation and imaging. The differential diagnosis of posttraumatic kyphotic cervical spine deformity includes infectious, neoplastic, Charcot degeneration, or compensatory changes as a result of trauma to contiguous and noncontiguous spinal levels.

The gold standard for diagnosis of posttraumatic kyphotic deformity of the cervical spine is lateral upright radiographs. Pertinent radiographic findings include the nature of the deformity, whether it is focal or global, the presence of translational deformities, overall alignment and horizontal gaze, and compensatory deformities. The etiology of the deformity may be identified more clearly with magnetic resonance imaging (MRI) or computed tomographic (CT) scan. MRI offers superior resolution of diskoligamentous injuries, which may guide treatment by illustrating the presence or absence of significant anterior thecal sac compression. MRI, due to its sensitivity, may also demonstrate injury to supportive soft tissue structures, such as the facet capsules, ligamentum flavum, or interspinous ligaments, and thereby allow for earlier treatment prior to the development of a spinal deformity. Lambiris et al. identified two cases of cervical flexion distraction injuries where an injury to the intervertebral disk would have been addressed if MRI had been used for diagnosis.[18] However, by the time the posttraumatic kyphotic deformity develops, usually the injury to the disk or facet capsules is manifested by morphological changes, such as desiccation, ankylosis, or subluxation. Superior bony resolution is well visualized with the use of CT.

The absolute indication for treatment of a posttraumatic kyphotic deformity is a progressive neurological deficit associated with spinal cord compression (**Fig. 19.1**). A relative indication for treatment of a kyphotic deformity involves progression of deformity over time. There is controversy over the best radiographic method to measure alignment and kyphosis.[19] Some authors define progression of the Cobb angle measurement of more than 5 degrees as a potential indication for treatment of a kyphotic deformity.[9,12] Based on White-Panjabi analysis, Johnson et al. defined radiographic failure of treatment operatively or nonoperatively as vertebral translation greater than 3.5 mm and/or a change in vertebral angulation greater than 11 degrees or device failure in the interval between the immediate postop film and the most recent follow-up radiograph.[13] However, a recent meta-analysis of the literature found that the interobserver reliability of Cobb angle measurement is 0.74 for evaluation of cervical arthrodesis success after ACDF, compared with 0.95 for spinous process tip distance measurement.[20] Thus, interspinous process distance may be a more reliable measurement technique for the assessment of posttraumatic kyphosis progression.

The principle of treatment of posttraumatic kyphotic deformity is avoidance of tension on the spinal cord. In the setting of a cervical kyphotic deformity that requires surgical correction, there are three approaches: anterior, posterior, or a combined anterior-posterior approach. Deformity correction may be effected by shortening of the posterior spinal column and lengthening of the anterior spinal column with an axis of rotation within or anterior to the spinal cord. The anterior approach allows for the direct removal of ventral compressive lesions via diskectomy and/or corpectomy as well as release on the concavity side of the deformity via resection of osteophytes and the joints of Luschka. However, in the presence of an incompetent posterior tension band, anterior decompression and reconstruction alone has been associated with graft complications, such as displacement, pseudarthrosis, and postoperative instability.[21,22] Reconstruction after diskectomy and fusion may be associated with improved lordosis and reduced risk of graft dislodgment compared with cervical corpectomy (**Fig. 19.2**). However, corpectomy offers an improved neural decompression, particularly in the setting of an ossified posterior longitudinal ligament behind the vertebral body, compared with diskectomy (**Fig. 19.3**). The posterior longitudinal ligament is preserved, if possible, to act as a hinge at the time of deformity correction so as to limit spinal cord lengthening.[23] Anterior instrumentation may prohibit any further realignment following a posterior procedure. If there is significant instability or soft bone quality, then an additional anterior approach should be considered to "lock in" the construct once the realignment is complete.

The main advantages of dorsal surgery are the relative ease of multilevel decompression and improved biomechanical strength of instrumentation. Reconstruction in the setting of kyphosis correction usually consists of posterior instrumentation two to three levels cephalad and caudad to the apex level of correction. Either cervical lateral mass screws, pedicle screws, or wiring may be used. Posterior instrumentation has been shown to be biomechanically stronger than anterior instrumentation in axial rotation and lateral bending. Pedicle screws extend anterior to the instant axis of rotation of the spine and may be biomechanically superior to anterior fixation in flexion and extension.[24] Abumi et al. demonstrated that mild degenerative kyphosis can be corrected entirely posteriorly with cervical pedicle screw fixation.[25] At follow-up, the average

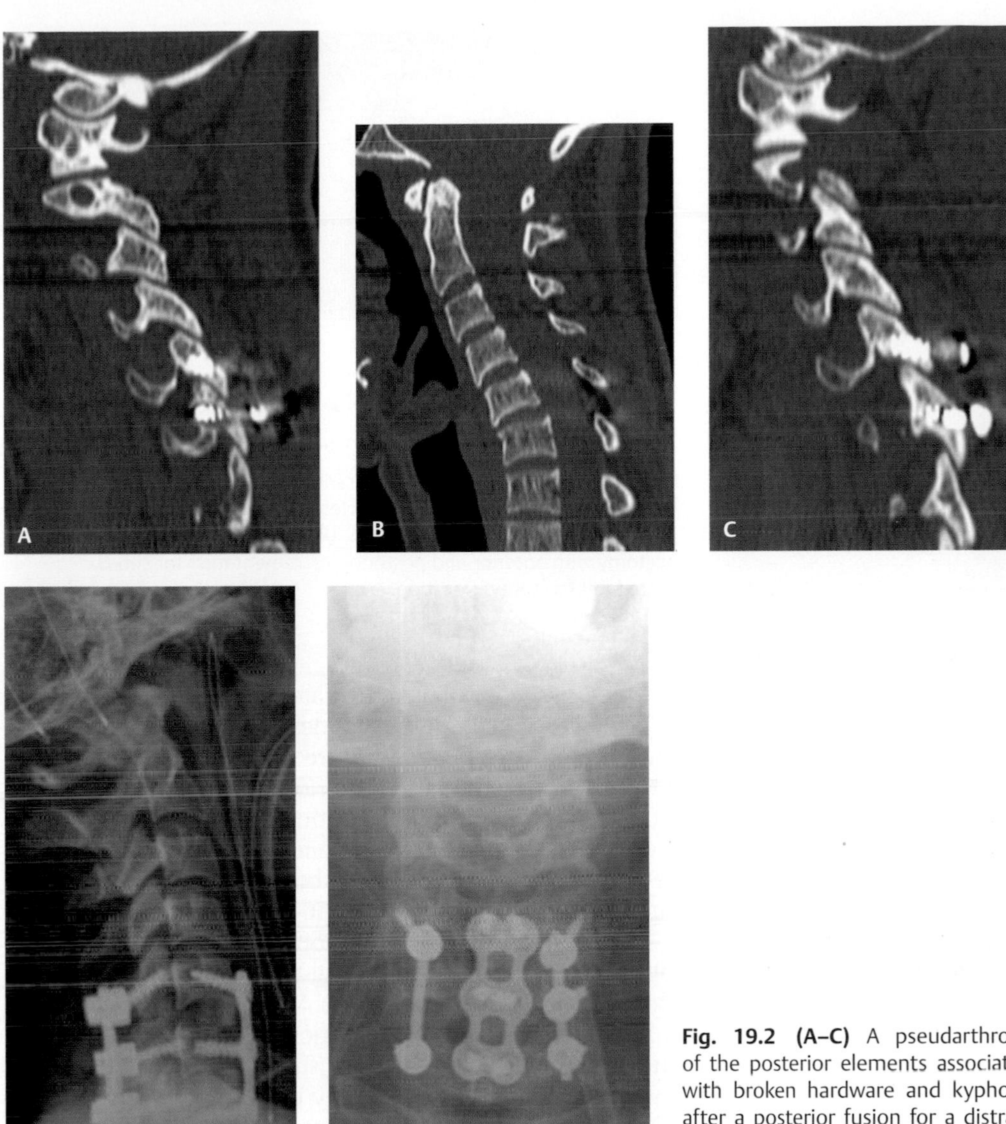

Fig. 19.2 (A–C) A pseudarthrosis of the posterior elements associated with broken hardware and kyphosis after a posterior fusion for a distraction injury. (D,E) The attainment of postoperative lordosis following anterior and posterior reconstruction.

correction went from 30.8 to 0.5 degrees of kyphosis.[26,27] **Figure 19.4** is an example of a patient with posttraumatic kyphosis from a chronic facet dislocation who underwent posterior correction with pedicle screws and a localized osteotomy.

Osteotomy and release of the spine are important components of correction of posttraumatic kyphosis. Provisional fixation using a provisional rod during the bony resection is advised to prevent unexpected changes in vertebral alignment.[28] Similar to thoracolumbar spine deformity surgery, a Smith-Peterson osteotomy may be considered to shorten the posterior column. A cervicothoracic junction osteotomy with and without instrumentation has been well described for the correction of the chin-on-chest deformity in ankylosing spondylitis.[29,30] The sequence of resection includes laminectomy at the level of correction, partial laminectomy of the cepha-

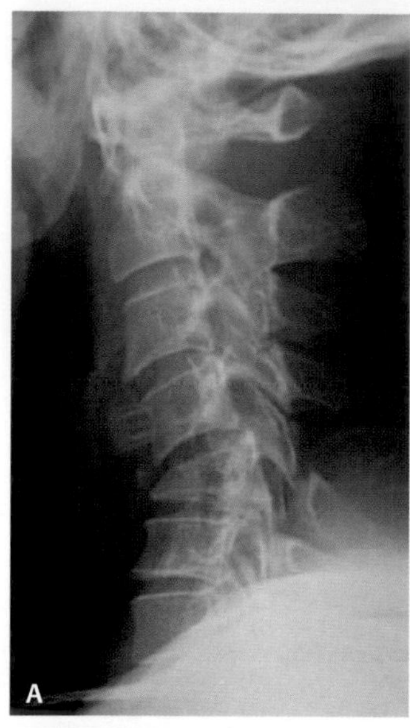

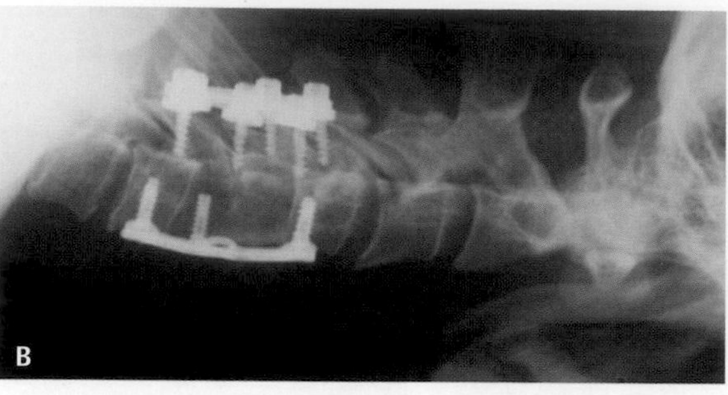

Fig. 19.3 **(A)** Preoperative lateral radiograph displays flexion compression injury resulting in vertebral body fracture with combined facet fracture dislocation. **(B)** Anterior cervical corpectomy with anterior and posterior instrumentation for subacute facet fracture dislocation.

lad and caudad levels, and facetectomy. **Figure 19.4** illustrates a superior facetectomy to facilitate reduction of a chronic facet dislocation. During resection, extreme care must be taken to avoid injury to the exiting spinal nerve root or vertebral artery. Transpedicular resection may also be indicated in rare cases of posttraumatic kyphotic cervical deformity.[31]

Realignment is actually performed once the osteotomy is complete. At the authors' institution, the surgeon breaks scrub and manipulates cervical alignment via the Mayfield head holder to improve the degree of cervical lordosis. The surgeon continuously watches the spinal cord over the drapes at the head of the table and controls the head once the circulating nurse has unlocked the Mayfield brake. The surgeon translates the head posteriorly while monitoring the spinal cord for excessive infolding as a result of lordosis. Care must be taken during an adjunctive posterior procedure in the absence of anterior instrumentation not to inadvertently dislodge an anterior graft. After realignment, motor evoked potentials are tested.

There are a myriad of complications associated with the surgical management of a cervical kyphotic deformity. The anterior approach commonly includes risks of dysphagia, dysphonia, hematoma, and infection. Representative examples of graft dislodgment (**Fig. 19.5**) and severe anterior hematoma (**Fig. 19.6**) after anterior cervical corpectomy are illustrated. To reduce the risk of graft dislodgment in the absence of anterior instrumentation, care must be taken to avoid extending the cervical spine during patient rotation to the prone position and also to avoid pushing anteriorly during the posterior dissection or instrumentation. Mummaneni et al. reported a 33% complication rate after combined anterior-posterior surgery for cervical kyphosis. The majority of the complications were related to the anterior approach. Significant anterior approach complications included a 13% percutaneous endoscopic gastrostomy tube/tracheostomy (PEG/Trach) rate and two deaths within 1 year after surgery. There were no new neurological deficits postoperatively.[32] Schultz et al. reviewed the outcomes of 78 patients who underwent single-stage anterior-posterior cervical decompression and fusion, of which 15 cases were performed for postlaminectomy kyphosis.[33] Although the immediate complication rate was high (32%), most problems were transient, yielding a long-term complication rate of only 5% related to the anterior approach. Neurological worsening was not observed in the trauma or postlaminectomy kyphosis patients.

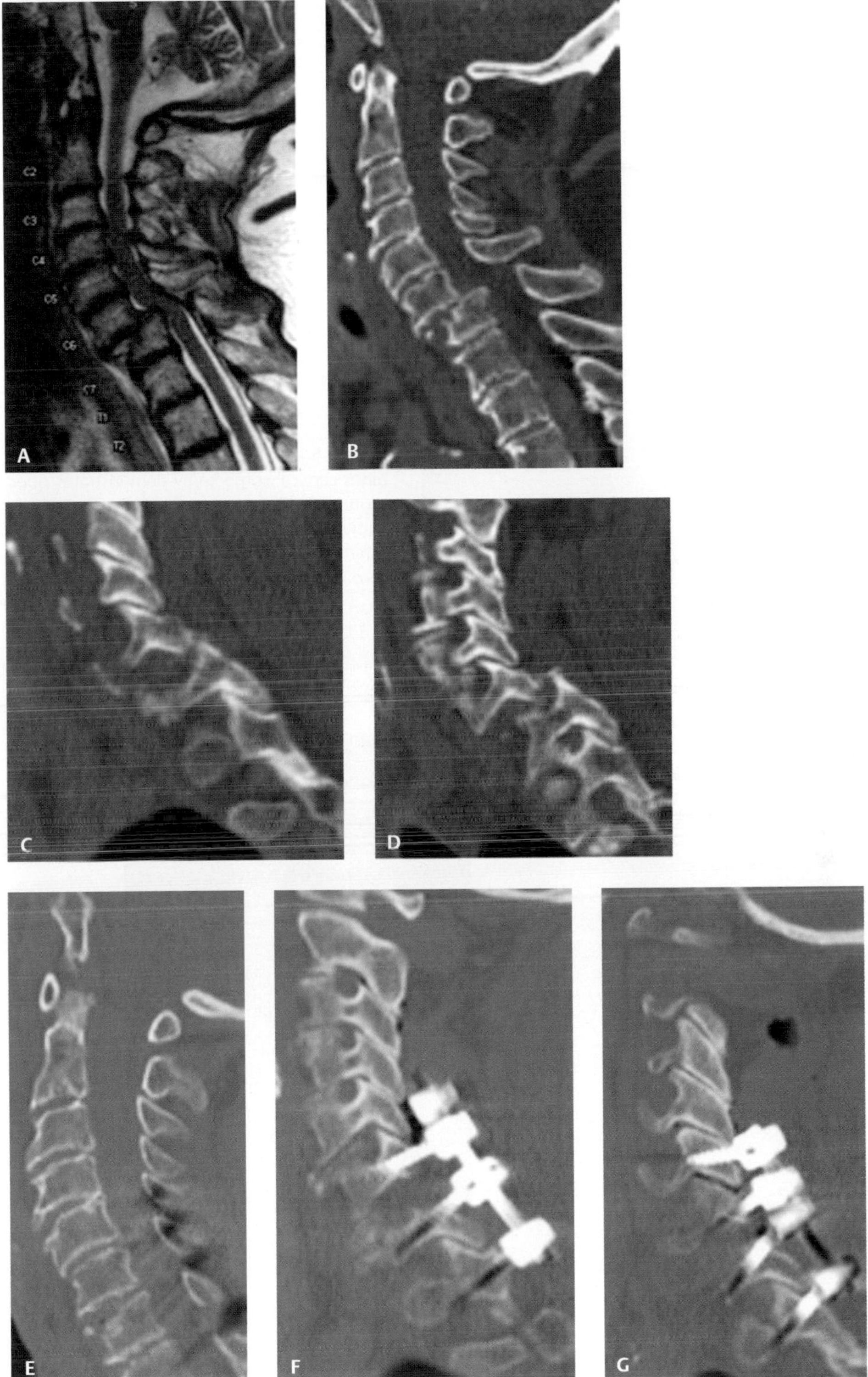

Fig. 19.4 The use of C6-T1 pedicle screws and facetectomy for mobilization of a chronic facet injury. **(A,B)** Spondylolisthesis and spinal cord compression. **(C, D)** Chronic facet subluxation and fracture. **(E–G)** Postoperative reconstruction.

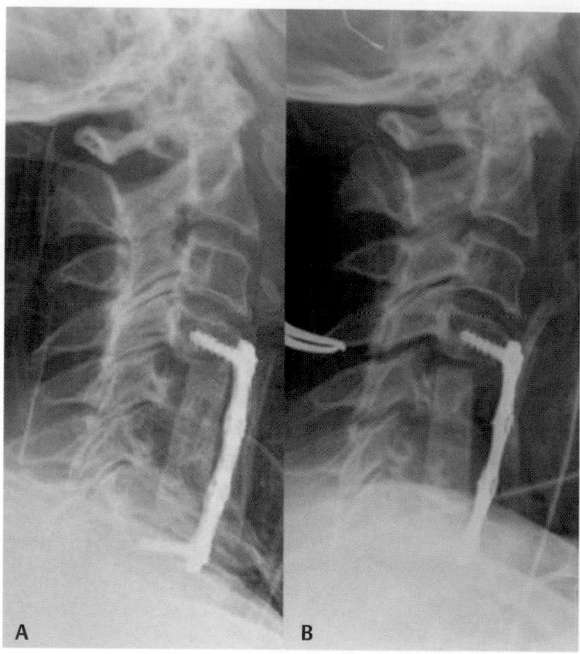

Fig. 19.5 **(A)** Lateral radiograph after an anterior cervical corpectomy demonstrates good alignment. **(B)** Lateral radiograph after intraoperative repositioning to prone position displays subluxation of bone graft resulting in spinal cord injury.

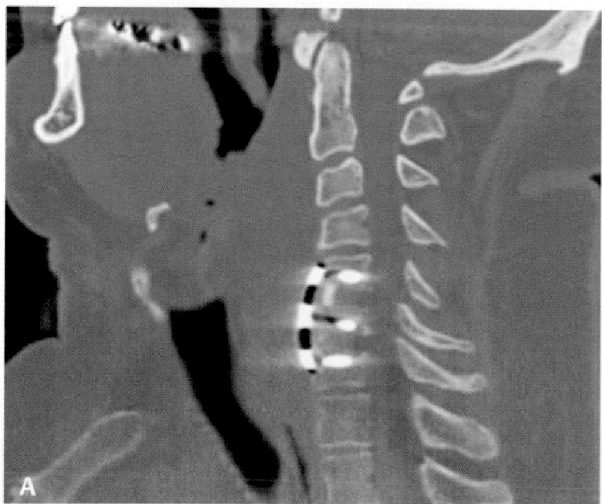

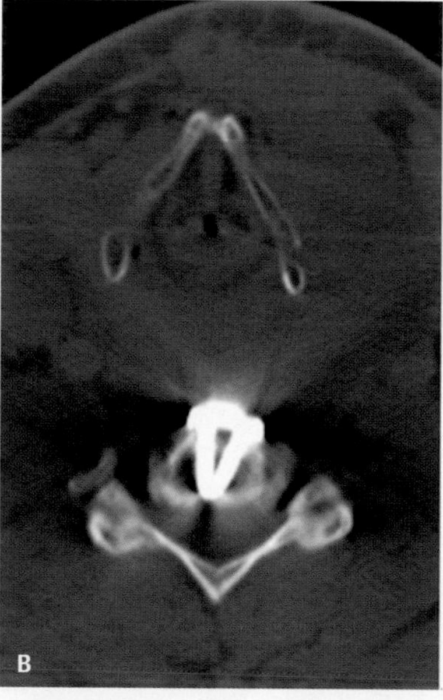

Fig. 19.6 **(A)** Midsagittal and **(B)** axial noncontrast CT scans demonstrating large hematoma anterior to a cervical diskectomy and fusion compromising the airway.

Spinal nerve root palsy may result from posterior drift of the spinal cord. **Figure 19.7** illustrates a patient with a severe posttraumatic kyphotic cervical deformity who developed profound C5 and C6 palsies after an anterior corpectomy with 15 mm of interbody distraction. It is possible that preservation of the posterior longitudinal ligament (PLL) as a fulcrum for angular correction, rather than distraction, may reduce the incidence of isolated nerve root palsy. Patients should be counseled about the increased risk of hardware complications after these cases.

In conclusion, posttraumatic kyphotic cervical deformity is a challenging clinical problem. The absolute indication for surgical intervention is a progressive neurological deficit associated with increasing kyphosis. Surgery is complex and usually involves combined anterior and posterior reconstructions. The complication rate is high and is more frequent with anterior approaches and often involves disturbance of anterior soft tissue function, such as swallowing and dysphagia. Neurological complications are fortunately rare. Modern posterior instrumentation systems with lateral mass and pedicle screws facilitate complex reconstruction of the spine and often result in satisfactory clinical outcomes.

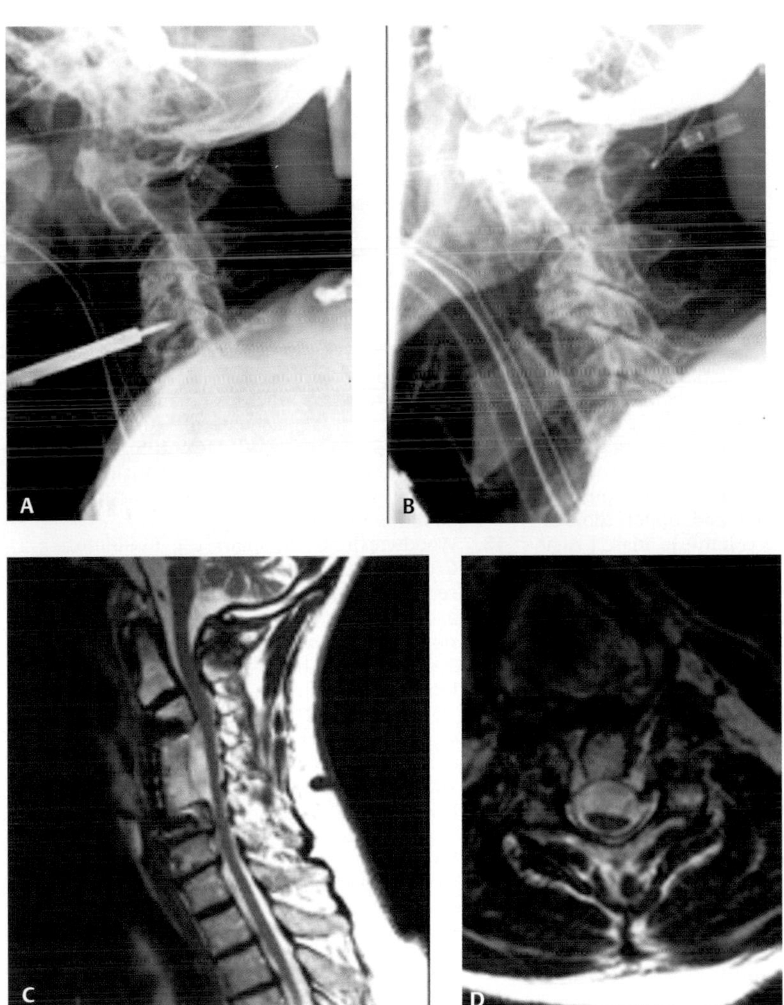

Fig. 19.7 **(A,B)** Patient who developed severe bilateral C5 and C6 palsy after lengthening of his anterior column with a cervical corpectomy. **(C)** Midsagittal and **(D)** axial images displaying decompression of the cord and dorsal cord drift.

Pearls

- Intraoperative neuromonitoring is essential to detect neurological injury.
- Spinal cord perfusion and temperature should be monitored carefully at all times.
- Cervical pedicle screws may facilitate posterior reduction more than lateral mass screws because they cross anterior to the axis of rotation of the osteotomy.

Pitfalls

- Anterior instrumentation may prevent posterior realignment and reconstruction.
- Excessive anterior distraction, even with an excellent decompression, may tension the spinal cord and result in neurological injury.
- Extension of the spine during the flip from supine to prone may result in graft displacement.
- The most dangerous portion of the procedure is intraoperative realignment of the head during the posterior portion of the procedure. It is essential to advise the anesthesiologist and nursing staff preoperatively to ensure a safe manipulation while the surgeon visually monitors the spinal cord in the setting of a laminectomy.
- Any complaints of respiratory distress after anterior cervical spine surgery should be immediately investigated.

References

1. Anderson DG, Albert TJ. Management of cervical kyphosis caused by surgery, degenerative disease, or trauma. In: CC, ed. The Cervical Spine. 4th ed. Philadelphia, PA: Lippincott Williams & Wilkins; 2005:1135–1146
2. Hardacker JW, Shuford RF, Capicotto PN, Pryor PW. Radiographic standing cervical segmental alignment in adult volunteers without neck symptoms. Spine 1997;22(13):1472–1480, discussion 1480
3. Pal GP, Routal RV. A study of weight transmission through the cervical and upper thoracic regions of the vertebral column in man. J Anat 1986;148:245–261
4. Masini M, Maranhão V. Experimental determination of the effect of progressive sharp-angle spinal deformity on the spinal cord. Eur Spine J 1997;6(2):89–92
5. McAfee PC, Bohlman HH, Ducker TB, Zeidman SM, Goldstein JA. One-stage anterior cervical decompression and posterior stabilization: a study of one hundred patients with a minimum of two years of follow-up. J Bone Joint Surg Am 1995;77(12):1791–1800
6. McAfee PC, Bohlman HH. One-stage anterior cervical decompression and posterior stabilization with circumferential arthrodesis: a study of twenty-four patients who had a traumatic or a neoplastic lesion. J Bone Joint Surg Am 1989;71(1):78–88
7. Breig A, el-Nadi AF. Biomechanics of the cervical spinal cord: relief of contact pressure on and overstretching of the spinal cord. Acta Radiol Diagn (Stockh) 1966;4(6):602–624
8. Dvorak MF, Fisher CG, Fehlings MG, et al. The surgical approach to subaxial cervical spine injuries: an evidence-based algorithm based on the SLIC classification system. Spine 2007;32(23):2620–2629
9. Koivikko MP, Myllynen P, Karjalainen M, Vornanen M, Santavirta S. Conservative and operative treatment in cervical burst fractures. Arch Orthop Trauma Surg 2000;120(7-8):448–451
10. Fisher CG, Dvorak MF, Leith J, Wing PC. Comparison of outcomes for unstable lower cervical flexion teardrop fractures managed with halo thoracic vest versus anterior corpectomy and plating. Spine 2002;27(2):160–166
11. Lifeso RM, Colucci MA. Anterior fusion for rotationally unstable cervical spine fractures. Spine 2000;25(16):2028–2034
12. Woodworth RS, Molinari WJ, Brandenstein D, Gruhn W, Molinari RW. Anterior cervical discectomy and fusion with structural allograft and plates for the treatment of unstable posterior cervical spine injuries. J Neurosurg Spine 2009;10(2):93–101
13. Johnson MG, Fisher CG, Boyd M, Pitzen T, Oxland TR, Dvorak MF. The radiographic failure of single segment anterior cervical plate fixation in traumatic cervical flexion distraction injuries. Spine 2004;29(24):2815–2820
14. Lonstein JE. Post-laminectomy kyphosis. Clin Orthop Relat Res 1977;(128):93–100
15. Mikawa Y, Shikata J, Yamamuro T. Spinal deformity and instability after multilevel cervical laminectomy. Spine 1987;12(1):6–11
16. Sim FH, Svien HJ, Bickel WH, Janes JM. Swan-neck deformity following extensive cervical laminectomy: a review of twenty-one cases. J Bone Joint Surg Am 1974;56(3):564–580
17. Deutsch H, Haid RW, Rodts GE, Mummaneni PV. Postlaminectomy cervical deformity. Neurosurg Focus 2003;15(3):E5
18. Lambiris E, Kasimatis GB, Tyllianakis M, Zouboulis P, Panagiotopoulos E. Treatment of unsta-

ble lower cervical spine injuries by anterior instrumented fusion alone. J Spinal Disord Tech 2008;21(7):500–507

19. Hipp JA, Reitman CA, Wharton N. Defining pseudoarthrosis in the cervical spine with differing motion thresholds. Spine 2005;30(2):209–210

20. Kaiser MG, Mummaneni PV, Matz PG, et al; Joint Section on Disorders of the Spine and Peripheral Nerves of the American Association of Neurological Surgeons and Congress of Neurological Surgeons. Radiographic assessment of cervical subaxial fusion. J Neurosurg Spine 2009;11(2):221–227

21. Herman JM, Sonntag VK. Cervical corpectomy and plate fixation for postlaminectomy kyphosis. J Neurosurg 1994;80(6):963–970

22. Zdeblick TA, Bohlman HH. Cervical kyphosis and myelopathy: treatment by anterior corpectomy and strut-grafting. J Bone Joint Surg Am 1989;71(2):170–182

23. Vaccaro AR, Silber JS. Post-traumatic spinal deformity. Spine 2001;26(24, Suppl):S111–S118

24. Kim SM, Lim TJ, Paterno J, Park J, Kim DH. A biomechanical comparison of three surgical approaches in bilateral subaxial cervical facet dislocation. J Neurosurg Spine 2004;1(1):108–115

25. Abumi K, Shono Y, Ito M, Taneichi H, Kotani Y, Kaneda K. Complications of pedicle screw fixation in reconstructive surgery of the cervical spine. Spine 2000;25(8):962–969

26. Abumi K, Shono Y, Taneichi H, Ito M, Kaneda K. Correction of cervical kyphosis using pedicle screw fixation systems. Spine 1999;24(22):2389–2396

27. Abumi K, Kaneda K, Shono Y, Fujiya M. One-stage posterior decompression and reconstruction of the cervical spine by using pedicle screw fixation systems. J Neurosurg 1999;90(1, Suppl):19–26

28. Mehdian SM, Freeman BJ, Licina P. Cervical osteotomy for ankylosing spondylitis: an innovative variation on an existing technique. Eur Spine J 1999;8(6):505–509

29. Simmons ED, DiStefano RJ, Zheng Y, Simmons EH. Thirty-six years experience of cervical extension osteotomy in ankylosing spondylitis: techniques and outcomes. Spine 2006;31(26):3006–3012

30. McMaster MJ. Osteotomy of the cervical spine in ankylosing spondylitis. J Bone Joint Surg Br 1997;79(2):197–203

31. Mummaneni PV, Mummaneni VP, Haid RW Jr, Rodts GE Jr, Sasso RC. Cervical osteotomy for the correction of chin-on-chest deformity in ankylosing spondylitis. Technical note. Neurosurg Focus 2003;14(1):e9

32. Mummaneni PV, Dhall SS, Rodts GE, Haid RW. Circumferential fusion for cervical kyphotic deformity. J Neurosurg Spine 2008;9(6):515–521

33. Schultz KD Jr, McLaughlin MR, Haid RW Jr, Comey CH, Rodts GE Jr, Alexander J. Single-stage anterior-posterior decompression and stabilization for complex cervical spine disorders. J Neurosurg 2000;93(2, Suppl):214–221

20

Posttraumatic Syringomyelia: Pathophysiology and Management

Mohammed Farid Shamji, Sung-Joo Yuh, and Eve C. Tsai

Key Points

1. Posttraumatic syringomyelia should be considered in patients experiencing subacute or chronic neurological deterioration after spinal cord injury.
2. Magnetic resonance imaging is the diagnostic modality of choice, with the syrinx most easily observed on sagittal T2-weighted sequences.
3. Comprehensive workup is required to rule out other causes of syringomyelia, including Chiari malformation, congenital tethered cord, and neoplastic disease.
4. Goal of posttraumatic syrinx treatment is disease stabilization, with therapeutic interventions ranging from simple spinal decompression, syrinx shunting, adhesiolysis and expansion duraplasty, to cord detethering.

Syringomyelia is characterized by the presence of abnormal fluid-filled cavities in the substance of the spinal cord. Syrinx etiology can be associated with a very diverse and heterogeneous group of diseases, ranging from hydrocephalus, associated structural malformations, infection or inflammation, spinal cord infarction or hemorrhage, to trauma. This chapter focuses on syringomyelia that occurs after spinal cord injury (SCI) and reviews the epidemiology, pathophysiology, and clinical management of posttraumatic syringomyelia (PTS).

Epidemiology

Radiographic and postmortem detection of syringomyelia occurs in up to 30% of patients with spinal cord trauma, with series variation based on the extent and pattern of injury.[1–5] Clinical presentation from such lesions occurs in fewer than 10% of the SCI population, most frequently in men, correlating with the trends in injury incidence.[3] In a prospective longitudinal study of 449 SCI patients, Schurch and coworkers observed the development of symptomatic syringomyelia in 4.5% of patients over 6 years. Of note, however, is that PTS can also occur in a delayed fashion at much longer follow-up.[4]

Vannemreddy and coworkers[6] retrospectively reviewed factors predisposing to the development of PTS in a series of 58 symptomatic patients. They found that onset of symptomatic PTS occurred earlier among patients with more advanced age, cervical- or thoracic-level injuries, complete neurological injury at the index level, and fracture-dislocations, especially if patients underwent surgery for deformity correction and stabilization. Advanced age may be associated with acquired canal stenosis, promoting the likelihood of syrinx formation in the traumatized cord.[5,6] The association of earlier syrinx development with greater neurological injury and fracture dislocations requiring surgical intervention may reflect the greater force severity applied to the spinal cord and consequent increased inflammatory activation.[6–8] Beyond injury to the neural tissue, deformity may contribute to PTS as a result of meningeal injury and adhesion, impaired circulation of cerebrospinal fluid (CSF), and altered vascular supply.[6,9,10] Cervical spine injury may promote syrinx development by local tethering at the naturally more mobile site, which is exacerbated in quadriplegics, for whom head and neck movement is the most significant remaining motor function.[6,8,11]

PTS location is expectedly most frequent at the injured level. Although rostral extension reportedly occurs in more than 96% of cases, isolated caudal extension rarely occurs (4%).[1,8] The remarkably low incidence of the latter may result from decreased detection because patients with extension below the level of injury may not develop symptoms to warrant investigation. Longitudinal extent of the syrinx is highly variable, with one of every six cases reportedly spanning more than 10 levels.[12]

Pathophysiology

The mechanism by which PTS develops remains speculative, although most theories support a two-step process by which the predisposing pathoanatomy is established at the time of initial injury, and propagation occurs by secondary mechanisms. The primary injury can cause an early cystic lesion by mechanical disruption of cord parenchyma, ischemic damage from arterial or venous obstruction, intraparenchymal hemorrhage with subsequent hematoma liquefaction, and proteolytic enzyme activity or excitatory amino acid activity.[13–16] Indeed, the mechanical deformation of the spinal column can also produce a variety of configurational abnormalities that may contribute to syrinx progression. Spinal stenosis, subarachnoid adhesions, and deformity are common among SCI patients who develop PTS, presumably reflecting the severity of the index injury and thereafter contributing to the generation of repeated microtrauma and impacting CSF circulation on an ongoing basis.

Posttraumatic syringes are associated with lesions localized to the dorsolateral and central gray matter, and dystrophic cavitations secondary to the ischemic or hemorrhagic insult. Unlike hydromyelia, wherein the cyst walls are lined by ependymal cells of the central canal, the cyst walls of PTS can be irregular in contour, with walls formed by compressed or gliotic tissue, containing microglia and hemosiderin-laden macrophages.[12,17,18] Cellular changes include Wallerian degeneration of the associated neurons, with demyelination of the white matter and neuronophagia in the gray matter.[12,18] Fibrotic thickening of the leptomeninges occurs, reflecting the underlying process of arachnoiditis observed during surgical management.[17]

The normal astroglial response to injury is reactive, with release of growth factors that promote neuronal survival[19]; however, any concomitant disturbance of this delicate healing balance can alternatively promote astrogliosis that generates both physical and biochemical barriers to neural regeneration.[20–22] Further consequences of an excessive healing response may be the initiation of an adhesive arachnoiditis at the level of the sustained injury.[7,23,24] In this setting, trauma to the arachnoid alone may cause progressive syringomyelia by spinal cord tethering and alteration of CSF circulation, with consequent expansion of intramedullary microcystic lesions into macroscopic syringomyelia lesions. Josephson and coworkers[25] describe this theory of CSF pulse pressure against an area of thecal sac constriction dividing the spinal canal into two separate hydrodynamic compartments, with consequent pulsatile activity against an area of high relative local pressure. This uncoupling of the pulse pressure in the CSF and spinal cord leads to higher intramedullary pressure directed centrifugally, with consequent macroscopic cyst formation and subsequent expansion as the proximal component is actively compressed and the distal portion is passively distended. Using a constriction model in Sprague-Dawley rats, edema was detectable by magnetic resonance imaging (MRI) within 3 weeks of injury, and cystic cavitation developed between 8 and 13 weeks postinjury. Similar computational studies by Bilston and coworkers[26] identify the peak pulsation pressure to depend on obstruction permeability, facilitating fluid flow into the spinal cord and consequent syrinx expansion. Although this mechanism of PTS development remains dependent on a primary process leading to microcystic cavitation, it underscores the value of surgical intervention to address the healing response as well as any primary bony and neural injury.

Clinical Presentation

Patients with PTS most commonly present with pain. Motor deficit and dissociated sensory loss are also common features.[4,8,27–29] Pain history is often variable, mild to severe, and intermittent to constant, reflecting injury to the spinothalamic pathway, and pain is consistently exacerbated by maneuvers that increase intracranial pressure and positional changes.[8,27,28] The classic dissociated sensory loss (loss of pain and temperature sensation with preservation of light touch and proprioception) reflects intact dorsal column functionality and is more common than a complete sensory loss.[8,27,28] Indeed, the selective loss of pain and temperature sensation in conjunction with an ascending sensory level is a very sensitive indicator for detecting progressive PTS.[4] Motor symptoms reflect injury to the neighboring lateral corticospinal tract, with an upper motor neuron pattern on clinical examination. Less common symptoms include hyperhidrosis, autonomic dysreflexia, Horner syndrome, and respiratory insufficiency. Bladder hyporeflexia and abnormalities of bowel function occur, normally in conjunction with other symptoms and signs, but have been reported to be the isolated presenting features.[18] Further, syrinx extension into the caudal medulla may also lead to cranial nerve involvement, and physical examination should include evaluating for signs of such involvement.

Diagnosis

The density of bone forming the spinal column makes plain computed tomography (CT) ineffective in establishing the diagnosis of PTS. Enhancement of this technique with contrast myelography provides for detection of associated adhesions, although with poor sensitivity, missing the diagnosis of PTS in up to half of cases. Excellent soft tissue discrimination afforded by MRI provides enhanced sensitivity and is the test of choice to establish the PTS diagnosis, demonstrating either a focal cystic lesion (**Fig. 20.1**) or a diffuse, longitudinal, expansile lesion (**Fig. 20.2**).[30,31] Additional information about syrinx pathoanatomy is also provided, such as lesion symmetry, loculation, and multiplicity. The presyrinx state, an entity evolving at present in the Chiari I malformation literature, may also be detected following SCI as a T1-hypointense, T2-hyperintense lesion that does not expand the spinal cord and can precede the development of radiographic PTS.[30,32–34] The value of cine MRI remains investigational, although the potential to identify sites of obstructed CSF flow and to observe normalization following intervention may be valuable in the future.[35]

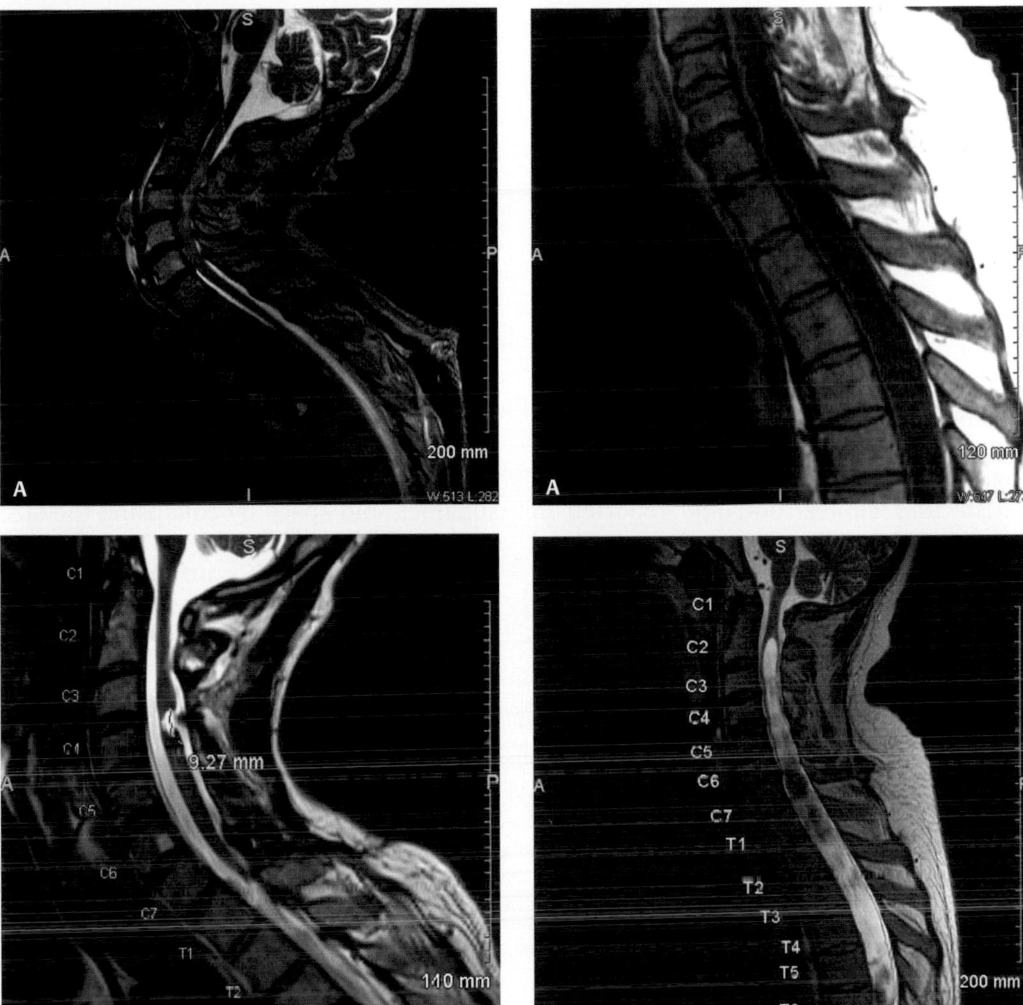

Fig. 20.1 Magnetic resonance imaging (MRI) study of a 50-year-old male patient who developed posttraumatic syringomyelia as a complication of an unstable C3-4 complex injury. **(A)** The preoperative T2-weighted MRI scan demonstrates the traumatic and degenerative changes, with **(B)** the postoperative T2-weighted scan showing a small posttraumatic cyst at the site of previous cord contusion.

Fig. 20.2 Magnetic resonance imaging (MRI) study of a 51-year-old male patient who developed posttraumatic syringomyelia as a complication of a T9-level injury. Symptoms include new onset of neck pain and stiffness in a previously T9-paraplegic patient. The expansile cystic lesion spans from C2 to T8 and is seen on both **(A)** T1-weighted and **(B)** T2-weighted MRI studies, with the syrinx contents having similar signal intensity to CSF.

Management

The need to intervene among patients with PTS is based on a consistent progression of neurological disability, with few reports of spontaneous resolution,[36–38] which presumably occurred consequent to spinal cord fissuring, with consequent syrinx decompression into the subarachnoid space. Medical management has a role only in the context of symptomatic treatment for patients with mild disability or who are not surgical candidates by choice or condition. Pharmacological options include antispasticity agents, tricyclic antidepressants and anticonvulsants targeting neuropathic pain, anticholinergic medications to treat excessive secretory activity, and narcotic analgesics for treatment of refractory pain.

Surgical indications include those with asymptomatic radiographic syrinx progression, new onset of symptoms following SCI with radiographic evidence of syrinx, or substantial neurological deterioration, pain, or autonomic dysreflexia in patients with known PTS.[4,8,28,39] The stated goal of surgical treatment for PTS should be disease stabilization, although variable reports of neurological recovery of neurological deficit have been described, with satisfactory clinical outcome reported in between 80 and 90% of patients.[4] Decreased pain and improved motor function are the most common improvements,[4] with recovery of disordered sensation and decrease in hyperhidrosis being less predictable.[27,29] Effect on limb spasticity is variable and the least improvement is noted in the clinical sign of deep tendon reflexes.[4,40]

Choices for surgical intervention are variable and highly dependent on the presenting pathoanatomy. Strategies that are commonly employed and that are technically accessible to most neurosurgeons include simple spinal decompression, percutaneous syrinx drainage, syrinx shunting, adhesiolysis and expansion duraplasty, and cord detethering. Limited symptomatic improvement in slightly more than half of patients has been reported for spinal decompression alone in small case series,[41] although this may represent a more limited operation that could be reasonably offered in the setting of substantial deformity or severe spinal stenosis. Although reduction of spinal column deformity has been reported,[13] with the conferred benefits of potentially treating local obstruction to CSF circulation, using a method that is entirely extradural must be balanced against the surgical trauma, particularly in cases requiring thoracotomy or thoracoabdominal exposures.

Simple syrinx fluid drainage without any mechanism for continued evacuation has been associated with only short-lived clinical effect and has been largely abandoned in favor of cyst fluid diversion strategies with more sustained results. Sudheendra and coworkers[42] review the literature surrounding this tactic and illustrate the case of a single patient who responded with both clinical and radiographic improvement to fluoroscopic syrinx aspiration, although repeated interventions were required three times over the span of 3 years. Nevertheless, such a technique may represent an adjunct to surgery, temporizing intervention among patients who are not optimized for surgery or improving operative access to the subarachnoid space by collapsing the size of the spinal cord.

Shunting of a PTS into the subarachnoid space (syringosubarachnoid) or into a low-pressure cavity, such as the pleural (syringopleural) or peritoneal (syringoperitoneal) regions, may provide effective and sustained diversion of cyst fluid to limit syrinx growth and afford neurological recovery. **Figure 20.3** illustrates steps involved in placement of a syringosubarachnoid shunt. Briefly, this involves laminectomy to provide access to the spinal canal, followed by a myelotomy over the thinnest rim of neural tissue surrounding the caudal syrinx, with preference given to the posterior median sulcus or dorsal root entry zone. The shunt is generally introduced in a caudal to cranial direction to minimize the risk of iatrogenic neurological injury. To minimize the possibility of shunt migration, a suture can be placed to secure the shunt to the pia or dura, or T-shaped shunts can be used. Syringosubarachnoid shunt failure can be associated with dense subarachnoid scarring that can lead to obstruction and reaccumulation of the cyst. Placement of the distal end of the syringosubarachnoid shunt in an area free of arachnoid adhesions may decrease the incidence of shunt failure.[8,43] Batzdorf and coworkers[43] critically appraised the success of the various shunting techniques, finding that half of the

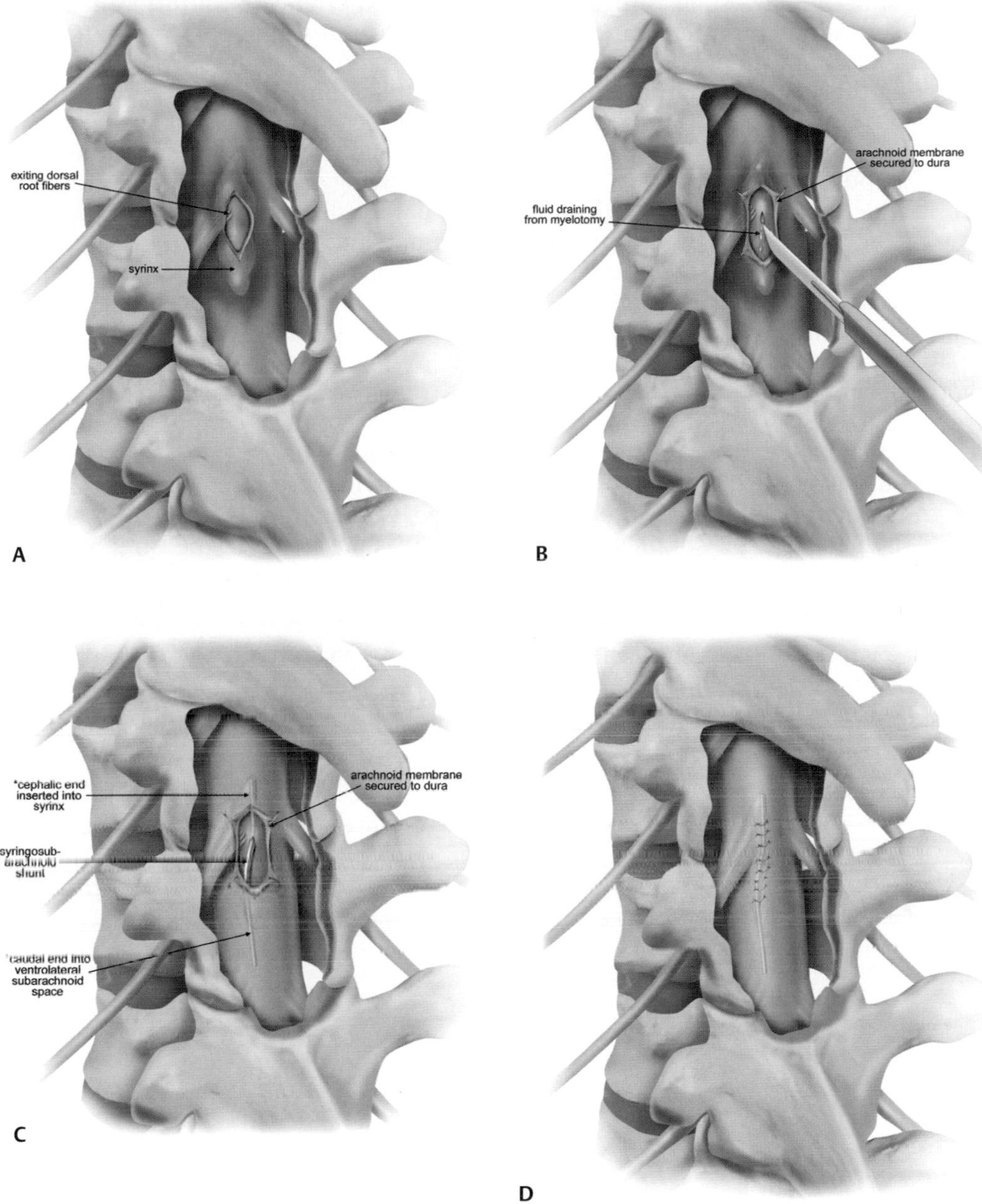

Fig. 20.3 (A) Technique for placement of syringosubarachnoid shunt. A laminectomy is performed to allow access to the dura, which is opened in the midline. **(B)** The pia is opened next, and pial sutures are placed and a midline myelotomy is performed to allow access to the syrinx. **(C)** The shunt is then inserted in a caudal to cranial direction into the syrinx. The distal end is placed in the adjacent subarachnoid space. **(D)** Following satisfactory placement and decompression of the syrinx, the dura is closed in a watertight fashion. For a syringopleural or syringoperitoneal shunt (not shown), the distal end is subcutaneously tunneled and placed in the pleural space or peritoneum, respectively.

patients undergoing such procedures experienced some complication of the procedure at a median of 9 years follow-up. Among those for whom the proximal shunt was removed because of obstruction, ingrowth of glial tissue was found to be the putative material. No difference in the incidence of complication was observed by the different shunting methods, a result previously reported by Umbach and Heilporn.[44] Over all, clinical improvement is reported in 12 to 89% of patients following shunt insertion, although these series report up to one third of patients exhibiting postoperative deterioration.[8,39,45] Various case series are summarized in **Table 20.1**, and the significant variability in results likely reflects the heterogeneity of the regional trauma experience with different severity, pattern of spinal column injury, and incidence of subarachnoid scarring.

Complications of syrinx shunting include direct spinal cord damage during the myelotomy, iatrogenic spinal instability following laminectomy, deafferentation pain, fistula formation, and surgical site infections ranging from meningitis to pyosyrinx. Asano and coworkers[46] report sustained clinical improvement in two patients subjected to midline myelotomy only, whose preoperative T2-weighted MRI scans revealed a positive flow void and whose intraoperative exploration revealed acute decompression of the syrinx following myelotomy with collapse of the expanded spinal cord. Such collapse was not noted in the three patients

Table 20.1 Summary of Results of Treatment for Posttraumatic Syringomyelia

Author	Number of patients	Management	Patient outcomes
Bleasel et al., 1991	2	Surgery: • Syringostomy[1] • Syringopleural shunt[1]	Surgery: • Improvement[2]
Schurch et al.,1996	20	Surgery: • Spine stabilization[2] • Syringostomia[2] • T-tube[3] Conservative[13]	Surgery: • Improvement[6] • Stable[1] Conservative: • Stable[10] • Progression[3]
el Masry et al., 1996	28	Surgery[22]: • Syringopleural shunt[13] • Syringosubarachnoid shunt[7] • Myelotomy[1] • Cordectomy[1] • Cord transection[1] • Omental grafting[1] Conservative[4]	Surgery: • Improvement[19] • Stable[3] Conservative: • Stable[4]
Bains et al., 2001	1	Surgery: • Decompression[1]	Surgery: • Improvement[1]
Lee et al., 2002	7	Surgery: • Decompression[3] • Decompression and stabilization[1] • Syringopleural shunt[1] • Syringosubarachnoid shunt[2] • Ventriculoperitoneal shunt[1]	Surgery: • Improvement[5] • Stable[2]

in whom such flow void was absent on preoperative imaging, and their surgical management was augmented by syringosubarachnoid shunting to provide for a fair clinical result.

Augmentation of surgical intervention with arachnoid adhesiolysis or detethering where such inflammatory change exists, typically at the level of injury, has been recommended to decrease strain on spinal tissue as well as to restore CSF circulation. Neurological recovery may be more substantial in the context of such intervention; however, this technique carries a higher risk of complication in patients with very extensive arachnoid adhesions or calcification.[47,48] In a series of 35 patients treated with additional adhesiolysis and duraplasty, Klekamp[49] reported 31% improved, 54% remained stable, and 15% worsened. Choice of duraplasty material remains controversial, but selected synthetic graft materials may decrease inflammatory scar tissue compared with autologous tissue.[50]

Intraoperative ultrasonographic techniques can be useful after initial decompressive laminectomy to delineate the precise syrinx site as well as the presence of septations that may require fenestration.[51] Similarly, endoscopic placement of a shunt catheter may ensure more effective drainage of all syrinx compartments, although there is no evidence of improved outcomes when compared with a nonendoscopic technique.[8]

In pregnant patients who have developed symptomatic PTS, elective cesarean section has been advocated, with the intention of avoiding surges in intrasyringeal pressures and the attendant risks of lesion expansion or hemorrhage associated with labor.[52,53]

Other Management Options

Other less common and investigational management options include cordectomy, transposition of vascularized omental grafts, and transplantation of fetal neural tissue. Cordectomy is typically only appropriate in patients with complete neurological injury and involves transection at the level of the syrinx below the functional level.[54–56] Vascularized omental grafts have the potential of enriching the local blood supply to damaged spinal cord and are used in the context of adhesive meningitis and cystic myelomalacia or in those who fail surgical treatment.[57] There is limited experience with this technique, and foreseeable complications include omental atrophy, visceral herniation through the transposition tract, and paradoxical increase in syrinx size. Fetal tissue grafts have been transplanted in patients with syringomyelia, and although they were found to obliterate cystic syrinx cavities, there was only limited neurological improvement.[58]

Development of posttraumatic syringomyelia represents one mechanism by which progressive neurological deterioration can occur following SCI. The surgeon must remain attuned to such possibility because surgical intervention can provide disease stabilization and offers the further possibility of neurological recovery. Further investigations into the mechanisms underlying the development of PTS will permit more specific and targeted therapy to optimize the likelihood of syrinx resolution and clinical improvement. Similarly, clinical and neuroimaging characteristics that are prognostic of recovery following surgical management of PTS will provide avenues for further clinical investigation.

Pearls

- Understanding the pathogenesis of posttraumatic syringomyelia will clarify surgical objectives, which include decompression of any neural tissue compression, reestablishment of normal CSF flow and patency of the subarachnoid space, and diversionary procedures as required when this is not possible.
- Intraoperative ultrasonography can be a valuable resource to help the surgeon delineate the appropriate myelotomy site once bony decompression has been performed.
- Endoscopic assistance can help ensure the adequacy of septation lysis within the syrinx and the appropriate placement of the syrinx shunt catheter if required.

Pitfalls

- Craniospinal neuroimaging is essential to rule out nontraumatic causes of syringomyelia, such as Chiari malformation, concomitant cord tethering, and spinal cord neoplastic disease.
- In contrast to hydromyelia, syringomyelia may ascend unilaterally, leading to asymmetry of clinical deficits. The clinician should be aware that evolution of myelopathy may not fit straightforward and symmetric clinical patterns, regardless of the initial posttraumatic deficit.
- Any progression of the initial posttraumatic deficit should warrant an evaluation for possible syringomyelia.

References

1. Backe HA, Betz RR, Mesgarzadeh M, Beck T, Clancy M. Post-traumatic spinal cord cysts evaluated by magnetic resonance imaging. Paraplegia 1991;29(9):607–612
2. Biyani A, el Masry WS. Post-traumatic syringomyelia: a review of the literature. Paraplegia 1994;32(11):723–731
3. Carroll AM, Brackenridge P. Post-traumatic syringomyelia: a review of the cases presenting in a regional spinal injuries unit in the north east of England over a 5-year period. Spine 2005;30(10):1206–1210
4. el Masry WS, Biyani A. Incidence, management, and outcome of post-traumatic syringomyelia. In memory of Mr. Bernard Williams. J Neurol Neurosurg Psychiatry 1996;60(2):141–146
5. Perrouin-Verbe B, Lenne-Aurier K, Robert R, et al. Post-traumatic syringomyelia and post-traumatic spinal canal stenosis: a direct relationship: review of 75 patients with a spinal cord injury. Spinal Cord 1998;36(2):137–143
6. Vannemreddy SS, Rowed DW, Bharatwal N. Posttraumatic syringomyelia: predisposing factors. Br J Neurosurg 2002;16(3):276–283
7. Cho KH, Iwasaki Y, Imamura H, Hida K, Abe H. Experimental model of posttraumatic syringomyelia: the role of adhesive arachnoiditis in syrinx formation. J Neurosurg 1994;80(1):133–139
8. Edgar R, Quail P. Progressive post-traumatic cystic and non-cystic myelopathy. Br J Neurosurg 1994;8(1):7–22
9. Williams B. Pathogenesis of post-traumatic syringomyelia. Br J Neurosurg 1994;8(1):114–115
10. Williams B, Terry AF, Jones F, McSweeney T. Syringomyelia as a sequel to traumatic paraplegia. Paraplegia 1981;19(2):67–80
11. Rothman RH, Simeone FA. The Spine. Philadelphia, PA: Saunders; 1992
12. Milhorat TH, Capocelli AL Jr, Anzil AP, Kotzen RM, Milhorat RH. Pathological basis of spinal cord cavitation in syringomyelia: analysis of 105 autopsy cases. J Neurosurg 1995;82(5):802–812
13. Brodbelt AR, Stoodley MA, Watling A, et al. The role of excitotoxic injury in post-traumatic syringomyelia. J Neurotrauma 2003;20(9):883–893
14. Kao CC, Chang LW, Bloodworth JM. The mechanism of spinal cord cavitation following spinal cord transection. Part 3: Delayed grafting with and without spinal cord retransection. J Neurosurg 1977;46(6):757–766
15. Kao CC, Chang LW, Bloodworth JM Jr. The mechanism of spinal cord cavitation following spinal cord transection. Part 2. Electron microscopic observations. J Neurosurg 1977;46(6):745–756
16. Koyanagi I, Tator CH, Theriault E. Silicone rubber microangiography of acute spinal cord injury in the rat. Neurosurgery 1993;32(2):260–268, discussion 268
17. Durward QJ, Rice GP, Ball MJ, Gilbert JJ, Kaufmann JC. Selective spinal cordectomy: clinicopathological correlation. J Neurosurg 1982;56(3):359–367
18. Foo D, Bignami A, Rossier AB. A case of post-traumatic syringomyelia. Neuropathological findings after 1 year of cystic drainage. Paraplegia 1989;27(1):63–69
19. Liberto CM, Albrecht PJ, Herx LM, Yong VW, Levison SW. Pro-regenerative properties of cyto-

kine-activated astrocytes. J Neurochem 2004; 89(5):1092–1100

20. Bilgen M, Rumboldt Z. Neuronal and vascular biomarkers in syringomyelia: investigations using longitudinal MRI. Biomarkers Med 2008;2:113–124

21. Menet V, Prieto M, Privat A, Giménez y Ribotta M. Axonal plasticity and functional recovery after spinal cord injury in mice deficient in both glial fibrillary acidic protein and vimentin genes. Proc Natl Acad Sci USA 2003;100(15):8999–9004

22. Ribotta MG, Menet V, Privat A. Glial scar and axonal regeneration in the CNS: lessons from GFAP and vimentin transgenic mice. Acta Neurochir Suppl (Wien) 2004;89:87–92

23. Klekamp J, Batzdorf U, Samii M, Bothe HW. Treatment of syringomyelia associated with arachnoid scarring caused by arachnoiditis or trauma. J Neurosurg 1997;86(2):233–240

24. Morikawa T, Takami T, Tsuyuguchi N, Sakamoto H, Ohata K, Hara M. The role of spinal tissue scarring in the pathogenesis of progressive posttraumatic myelomalacia. Neurol Res 2006;28(8): 802–806

25. Josephson A, Greitz D, Klason T, Olson L, Spenger C. A spinal thecal sac constriction model supports the theory that induced pressure gradients in the cord cause edema and cyst formation. Neurosurgery 2001;48(3):636–645, discussion 645–646

26. Bilston LE, Fletcher DF, Stoodley MA. Focal spinal arachnoiditis increases subarachnoid space pressure: a computational study. Clin Biomech (Bristol, Avon) 2006;21(6):579–584

27. Rossier AB, Foo D, Shillito J, Dyro FM. Posttraumatic cervical syringomyelia. Incidence, clinical presentation, electrophysiological studies, syrinx protein and results of conservative and operative treatment. Brain 1985;108(Pt 2):439–461

28. Schurch B, Wichmann W, Rossier AB. Posttraumatic syringomyelia (cystic myelopathy): a prospective study of 449 patients with spinal cord injury. J Neurol Neurosurg Psychiatry 1996; 60(1):61–67

29. Vernon JD, Silver JR, Ohry A. Post-traumatic syringomyelia. Paraplegia 1982;20(6):339–364

30. Demaerel P. Magnetic resonance imaging of spinal cord trauma: a pictorial essay. Neuroradiology 2006;48(4):223–232

31. Dowling RJ, Tress BM. MRI—the investigation of choice in syringomyelia? Australas Radiol 1989;33(4):337–343

32. Fischbein NJ, Dillon WP, Cobbs C, Weinstein PR. The "presyrinx" state: a reversible myelopathic condition that may precede syringomyelia. AJNR Am J Neuroradiol 1999;20(1):7–20

33. Jinkins JR, Reddy S, Leite CC, Bazan C III, Xiong L. MR of parenchymal spinal cord signal change as a sign of active advancement in clinically progressive posttraumatic syringomyelia. AJNR Am J Neuroradiol 1998;19(1):177–182

34. Levy EI, Heiss JD, Kent MS, Riedel CJ, Oldfield EH. Spinal cord swelling preceding syrinx development. Case report. J Neurosurg 2000;92(1, Suppl):93–97

35. Menick BJ. Phase-contrast magnetic resonance imaging of cerebrospinal fluid flow in the evaluation of patients with Chiari I malformation. Neurosurg Focus 2001;11(1):E5

36. Birbamer G, Buchberger W, Felber S, Posch A, Russegger L. Spontaneous collapse of posttraumatic syringomyelia: serial magnetic resonance imaging. Eur Neurol 1993;33(5):378–381

37. Olivero WC, Dinh DH. Chiari I malformation with traumatic syringomyelia and spontaneous resolution: case report and literature review. Neurosurgery 1992;30(5):758–760

38. Ozisik PA, Hazer B, Ziyal IM, Ozcan OE. Spontaneous resolution of syringomyelia without Chiari malformation. Neurol Med Chir (Tokyo) 2006;46(10):512–517

39. Hida K, Iwasaki Y, Imamura H, Abe H. Posttraumatic syringomyelia: its characteristic magnetic resonance imaging findings and surgical management. Neurosurgery 1994;35(5):886–891, discussion 891

40. Umbach I, Heilporn A. Evolution of post-traumatic cervical syringomyelia: case report. Paraplegia 1988;26(1):56–61

41. Lee JH, Chung CK, Kim HJ. Decompression of the spinal subarachnoid space as a solution for syringomyelia without Chiari malformation. Spinal Cord 2002;40(10):501–506

42. Sudheendra D, Bartynski WS. Direct fluoroscopic drainage of symptomatic post-traumatic syringomyelia. A case report and review of the literature. Interv Neuroradiol 2008;14(4):461–464

43. Batzdorf U, Klekamp J, Johnson JP. A critical appraisal of syrinx cavity shunting procedures. J Neurosurg 1998;89(3):382–388

44. Umbach I, Heilporn A. Review article: post-spinal cord injury syringomyelia. Paraplegia 1991; 29(4):219–221

45. Sgouros S, Williams B. A critical appraisal of drainage in syringomyelia. J Neurosurg 1995;82(1): 1–10

46. Asano M, Fujiwara K, Yonenobu K, Hiroshima K. Post-traumatic syringomyelia. Spine 1996; 21(12):1446–1453

47. Lee TT, Alameda GJ, Camilo E, Green BA. Surgical treatment of post-traumatic myelopathy associated with syringomyelia. Spine 2001;26(24, Suppl):S119–S127

48. Schaller B, Mindermann T, Gratzl O. Treatment of syringomyelia after posttraumatic paraparesis or tetraparesis. J Spinal Disord 1999;12(6): 485–488

49. Klekamp JSM, ed. Syringomyelia: Diagnosis and Management. 2002

50. Brodbelt AR, Stoodley MA. Post-traumatic syringomyelia: a review. J Clin Neurosci 2003; 10(4):401–408

51. Dohrmann GJ, Rubin JM. Intraoperative ultrasound imaging of the spinal cord: syringomyelia, cysts, and tumors—a preliminary report. Surg Neurol 1982;18(6):395–399

52. Daskalakis GJ, Katsetos CN, Papageorgiou IS, et al. Syringomyelia and pregnancy-case report. Eur J Obstet Gynecol Reprod Biol 2001;97(1): 98–100

53. Murayama K, Mamiya K, Nozaki K, et al. Cesarean section in a patient with syringomyelia. Can J Anaesth 2001;48(5):474–477
54. Kasai Y, Kawakita E, Morishita K, Uchida A. Cordectomy for post-traumatic syringomyelia. Acta Neurochir (Wien) 2008;150(1):83–86, discussion 86
55. Laxton AW, Perrin RG. Cordectomy for the treatment of posttraumatic syringomyelia. Report of four cases and review of the literature. J Neurosurg Spine 2006;4(2):174–178
56. Lyons BM, Brown DJ, Calvert JM, Woodward JM, Wriedt CH. The diagnosis and management of post traumatic syringomyelia. Paraplegia 1987;25(4):340–350
57. Williams B. Pathogenesis of post-traumatic syringomyelia. Br J Neurosurg 1992;6(6):517–520
58. Wirth ED III, Reier PJ, Fessler RG, et al. Feasibility and safety of neural tissue transplantation in patients with syringomyelia. J Neurotrauma 2001;18(9):911–929

21

Rehabilitation of the Individual with Spinal Cord Injury

Aria Fallah, Derry Dance, and Anthony S. Burns

Key Points

1. Until World War II, severe spinal cord injury (SCI) was almost universally fatal during the initial 2 years following injury.
2. The development of specialized SCI centers has dramatically improved survival rates, health, and functional outcomes of individuals with SCI.
3. SCI rehabilitation is ideally delivered by an interdisciplinary team.
4. Goal setting is a fundamental component of rehabilitation and facilitates the achievement of desired functional outcomes.
5. SCI rehabilitation should embrace and plan for community reintegration to maximize long-term outcomes.

The History of Spinal Cord Rehabilitation

For the majority of humankind's history, SCI has carried a grave prognosis. The Edwin Smith Surgical Papyrus, dating to ancient Egypt (2500 BC) and named after Egyptologist Edwin Smith, is a medical text containing 48 detailed case histories. In this early document, SCI is referred to as "an ailment not to be treated."[1] Hippocrates, the ancient Greek physician, also believed that individuals with SCIs were destined to die.[2] During World War I, 80% of individuals with severe SCIs typically died within 2 weeks of injury, and even up to 1934, the mortality rate for paraplegia in the United States exceeded 80% during the first 1 to 2 years postinjury,[3,4] with the majority of patients succumbing to sepsis from urinary tract infections and pressure ulcers. Individuals who survived were largely relegated to institutional care with little hope of reintegration into the community. The picture remained bleak until World War II (WWII).

In 1936, Dr. Donald Munro, with the sponsorship of the Liberty Mutual Insurance Company, established the first civilian SCI unit (10 beds) in the United States at Boston City Hospital. He was able to demonstrate a 200 to 300% reduction in medical and hospital costs.[3] The challenges posed by the large number of SCIs related to WWII would inspire the development of additional dedicated SCI units around the globe. In February 1944, the National Spinal Injuries Centre was established at Stoke Mandeville Hospital in Aylesbury, England. The SCI unit at Stoke Mandeville employed a comprehensive, multidisciplinary approach and was a response to the large number of injured servicemen and ex-servicemen. Sir Ludwig Guttmann was the first medical director and is considered by many to be the father of SCI medicine. He had been one of Germany's leading neurosurgeons at the Jewish Hospital in Breslau before he fled to England in 1939. Guttman espoused some fundamental principles for SCI units.[3]

- Management of a unit by an experienced physician who is prepared to give up part, or all, of his own specialty
- Sufficient allied health professionals (e.g., nurses and therapists) to cope with details of care
- Technical facilities to establish workshops and vocational outlets
- Attention to social, domestic, and industrial resettlement
- Regular aftercare, or extended care, over the lifetime of each individual.

Employing these principles, Stoke Mandeville enjoyed great success and served as an example for the rest of the world.

At the conclusion of WWII, Dr. E. Harry Botterell, consultant neurosurgeon to the Canadian army, worked with John Counsell, an injured veteran, to convince the Canadian Veterans' Affairs Department to establish a dedicated facility for individuals with SCI. As a result, on January 15, 1945, the Lyndhurst Lodge was established in Toronto, Ontario. The first medical director was Dr. Al Jousse. The same year, the US Department of Veterans Affairs followed suit and established six SCI units. In Australia, the Royal Perth Hospital in Western Australia established an SCI unit in 1954, led by Dr. G. M. Bedbrook. Other Australian centers would follow.

In 1970, the first model SCI system was awarded by the US Rehabilitation Services Administration to Good Samaritan Hospital in Phoenix, Arizona. The success of this demonstration project led to the establishment of six additional centers in 1972. The Model SCI Systems (MSCIS) program is now administered by the National Institute on Disability and Rehabilitation Research (NIDRR) within the Office of Special Education and Rehabilitation Services in the US Department of Education. The program has included 26 SCI centers over the years, and currently there are 14 Model SCI Systems dispersed throughout the United States. Model SCI Systems are capable of providing the entire continuum of care, from acute medical management to rehabilitation and lifelong follow-up. Grantees also contribute data to a National Spinal Cord Injury Database. Today, dedicated SCI units exist around the world.

Spinal cord medicine continues to mature and develop as a medical subspecialty. In 1980, the US Department of Veterans Affairs established fellowship programs for SCI. In 1996, the US Accreditation Council for Graduate Medical Education (ACGME) approved spinal cord medicine as a subspecialty, and the first examination was subsequently given in October 1998. Subspecialty certification is conferred through the American Board of Physical Medicine and Rehabilitation; however, any current diplomates in good standing with a member of the American Board of Medical Specialties (ABMS) are eligible, if they otherwise meet training requirements.

Rehabilitation Setting and Team

Advantages of Cohorting and Regionalized Centers

Given the multisystem, multifactorial nature of SCI, in 1984 Donovan and colleagues postulated that SCI patients would experience improved outcomes if treated in a "coordinated" (specialized) system.[5] It has now been demonstrated that specialist spinal injury units, which encompass rehabilitation, are associated with improved health, functional, and social outcomes. Smith in the United Kingdom found that individuals who received their rehabilitation through dedicated SCI programs experienced fewer health complications, such as pressure-related skin injury, chest infections, urinary tract infections, constipation, uncontrolled autonomic dysreflexia, problematic spasms, disrupted sleep, and depression.[6] Significant differences were also observed for functional activities, such as eating, drinking, grooming, dressing, showering, transfers, wheelchair mobility, and managing bowel and bladder function.[6] These individuals were also less likely to report relationship problems with partners, family, and friends, and were more likely to have a partner, paid employment, voluntary employment, and satisfaction with sex.[6]

The establishment of the Model Systems for SCI in the United States has also yielded important clinical benefits.[7] Patients admitted to Model Systems experience fewer medical complications, such as pressure ulcers. Other benefits include greater efficiency, as evidenced by increased functional index measure (FIM) gain per day, and a greater likelihood of discharge to the home or community.[7] Survival rates followed a similar pattern, with reduced mortality demonstrated for Model Systems.[8] Furthermore, there have been significant reductions in mean length of hospital stay and associated cost savings for both acute care and rehabilitation.[7]

Cohorting of patients in dedicated facilities helps accrue the critical mass of individuals required to perform meaningful research studies and further improve outcomes.[6] In summary, care provided in a setting dedicated to SCI can minimize complications while enhancing functional outcomes, resulting in shorter hospitalization times and lower economic costs.

Composition of Rehabilitation Team and Interdisciplinary Care

Rehabilitation of the individual with SCI focuses on achieving and maintaining good health, maximizing function, and promoting good quality of life. Medical and rehabilitation needs are extensive following a severe SCI, and routinely extend beyond the scope of any one clinical discipline. For these reasons, rehabilitation is ideally delivered by an interdisciplinary team working in a collaborative fashion. Traditionally, the core rehabilitation team has consisted of physical therapy, occupational therapy, rehabilitation nursing, rehabilitation psychology, social work or case management, and a physician. Other common members of the team include speech language pathology, recreational therapy, respiratory therapy, and rehabilitation aides.

- Occupational therapy typically focuses on upper-extremity function for the performance of activities of daily living (ADLs). Strategies address strengthening, active-assisted range-of-motion, and fine motor control, as well as accessibility of the environment both at home and in the community. Assistive devices and splints can also be incorporated into the treatment plan to facilitate and promote functional independence.
- Physical therapy has traditionally focused on aspects of mobility, such as ambulation, wheel chair mobility, and the performance of transfers. Maximizing mobility often requires one to address strength, balance, coordination, and endurance. Bracing and other orthotics are often incorporated into the treatment plan.
- Rehabilitation nurses provide daily care, monitor health, participate in patient education, and collaborate with the rehabilitation team to maximize patient independence with self-care activities.
- Social work can provide emotional support and adjustment counseling related to illness or disability, identify community resources and supports, help address important social needs (e.g., finances, housing), and facilitate community reintegration through discharge planning. Case managers can also serve many of these functions but typically do not provide counseling.
- Physicians diagnose conditions and underlying impairments, participate

in goal setting and formulation of treatment plans, monitor and manage medical issues, and contribute to educational needs. Physicians have also typically served as the lead of the rehabilitation team.

- Rehabilitation psychology provides important mental and emotional support. Examples of activities include the screening and treatment of depression, addressing substance abuse, assessing cognition (particularly with comorbid brain injury), and facilitating client adjustment to new impairments and limitations.

The composition of the rehabilitation team varies depending on the characteristics and impairments of the individual patient and is dynamic in nature because it must constantly adjust to the needs of the patient. Regular meetings and good communication by all team members ensure the optimal environment for rehabilitation.[9] The ultimate goal is to achieve the best functional outcome in the most efficient manner. The team approach is also beneficial to clarify goals, coordinate treatment plans, reduce redundancy in efforts, and lessen or avoid secondary medical complications.[9]

Goal Setting

An important and fundamental component of the rehabilitation process is goal setting. The articulated goals to a large extent determine the nature and focus of clinical interventions. For these reasons, it is important that goals be realistic and progress measurable. The assessment of goals should also be multidisciplinary to ensure that important needs are not overlooked.

One approach that has been described is the performance of a comprehensive needs assessment following initial mobilization out of bed.[10] The National Spinal Injuries Centre at Stoke Mandeville Hospital has developed a formal Needs Assessment Checklist (NAC).[11]

A fundamental principle of goal planning is to target and plan the rehabilitation program in accordance with the individualized needs of the patient.[10] Within the framework of identified needs, rehabilitation goals are then defined in partnership with the patient. Often a specific individual or lead is appointed to oversee and coordinate goal setting for the team. Global goals should also be operationalized. As an example, achieving independence with bladder management can be operationalized into learning how to perform intermittent self-catheterization.

Functional Outcomes of Rehabilitation

Although a detailed description of specific interventions (e.g., body weight support treadmill training) is beyond the scope of this chapter, functional improvements during rehabilitation are typically achieved through compensatory strategies (e.g., driving with hand controls) or the facilitation of improvement in an underlying impairment (e.g., paraparesis) and its accompanying functional activity (e.g., walking). Relatively recent approaches, such as the utilization of weight-supported gait training (**Fig. 21.1**), are increasingly based on presumed physiology and accompanying concepts, such as the existence of a central pattern generator in the lumbosacral spinal cord. Mechanisms of recovery are addressed in depth in Section V.

Projected functional outcomes are often based on a neurological assessment performed within 72 hours to 1 month following SCI,[12] and long-term outcomes are largely dependent on the level and completeness of the injury. It is important to note that, although the lesion level provides some insight into anticipated recovery, the unique characteristics of each case also have to be taken into account. Patient recovery and accompanying function are influenced by differences in injury characteristics; the course of medical events and comorbidities; psychological, social, and environmental supports; and cognitive abilities. Highly motivated patients may exceed the expected functional outcomes for their level of injury.[13]

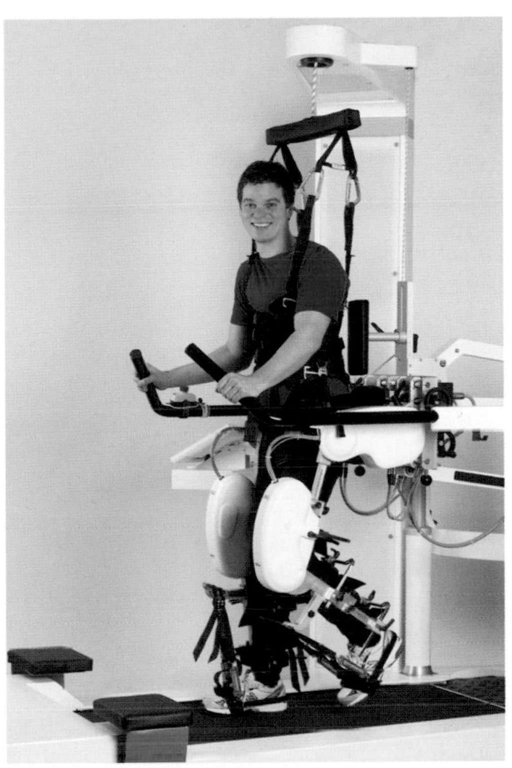

Fig. 21.1 Lokomat Pro automated gait training device (Hocoma AG, Switzerland).

Compared with the neurological level, the motor level is a better predictor of independence with self-care.[14] The neurological level of injury is the most caudal level with normal sensory and motor function on both sides of the body while the motor level corresponds to the most caudal segment with normal motor function on both sides of the body.[15] For the purposes of a discussion on expected functional outcomes, it is simplest to regard injuries as complete and sharply demarcated at their respective motor level (**Table 21.1**).[16] The following levels of independence can be expected given optimal circumstances.

Patients with high cervical injuries (i.e., C1–4) require complete assistance with ADLs, bed mobility, and transfers. They require 24-hour attendant care. They require a power wheelchair using head, chin, or breath control. C1–3 patients usually require permanent mechanical ventilation and suctioning to clear secretions.[17] Ventilator dependence may or may not be present for patients with C4 injuries.

Patients with C5 injuries demonstrate active elbow flexion and can therefore perform some simple tasks (e.g., grooming) pertaining to ADLs with the aid of special devices. However, they still require an attendant for most other ADLs and transfers. They are unable to independently roll over or come to a sitting position. They benefit from a motorized wheelchair with hand controls. These patients typically require 10 hours a day of personal care.[18]

Patients with C6 injuries demonstrate active wrist extension, passive finger flexion, and opposition of the second digit and the thumb, in addition to full innervation of the rotator cuff providing shoulder stability. The accompanying passive grip is referred to as tenodesis and allows them to grasp and manipulate objects following appropriate training with occupational therapy. Grip strength can be improved using a wrist-driven flexor-hinge orthosis. These patients require assistance for some ADLs, bed mobility, and transfers. Often eating but not cutting can be performed independently following setup. They are able to bathe and dress the upper body independently, although this may require considerable effort and time. Manual wheelchair propulsion is often possible on smooth surfaces and can be facilitated by the use of pushrim projections (knobs). A motorized wheelchair is often required for mobility in the community. These patients typically require 6 hours a day of personal care.[18]

Patients with C7 injuries have retained strength of the triceps. The forceful extension of this muscle allows these patients to lift their body weight. Motivated patients are able to transfer independently. In addition, they can roll over, sit up in bed, and transfer to a sitting position. Some assistance may be required for toileting and dressing activities, particularly for the lower extremities. However, eating, grooming, and communicating, as well as dressing and bathing of the upper extremities can be performed independently. In addition,

Table 21.1 Functional Significance of Spinal Cord Injury Based on Motor Level

Activities	C5	C6	C7	T1	T6	T12	L4
Self-care							
Eating	–	±	+	+	+	+	+
Dressing	–	–	±	+	+	+	+
Toileting	–	–	±	+	+	+	+
Bed mobility							
Rolling over/sitting up	–	±	+	+	+	+	+
Moving about in bed; supine and sitting	–	–	±	+	+	+	+
Wheelchair independence (includes transfer from/to wheelchair)	–	±	±	+	+	+	+
Functional ambulation (includes to standing position)	–	–	–	–	±	+	+
Attendant							
Lifting	+	+	±	–	–	–	–
Assisting	+	+	+	±	±	–	–
Working from home (using upper extremities)	–	–	–	+	+	+	+
Outside job	–	–	–	±	±	+	+
Private car	–	–	–	±	+	+	+
Public transportation	–	–	–	–	–	±	+

Source: This table was published in Long CI, Lawton EB. Functional significance of spinal cord lesion level. Arch Phys Med Rehab, 1955;36(4):249–255. Copyright Elsevier 1955.

manual wheelchair propulsion can be used for longer distances.

Patients with C8 or T1 injuries have increasingly greater intrinsic hand function, which results in improved grasp strength and dexterity. This allows for independence with bed mobility, transfers, and all ADLs. They often require some assistance with toileting and lower body care due to truncal impairments and instability. All patients are wheelchair dependent at a minimum. For individuals with paraplegia (T2–L1), sitting balance progressively improves with descending levels and worsens with higher levels. Respiratory function and the ability to cough and clear secretions are also improved with lower levels, due to increased volitional function of the abdominal and intercostal muscles. Augmented mobility is a major focus following thoracic SCI, and driving is possible with hand controls. Homemaking is largely independent. These patients typically require 3 hours a day of homemaking assistance.[18] Patients with injuries below L1 often have some capacity to ambulate.

In addition to the level, the completeness of SCI is also an important determinant of neurological recovery and function. In the foregoing scenarios, patients were presumed to have a complete SCI. There is little chance of functional motor recovery if a patient exhibits complete SCI (motor and sensory) 1 month postinjury, excluding cauda equina/conus medullaris injuries.[19,20] Neurorecovery in the upper extremities is of paramount importance because each level can determine the degree of functional independence. For both complete and incomplete injuries, the majority of recovery occurs in the first 6 to 9 months postinjury, with a plateau typically reached at 12 to 18 months, after which little additional improvement is anticipated.[21] Incomplete injuries demonstrate considerably more neurorecovery than complete injuries. Greater than 90% of incomplete injuries gain an additional motor level in cervical injuries compared with 70 to 85% of complete injuries.[12,22] Only 30% of individuals with complete SCI gain two or more motor levels,[22] although ability to distinguish pinprick versus light-touch in a dermatome is a good prognostic sign because it is associated with a 92% chance of motor recovery for the same level.[23] Up to 46 and 76% of individuals with incomplete tetraplegia and paraplegia, respectively, will ambulate in some capacity, with the difference often being attributed to greater trunk and upper extremity impairments for cervical injuries.[24,25]

Community Reintegration and Health Maintenance

Timely access to health care services is essential to the long-term health of persons with SCI. Individuals are particularly vulnerable during the initial weeks and months following inpatient rehabilitation, when vital community supports are still being established and there might not be a full appreciation for one's susceptibility to secondary complications. Compared with the able-bodied population, individuals demonstrate higher rates of health care utilization largely due to secondary complications.[26,27] Reported rates of rehospitalization during the first year after initial rehabilitation have ranged from 19 to 57%.[28–30] Furthermore, access to vital preventative services (mammography, bone density studies, pap smears, etc.) is often compromised, particularly if it involves the availability of accessible imaging equipment or adjustable exam tables.[31] Wheelchair users also require additional time, and there is often a financial disincentive for busy office practices to see such individuals.

Approaches to address health maintenance have included (1) patient education and health behavior change, (2) improving the transition from rehabilitation care to community care, and (3) improving systems of health care for individuals with disabilities.[32] Telehealth and the Internet are also being increasingly used to promote and maintain health in individuals with disabilities. Ultimately, health maintenance requires the existence of effective community-based health delivery systems. Successful community-based health care for vulnerable populations has tended to embrace the following concepts:[32]

1. Incorporate care coordination and case management principles, including consumer involvement in care management and design.
2. Use clinical protocols and pathways to address common problems among enrollees.
3. Use clinical information systems that can track patient needs and progress.
4. Use evaluation protocols that emphasize in varying degrees the following: enrollee satisfaction, prevention of secondary complications, and prevention of readmissions.
5. Dovetail services, where possible, with personal assistance, assisted living, and long-term care service needs of their target populations.
6. Maintain linkages, partnerships, or other relationships with organized disability groups and other community stakeholders.
7. Use physician extenders, such as physician assistants or nurse practitioners.
8. Use home visits as well as office visits.

9. Provide 24/7 availability.
10. Tackle transportation issues related to office visits.
11. Respect patient self-determination and the independent living aspirations of target populations.
12. Encourage self-management and responsibility for maintaining health.
13. Take into account the patient's mental and behavioral health needs (e.g., depression) that might otherwise compromise the medical management of other health conditions.

Meeting the preceding requirements is a daunting challenge and not surprisingly the provision of primary care to individuals with SCI has often been limited. Innovative funding models and the presence of a local champion are a must.

Longitudinal care for SCI could also benefit by emulating chronic care models developed for conditions like diabetes, congestive heart failure, and the like.[33,34] The chronic care model is based on the following six components: self-management support, clinical information systems, delivery system redesign, decision support, health care organization, and community resources.[32] Periodic evaluation, every 1 to 2 years, by an SCI specialist also has value for the surveillance and prevention of SCI-specific secondary conditions.

Pearls

- SCI medicine traces its roots to World War II.
- Dedicated SCI programs reduce secondary complications and improve functional outcomes.
- Rehabilitation needs following SCI require a coordinated, interdisciplinary approach.

Pitfalls

- Health care utilization is greater following SCI, and requirements for specialized care do not end at rehabilitation discharge.
- Financial disincentives for health care providers and lack of accessible facilities are common barriers to health maintenance following SCI.

References

1. Lifshutz J, Colohan A. A brief history of therapy for traumatic spinal cord injury. Neurosurg Focus 2004;16(1):E5
2. Marketos SG, Skiadas P. Hippocrates: the father of spine surgery. Spine 1999;24(13):1381–1387
3. Bedbrook GM. The development and care of spinal cord paralysis (1918 to 1986). Paraplegia 1987;25(3):172–184
4. Guttman L. Spinal Cord Injuries: Comprehensive Management and Research. 2nd ed. Oxford, UK: Blackwell Scientific; 1976
5. Donovan WH, Carter RE, Bedbrook GM, Young JS, Griffiths ER. Incidence of medical complications in spinal cord injury: patients in specialised, compared with non-specialised centres. Paraplegia 1984;22(5):282–290
6. Smith M. Efficacy of specialist versus non-specialist management of spinal cord injury within the UK. Spinal Cord 2002;40(1):10–16
7. Stover SL, DeLisa JA, Whiteneck GG. Spinal Cord Injury: Clinical Outcomes from the Model Systems. Gaithersburg, MD: Aspen; 1995
8. DeVivo MJ, Kartus PL, Stover SL, Fine PR. Benefits of early admission to an organised spinal cord injury care system. Paraplegia 1990;28(9):545–555
9. Flood KEM, ed. Physiatry: Interdisciplinary Management. Washington, DC: TMM Publications; 1999
10. Duff J, Evans MJ, Kennedy P. Goal planning: a retrospective audit of rehabilitation process and outcome. Clin Rehabil 2004;18(3):275–286
11. Kennedy P, Hamilton LR. The needs assessment checklist: a clinical approach to measuring outcome. Spinal Cord 1999;37(2):136–139
12. Burns AS, Ditunno JF. Establishing prognosis and maximizing functional outcomes after spinal cord injury: a review of current and future directions in rehabilitation management. Spine 2001;26(24, Suppl):S137–S145
13. Rintala DH, Willems EP. Behavioral and demographic predictors of postdischarge outcomes in spinal cord injury. Arch Phys Med Rehabil 1987;68(6):357–362
14. Marino RJ, Rider-Foster D, Maissel G, Ditunno JF. Superiority of motor level over single neurological level in categorizing tetraplegia. Paraplegia 1995;33(9):510–513
15. Kirshblum SC, O'Connor KC. Predicting neurologic recovery in traumatic cervical spinal cord injury. Arch Phys Med Rehabil 1998;79(11):1456–1466
16. Long CI, Lawton EB. Functional significance of spinal cord lesion level. Arch Phys Med Rehabil 1955;36(4):249–255

17. Lanig IS, Peterson WP. The respiratory system in spinal cord injury. Phys Med Rehabil Clin N Am 2000;11(1):29–43, vii
18. Consortium for Spinal Cord Medicine. Outcomes following traumatic spinal cord injury: clinical practice guidelines for health-care professionals. J Spinal Cord Med 2000;23(4):289–316
19. Waters RL, Yakura JS, Adkins RH, Sie I. Recovery following complete paraplegia. Arch Phys Med Rehabil 1992;73(9):784–789
20. Waters RL, Adkins RH, Yakura JS, Sie I. Motor and sensory recovery following complete tetraplegia. Arch Phys Med Rehabil 1993;74(3):242–247
21. Waters RL, Adkins R, Yakura J, Sie I. Donal Munro Lecture: functional and neurologic recovery following acute SCI. J Spinal Cord Med 1998;21(3):195–199
22. Steeves JD, Kramer JK, Fawcett JW, et al; EMSCI Study Group. Extent of spontaneous motor recovery after traumatic cervical sensorimotor complete spinal cord injury. Spinal Cord 2011;49(2):257–265
23. Poynton AR, O'Farrell DA, Shannon F, Murray P, McManus F, Walsh MG. Sparing of sensation to pin prick predicts recovery of a motor segment after injury to the spinal cord. J Bone Joint Surg Br 1997;79(6):952–954
24. Waters RL, Adkins RH, Yakura JS, Sie I. Motor and sensory recovery following incomplete tetraplegia. Arch Phys Med Rehabil 1994;75(3):306–311
25. Waters RL, Adkins RH, Yakura JS, Sie I. Motor and sensory recovery following incomplete paraplegia. Arch Phys Med Rehabil 1994;75(1):67–72
26. Dryden DM, Saunders LD, Rowe BH, et al. Utilization of health services following spinal cord injury: a 6-year follow-up study. Spinal Cord 2004;42(9):513–525
27. Munce SE, Guilcher SJ, Couris CM, et al. Physician utilization among adults with traumatic spinal cord injury in Ontario: a population-based study. Spinal Cord 2009;47(6):470–476
28. Cardenas DD, Hoffman JM, Kirshblum S, McKinley W. Etiology and incidence of rehospitalization after traumatic spinal cord injury: a multicenter analysis. Arch Phys Med Rehabil 2004;85(11):1757–1763
29. Jaglal SB, Munce SE, Guilcher SJ, et al. Health system factors associated with rehospitalizations after traumatic spinal cord injury: a population-based study. Spinal Cord 2009;47(8):604–609
30. Middleton JW, Lim K, Taylor L, Soden R, Rutkowski S. Patterns of morbidity and rehospitalisation following spinal cord injury. Spinal Cord 2004;42(6):359–367
31. Ramirez A, Farmer GC, Grant D, Papachristou T. Disability and preventive cancer screening: results from the 2001 California Health Interview Survey. Am J Public Health 2005;95(11):2057–2064
32. The Special Interest Group on SCI Model System Innovation. Toward a Model System of Post-rehabilitation Health Care for Individuals with SCI. 2010. http://www.ncscims.org/SCIModelSystemInnovationReport.pdf. Accessed June 4, 2012
33. Bodenheimer T, Wagner EH, Grumbach K. Improving primary care for patients with chronic illness: the chronic care model, Part 2. JAMA 2002;288(15):1909–1914
34. Bodenheimer T, Wagner EH, Grumbach K. Improving primary care for patients with chronic illness. JAMA 2002;288(14):1775–1779

22

The Management of Secondary Complications Following Spinal Cord Injury

Anthony S. Burns, Jefferson R. Wilson, and B. Catharine Craven

Key Points

1. A severe spinal cord injury affects every major organ system.
2. Secondary complications lead to increased health care utilization and costs.
3. Specialized medical care and ongoing support are required to prevent secondary complications and maintain long-term health.
4. The management of the following medical complications is reviewed—heterotopic ossification, neurogenic bladder dysfunction, neurogenic bowel dysfunction, osteoporosis, respiratory management, spasticity, and upper extremity preservation.

A spinal cord injury (SCI) is a devastating event. In addition to the accompanying loss of function and independence, the affected individual is predisposed to a constellation of secondary complications. A severe SCI affects every major organ system (e.g., pressure ulcers, neurogenic bowel and bladder dysfunction, sublesional osteoporosis, neuropathic pain, cardiovascular dysfunction), and individuals remain at risk for secondary complications for the remainder of their lives. The complications are distinct from those associated with normal aging. One study from the US Model SCI System found that 96% of clients had a medical complication when seen for routine annual follow-up.[1] A Canadian study reported that 56% of individuals had experienced a urinary tract infection during the previous year, with another 28% reporting a pressure ulcer.[2]

Secondary complications ultimately lead to increased health care utilization and costs. Dryden and colleagues reported that, compared with controls, individuals with SCI were rehospitalized 2.6 times more often and were 2.7 times more likely to have physician contact during a 6-year follow-up period postinjury.[3] Fifty-seven percent were hospitalized at least once during this period, with 32% admitted between three and nine times. Four percent were hospitalized on 10 or more occasions. Recent studies continue to confirm increased health care utilization following SCI. During the first year postdischarge, the mean number of physician visits was ~30, and 27.5% of individuals required at least one rehospitalization.[4,5]

The responsibility of the health care system therefore does not end when the individual with SCI leaves the acute care or rehabilitation center to reenter the community. Health care providers must remain proactive and vigilant; and specialized and ongoing medical care is required to prevent secondary complications, maintain long-term health, and maximize overall health and quality of life. This chapter reviews the management of common complications following SCI.

Autonomic Dysreflexia

Autonomic dysreflexia (AD) is a condition characterized by episodes of malignant hypertension, which, when severe, can lead to potentially life-threatening complications, such as stroke. AD occurs in individuals with SCI at or above T6. It increases with ascending level and injury severity[6,7] and is three times more common following complete compared with incomplete injuries.[6] The pathophysiology and treatment of this condition are discussed in detail in Chapter 16.

Cardiovascular Disease

The prevalence of risk factors for coronary artery disease (CAD) increases following SCI. Specific risk factors include elements of the metabolic syndrome (hyperlipidemia, abdominal obesity, glucose intolerance, insulin resistance), elevated homocysteine, elevated C-reactive protein (CRP), and low physical activity/fitness levels. The prevalence of CAD risk factors translates into a higher incidence of CAD following SCI. Cardiovascular morbidity and mortality occur earlier and more often than in the able-bodied population. As a result, CAD is the leading cause of death for individuals living with chronic SCI.[8]

CAD can also be asymptomatic ("silent"). Visceral afferent fibers from the heart enter the spinal cord at T1–4, and individuals with neurological levels at and above these segments might not experience cardiac pain. The exact prevalence of asymptomatic CAD among people with SCI is unclear, with reported rates ranging from 25 to 65%.[9] Because CAD can be relatively asymptomatic following SCI, the diagnosis requires vigilance and a high index of suspicion on the part of the clinician. A comprehensive review of cardiovascular health following SCI is provided in Chapter 16.

Heterotopic Ossification

Heterotopic ossification (HO) is a condition characterized by the formation of mature ectopic bone in the periarticular soft tissues of joints. HO occurs after SCI, traumatic brain injury, burns, and acetabular fractures. Although our understanding of the underlying pathophysiology is limited, the differentiation of primitive mesenchymal stem cells into osteogenic cells plays a prominent role. In the setting of SCI, HO always occurs at joints below the neurological level of the injury, with the most common site being the hips, followed in descending order of frequency by the knees, shoulders, elbows, and hands. Although severe cases can lead to a loss of range of motion and even joint ankylosis, most cases are asymptomatic and often diagnosed incidentally. Loss of hip range of motion can interfere with seated posture and independence during transfers.

Signs of earlier HO are nonspecific and inflammatory—erythema, swelling, low-grade fever. Calcified HO is visible with plain x-ray but triple-phase bone scan remains the gold standard for the diagnosis of earlier HO prior to maturation and calcification. HO becomes evident on plain radiography ~2 to 6 weeks after diagnosis using triple-phase bone scan.[10,11] Early diagnosis is critical because treatment is more effective when initiated prior to the formation of visible calcification. Serum alkaline phosphatase rises prior to radiographic evidence of HO and may be used for monitoring the activity of HO. Urinary excretion of prostaglandin E2 has also been reported to be elevated in individuals with acute SCI who later develop HO.[12]

The mainstays of treatment are nonsteroidal antiinflammatories (selective and nonselective cyclooxygenase-2 inhibitors) and bisphosphonates (e.g., etidronate). Antiinflammatories are believed to inhibit the differentiation of primitive mesenchymal cells into osteogenic cells, whereas bisphosphonates prevent the calcification and maturation of existing osteoid. Indomethacin and rofecoxib have both been evaluated post-SCI and demonstrated to be effective for primary prevention of HO when given early after injury.[13,14] Two bisphosphonates, etidronate and pamidronate, have been studied for the treatment of diagnosed HO post-SCI. Bisphosphonates inhibit the transformation of amorphous calcium phosphate into crystalline hydroxyapatite. Etidronate can inhibit progression of HO when given early, meaning a positive bone scan in the setting of negative radiographs.[15,16] One study also suggests that pamidronate can halt the progression of HO following surgical resection.[17] Surgery is sometimes necessary to regain range of motion, but recurrence is common, especially if resection is done during the inflammatory phase of active ossification.

Neurogenic Bladder Dysfunction

The full impact of SCI on voiding and the genitourinary system is underappreciated by many clinicians. Failure to address these issues can lead to significant social isolation as well as patient morbidity and mortality. In the past, renal failure was the leading cause of death following SCI.[18] Fortunately, this is no longer the case, due to improved awareness, management, and surveillance of neurogenic bladder dysfunction following SCI. Today there are practice guidelines and systematic evidence-based reviews [Spinal Cord Injury Rehabilitation Evidence (SCIRE)] to guide clinical management.[18,19]

Physiological Alterations after Spinal Cord Injury

Bladder dysfunction after SCI can be classified as either a lower motor neuron (LMN) or an upper motor neuron (UMN) syndrome.[20] LMN syndrome occurs following injury to either the conus medullaris or cauda equina. The accompanying injury to sacral (S2–4) motor neurons or their associated axons compromises motor output to the bladder, resulting in decreased or absent detrusor contractility (flaccidity). Clinical manifestations of this include urinary retention or incomplete emptying postvoid or both.

UMN syndrome occurs with SCIs cephalad to the conus medullaris and is characterized by disruption of the descending spinal pathways and a loss of cortical inhibition over reflexive voiding. Immediately after SCI, the distinction between LMN and UMN syndromes can be clouded by the presence of spinal shock because the transient loss or depression of neural activity below an acute spinal cord lesion leads to initial bladder flaccidity.

Upper Motor Neuron Syndrome

The majority of SCIs will exhibit UMN dysfunction due to the anatomical location of the lesion. Individuals with complete SCIs are expected to have involuntary, reflexive emptying with filling of the bladder. In comparison, many persons with incomplete SCI will have detrusor disinhibition (hyperreflexia) and urge incontinence. Communication between the pontine (brain stem) micturition center and the sacral micturition center is also disrupted or compromised. This leads to poor coordination between reflexive detrusor contractions and accompanying brain stem–mediated events, such as relaxation of the bladder neck, internal sphincter, and external sphincter. The terms used to describe this discoordination are *bladder–sphincter* or *detrusor–sphincter dyssynergia* (*DSD*). The net result is that the bladder reflexively contracts against the relative outlet obstruction of a closed bladder neck, internal sphincter, or external sphincter. In turn, this leads to elevated bladder pressures with micturition. Over time, elevated detrusor pressures can predispose to vesicoureteral reflux, hydronephrosis, recurrent pyelonephritis, and progressive deterioration in renal function.

When reflexive voiding returns post–spinal shock, urodynamic studies should be performed to exclude occult DSD. If reflex voiding fails to return by 6 months post-SCI in a patient expected to have a UMN syndrome, urodynamic testing should also be performed. Urodynamic testing can include the following components: cystometrography, electromyography, urethral pressure profiling, and fluoroscopy. Cystometrography provides information about pressure–volume relationships in the bladder. Electromyography, using needle or surface electrodes, clarifies the function of the external sphincter and its coordination with the detrusor. Urethral pressure profiling gives information about the resistance to outflow. Fluoroscopy allows actual visualization of the bladder during voiding. An elevated voiding pressure in the face of increased sphincter electromyography activity during a detrusor contraction is diagnostic of DSD.

DSD requires intervention to prevent long-term complications like vesicoureteral reflux. Goals of management focus on achieving adequate drainage, low-pressure urine storage, and low-pressure voiding. After any therapeutic intervention, follow-up testing should be performed to confirm that bladder pressures have been effectively lowered. To lower bladder pressures, reflexive contractions can be suppressed with anticholinergic agents, such as oxybutynin chloride and tolterodine tartrate. If needed, anticholinergic suppression can be augmented further with a tricyclic antidepressant. Another option is the intramuscular injection of botulinum A toxin into the detrusor body. Botulinum A toxin paralyzes muscle by blocking the release of acetylcholine at the neuromuscular junction. Disadvantages of botulinum A include expense and the fact that it has to be periodically repeated (approximately every 3 to 6 months). Following the pharmacological inhibition of detrusor contractions, bladder emptying can be safely accomplished with intermittent catheterization. Many patients with motor levels of C7 and below can be taught to perform self-catheterization. If conservative management with medications fails to work, bladder augmentation can facilitate low-pressure storage in small, noncompliant bladders. Bladder augmentation procedures with urinary diversion can also facilitate intermittent catheterization via an easier to reach abdominal stoma.

In men, an alternative approach is the use of α-blockers (i.e., prazosin, terazosin, doxazosin, tamsulosin) to reduce resistance to outflow at the α-adrenergically innervated bladder neck and internal sphincter. This can lower peak bladder pressures during contractions and allow the safe use of a condom (external) catheter and collection bag attached to the leg. Transurethral and transperineal injections of botulinum A toxin have also been to used to treat dyssynergia by lowering resistance to urine outflow. Outlet obstruction can also be reduced by transurethral sphincterotomy or placement of a urethral stent. Afterward, reflexive voiding can then be managed by wearing a condom (external) catheter.

For SCI patients without significant dyssynergia but with detrusor hyperreflexia, urge incontinence has been traditionally treated with systemic anticholinergic agents. Local pharmacological interventions include the intravesicular administration of capsaicin and botulinum toxin A. Capsaicin desensitizes afferent c-fibers through the depletion of substance P. In chronic SCI, the c-fibers are thought to mediate the afferent limb of the micturition reflex.

Another approach to the management of UMN bladder dysfunction is the use of electrical stimulation. First, a posterior rhizotomy of the sacral nerve roots is performed to prevent reflex incontinence. Electrodes are then attached to the anterior nerve roots. Electrical stimulation of these roots causes simultaneous contraction of the detrusor and sphincters. Because the striated-muscle external sphincter fatigues before the smooth-muscle detrusor, voiding occurs in short spurts when the sphincter intermittently relaxes.

Long-term management with an indwelling catheter should be the choice of last resort because it increases the risk of bladder cancer, recurrent bladder infections, and bladder stones. Nevertheless, it is sometimes indicated for the individual who lacks the manual dexterity to independently perform intermittent catheterization and/or does not have additional assistance available. This is more commonly an issue in women because external catheters are not an option and intermittent catheterization is more difficult due to anatomical considerations. In men who require a long-term indwelling catheter, consideration should be given to converting to a suprapubic catheter to prevent complications such as improper insertion and placement, urethral strictures and fistulas, and urethral erosions. Indwelling catheters should be replaced every 3 to 4 weeks.

Lower Motor Neuron Syndrome

LMN bladder syndrome is associated with conus medullaris and cauda equina injuries. The anatomical location of the lesion interrupts the sacral reflex arc, which consists of afferent input from the detrusor, the sacral micturition center (S2–4), and efferent input to the detrusor. The end result is detrusor areflexia (hypocontractility). Other clinical findings that accompany detrusor areflexia include saddle anesthesia, reduced anal sphincter tone, loss of voluntary sphincter control, and permanent absence of the bulbocavernosus reflex. Long-term bladder management of this patient population is straightforward and ideally consists of intermittent, clean self-catheterization timed to regularly empty the bladder and prevent bladder overdistention. If intermittent catheterization is not possible, adequate drainage can be achieved with a chronic, indwelling catheter.

Other Genitourinary Issues after Spinal Cord Injury

Recurrent urinary tract infections (UTIs) are common after SCI; however, colonization with bacteria should be expected. The presence of bacteria in the urine therefore does not warrant treatment unless the patient is clinically symptomatic (e.g., febrile) or there is laboratory evidence of tissue invasion, such as significant pyuria. The cornerstones of preventing UTIs are clean technique and regular, complete bladder drainage, because residual urine is an ideal medium for bacterial overgrowth. In addition, recurrent UTIs can be a manifestation of underlying pathology, such as kidney or bladder stones, poor hygiene, and detrusor–sphincter dyssynergia with outlet obstruction. Evaluation should therefore exclude the possibility of underlying causes. Prophylactic antibiotics should be avoided because they only serve to promote the emergence of drug-resistant organisms. Patients with SCI are also at increased risk for renal and bladder calculi secondary to factors like hypercalciuria, recurrent UTIs, and indwelling catheters. Stones in the urinary tract can present with increased lower limb spasticity, recurrent UTIs, or refractory autonomic dysreflexia. Calcified stones can often be visualized with abdominal plain films, but ultrasonography remains the gold standard for diagnosis. Bladder calculi can also be directly visualized with endoscopy. In susceptible patients, overdistention can lead to the potentially life-threatening condition of AD. To prevent this condition, most patients are advised to perform self-catheterization every 4 to 6 hours. The goal is to keep catheterization volumes less than ~500 mL in men and less than 400 mL in women to minimize the risk of UTIs and other complications.

Long-Term Screening and Follow-Up

Long-term follow-up is essential to maintain health and prevent complications. Although no studies have been done on the optimum frequency of follow-up evaluations, many medical centers evaluate upper and lower tract functioning on an annual basis. To guide clinicians, the American Paraplegia Society (APS) published guidelines for the urological evaluation of patients with SCI.[19] Annual follow-up is recommended for the first 5 to 10 years after injury. If the patient continues to do well, the follow-up interval can be reduced to every other year. Serum creatinine should be evaluated initially and then every 1 to 2 years. The upper (kidneys, ureters) and lower (bladder, urethra) urinary tracts should also be assessed initially and then annually for the first 5 to 10 years and afterward every other year.

Options for upper urinary tract evaluation include nuclear renal scans, renal ultrasound, intravenous pyelography, and high-resolution computed tomography (CT). The nuclear renal scan is probably the most effective test with the fewest adverse effects for monitoring renal function. A decrease of more than 20% in renal plasma flow warrants further investigation. The lower urinary tract can be assessed with cystoscopy, and annual cystoscopy is recommended in those with an indwelling suprapubic or urethral catheter due to the risk of squamous cell carcinoma. Urodynamics should be performed at the same intervals as upper and lower urinary tract screening.

Neurogenic Bowel Dysfunction

Following SCI, alterations in bowel function are a significant source of morbidity and an impediment to quality of life. Neurogenic bowel dysfunction impacts the majority of individuals with SCI, and one survey of ~1300 patients found that only 1.5% reported having no bowel problems, with most patients reporting at least two significant gastrointestinal complications.[21] Impaired abdominal and pelvic sensation, decreased gastrointestinal mobility, and compromised autonomic control of the alimentary tract all contribute to observed problems. The specific characteristics of neurogenic bowel dysfunction depend on the anatomical location of the injury. Injury cephalad to the conus medularis leads to a UMN bowel syndrome, whereas injury to the conus medullaris or cauda equina produces an LMN bowel syndrome. UMN and LMN syndromes require distinct management strategies, and clinicians should have a basic understanding of the underlying pathophysiology. Both UMN and LMN syndromes can be associated with prolonged gastrointestinal transit times, constipation or impaction, and incontinence. The management strategies, however, differ significantly.

UMN Bowel Syndrome

The UMN bowel syndrome is characterized by preserved reflexive contractions of the gut (peristalsis) allowing for continued stool propulsion; however, loss of cortical control impairs or prevents volitional defecation. This is due to the inability to voluntarily contract and relax striated pelvic floor muscles, including the external rectal sphincter, which in turn leads to prolonged constipation followed by episodes of bowel incontinence in the absence of intervention.

LMN Bowel Syndrome

Conversely, for LMN bowel syndrome, or "areflexic bowel disorder," the accompanying injury at the level of the conus medullaris or cauda equina abolishes autonomic and somatic reflex arcs that receive their innervation from sacral segments. The absence of reflexive spinal–colonic connections to the descending colon and rectum leads to flaccidity and compromised stool propulsion and expulsion. Sphincter tone is also diminished or absent. On examination, sacral reflexes (e.g., bulbocavernosus, anal wink) are often absent.

Goals of a Bowel Program

An effective bowel program should promote effective gastrointestinal transport, achieve regular and complete rectal evacuation, eliminate incontinence, avoid anorectal injury, and occur within a reasonable time frame in a safe, comfortable setting. This typically means employing a multifaceted approach to trigger a bowel movement at the desired time and avoid incontinence in between. Timing and a consistent schedule are the cornerstones of a bowel program, and it should be performed at the same time, typically in the morning or evening depending on individual preference. Common frequencies of bowel programs include daily or every other day, and decisions regarding the optimal frequency for an individual can be guided by preinjury bowel habits, patient lifestyle, and individual response.

Fluid and Fiber Intake

Typical treatment algorithms incorporate baseline recommendations for adequate fiber (15 to 30 g daily) and fluid intake (1.5 to 2 L of clear fluid daily) to promote ideal stool consistency and regularity. A primary function of the colon is water absorption and without adequate fluid intake, increased colon transit times can predispose to small hard stools and impaction. Fiber is an effective bulking agent that promotes water retention and improves peristalsis by maintaining ideal stool girth and consistency. Existing guidelines suggest starting with at least 15 mg daily.[22] Thereafter, fiber intake should be individualized and titrated accordingly. Stool softeners, such as docusate sodium, can also be a helpful adjunct for managing stool consistency.

Additional Aspects of Bowel Management

In addition to promoting the consistent transport of stool through the gastrointestinal tract, a neurogenic bowel program should incorporate strategies for achieving regular and predictable stool expulsion. Here the strategies differ for UMN and LMN syndromes. Individuals with UMN syndrome can take advantage of both gastrocolic and anorectal reflexes. Distention of the stomach increases peristalsis (gastrocolic reflex); therefore, bowel evacuation is best completed 20 to 30 minutes after a meal—breakfast for a morning schedule and dinner for an evening schedule. The anorectal reflex can then be triggered following a transfer to an appropriate commode or raised toilet, or alternatively lying on the left side. The anorectal reflex increases peristaltic waves in the descending colon and rectum following rectal stimulation, thereby facilitating stool expulsion. Rectal stimulation can be achieved with digital stimulation, suppository insertion, or use of a mini-enema. The gastrocolic and anorectal reflexes are absent in the setting of LMN syndrome. Due to accompanying rectal flaccidity, individuals need to be taught to perform regular manual disimpaction to achieve evacuation, prevent incontinence, and avoid long-term complications from overdistention.

If an existing bowel program proves ineffective, one variable should be changed at a time and continued for three to five cycles prior to making additional changes.[22] When the time between rectal stimulation and evacuation becomes excessive or an individual fails to have a bowel movement within 24 hours of a planned evacuation, one can consider a trial of a lubricant, osmotic, or stimulant laxative. Alternatively, the form of rectal stimulation can also be changed. Polyethylene glycol based bisacodyl suppositories and mini-enemas are more effective than hydrogenated vegetable oil–based bisacodyl suppositories.[23,24] For refractory chronic constipation, consideration can be given to adding a prokinetic agent. Options include cisapride, metoclopramide, and neostigmine. In spite of differences in their mechanism of action, there is level 1 evidence that both cisapride and neostigmine reduce intestinal transit times and improve bowel evacuation in the SCI population.[25] Unfortunately, cisapride has been withdrawn from the United States and many other markets due to side effects. Metoclopromide acts primarily on the stomach and has been shown to be effective at promoting gastric emptying.[26] Each of these medications has unique pharmacokinetic and side effect profiles that must be considered prior to prescribing. Other interventions that improve bowel motility and evacuation, include increased activity levels and warm caffeinated beverages (e.g., coffee or tea). Warm tea or coffee has the additional benefit of activating the gastrocolic reflex.

If conservative management fails, more invasive therapeutic options exist. Pulsed transanal irrigation involves instilling intermittent rapid pulses of warm irrigation within the rectum with an aim to break up impacted stool and stimulate peristalsis. This therapy is administered in a retrograde fashion through an enema continence catheter secured in the anorectum with an inflatable balloon. In more extreme cases, colonic irrigation has been delivered in an anterograde fashion through an ostomy created surgically with the appendix, known as an "appendecostomy." Although currently not routine practice, some authors advocate colostomy as a safe and effective treatment for severe, chronic gastrointestinal problems and perianal pressure ulcers in persons with SCI.[27] Magnetic and electrical stimulation have also been evaluated in individuals with SCI[25,28] and have been shown to reduce mean colonic transit time.

In summary, mitigating gastrointestinal complications after SCI requires the institution of an individually tailored bowel routine centered on diet (e.g., fiber), hydration, postinjury physiology, and administration of local and systemic drug therapies as needed. In addition, it is common for persons with motor complete injuries to develop hemorrhoids, anusitis, and rectal prolapse as they age. Treatment of these conditions is analogous to that for the able-bodied population. For refractory or more complicated situations, pulse irrigation techniques and colostomy can be considered. On the horizon are functional magnetic and electrical stimulation techniques to stimulate peristalsis and reduce colonic transit time.

Pain Following Spinal Cord Injury

Chronic pain is defined as pain persisting for 6 months or more and having the potential to disrupt physical functioning beyond the parameters imposed by the SCI.[29] It is a common and debilitating condition following SCI, as well as one of the most challenging medical problems associated with SCI.[30] Due to differences in methodology and definitions, the reported prevalence has varied widely—from 26 to 96%.[31] Chronic pain is also perceived as difficult to deal with by the person experiencing it,[32] as well as by the health care providers managing it.[29] Furthermore, chronic pain negatively impacts quality of life and interferes with valued life activities, such as employment, sleep, recreational and social activities, therapy, and ability to engage in household chores.[33]

Pain following SCI is typically divided into neuropathic and nociceptive pain.[34] *Nociceptive pain* is the result of the normal processing of stimuli that damage or disturb normal tissues. Nociceptive pain typically occurs above the level of the spinal cord lesion, has an identifiable cause, and may result from musculoskeletal problems such as fractures or rotator cuff tears. *Neuropathic pain* is more complex and results from the abnormal processing of sensory input due to damage to the nervous system.[35] Although neuropathic pain can be identified by site (region of sensory disturbance) and by features (sharp, shooting, electric, burning, stabbing), it is difficult to identify a specific stimulus or cause, and patients may find it difficult to describe the quality of neuropathic pain.[35] Typically, neuropathic pain is present at or below the level of the spinal cord lesion and can fluctuate in intensity depending on the individual's emotional state or level of fatigue.[36]

The evaluation and management of chronic pain following SCI are addressed in Chapter 17.

Osteoporosis

Osteoporosis following SCI is a significant source of morbidity and mortality. When it occurs below the neurological level of injury, it is referred to as sublesional osteoporosis (SLOP). As many as 25 to 46% of individuals with chronic SCI will sustain fragility fractures,[37,38] most commonly of the distal femur and proximal tibia. Fragility fractures occur with events one would not typically associate with fractures, such as transfers (torsion) or low-velocity falls (compression),[38,39] and frequently result in delayed union, nonunion, malunion, or lower extremity amputation.[38]

Twelve to eighteen months following a motor complete SCI, bone mineral density (BMD) of the hips, distal femur, and proximal tibia decline to 28%, 37 to 43%, and 36 to 50% of age-matched peers, respectively.[40] The decline of BMD in persons with motor incomplete injuries (American Spinal Injury Association Impairment Scale [AIS] C and D) is less predictable, and there is controversy regarding whether hip and knee BMD stabilizes or continues to decline with chronic injury.[41–45]

Identifying Sublesional Osteoporosis and Assessing Fracture Risk

SLOP is unique to persons with SCI and is characterized by lower extremity bone resorption, changes in hip and knee region bone architecture, and increased risk of lower extremity fractures. Diagnosing SLOP and assessing fracture risk entail measuring BMD and reviewing risk factors. Risk factors after SCI include SCI before age 16, duration of SCI > 10 years, paraplegia (vs tetraplegia), body mass index (BMI) ≤ 19, alcohol intake > five servings per day, motor complete SCI (AIS A or B), female gender, prior history of fracture, and maternal family history of fracture.[40]

Dual x-ray absorptiometry (DXA) is the standard clinical tool for diagnosing SLOP and monitoring treatment effectiveness; although peripheral quantitative CT (p-QCT) is increasingly available. DXA measures areal BMD [aBMD = bone mineral content (BMC)(g)/area (cm^2)], whereas p-QCT measures volumetric BMD [vBMD = BMC(g)/volume (cm^3)]. BMD T-scores or Z-scores of the hip or knee regions can identify patients with SLOP based on their gender and age at scan acquisition (**Table 22.1**). Assessment of knee region BMD is crucial because it is the best predictor of knee region fracture risk after SCI.[45,46] BMD fracture thresholds are values below which fragility fractures begin to occur, whereas fracture breakpoints are values below which the majority of fractures occur.[47] Knee region aBMD and vBMD thresholds for fracture and breakpoint have been identified.[46,48] Knee fracture thresholds are ≤ 0.78 g/cm^2 (aBMD), < 114 mg/cm^3 (vBMD-femur), and < 72 mg/cm^3 (vBMD-tibia), whereas the accompanying fracture breakpoint is < 0.49 g/cm^2 (aBMD). Increases in BMD are presumed to be a suitable surrogate outcome for fracture risk reduction.

Lifestyle or Metabolic Causes of Low/Declining Bone Mineral Density Unrelated to Spinal Cord Injury

Identification of lifestyle behaviors and secondary metabolic causes of low or declining BMD can be accomplished via serum screening and simple questions regarding daily or weekly caffeine or alcohol intake and smoking history (**Fig. 22.1**). Hypothyroidism, secondary hyperparathyroidism, renal insufficiency, vitamin D deficiency, hypogonadism (men), and amenorrhea (women) are frequently identified secondary causes of decreased BMD. Smoking cessation, caffeine intake (≤ 3 servings/day) and alcohol intake (≤ 2 servings/day) are targets for behavioral interventions.

Table 22.1 Definition of Sublesional Osteoporosis (SLOP)

Age range	Definition
Men ≥ 60 years or postmenopausal women	Hip or knee region *T* score ≤ −2.5
Men < 59 years or premenopausal women	Hip or knee region *Z* score ≤ −2.0 with ≥ 3 fracture risk factors
Men or women age 16–90	Prior fragility fracture and no identifiable etiology of osteoporosis other than spinal cord injury

Note: The *T* score is the number of standard deviations (SDs) BMD is above or below gender-specific young adult mean peak bone mass. The *Z* score is the number of SDs BMD is above or below that expected for individuals of the same age and gender.
Source: Craven BC, Robertson LA, McGillivray CF, Adachi JD. Detection and treatment of sublesional osteoporosis among patients with chronic spinal cord injury: proposed paradigms. Top Spinal Cord Inj Rehabil 2009;14:9 © 2009. Reprinted with permission.

Paradigm	Clinical Questions
Health Status	•Does my patient have secondary causes of osteoporosis unrelated to their SCI? •Does my patient have causes of low BMD amenable to treatment?
Lifestyle	•Does my patient consume excessive amounts of alcohol or caffeine? •Does my patient smoke? •Does my patient participate in high risk activity or contact sport? •Has there been an interim decline in my patient's mobility or transfers?
Nutrition	•Does my patient's nutrition status contribute to their SLOP? •Does my patient have an adequate, but not excessive calcium intake? •Does my patient have an adequate serum 25-OH vitamin D level?
Bone Factors	•How many SCI fracture risk factors does my patient have? •Does my patient meet the WHO criteria for osteoporosis or SLOP definition? •Does my patient have a knee region BMD below the fracture threshold?

Fig. 22.1 Framework for clinical history and risk assessment for sublesional osteoporosis after spinal cord injury. (From Craven BC, Giangregorio LM, Robertson LA, Delparte JJ, Ashe MC, Eng JJ. Sublesional osteoporosis prevention, detection and treatment: a decision guide for rehabilitation clinicians treating patients with spinal cord injury. Crit Rev Phys Rehabil Med 2008;20(4):10. Reprinted with permission.)

Calcium and Vitamin D Intake

Assessment of the patient's diet is necessary to ensure sufficient but not excessive calcium and vitamin D intake (diet or supplements), because excessive calcium intake may precipitate bladder or kidney stones, while some clinicians are concerned that excessive vitamin D intake may precipitate heterotopic ossification.

Vitamin D insufficiency or deficiency is prevalent among persons with SCI,[49,50] and serum 25-hydroxyvitamin D levels should be monitored to ensure serum levels are in the therapeutic range. Factors that decrease calcium absorption include dietary fiber, phytates (in unleavened bread), oxalate found in green leafy vegetables (spinach, okra, celery), fruit (berries, currants), nuts (peanuts, pecans), and caffeinated beverages (tea, cocoa).[51] Given the theoretical risk of renal or bladder stones, a dietary calcium intake of 1000 mg daily is a reasonable target for patients with SCI and SLOP and no premorbid history of stones.

Therapeutic Interventions: Pharmacological and Rehabilitation

A decision tree for evaluation and treatment is provided in **Fig. 22.2**. Several systematic reviews have summarized the drug and rehabilitation interventions available for SLOP treatment.[52–54] Of the rehabilitation intervention studies reviewed, no intervention led to sustained increases in hip or knee region BMD. FES cycle-ergometry or passive standing may be offered as therapy provided patients understand it is a lifetime prescription because the therapeutic benefit abates with cessation of therapy.

There is evidence supporting the efficacy of alendronate for SLOP among patients with motor complete paraplegia. In a randomized open-label trial, Zehnder et al.[55] evaluated the effectiveness of alendronate 10 mg daily combined with elemental calcium 500 mg daily versus elemental calcium 500 mg daily (alone). Fifty-five men with motor complete SCI were treated for 24 months. Injury duration ranged from 1 month to 29 years post-SCI, with a group mean of 10 years postinjury. Key findings included an 8.0% decline in tibia epiphysis BMD in the control group and relative maintenance of tibia epiphysis BMD (–2.0%) in the treatment group ($p < 0.001$). Reported side effects of alendronate in the general population include: hypocalcemia (>10%); abdominal pain, reflux, flatulence, and dyspepsia (1 to 19%); and rare but serious events, including osteonecrosis of the jaw, atrial fibrillation (1.5%), and hepatotoxicity.[56] There are no clinical trials evaluating drug treatments of SLOP among patients with motor incomplete

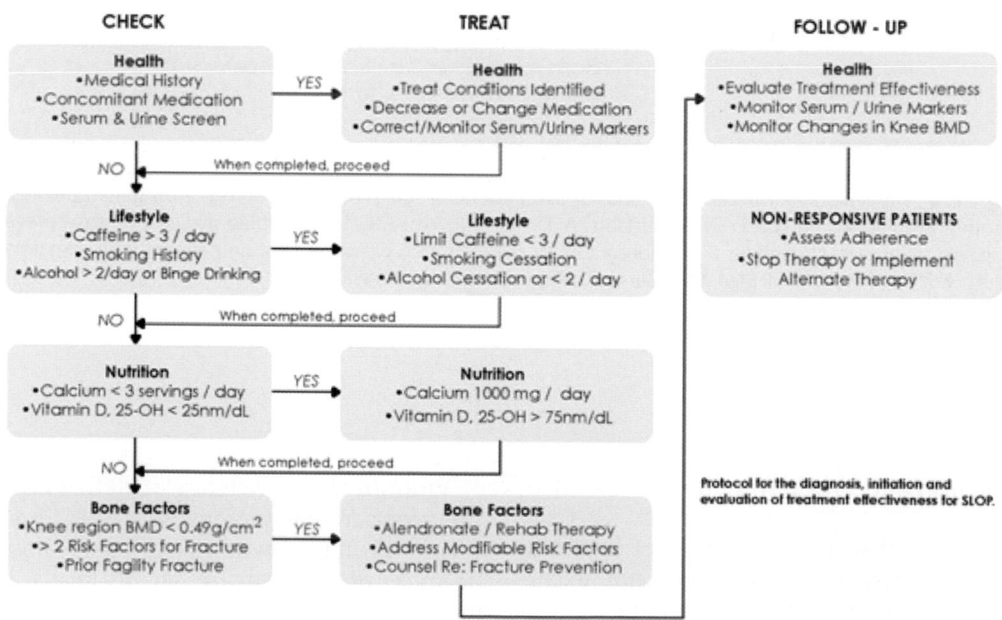

Fig. 22.2 Decision Tree for Treatment of sublesional osteoporosis following spinal cord injury. (From Craven BC, Robertson LA, McGilllivray CF, Adachi JD. Detection and Treatment of sublesional Osteoporosis among patients with chronic spinal cord injury: proposed paradigms. Top Spinal Cord Inj Rehabil. 2009;14(4):1–22. Reprinted with permission.)

injuries (AIS C to D). Recently, p-QCT suggests there is a therapeutic window (2 to 8 years postinjury) during which antiresorptive therapies are most likely to be effective for individuals with SCI.[43]

Monitoring Treatment Adherence and Evaluating Treatment Effectiveness

Changes in BMD from serial scans must be equivalent to or exceed the least significant change (LSC) of the densitometer to be valid.[57] The current International Society of Clinical Densitometry (ISCD) recommendation is to monitor treatment response by measuring BMD every 1 to 2 years at the same facility with the same densitometer.[57] In clinical practice, an increase in BMD above the LSC supports a therapeutic response. Lack of a therapeutic response should prompt a review of patient adherence followed by consideration of therapy cessation. Among postmenopausal women, adherence to bisphosphonate therapy has been shown to be greater with weekly (69.2%) versus daily (57.6%) administration.[58] Following SCI, a minimum of 60% adherence for 18 months with oral bisphosphonate therapy is recommended prior to abandoning therapy,[40] and an interim fragility fracture should prompt a review of treatment adherence and consideration of alternate treatment(s).

Pressure Ulcers

Pressure ulcers are one of the most common and costly complications of SCI. A severe pressure ulcer can be life threatening, can compromise quality of life and independence, and can confine the affected individual to weeks or months of bed rest. The prevalence rate for pressure ulcers among individuals living with SCI in the community has been reported to be up to 33%,[59] and pressure ulcers occur more commonly in individuals with complete paralysis, longer duration of injury, and less independence. The pathophysiology, prevention, and treatment of pressure ulcers are addressed in detail in Chapter 15.

Respiratory Management

Respiratory complications are a leading cause of morbidity and mortality during the first year postinjury as well as during long-term follow-up.[8] Proper pulmonary care following a traumatic cervical SCI begins with the performance of an initial history and physical. Relevant issues that the health care provider should be aware of include a prior history of lung disease, smoking history, current medications, substance abuse, extent of neurological impairment, and coexisting injuries. The primary muscle of respiration, the diaphragm, is innervated by C3–4–5 via the phrenic nerve. In the absence of preexisting disease or other medical complications, the majority of individuals with complete SCI and neurological levels at and below C4 can be expected to be ventilator independent, although they may require a transient period of ventilator support initially after the injury.

Pulmonary function can be followed over time using parameters such as serial vital capacities (VCs) and negative inspiratory forces (NIFs). As an individual ages following an SCI, pulmonary function can be expected to decline,[60] and these parameters can alert the clinician to impending respiratory insufficiency. Parameters can be assessed annually, with the goal of identifying early deterioration in pulmonary function before it becomes clinically urgent.

Pulmonary function can also be compromised transiently by a superimposed infection (e.g., influenza, pneumonia). In an individual with borderline respiratory insufficiency, this might be enough to necessitate a period of respiratory support. Signs and symptoms that should prompt further investigation include fevers, increased respiratory rate and shortness of breath, increased anxiety, and changes in secretion characteristics, such as increased volume, increased tenacity, or more frequent suctioning. Consideration should be given to elective intubation for rapidly diminishing NIFs or VCs or failure to achieve –30 to –40 cm H_2O for the NIF or 10 to 15 cc/kg of ideal body weight for the VC. In some patients, assistance can be provided and intubation avoided through the utilization of continuous positive airway pressure (CPAP) or bilevel positive airway pressure (BiPAP), with either a facemask or a mouthpiece.

Maintaining secretion clearance requires constant vigilance. Pneumonia and atelectasis occur more often in the left than in the right lung.[61] This has been attributed to the acute angle of takeoff of the left mainstem bronchus, resulting in difficulty in accessing this airway for suctioning and secretion clearance. In cervical and high thoracic injuries, expiratory flow rates are inadequate for coughing due to the absence of volitional abdominal contractions. Expiratory capacity can be documented and followed with peak expiratory flow rates.[62] Sympathetic innervation to the lungs is commonly compromised but parasympathetic innervation via the vagal nerve remains intact. This results in airway hyperreactivity and increased secretion production. Due to the foregoing, bronchodilators and mucolytic agents (i.e., guaifenesin) are often helpful. Chest physiotherapy and assisted coughing also help to mobilize secretions effectively. The latter involves either compressing the costophrenic margin bilaterally or exerting upward pressure inferior to the xyphoid process in a timed fashion with expiration. These maneuvers augment expiratory airflow and substitute for paralyzed abdominal muscles. The CoughAssist insufflator-exsufflator (Philips Respironics, Andover, MA) is a device that rapidly generates positive pressures up to +40 mmHg followed by a rapid reversal of airflow to −40 mmHg accompanied by the removal of airway secretions. Most patients prefer it to endotracheal suctioning because it avoids irritation associated with endotracheal suctioning, and it can be attached to a tracheotomy or alternatively utilized with a mouthpiece.

Long-term, preventative care also involves the regular provision of influenza and pneumococcal vaccinations. Individuals with SCI fall into the high-risk category. Influenza vaccinations can be administered annually and pneumococcal once after injury followed by a possible booster in the future.

Spasticity

Spasticity is one of many complications that can contribute to further impairment following an SCI. Lance defined spasticity as "a motor disorder characterized by a velocity dependent increase in tonic stretch reflexes (muscle tone) with exaggerated tendon jerks, resulting from hyperexcitability of the stretch reflex, as one component of the upper motor neuron syndrome."[63] To the patient, the development of this complication can mean unpredictable jerking movements of the extremities, painful muscle spasms, and impaired range of motion in the limbs, leading to joint contractures. Aside from causing pain, spasticity can diminish patient quality of life by interfering with sleep, preventing grooming and performance of personal hygiene, interfering with the safety of transfers, and ultimately impeding rehabilitation efforts and function.

Sixty-five to eighty percent of patients develop symptoms of spasticity 1 year after injury[64]; however, the incidence can vary depending on the initial injury characteristics, with a higher neurological level of injury and complete lesions portending higher rates of spasticity. Treatment and prevention of this complication remain problematic. Current therapeutic strategies employ a combination of physical therapy, oral pharmaceuticals, local injections, and as a last resort, surgery, which can include the placement of intrathecal drug delivery systems.

Oral Agents

Oral agents used to combat this complication fall into one of three categories depending on mechanism of action: (1) drugs that act to mimic or compound the effects of gamma aminobutyric acid (GABA), (2) α-2-adrenergic agonists, and (3) agents acting directly on skeletal muscle. Benzodiazepines and baclofen mimic or enhance the activity of GABA, a neurotransmitter released from spinal interneurons that inhibits motor neuron action potential transmission. Diazepam is the most commonly administered benzodiazepine in the treatment of spasticity. Instead of binding directly to receptors it binds near postsynaptic GABA(A), potentiating GABA-mediated chloride influx, leading to cellular hyperpolarization. Diazepam has been shown to be efficacious for reducing flexor spasticity, muscle spasms, and hyperactive reflexes; however, with higher dosing and frequent administration, sedation can limit its efficacy.[65] In contrast to diazepam, baclofen is a structural analogue of GABA and binds directly to GABA(B) receptors on pre- and postsynaptic receptors. Although there is minimal evidence that baclofen improves walking ability or the performance of activities of daily living (ADLs), it has been shown to be particularly effective at reducing the frequency and severity of flexor spasms and reducing flexor tone.[65] The incidence of adverse effects with oral administration ranges from 10 to 75%, with reported symptoms including drowsiness, insomnia, dizziness, and ataxia. Gabapentin, a structural analogue of GABA, has also shown promise in the treatment of spasticity post-SCI.

Tizanidine and clonidine are centrally acting α-2-adrenergic agonists that inhibit the release of epinephrine and norepinephrine from spinal interneurons. Tizanidine may also potentiate the inhibitory action of the neurotransmitter glycine. Both agents have been found to reduce spasticity and muscle spasms in individuals with SCI; however, clonidine, unlike tizanidine, has been shown to improve walking and functional ability in individuals with incomplete SCI.[65,66] Clonidine, at present, is rarely used as monotherapy in treatment of spasticity following SCI, with reported side effects of bradycardia, hypotension, and depression.

In contrast to the agents discussed thus far, which exert their effects centrally, dantrolene acts peripherally on skeletal muscle. Also used in malignant hyperthermia, dantrolene targets the sarcoplasmic reticulum of skeletal muscle, reducing calcium release and thereby mitigating muscular contraction. Clinical trials evaluating dantrolene versus placebo have shown a treatment-related reduction of hyperreflexia and muscle tone. Unfortunately, the reduction in spasticity seen with this drug is often accompanied by the development of muscle weakness, which can compromise function and rehabilitation efforts. A recent trial ($n = 11$) of nabilone, a synthetic cannabinoid, also reported a reduction in spasticity following SCI.[67]

Focal, Intramuscular Injections

In addition to oral pharmaceuticals, focal intramuscular injections are commonly administered for treatment of spasticity. These focal therapies treat the spastic symptoms of an upper motor neuron syndrome by creating a lower motor neuron lesion. Botulinum, a potent neurotoxin, spreads to a radius of 30 mm within muscle and fascia when injected locally. It acts principally at the neuromuscular junction to inhibit the presynaptic release of acetylcholine, effectively resulting in chemical denervation of muscle. After injection, muscle paralysis begins within 24 to 72 hours and typically persists for 12 to 16 weeks. In individuals with SCI, botulinum has been shown to effectively reduce pain and tone as well as to improve range of motion, functionality, and walking ability.[68] Phenol and ethanol are additional chemodenervation agents used to treat focal spasticity.[69] Acutely, these agents act as sodium channel blockers, preventing presynaptic depolarization at the neuromuscular junction and resulting in focal paralysis. Their chronic effects, compounded by repeat administration, involve neural protein denaturation and fibrosis leading to permanent denervation. In comparison to phenol, ethanol has a lower rate of reported complications, including skin necrosis, sensory dysesthesias, and muscular weakness. A practical limitation of focal agents is that they are only effective for injected muscles, whereas spasticity is often generalized, and addressing all involved muscles is not feasible.

Intrathecal Drug Administration

When spasticity proves refractory to a combination of oral medication and focal injections, or for those who have had intolerable side effects related to medications, the current gold standard for treatment is the direct delivery of baclofen into the cerebrospinal fluid through an implanted intrathecal drug delivery device.[69] A programmable drug reservoir pump is implanted subcutaneously in the abdominal wall and connected to the intrathecal space by a circumferentially tunneled catheter. With this targeted approach, the drug doses are significantly lower, largely eliminating the sedative and cognitive side effects seen with systemic administration. In addition, the programmable nature of the system enables clinicians to precisely titrate the rate of drug delivery depending on the specific needs of the patient throughout the day.

Assessing Severity and Monitoring Treatment Efficacy

The reliable clinical measurement of spasticity has been, and continues to be, a significant limitation. Currently, the Modified Ashworth Scale (MAS) is the predominant instrument used in the clinic. The MAS is a six-category ordinal scale (0 to 5), with 5 being most severe. Despite this, as reviewed in a recent article, the intrarater, interrater, and intrasession reliability is far from ideal.[70] Until new practical instruments are available for clinical care, a practical approach is the titration of interventions based on their effect on the targeted symptom and side effects. Although we lack a "silver bullet," effective treatment of spasticity is attainable through the use of the therapies tailored to individual patient needs and specific clinical scenarios.

Sexuality Following Spinal Cord Injury

Following an SCI, physiological changes and psychological ramifications can compromise the person's ability to express sexuality and participate in satisfying sexual activity. Cultural attitudes toward, and beliefs about, individuals with disabilities also impact the nature of sexuality following SCI.[71,72] Strategies to address sexual dysfunction and health are reviewed in Chapter 14.

Syringomyelia

Syringomyelia is a cyst or cavitation of the spinal cord that can extend above or below the original site of injury and is characterized by expanding enlargement of the central canal. Accompanying compression of the parenchyma can lead to significant neurological deterioration. Clinical features include progressive functional motor loss, progressive sensory loss, increasing spasticity, hyperhidrosis (increased sweating), changes in bowel and bladder status, and late-onset burning, tingling pain. Diagnosis and treatment of syringomyelia are presented in Chapter 20.

Upper Extremity Preservation

Following an SCI, the presence of lower extremity impairments often necessitates that individuals compensate by using the upper extremities for instrumental ADLs and mobility (e.g., transfers, wheelchair propulsion). Over time, increased and repetitive use of the upper extremities can lead to overuse syndromes, such as shoulder impingement and rotator cuff pathology, as well as carpal tunnel syndrome. In a study encompassing all etiologies of upper limb pain, Sie and colleagues[73] reported significant pain was present in 59% of individuals with tetraplegia and 41% of individuals with paraplegia. Secondary musculoskeletal problems can produce pain, loss of range of motion, and loss of function, creating further disability. Upper extremity pain interferes with transfers in as many as 65% of those who transfer, and about a fourth of those with upper extremity pain will need additional help with functional activities.[74]

Shoulder pain is the most common upper extremity complaint following SCI, with a reported prevalence ranging from 30 to 60%.[75] The glenohumeral joint maximizes range of motion and placement of the upper extremity in space at the expense of joint stability and the ability to accommodate weight bearing. Following an SCI, imbalance in the strength of rotator cuff muscles can lead to conditions like glenohumeral subluxation or muscular imbalance. Chronic use during wheeling, reaching, and transfers often leads to anterior shoulder muscles that are tight and comparatively stronger than posterior shoulder stabilizers. Partial- or full-thickness tears of the rotator cuff are a common problem. Other conditions associated with shoulder pain include impingement syndrome, capsulitis, osteoarthritis, recurrent dislocations, bicipital tendonitis, acromioclavicular arthropathy, and myofascial pain syndrome involving the cervical and thoracic paraspinal muscles

Other commonly encountered sites of upper extremity pain following SCI include the elbow, wrist, and hand. Common etiologies of elbow pain include medial or lateral epicondylitis, olecranon bursitis, and ulnar nerve entrapment. The reported prevalence of elbow pain following SCI is 5 to 16%, and the prevalence of ulnar mononeuropathy is 22 to 45%, although this is not necessarily symptomatic.[75] Elbow pads may be helpful to prevent recurrent olecranon bursitis.

The prevalence of hand and wrist pain following SCI ranges from 15 to 48%[75] and interferes with transfers, ability to perform ADLs, and wheelchair propulsion.[74,70,77] Carpal tunnel syndrome (CTS) is the most studied etiology of hand and wrist pain and is more common in persons with paraplegia than in those with tetraplegia. CTS incidence increases with time from injury. The reported prevalence of CTS following SCI has ranged from 40 to 66%,[75] although many individuals can be asymptomatic. The pathogenesis may be related to pushrim forces as the person propels a wheelchair. Other contributing factors include the person's weight and height. Management for CTS typically includes steroid injections and sometimes surgery. Splints at night may be tolerated, but splints usually interfere too much with ADLs to prove of much value during the day. Although carpal tunnel release may be required, the time to heal after surgery will reduce function, and more assistance will be needed temporarily. Additional causes of hand and wrist pain following SCI include ulnar nerve entrapment at the Guyon canal, tendinitis, carpal instability, and arthritis.

The cornerstone of managing overuse syndromes is the reduction of repetitive activities and the incorporation of adaptations that minimize associated stress on the upper extremity. Specific activities include minimizing overhead reaching and the incorporation of assistive devices (e.g., transfer board) into the performance of everyday activities. Attention should also be paid to ergonomics and proper wheelchair seating positioning. Daily stretching to maintain range-of-motion and strengthening exercises are also important. For wheelchair users, a general principle is the lighter the chair, the better. Reviewing proper technique for wheelchair propulsion and transfers with an experienced physiotherapist can also be helpful. Long smooth strokes are preferred for wheelchair propulsion, as opposed to short choppy strokes, due to fewer cumulative strokes and less wear and tear. The hands should drop below the pushrim during the recovery phase between pushes. Smooth strokes also lessen the impact of the hands on the pushrim.

Despite the exercise benefits and increased independence associated with a lightweight wheelchair, recalcitrant arm pain may require an individual to transition from a manual to a power wheelchair, or in select cases, from a manual wheelchair to a manual wheelchair with power-assisted wheels. Power-assisted wheelchairs have a traditional frame but the standard rear wheels are replaced with wheels that incorporate small battery-powered motors into the hubs. The motors are activated automatically when the user exerts force on the pushrim. Power-assisted wheelchairs maintain many of the benefits of conventional manual wheelchairs, such as small size, light weight, and small turning radius, and they are particular helpful for uneven terrain or slopes.

Rotator cuff pathology can be addressed conservatively with steroid injections, compensatory strengthening exercises, and the lifestyle modifications already reviewed. Surgical decompression or repair is a last resort, which temporarily decreases function and increases dependence; these factors should be considered during preoperative planning.

Pearls

- SCI impacts every major organ system.
- Ongoing surveillance and management are essential following community reintegration.
- Health maintenance following SCI requires a multispecialty, interdisciplinary approach.
- Many secondary complications of SCI can be reduced in frequency and severity through primary and secondary prevention strategies and tertiary treatment.

Pitfalls

- Secondary complications following SCI are a major source of morbidity and mortality.
- Some complications can be clinically asymptomatic (e.g., osteoporosis, vesicoureteral reflux) until advanced and therefore require proactive screening and management.
- A single secondary health condition can lead to a cascade of complications, which in turn can necessitate months of intervention to restore patients to their premorbid function (e.g., nonhealing pressure ulcer complicated by cellulitis, osteomyelitis, sepsis, surgery, and deconditioning).

References

1. Anson CA, Shepherd C. Incidence of secondary complications in spinal cord injury. Int J Rehabil Res 1996;19(1):55–66
2. Noreau L, Proulx P, Gagnon L, Drolet M, Laramée MT. Secondary impairments after spinal cord injury: a population-based study. Am J Phys Med Rehabil 2000;79(6):526–535
3. Dryden DM, Saunders LD, Rowe BH, et al. Utilization of health services following spinal cord injury: a 6-year follow-up study. Spinal Cord 2004;42(9):513–525
4. Guilcher SJT, Munce SEP, Couris CM, et al. Health care utilization in non-traumatic and traumatic spinal cord injury: a population-based study. Spinal Cord 2010;48(1):45–50
5. Jaglal SB, Munce SEP, Guilcher SJ, et al. Health system factors associated with rehospitalizations after traumatic spinal cord injury: a population-based study. Spinal Cord 2009;47(8):604–609
6. Curt A, Nitsche B, Rodic B, Schurch B, Dietz V. Assessment of autonomic dysreflexia in patients with spinal cord injury. J Neurol Neurosurg Psychiatry 1997;62(5):473–477
7. Helkowski WM, Ditunno JF Jr, Boninger M. Autonomic dysreflexia: incidence in persons with neurologically complete and incomplete tetraplegia. J Spinal Cord Med 2003;26(3):244–247
8. DeVivo MJ, Krause JS, Lammertse DP. Recent trends in mortality and causes of death among persons with spinal cord injury. Arch Phys Med Rehabil 1999;80(11):1411–1419
9. Bauman WA, Raza M, Chayes Z, Machac J. Tomographic thallium-201 myocardial perfusion imaging after intravenous dipyridamole in asymptomatic subjects with quadriplegia. Arch Phys Med Rehabil 1993;74(7):740–744
10. Freed JH, Hahn H, Menter R, Dillon T. The use of the three-phase bone scan in the early diagnosis of heterotopic ossification (HO) and in the evaluation of Didronel therapy. Paraplegia 1982;20(4):208–216
11. Orzel JA, Rudd TG. Heterotopic bone formation: clinical, laboratory, and imaging correlation. J Nucl Med 1985;26(2):125–132
12. Schurch B, Capaul M, Vallotton MB, Rossier AB. Prostaglandin E2 measurements: their value in the early diagnosis of heterotopic ossification in spinal cord injury patients. Arch Phys Med Rehabil 1997;78(7):687–691
13. Banovac K, Williams JM, Patrick LD, Haniff YM. Prevention of heterotopic ossification after spinal cord injury with indomethacin. Spinal Cord 2001;39(7):370–374
14. Banovac K, Williams JM, Patrick LD, Levi A. Prevention of heterotopic ossification after spinal cord injury with COX-2 selective inhibitor (rofecoxib). Spinal Cord 2004;42(12):707–710
15. Banovac K, Gonzalez F, Renfree KJ. Treatment of heterotopic ossification after spinal cord injury. J Spinal Cord Med 1997;20(1):60–65
16. Banovac K. The effect of etidronate on late development of heterotopic ossification after spinal cord injury. J Spinal Cord Med 2000;23(1):40–44
17. Schuetz P, Mueller B, Christ-Crain M, Dick W, Haas H. Amino-bisphosphonates in heterotopic ossification: first experience in five consecutive cases. Spinal Cord 2005;43(10):604–610
18. Consortium for Spinal Cord Medicine. Bladder management for adults with spinal cord injury: a clinical practice guideline for health-care providers. J Spinal Cord Med 2006;29(5):527–573
19. Linsenmeyer TA, Culkin D. APS recommendations for the urological evaluation of patients with spinal cord injury. J Spinal Cord Med 1999;22(2): 139–142
20. Burns AS, Rivas DA, Ditunno JF. The management of neurogenic bladder and sexual dysfunction after spinal cord injury. Spine 2001;26(24, Suppl):S129–S136
21. Coggrave M, Norton C, Wilson-Barnett J. Management of neurogenic bowel dysfunction in the community after spinal cord injury: a postal survey in the United Kingdom. Spinal Cord 2009; 47(4):323–330, quiz 331–333

22. Spinal Cord Medicine Consortium. Clinical practice guidelines: neurogenic bowel management in adults with spinal cord injury. J Spinal Cord Med 1998;21(3):248–293
23. Dunn KL, Galka ML. A comparison of the effectiveness of Therevac SB and bisacodyl suppositories in SCI patients' bowel programs. Rehabil Nurs 1994;19(6):334–338
24. House JG, Stiens SA. Pharmacologically initiated defecation for persons with spinal cord injury: effectiveness of three agents. Arch Phys Med Rehabil 1997;78(10):1062–1065
25. Krassioukov A, Claxton G, Abramson C, Shum S. Bowel Management. Spinal Cord Injury Rehabilitation Evidence (SCIRE). http://www.icord.org/scire/home.php
26. Segal JL, Milne N, Brunnemann SR, Lyons KP. Metoclopramide-induced normalization of impaired gastric emptying in spinal cord injury. Am J Gastroenterol 1987;82(11):1143–1148
27. Munck J, Simoens Ch, Thill V, et al. Intestinal stoma in patients with spinal cord injury: a retrospective study of 23 patients. Hepatogastroenterology 2008;55(88):2125–2129
28. Mentes BB, Yüksel O, Aydin A, Tezcaner T, Leventoğlu A, Aytaç B. Posterior tibial nerve stimulation for faecal incontinence after partial spinal injury: preliminary report. Tech Coloproctol 2007;11(2):115–119
29. Ehde DM, Jensen MP, Engel JM, Turner JA, Hoffman AJ, Cardenas DD. Chronic pain secondary to disability: a review. Clin J Pain 2003;19(1):3–17
30. Siddall PJ, McClelland JM, Rutkowski SB, Cousins MJ. A longitudinal study of the prevalence and characteristics of pain in the first 5 years following spinal cord injury. Pain 2003;103(3):249–257
31. Dijkers M, Bryce T, Zanca J. Prevalence of chronic pain after traumatic spinal cord injury: a systematic review. J Rehabil Res Dev 2009;46(1):13–29
32. Widerström-Noga EG, Felipe-Cuervo E, Broton JG, Duncan RC, Yezierski RP. Perceived difficulty in dealing with consequences of spinal cord injury. Arch Phys Med Rehabil 1999;80(5):580–586
33. Jensen MP, Chodroff MJ, Dworkin RH. The impact of neuropathic pain on health-related quality of life: review and implications. Neurology 2007;68(15):1178–1182
34. Teasell RW, Aubut J, Wolfe DL, Hsieh JTC, Townson AF. Pain following spinal cord injury. In: Eng JJ, Teasell RW, Miller WC, et al, eds. Spinal Cord Injury Rehabilitation Evidence. Vancouver; 2006:14.1–14.32
35. Jadad A, O'Brien MA, Wingerchuk D, et al. Management of Chronic Central Neuropathic Pain following Traumatic Spinal Cord Injury. AHRQ Evidence Reports and Summaries. 2001;45. http://www.ncbi.nlm.nih.gov/books/bv.fcgi?rid=hstat1.chapter.64890
36. Scadding J. Neuropathic pain. Adv Clin Neurosci and Rehabil 2003;3(2):8–14
37. Vestergaard P, Krogh K, Rejnmark L, Mosekilde L. Fracture rates and risk factors for fractures in patients with spinal cord injury. Spinal Cord 1998;36(11):790–796
38. Comarr AE, Hutchinson RH, Bors E. Extremity fractures of patients with spinal cord injuries. Top Spinal Cord Inj Rehabil 2005;11(1):1–10
39. Freehafer AA. Limb fractures in patients with spinal cord injury. Arch Phys Med Rehabil 1995;76(9):823–827
40. Craven BC, Giangregorio L, Robertson L, Delparte JJ, Ashe MC, Eng JJ. Sublesional osteoporosis prevention, detection, and treatment: a decision guide for rehabilitation clinicians treating patients with spinal cord injury. Crit Rev Phys Rehabil Med 2008;20(4):277–321
41. Eser P, Schiessl H, Willnecker J. Bone loss and steady state after spinal cord injury: a cross-sectional study using pQCT. J Musculoskelet Neuronal Interact 2004;4(2):197–198
42. Biering-Sørensen F, Bohr H, Schaadt O. Bone mineral content of the lumbar spine and lower extremities years after spinal cord lesion. Paraplegia 1988;26(5):293–301
43. Frotzler A, Berger M, Knecht H, Eser P. Bone steady-state is established at reduced bone strength after spinal cord injury: a longitudinal study using peripheral quantitative computed tomography (pQCT). Bone 2008;43(3):549–555
44. Frey-Rindova P, de Bruin ED, Stüssi E, Dambacher MA, Dietz V. Bone mineral density in upper and lower extremities during 12 months after spinal cord injury measured by peripheral quantitative computed tomography. Spinal Cord 2000;38(1):26–32
45. Eser P, Frotzler A, Zehnder Y, Denoth J. Fracture threshold in the femur and tibia of people with spinal cord injury as determined by peripheral quantitative computed tomography. Arch Phys Med Rehabil 2005;86(3):498–504
46. Garland DE, Adkins RH, Stewart CA. Fracture threshold and risk for osteoporosis and pathologic fractures in individuals with spinal cord injury. Top Spinal Cord Inj Rehabil 2005;11(1):61–69
47. Mazess RB. Bone densitometry of the axial skeleton. Orthop Clin North Am 1990;21(1):51–63
48. Eser P, Frotzler A, Zehnder Y, Schiessl H, Denoth J. Assessment of anthropometric, systemic, and lifestyle factors influencing bone status in the legs of spinal cord injured individuals. Osteoporos Int 2005;16(1):26–34
49. Bauman WA, Morrison NG, Spungen AM, Vitamin D. Vitamin D replacement therapy in persons with spinal cord injury. J Spinal Cord Med 2005;28(3):203–207
50. Nemunaitis GA, Mejia M, Nagy JA, Johnson T, Chae J, Roach MJ. A descriptive study on vitamin D levels in individuals with spinal cord injury in an acute inpatient rehabilitation setting. PM R 2010;2(3):202–208, quiz 228
51. Craven BC, Robertson LA, McGillivray CF, Adachi JD. Detection and treatment of sublesional osteoporosis among patients with chronic spinal cord injury: proposed paradigms. Top Spinal Cord Inj Rehabil 2009;14(4):1–22
52. Craven BC, Ashe MC, Krassioukov A, Eng JJ. Bone health following spinal cord injury. In: Eng J, Teasell R, Miller W, et al, eds. Spinal Cord Injury Rehabilitation Evidence. Version 2.0. Vancouver: ICORD; 2008b:9.1–9.23

53. Bryson JE, Gourlay ML. Bisphosphonate use in acute and chronic spinal cord injury: a systematic review. J Spinal Cord Med 2009;32(3): 215–225
54. Biering-Sørensen F, Hansen B, Lee BS. Non-pharmacological treatment and prevention of bone loss after spinal cord injury: a systematic review. Spinal Cord 2009;47(7):508–518
55. Zehnder Y, Risi S, Michel D, et al. Prevention of bone loss in paraplegics over 2 years with alendronate. J Bone Miner Res 2004;19(7):1067–1074
56. Papapetrou PD. Bisphosphonate-associated adverse events. Hormones (Athens) 2009;8(2): 96–110
57. Baim S, Wilson CR, Lewiecki EM, Luckey MM, Downs RW Jr, Lentle BC. Precision assessment and radiation safety for dual-energy X-ray absorptiometry: position paper of the International Society for Clinical Densitometry. J Clin Densitom 2005;8(4):371–378
58. Cramer JA, Amonkar MM, Hebborn A, Altman R. Compliance and persistence with bisphosphonate dosing regimens among women with postmenopausal osteoporosis. Curr Med Res Opin 2005;21(9):1453–1460
59. Consortium for Spinal Cord Medicine Clinical Practice Guidelines. Pressure ulcer prevention and treatment following spinal cord injury: a clinical practice guideline for health-care professionals. Paralyzed Veterans of America, 2000. Washington, DC. www.pva.org
60. Tow AM, Graves DE, Carter RE. Vital capacity in tetraplegics twenty years and beyond. Spinal Cord 2001;39(3):139–144
61. Fishburn MJ, Marino RJ, Ditunno JF Jr. Atelectasis and pneumonia in acute spinal cord injury. Arch Phys Med Rehabil 1990;71(3):197–200
62. Wang AY, Jaeger RJ, Yarkony GM, Turba RM. Cough in spinal cord injured patients: the relationship between motor level and peak expiratory flow. Spinal Cord 1997;35(5):299–302
63. Lance JW. The control of muscle tone, reflexes, and movement: Robert Wartenberg Lecture. Neurology 1980;30(12):1303–1313
64. Sköld C, Levi R, Seiger A. Spasticity after traumatic spinal cord injury: nature, severity, and location. Arch Phys Med Rehabil 1999;80(12): 1548–1557
65. Kita M, Goodkin DE. Drugs used to treat spasticity. Drugs 2000;59(3):487–495
66. Elovic E. Principles of pharmaceutical management of spastic hypertonia. Phys Med Rehabil Clin N Am 2001;12(4):793–816, vii
67. Pooyania S, Ethans K, Szturm T, Casey A, Perry D. A randomized, double-blinded, crossover pilot study assessing the effect of nabilone on spasticity in persons with spinal cord injury. Arch Phys Med Rehabil 2010;91(5):703–707
68. Ward AB. Long-term modification of spasticity. J Rehabil Med 2003;41(41, Suppl):60–65
69. Adams MM, Hicks AL. Spasticity after spinal cord injury. Spinal Cord 2005;43(10):577–586
70. Craven BC, Morris AR. Modified Ashworth scale reliability for measurement of lower extremity spasticity among patients with SCI. Spinal Cord 2010;48(3):207–213
71. Sakellariou D, Sawada Y. Sexuality after spinal cord injury: the Greek male's perspective. Am J Occup Ther 2006;60(3):311–319
72. Sharma SC, Singh R, Dogra R, Gupta SS. Assessment of sexual functions after spinal cord injury in Indian patients. Int J Rehabil Res 2006; 29(1):17–25
73. Sie IH, Waters RL, Adkins RH, Gellman H. Upper extremity pain in the postrehabilitation spinal cord injured patient. Arch Phys Med Rehabil 1992;73(1):44–48
74. Dalyan M, Cardenas DD, Gerard B. Upper extremity pain after spinal cord injury. Spinal Cord 1999;37(3):191–195
75. Paralyzed Veterans of America Consortium for Spinal Cord Medicine. Preservation of upper limb function following spinal cord injury: a clinical practice guideline for health-care professionals. J Spinal Cord Med 2005;28(5):434–470
76. Blankstein A, Shmueli R, Weingarten I, et al. Hand problems due to prolonged use of crutches and wheelchairs. Orthop Rev 1985;14:29–34
77. Subbarao JV, Klopfstein J, Turpin R. Prevalence and impact of wrist and shoulder pain in patients with spinal cord injury. J Spinal Cord Med 1995;18(1):9–13

II

Controversies in Management

23

Timing of Surgery for Acute Spinal Cord Injury: From Basic Science to Clinical Application

David W. Cadotte and Michael G. Fehlings

Key Points

1. A systematic review was conducted to evaluate the evidence relating to the timing of decompression for spinal cord injury.
2. Although animal evidence largely supports early decompression after spinal cord injury, the preclinical and clinical evidence in humans is less clear.
3. Early decompression—within 24 hours of injury—should be strongly considered as an option for patients who are medically stable without major comorbidities or multiple traumas

Spinal cord injury (SCI) is a devastating condition with immense physical, emotional, and economic costs for the patient, family, and health care system. Treatments that can increase recovery and decrease complications could address these issues. To this end, the rate of discovery in basic, translational, and clinical research in neurotrauma has been increasing over many years, particularly with regard to the pathophysiology of traumatic SCI. The focus of treatment strategies for SCI has aimed to minimize the deleterious effects of secondary injury and to lead to an environment conducive to recovery. Several such translational strategies have either made their way into clinical practice or are the focus of ongoing clinical trials to determine their safety and efficacy in patients with SCI. Despite this progress, pharmacological therapies have yet to affect outcomes in a predictable and consistent fashion. Furthermore, the current standard of care for a patient with a new spinal cord injury varies from hospital to hospital.

Surgical decompression, however, is a treatment option that aims to reduce neurological deficit occurring as a result of secondary damage and is currently widely practiced. Persistent compressive forces from the injured spinal column contribute to ongoing secondary damage. This issue leads to the theory behind decompressive surgery, that removing compression will reduce secondary damage. There may be several indications for surgery following traumatic SCI. Although there is little controversy over the need for surgical stabilization for spinal instability caused by torn ligaments and bony fracture, there remain some questions about surgical decompression that aims to improve neurological outcome without a strong indication for the treatment of spinal column instability. This chapter discusses this issue. As already mentioned, physical compression of the spinal cord is responsible for triggering an ongoing series of deleterious cascades; surgical decompression aims to relieve this compression. Evidence is also mounting for improved outcomes with decompressive surgery and the timing threshold associated with these improved outcomes. Recent systematic reviews of the literature suggest that there is a biological basis for surgical decompression of the spinal cord within 24 hours of injury.[1–4] Furthermore, results from the Surgical Treatment of Acute Spinal Cord Injury Study (STASCIS) indicate that decompression within 24 hours of injury improves outcome in patients with isolated SCI.[5] This chapter reviews the current evidence for early decompression.

■ Systematic Review Methods

Given the background information presented earlier, a knowledge gap was identified that has been addressed by several preclinical and clinical research studies. The results of these studies are varied and focus on many different aspects of surgical treatment for SCI. Two questions were developed to frame the literature search and address this aim:

1. Do preclinical studies confirm the biological basis for surgical decompression after SCI?
2. What are the neurological and functional outcome effects of early surgical decompression in the clinical setting?

The MEDLINE database (1950–May 2010) and the EMBASE database (1980–2010) were searched. The search terms were "timing" AND "decompression" AND "spinal cord injury." This search strategy revealed 66 results. After application of the inclusion and exclusion criteria to eliminate irrelevant articles, 38 studies remained for analysis. All original research papers in the English language were included. All clinical case reports, in vitro experiments, photochemically induced injury models, and nerve root or peripheral nervous system injury models were excluded. Lastly, review articles were read and the references hand searched to ensure that all relevant studies were captured, but the review papers themselves were not included in the results. Review articles provided an additional three articles that were not captured by our original search, bringing the total to 41 studies.

■ Results

After narrowing the search results using the inclusion and exclusion criteria, 19 preclinical and 22 clinical studies were identified. The timing of decompression in animal models ranges from minutes to 24 hours postinjury, with earlier decompression usually associated with greater neurological improvement. Clinically, the definition of early surgery is generally accepted as that which is undertaken within 24 hours of the initial injury. The evidence available for both preclinical and clinical studies is reviewed here.

Preclinical Literature

The majority of these studies showed that either the degree or the duration of compression directly correlated to the degree of recovery. The preclinical literature was reviewed, focusing particularly on (1) histopathological correlation between the injury model and the damage caused to the spinal tissue, (2) animal models that did not show a functional benefit following early decompression, and (3) animal models that showed a functional benefit following early decompression. These studies are summarized in **Table 23.1**.

Histopathological Correlation

Three studies examined either the electrophysiological or the histological consequences of spinal cord compression with a fixed duration of time.[6–8] The collective results of these early investigations into SCI suggest that direct pressure to the spinal cord, likely resulting in direct damage to the neural cell membranes, combined with hypotension and resultant ischemia, causes a loss of neurological function. Animals that showed recovery following injury demonstrated either a normal microscopic examination of the spinal cord or evidence of central gray necrosis, peripheral demyelination, or laceration. Animals that failed to recover showed more pronounced evidence of damage to the neuroanatomical circuits of the spinal cord at the level of the anterior horn cells or laceration of either the gray or the white matter.

Animal Models That Showed No Benefit from Early Decompression

Five studies failed to demonstrate a benefit of early decompression following SCI. This generalized conclusion is closely linked to the experimental design of each of these studies. Of those that compared time of compression to outcome,[9–11] the maximum time of compression was 2 hours. To elaborate, Croft et al.[10] showed that, with a graded pressure and time up to a maximum of 58 g for 20 minutes, the electrophysiological changes observed (somatosensory evoked potentials, SSEP) were completely reversible. The weakness of this investigation was that no statistical analysis was performed. Thienprasit et al.[11] subjected a group of cats to a compression model of SCI and then stratified the animals into those that demonstrated electrophysiological recovery within 6 hours and those that did not. Each group would then be stratified to receive decompression or decompression + hypothermia. Of the animals that showed electrophysiological recovery, there was no difference between the control group and the groups that received decompression or decompression + cooling. Of the animals that showed no electrophysiological recovery, there was no difference between the control group and the group that received early decompression; however, the early decompression + cooling did show better behavioral outcomes, suggesting a possible neuroprotective role for hypothermia after SCI. Aki and Toya,[9] using a dog model, showed that compression for either 30 minutes or 60 minutes resulted in similar electrophysiological and histological outcomes. The remaining two studies that failed to demonstrate a correlation between the time of compression and outcome attempted to model cauda equina injury[12] and studied a novel hydrogel[13] with the hypothesis that this agent would act as a scaffold for neural repair following transection. Neither demonstrated an effect of early treatment.

Animal Models That Showed Benefit from Early Decompression

The number of animal studies that showed benefit from early decompression far outweighed those that did not. Using a primate model of SCI, Kobrine and others[14] showed that the duration of compression correlated to the neurological outcome of these animals and that physical injury to the neuronal membrane could account for a lack of recovery. In a rat model that used five times as many animal subjects, Dolan et al.[15] showed that the degree of functional recovery was directly proportional to the duration and force of compression, whereby greater recovery was observed with lower forces and less time of compression. Guha et al.[16] further delineated this observation using a rat model and concluded that the major determinant of recovery was the intensity of the compression, and that the time of compression was important only with lighter compressive forces. These results were echoed by a similar study conducted 1 year later.[17] Zhang et al.[18] expanded on this notion by measuring concentrations of energy-related metabolites in the spinal cord after injury. They concluded that animals with a larger compressive force showed higher concentrations of lactate and inosine in the extracellular compartment of the spinal cord and that these higher concentrations were associated with less neurological recovery. Delamarter et al.[19] used a canine model to show that compression of the cauda equina for 6 hours or longer resulted in a lack of significant motor recovery despite decompression. This lack of recovery was associated with central necrosis of the spinal cord. In a set of two experiments using a canine model of SCI, Carlson et al.[20] showed

Table 23.1 An Overview of the Preclinical Studies Addressing the Timing of Surgical Decompression after Spinal Cord Injury

Reference	Species, N	Injury model
Brodkey et al., 1972[7]	Cats, $n = 5$	Weight was applied over the dorsal surface of the spinal cord and intact dura
Croft et al., 1972[10]	Cats, $n = 15$	Weight was applied over the dorsal surface of the spinal cord and intact dura
Thienprasit et al., 1975[11]	Cats, $n = 28$	A no. 3 French Fogarty catheter was passed through an L2-laminectomy extradurally in the cephalic direction for 6 cm and inflated with 0.6–0.9 cc of air and immediately deflated
Kobrine et al., 1978[8]	Macaque monkeys, $n = 10$	Spinal cord compression (right, lateral) using Fogarty catheter in the epidural space
Kobrine et al., 1979[14]	Macaque monkeys, $n = 18$	Spinal cord compression (right, lateral) using Fogarty catheter in the epidural space
Bohlman et al., 1979[6]	Dogs, $n = 14$	Compression model: transducer Contusion model: Allen weight-drop device
Dolan et al., 1980[15]	Rats, $n = 91$	Spinal cord clip compression
Aki and Toya, 1984[9]	Dogs, $n = 33$	Spinal cord compression: weight placement
Guha et al., 1987[16]	Rats, $n = 75$	Spinal cord clip compression
Nyström and Berglund, 1988[17]	Rats, $n = 81$	Spinal cord compression: weight placement

Timing of decompression	Study conclusions
Time since spinal cord compression and/or aortic clamping to CEP effects	Direct pressure to the spinal cord and hypotension result in additive deficits as recorded by CEP
Graded weight (18–58 g) and graded time (5–20 min)	Graded pressure (38 g for 5 to 20 min and 58 g for 20 min) on the spinal cord produced reversible blocking of SSEPs
No treatment vs laminectomy at 6 h after SCI vs laminectomy at 6 h after SCI + cooling of spinal cord for 2 h	In more severely injured animals (based on return of CEP), surgical decompression and cooling offered improved outcome
1 h	Results suggested that mechanical forces of compression, rather than ischemia, are mainly responsible for the loss of neural conduction in such a model
1, 3, 5, 7, or 15 min	These data suggest that the cause for neural dysfunction after balloon compression is physical injury of the neural membrane, irrespective of blood flow changes; recovery is related to length of time of compression
4 to 8 wk until neurological recovery ceased to improve	• Of the eight pressure-induced SCIs that recovered, microscopic examination was normal in two, central gray necrosis occurred in two, peripheral demyelinization occurred in two, and lacerations occurred in three • Pathological findings associated with significant paralysis: mild anterior horn gray matter necrosis in two, laceration of the ventral white and gray matter in three, and no microscopic evidence of cord damage in one • In this study, the CEP response closely paralleled the degree of initial SCI either from contusion or from compression as well as the neurological recovery of the animals
3 s, 30 s, 60 s, 300 s or 900 s (15 min)	Functional recovery decreased as the duration of compression increased and the force of compression increased
30 or 60 min	• With increasing compressive weights (6–60 g), SEP amplitudes were progressively more reduced and latencies more prolonged • Following release of compression, amplitudes and latencies recovered at the lower weights but were more likely to reflect greater conduction deficits with progressively greater weights • Pathological findings: hemorrhage and necrosis were not found in the gray and white matter in the groups weighted with 6 and 16 g, whereas small petechial hemorrhages and tissue necrosis were observed in the center of the gray matter in the groups weighted with 36 and 60 g • However, there were no distinct findings in the white matter with these higher weights
15 min, 60 min, 120 min, or 240 min	The major determinant of recovery was the intensity of compression applied to the spinal cord; the time until decompression also affected recovery, but only for the lighter compression forces (2.3 and 16.9 g)
1 min, 5 min, and 10 min	Both the amount of weight and the duration of placement affect the animal's ability to recover—whereby a heavier weight and longer duration of placement are associated with less recovery

(Continued on page 270)

Table 23.1 An Overview of the Preclinical Studies Addressing the Timing of Surgical Decompression after Spinal Cord Injury *(Continued)*

Reference	Species, N	Injury model
Delamarter et al., 1991[12]	Dogs, *n* = 30	Circumferential constriction of the cauda equina with a nylon electrical cable
Zhang et al., 1993[18]	Rats, *n* = not disclosed	Spinal cord compression (graded weight compression)
Delamarter et al., 1995[19]	Dogs, *n* = 30	Circumferential constriction of the caudal spinal cord with a nylon electrical cable to 50% of the diameter of the spinal canal
Carlson et al., 1997a[20]	Dogs, *n* = 12	Spinal cord compression: hydraulic loading piston
Carlson et al., 1997b[21]	Dogs, *n* = 21	Cord compression

Timing of decompression	Study conclusions
2–3 s, 1 h, 6 h, 24 h, and 1 wk	• All 30 dogs developed cauda equina syndrome after constriction, and all dogs recovered significant motor function 6 wk after decompression (recovered to walking (Tarlov grade 5) with bladder and tail control at 6 wk after SCI) • Immediately after compression, all five groups demonstrated > 50% deterioration of the posterior tibial nerve SSEP amplitudes; at 6 wk after decompression, all five groups had a mean amplitude recovery of 20–30%; there was no difference in recovery of SSEPs among the groups • All groups demonstrated scattered Wallerian degeneration and axonal regeneration; there were no significant differences in the histological findings among the five groups
5 min compression with varied weight: group 1 (no compression, control), group 2 (9 g weight), group 3 (35 g weight), and group 4 (50 g weight)	• In groups 2 and 3, lactate levels increased 6 to 7 times the basal levels in the first fraction; group 2 levels normalized within ~ 30 minutes, whereas group 3 levels were a lot slower in recovering • Group 4 lactate levels increased 10× in the second fraction; only partial recovery was seen in the 2 hour period • No significant change in pyruvate levels was seen in any of the groups • Inosine levels rose 0.7–0.9 μM in groups 2 and 3 and 1.4 μM in group 4 • Inosine recovery was faster than lactate, with group 4 recovering completely in ~ 40 min • Recovery of hypoxanthine was more delayed compared with other metabolites; complete recovery took almost 80 min
2–3 s, 1 h, 6 h, 24 h, and 1 wk	• The dogs with immediate decompression generally recovered neurological function within 2 to 5 days; animals that were compressed for 6 hours or more showed no significant motor recovery after decompression of spinal cord • Discrete areas of Wallerian degeneration and demyelination were seen in the spinal cord of animals decompressed either immediately or at 1 h; in contrast, there was severe central necrosis in the spinal cord of animals that were decompressed at 6 h or later
5 min, 3 h	Regional spinal cord blood flow was reduced at the site of piston compression. In the sustained compression group, no recovery of SSEP occurred, and blood flow remained significantly lower than baseline at 30 and 180 min after maximum compression; spinal cord decompression was associated with an early recovery of blood flow and SSEP recovery; by 3 h, blood flow was similar in both the compressed and the decompressed groups, even though SSEP recovery occurred only in the decompressed group
Spinal cord displacement was maintained for 30 min ($n = 7$), 60 min ($n = 8$), or 180 min ($n = 6$) after lower extremity SEP amplitudes were reduced by 50% of baseline	• SEP recovery was seen in 6/7 dogs in 30 min, 5/8 dogs in 60 min, and 0/6 dogs in 180 min compression group • Regional spinal cord blood flow at baseline decreased after stopping dynamic compression; reperfusion flows after decompression were inversely related to duration of compression • Reperfusion flows, measured as the interval change in blood flow between the time dynamic compression was stopped to 5, 15, or 180 min after decompression, were significantly greater in those dogs that recovered SEP ($p < 0.05$) • Spinal cord decompression within 1 h of SEP loss resulted in significant electrophysiological recovery after 3 h of monitoring

(Continued on page 272)

Table 23.1 An Overview of the Preclinical Studies Addressing the Timing of Surgical Decompression after Spinal Cord Injury *(Continued)*

Reference	Species, N	Injury model
Dimar et al., 1999[22]	Rats, *n* = 42	Contusion injury: impactor
Carlson et al., 2003[23]	Dogs, *n* = 16	Spinal cord compression: hydraulic piston
Hejcl et al., 2008[13]	Rats, *n* = 23	Spinal cord transection
Rabinowitz et al., 2008[24]	Dogs, *n* = 18	Circumferential constriction of the thoracolumbar junction with a nylon electrical cable

Abbreviations: BBB, Basso; Beattie; Bresnahan; CEP, cortical evoked potentials; MRI, magnetic resonance imaging; SCI, spinal cord injury; SEP, sensory evoked potential; SSEP, somatosensory evoked potentials.

that the duration of compression could be correlated to electrophysiology recordings and spinal cord blood flow, whereby a shorter duration of compression was associated with return of blood flow and SSEP recovery. Dimar et al.[22] added the fact that longer duration of compression was associated with an extension of the injury in a cephalad and caudal direction, resulting in more pronounced cavitation and necrosis of the spinal cord. As technology improved, Carlson and others made use of magnetic resonance imaging (MRI) to further our knowledge with regard to lesion volumes relative to the time of spinal compression.[23] They demonstrated a significant difference in MRI-based lesion volumes between a 30 minute compression group and a 180 minute compression group. Perhaps the most hypothesis-driven study of recent times was performed by Rabinowitz et al.,[24] who compared not only the timing of decompression but also the use of methylprednisolone. Using a randomized design, the authors demonstrated that dogs randomized to surgical decompression, with or without methylprednisolone administration showed greater neurological improvement than with the use of methylprednisolone alone. The use of steroids, including methylprednisolone, is discussed thoroughly in Chapter 10. This is an important study that compared two therapies at the forefront of human treatment that had not yet been compared. The authors rightfully comment on the value of such a trial. In summary, this collection of animal studies represents a significant body of evidence, across many species, that both the degree of initial force and the duration of compression are related to the degree of neurological improvement.

Timing of decompression	Study conclusions
0, 2 h, 6 h, 24 h, and 72 h	• There was progressively more severe central and dorsal cavitation as the time of spinal cord compression increased • Midsagittal sections demonstrated progressive cephalad and caudal cord necrosis and cavitation, which worsened the longer the duration of compression; these changes were most severe in the 24 and 72 h specimens
Spinal cord displacement was maintained for 30 min ($n = 8$) or 180 min ($n = 8$) after SSEP amplitudes were reduced by 50% of baseline	• A shorter time of compression was associated with better neurological function at both early and late time points • Lesion volumes as assessed with MRI were smaller in the 30 min compression group than in the 180 min compression group ($p = 0.04$) • The 30 min compression group showed smaller lesion volume ($p < 0.001$) and greater percentage of residual white matter ($p = 0.005$) than the 180 min compression group
HEMA-MOETACl hydrogel* was inserted right away after SCI (acute group) or 1 wk after SCI (delayed group)	There was no significant difference in histopathological examination of spinal cord between the acute and delayed implantation groups; there were no significant differences between the two treatment groups with regard to the BBB scores
Group 1: decompression at 6 h + methylprednisolone Group 2: decompression at 6 h + sham Group 3: methylprednisolone only	Decompression within 6 h (groups 1 and 2) showed significant neurological improvement when compared with no decompression (group 3), methylprednisolone did not significantly affect outcome; there was no statistical difference in the percentage of cord involvement histologically between the three groups; group 3 did show greater involvement below the level of the lesion

*Macroporous hydrogels based on 2-hydroxyethyl methacrylate (HEMA)–[2-(methacryloyloxy)ethyl]trimethylammonium chloride (MOETACl) copolymer, HEMA-MOETACl—methacrylic acid.

Human Clinical Trials

Although the neurological outcomes after early decompressive surgery in human clinical studies have been less conclusive than those in animal models, recent work[25,26] adds weight to the growing clinical consensus that favors early surgical decompression for patients with an acute traumatic SCI. Studies have focused on the safety and feasibility of early surgery in addition to improvement in neurological function. The clinical evidence, according to the level of evidence of each study, is reviewed here. The studies are summarized in **Table 23.2**.

Level I

No level I evidence exists to guide clinicians with regard to the timing of surgical decompression following SCI.

Level II

Three level II studies were identified.[27,28] Vaccaro and others[28] studied 62 patients who presented with a spinal injury between C3 and T1. They defined the early surgery group as those who were treated within 72 hours and the late surgery group as those who were treated after 5 days. These authors found no difference between groups with regard to the length of stay in the intensive care unit or inpatient rehabilitation and no difference with regard to the American Spinal Injury Association (ASIA) motor score. In contrast, Cengiz et al.[27] studied 27 patients who sustained a traumatic SCI from T8 to L2. They defined early surgery as that occurring within 8 hours of injury and late surgery as that occurring from 3 to 15 days after surgery. There were several differences between the groups at follow-up. The early

Table 23.2 An Overview of the Clinical Studies Addressing the Timing of Surgical Decompression after Spinal Cord Injury

Reference	Study population	Timing of intervention
Levi et al., 1991[29]	*N* =103 Cervical SCI • Incomplete deficit, early surgery: ◦ *N* = 35 ◦ Median age: 30.4 years ◦ Males: 80% • Incomplete deficit, delayed surgery: ◦ *N* = 18 ◦ Median age: 33 years ◦ Males: 80% • Complete deficit, early surgery: ◦ *N* = 10 ◦ Median age: 24.9 years ◦ Males: 85.7% • Complete deficit, delayed surgery: ◦ *N* = 40 ◦ Median age: 27.6 years ◦ Males: 83.3%	Early surgery ≤ 24 h Delayed surgery > 24 h Procedure: anterior cervical decompression and stabilization were included
Clohisy et al., 1992[30]	*N* = 20 Thoracolumbar SCI Mean age: 33 years (15–66 years) Males/Females: 12:8	Group A: anterior decompression ≤ 48 h Group B: Anterior decompression > 48 h
Krengel et al., 1993[31]	*N* = 14 T2-11 SCI *N* (early surgery group) = 12 *N* (late surgery group) = 2 Mean age: 35 years (14–75 years) Males: 14	Early surgery ≤ 24 h Late surgery > 24 h
Duh et al., 1994[32]	*N* = 487 All levels SCI Demographic data not reported in this paper but available in the original publication: Second National Spinal Cord Injury Study (NASCIS-II) in N Engl J Med 1990;322(20):1405–1411.	Early surgery ≤ 25 h Intermediate surgery group: from 26 to 200 h Late surgery > 200 h
Botel et al., 1997[33]	*N* = 255 *N* (traumatic SCI) = 205 All levels SCI Tetraplegia: 31.4% Paraplegia: 68.6% Mean age: 39.3 years (2–82 years) Males/Females: 72%:28%	Early surgery: ≤ 24 h

Study conclusions	Level of evidence	Quality assessment
• There was a significant difference in the hospital LOS between the early and delayed surgery groups (38.7 vs 45.2 d; $p < 0.05$) • Respiratory care was significantly more required in the early surgery group than the delayed surgery group ($p < 0.05$) • There were no significant differences between early and delayed surgery groups with regard to the frequency of complications ($p > 0.05$) • Early surgery group was not significantly different from delayed surgery group regarding neurological and functional recovery (no *p* value was reported)	3	10
• Although four patients had neurological deterioration prior to surgery (three in group A; one in group B), no patients had any deterioration in neurological function after surgery • Group A had significant mean modified Frankel grade improvement when compared with group B ($p < 0.04$) • The mean ASIA motor score improvement among patients in group A was greater than the motor improvement among patients in group B ($p = 0.01$) • Whereas four of nine patients in group A completely recovered from a conus medullaris syndrome, six of nine patients in group B partially recovered ($p = 0.1$)	3	13
• All 12 patients who underwent early surgery recovered at least one Frankel grade • No patient showed neurological deterioration after surgery • There were no wound infections or pseudarthrosis • One patient had his rod removed earlier because the hook dislodged	3	7
• The results suggest that either early surgery or late surgery may be associated with increased neurological recovery, particularly motor function, but these results were equivocal • Logistic regression analysis adjusted for severity of SCI indicated that the timing of surgery was not significantly associated with neurological improvement of at least 5 points in the NASCIS-II motor scores from baseline to 6 wk ($p > 0.31$), 6 months ($p > 0.7$), or 1 year following SCI ($p > 0.67$). • Early surgery group and intermediate/late surgery group (>25 h) did not differ regarding the improvement in the NASCIS-II motor score at 6 wk ($p = 0.43$), at 6 months ($p = 0.16$), or at 1 year after SCI ($p = 0.14$) after adjusting for age and severity of SCI	3	18
• 42.2% of patients reached the hospital within the first 24 h; of these, 64.4% were admitted within the first 8 h of SCI; of the remaining 23.6% cases from other centers, 45.2% had to undergo corrective reoperations • 178 of 255 patients required spine surgery; of those 178 patients, 92 (51.4%) could be stabilized within 24 h after SCI • "The time of operation depended on the day of admission on the one hand but on the state of the patient at the other, especially regarding patients with severe polytrauma and thoracic injuries"	3	11

(Continued on page 276)

Table 23.2 An Overview of the Clinical Studies Addressing the Timing of Surgical Decompression after Spinal Cord Injury *(Continued)*

Reference	Study population	Timing of intervention
Campagnolo et al., 1997[34]	*N* = 64 All levels SCI Early surgery group: • *N* = 37 • Mean age: 32.4 years • Males/Females: 35:2 • Paraplegic complete: 7 • Paraplegic incomplete: 7 • Tetraplegic complete: 12 • Tetraplegic incomplete: 11 Late surgery group: • *N* = 27 • Mean age: 41.9 years • Males/Females: 23:4 • Paraplegic complete: 8 • Paraplegic incomplete: 4 • Tetraplegic complete: 8 • Tetraplegic incomplete: 7	Early spinal stabilization group: ≤24 h Late spinal stabilization group: >24 h
Vaccaro et al., 1997[28]	*N* (all cases) = 62 Level of injury: C3-T1 Early surgery group: • *N* = 34 • Mean age: 39.79 years • Males/Females: 24:10 Late surgery group: • *N* = 28 • Mean age: 39 years • Males/Females: 22:6	Early surgery group: ≤72 h Late surgery group: >5 d
McLain and Benson, 1999[35]	*N* (all cases) = 27 Level of injury: • Thoracic: 9 • Lumbar: 18 *N* (urgent surgery group): 14 *N* (early surgery group): 13 Mean age (urgent surgery group): 27.5 years (16–46 years) Mean age (early surgery group): 30 years (18–58 years) Males/Females: 21:6	Urgent surgery group: ≤24 h Early surgery group: 24–72 h
Mirza et al., 1999[36]	*N* (all cases) = 30 Level of injury: C2-7 Age range: 14–56 years Males/Females: 26:4 Early surgery group • *N* = 15 • ISS = 24.8 Late surgery group • *N* = 15 • ISS = 26.2	Early surgery group: ≤72 h Late surgery group: >72 h

Study conclusions	Level of evidence	Quality assessment
• Mean LOS in the early surgery group (37.5 d) was smaller than in the late surgery group (54.7 d; $p = 0.01$) • The early surgery group did not differ from the late surgery group regarding the mean ISS (17.9 vs 21.3, respectively; $p = 0.10$) • Groups did not differ regarding the frequency of need for mechanical ventilation ($p = 0.66$), decubitus ulcers ($p = 0.33$), atelectasis/pneumonia ($p = 0.56$), wound infections ($p = 0.63$), autonomic dysreflexia ($p = 0.64$), DVT ($p = 0.64$), cardiac arrest ($p = 1$), urinary calculus ($p = 0.43$), gastrointestinal hemorrhage ($p = 0.43$), spasticity ($p = 0.43$), heterotopic ossification ($p = 0.56$) or UTI ($p = 0.99$)	3	12
No significant differences were seen in LOS in the acute postoperative ICU, length of inpatient rehabilitation, or improvement in AIS or ASIA motor score between the early versus late surgery groups (no *p* values were reported)	2	12
• The mean ISS was 36 for early surgery group and 42 for urgent surgery group (no *p* was reported) • One patient died in each group • Urgent group showed a higher mean neural improvement (1.12 vs 0.65) and percent with neurological improvement (88 vs 50) than the early group (no *p* was reported) • Blood loss for anterior procedures was significantly higher in the urgent group but estimated blood losses for posterior procedures were similar for both groups (no *p* was reported) • At 49 months follow-up time, no revisions were necessitated by the urgent spinal treatment	3	10
• The duration of acute LOS was longer in the late surgery group than in the early surgery group (36.8 vs 21.9 d; $p = 0.04$) • The postoperative motor index scores were significantly different for the two groups ($p = 0.01$) • The change in the motor score from preoperative assessment to postoperative assessment was significant in the early surgery group ($p = 0.006$) but not in the late surgery group ($p = 0.14$) • Although the early surgery group showed significant improvement in the Frankel grade after surgery ($p = 0.003$), there were no significant differences between preoperative and postoperative assessments using Frankel grade in the late surgery group ($p = 0.3$) • The number of total complications was significantly greater in the late surgery group than in the early surgery group ($p = 0.05$)	3	10

(Continued on page 278)

Table 23.2 An Overview of the Clinical Studies Addressing the Timing of Surgical Decompression after Spinal Cord Injury *(Continued)*

Reference	Study population	Timing of intervention
Ng et al., 1999[37]	*N* = 26 Cervical (C3-T1) SCI Mean age: 30.3 years (18–68 years) Males/Females: 22:4 ASIA • A: 13 • B: 4 • C: 2 • D: 7	Early surgery group: ≤8 h Late surgery group: >8 h
Tator et al., 1999[38]	*N* = 585 Level of injury: • C1-7: 64.6% • T1-11: 18.7% • T11-L2: 11% • L2-S5: 5.6% Mean age: 40 years	Surgery • ≤24 h • between 25 and 48 h • between 48 and 96 h • >5 d
Guest et al., 2002[39]	*N* = 50 Central cord syndrome Mean age: 45 years (14–77 years) Males/Females: 31:19	Early surgery group: ≤24 h Late surgery group: >24 h
Croce et al., 2001[40]	N = 291 Level of injury: • Cervical: 56% • Thoracic: 27% • Lumbar: 15% Mean age: 34 years Males/Females: 212:79	Early surgical fixation: ≤3 d Late surgical fixation: >3 d

Study conclusions	Level of evidence	Quality assessment
• Decompression by traction required an average of 10.9 h; only six out of the 11 were able to get the procedure within 8 h of injury • Only two patients underwent a surgical decompressive procedure within 8 h postinjury • After surgery, 84.6% of patients remained as ASIA grade A • 19.2% improved from grade D to E in 6 months and had an average time of decompressive treatment of 30.8 h postinjury. • Only one patient died, of sepsis and pneumonia	3	11
• The timing of surgery varied: less than 24 h postinjury in 23.5%, between 25 and 48 h postinjury in 15.8%, between 48 and 96 h in 19%, and more than 5 d post-injury in 41.7% of patients	3	9
• Both groups were statistically comparable with regard to the PSIMFS (p = 0.3), mean admission ASIA motor score (p = 0.45), and mean follow-up ASIA motor score (p = 0.23) • Whereas four of 16 patients in the early surgery group had preoperative bladder dysfunction and all recovered, 11 of 15 patients with bladder dysfunction in the late surgery group (n = 34) regained bladder control • Patients in the early surgery group showed shorter ICU LOS and hospital LOS than patients in the late surgery group (no p value was reported)	3	9
• Both groups did not differ regarding ISS, admission systolic blood pressure, 48 h transfusions, frequency of SCI, cervical and lumbar fractures, but patients in the early fixation group were younger (p = 0.01) and had higher GCS (p = 0.02), lower chest abbreviated injury score (p = 0.01), and lower frequency of thoracic fracture (p = 0.01) • Although both groups did not differ regarding the time in mechanical ventilation and mortality rates, the early fixation group showed lower ICU LOS (p = 0.001), lower hospital LOS (p = 0.001), lower frequency of pneumonia (p = 0.03), and lower total hospital charges (p = 0.003) • There was no difference between the groups regarding FIM ($p > 0.05$) • For patients with ISS > 25, early spine fracture fixation was associated with shorter ICU LOS and hospital LOS, a lower frequency of pneumonia, and less resource utilization but a significantly increased death rate (no p values were reported) • In patients with ISS < 25, patients in the early surgery group had lower number of ventilator days ($p < 0.02$), ICU LOS ($p < 0.001$), hospital LOS ($p < 0.001$), and hospital charges ($p < 0.001$) than the late surgery group • In patients with significant pulmonary injury, patients in the early surgery group had lower ICU LOS ($p < 0.003$), hospital LOS ($p < 0.02$), hospital charges ($p < 0.02$), and frequency of pneumonia ($p < 0.003$) • The frequency of DVT was lower in the early group ($p < 0.04$) • There were eight deaths in the early fixation group and four in the late fixation group ($p > 0.05$)	3	14

(Continued on page 280)

Table 23.2 An Overview of the Clinical Studies Addressing the Timing of Surgical Decompression after Spinal Cord Injury *(Continued)*

Reference	Study population	Timing of intervention
Papadopoulos et al., 2002[41]	*N* (all cases) = 91 Level of injury: C2-8, T1 Protocol group: • *N* = 66 • Mean age: 32 years (2–92 years) • Males: 68% Reference group: • *N* = 25 • Mean age: 42 years (9–75 years) • Males: 76%	• *Protocol group:* patients who followed the University of Michigan Acute SCI Protocol that recommends early surgical decompression of spinal cord • Time from SCI to operative decompression (protocol group): 12.6 ± 1.3 h • *Reference group:* patients not included in the above group due to contraindication to MRI, need for other emergency procedures, or admitting surgeon preference
Pollard and Apple, 2003[42]	*N* = 412 Traumatic incomplete cervical SCI admitted within 90 days of injury Specific characteristics not reported	Early surgery group: <24 h Late surgery group: >24 h
Chipman et al., 2004[43]	*N* = 146 Thoracolumbar spinal column injury Early surgery and low ISS (<15): • *N* = 32 • Mean age: 34.3 years • Males: 84.4% • Mean ISS: 10 Late surgery and low ISS: • *N* = 26 • Mean age: 46.2 years • Males: 65.4% • Mean ISS: 10.6 Early surgery and high ISS (≥ 15): • *N* = 37 • Mean age: 29.9 years • Males: 64.9% • Mean ISS: 25.8 Late surgery and high ISS: • *N* = 51 • Mean age: 35.7 years • Males: 66.7% • Mean ISS: 29.1	Group 1: surgery before 72 h and low ISS (<15) Group 2: surgery after 72 h and low ISS Group 3: surgery before 72 h and high ISS (≥ 15) Group 4: surgery before 72 h and high ISS

Study conclusions	Level of evidence	Quality assessment
• Patients treated using the protocol showed a significantly greater neurological improvement than patients in the reference group ($p < 0.006$) • Using a multiple regression analysis, early spinal cord decompression was significantly correlated with change in Frankel grade from admission to the latest follow-up assessment ($p = 0.048$) • There were no significant differences between both groups regarding in-hospital mortality ($p > 0.05$)	3	10
• Both groups did not significantly differ with regard to change in the ASIA motor score ($p = 0.42$), follow-up ASIA motor scores ($p = 0.73$), change in the ASIA sensory score ($p = 0.49$) and follow-up ASIA sensory score ($p = 0.5$)	3	11
• Although groups 1 and 2 were comparable regarding ISS, group 1 showed lower frequency of anterior fusion ($p = 0.047$) and younger age at the time of injury ($p = 0.01$); there was a trend for higher proportion of males in group 1 than in group 2 ($p = 0.04$) • There were no significant differences between groups 3 and 4 regarding ISS ($p = 0.12$), proportion of males ($p = 0.86$), and frequency of anterior fusion ($p = 0.97$); there was a trend toward a younger age in group 3 compared with group 4 ($p = 0.08$) • No differences were seen between groups 1 and 2 with regard to the frequency of infectious complications ($p = 0.44$), respiratory failure ($p = 0.83$), and all complications ($p = 0.59$) and the LOS in the ICU ($p = 0.14$) • Patients in group 2 stayed significantly longer in the hospital than patients in group 1 ($p < 0.001$) • While groups 3 and 4 did not differ regarding the frequency of infectious complications ($p = 0.11$) and respiratory failure ($p = 0.6$), patients in group 3 showed significantly lower frequency of all complications ($p = 0.03$), shorter hospital LOS ($p < 0.001$), and shorter LOS in the ICU ($p = 0.003$) than patients in group 4 • Groups 3 and 4 were statistically comparable regarding the lowest systolic blood pressure ($p = 0.42$), resuscitation volume in crystalloid ($p = 0.68$), total resuscitation volume ($p = 0.91$), volume of packed red blood cells ($p = 0.24$), volume of platelets ($p = 0.26$), and volume of other colloids ($p = 0.64$); however, group 4 received a greater volume of fresh frozen plasma than group 3 ($p = 0.055$)	3	15

(Continued on page 282)

Table 23.2 **An Overview of the Clinical Studies Addressing the Timing of Surgical Decompression after Spinal Cord Injury** *(Continued)*

Reference	Study population	Timing of intervention
McKinley et al., 2004[44]	*N* (all cases) = 779 All levels SCI Level and severity of injury: • Paraplegia, incomplete: 17.8% • Paraplegia, complete: 27.2% • Tetraplegia, incomplete: 32.9% • Tetraplegia, complete: 22.1% *N* (early surgery group) = 307 *N* (late surgery group) = 296 *N* (nonsurgery group) = 176 Mean age: 37.65 years Males/Females: 78.8%:21.2%	Early surgery group (≤72 h after SCI) Late surgery group (>72 h) Nonsurgery group In addition, patients who underwent surgery were classified into • surgery on day of injury (group 1): ≤24 h after SCI; • surgery on day 1 (group 1.A): <48 h after SCI; • surgery on day 2 (group 2): 24–72 h after injury
Kerwin et al., 2005[45]	*N* (all cases): 299 Level of injury: • Cervical: 150 • Thoracic: 90 • Lumbar: 68 • Multiple levels: 9 *N* (early surgery group): 174 *N* (late surgery group): 125 Males/Females: 217:82	Early surgery group: ≤3 d of injury Late surgery group: >3 d
Schinkel et al., 2006[46]	*N* (all cases) = 298 Thoracic spine injuries Early surgery group: • *N* = 156 • Mean age: 36.7 years • Median age: 28 years • Mean ISS: 28.5 • Mean GCS: 9.7 Late surgery group: • *N* = 49 • Mean age: 38.1 years • Median age: 34 years • Mean ISS: 30.9 • Mean GCS: 9.1 Control group: • *N* = 93 • Mean age: 31.7 years • Mean ISS: 28.4 • Mean GCS: 8.4	Group I (early surgery group): ≤72 h Group II (late surgery group): >72 h Group III (control group): no surgery

Study conclusions	Level of evidence	Quality assessment
• All three groups were comparable regarding the FIM motor efficiency ($p = 0.38$), FIM motor change from admission to follow-up ($p = 0.81$), and from discharge to follow-up ($p = 0.99$) • Patients without spinal surgeries or early spine surgery had shorter acute care and total LOS than those with later surgery ($p < 0.01$); there were no differences among groups regarding the LOS in rehabilitation ($p = 0.31$) • Patients receiving no spinal surgery or early spine surgery had lower hospital costs in the acute care ($p < 0.01$) and in the rehabilitation ($p = 0.055$) than patients who underwent late surgery • The ASIA motor index did not differ among the three groups from acute care admission to rehabilitation ($p = 0.87$), from rehab admission to discharge ($p = 0.42$), and from discharge to follow-up ($p = 0.21$) • No significant differences between groups were found for changes in neurological, motor, or sensory levels or AIS grade ($p > 0.15$) • Late surgery group had a higher occurrence of pneumonia and atelectasis in acute care ($p = 0.004$) but not in rehabilitation ($p = 0.62$) • The frequencies of DVT, pulmonary embolism, autonomic dysreflexia, and pressure ulcers were similar among the three groups in both settings ($p > 0.11$) • However, the occurrence of autonomic dysreflexia at 1 year after SCI was higher in the late surgery group ($p = 0.03$) • The groups were comparable regarding rehospitalizations ($p = 0.82$) and rehospitalization days ($p = 0.13$)	3	18
• Both groups were comparable regarding mean age, GCS, and ISS ($p > 0.05$) • The mortality was higher in the early group compared with the late group (6.9% vs 2.5%); however, it was not statistically significant ($p > 0.05$) • The hospital LOS was significantly shorter ($p = 0.0005$) for patients with early spine fixation, but no significant difference between the two groups with regard to ICU LOS ($p > 0.05$), frequency of pneumonia ($p > 0.05$), or number of days in mechanical ventilator ($p > 0.05$) • Both study groups were statistically comparable with regard to feeding, motor, and independence components of the modified FIM scores ($p > 0.05$)	3	12
• Groups I and II were statistically comparable regarding the PaO_2:FiO_2 ratio (Horowitz-Ratio) ($p > 0.05$), frequency of sepsis ($p > 0.05$), and mortality by TRISS ($p > 0.05$); however, the mortality rate in group II was significantly higher than that in group I ($p < 0.05$) • Patients in group I had significantly shorter ICU LOS ($p = 0.001$), dependence on mechanical ventilation ($p = 0.02$), and hospital LOS ($p = 0.048$) than did group II • When groups I and II were subdivided into three further groups: (a) ISS < 26; (b) 26 < ISS < 38; (c) ISS > 38; mortality rate was higher in group II subgroups than in group I (Ia vs IIa = 3% vs 13%; Ib vs IIb = 5% vs 9%; Ic vs IIc = 10% vs 27%)	3	12

(Continued on page 284)

Table 23.2 **An Overview of the Clinical Studies Addressing the Timing of Surgical Decompression after Spinal Cord Injury** *(Continued)*

Reference	Study population	Timing of intervention
Sapkas and Papadakis, 2007[47]	*N* = 67 Lower cervical spine injury (C3-7) Severity of SCI: • A: 20 • B: 10 • C: 11 • D: 17 • E: 9 Mean age: 36 years (16–72 years) M/F: 49:18	Early surgery group: ≤72 h Delayed surgery group: >72 h
Cengiz et al., 2008[27]	*N* (all cases) = 27 Level of injury: T8-L2 Mean age: 41.4 years (23–68 years) M/F=18:9 Early surgery group: • *N* = 12 • Mean age: 39.7 years • M/F: 8:4 Late surgery group: • *N* = 15 • Mean age: 41.4 years • M/F: 10:5	Early surgery group: ≤8 h Late surgery group: 3–15 d
Chen et al., 2009[48]	*N* = 49 Cervical SCI (central cord syndrome) Age = 55.9 years Males/Females = 40:9 *N* (early surgery group) = 21 *N* (late surgery group) = 28	Early surgery group: ≤4 d Late surgery group: >4 d
Lenehan et al., 2010[26]	Survey study: 77 spine surgeons	N/A
Fehlings et al., 2010[25]	Survey study: 971 spine surgeons	N/A
Fehlings et al., 2012[5]	N = 313 Cervical SCI Mean age = 47.46±16.9 (range = 16–80) Males/Females = 236:77	Early surgery: <24 hr Late surgery: ≥24 hr

Abbreviations: AIS, ASIA Impairment Scale; ASIA, American Spinal Injury Association; DVT, deep vein thrombosis; FIM, Functional Independence Measure; GCS, Glasgow Coma Scale score; ICU, intensive care unit; ISS, Injury Severity Score; LOS, length of stay; N/A, not applicable; NASCIS, National Spinal Cord Injury Study; PSIMFS, Post-Spinal Injury Motor Function Scale; SCI, spinal cord injury; TRISS, Trauma Injury Severity Score; UTI, urinary tract infection.

Study conclusions	Level of evidence	Quality assessment
• Patients with preoperative Frankel grade A did not improve in neurological status • Both groups were comparable regarding the neurological improvement among patients with incomplete SCI ($p = 0.44$) • Two patients with grade A injury died within 2 to 4 months of surgery	3	8
• Both groups were comparable regarding AIS ($p = 0.9$) and type of fracture ($p \geq 0.05$) • Postoperative AIS significantly increased from the preoperative AIS in the early surgery group ($p = 0.004$) and in the late surgery group ($p = 0.046$), but postoperative AIS of the early surgery group was better than the late surgery group ($p < 0.011$) • However, 83.3% of individuals in the early surgery group showed improvement in the AIS, whereas only 26.6% in the late surgery group improved their AIS • The early surgery group had no complications, whereas the late surgery group had three cases of lung failure and one case of sepsis; there were no deaths in both groups • The early surgery group had significantly shorter LOS in the hospital ($p < 0.001$) and ICU ($p = 0.005$) than the late surgery group	2	25
Both early and late surgery groups had similar ASIA motor scores in the final follow-up (88.7 vs 90.3, respectively)	3	16
The authors conclude that there is a lack of consensus among highly qualified spine surgeons with regard to operative care, nonoperative care, and postinjury patient management	4	N/A
The majority of spine surgeons surveyed prefer to decompress the acutely injured spinal cord within 24 h of injury; this was emphasized in the cervical SCI population; in persons with an incomplete cervical SCI, the survey respondents chose to perform decompressive surgery within 12 h when possible; central cord syndrome remains an area of uncertainty with regard to necessity or timing of surgery	4	N/A
• At 6 months postinjury, 19.8% of patients undergoing early surgery showed a ≥2 grade improvement in AIS compared to 8.8% in the late decompression group • In multivariate analysis adjusted for preoperative neurological status, the odds of at least a 2 grade AIS improvement were 2.8 times higher among those who underwent early surgery as compared to those who underwent late surgery • Decompression prior to 24 hours after SCI can be performed safely and is associated with improved neurologic outcome, defined as at least a 2 grade AIS improvement at 6 months follow-up	2	20

surgery group showed more improvement on the ASIA Impairment Scale, no in-hospital complications, and a shorter length of stay both in hospital and in the intensive care unit (ICU). The later surgery group had four complications: three cases of lung failure and one case of sepsis. The authors concluded that there are statistical differences between patients treated early and those treated late, with regard to both neurological improvement and overall morbidity. There were no mortalities in either group.

The third and most recent study, by the senior author of this chapter, studied over 300 patients and employed multivariate analysis to control for baseline neurological status. They found that the odds of at least a 2 grade AIS improvement were 2.8 times higher among those who underwent early surgery (defined as <24 hours) as compared to those who underwent late surgery (≥24 hours). They also found significantly fewer complications in the early surgery group, with the majority, for both groups, being cardiopulmonary complications. The mortality rate was the same in both groups (one in each). The authors conclude that decompression prior to 24 hours after SCI can be performed safely and is associated with improved neurologic outcome.

Level III

The majority of clinical studies that attempt to address the question of timing of decompression following traumatic SCI provide level III evidence. Although space constraints prevent a detailed discussion of each study, a general overview of investigations is provided that outlines (1) length of stay in hospital, (2) medical complications following SCI, and (3) neurological outcome.

Length of Stay in Hospital following Spinal Cord Injury

When attempting to study the effect of early surgery on SCI, a relatively easy metric to follow is the length of time a patient spends in the ICU or in-patient unit. This measurement encompasses not only the severity of injury but also the efficacy of the medical system in stabilizing patients and allowing them to proceed with rehabilitation. Of the 22 clinical studies identified in this review, nine level IV studies measured the length of stay.[27,29,34,36,40,43–46] Early surgical decompression offered a statistically significant shorter hospital stay in eight studies[29,34,36,39,40,43–45] (although Guest et al.[39] reported no *p* values), whereas the others recorded only the length of stay in the ICU.[46] A subset of these studies further divided overall length of stay with the duration of stay in the ICU[39,40,43,45] and found that this was also less in patients receiving early decompressive surgery. Only one study that measured these values found no correlation between timing of surgical decompression and the length of stay in the ICU.[45] An obvious extension to this measurement is the rate at which patients are readmitted to the hospital. This was measured in only one study and the authors found no difference between the early and late surgical intervention group.[44]

Medical Complications Following Spinal Cord Injury

The following complications were recorded in eight of the 22 studies: respiratory care, wound infections, decubitus ulcers, cardiac complications, urinary tract infections, gastrointestinal hemorrhage, deep vein thrombosis (DVT), and death. Four studies[29,31,34,35] showed no difference in the rate of medical complications between the early and late surgical groups, whereas four studies showed fewer complications overall in the persons receiving early surgical decompression. Specifically, Mirza et al.[36] reported significantly fewer complications in persons receiving surgery within 72 hours of injury; Croce et al.[40] reported lower rates of pneumonia and DVT in persons receiving surgery within 24 hours; Chipman et al.[43] reported a lower frequency of all complications in patients with an Injury Severity Score (ISS) >15 and receiving surgery within 72 hours of injury (although this same group reports equal medical complications in persons with low ISS <15 regardless of the time of decompression); McKinley et al.[44] report higher rates of pneumonia in the late surgery group but equal rates of other complications (DVT, pulmonary embolism, ulcers).

Degree of Neurological Improvement

All studies reported whether or not patients recovered neurological function after surgical intervention and the majority of studies attempt to relate the effect of early treatment on neurological improvement and functional outcomes. Four studies demonstrated that early surgical decompression afforded better neurological outcomes: Clohisy et al.[30] report that surgical decompression within 48 hours resulted in improvement in the modified Frankel scale; McLain and Benson[35] report better neurological improvement (no *p* value reported) with surgical decompression within 24 hours; Mirza et al.[36] showed that surgery within 72 hours resulted in significant improvements in the American Spinal Injury Association motor score, whereas surgery after 72 hours resulted in no significant improvement in the mean motor score; lastly, Papadopoulos et al.[41] showed that patients who received surgical decompression within 12 hours (± 1.3 h) had significantly better neurological improvement than those with surgery outside this time window. In a similar fashion, seven of the other studies with the same level of evidence reported no neurological benefit to early surgical decompression.[29,39,40,42,44,47,48] Two studies showed equivocal results.[31,32]

Level IV

Two recent studies have provided level IV evidence suggesting that early intervention is supported by surgeons. These surveys of spine surgeons' treatment preferences have differing conclusions, however. There was a lack of consensus among 77 surgeons surveyed by Lenehan et al.[26] while the Fehlings et al.[25] survey of 971 surgeons showed that the majority of spine surgeons surveyed prefer to decompress the acutely injured spinal cord within 24 hours of injury. This preference was particularly significant when discussing cervical SCI. In persons with an incomplete cervical SCI, the survey respondents chose to perform decompressive surgery within 12 hours when possible. Central cord syndrome remains an area of uncertainty with regard to necessity or timing of surgery.

■ Conclusion

Surgical decompression after SCI is founded on a solid basis of animal studies demonstrating improved neurological outcomes with early decompression. Not surprisingly, human clinical trials have been less convincing, most likely due to the complexity of caring for acutely injured patients.

Although somewhat limited in their ability to directly answer clinically relevant questions regarding human SCI, animal models provide overwhelming evidence for two aspects of injury pathophysiology: both the degree of spinal cord compression and the duration of that compression have an impact on the possibility of recovering neurological function. Early surgical decompression following SCI has also been demonstrated to be feasible in humans. It is associated with shorter hospital stays and fewer medical complications than delayed surgery.

As shown by this review, the evidence for neurological improvement after early surgical decompression is mixed. However, evidence is mounting for its safety and clinical and neurological outcomes, and surgical opinion is now favoring early intervention. Early surgical decompression is, therefore, playing an increasing role in the treatment of acute SCI. **Figure 23.1** outlines a clinical vignette whereby early surgical decompression was performed in an 18-year-old male who sustained injuries in a high-speed motor vehicle accident. This case illustrates compression of the spinal cord immediately following the traumatic accident (**Fig. 23.1B**) with T2-weighted signal changes in the spinal cord. Surgical decompression relieved compression of the spinal cord and restored normal alignment of the vertebral column. At 1 year follow-up, this patient improved one grade on the American Spinal Injury Association scale.

The definition of early surgery is not fixed, but most consider early to be less than 24 hours. In terms of safety, the treating surgeon must balance the potential benefits of early surgery versus the risk. The benefits include relieving cord compression and therefore limiting secondary injury. The risks include aggravating secondary injury by hypotensive episodes or blood loss. Several studies point out that patients should be treated with early surgery if medically stable.[27,49] Clinical benefits of early surgery possibly include shorter length of both ICU and overall hospital stay with fewer medical complications (such as pneumonia and DVT).[50] This claim has been challenged by other studies. In terms of neurological outcome, the field of SCI research is torn between substantive evidence from preclinical animal models favoring early surgery[41,51,52] and mixed evidence from human clinical trials. Finally, as previously mentioned, recently published results from the multicenter Surgical Timing for Acute Spinal Injury Study suggest that decompression of the spinal cord within 24 hours of injury is associated with improved neurological recovery in persons with cervical injury.[37]

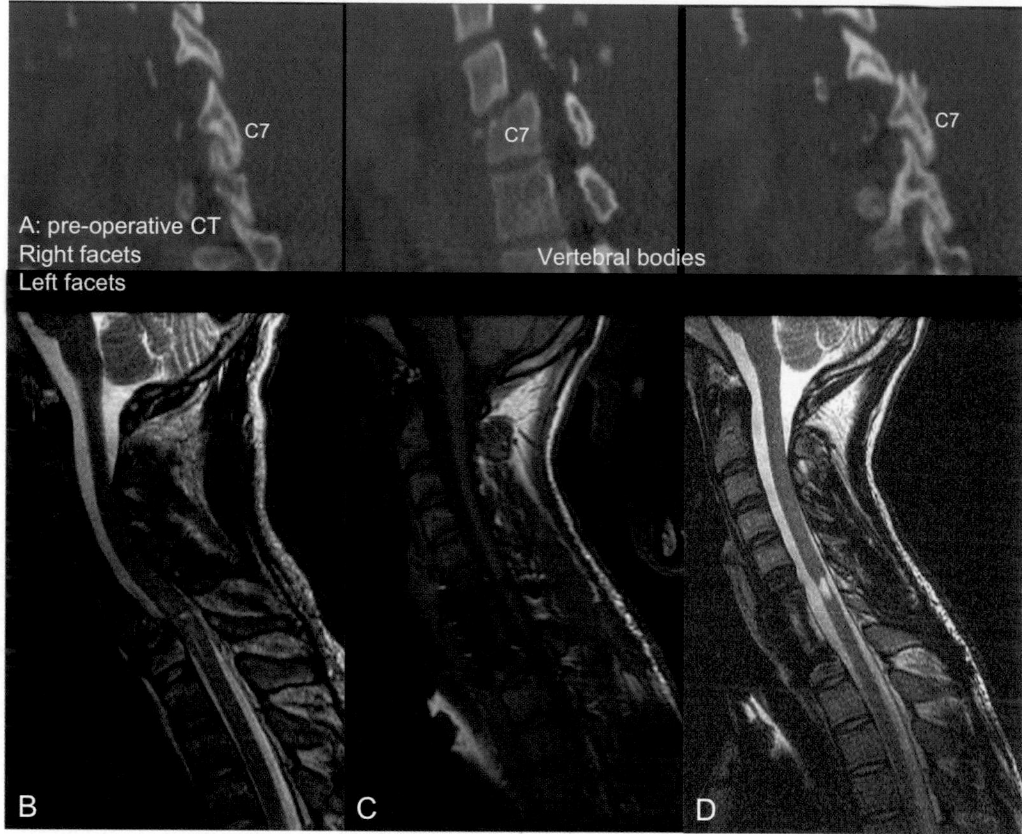

Fig. 23.1 **(A)** The preoperative computed tomographic (CT) scan with sagittal reconstructions outlining the posterior facets and vertebral bodies along with **(B)** a preoperative T2-weighted midsagittal magnetic resonance imaging (MRI) scan and **(C)** postoperative T1-weighted and **(D)** T2-weighted MRI scans. These images were obtained from an 18-year-old male who was involved in a high-speed motor vehicle accident. Neurological examination immediately following the injury revealed C5: 5/5 power, C6 4/5 power bilaterally, C7 3/5 power bilaterally and 0/5 power below the level of C7. Pinprick and soft touch sensation were preserved to the level of L3 and absent below this level. Rectal tone and sensation were preserved. His admission examination can be summarized as an American Spinal Injury Association (ASIA) B incomplete injury. **(B)** MRI scans reveal a grade I anterolisthesis of C6 on C7. There is increased signal within the C7 vertebral body. There is mild compression of the spinal cord at this level. In addition, there is apparent swelling of the cord at this level and increased T2 signal. An urgent anterior decompression and both anterior and posterior stabilizations were preformed. The patient was taken to the operating room within 24 hours. An anterior C7 corpectomy with C6-T1 fusion and posterior cervical instrumentation from C6 to T1 was completed. **(C,D)** Postoperative MRI scans reveal restored alignment of the vertebral column and no compression of the spinal cord; there is persistent T2 hyperintensity within the spinal cord. On follow-up at 1 year, the patient had improved neurologically: C7 was graded as 5/5 bilaterally and C8/T1 was 2–3 in most muscle groups bilaterally. The lower extremity muscle groups also improved to 3 to 4/5 in most muscle groups on the right and 2 to 3/5 in most muscle groups on the left. This examination remained stable beyond the 2 year mark, and the overall improvement was graded from an ASIA B at admission to ASIA C at 1 and 2 year follow-up.

Pearls

- Preclinical literature favors early surgical decompression following traumatic spinal cord injury on the basis of attenuating the cascade of secondary injury events.
- The weight of clinical evidence and the STASCIS study, as well as expert opinion, would favor early surgical decompression for individuals with acute cervical SCI with contining compression.

Pitfalls

- Early surgical decompression should be considered as a treatment option only for those who are medically stable without life-threatening multisystem trauma or major medical comorbidities.
- Avoidance of perioperative hypotension is particularly critical when undertaking early surgical intervention, particularly in the setting of acute cervical SCI.

References

1. Gunnarsson T, Fehlings MG. Acute neurosurgical management of traumatic brain injury and spinal cord injury. Curr Opin Neurol 2003;16(6): 717–723
2. Fehlings MG, Perrin RG. The role and timing of early decompression for cervical spinal cord injury: update with a review of recent clinical evidence. Injury 2005;36(Suppl 2):B13–B26
3. Fehlings MG, Perrin RG. The timing of surgical intervention in the treatment of spinal cord injury: a systematic review of recent clinical evidence. Spine 2006;31(11, Suppl):S28–S35, discussion S36
4. Fehlings MG, Tator CH. An evidence-based review of decompressive surgery in acute spinal cord injury: rationale, indications, and timing based on experimental and clinical studies. J Neurosurg 1999;91(1, Suppl):1–11
5. Fehlings MG, Vaccaro A, Wilson JR, et al. Early versus delayed decompression for traumatic cervical spinal cord injury. Results of the Surgical Timing in Acute Spinal Cord Injury Study (STASCIS). PLoS ONE 2012;7(2):e32037
6. Bohlman HH, Bahniuk E, Raskulinecz G, Field G. Mechanical factors affecting recovery from incomplete cervical spinal cord injury: a preliminary report. Johns Hopkins Med J 1979;145(3):115–125
7. Brodkey JS, Richards DE, Blasingame JP, Nulsen FE. Reversible spinal cord trauma in cats: additive effects of direct pressure and ischemia. J Neurosurg 1972;37(5):591–593
8. Kobrine AI, Evans DE, Rizzoli H. Correlation of spinal cord blood flow and function in experimental compression. Surg Neurol 1978;10(1): 54–59
9. Aki T, Toya S. Experimental study on changes of the spinal-evoked potential and circulatory dynamics following spinal cord compression and decompression. Spine 1984;9(8):800–809
10. Croft TJ, Brodkey JS, Nulsen FE. Reversible spinal cord trauma: a model for electrical monitoring of spinal cord function. J Neurosurg 1972; 36(4):402–406
11. Thienprasit P, Bantli H, Bloedel JR, Chou SN. Effect of delayed local cooling on experimental spinal cord injury. J Neurosurg 1975;42(2):150–154
12. Delamarter RB, Sherman JE, Carr JB. 1991 Volvo Award in experimental studies: cauda equina syndrome: neurologic recovery following immediate, early, or late decompression. Spine 1991; 16(9):1022–1029
13. Hejcl A, Urdzikova L, Sedy J, et al. Acute and delayed implantation of positively charged 2-hydroxyethyl methacrylate scaffolds in spinal cord injury in the rat. J Neurosurg Spine 2008;8(1): 67–73
14. Kobrine AI, Evans DE, Rizzoli HV. Experimental acute balloon compression of the spinal cord: factors affecting disappearance and return of the spinal evoked response. J Neurosurg 1979;51(6):841–845
15. Dolan EJ, Tator CH, Endrenyi L. The value of decompression for acute experimental spinal cord compression injury. J Neurosurg 1980;53(6): 749–755
16. Guha A, Tator CH, Endrenyi L, Piper I. Decompression of the spinal cord improves recovery after acute experimental spinal cord compression injury. Paraplegia 1987;25(4):324–339
17. Nyström B, Berglund JE. Spinal cord restitution following compression injuries in rats. Acta Neurol Scand 1988;78(6):467–472
18. Zhang Y, Hillered L, Olsson Y, Holtz A. Time course of energy perturbation after compression trauma to the spinal cord: an experimental study in the rat using microdialysis. Surg Neurol 1993;39(4):297–304
19. Delamarter RB, Sherman J, Carr JB. Pathophysiology of spinal cord injury. Recovery after immediate and delayed decompression. J Bone Joint Surg Am 1995;77(7):1042–1049
20. Carlson GD, Minato Y, Okada A, et al. Early time-dependent decompression for spinal cord injury: vascular mechanisms of recovery. J Neurotrauma 1997a;14(12):951–962
21. Carlson GD, Warden KE, Barbeau JM, Bahniuk E, Katina-Nelson KL, Biro CL, et al. Viscoelastic relaxation and regional blood flow response to spinal cord compression and decompression. JC Spine 1997b;22(12):1285–1291
22. Dimar JR II, Glassman SD, Raque GH, Zhang YP, Shields CB. The influence of spinal canal narrowing and timing of decompression on neurologic recovery after spinal cord contusion in a rat model. Spine 1999;24(16):1623–1633
23. Carlson GD, Gorden CD, Oliff HS, Pillai JJ, LaManna JC. Sustained spinal cord compression: part I: time-dependent effect on long-term pathophysiology. J Bone Joint Surg Am 2003;85-A(1): 86–94

24. Rabinowitz RS, Eck JC, Harper CM Jr, et al. Urgent surgical decompression compared to methylprednisolone for the treatment of acute spinal cord injury: a randomized prospective study in beagle dogs. Spine 2008;33(21):2260–2268
25. Fehlings MG, Rabin D, Sears W, Cadotte DW, Aarabi B. Current practice in the timing of surgical intervention in spinal cord injury. Spine 2010;35(21, Suppl):S166–S173
26. Lenehan B, Dvorak MF, Madrazo I, Yukawa Y, Fisher CG. Diversity and commonalities in the care of spine trauma internationally. Spine 2010;35(21, Suppl):S174–S179
27. Cengiz SL, Kalkan E, Bayir A, Ilik K, Basefer A. Timing of thoracolomber spine stabilization in trauma patients; impact on neurological outcome and clinical course: a real prospective (rct) randomized controlled study. Arch Orthop Trauma Surg 2008;128(9):959–966
28. Vaccaro AR, Daugherty RJ, Sheehan TP, et al. Neurologic outcome of early versus late surgery for cervical spinal cord injury. Spine 1997; 22(22):2609–2613
29. Levi L, Wolf A, Rigamonti D, Ragheb J, Mirvis S, Robinson WL. Anterior decompression in cervical spine trauma: does the timing of surgery affect the outcome? Neurosurgery 1991;29(2):216–222
30. Clohisy JC, Akbarnia BA, Bucholz RD, Burkus JK, Backer RJ. Neurologic recovery associated with anterior decompression of spine fractures at the thoracolumbar junction (T12-L1). Spine 1992;17(8, Suppl):S325–S330
31. Krengel WF III, Anderson PA, Henley MB. Early stabilization and decompression for incomplete paraplegia due to a thoracic-level spinal cord injury. Spine 1993;18(14):2080–2087
32. Duh MS, Shepard MJ, Wilberger JE, Bracken MB. The effectiveness of surgery on the treatment of acute spinal cord injury and its relation to pharmacological treatment. Neurosurgery 1994; 35(2):240–248, discussion 248–249
33. Botel U, Glaser E, Niedeggen A. The surgical treatment of acute spinal paralysed patients. Spinal Cord 1997;35:420–428
34. Campagnolo DI, Esquieres RE, Kopacz KJ. Effect of timing of stabilization on length of stay and medical complications following spinal cord injury. J Spinal Cord Med 1997;20(3):331–334
35. McLain RF, Benson DR. Urgent surgical stabilization of spinal fractures in polytrauma patients. Spine 1999;24(16):1646–1654
36. Mirza SK, Krengel WF III, Chapman JR, et al. Early versus delayed surgery for acute cervical spinal cord injury. Clin Orthop Relat Res 1999; (359):104–114
37. Fehlings MG, Vaccaro A, Wilson JR, et al. Early versus delayed decompression for traumatic cervical spinal cord injury: results of the Surgical Timing in Acute Spinal Cord Injury Study (STASCIS). PLos ONE 2012;7(2):e32037
38. Tator CH, Fehlings MG, Thorpe K, Taylor W. Current use and timing of spinal surgery for management of acute spinal cord injury in North America: results of a retrospective multicenter study. J Neurosurg 1999;91(1, Suppl):12–18
39. Guest J, Eleraky MA, Apostolides PJ, Dickman CA, Sonntag VK. Traumatic central cord syndrome: results of surgical management. J Neurosurg 2002;97(1, Suppl):25–32
40. Croce MA, Bee TK, Pritchard E, Miller PR, Fabian TC. Does optimal timing for spine fracture fixation exist? Ann Surg 2001;233(6): 851–858
41. Papadopoulos SM, Selden NR, Quint DJ, Patel N, Gillespie B, Grube S. Immediate spinal cord decompression for cervical spinal cord injury: feasibility and outcome. J Trauma 2002;52(2): 323–332
42. Pollard ME, Apple DF. Factors associated with improved neurologic outcomes in patients with incomplete tetraplegia. Spine 2003;28(1):33–39
43. Chipman JG, Deuser WE, Beilman GJ. Early surgery for thoracolumbar spine injuries decreases complications. J Trauma 2004;56(1):52–57
44. McKinley W, Meade MA, Kirshblum S, Barnard B. Outcomes of early surgical management versus late or no surgical intervention after acute spinal cord injury. Arch Phys Med Rehabil 2004;85(11): 1818–1825
45. Kerwin AJ, Frykberg ER, Schinco MA, Griffen MM, Murphy T, Tepas JJ. The effect of early spine fixation on non-neurologic outcome. J Trauma 2005;58(1):15–21
46. Schinkel C, Frangen TM, Kmetic A, Andress HJ, Muhr G; German Trauma Registry. Timing of thoracic spine stabilization in trauma patients: impact on clinical course and outcome. J Trauma 2006;61(1):156–160, discussion 160
47. Sapkas GS, Papadakis SA. Neurological outcome following early versus delayed lower cervical spine surgery. J Orthop Surg (Hong Kong) 2007;15(2):183–186
48. Chen L, Yang H, Yang T, Xu Y, Bao Z, Tang T. Effectiveness of surgical treatment for traumatic central cord syndrome. J Neurosurg Spine 2009;10(1):3–8
49. Albin MS, White RJ. Epidemiology, physiopathology, and experimental therapeutics of acute spinal cord injury. Crit Care Clin 1987;3(3): 441–452
50. Tator CH, Koyanagi I. Vascular mechanisms in the pathophysiology of human spinal cord injury. J Neurosurg 1997;86(3):483–492
51. Harvey C, Wilson SE, Greene CG, Berkowitz M, Stripling TE. New estimates of the direct costs of traumatic spinal cord injuries: results of a nationwide survey. Paraplegia 1992;30(12):834–850
52. Kakulas BA. Neuropathology: the foundation for new treatments in spinal cord injury. Spinal Cord 2004;42(10):549–563

24

Hypothermia: Evidence-Based Review

David M. Benglis Jr., Allan D. Levi, and Michael Y. Wang

Key Points

1. A vast body of literature exists reporting the effects of experimentally induced spinal cord injury in animals and the effects of hypothermia as a neuroprotective agent (**Tables 24.1** and **24.2**). The two methods of cooling include systemic and local. The results are highly variable, with some studies showing benefit and others not.
2. There have been at least four multicenter, large, randomized trials examining the effects of hypothermia as a neuroprotective agent in TBI, which have either been completed or are ongoing. To date there have been no large, multicenter, randomized, controlled clinical trials examining the benefits and side effects of modest hypothermia following spinal cord injury.
3. Common definitions of hypothermia temperature ranges utilized in both experimental and clinical research include moderate hypothermia (28 to 32°C), modest hypothermia (32 to 34°C), and mild hypothermia (33 to 36°C).
4. There is evidence in various animal models of stroke, epilepsy, TBI, and SCI that supports the statement that hyperthermia is deleterious to the healing nervous system.

More than 12,000 persons each year are affected by spinal cord injury (SCI) in the United States (National Spinal Cord Injury Statistical Center). Although several neuroprotective strategies exist for the treatment of SCI, none of them has been established as the standard of care.[1] Recent reports in the literature have focused primarily on hypothermia as a treatment following stroke, traumatic brain injury (TBI), cardiac arrest, and intracerebral and aortic aneurysm repair.[2–7] Two recent studies found a benefit in mortality and functional outcomes following cardiac arrest.[2,8] There also exists a vast history and a relatively recent growing body of literature in both animal and clinical studies examining the effects of hypothermia on the injured spinal cord.[9] There is also evidence in various animal models of stroke, epilepsy, TBI, and SCI that hyperthermia is deleterious to the healing nervous system.[10–13]

This chapter presents the current evidence-based knowledge concerning the use of hypothermia as a neuroprotective agent following SCI in animals and humans. It also covers the history of the use of hypothermia and examines its biological effects on the nervous system from the work of in vitro, in vivo, and clinical studies. The different methods of cooling and modern cooling devices are also briefly discussed. The chapter concludes with a focus on future directions and challenges in clinical trial designs.

■ History of Hypothermia-Based Treatments for Spinal Cord Injury (1940s to 1980s)

The first mention of hypothermia for central nervous system-based pathology in the literature dates back to 1938, when Dr. Temple Fay documented his experience of its use in a cancer patient.[14] Fay then followed with a larger study of 120 patients, and reported that surface cooling improved outcomes in TBI. In addition to Dr. Fay, Dr. Rosamoff also pioneered some of the early work in the field of hypothermia for the treatment of TBI.[15–17] More recently, ischemic SCI, a common potentially devastating complication following aortic aneurysm surgery, has been an area of interest for cardiovascular surgeons, many having instituted deep hypothermia (18 to 25°C) to prevent this complication.

Early Animal Models of Hypothermia and Spinal Cord Injury

Experimentally induced hypothermia for the treatment of SCI was studied extensively in the 1960s and 1970s. Albin and White were the first to report on the effects of local cooling both intradurally and extradurally on the injured spinal cord in both primate and canine models. Their results indicated a useful beneficial effect of hypothermia in improving neurological outcomes.[18–20] Albin and White's early findings were followed by several other groups, who over the next 10 years utilized various animal models to examine the effects of local hypothermia in SCI (**Table 24.1**).[21–27] However, enthusiasm for pharmacological neuroprotection during the 1980s and 1990s resulted in waning interest in hypothermia as a neuroprotectant for SCI.

In the contemporary scientific literature, several groups reported on the positive effects of hypothermia on histopathology or motor function. Green et al. observed histopathological differences between control and hypothermia-treated animals when they analyzed posttraumatic feline spinal cords. These effects were reduced with a delay in the time that hypothermia was begun (i.e., 1 h vs 5 h following injury).[22] Wells and Hansebout and Hansebout et al. documented motor outcome improvements in their canine compressive SCI model when hypothermia was administered epidurally for 4 hours either 15 minutes or 4 hours postinjury.[21,26] Kuchner and Hansebout found an additive effect when steroids and hypothermia were used together, compared with either therapy alone, in canine motor function.[27]

These beneficial effects were met by an equal number of groups showing minimal benefit or negative effects of local hypothermia in experimental SCI. Black and Markowitz demonstrated that hypothermia actually slowed neurological recovery, albeit not significantly, in a primate model of SCI when 4 to 8°C saline was placed epidurally for 5 hours following injury.[23] Tator and Deecke also showed that primates treated with normothermia and saline perfusion following SCI fared better in motor function than hypothermia-treated groups, whereas Howitt and Turnbull found no difference in hindlimb motor function improvement between rabbits treated with epidural cooling compared with controls.[24,28]

Early Human Research in Hypothermia and Spinal Cord Injury

Epidural saline application following SCI in humans was utilized to a limited extent during the 1960s and 1970s. Most of this early work, although novel, failed to show efficacy due to low sample numbers and the lack of control populations, as well as highly variable time intervals from the actual time of injury until the initiation of cooling.[29–36] Perfusion devices used for continuous cooling of the epidural space also required that an acute multilevel posterior surgery be performed. Kwon et al. also listed them in a concise table in a recent review article.[14] As also pointed out by Kwon et al. in their recent comprehensive review on hypothermia and SCI, many of these early researchers understood the limitations of these studies, and they were careful to note that no major adverse events occurred.[14]

Research on hypothermia for various neurological injuries declined in the early 1980s. In the SCI literature, this may have been due to several factors, including (1) the wide variation of results negating or supporting hypothermia in experimental SCI models, (2) the logistical challenges of local hypothermia application and maintenance in open surgery, and (3) complications encountered with profound systemic hypothermia (24 to 33°C) (discussion follows).[37]

Complications Encountered with Hypothermia

Complications reported with the use of hypothermia include bradycardia, hypothermia, increased risk of deep venous thrombosis (DVT), respiratory infection, lower leukocyte counts, hypotension, coagulopathy, altered drug pharmacokinetics, and skin injury with direct cooling methods.[38–43] Of note, many of these adverse events were observed in early studies, where temperatures often ran below 30°C.

Hypothermia induces reversible platelet dysfunction and resultant increases in bleeding times as well as disturbances in the coagulation cascades.[44,45] Hypothermia-treated patients in the Hypothermia after Cardiac Arrest (HACA) trial developed a higher incidence of bleeding complications, although they were not statistically significant.[8]

Dysfunction of the immune response under the influence of hypothermia has been reported in both animals and humans.[46,47] Russwurm et al., in an in vitro model, were able to link decreased cytokine expression and release, for example, interleukin (IL)-2, in human peripheral blood mononuclear cells. They noted this finding as a potential cause of increased infection risk due to an impaired immune response.[48] In the HACA trial, patients in the experimental group had a higher incidence of sepsis and pneumonia (not significant).[8] Todd et al. reported a higher incidence of bacteremia in their series on mild intraoperative hypothermia in aneurysm surgery.[49] Intravascular devices also pose risks associated with vessel access, including hemorrhage, infection, and thrombosis.

Thermoregulatory responses, such as shivering, can also present obstacles to temperature management because this physiological response results in increased metabolic demands, patient discomfort, and elevated temperature. Meperidine-based medical therapies represent the current best methods of treatment of shivering; however, they tend to cause sedation, nausea, and respiratory suppression at high doses.[50]

Resurgence of Mild/Modest Hypothermia

A resurgence of interest in the use of therapeutic hypothermia in TBI over the last 15 years has necessitated many scientists to take a "second look" at its potential benefits in SCI.[51] A publication by Busto et al. changed the perception that hypothermia could only be effective if administered between 24 and 33°C.[52] They found that mild hypothermia (34°C) conferred a protective effect in a rat brain ischemia model. This reinvigorated the modern era of hypothermia research and subsequently led to various animal hypothermia trials in SCI.

The manner in which cooling is delivered has also advanced when compared with past methods. Systemic and local

Table 24.1 Description of Animal Experiments That Examined Administration of Local Hypothermia following Experimentally Induced Spinal Cord Injury

Authors, year	Animals, injury	Mode of HT
Albin et al., 1967[20]	Canine, T10, Imp	L-HT postinjury 400 g • cm Imp, epidural (5°C) saline for 2.5 h
Albin et al., 1969[53]	Primate, T10, Imp	L-HT 4 h or 8 h postinjury, intradural (2–5°C) saline for 3 h
Black and Markowitz, 1971[23]	Primate, T10, Imp	L-HT 1 h postinjury, epidural (4–8°C) saline for 5 h*
Howitt and Turnbull, 1972[24]	Rabbit, TL junction, Imp	L-HT preinjury or 15 min postinjury, epidural cooling (7°C) saline for 1–3 h
Tator and Deecke, 1973[25]	Primate, T9, Bal	L-HT/normothermia no perfusion, HT (5°C) and normothermia (36°C) perfusion, 3 h postinjury
Green et al., 1973[22]	Feline, T10, weight drop	L-HT (3°C) epidural infusion for 3 h, 1 h, or 5 h postinjury
Hansebout et al., 1975[26]	Canine, T13, Bal	L-15 min postinjury, epidural cooling (6°C) saline for 4 h**
Kuchner and Hansebout, 1976[27]	Canine, T13, Bal	L-15 min postinjury or 3.5 h postinjury, epidural cooling (6°C) saline for 4 h***
Wells and Hansebout, 1978[21]	Canine, T13, Bal	L-4 h postinjury, epidural cooling (6°C) for 1 h, 4 h, or 18 h
Tuzgen et al., 1998[54]	Rat, C7/T1, Clip	L-30 min postinjury, cord T of (24–26°C) for 30 min
Kuchner et al., 2000[55]	Canine, T13, Bal	L-15 min postinjury for HT, 3.5 h postinjury for HT/dexamethasone, epidural cooling (6°C) for 4 h***
Dimar et al., 2000[56]	Rat, T10, Spacer and Imp	L-immediately postinjury, epidural perfusion cooling to (19°C) for 2 h****
Casas et al., 2005[57]	Rat, T10, Imp	L-30 min postinjury, epidural perfusion cooling normothermic, 35.3°C (mild); 30.5°C (moderate); and 24.1°C (severe) for 3 h
Ha and Kim, 2008[58]	Rat, T9, Imp	L-(30°C) immediately postinjury epidural perfusion cooling for 48 h
Morochovic et al., 2008[59]	Rat, T8/9, Bal	L-25 min postinjury, epidural perfusion cooling to (28.5°C) for 1 h

Source: Inamasu J, Nakamura Y, Ichikizaki K. Induced hypothermia in experimental traumatic spinal cord injury: an update. J Neurol Sci 2003;209(1–2):55–60; Kwon BK, Mann C, Sohn HM, et al.. Hypothermia for spinal cord injury. Spine J 2008;8(6):859–874. Adapted with permission.

Abbreviations: Bal, Balloon; BBB, Basso, Beattie, Bresnahan; h, hour; HP, histopathology; HT, hypothermia; Imp, impactor; L, local; min, minute; MDA, malonyl dialdehyde; MF, motor function; MMEP, magnetic motor evoked potential; T, temperature

Parameters measured	Benefit	Outcome
MF	Yes	Experimental 400 g • cm Imp HT group had "marked" recovery when compared with control
MF	Yes	Qualitative description of complete neurological recovery in HT-treated animals after 4 h delay compared with controls; no benefit when HT delayed to 8 h
MF	No	HT slowed neurological recovery but difference not significant
MF	No	No difference between hindlimb function in either HT experimental groups when compared with control
MF	No	Intradural perfusion with normothermia group did better than intradural perfusion with HT
HP	Yes	HT resulted in beneficial effects limited to the dorsal third of the SC in groups receiving therapy 1 h postinjury; a delay of 5 h in HT resulted in benefit localized only to dorsal sixth of spinal cord
MF	Yes	HT resulted in significantly improved motor scores when compared with normothermia
MF	Yes	Additive effect when steroids and HT used together; these animals did better than with either therapy alone
MF	Yes	HT for 4 h resulted in significant improvement in hindlimb function versus normothermia
Lipid peroxidation (tissue content of MDA)	Yes	2 h postinjury, tissue MDA in HT decreased compared with control normothermia
MF, HP, and tissue electrolyte content	Yes	HT and dexamethasone improved hindlimb motor function compared with normothermia; no benefit to combination Rx; HT was ineffective at reducing cord edema at 6 d postinjury; at 7 wk postinjury, HT alone or with dexamethasone had no effect on dry weight or Na and K concentrations
MF, HP, and transcranial MMEP	Yes	Significant improvement of BBB motor scores at 6 wk, MMEPs, and secondary damage (not quantified) in HT group with cord injury from epidural spacer only
MF, HP	No	No significant improvement of BBB of experimental groups at any temperature at 6 wk, no HP difference from experimental and control
MF, HP	Yes	HT significantly reduced the apoptosis of neurons and glial cells and improved functional recovery at 7 d when compared with controls
MF, HP	No	No differences in BBB scores and preserved volumes after 4 wk survival; HT-treated animals had significantly more preserved white matter at cranial periphery of lesion

*Included experimental steroid group with benefit when compared with control animals.
**Included experimental steroid group, which fared better in MF than hypothermia at weeks 3 and 4.
***Included experimental steroid group and a steroid + hypothermia group.
****Included groups with cord injury from impactor, epidural spacer, and impactor + epidural spacer.

cooling are two methods that have been implemented in current animal studies examining the effects of hypothermia in SCI (see **Table 24.1** and **Table 24.2** for a listing of experimental SCI studies).[51] Modern devices such as subcutaneous or epidural heat exchangers have been developed for use in animal models.[60] The majority of the animal studies, however, utilize noninvasive external systemic cooling. Rodents, given their smaller body surface areas, can more easily reach target temperatures with systemic external cooling.[51] These groups in general have not reported abnormal changes in physiological parameters with hypothermia. This disparity in the reporting of adverse events between animal models and humans in studies of hypothermia could be due to trial design. Most animal studies utilize a lower injury to the thoracic region (e.g., reduces animal care needs), whereas human trials that often include patients with cervical injuries.[61]

The question of whether systemic temperatures reflect actual temperatures within the spinal cord parenchyma was addressed by Westergren et al.[62] They found that in rat models of SCI, esophageal temperatures, although not exact, more accurately reflected intramedullary and epidural temperatures during hypothermia than rectal temperatures. Other methods of experimental temperature monitoring include paravertebral muscle or epidural probes.

Histopathological and Neurochemical Effects of Hypothermia

The physiological effects of hypothermia on the injured spinal cord have been theorized to be due to (1) a decrease in metabolic demand and oxygen consumption, (2) reduction of edema and hemorrhage, and (3) cellular membrane stabilization.[51,63,64] Some groups have focused on the histological or neurochemical effects of hypothermia following experimentally induced SCI in animals. Chatzipanteli and colleagues demonstrated attenuation of posttraumatic inflammation measured by decreased myeloperoxidase activity (e.g., neutrophil accumulation) in rats following weight drop and treatment with moderate hypothermia (32°C) for 3 hours when compared with those treated with normothermia.[65] Kuchner and colleagues, using a canine balloon compression SCI model, found no differences in electrolyte content or edema in the spinal cords of hypothermia-treated animals versus controls. They did, however, observe improved hindlimb motor function in the hypothermia-treated group (epidural cooling [6°C] begun 15 minutes after injury for 4 hours).[55]

Yu et al. and Westergren et al. demonstrated an increased number of functional spinal axons and dendrites in a rat weight compression model of SCI when the animals were maintained at 30°C for 2 hours following injury.[66,67] Lower ubiquitin and β-amyloid protein precursor (axons) and higher microtubule associated protein 2 (MAP-2) (dendrites) were used as a measure of cellular integrity. This group also confirmed that hypothermia suppressed proliferation of capillaries and astrocytes proximal to injury zones, via reduced vimentin and glial fibrillary acid protein (GFAP), respectively, induced by hypothermia.[68]

Increased excitatory amino acids (EAAs) (e.g., glutamate, aspartate) and free radicals (e.g., superoxides, nitric oxides) as well as disruption of cell membranes have been shown to occur following experimental SCI and may contribute to secondary injury processes. Two groups, however, have reported conflicting results of the effect of hypothermia on these pathways. In a rat balloon compression model of SCI (L1, 33°C for 4 h preinjury), Yamamoto et al. showed suppression of EAA, whereas Farooque et al. reported an increase in EAA in hypothermia-treated animals (T8, 31°C for the preinjury period).[69,70] These differences could potentially be explained by variances in model design and injury level. Tuzgen et al. examined the effect of epidural hypothermia on lipid peroxidation via measurement of the tissue content of malonyl dialdehyde (MDA) in a rat SCI model (C7 clip, 24 to 26°C for 30 min beginning 30 min postinjury) at one time point.[54] They found decreased levels of MDA in the hypothermia-treated group yet did not correlate these findings with histological or functional improvements.

Functional Outcomes of Hypothermia in Experimental Models

From 1992 through 2009 there have been five animal studies examining functional recovery following induced SCI and subsequent systemic hypothermia, whereas five have focused on epidural cooling administration. The results in these 10 experimental studies are variable, involving different cooling methods, injury levels, devices, severity, species of animal, and variations in timing, duration, and extent of hypothermia.[14] This information was derived from two recent comprehensive reviews.[14,31]

Morochovic et al., in a rat T8/9 balloon compression model (28.5°C beginning 25 min postinjury for 1 h), reported similar negative results.[59] Westergren and colleagues, using a rat weight/compression model (T8), observed no functional benefit to hypothermia (30°C for 2 h following SCI) versus control therapy, whereas Casas et al. also found no functional or histopathological improvement after 6 weeks at four different temperatures 30 minutes postcontusive injury for 3 hours (e.g., normothermic, mild hypothermia 35.3°C, moderate 30.5°C, severe 24.1°C) in their rat T10 injury model.[57,71]

Yu et al., on the other hand, reported motor function improvement in animals at both 9 days and 6 weeks postinjury (T8, weight-drop contusion, 32°C for 4 h immediately after SCI).[72] Specific physiological parameters, such as mean arterial blood pressure (MABP), blood pH, pCO_2, and PO_2 were well matched at all time points (pretrauma and 2 or 4 h posttrauma) in both the experimental hypothermia (n = 9) and control groups (n = 7).

The normothermia-treated group also showed some recovery of function, suggesting that their model created a partial or subthreshold injury versus prior studies. Functional motor recovery in the control group progressed gradually over a period of 2 to 3 weeks, even though in the first 5 days following injury relatively no movement was noted. After 3 weeks, no further improvement in motor function was observed. In contrast, hypothermia-treated animals demonstrated a continuous improvement in functional scales, such as the Basso, Beattie, Bresnahan (BBB), beginning on day 9, that was significantly better than that of normothermia-treated animals at 6 weeks. The mean area of histopathological damage was also noted to be significantly less in the experimental hypothermia group.

Dimar et al., in their rat SCI injury model, created a range of severity of injuries utilizing a compression SCI device, impactor, or both. A local cooling device (T10, 19°C for 2 h immediately after SCI) effectively improved ambulatory function after 5 weeks in the moderate injury group but failed in the other two groups, supporting the idea that there may be certain subthreshold injuries where hypothermia becomes effective.[56] Another explanation suggested by Kwon et al. is that regional cooling may be effective for ischemic compression of the spinal cord but somewhat limited when the injury includes a contusive component.[14] This statement is also supported by the work of Casas et al., where the authors found no improvement in rat BBB scores at four different temperatures in a contusive SCI model (see earlier discussion).[57]

Kuchner et al. also found a positive effect of local hypothermia (6°C for 4 h 15 min after injury) that was comparable to postinjury steroid treatment following balloon compression in a canine T13 injury model.[55] This study was divided among four groups: (1) dexamethasone-treated (n = 16), (2) local hypothermia (n = 16), (3) dexamethasone + local hypothermia (n = 17),

Table 24.2 Description of Animal Experiments That Examined Administration of Systemic Hypothermia Following Experimentally Induced Spinal Cord Injury

Authors, year	Animals, injury	Mode of HT
Farooque et al., 1997[70]	Rat, T8, cord compression	S-(30–31°C) during entire observation period preinjury
Yamamoto et al., 1998[69]	Rat, L1, Bal	S-(33°C) 4 h preinjury*
Westergren et al., 1999[66]	Rat, T8	S-(30°C) 20 min immediately postinjury**
Yu et al., 1999[68]	Rat, T8, weight +5 min compression	S-(30°C) 20 min immediately postinjury**
Yu et al., 1999[68]	Rat, T8, weight +5 min compression	S-(30°C) 20 min immediately postinjury**
Yu et al., 2000[72]	Rat, T10, weight +5 min compression	S-(32°C) 30 min postinjury for 4 h
Yu et al., 2000[67]	Rat, T8, weight +5 min compression	S-(30°C) 20 min immediately postinjury**
Jou, 2000[73]	Rat,C6/7, clip	S-(30°C) or (34°C) 1 h preinjury
Westergren et al., 2000[71]	Rat, T8, weight +5 min compression	S-(30°C) for 2 h immediately postinjury
Chatzipanteli et al., 2000[65]	Rat, T10, Imp	S-(32°C) for 3 dh immediately postinjury***
Westergren et al., 2001[74]	Rat, T8, weight + 5 min compression	S-(30°C) 15 min postinjury maintained during measurements***
Shibuya et al., 2004[75]	Rat, T11, compression10 min	S-(32°C) immediately 4 h postinjury****
Nishi et al., 2007[76]	Rat SC sections, L1-S3	(32–24°C), time of hypothermia not applicable
Duz et al.., 2009[77]	Rat, T8-10, clip	S-(27–29°C) 5 min postinjury for 1 h; 1a,1b-control/experimental sacrificed after 1 h, 2a,2b control/experimental sacrificed after 24 h
Lo et al., 2009[78]	Rat, cervical, Imp	S-(33°C) 5 min postinjury for 4 h

Source: Inamasu J, Nakamura Y, Ichikizaki K. Induced hypothermia in experimental traumatic spinal cord injury: an update. J Neurol Sci 2003;209(1–2):55–60; Kwon BK, Mann C, Sohn HM, et al. Hypothermia for spinal cord injury. Spine J 2008;8(6):859–874. Adapted with permission.

Abbreviations: AA, amino acids; Bal, balloon; BBB, Basso, Beattie, Bresnahan; CSF, cerebrospinal fluid; EC, extracellular; GFAP, glial fibrillary acidic protein; GSH-Px, glutathione peroxidase; h, hour; HP, histopathology; HT, hypothermia; IHC, immunohistochemistry; Imp, impactor; L, local; min, minutes; MAP-2, microtubule-associated protein 2; MDA, malonyl dialdehyde; MD, microdialysis; MF, motor function; MP, myeloperoxidase; MMEP, magnetic motor evoked potential; PMNL, polymorphonuclear leukocyte; S, systemic; SC, spinal cord; SCBF, spinal cord blood flow; SSEP, spinal somatosensory evoked potentials; T, temperature; TBARS, thiobarbituric acid reactive substances

Parameters measured	Benefit	Outcome
EC lactate and AA by MD	No	No difference in lactate levels, increased glutamate and aspartate in experimental group
CSF glutamate by MD	Yes	Significantly lower glutamate levels in experimental group
Expression of β-APP, ubiquitin, and PGP 9.5 by IHC	Yes	Semiquantitative analysis revealed decreased β-APP, ubiquitin, and PGP 9.5 in experimental group
Expression of vimentin and GFAP	Yes	Semiquantitative analysis revealed decreased vimentin and GFAP in experimental group
Extravasation of plasma protein by IHC	Yes	Semiquantitative analysis revealed decreased plasma proteins and SC cross-sectional area in experimental group suggesting decreased edema
MF, HP	Yes	BBB scores significantly better in experimental group by 9 d postinjury and at 6 wk; decreased lesion size on HP in experimental group
HP, MAP-2	Yes	Smaller SC cross-sectional area in experimental group (suggestive of less edema), significant reduction in MAP-2 immunostaining in controls
MF, HP, spinal SSEP	Yes	Significant differences of moderate hypothermia when compared with mild and control, with (1) improved SSEP during cord compression, (2) improved MF hindlimb 3 d postinjury, and (3) decreased gross tissue destruction at injury site
MF, HP	No	No improvement in hindlimb motor scores or inclined plane performance in experimental group at 2 wk postinjury
Tissue MP (neutrophil accumulation) assay, and PMNL count	Yes	MP assay significantly decreased in experimental group
SCBF changes by laser Doppler	No	Trend toward hypothermia and reduced SCBF but not significant
TUNEL (apoptosis)	Yes	Significantly less TUNEL positive cells around injury site 3 and 7 d postinjury in experimental group
Patch clamp of ventral horn neurons with an ischemic perfusion model	Yes	Progressive decrease in spontaneous excitatory postsynaptic currents with decreasing T (32–24°C)
TBARS, GSH-Px (lipid peroxidation)	Yes	Hypothermia was effective in the early stages of treatment (1 h) in reducing lipid peroxidation, but had a negative effect over control on lipid peroxidation after (24 h)
MF, HP	Yes	Improved BBB at 1–3 wk, increase in forelimb strength, 31% increase in normal white matter and 38% increase in normal gray matter; preservation of neurons (quantitatively four times greater) rostral and caudal to the injury

*Included nicaraven (free radical scavenger) group alone and with hypothermia that showed no significant benefit of nicaraven.
**This study also had a hypothermia sham group in addition to control and experimental groups.
***This study also had a hypothermia sham and a normothermia sham in addition to control and experimental groups.
****This study also had a normothermia sham in addition to control and experimental groups.

(4) lesion with no therapy ($n = 24$). A modified Tarlov rating system was used to evaluate clinical motor recovery.[79]

There was a significant marked difference in the motor recovery (beginning at day 5 postinjury) of the treated (dexamethasone or hypothermia) versus the nontreated groups. These motor findings also correlated with significant differences in measures of spinal cord dry weights at 6 days and 7 weeks postinjury (signifying less edema in treated animals). They also found a trend toward even more improved motor outcomes with combination therapy; however, these findings were not significant.

Jou[73] divided 36 rats into three different temperature groups (moderate hypothermia 30°C, mild hypothermia 34°C, normothermia 38°C). Somatosensory evoked potential measurements (SSEPs) were recorded in the upper cervical spine by median nerve stimulation. Gross motor and sensory status of both forelimbs were examined according to a modified scale by Kai et al. 3 days following the injury.[80] The animals were then sacrificed.

Following a C6/7 clip injury, this group found a significant benefit in hindlimb motor functional recovery (after 3 days) when moderate (30°C) epidural cooling was used for 1 hour preinjury versus mild (34°C) or normothermia. They also observed correlative improvements in histology and SSEPs (e.g., significantly greater preservation of posttraumatic amplitudes noted 60 minutes following injury) in the experimental moderate hypothermia arm.[73] This study was important because it introduced an alternate method (i.e., SSEP) of quantifying the effects of hypothermia on the injured spinal cord. Ha and Kim also noted improved functional recovery (at 7 days) when saline was perfused epidurally in a T9 rat impactor SCI model (30°C, postinjury for 48 h).[58]

Lo and colleagues, using a rat cervical model of contusive SCI, investigated the efficacy of transient hypothermia (beginning 5 minutes postinjury for 4 h, 33°C) for the preservation of neural tissue and improved functional recovery. The experimental group had significant increases in normal-appearing white and gray matter volumes, as well as greater preservation of neurons proximal to the injury epicenter (**Fig. 24.1**). They observed a faster rate of recovery in open-field locomotor ability (BBB score, weeks 1 to 3) and forelimb strength.[78]

Human Hypothermia Spinal Cord Injury Trials and Current Cooling Devices

Modern Cooling Devices

Over the past few years, technological advances in intravascular and surface cooling delivery have enabled caregivers to more accurately manage this form of treatment.[41] Two categories of cooling devices available for human use are external and internal. These devices differ in both their safety and their cooling profiles. External cooling methods have been used more commonly in human trials.[41] Methods of external cooling include, in the simplest form, ice packs applied to the body surface, along with bladder and gastric irrigation. More complex external systems include hydrogel pads with continuous feedback mechanisms depending on the patient's temperature status (**Fig. 24.2**) (Arctic Sun, Medivance, Inc., Louisville, CO or Cincinnati Subzero Hypothermia System, Cincinnati Subzero Products Inc., OH). Air circulation systems, such as the Bair Hugger (Arizant, Eden Prairie, MN) or TheraKool (Kinetic Concepts, Wareham, England), blow temperature-controlled air across the body surface and are set manually to achieve a core body temperature. Mean time to target temperature, however, for these air-cooling devices in one study was significantly greater (8 h) when compared with other studies that used either intravascular or hydrogel-based systems (1.9–3.5 h).[8,81–83]

Internal or intravascular cooling devices require that a catheter be inserted into a central vein. These systems utilize a closed system of circulating saline to achieve a particular core temperature.

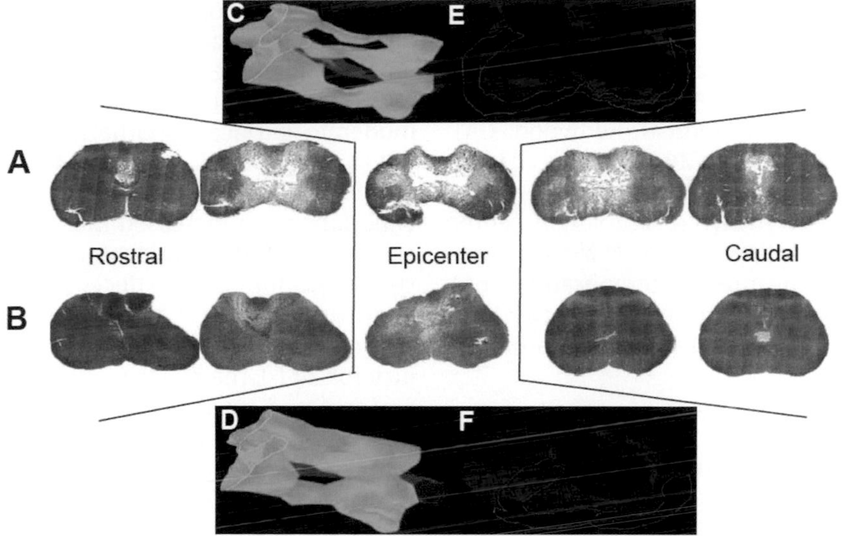

Fig. 24.1 Coronal section series showing improved tissue preservation following hypothermia with three-dimensional (3-D) models of preserved gray and white matter volumes. Hematoxylin & eosin, and luxol fast blue stained 10 mm transverse sections from the injury epicenter, and at 900 and 1500 mm rostral and caudal from a representative spinal cord at 10 weeks after spinal cord injury (SCI) and either **(A)** normothermia or **(B)** hypothermia. A significant reduction in the lateral and longitudinal extension of tissue damage can be observed with hypothermia treatment. **(C,D)** Reconstructed 3-D tissue volumes of normal-appearing gray and **(E,F)** white matter after normothermia or hypothermia treatment, respectively, using Neuroleucida software, show greater tissue preservation with the application of mild systemic hypothermia following SCI. Scale bar = 1 mm. (Courtesy of Damien Pearse, PhD, University of Miami, Miami Project to Cure Paralysis.)

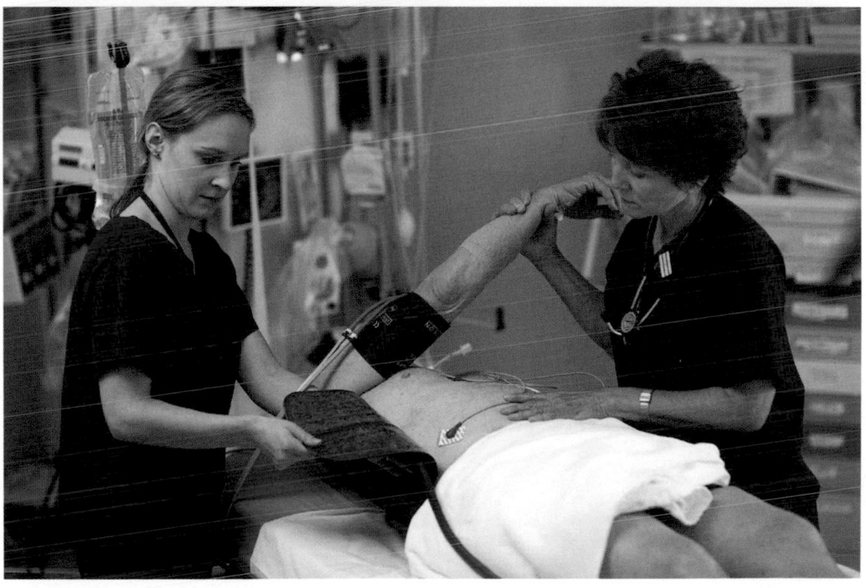

Fig. 24.2 Application of Arctic Sun device. (With permission from Medivance, Louisville, CO)

Two devices with recent US Food and Drug Administration (FDA) approval are the Celsius Control System (Innercool Therapies, San Diego, CA) and the Repreive System (Radiant Medical, Redwood, CA). The Coolguard (**Fig. 24.3**) (Alsius, Irvine, CA) intravascular catheter cooling system was also used in two recent single-center safety trials following SCI.[1,84] Newer models contain an internal temperature control system that eliminates the need for placement of rectal or bladder temperature probes.

■ Challenges in Human Trial Design

Human Trials

Non–Spinal Cord Injury Human Trials

Recent randomized trials analyzing hypothermia in traumatic brain injury (TBI) and intracranial aneurysm surgery have failed to show clear benefits of moderate hypothermia (e.g., the results were not statistically significant or the benefits were only observed in a particular subgroup).[85,86] A large, multicenter, randomized trial followed in 2001 did not show a benefit for moderate surface hypothermia following TBI (n = 392, 33°C, initiation 4 h after injury for 48 h).[42] The experimental arm also experienced an increased rate of hypotension. In another multicenter, randomized study examining the effects of hypothermia in the pediatric population following TBI (n = 225, 33°C, initiation 6.3 h after injury for 24 h), the experimental group had an increased mortality rate as well as an increase in hypotension.[87]

A third multicenter, randomized TBI trial was designed in response to lessons learned from the two prior studies: (1) treating patients within a shorter time window (e.g., mild hypothermia 35°C as soon as possible after injury followed by moderate 33°C within 4 h of injury for 48 h), as well as (2) stricter management of systemic problems with hypotension. To facilitate shortened time-to-treatment, patients could also be enrolled by emergency

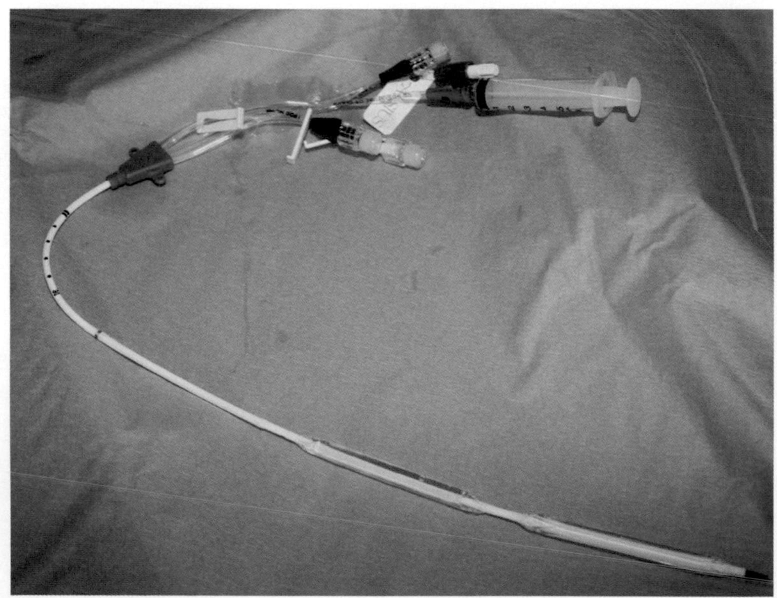

Fig. 24.3 The Coolguard catheter. (With permission from Alsius, Irvine, CA.)

medical services (EMS) in the field or in the emergency room. The trial was ultimately terminated in 2009 and did not confirm the utility of hypothermia as a neuroprotective strategy in TBI.[88] Another pediatric trial addressing many of the concerns of the prior pediatric TBI hypothermia study is also under way (ClinicalTrials.gov identifier NCT00222742).

The Cochrane Database review of TBI and hypothermia by Sydenham et al. noted 22 trials with a total of 1589 randomized patients. The authors cited fewer deaths in patients treated with hypothermia than in the control groups, as well as treated patients' being less likely to have an unfavorable outcome, yet both of these findings were not significant. Hypothermia was also associated with a slightly higher incidence of pneumonia. Their conclusion was that, currently, hypothermia in TBI should only be used in the context of a high-quality randomized, controlled trial.[89]

Spinal Cord Injury Human Trials

There has been a recent study published on the safety and feasibility of intravascular cooling for SCI. To date, however, no large, randomized, prospective trials exist examining the effects of systemic hypothermia following SCI. Levi et al. reported on a small series of 14 patients with American Spinal Injury Association (ASIA) A complete cervical cord injuries who underwent a protocol to achieve a modest 33°C temperature with good correlation between intravascular and intrathecal cerebrospinal fluid temperature via a closed-loop delivery system. Their average time between induction of hypothermia was 9.17 ± 2.24 h (mean ± standard error of mean); the time to target temperature was 2.72 ± 0.42 h; the duration of cooling at target was 47.6 ± 3.1 h; and the average total time of cooling was 93.6 ± 4 h.

This pilot study suggested that systemic intravascular cooling can be accomplished with minimal variations in temperature and few adverse events, and it may pave the way for larger multicenter SCI trials to test the efficacy of modest hypothermia in SCI.[84] Time course of total therapy in this study typically included 3 hours for induction and a 48 hour cooling period followed by one and a half days of rewarming. Further outcome measurements of these patients are to be published at a later date.[1] Using hypothermia as a neuroprotective strategy may add time to the hospital stay, however, and the authors recommended that it should only be used when neuroprotection is warranted and not in cases of cord transection, where the hope of any motor recovery is nil.

■ Conclusion

Widespread adoption of hypothermia protocols within hospitals and emergency settings for SCI will likely remain limited until a large, randomized human trial shows evidence supporting its use in SCI. To date there have been no large, multicenter, randomized, controlled clinical trials examining the benefits and side effects of modest hypothermia following SCI. Existing experimental and human studies have a wide range of variables, including (1) the method of cooling, (2) the time from injury until initiation of hypothermia, (3) the target temperature (e.g., moderate [28 to 32°C], modest [32 to 34°C], and mild [33 to 36°C]), and (4) the time spent at that target temperature. Other pitfalls encountered in human studies currently available include small patient numbers and lack of control populations. The cost to develop a study of this magnitude will also be significant, but great enthusiasm exists, given the potential impact of any neuroprotective therapy that improves neurological outcomes in humans.

Pearls

- Two methods of cooling available to humans include intravascular and external cooling. Recent technological advances in these devices have enabled clinicians to deliver consistent feedback-regulated therapy within shorter time-to-target windows.
- One pilot study on the effects of systemic intravascular cooling in humans suggested that it can be accomplished with minimal variations in temperature and few adverse events, and this study may pave the way for larger, multicenter SCI trials to test the efficacy of modest hypothermia in SCI.

Pitfalls

- Hypothermia is not a completely benign therapy. Its use has been associated with several complications, including bradycardia, increased risk of DVT, respiratory infection, lower leukocyte counts, hypotension, coagulopathy, altered drug pharmacokinetics, skin injury, and infectious complications of intravascular catheters.
- The majority of the literature examining the use of hypothermia as a neuroprotective agent in SCI in humans, although innovative for its time, lacks the appropriate sample numbers and control populations to demonstrate efficacy. There are also highly variable time intervals from the actual time of injury until the initiation of cooling.
- Widespread adoption of hypothermia protocols within hospitals and emergency settings for SCI will likely remain limited until a large, randomized human trial shows evidence supporting its use in SCI.

References

1. Levi AD, Casella G, Green BA, et al. Clinical outcomes using modest intravascular hypothermia after acute cervical spinal cord injury. Neurosurgery 2010;66(4):670–677
2. Bernard SA, Gray TW, Buist MD, et al. Treatment of comatose survivors of out-of-hospital cardiac arrest with induced hypothermia. N Engl J Med 2002;346(8):557–563
3. Clifton GL, Choi SC, Miller ER, et al. Intercenter variance in clinical trials of head trauma—experience of the National Acute Brain Injury Study: Hypothermia. J Neurosurg 2001;95(5):751–755
4. Conrad MF, Crawford RS, Davison JK, Cambria RP. Thoracoabdominal aneurysm repair: a 20-year perspective. Ann Thorac Surg 2007;83(2):S856–S861, discussion S890–S892
5. Fehrenbacher JW, Hart DW, Huddleston E, Siderys H, Rice C. Optimal end-organ protection for thoracic and thoracoabdominal aortic aneurysm repair using deep hypothermic circulatory arrest. Ann Thorac Surg 2007;83(3):1041–1046
6. Krieger DW, De Georgia MA, Abou-Chebl A, et al. Cooling for acute ischemic brain damage (cool aid): an open pilot study of induced hypothermia in acute ischemic stroke. Stroke 2001; 32(8):1847–1854
7. Steinberg GK, Ogilvy CS, Shuer LM, et al. Comparison of endovascular and surface cooling during unruptured cerebral aneurysm repair. Neurosurgery 2004;55(2):307–314, discussion 314–315
8. Hypothermia after Cardiac Arrest Study Group. Mild therapeutic hypothermia to improve the neurologic outcome after cardiac arrest. N Engl J Med 2002;346(8):549–556
9. Guest JD, Vanni S, Silbert L. Mild hypothermia, blood loss and complications in elective spinal surgery. Spine J 2004;4(2):130–137
10. Chen H, Chopp M, Welch KM. Effect of mild hyperthermia on the ischemic infarct volume after middle cerebral artery occlusion in the rat. Neurology 1991;41(7):1133–1135
11. Dietrich WD, Alonso O, Halley M, Busto R. Delayed posttraumatic brain hyperthermia worsens outcome after fluid percussion brain injury: a light and electron microscopic study in rats. Neurosurgery 1996;38(3):533–541, discussion 541
12. Yu CG, Jagid J, Ruenes G, Dietrich WD, Marcillo AE, Yezierski RP. Detrimental effects of systemic hyperthermia on locomotor function and histopathological outcome after traumatic spinal cord injury in the rat. Neurosurgery 2001;49(1):152–158, discussion 158–159
13. Lundgren J, Smith ML, Blennow G, Siesjö BK. Hyperthermia aggravates and hypothermia ameliorates epileptic brain damage. Exp Brain Res 1994;99(1):43–55
14. Kwon BK, Mann C, Sohn HM, et al; NASS Section on Biologics. Hypothermia for spinal cord injury. Spine J 2008;8(6):859–874
15. Fay T. Observations on prolonged human refrigeration. N Y State J Med 1945;4:1351–1354
16. Rosomoff HL, Holaday DA. Cerebral blood flow and cerebral oxygen consumption during hypothermia. Am J Physiol 1954;179(1):85–88
17. Fay T. Early experiences with local and generalized refrigeration of the human brain. J

Neurosurg 1959;16(3):239–259, discussion 259–260
18. Albin MS, White RJ, Acosta-Rua G, Yashon D. Study of functional recovery produced by delayed localized cooling after spinal cord injury in primates. J Neurosurg 1968;29(2):113–120
19. Albin MS, White RJ, Locke GE. Treatment of spinal cord trauma by selective hypothermic perfusion. Surg Forum 1965;16:423–424
20. Albin MS, White RJ, Locke GS, Massopust LC Jr, Kretchmer HE. Localized spinal cord hypothermia—anesthetic effects and application to spinal cord injury. Anesth Analg 1967;46(1):8–16
21. Wells JD, Hansebout RR. Local hypothermia in experimental spinal cord trauma. Surg Neurol 1978;10(3):200–204
22. Green BA, Khan T, Raimondi AJ. Local hypothermia as treatment of experimentally induced spinal cord contusion: quantitative analysis of beneficient effect. Surg Forum 1973;24:436–438
23. Black P, Markowitz RS. Experimental spinal cord injury in monkeys: comparison of steroids and local hypothermia. Surg Forum 1971;22:409–411
24. Howitt WM, Turnbull IM. Effects of hypothermia and methysergide on recovery from experimental paraplegia. Can J Surg 1972;15(3):179–186
25. Tator CH, Deecke L. Value of normothermic perfusion, hypothermic perfusion, and durotomy in the treatment of experimental acute spinal cord trauma. J Neurosurg 1973;39(1):52–64
26. Hansebout RR, Kuchner EF, Romero-Sierra C. Effects of local hypothermia and of steroids upon recovery from experimental spinal cord compression injury. Surg Neurol 1975;4(6):531–536
27. Kuchner EF, Hansebout RR. Combined steroid and hypothermia treatment of experimental spinal cord injury. Surg Neurol 1976;6(6):371–376
28. Tator CH, Deecke L. Studies of the treatment and pathophysiology of acute spinal cord injury in primates. Paraplegia 1973;10(4):344–345
29. Tator C. Spinal cord cooling and irrigation for treatment of acute cord injury. In: Press R, ed. Popp Neural Trauma. New York: Raven Press; 1979:363–370
30. Bricolo A, Ore GD, Da Pian R, Faccioli F. Local cooling in spinal cord injury. Surg Neurol 1976;6(2):101–106
31. Koons DD, Gildenberg PL, Dohn DF, Henoch M. Local hypothermia in the treatment of spinal cord injuries. Report of seven cases. Cleve Clin Q 1972;39(3):109–117
32. Demian YK, White RJ, Yashon D, Kretchmer HE. Anaesthesia for laminectomy and localized cord cooling in acute cervical spine injury. Report of three cases. Br J Anaesth 1971;43(10):973–979
33. Selker RG. Icewater irrigation of the spinal cord. Surg Forum 1971;22:411–413
34. Meacham WF, McPherson WF. Local hypothermia in the treatment of acute injuries of the spinal cord. South Med J 1973;66(1):95–97
35. Negrin J Jr. Spinal cord hypothermia. Neurosurgical management of immediate and delayed posttraumatic neurologic sequelae. N Y State J Med 1975;75(13):2387–2392
36. Hansebout RR, Tanner JA, Romero-Sierra C. Current status of spinal cord cooling in the treatment of acute spinal cord injury. Spine 1984;9(5):508–511
37. Inamasu J, Ichikizaki K. Mild hypothermia in neurologic emergency: an update. Ann Emerg Med 2002;40(2):220–230
38. Leslie K, Sessler DI, Bjorksten AR, Moayeri A. Mild hypothermia alters propofol pharmacokinetics and increases the duration of action of atracurium. Anesth Analg 1995;80(5):1007–1014
39. Simosa HF, Petersen DJ, Agarwal SK, Burke PA, Hirsch EF. Increased risk of deep venous thrombosis with endovascular cooling in patients with traumatic head injury. Am Surg 2007;73(5):461–464
40. Wu ET, Huang SC, Chi NH, et al. Idioventricular rhythm induced by therapeutic hypothermia. Resuscitation 2008;76(3):471–473
41. Jordan JD, Carhuapoma JR. Hypothermia: comparing technology. J Neurol Sci 2007;261(1-2):35–38
42. Clifton GL, Miller ER, Choi SC, et al. Lack of effect of induction of hypothermia after acute brain injury. N Engl J Med 2001;344(8):556–563
43. Ishikawa K, Tanaka H, Shiozaki T, et al. Characteristics of infection and leukocyte count in severely head-injured patients treated with mild hypothermia. J Trauma 2000;49(5):912–922
44. Valeri CR, Feingold H, Cassidy G, Ragno G, Khuri S, Altschule MD. Hypothermia-induced reversible platelet dysfunction. Ann Surg 1987;205(2):175–181
45. Rohrer MJ, Natale AM. Effect of hypothermia on the coagulation cascade. Crit Care Med 1992;20(10):1402–1405
46. Beilin B, Shavit Y, Razumovsky J, Wolloch Y, Zeidel A, Bessler H. Effects of mild perioperative hypothermia on cellular immune responses. Anesthesiology 1998;89(5):1133–1140
47. Cheng GJ, Morrow-Tesch JL, Beller DI, Levy EM, Black PH. Immunosuppression in mice induced by cold water stress. Brain Behav Immun 1990;4(4):278–291
48. Russwurm S, Stonāns I, Schwerter K, Stonāne E, Meissner W, Reinhart K. Direct influence of mild hypothermia on cytokine expression and release in cultures of human peripheral blood mononuclear cells. J Interferon Cytokine Res 2002;22(2):215–221
49. Todd MM, Hindman BJ, Clarke WR, Torner JC; Intraoperative Hypothermia for Aneurysm Surgery Trial (IHAST) Investigators. Mild intraoperative hypothermia during surgery for intracranial aneurysm. N Engl J Med 2005;352(2):135–145
50. Mahmood MA, Zweifler RM. Progress in shivering control. J Neurol Sci 2007;261(1-2):47–54
51. Inamasu J, Nakamura Y, Ichikizaki K. Induced hypothermia in experimental traumatic spinal cord injury: an update. J Neurol Sci 2003;209(1-2):55–60
52. Busto R, Globus MY, Dietrich WD, Martinez E, Valdes I, Ginsberg, MD. Effect of mild hypothermia on ischemia-induced release of neurotransmitters and free fatty acids in rat brain. Stroke 1989;20(7):904–910

53. Albin MS, White RJ, Yashon D, Harris LS. Effects of localized cooling on spinal cord trauma. J Trauma 1969;9(12):1000–1008
54. Tüzgen S, Kaynar MY, Güner A, Gümüştaş K, Belce A, Etuş V, et al. The effect of epidural cooling on lipid peroxidation after experimental spinal cord injury. Spinal Cord 1998;36(9):654–657
55. Kuchner EF, Hansebout RR, Pappius HM. Effects of dexamethasone and of local hypothermia on early and late tissue electrolyte changes in experimental spinal cord injury. J Spinal Disord 2000;13(5):391–398
56. Dimar JR II, Shields CB, Zhang YP, Burke DA, Raque GH, Glassman SD. The role of directly applied hypothermia in spinal cord injury. Spine 2000;25(18):2294–2302
57. Casas CE, Herrera LP, Prusmack C, Ruenes G, Marcillo A, Guest JD. Effects of epidural hypothermic saline infusion on locomotor outcome and tissue preservation after moderate thoracic spinal cord contusion in rats. J Neurosurg Spine 2005;2(3):308–318
58. Ha KY, Kim YH. Neuroprotective effect of moderate epidural hypothermia after spinal cord injury in rats. Spine 2008;33(19):2059–2065
59. Morochovic R, Chudá M, Talánová J, Cibur P, Kitka M, Vanický I. Local transcutaneous cooling of the spinal cord in the rat: effects on long-term outcomes after compression of spinal cord injury. Int J Neurosci 2008;118(4):555–568
60. Marsala M, Galik J, Ishikawa T, Yaksh TL. Technique of selective spinal cord cooling in rat: methodology and application. J Neurosci Methods 1997;74(1):97–106
61. Amar AP, Levy ML. Surgical controversies in the management of spinal cord injury. J Am Coll Surg 1999;188(5):550–566
62. Westergren H, Holtz A, Farooque M, Yu WR, Olsson Y. Systemic hypothermia after spinal cord compression injury in the rat: does recorded temperature in accessible organs reflect the intramedullary temperature in the spinal cord? J Neurotrauma 1998;15(11):943–954
63. Anderson DK, Hall ED. Pathophysiology of spinal cord trauma. Ann Emerg Med 1993;22(6): 987–992
64. Janssen L, Hansebout RR. Pathogenesis of spinal cord injury and newer treatments. A review. Spine 1989;14(1):23–32
65. Chatzipanteli K, Yanagawa Y, Marcillo AE, Kraydieh S, Yezierski RP, Dietrich WD. Posttraumatic hypothermia reduces polymorphonuclear leukocyte accumulation following spinal cord injury in rats. J Neurotrauma 2000;17(4):321–332
66. Westergren H, Yu WR, Farooque M, Holtz A, Olsson Y. Systemic hypothermia following spinal cord compression injury in the rat: axonal changes studied by beta-APP, ubiquitin, and PGP 9.5 immunohistochemistry. Spinal Cord 1999;37(10): 696–704
67. Yu WR, Westergren H, Farooque M, Holtz A, Olsson Y. Systemic hypothermia following spinal cord compression injury of rat spinal cord: reduction of plasma protein extravasation demonstrated by immunohistochemistry. Acta Neuropathol 1999;98(1):15–21
68. Yu WR, Westergren H, Farooque M, Holtz A, Olsson Y. Systemic hypothermia following compression injury of rat spinal cord: an immunohistochemical study on the expression of vimentin and GFAP. Neuropathology 1999;19:172–180
69. Yamamoto K, Ishikawa T, Sakabe T, Taguchi T, Kawai S, Marsala M. The hydroxyl radical scavenger Nicaraven inhibits glutamate release after spinal injury in rats. Neuroreport 1998;9(7): 1655–1659
70. Farooque M, Hillered L, Holtz A, Olsson Y. Effects of moderate hypothermia on extracellular lactic acid and amino acids after severe compression injury of rat spinal cord. J Neurotrauma 1997;14(1):63–69
71. Westergren H, Farooque M, Olsson Y, Holtz A. Motor function changes in the rat following severe spinal cord injury. Does treatment with moderate systemic hypothermia improve functional outcome? Acta Neurochir (Wien) 2000;142(5):567–573
72. Yu CG, Jimenez O, Marcillo AE, et al. Beneficial effects of modest systemic hypothermia on locomotor function and histopathological damage following contusion-induced spinal cord injury in rats. J Neurosurg 2000;93(1, Suppl):85–93
73. Jou IM. Effects of core body temperature on changes in spinal somatosensory-evoked potential in acute spinal cord compression injury: an experimental study in the rat. Spine 2000;25(15): 1878–1885
74. Westergren H, Farooque M, Olsson Y, Holtz A. Spinal cord blood flow changes following systemic hypothermia and spinal cord compression injury: an experimental study in the rat using Laser-Doppler flowmetry. Spinal Cord 2001;39(2):74–84
75. Shibuya S, Miyamoto O, Janjua NA, Itano T, Mori S, Norimatsu H. Post-traumatic moderate systemic hypothermia reduces TUNEL positive cells following spinal cord injury in rat. Spinal Cord 2004;42(1):29–34
76. Nishi H, Nakatsuka T, Takeda D, Miyazaki N, Sakanaka J, Yamada H, et al. Hypothermia suppresses excitatory synaptic transmission and neuronal death induced by experimental ischemia in spinal ventral horn neurons. Spine 2007;32(25): E741–E747
77. Duz B, Kaplan M, Bilgic S, Korkmaz A, Kahraman S. Does hypothermic treatment provide an advantage after spinal cord injury until surgery? An experimental study. Neurochem Res 2009;34(3):407–410
78. Lo TP Jr, Cho KS, Garg MS, et al. Systemic hypothermia improves histological and functional outcome after cervical spinal cord contusion in rats. J Comp Neurol 2009;514(5):433–448
79. Tarlov I. Spinal Cord Compression. Mechanisms of Paralysis and Treatment. Springfield, IL: Thomas CC; 1957
80. Kai Y, Owen JH, Allen BT, Dobras M, Davis C. Relationship between evoked potentials and clinical status in spinal cord ischemia. Spine 1994;19(10):1162–1167, discussion 1167–1168
81. El-Feky W, Baird R, Baldrige S, Bercen J. Establishing a mild hypothermia induction protocol for patients following cardiac arrest using conventional cooling blankets and the Arctic Sun 2000 cooling system. Neurocrit Care 2004;1(2):2

82. Holzer M, Müllner M, Sterz F, et al. Efficacy and safety of endovascular cooling after cardiac arrest: cohort study and Bayesian approach. Stroke 2006;37(7):1792–1797
83. Al-Senani FM, Graffagnino C, Grotta JC, et al. A prospective, multicenter pilot study to evaluate the feasibility and safety of using the CoolGard System and Icy catheter following cardiac arrest. Resuscitation 2004;62(2):143–150
84. Levi AD, Green BA, Wang MY, et al. Clinical application of modest hypothermia after spinal cord injury. J Neurotrauma 2009;26(3):407–415
85. Hindman BJ, Todd MM, Gelb AW, et al. Mild hypothermia as a protective therapy during intracranial aneurysm surgery: a randomized prospective pilot trial. Neurosurgery 1999;44(1):23–32, discussion 32–33
86. Marion DW, Penrod LE, Kelsey SF, et al. Treatment of traumatic brain injury with moderate hypothermia. N Engl J Med 1997;336(8):540–546
87. Hutchison JS, Ward RE, Lacroix J, et al; Hypothermia Pediatric Head Injury Trial Investigators and the Canadian Critical Care Trials Group. Hypothermia therapy after traumatic brain injury in children. N Engl J Med 2008;358(23):2447–2456
88. Clifton GL, Valadka A, Zygun D, Coffey CS, Drever P, Fourwinds S, et al. Very early hypothermia induction in patients with severe brain injury (the National Acute Brain Injury Study: Hypothermia II): a randomised trial. Lancet Neurol 2011;10(2):131–139
89. Sydenham E, Roberts I, Alderson P. Hypothermia for traumatic head injury. Cochrane Database Syst Rev 2009;(2):CD001048

25

Management of Cervical Facet Dislocation

Ishaq Y. Syed and Joon Y. Lee

Key Points

1. High index of suspicion, strict cervical spine precautions, and complete clinical and radiographic evaluation are vital in patients presenting after trauma.
2. High-resolution multidetector CT scan is the study of choice in initial evaluation for cervical spine injury.
3. Timing of obtaining an MRI scan in patients with cervical facet dislocation is multifactorial and controversial.
4. Surgical technique is dependent on fracture stability, neurological status, presence of disk herniation, and whether a closed reduction is possible.

Approximately 15,000 patients sustain spinal cord injury in the United States and Canada per year.[1] Up to half of these injuries can be associated with neurological deficits, with initial mortality approaching 10%.[2] Management of patients with cervical spine injury is a complex interdisciplinary process that requires efficient and accurate assessment and initiation of care.

Cervical facet dislocations result from flexion-distraction forces with or without a rotational component acting on the subaxial cervical spine. Flexion may result from a force onto the occiput or from a deceleration mechanism associated with a motor vehicle collision. The flexion moment occurs around the center of rotation thought to be anterior to the vertebral body, resulting in progressive tension failure. This injury pattern is thought to be a continuum of pathology, with sequential disruption of various osseous and ligamentous structures. Imaging studies reveal that both unilateral and bilateral facet dislocations result from disruption of the posterior musculature, interspinous ligament, supraspinous ligament, facet capsule, ligamentum flavum, and annulus. Bilateral facet dislocations are associated with a statistically significant increase in disruption of both anterior and posterior longitudinal ligaments compared with unilateral facet dislocation.[3] Disruption of the annulus raises the potential for extrusion of nucleus pulposus into the spinal canal and may have important implications in the patient management strategy.[4]

Based on the spectrum of severity, Allen et al. classified these injuries into four stages: (1) facet subluxation, (2) unilateral facet dislocation with 25% displacement, (3) bilateral facet dislocation with 50% displacement, and (4) complete dislocation.[5] Patients with unilateral facet dislocations often have either an intact neurological exam or a nerve root injury, whereas bilateral facet dislocations more commonly result in neurological deficit.

Among spine surgeons, much controversy surrounds appropriate management of cervical spine dislocations. Traditionally, rapid realignment of the spine through closed traction reduction followed by posterior spinal fixation has been recommended. Others have recommended obtaining an initial magnetic resonance imaging (MRI) scan followed by treatment decisions based on findings of this study. This chapter reviews recent evidence-based literature surrounding various controversies in the evaluation and management of cervical facet dislocations to help guide treatment recommendations.

Evaluation

History and Physical Exam

Missed cervical spine injury on initial evaluation has the potential to lead to catastrophic, permanent disability. Therefore, a careful clinical and radiographic evaluation is essential. All trauma patients should be treated as potentially having a cervical spine injury and be initially immobilized in a hard cervical collar. Management of all patients with suspected cervical spine injury should begin with primary survey and resuscitation as outlined by the Advanced Trauma Life Support protocol. Care must be taken to maintain cervical spine precautions throughout the trauma evaluation until appropriate cervical spine clearance can be obtained. Once the patient has been physiologically stabilized, a thorough spine and neurological assessment can be conducted as part of the secondary survey. A well-done history is vital in helping elucidate the mechanism of injury and may help direct evaluation for other concomitant injuries and provide insight on how forces were imparted on the cervical spine. In addition to documenting details of the actual trauma, it is important to inquire regarding associated conditions and comorbidities that may be relevant in a patient suspected of having cervical spine injury (e.g., ankylosing spondylitis).

The patient should be logrolled and each individual spinous process should be inspected and palpated to detect posterior midline tenderness and to detect step-off. While the patient is in a logrolled position, a rectal examination can assess for presence or loss of tone. The patient should be inspected for rotational or angular deformity that may point to a unilateral facet dislocation. A complete motor, sensory, and reflex examination should be done and should be clearly documented prior to the initiation of any treatment. A more detailed review of evaluating patients with spinal cord injury is presented in Chapter 2. Controversy about pharmacological treatment of patients with spinal cord injury, including methylprednisolone, is discussed in Chapter 10.

Screening Radiographic Studies

Despite efforts to standardize radiographic evaluation in patients with suspected cervical spine injury, protocols remain highly debated and variable across institutions. Two large, prospective, multicenter studies have attempted to clarify the criteria for obtaining radiographs in patients presenting with possible cervical spine injury.[6,7] These studies have become the cornerstone for emergency room trauma spine evaluation and been incorporated into triage trauma protocols at many institutions to determine the need for cervical spine screening imaging. Specific guidelines exist for clearance of cervical spine injuries in patients who are awake, alert, and without distracting injury or evidence of intoxication.[7]

No consensus, however, exists on evaluation of obtunded or unreliable patients with suspected cervical spine injury. This can often lead to prolonged use of rigid cervical collars until patients can safely be imaged or they regain the capacity to participate in an appropriate clinical examination. Prolonged rigid cervical collar can have significant associated morbidity, including compromised airway management, skin ulceration, limited central venous access, increased intracranial pressure, pneumonia, and deep venous thrombosis.[8,9] The lack of consensus has led trauma centers to develop individualized algorithms for clearing cervical spines in obtunded patients. The imaging studies most commonly used include plain radiographs, dynamic radiographs, dynamic fluoroscopy, computed tomography (CT), and MRI.

In the past 15 years, helical CT has replaced traditional cervical spine radiography at most large US trauma centers.[10] An updated consensus document published by the Eastern Association for the Surgery of Trauma in 2009 reported that plain radiography has been supplanted by CT as the primary screening modality in patients requiring imaging of suspected cervical spine injury.[11] The helical CT scan is especially useful for closer examination of suspicious or poorly visualized areas in the upper cervical spine or cervical thoracic junction. These images can also be reformatted into two- and three-dimensional reconstructions to assist the spine surgeon in evaluating complex injuries and in preoperative planning. Studies also show that helical CT scan of the cervical spine requires half the time of obtaining the standard six views of the cervical spine.[12] If the rate of missed fracture is incorporated into the analysis, helical CT has been shown to be more cost-effective in the long run. Widder et al. performed a prospective study comparing plain radiographs and CT scans in detecting cervical spine injuries in obtunded patients and found the sensitivity, specificity, and accuracy of plain radiographs to be 39%, 98%, and 88%, while CT scans had a sensitivity of 100%.[13] McCulloch and colleagues prospectively analyzed over 400 consecutive trauma patients and found plain radiographs to have a sensitivity of only 52% in detecting cervical spine fractures, compared with 98% for CT scans.[14] There has been a recent trend in high-risk level 1 trauma patients toward using helical CT scans alone as a primary screening tool.[15] Some potential pitfalls exist in exclusive use of helical CT. One caveat is that standard lower-resolution multislice helical CT may miss subtle spinal fractures, and not all institutions are equipped with a higher-resolution CT scanner. The downside to high-resolution multidetector CT scans is that they expose the patient to higher levels of radiation than a standard CT scan. No current studies compare sensitivity and specificity of various types of CT scanners in detecting cervical spine injuries. **Figure 25.1** displays an example of a sagittal CT scan obtained in a blunt trauma patient presenting with a cervical facet dislocation.

MRI offers a method of assessing soft tissues and often complements the bony detail provided by CT scans with enhanced depiction of soft-tissue pathology. The use of MRI to identify potential cervical spine trauma missed by CT scan remains controversial. Tomycz and colleagues performed a retrospective analysis of 690 obtunded trauma patients who had undergone both cervical CT and MRI.[16] Of the 180 patients (26.2%) with normal CT scans, MRI detected acute traumatic injury in 38 (21.1%). None of the injuries identified by MRI, however, was unstable or required additional surgical intervention. On the contrary, Menaker et al.[17] performed a similar analysis of 734 obtunded trauma patients and found a change in management of 7.9% of patients with additional findings on MRI.

The incidence of vertebral artery injury in patients with major blunt cervical spine trauma is estimated to be between 24 and 46%.[18] Most vertebral artery injuries are asymptomatic due to ample collateral circulation, and it is important to determine which patients should be screened for clinically significant injuries. Insufficient evidence currently exists to support standards or guidelines for either the diagnosis or treatment of these injuries.[19] Screening of all cervical spine injuries is not generally recommended because these imaging stud-

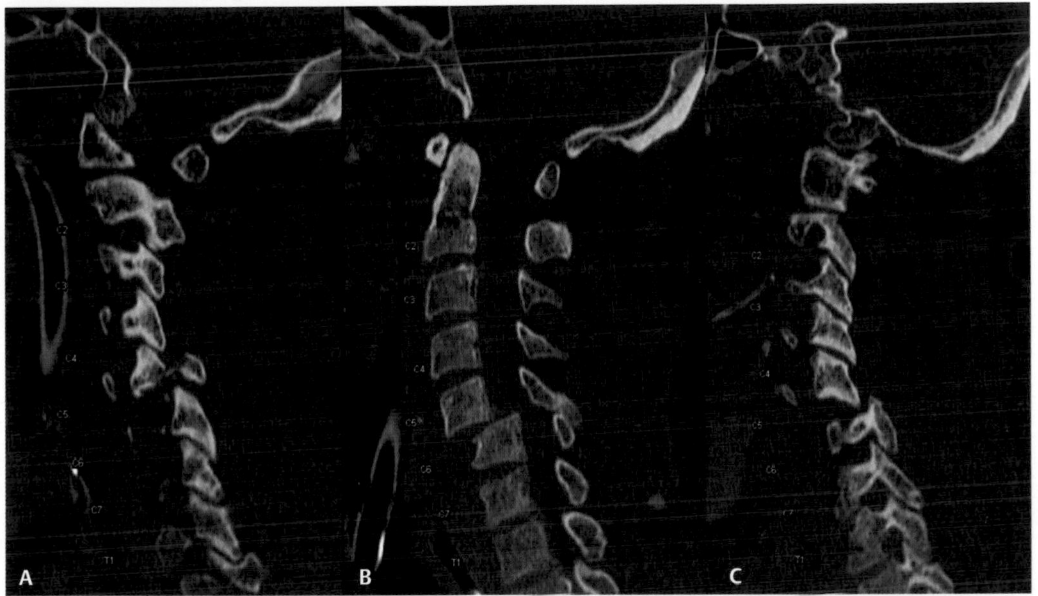

Fig. 25.1 Sagittal computed tomography scan revealing bilateral facet fracture dislocation at the C5-6 level. **(A)** Scan demonstrating the left facet fracture dislocation. **(B)** Midline of the scan demonstrating greater than 50% anterior translation of C5 on C6 consistent with bilateral facet dislocation. **(C)** Scan demonstrating the right facet dislocation.

ies can be associated with complications of their own as well as added financial and technical resource use with no clear clinical benefit. Most spine surgeons advocate obtaining vascular imaging studies when the patient's neurological findings are suggestive of vascular etiology. Others recommend screening patients with high-risk injury patterns, such as fractures through the foramen transversarium, vertebral dislocations, and upper cervical spine injuries.[20] Patients with evidence of posterior ischemia can be managed with either anticoagulation or observation, whereas observation alone is recommended in those with no evidence of posterior circulation compromise.

When to Obtain a Magnetic Resonance Imaging Scan

The next step in patients presenting with cervical facet dislocation is to quickly and safely realign the spine. Cervical facet dislocations are often associated with soft-tissue injury, including the presence of possible disk herniation. The presence of a disk herniation does not necessarily result in neurological deficit. Eismont et al.[4] and Vaccaro et al.[21] define a disk herniation as potentially dangerous when the disk protrudes behind the cephalad vertebral body (**Fig. 25.2**). Whether an MRI scan is necessary prior to reduction has been a topic of debate since the early 1990s. Some advocate that all patients with bilateral facet dislocation undergo MRI evaluation prior to attempted reduction, due to the fear of neurological deterioration secondary to further posterior disk migration into the canal with a reduction maneuver. Eismont et al. highlighted the danger of closed reduction in a case series of six patients in 1991 with associated cervical disk herniation and facet dislocation or subluxation.[4] One of the patients in the series sustained neurological deterioration after reduction was performed under general anesthesia. Other small retrospective case series have recommended MRI prior to reduction secondary to potential neurological deficit as a result of disk herniation during closed reduction.[22–24]

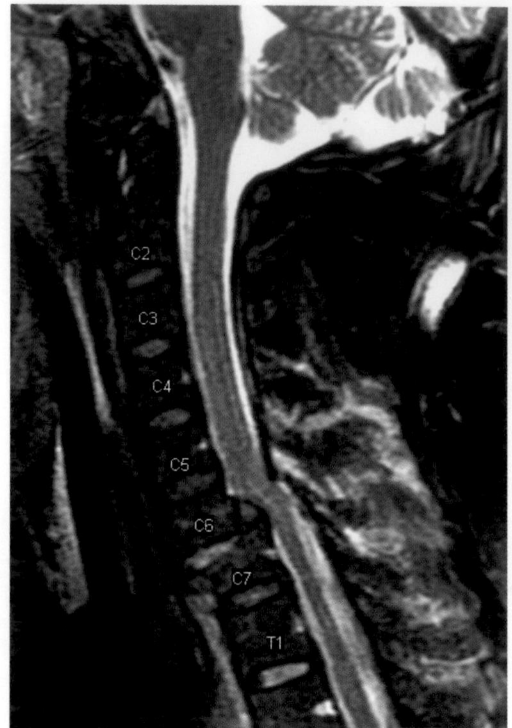

Fig. 25.2 Prereduction sagittal T2-weighted magnetic resonance imaging demonstrating an associated disk herniation behind the body of C6 in a patient with bilateral facet dislocation. An anterior C6-7 diskectomy was performed prior to intraoperative open reduction.

Several subsequent studies, including a prospective clinical trial by Vaccaro et al., suggest that closed reduction in an awake, alert, cooperative patient can be performed safely without a prereduction MRI scan.[21] Eleven patients with cervical spine dislocations were prospectively evaluated with pre- and postreduction MRI. Two patients were noted to have a disk herniation prior to reduction. Closed reduction was attempted in all 11 patients, nine of which were successful. Five disk herniations were found postreduction, none had worsening neurological exams postreduction. Though disk herniations may be increased, the investigators concluded that closed reduction could be safely performed in awake, cooperative patients. Similarly, Cotler and colleagues reviewed a series of 24 neurologically normal patients awake and able to cooperate with an exam. All patients were successfully reduced with increasing traction weight without neurological deterioration. A recent study by Darsaut et al. presented 17 patients with cervical fracture-dislocations treated with closed reduced with in-line axial traction under MRI guidance.[25] All patients tolerated traction without neurological worsening; interestingly, the investigators illustrated with a sequential MRI-aided reduction technique that a herniated disk could reconstitute itself into its respective disk space. A survey analysis of the Spine Trauma Study Group (STSG) resulted in highly variable opinions and no consensus on timing or utilization of MRI in cervical facet dislocations.[26] There are also no radiological studies to date that explore differentiating disk material from hematoma or that delineate how large a disk herniation must be to cause cord impingement. Surgeon interpretation of a significant anterior lesion is highly subjective, with no clear literature to guide treatment.

In the case of an obtunded patient who cannot cooperate with a clinical exam, a prereduction MRI is recommended to gain better understanding of the status of the spinal cord and to delineate any potential soft-tissue or bony structure that may place the spinal cord at risk during reduction. Patients who present with complete or near complete neurological deficit should undergo immediate closed reduction, given that the patient has little to lose and the greatest possibility of neurological functional recovery.[27] **Figure 25.3** summarizes a general algorithm on how to approach imaging of cervical facet dislocation, along with some of the supporting literature.

Reduction and Realignment

Reduction and realignment of cervical facet dislocation can either be done with a closed or open technique. If the patient is examinable and a prereduction MRI scan does not show a significant anterior space–occupying lesion, a closed reduction may be considered safe. Without a clear defini-

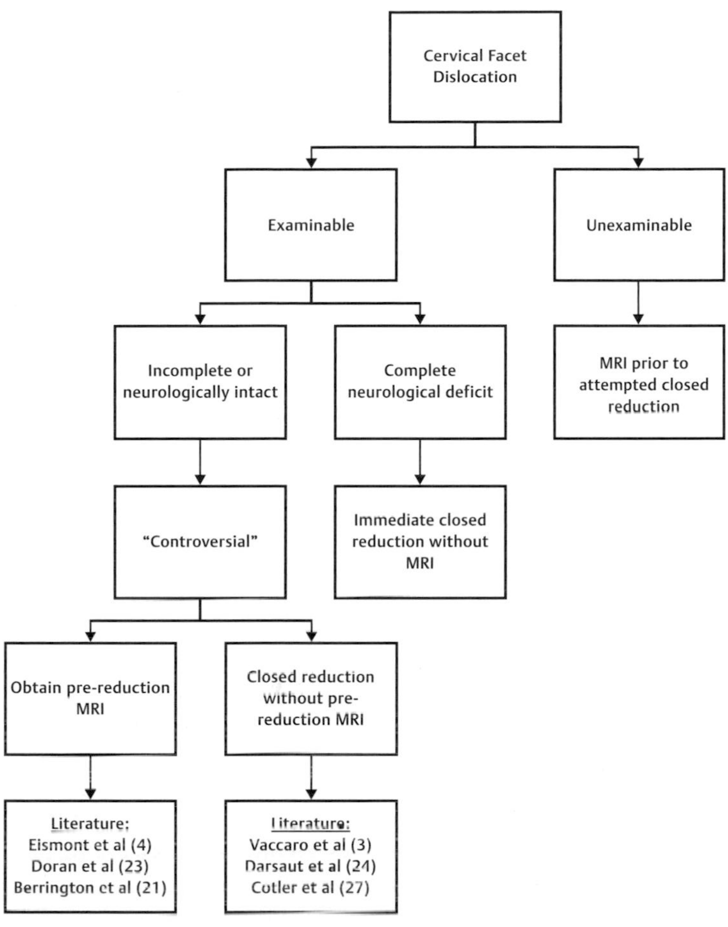

Fig. 25.3 General algorithm for evaluation of cervical facet dislocation.

tion of what constitutes a dangerous disk fragment, whether a closed reduction is safe can be debatable. Several articles present level IV evidence that closed reduction in an awake, alert patient can be performed relatively safely.[21,28,29] Conversely, no consensus exists on the safety of such a maneuver in obtunded, unexaminable patients. Most would agree that a closed reduction should not be attempted in obtunded unexaminable patients in most circumstances. An open reduction with or without decompression can be considered in patients having undergone a failed attempted closed reduction after an MRI scan is obtained or when a dangerous herniated disk is present on prereduction MRI. When an open reduction is deemed necessary, a preoperative MRI should be obtained to assess the status of the disk and would help dictate surgical approach.

Attempted closed reduction remains the most common initial treatment strategy. Timing appears to be important in overall success of obtaining a reduction and potential neurological recovery. Successful closed reduction accomplished within 8 hours of injury has been shown to lead to greater neurological improvement.[30] The goal of closed reduction is to restore the overall normal alignment of the spine and to decompress the neural elements. Walton first described closed manipulation of the cervical spine in 1893. In 1933, Crutchfield described using skull tongs with inline traction. Gardner modified the tong design in 1973 to include a spring-loaded tensioning component and it is still in use today.

Spinal reduction and immobilization can be accomplished by using either Gardner-Wells skull tongs or a halo ring. The details of halo application and closed reduction are outlined in Chapter 11. Many authors advocate starting with ~10 lb to account for the weight of the head and sequentially adding increments of 10 lb every 10 to 15 minutes up to 5 to 10 lb per level of injury. The literature is unclear as to what constitutes a safe weight limit to achieve a closed reduction[31]; however, safe closed reductions have been reported using weight up to 140 lb.[28] Neurological examination should be followed and documented closely, along with serial radiographs to confirm when closed reduction has been accomplished and to avoid overdistraction. Gentle neck flexion and rotation may be necessary to disengage locked facets. Once closed reduction is accomplished, all but 10 to 15 lb of traction is removed for continued immobilization. Closed reduction should be immediately discontinued and reversed if neurological deterioration is observed, overdistraction without reduction is seen on radiography, or the patient becomes clinically intolerant of the procedure.[32]

A failed attempt at closed reduction typically necessitates open reduction. If MRI has not already been obtained, most would acquire an MRI scan prior to an open reduction and definitive surgical management. Information interpreted from the MRI scan often influences the chosen surgical management.

■ Surgical Approach and Fixation

Nonoperative management of cervical facet dislocation with cervical orthosis or halo brace treatment has been shown to result in poorer outcome than with surgical intervention, with ~30% of patients treated conservatively presenting with late deformities, persistent pain, instability, and loss of reduction.[33,34] Open reduction of facet injury is indicated if closed reduction fails or in the presence of neurological worsening. The choice of surgical approach, fixation, and type of graft remains controversial. The options for surgical approach include anterior approach alone, posterior approach alone, a combined anterior and posterior approach, or a staged anterior/posterior/anterior approach. The chosen approach is dependent on several factors: (1) stability of the fracture/dislocation, (2) neurological status, (3) presence of a disk herniation, and (4) whether the dislocation is reducible either closed or through an anterior approach. Often the divergence of opinion stems from interpretation of the MRI scan that is used to assess these factors. A survey analysis of the STSG showed extreme variations in choice of approach for unilateral or bilateral facet fracture dislocations, with the kappa value of less than 0.1.[35] Neurologically intact patients were more commonly treated with an anterior approach; a combined approach was chosen more often in bilateral facet injuries.

The anterior approach has the advantage of giving direct access to potential disk pathology and the ability to perform a direct decompression. Open reduction performed from an anterior approach can, however, be more technically demanding. Reduction can be performed with a distractor placed within the disk space or with distraction pins inserted into the vertebral bodies.[36,37] With sufficient distraction, the anteriorly displaced vertebral body can then be levered back into position. Stabilization involves performing a diskectomy, placement of a structural graft, and plate fixation. Reindl and colleagues demonstrated that the anterior approach with tricortical iliac crest autograft and plate fixation can result in successful reduction, stabilization, and fusion.[38] A recent study by Woodworth et al. reviewed isolated anterior stabilization of unstable posterior subaxial cervical spine fractures with structural allograft and plate fixation that resulted in low intraoperative blood loss, short operating times, brief length of stay, excellent segmental stability, and high fusion rate.[39] The authors did exclude patients who had concomitant anterior vertebral fractures. Johnson et al. reported radiographic failure with loss of fixation in 13% of patients treated anteriorly in the presence of end plate compression fracture and facet fractures. They suggest that patients with these associated injuries be treated with posterior instrumentation and fusion.[40] Brodke and colleagues conducted a prospective randomized study comparing an anterior and posterior approach after successful closed reduction had been achieved. They found no statistically significant difference in the two groups in regard to neurological outcomes, fusion rates, alignment, or long-term complaints of pain.[41]

The advantage of the posterior approach is that it allows direct access and ease of reduction. Open posterior reduction can be achieved by applying distractive forces across the spinous processes or the lamina by using a modified laminar spreader.[42] It may be necessary to burr away part of the superior facet to help disengage the locked facets. Definitive stabilization can be achieved with segmental posterior instrumentation with arthrodesis. Several retrospective studies of posterior techniques have reported successful stabilization and fusion in treatment of unstable cervical spine injuries.[43,44] New cervical polyaxial screw and rod systems appear to be safe and reliable and have the advantage of multiplanar rod contouring and offset attachments with successful posterior cervical arthrodesis without significant complications.[45,46] In addition, lateral mass screw placement is more precise without being constrained by screw hole spacing of the plate. The screw–rod system can more easily be extended across the occiput and cervicothoracic junction. It also permits the selective application of compression, distraction, and reduction forces within the construct greater than plate systems.[47]

Combined approaches in most instances are utilized in patients who require an anterior approach to address a disk herniation and have failed both closed reduction as well as attempted open reduction from the anterior approach (**Fig. 25.4**). This necessitates a subsequent posterior reduction and stabilization. A second anterior approach may then be utilized to place a bone graft anteriorly, or an undersized graft can be used on the first approach with a buttress plate to prevent the graft from dislodging during posterior reduction. Circumferential fusion can also be utilized when there is concern about fracture stability due to fracture comminution or presence of significant ligamentous disruption (i.e., bilateral facet fracture-dislocation), or when fixation via one approach is judged to be marginal. **Figure 25.5** outlines a proposed general treatment algorithm.

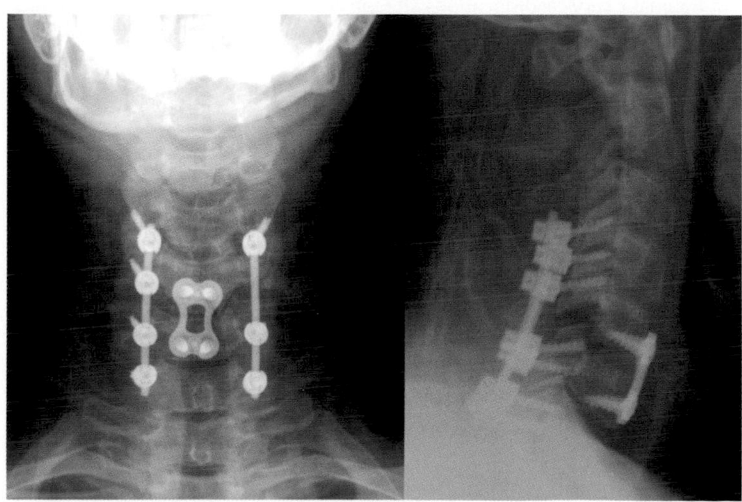

Fig. 25.4 Postoperative anteroposterior and lateral radiographs of a patient with bilateral facet fracture dislocation and associated disk herniation who underwent a combined anterior/posterior circumferential fusion.

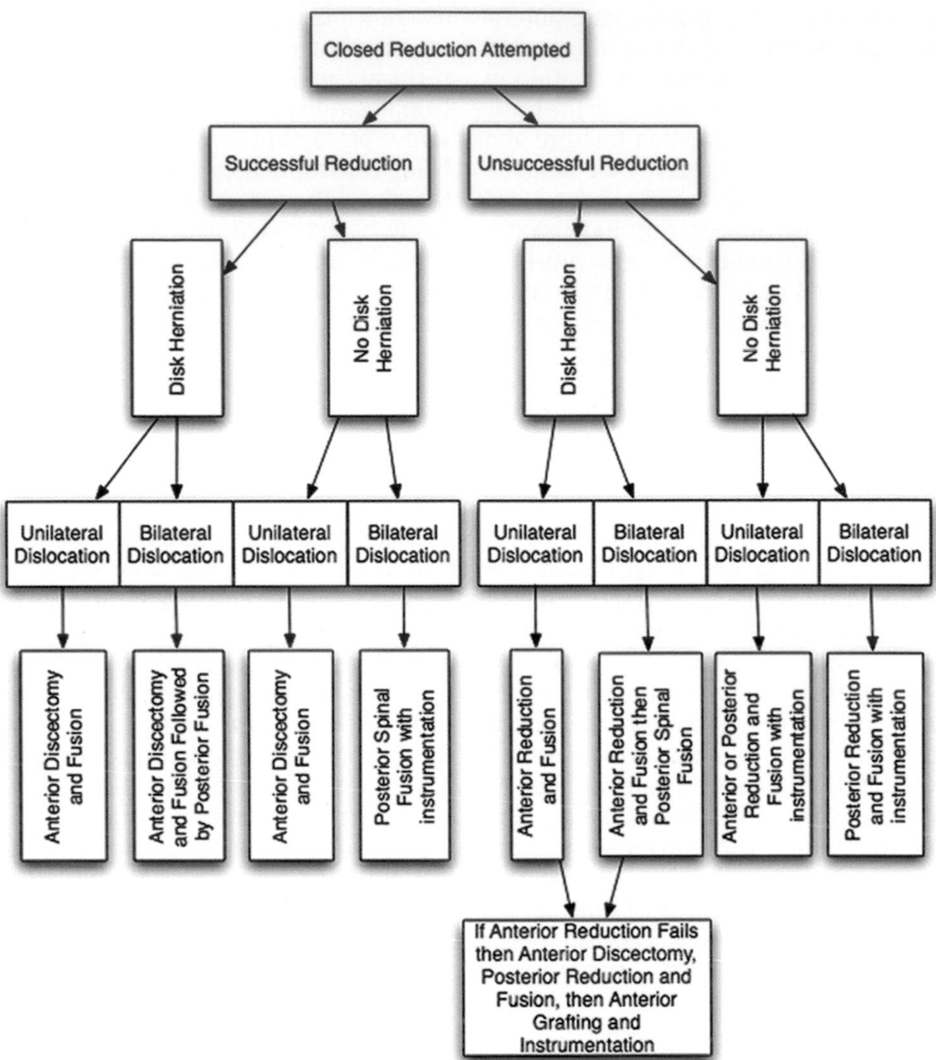

Fig. 25.5 Treatment algorithm for traumatic cervical dislocations after an attempted closed reduction. (Reproduced from Nassr A, Lee JY, Dvorak MF, et al. Variations in surgical treatment of cervical facet dislocations. Spine 2008;33(7):E188–E193.)

■ Conclusion

The current literature provides little in the way of level I evidence to help guide the treating surgeon on the management of cervical facet dislocations. Careful clinical and radiographic evaluation is necessary to avoid catastrophic neurological consequences. High-resolution multidetector CT scans appear to have supplanted plain radiographs as the screening modality for cervical spine injuries. In general, patients are recommended to have an MRI scan prior to reduction if a neurological examination cannot be obtained. Closed reduction without an MRI scan appears to be safe in an alert, cooperative, and examinable patient. Definitive treatment is often dictated by the interpretation of available imaging, detection of specific pathology (such as disk herniation), neurological status, and stability of the injury pattern. Either an anterior or a posterior approach appears to be efficacious in the treatment of cervical facet dislocations as long as the spine is appropriately reduced and stabilized. Posterior stabilization or a combined approach appears to be favored in the presence of a facet fracture, endplate fracture, or vertebral comminution. Many of the current treatment algorithms are at the discretion of the treating physician due to the lack of evidence-based research.

Pearls

- When patients meet the criteria to warrant radiographic screening for suspected cervical spine injury, high-resolution multidetector CT scans appear to be efficient, accurate, and cost-effective.
- An examinable patient who has complete neurological deficit should undergo immediate closed reduction without MRI. Obtunded, unexaminable patients should have an MRI scan prior to attempted closed reduction to evaluate for the presence of a disk herniation. The need for a prereduction MRI continues to be a topic of debate in examinable incomplete or neurologically intact patients.
- Surgical approach and fixation are dependent on fracture stability, neurological status, the presence of disk herniation, and whether a closed reduction is possible. Both anterior and posterior approaches can result in good clinical and radiographic outcomes in an appropriately chosen fracture pattern.

Pitfalls

- A high index of suspicion and strict cervical spine precautions throughout the trauma evaluation are necessary until complete clinical and radiographic evaluation to avoid catastrophic iatrogenic neurological injury.
- The goal in treating cervical facet dislocations is to quickly and safely realign the spine. Closed reduction should be immediately discontinued and reversed if neurological deterioration is observed, overdistraction without reduction is seen on radiography, or the patient becomes clinically intolerant of the procedure.
- Unstable, comminuted fractures with severe ligamentous disruption should likely undergo circumferential arthrodesis. Patients should be followed carefully postoperatively with serial radiographs to monitor fracture healing and should be observed for development of secondary deformity.

References

1. Sekhon LH, Fehlings MG. Epidemiology, demographics, and pathophysiology of acute spinal cord injury. Spine 2001;26(24, Suppl):S2–S12
2. Hills MW, Deane SA. Head injury and facial injury: is there an increased risk of cervical spine injury? J Trauma 1993;34(4):549–553, discussion 553–554
3. Vaccaro AR, Madigan L, Schweitzer ME, Flanders AE, Hilibrand AS, Albert TJ. Magnetic resonance imaging analysis of soft tissue disruption after flexion-distraction injuries of the subaxial cervical spine. Spine 2001;26(17):1866–1872
4. Eismont FJ, Arena MJ, Green BA. Extrusion of an intervertebral disc associated with traumatic subluxation or dislocation of cervical facets. Case report. J Bone Joint Surg Am 1991;73(10): 1555–1560
5. Allen BL Jr, Ferguson RL, Lehmann TR, O'Brien RP. A mechanistic classification of closed, indirect fractures and dislocations of the lower cervical spine. Spine 1982;7(1):1–27
6. Stiell IG, Wells GA, Vandemheen KL, et al. The Canadian C-spine rule for radiography in alert and stable trauma patients. JAMA 2001;286(15): 1841–1848
7. Hoffman JR, Mower WR, Wolfson AB, Todd KH, Zucker MI; National Emergency X-Radiography Utilization Study Group. Validity of a set of clinical criteria to rule out injury to the cervical spine in patients with blunt trauma. N Engl J Med 2000;343(2):94–99
8. Davies G, Deakin C, Wilson A. The effect of a rigid collar on intracranial pressure. Injury 1996;27(9): 647–649
9. Richards PJ. Cervical spine clearance: a review. Injury 2005;36(2):248–269, discussion 270
10. Berne JD, Velmahos GC, El-Tawil Q, et al. Value of complete cervical helical computed tomographic scanning in identifying cervical spine injury in the unevaluable blunt trauma patient with mul-

tiple injuries: a prospective study. J Trauma 1999;47(5):896–902, discussion 902–903

11. Como JJ, Diaz JJ, Dunham CM, et al. Practice management guidelines for identification of cervical spine injuries following trauma: update from the Eastern Association for the Surgery of Trauma Practice Management Guidelines Committee. J Trauma 2009;67(3):651–659
12. Daffner RH. Helical CT of the cervical spine for trauma patients: a time study. AJR Am J Roentgenol 2001;177(3):677–679
13. Widder S, Doig C, Burrowes P, Larsen G, Hurlbert RJ, Kortbeek JB. Prospective evaluation of computed tomographic scanning for the spinal clearance of obtunded trauma patients: preliminary results. J Trauma 2004;56(6):1179–1184
14. McCulloch PT, France J, Jones DL, et al. Helical computed tomography alone compared with plain radiographs with adjunct computed tomography to evaluate the cervical spine after high-energy trauma. J Bone Joint Surg Am 2005;87(11): 2388–2394
15. Barba CA, Taggert J, Morgan AS, et al. A new cervical spine clearance protocol using computed tomography. J Trauma 2001;51(4):652–656, discussion 656–657
16. Tomycz ND, Chew BG, Chang YF, et al. MRI is unnecessary to clear the cervical spine in obtunded/comatose trauma patients: the four-year experience of a level I trauma center. J Trauma 2008;64(5):1258–1263
17. Menaker J, Philip A, Boswell S, Scalea TM. Computed tomography alone for cervical spine clearance in the unreliable patient—are we there yet? J Trauma Acute Care Surg 2008;64(4):898–904
18. Fassett DR, Dailey AT, Vaccaro AR. Vertebral artery injuries associated with cervical spine injuries: a review of the literature. J Spinal Disord Tech 2008;21(4):252–258
19. Management of vertebral artery injuries after nonpenetrating cervical trauma. Neurosurgery 2002;50(3, Suppl):S173–S178 PubMed
20. Cothren CC, Moore EE, Ray CE Jr, Johnson JL, Moore JB, Burch JM. Cervical spine fracture patterns mandating screening to rule out blunt cerebrovascular injury. Surgery 2007;141(1):76–82
21. Vaccaro AR, Falatyn SP, Flanders AE, Balderston RA, Northrup BE, Cotler JM. Magnetic resonance evaluation of the intervertebral disc, spinal ligaments, and spinal cord before and after closed traction reduction of cervical spine dislocations. Spine 1999;24(12):1210–1217
22. Berrington NR, van Staden JF, Willers JG, van der Westhuizen J. Cervical intervertebral disc prolapse associated with traumatic facet dislocations. Surg Neurol 1993;40(5):395–399
23. Burke DC, Berryman D. The place of closed manipulation in the management of flexion-rotation dislocations of the cervical spine. J Bone Joint Surg Br 1971;53(2):165–182
24. Doran SE, Papadopoulos SM, Ducker TB, Lillehei KO. Magnetic resonance imaging documentation of coexistent traumatic locked facets of the cervical spine and disc herniation. J Neurosurg 1993;79(3):341–345
25. Darsaut TE, Ashforth R, Bhargava R, et al. A pilot study of magnetic resonance imaging-guided closed reduction of cervical spine fractures. Spine 2006;31(18):2085–2090
26. Grauer JN, Vaccaro AR, Lee JY, et al. The timing and influence of MRI on the management of patients with cervical facet dislocations remains highly variable: a survey of members of the Spine Trauma Study Group. J Spinal Disord Tech 2009; 22(2):96–99
27. Hart RA. Cervical facet dislocation: when is magnetic resonance imaging indicated? Spine 2002; 27(1):116–117
28. Cotler JM, Herbison GJ, Nasuti JF, Ditunno JF Jr, An H, Wolff BE. Closed reduction of traumatic cervical spine dislocation using traction weights up to 140 pounds. Spine 1993;18(3):386–390
29. Grant GA, Mirza SK, Chapman JR, et al. Risk of early closed reduction in cervical spine subluxation injuries. J Neurosurg 1999;90(1, Suppl): 13–18
30. Rizzolo SJ, Vaccaro AR, Cotler JM. Cervical spine trauma. Spine 1994;19(20):2288–2298 PubMed
31. Initial closed reduction of cervical spine fracture-dislocation injuries. Neurosurgery 2002;50(3, Suppl):S44–S50
32. Hadley MN, Walters BC, Grabb PA, et al. Guidelines for the management of acute cervical spine and spinal cord injuries. Clin Neurosurg 2002; 49:407–498
33. Koivikko MP, Myllynen P, Santavirta S. Fracture dislocations of the cervical spine: a review of 106 conservatively and operatively treated patients. Eur Spine J 2004;13(7):610–616
34. Hadley MN, Fitzpatrick BC, Sonntag VK, Browner CM. Facet fracture-dislocation injuries of the cervical spine. Neurosurgery 1992;30(5):661–666
35. Nassr A, Lee JY, Dvorak MF, et al. Variations in surgical treatment of cervical facet dislocations. Spine 2008;33(7):E188–E193
36. de Oliveira JC. Anterior reduction of interlocking facets in the lower cervical spine. Spine 1979; 4(3):195–202
37. Ordonez BJ, Benzel EC, Naderi S, Weller SJ. Cervical facet dislocation: techniques for ventral reduction and stabilization. J Neurosurg 2000;92(1, Suppl):18–23
38. Reindl R, Ouellet J, Harvey EJ, Berry G, Arlet V. Anterior reduction for cervical spine dislocation. Spine 2006;31(6):648–652
39. Woodworth RS, Molinari WJ, Brandenstein D, Gruhn W, Molinari RW. Anterior cervical discectomy and fusion with structural allograft and plates for the treatment of unstable posterior cervical spine injuries. J Neurosurg Spine 2009; 10(2):93–101
40. Johnson MG, Fisher CG, Boyd M, Pitzen T, Oxland TR, Dvorak MF. The radiographic failure of single segment anterior cervical plate fixation in traumatic cervical flexion distraction injuries. Spine 2004;29(24):2815–2820
41. Brodke DS, Anderson PA, Newell DW, Grady MS, Chapman JR. Comparison of anterior and posterior approaches in cervical spinal cord injuries. J Spinal Disord Tech 2003;16(3):229–235

42. Fazl M, Pirouzmand F. Intraoperative reduction of locked facets in the cervical spine by use of a modified interlaminar spreader: technical note. Neurosurgery 2001;48(2):444–445, discussion 445–446
43. Fehlings MG, Cooper PR, Errico TJ. Posterior plates in the management of cervical instability: long-term results in 44 patients. J Neurosurg 1994; 81(3):341–349
44. Anderson PA, Henley MB, Grady MS, Montesano PX, Winn HR. Posterior cervical arthrodesis with AO reconstruction plates and bone graft. Spine 1991;16(3, Suppl):S72–S79
45. Mummaneni PV, Haid RW, Traynelis VC, et al. Posterior cervical fixation using a new polyaxial screw and rod system: technique and surgical results. Neurosurg Focus 2002;12(1):E8
46. Hwang IC, Kang DH, Han JW, Park IS, Lee CH, Park SY. Clinical experiences and usefulness of cervical posterior stabilization with polyaxial screw-rod system. J Korean Neurosurg Soc 2007;42(4): 311–316
47. Deen HG, Birch BD, Wharen RE, Reimer R. Lateral mass screw-rod fixation of the cervical spine: a prospective clinical series with 1-year follow-up. Spine J 2003;3(6):489–495

26

Management of Acute Spinal Cord Injury in Thoracolumbar Burst Fractures Including Cauda Equina Syndrome

Marcel F. Dvorak and Brian Lenehan

Key Points

1. Careful examination of the lowest sacral segments is necessary to identify neurological injury and determine prognosis in thoracolumbar burst fractures with neurological injury.
2. Neurological recovery varies with the anatomical structure at the site of the fracture (spinal cord, conus medullaris, or cauda equina). It may also be influenced by timely stabilization and decompression.
3. Early posterior stabilization and realignment may be followed by anterior decompression at a later date (within the first 1 to 2 weeks following injury) if ongoing bony or soft tissue compression of neurological elements persists and is demonstrated on imaging.
4. Profound neurological injury may lead to "walking paraplegia," wherein the patient regains the ability to ambulate but is plagued by significant weakness and poor balance, as well as profound bladder, bowel, and sexual dysfunction.

The thoracolumbar region comprises the 11th and 12th thoracic, and first and second lumbar, vertebrae (T11 to L2). At these motion segments, the rigid thoracic kyphosis transitions into the mobile lumbar lordosis, making this region susceptible to traumatic injuries.[1–4] The patterns of injury to the spinal column include compressive injuries, such as burst fractures of the vertebral body, as well as distraction (Chance-type fractures) and translational/rotational injuries, such as fracture-dislocations.[5–7] There are also a variety of neurological structures that can be injured, including the lower portion of the thoracic spinal cord, the conus medullaris, and the cauda equina. This chapter describes the nature, evaluation, and management of compressive burst fractures that result in neurological injury to the distal spinal cord, conus medullaris, and cauda equina. The complexity of the neuroanatomy in this region influences the prognosis and should influence therapeutic decision making as well.

Neuroanatomy

The spinal cord terminates as the conus medullaris in a variable location relative to the vertebral segments.[8,9] Although there is no defined anatomical landmark that identifies the distal extent of the conus medullaris, its tip has a variable location between the T11–12 disk space and the L4 vertebra, with its most common location being the L1–2 disk space.

The conus medullaris morphologically represents a transition from the central to the peripheral nervous system.[10] At the T12–L1 disk space, the spinal cord tapers and the L1–5 nerve roots form a peripheral rim around the distal spinal cord. At the L1–2 disk space, the lumbar nerve roots are somatotopically oriented from lateral (L2) to medial (L5).[11–13] The lumbar sympathetic, sacral parasympathetic, and sacral somatic nerves originate within the conus medullaris and are carried within the nerve roots of the cauda equina. Although many of these lumbar roots descend over several vertebral segments within the thecal sac, the formal designation of the cauda equina begins below the termination of the conus medullaris.

One of the unique features of the thoracolumbar region is the disparity between the location of the spinal cord segment and the vertebrae; for example; the L5 vertebra is very distant from the segment of the spinal cord from which the L5 dorsal and ventral roots emanate.

The very practical impact of the variation in segmental location and variable neuroanatomy is that the description of a burst fracture resulting in a neurological injury at the L1 vertebral level tells us very little about the precise neurological structure that has been injured.

Demographics

Thoracolumbar burst fractures account for up to 17% of major spinal fractures, and males are at a fourfold greater risk than females. The incidence of neurological deficit resulting from thoracolumbar burst fractures is estimated to be 50 to 60%.[3,4,14]

Natural History of Conus and Cauda Injuries

Neurological recovery from injury to the conus medullaris or cauda equina is unpredictable. Variables that influence prognosis are thought to include age, comorbidities that influence vascularity (diabetes, etc.), magnitude of energy absorbed, secondary injuries, and possibly the timing of neural decompression.[1,15–24] Traumatic lesions of the cauda equina causing sudden, acute neurological deterioration generally have a poorer prognosis when compared with the gradual onset of lower motor neuron dysfunction in chronic or acute nontraumatic cauda equina syndrome.

Neurological recovery for injuries to the termination of the spinal cord, and particularly to the cauda equina, carries a better prognosis than does recovery for injuries to the midthoracic spinal cord.[25] In conus medullaris injuries, if there is some residual motor sparing, it is most likely to occur in the more proximal lower extremity muscle groups (hip flexors, adductors, and knee extensors) because these more cephalad nerve roots will be most likely to have escaped injury. Greater motor score improvement in patients with spinal cord injuries compared with conus medullaris and cauda equina injuries has been reported by Kaneda et al., who also noted the highest final motor scores in the cauda equina patients. The dramatic neurological recovery reported in Kaneda et al.'s series has not been duplicated.[26,27]

Very little is known about the specific motor recovery patterns in lower thoracic spinal cord, conus medullaris, and cauda equina injuries and how patient factors, injury patterns, and perioperative variables affect neurological recovery. In a recent study from our center,[25] the neural axis level of injury, identified with magnetic resonance imaging (MRI), and not the vertebral column level of injury, was predictive of neurological motor recovery. The initial motor score also influenced recovery. Identification of the precise level of neural axis injury utilizing MRI was one of the key determinants with respect to the prognosis for patients that sustain these common injuries.

■ Clinical and Neurological Evaluation

A thorough Advanced Trauma Life Support (ATLS) approach is required when evaluating these patients, and a precise neurological exam is critical for characterizing the type of clinical syndrome that the patient has sustained.[28,29]

The neurological structures at the level of the thoracolumbar spine are critical for lower extremity motor and sensory function as well as bowel, bladder, and sexual function.

Examination may reveal variable lower extremity weakness, absent lower limb reflexes, and anesthesia ranging from the waistline down to the lowest sacral segments in the perianal region. Preservation or early return of the bulbocavernosus reflex (BCR) and anal reflex is more commonly observed with spinal cord injuries, whereas they are typically permanently abolished with either conus or cauda injuries. Because of this, injuries of the cauda equina cannot be strictly assigned an American Spinal Injury Association (ASIA) grade.[30] Cauda equina injuries are pure lower motor neuron injuries, and as such they are associated with absent deep tendon reflexes and BCR, a flaccid urinary bladder, and flaccid lower extremity paralysis.

■ Spinal Imaging

Although plain films provide useful information, particularly to assess the effects of gravity on spinal alignment in patients without a neurological deficit and questionable stability, their utility in the evaluation of an acute neurological deficit at the thoracolumbar spine is superseded by advanced imaging modalities. A computed tomographic (CT) scan with sagittal and coronal reformats is crucial for characterizing the bony injury as well as the resultant bony canal compromise (**Fig. 26.1**).

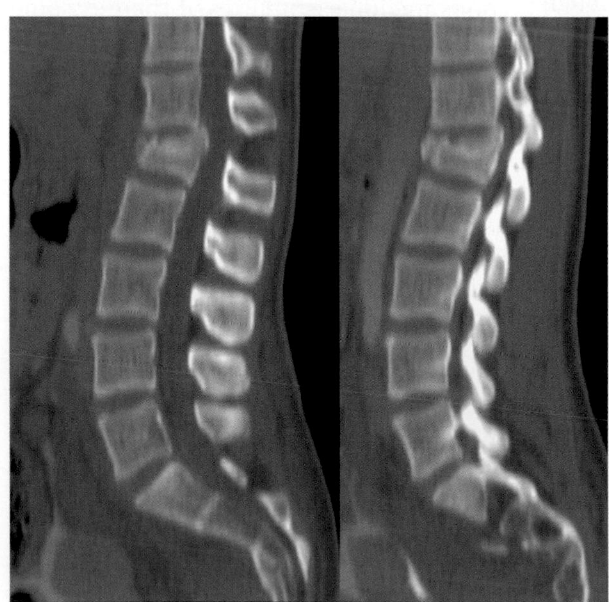

Fig. 26.1 Paramedian reformatted CT scans from a 56-year-old male with an L1 burst fracture.

There is no difference in neural recovery based on the final spinal canal area or spinal level of injury (T11–L2).[31] No association between initial canal encroachment and neurological recovery has been shown.[21,32,33]

In the setting of a neurological deficit attributable to a traumatic thoracolumbar spine injury, MRI is almost always advisable. MRI may not be appropriate, due to medical instability, patient size, or other contraindications related to metallic implants. The value of MRI includes the assessment of spinal cord signal change, the precise location of the conus medullaris, and evaluation of the posterior ligamentous complex (PLC).[7,34] The integrity of the PLC is an important consideration in the management of thoracolumbar burst fractures, and it is best evaluated with short tau inversion recovery (STIR) or fat-suppressed T2 sequences on MRI (**Fig. 26.2**). MRI may also be of value in anticipating treatment complexities, such as identifying the presence and location of disk or bone fragments in the spinal canal; anticipating the location of maximal spinal cord compression, traumatic durotomy, and cerebrospinal fluid (CSF) leaks; and planning surgical approaches. The extent of abnormal signal change in the spinal cord may have prognostic significance.

The most common spinal column injuries resulting in codus medullaris injury (CMI) or cauda equina injury (CEI) are burst fractures (**Fig. 26.3**) and fracture-dislocations. Flexion-distraction injuries may also lead to neurological deficits at these levels, although they are less common and have less risk of an associated neurological lesion.[1,3,4,10]

Combining the assessment of spinal stability, neurological status, and unique patient factors, the surgeon is now able to develop an appropriate management plan.

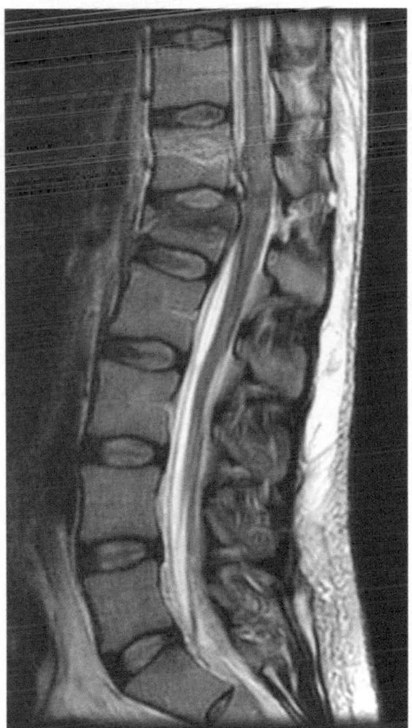

Fig. 26.2 Magnetic resonance imaging revealing increased signal change and swelling in the conus medullaris and terminal spinal cord and posterior ligament injury.

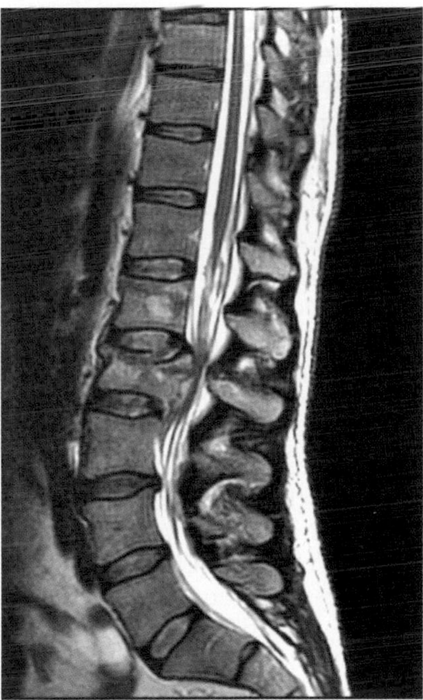

Fig. 26.3 Magnetic resonance imaging of an L2 burst fracture demonstrating bony compression of the cauda equina.

Factors Influencing Clinical and Neurological Outcome

Neurological Outcome and Operative versus Nonoperative Treatment

In the setting of CMI and CEI secondary to spinal column trauma, the treating surgeon must decide whether surgical treatment is indicated and, if so, what the surgical plan should entail. Ideally, the analysis should be evidence based and consider the balance of harms, benefits, and costs of a proposed intervention. Treatment options include bed rest, orthoses, and various surgical approaches, construct lengths, and instrumentation alternatives.[4,28,35–42] In the case of traumatic CMI or CEI where the patient will likely benefit from early expert management related to bowel and bladder function, treatment in a specialized center may be of benefit.

A review of published literature involving traumatic neurological deficits at the thoracolumbar and lumbar spine reveals generally low-quality retrospective studies of heterogeneous patients and treatment approaches. Results specifically cited as relating to CMI or CEI may not be precisely applicable to these injuries because these syndromes are typically inferred based on the spinal level of injury or the neurological presentation.

A systematic review on the effectiveness of surgical decompression for thoracolumbar burst fractures with a neurological deficit showed a weak trend toward improved recovery in the nonsurgical group but involved heterogeneous surgical techniques.[16] Patients with incomplete neurological deficits fared better with surgical stabilization and decompression.

Based on the population-based study by Daniels et al. it would appear that patients with traumatic CMI, CEI, and spinal cord injuries are frequently treated nonsurgically.[37] Only 61.4% of patients with a thoracolumbar fracture and a neurological injury are treated surgically. The percentage is only slightly greater in the highest-volume centers. Daniels et al.'s conclusions are drawn from a review of treatment codes and may be inherently flawed due to the potential inaccuracies in this type of administrative data. This literature supports the assertion that nonsurgical treatment is a viable alternative.

Several studies have shown no correlation between neurological recovery and nonoperative or surgical treatment, canal compromise, or fracture pattern.[22,23,43,44]

Other authors have suggested that patients with neurological deficits secondary to thoracolumbar and lumbar spinal injuries may benefit from surgical treatment in terms of shorter hospital stays, which often leads to more timely active rehabilitation.[17,38,45,46]

It is the authors' opinion that the specific expertise and resources necessary to provide safe, effective nonoperative care to patients with a spinal cord injury are diminishing, particularly in North America and Europe. Although nonsurgical care of traumatic CMI and CEI will likely result in some degree of neurological improvement, the vast majority of these injuries should be treated with surgical stabilization and, when necessary, with a concomitant decompression. Not only is this likely to reduce the patient's hospital stay and facilitate nursing and rehabilitation but also it is clearly safe from a neurological perspective and may optimize neurological recovery.

Neurological Outcome and Surgical Approach/Timing

Studies of anterior decompression for thoracolumbar fractures with incomplete neurological deficits have demonstrated that neurological recovery was not associated with the timing of anterior decompression. Generally, patients improve by at least one motor grade after even delayed decompression, particularly those with CEI. There also appears to be substantial improvement in bladder function following decompression for injuries at T12–L1.[26,47,48] The quality of decompression may be improved in patients treated with anterior decompression, and this may influence bladder/bowel recovery.

Decompression and stabilization, as opposed to posterior fusion alone, appear to lead to a more substantial motor improvement in patients with lumbar fractures and incomplete cauda equina neurological deficits.[49]

Other authors report satisfactory neurological outcomes with motor improvement in up to half of the patients and bladder functional improvement in two thirds, suggesting that posterior surgery alone is safe and acceptable in patients with CMI and CEI. Delayed anterior vertebrectomy can often be performed within a subacute timeframe depending upon stability or neurological indications.[50,51]

Most studies looking at the timing of surgery are underpowered, and the only conclusions that can be drawn are that it is likely safe to perform early surgery and early surgery does not appear to be associated with a profound risk of neurological deterioration.[20,52] There is some suggestion that early fixation results in improved clinical outcome in terms of complications and hospital stay, but it has an unclear effect on neurological outcome.[52,53]

Neurological Outcome and Bladder/Sexual Function

Lower spinal cord injuries result in an upper motor neuron spastic bladder where the sacral micturition center and sacral reflex arcs continue to respond, although they are deprived of brain stem and cortical micturition control. This syndrome may lead to detrusor hyperreflexia, increased pressure within the bladder, and the potential risk of retrograde urine flow.[52,54–57]

Injuries to the cauda equina, on the other hand, result in a lower motor neuron flaccid bladder, as do injuries located within the conus medullaris. Lower motor neuron disruption typically results in a flaccid bladder, urinary retention, and overflow incontinence. Treatment consists of clean intermittent catheterization to ensure complete bladder emptying. Management goals include avoidance of bladder overdistension and retrograde urine flow, which may lead to pyelonephritis and secondary renal failure.

With respect to sexual function, men with a lower motor neuron lesion will have more difficulty achieving a reflexive erection. The pharmacological treatment of erectile dysfunction is dependent on the level and extent of the spinal cord injury. Fertility issues, for female and male patients, should be specifically addressed by urologists and gynecologists with a specific interest in spinal cord injury because most patients will retain the ability to have children.

■ Conclusion

Thoracolumbar burst fractures may be associated with injury to the lower spinal cord, the conus medullaris, or the cauda equina. When injured, each of these neuroanatomical structures carries with it a unique spectrum of functional impairment and prognosis for neurological recovery.

Greater motor score improvement occurs following cauda equina injury than following a low thoracic spinal cord injury. Other predictors of favorable neurological recovery include the presence of sacral sensation and higher initial motor score at the time of initial assessment. From a prognostic point of view, it is important to visualize the exact location of the conus medullaris in relation to the level of injury and report on the MRI-determined neural axis level of injury as opposed to the vertebral level of injury.

Surgical decompression for incomplete thoracolumbar injuries has become common practice and is supported by poor quality evidence in the literature. Nonsurgical treatment results in neurological improvement as well; however, the comparative efficacy or effectiveness of surgery and nonsurgical treatment cannot be assessed by the available evidence specific to CMI or CEI.

Regardless of the potential influence of surgical treatment on neurological improvement, surgical treatment may be preferred due to shorter hospital stays, earlier rehabilitation, availability of equipment, and expert nursing care, as well as patient preference. When surgical treatment is selected, posterior stabilization with or without posterolateral decompression appears to offer good neurological outcomes and has the benefit of being familiar to the surgeon and avoiding the additional morbidity of an anterior approach. Anterior decompression, however, may offer potential benefits in terms of bladder recovery, and it can always be performed in a subacute time frame after initial posterior stabilization and after the patient is less acute. Indications for a secondary anterior decompression and stabilization would include (1) stability in those patients who have extremely comminuted fractures and (2) persistent neural element compression after posterior surgery, particularly in the presence of a profound or incomplete neurological deficit. From the available evidence, timing of surgery for traumatic CMI or CEI does not improve neurological recovery, although there does not appear to be any evidence of a deleterious effect from early surgical stabilization or decompression.

Pearls

- Thoracolumbar injuries have a variable prognosis that is dependent upon the neuroanatomical structure located at the level of the fracture.
- Sacral sensory preservation and injury at the level of the cauda equina are favorable prognostic indicators.
- In the severely traumatized patient, posterior stabilization can be performed to facilitate nursing care, and then the patient can be reimaged with MRI or CT scanning to assess the need for a subacute anterior vertebral body resection and reconstruction.

Pitfalls

- Injuries to the conus medullaris may result in profound loss of motor function and sensation in the most caudal segments (flaccid anus, absent BCR, etc.), and there may still be substantial opportunity for motor recovery in the legs. At follow-up examination, even though the patient appears to be walking quite normally, there may still be profound weakness of the foot plantar-flexion and a profound neurogenic bowel and bladder with complete loss of sexual function. Careful questioning and examination are necessary in follow-up.
- Anterior decompression (vertebrectomy) in the first 24 hours may be associated with massive blood loss.
- When translation or posterior distraction is a feature of the injury morphology, posterior open reduction and instrumentation are required because the translation and posterior distraction cannot be reduced through an anterior approach.

References

1. Aebi M, Mohler J, Zäch G, Morscher E. Analysis of 75 operated thoracolumbar fractures and fracture dislocations with and without neurological deficit. Arch Orthop Trauma Surg 1986;105(2): 100–112
2. Denis F, Burkus JK. Shear fracture-dislocations of the thoracic and lumbar spine associated with forceful hyperextension (lumberjack paraplegia). Spine 1992;17(2):156–161
3. Gertzbein SD. Scoliosis Research Society. Multicenter spine fracture study. Spine 1992;17(5): 528–540
4. Magerl F, Aebi M, Gertzbein SD, Harms J, Nazarian S. A comprehensive classification of thoracic and lumbar injuries. Eur Spine J 1994;3(4): 184–201
5. Lenarz CJ, Place HM, Lenke LG, Alander DH, Oliver D. Comparative reliability of 3 thoracolumbar fracture classification systems. J Spinal Disord Tech 2009;22(6):422–427
6. Sethi MK, Schoenfeld AJ, Bono CM, Harris MB. The evolution of thoracolumbar injury classification systems. Spine J 2009;9(9):780–788
7. Vaccaro AR, Lehman RA Jr, Hurlbert RJ, et al. A new classification of thoracolumbar injuries: the importance of injury morphology, the integrity of

the posterior ligamentous complex, and neurologic status. Spine 2005;30(20):2325–2333
8. Saifuddin A, Burnett SJ, White J. The variation of position of the conus medullaris in an adult population: a magnetic resonance imaging study. Spine 1998;23(13):1452–1456
9. Soleiman J, Demaerel P, Rocher S, Maes F, Marchal G. Magnetic resonance imaging study of the level of termination of the conus medullaris and the thecal sac: influence of age and gender. Spine 2005;30(16):1875–1880
10. Harrop JS, Hunt GE Jr, Vaccaro AR. Conus medullaris and cauda equina syndrome as a result of traumatic injuries: management principles. Neurosurg Focus 2004;16(6):e4
11. Kesler H, Dias MS, Kalapos P. Termination of the normal conus medullaris in children: a whole-spine magnetic resonance imaging study. Neurosurg Focus 2007;23(2):E7
12. Wall EJ, Cohen MS, Abitbol JJ, Garfin SR. Organization of intrathecal nerve roots at the level of the conus medullaris. J Bone Joint Surg Am 1990;72(10):1495–1499
13. Wall EJ, Cohen MS, Massie JB, Rydevik B, Garfin SR. Cauda equina anatomy, I: Intrathecal nerve root organization. Spine 1990;15(12):1244–1247
14. Aebi M. Classification of thoracolumbar fractures and dislocations. Eur Spine J 2010;19(Suppl 1):S2–S7
15. Benzel EC, Larson SJ. Functional recovery after decompressive operation for thoracic and lumbar spine fractures. Neurosurgery 1986;19(5):772–778
16. Boerger TO, Limb D, Dickson RA. Does 'canal clearance' affect neurological outcome after thoracolumbar burst fractures? J Bone Joint Surg Br 2000;82(5):629–635
17. Braakman R, Fontijne WP, Zeegers R, Steenbeek JR, Tanghe HL. Neurological deficit in injuries of the thoracic and lumbar spine. A consecutive series of 70 patients. Acta Neurochir (Wien) 1991;111(1-2):11–17
18. Bravo P, Labarta C, Alcaraz MA, Mendoza J, Verdu A. Outcome after vertebral fractures with neurological lesion treated either surgically or conservatively in Spain. Paraplegia 1993;31(6):358–366
19. Bravo P, Labarta C, Alcaraz MA, Mendoza J, Verdú A. An assessment of factors affecting neurological recovery after spinal cord injury with vertebral fracture. Paraplegia 1996;34(3):164–166
20. Clohisy JC, Akbarnia BA, Bucholz RD, Burkus JK, Backer RJ. Neurologic recovery associated with anterior decompression of spine fractures at the thoracolumbar junction (T12-L1). Spine 1992;17(8, Suppl):S325–S330
21. Dai LY, Wang XY, Jiang LS. Neurologic recovery from thoracolumbar burst fractures: is it predicted by the amount of initial canal encroachment and kyphotic deformity? Surg Neurol 2007;67(3):232–237, discussion 238
22. Dall BE, Stauffer ES. Neurologic injury and recovery patterns in burst fractures at the T12 or L1 motion segment. Clin Orthop Relat Res 1988;(233):171–176
23. Kim NH, Lee HM, Chun IM. Neurologic injury and recovery in patients with burst fracture of the thoracolumbar spine. Spine 1999;24(3):290–293, discussion 294
24. Weyns F, Rommens PM, Van Calenbergh F, Goffin J, Broos P, Plets C. Neurological outcome after surgery for thoracolumbar fractures. A retrospective study of 93 consecutive cases, treated with dorsal instrumentation. Eur Spine J 1994;3(5):276–281
25. Kingwell SP, Noonan VK, Fisher CG, et al. Relationship of neural axis level of injury to motor recovery and health-related quality of life in patients with a thoracolumbar spinal injury. J Bone Joint Surg Am 2010;92(7):1591–1599
26. Kaneda K, Abumi K, Fujiya M. Burst fractures with neurologic deficits of the thoracolumbar-lumbar spine. Results of anterior decompression and stabilization with anterior instrumentation. Spine 1984;9(8):788–795
27. Kaneda K, Taneichi H, Abumi K, Hashimoto T, Satoh S, Fujiya M. Anterior decompression and stabilization with the Kaneda device for thoracolumbar burst fractures associated with neurological deficits. J Bone Joint Surg Am 1997;79(1):69–83
28. Harris MB, Shi LL, Vacarro AR, Zdeblick TA, Sasso RC. Nonsurgical treatment of thoracolumbar spinal fractures. Instr Course Lect 2009;58:629–637
29. Harrop JS, Vaccaro AR, Hurlbert RJ, et al; Spine Trauma Study Group. Intrarater and interrater reliability and validity in the assessment of the mechanism of injury and integrity of the posterior ligamentous complex: a novel injury severity scoring system for thoracolumbar injuries. Invited submission from the Joint Section Meeting on Disorders of the Spine and Peripheral Nerves, March 2005. J Neurosurg Spine 2006;4(2):118–122
30. Ertekin C, Reel F, Mutlu R, Kerküklü I. Bulbocavernosus reflex in patients with conus medullaris and cauda equina lesions. J Neurol Sci 1979;41(2):175–181
31. Herndon WA, Galloway D. Neurologic return versus cross-sectional canal area in incomplete thoracolumbar spinal cord injuries. J Trauma 1988;28(5):680–683
32. Dai LY. Remodeling of the spinal canal after thoracolumbar burst fractures. Clin Orthop Relat Res 2001;(382):119–123
33. Mohanty SP, Venkatram N. Does neurological recovery in thoracolumbar and lumbar burst fractures depend on the extent of canal compromise? Spinal Cord 2002;40(6):295–299
34. Vaccaro AR, Rihn JA, Saravanja D, et al. Injury of the posterior ligamentous complex of the thoracolumbar spine: a prospective evaluation of the diagnostic accuracy of magnetic resonance imaging. Spine 2009;34(23):E841–E847
35. Been HD, Bouma GJ. Comparison of two types of surgery for thoraco-lumbar burst fractures: combined anterior and posterior stabilisation vs. posterior instrumentation only. Acta Neurochir (Wien) 1999;141(4):349–357
36. Burke DC, Murray DD. The management of thoracic and thoraco-lumbar injuries of the spine with neurological involvement. J Bone Joint Surg Br 1976;58(1):72–78
37. Daniels AH, Arthur M, Hart RA. Variability in rates of arthrodesis for patients with thoracolumbar

spine fractures with and without associated neurologic injury. Spine 2007;32(21):2334–2338

38. Davies WE, Morris JH, Hill V. An analysis of conservative (non-surgical) management of thoracolumbar fractures and fracture-dislocations with neural damage. J Bone Joint Surg Am 1980;62(8):1324–1328

39. Durward QJ, Schweigel JF, Harrison P. Management of fractures of the thoracolumbar and lumbar spite. Neurosurgery 1981;8(5):555–561

40. Geisler WO, Wynne-Jones M, Jousse AT. Early management of the patient with trauma to the spinal cord. Med Serv J Can 1966;22(7): 512–523

41. Hitchon PW, Torner JC, Haddad SF, Follett KA. Management options in thoracolumbar burst fractures. Surg Neurol 1998;49(6):619–626, discussion 626–627

42. Rechtine GR II, Cahill D, Chrin AM. Treatment of thoracolumbar trauma: comparison of complications of operative versus nonoperative treatment. J Spinal Disord 1999;12(5):406–409

43. Dendrinos GK, Halikias JG, Krallis PN, Asimakopoulos A. Factors influencing neurological recovery in burst thoracolumbar fractures. Acta Orthop Belg 1995;61(3):226–234

44. Lifeso RM, Arabie KM, Kadhi SK. Fractures of the thoraco-lumbar spine. Paraplegia 1985;23(4): 207–224

45. Braakman R. The value of more aggressive management in traumatic paraplegia. Neurosurg Rev 1986;9(1-2):141–147

46. Jodoin A, Dupuis P, Fraser M, Beaumont P. Unstable fractures of the thoracolumbar spine: a 10-year experience at Sacré-Coeur Hospital. J Trauma 1985;25(3):197–202

47. Bradford DS, McBride GG. Surgical management of thoracolumbar spine fractures with incomplete neurologic deficits. Clin Orthop Relat Res 1987;(218):201–216

48. McAfee PC, Bohlman HH, Yuan HA. Anterior decompression of traumatic thoracolumbar fractures with incomplete neurological deficit using a retroperitoneal approach. J Bone Joint Surg Am 1985;67(1):89–104

49. Hu SS, Capen DA, Rimoldi RL, Zigler JE. The effect of surgical decompression on neurologic outcome after lumbar fractures. Clin Orthop Relat Res 1993;(288):166–173

50. Boriani S, Palmisani M, Donati U, et al. The treatment of thoracic and lumbar spine fractures: a study of 123 cases treated surgically in 101 patients. Chir Organi Mov 2000;85(2):137–149

51. Rahimi-Movaghar V, Vaccaro AR, Mohammadi M. Efficacy of surgical decompression in regard to motor recovery in the setting of conus medullaris injury. J Spinal Cord Med 2006;29(1): 32–38

52. Rutges JP, Oner FC, Leenen LP. Timing of thoracic and lumbar fracture fixation in spinal injuries: a systematic review of neurological and clinical outcome. Eur Spine J 2007;16(5):579–587

53. Rath SA, Kahamba JF, Kretschmer T, Neff U, Richter HP, Antoniadis G. Neurological recovery and its influencing factors in thoracic and lumbar spine fractures after surgical decompression and stabilization. Neurosurg Rev 2005;28(1):44–52

54. Benevento BT, Sipski ML. Neurogenic bladder, neurogenic bowel, and sexual dysfunction in people with spinal cord injury. Phys Ther 2002; 82(6):601–612

55. Burchiel KJ, Burns AS. Summary statement: pain, spasticity, and bladder and sexual function after spinal cord injury. Spine 2001;26(24, Suppl): S161

56. Burns AS, Rivas DA, Ditunno JF. The management of neurogenic bladder and sexual dysfunction after spinal cord injury. Spine 2001;26(24, Suppl):S129–S136

57. Samson G, Cardenas DD. Neurogenic bladder in spinal cord injury. Phys Med Rehabil Clin N Am 2007;18(2):255–274, vi

27

Management of Central Cord Syndrome

Harvey E. Smith and Todd J. Albert

Key Points

1. Most spinal injuries in the elderly are cervical, and over 50% of those injuries occur without fracture; the relative proportion of these injuries in the population is increasing.
2. Fractures may not be readily apparent in the spondylotic or spondylitic spine, and the clinician must maintain a high index of suspicion for extension/distraction injury in the setting of advanced degenerative spondylosis.
3. The indications for, and timing of, surgical intervention are controversial, but it is generally agreed that imaging-confirmed spinal cord compression should be decompressed. Early decompression (within 24 hours of injury) is feasible and safe, but prospective data are needed to ascertain the effect of early decompression on long-term outcomes.

Spinal Cord Injury Epidemiology

The reported incidence of spinal cord injury (SCI) in North America varies from 25 to 93 per million population.[1–5] The distribution of spinal cord injuries is bimodal, with younger patients generally sustaining injury from motor vehicle accidents and other high-energy mechanisms, and older patients predominantly incurring injury via lower-energy mechanisms, such as falls.[6] Accordingly, in the elderly, most injuries are cervical spinal cord injuries, and over 50% of cervical spinal cord injuries in the older population occur without fracture.[2] The size of the elderly population is increasing, and this corresponds to an increased incidence of elderly patients presenting with acute SCI: the National Spinal Cord Injury Statistical Center data indicate an increase in the relative proportion of spinal cord injuries that occur in the elderly.[6] Given the increasing relative proportion of the elderly in the population, coupled with the increased survival rates for spinal injuries,[6,7] it is likely that the management of cervical spine trauma in the elderly will become an issue of increasing relevance in the future.

■ Central Cord Syndrome: Definition, Mechanism, Pathophysiology

Central cord syndrome describes a neurological presentation of disproportionate weakness of the upper relative to the lower extremities in the setting of cervical spine trauma; the injury mechanism is classically described as that of hyperextension in the setting of a congenitally narrow or spondylotic spine. First described by Schneider et al.,[8] the clinical presentation of central cord syndrome was initially hypothesized to be due to injury and subsequent hematoma at the center of the cord (gray matter), with associated damage to the medial fibers of the corticospinal tract. The clinical presentation was hypothesized to be due to the somatotopic organization of the corticospinal tract, in which the fibers for the lower extremities and sacrum were hypothesized to be more superficial and lateral than the fibers corresponding to the upper extremities. Historically, it was hypothesized that the forces resulting from in-buckling of the posterior ligamentum flavum coupled with anterior compression from a spondylotic disk-osteophyte complex (the spinal canal is narrowed by up to 30% in hyperextension)[9,10] yielded a net compressive force that was maximal in the center of the spinal cord. Thus, the nidus of injury has historically been described as being in the central gray matter, with subsequent expanding hematoma. More recently, the attribution of the clinical presentation of central cord syndrome to a somatotopic organization of the corticospinal tract (with the upper extremity fibers more centrally located) has been criticized, due in large part to the lack of published literature establishing such an organization of the corticospinal tract in humans and primates.[11,12] Jimenez et al.[11] examined the cervical spinal cords of five patients with acute traumatic central cord syndrome or Bell cruciate paralysis compared with age-matched controls and found degeneration of the corticospinal axonal tracts, with Wallerian degeneration distal to the injury. The identified loss of motor neurons supports a hypothesis that the disproportionate upper extremity dysfunction in central cord syndrome may be due to injury involving the large fibers of the lateral corticospinal tract,[11] and suggests that the corticospinal tracts may be disproportionately involved in upper, relative to lower, extremity function.

■ Initial Evaluation and Management Strategies

The patient presenting with new-onset neurological deficit is in neurological and physiological extremis. Standard trauma protocols should be followed, first securing the airway, and then supporting respiratory and cardiovascular status. Initial trauma films should be obtained as per institutional protocols. Particularly in the older patient with significant spondylosis, a high index of suspicion should be maintained for possible fracture, and there should be a low threshold for obtaining advanced imaging studies. Adequate imaging of the cervical spine is crucial, including the C7–T1 junction. Depending on the mechanism of injury and associated clinical suspicion, one should also consider obtaining imaging studies of the thoracic and lumbar spine because noncontiguous injuries in the cervical spine or cervicothoracic junction have been identified in up to 28% of patients with cervical spine trauma.[13,14] In the setting of a neurological deficit or suspicion of diskoligamentous injury, a magnetic resonance imaging (MRI) scan should be obtained of the appropriate spinal regions. Any area of clinical suspicion or where fracture or dislocation cannot be excluded with x-ray studies should be considered for evaluation with computed tomographic (CT) imaging. In the older patient presenting with a neurological deficit in the setting of advanced degenerative spondylosis, the clinician should maintain a high index of suspicion for an extension/distraction injury.[15] Soft-tissue swelling in the prevertebral space or distraction in a spondylitic disk space is suggestive of a possible extension/distraction mechanism, and MRI should be considered to further evaluate the anterior soft tissues and diskoligamentous complex.[15]

At the time of presentation to the physician, the primary injury has occurred, and the goal of management is to mitigate the secondary injury cascade and to provide physiological support that maximizes the potential for recovery. Paramount to this goal is the maintenance of adequate perfusion pressures. One should consider prompt placement of an arterial line at the time of initial evaluation to facilitate the maintenance of the mean arterial pressure; a central line may need to be considered if there is concern about cardiovascular instability or the possible need for pressors to maintain central perfusion. As will be discussed, there is significant controversy regarding the role and timing of surgical decompression of any compressive pathology. The rationale for decompression and the debate regarding the timing of decompression are based in part on mitigating the ischemic insult due to vascular compromise. Maintaining spinal cord perfusion pressures is readily accomplished in the trauma bay with medical management and monitoring; constant attention to the mean arterial pressure should be stressed. The clinician should also be aware of the possibility of spinal shock in the setting of a significant SCI and maintain it[16] in the differential diagnosis of any hemodynamic instability.

The role of steroids in the acute SCI patient is controversial,[17–19] and there is no clear consensus. Steroids may be considered as a management option if the patient meets appropriate National Acute Spinal Cord Injury Study (NASCIS) inclusion criteria, but the physician must also consider patient-specific factors when weighing the potential comorbidities of high-dose steroid treatment.

Management strategy is dictated, in large part, by the injury mechanism. A high-energy injury in a younger patient population is more likely to present with a fracture or dislocation, with spinal cord compression in the setting of mechanical instability. In this scenario, the surgical management will be aimed at restoring spinal stability, with a concomitant decompression of the neural elements, and in the setting of traumatic fracture-dislocation with neural element compression, the spine should be decompressed and stabilized as expeditiously as possible given patient-specific factors; closed reduction may be a management option to facilitate rapid decompression. The role of closed reduction for specific fracture types is beyond the scope of this chapter, but it is mentioned to stress that, although central cord syndrome is typically discussed as a separate entity in cervical spine trauma, a central cord presentation in the setting of a fracture-dislocation should be managed as appropriate for the given injury mechanism.

The elderly patient presenting after a relatively low-energy hyperextension mechanism, such as a fall from standing, without a fracture is the more classic presentation of a central cord syndrome. As is discussed in this chapter, there is considerable controversy regarding the role and timing of surgical decompression in this patient population. This is due in part to the fact that the natural history of central cord syndrome is one of relatively significant motor improvement. Several treatment algorithms[19] advocate for observation during this phase of improvement, with intervention only if there is a plateau in improvement or a neurological decline. This creates a selection bias in the literature because patients historically operated on as the initial treatment are those that had a more severe neurological injury, failure to improve, or new deterioration; given that the most important predictor of neurological outcome is initial neurological status, this may bias against positive outcomes in the historical operative cohorts.

■ Prognostic Factors for Clinical Outcome

The literature regarding clinical outcomes of central cord syndrome is diverse. Although it is generally thought that patients with central cord syndrome have a reasonable prognosis for some degree of recovery, the majority of published studies are Class III data with differing outcomes measures.[20] The single greatest prognostic indicator of final neurological outcome is the initial neurological status. As reviewed by Dvorak et al., other prognostic variables described have included patient age, spasticity, and hyperpathia.[20] However, the majority of published studies have not linked given outcome indices to generic health-related quality of life (HRQoL). Although many patients with central cord syndrome have improvement in their motor function, improvement of motor function has been correlated with increased spasticity,[20] and spasticity negatively correlates with functional status[21,22] and HRQoL.[20] Dvorak et al.[20] utilized a prospectively collected database to analyze American Spinal Injury Association (ASIA) motor scores at the time of injury and at follow-up, and they evaluated the short form (SF)-36 and the Functional Independence Measure (FIM) at follow-up. Level of education was found to directly correlate with HRQoL and motor recovery, and spasticity was found to correlate with degree of motor recovery. The degree of spasticity was confirmed to adversely affect outcome measures, and age was found to adversely affect the FIM. Aito et al.[23] similarly found that age >65 was a negative prognostic factor for recovery but did not find any correlation between patient age and bladder function or spasticity; spasticity developed in 54% of patients in Aito et al.'s cohort; Perkash[24] reported a 48% incidence of spasticity.

Case Example

A 37-year-old male with acquired and congenital cervical stenosis incurred a hyperextension injury due to a fall. At the time of presentation, the patient had an incomplete spinal cord injury, and was classified as ASIA C (**Fig. 27.1** and **27.2**). Due to the patient's neurologic status in the setting of neural element compression, it was elected to perform a posterior cervical decompression and fusion procedure (**Fig. 27.3**).

Management Controversies

The issue of the acute management of SCI is controversial, particularly with respect to traumatic central cord syndrome (TCCS). To date, the majority of published stud-

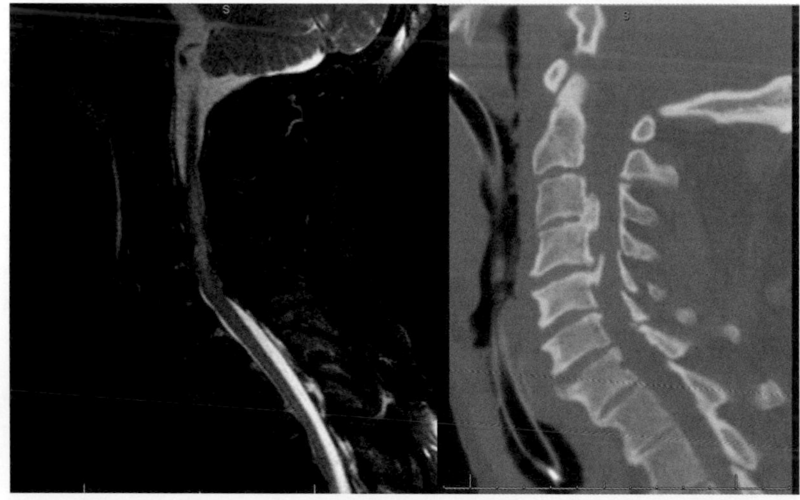

Fig. 27.1 Sagittal magnetic resonance imaging (short tau inversion recovery) and CT reconstruction of the cervical spine of a 37-year-old male with congenital and acquired cervical stenosis who fell, striking his head, with a resulting hyperextension injury. Note the posterior osteophytes at C3–4 and C4–5, and the significant cord edema from C3–6. The patient presented as an incomplete spinal cord injury (American Spinal Injury Association C).

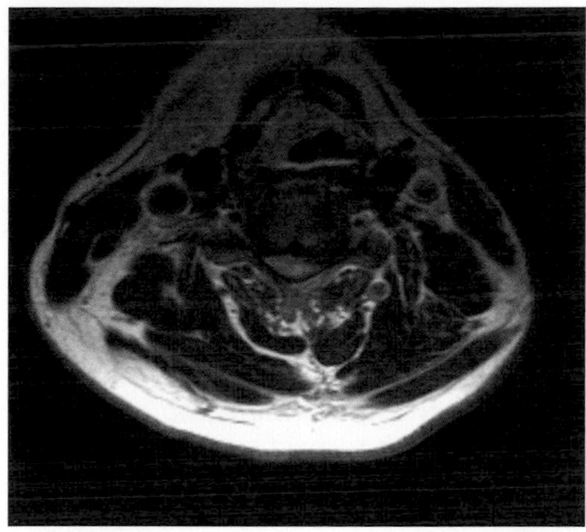

Fig. 27.2 Axial magnetic resonance imaging (short tau inversion recovery) demonstrating significant canal narrowing and spinal cord compression.

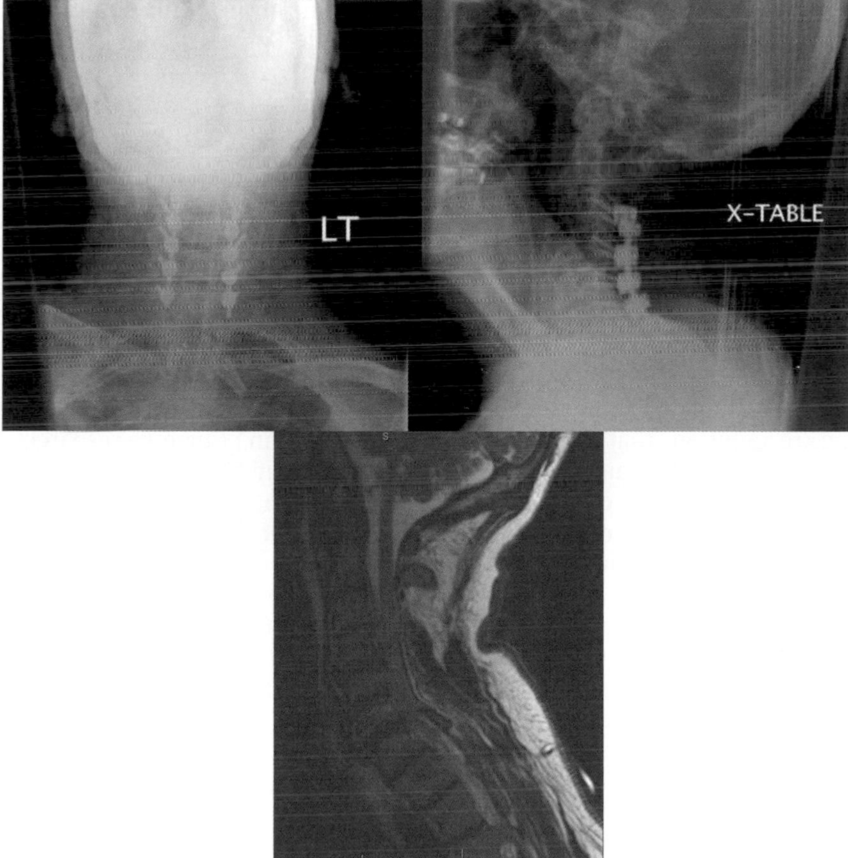

Fig. 27.3 A posterior laminectomy and fusion was performed to decompress the cord. Postoperative magnetic resonance imaging demonstrates decompression of the spinal cord with significant remaining spinal cord edema.

ies on the timing of surgical decompression of SCI have been retrospective, level III evidence. There is wide variation in the definition of *early* versus *late* decompression in the literature. Ethical considerations pose a considerable challenge to the design and execution of a prospective randomized trial. The Surgical Treatment for Acute Spinal Cord Injury Study (STASCIS) outcomes suggest that there may be a significant benefit to neurological outcome with early (within 24 hours) decompression; patients that were decompressed early (mean 14.2 hours) had odds of improving at least 2 AIS grades that were 2.8 times higher than patients that were decompressed later (mean 48.3 hours).[25] The management of TCCS is perhaps more complicated than other aspects of SCI because some authors consider it separately from other cervical SCI, and in fact, some authors have specifically excluded the condition when reporting their cohorts.[26] Central cord syndrome occurs more commonly in an older population, which has an associated higher incidence of medical comorbidities to consider in treatment.[27]

The majority of central cord SCI patients have some degree of recovery of their function, and this, coupled with what was historically a significant surgical morbidity, led to initial recommendations against surgical management. However, there is increasing recognition that with longer follow-up there is a significant incidence of spasticity,[23,24] as well as late-onset progressive myelopathy and neurological deterioration in a portion of patients managed nonoperatively.[21]

It is increasingly recognized that, with modern surgical techniques, in concert with advances in perioperative management, surgical management in the TCCS population is feasible and has acceptable perioperative morbidity.[9] With respect to surgical management of central cord syndrome, Chen et al. found that surgical decompression resulted in faster recovery and fewer complications than nonoperative management.[28] Duh et al. found that surgical management resulted in earlier rehabilitation and suggested that stabilization may protect against late-onset progressive deterioration.[29] Most authors now advocate for surgical decompression of imaging-confirmed spinal cord compression[9,30,31]; what remains unresolved is if one should defer surgical management during a period of initial recovery until there is a plateau or deterioration, or if one should operate acutely. Chen et al.[32] recently reported a cohort of 49 patients with TCCS managed surgically; although surgical management was found to be feasible, safe, and with neurological improvement, no difference was noted with respect to time of decompression (earlier or later than 4 days.) Similar to other reports, Chen et al. also noted that age was a negative prognostic factor. Studies investigating outcomes relative to timing of decompression have been inconsistent in the definition of early versus late.[25] The Spine Trauma Study Group has recommended that 24 hours be considered the definition of early versus late decompression when considering outcomes.[25,33]

■ Future Research

There are several areas of ongoing research and clinical trials aimed at investigating potential therapeutic modalities to modulate glial scar formation after SCI and to promote axon regeneration and remyelination. Current research involves both cellular therapy with neural stem cells, pharmacological therapy, and combinations of both.[34] Clinical studies investigating the neuroprotective agents minocycline and Cethrin are under way, and the US Food and Drug Administration (FDA) recently approved the first stem-cell therapy trial for SCI in humans.

■ Conclusion

Central cord syndrome refers to an incomplete cervical SCI that occurs in the subaxial cervical spine; the classic mechanism is hyperextension of a congenitally or acquired stenotic neck. The pathophysiology underlying the clinical presentation has historically been attributed to a central nidus of injury in the gray matter, there is emerging evidence that the neural injury may largely be due to axonal damage in the corticospinal tracts. Treatment algorithms should follow the same rationale as other cervical SCI patterns, and literature supports the decompression of anatomical cord compression or fracture-dislocation with appropriate stabilization. There is an increasing recognition of the deleterious effects of spasticity on long-term outcomes, and a sole reliance on motor score improvement as an outcome indicator may not be appropriate. Early decompression is feasible and safe from a medical standpoint, but prospective data are needed to ascertain what role, if any, early decompression may play with respect to long-term outcomes. It is anticipated that the STASCIS study will make a significant contribution to developing an evidence-based rationale regarding the role and timing of decompression.

Pearls

- Maintain a high index of suspicion for extension-distraction injury in the spondylotic spine.
- Medical management stressing the maintenance of spinal cord perfusion pressure is critical.
- The role (and timing) of surgical decompression remains controversial, but emerging evidence supports that early decompression can be done safely; the relative benefits of early decompression remain to be defined.

Pitfalls

- The elderly patient with central cord syndrome is at high risk of medical complications.
- New studies indicate that with time there is increasing spasticity in patients recovering from central cord syndrome, and this spasticity inversely correlates with quality of life measures.
- The natural course of TCCS is generally that of slow recovery—a plateau in recovery or loss of function merits immediate evaluation.

References

1. Burke DA, Linden RD, Zhang YP, Maiste AC, Shields CB. Incidence rates and populations at risk for spinal cord injury: a regional study. Spinal Cord 2001;39(5):274–278
2. Pickett GE, Campos-Benitez M, Keller JL, Duggal N. Epidemiology of traumatic spinal cord injury in Canada. Spine 2006;31(7):799–805
3. Price C, Makintubee S, Herndon W, Istre GR. Epidemiology of traumatic spinal cord injury and acute hospitalization and rehabilitation charges for spinal cord injuries in Oklahoma, 1988-1990. Am J Epidemiol 1994;139(1):37–47
4. Sekhon LH, Fehlings MG. Epidemiology, demographics, and pathophysiology of acute spinal cord injury. Spine 2001;26(24, Suppl):S2–S12
5. Wyndaele M, Wyndaele JJ. Incidence, prevalence and epidemiology of spinal cord injury: what learns a worldwide literature survey? Spinal Cord 2006;44(9):523–529
6. Sokolowski MJ, Jackson AP, Haak MH, Meyer PR Jr, Sokolowski MS. Acute mortality and complications of cervical spine injuries in the elderly at a single tertiary care center. J Spinal Disord Tech 2007;20(5):352–356
7. Tan HB, Sloan JP, Barlow IF. Improvement in initial survival of spinal injuries: a 10-year audit. Injury 2005;36(8):941–945
8. Schneider RC, Cherry G, Pantek H. The syndrome of acute central cervical spinal cord injury; with special reference to the mechanisms involved in hyperextension injuries of cervical spine. J Neurosurg 1954;11(6):546–577
9. Guest J, Eleraky MA, Apostolides PJ, Dickman CA, Sonntag VK. Traumatic central cord syndrome: results of surgical management. J Neurosurg 2002;97(1, Suppl):25–32
10. Taylor AR, Blackwood W. Paraplegia in hyperextension cervical injuries with normal radiographic appearances. J Bone Joint Surg Br 1948;30B(2):245–248
11. Jimenez O, Marcillo A, Levi AD. A histopathological analysis of the human cervical spinal cord in patients with acute traumatic central cord syndrome. Spinal Cord 2000;38(9):532–537
12. Pappas CT, Gibson AR, Sonntag VK. Decussation of hind-limb and fore-limb fibers in the monkey corticospinal tract: relevance to cruciate paralysis. J Neurosurg 1991;75(6):935–940
13. Choi SJ, Shin MJ, Kim SM, Bae SJ. Non-contiguous spinal injury in cervical spinal trauma: evaluation with cervical spine MRI. Korean J Radiol 2004;5(4):219–224
14. Vaccaro AR, An HS, Lin S, Sun S, Balderston RA, Cotler JM. Noncontiguous injuries of the spine. J Spinal Disord 1992;5(3):320–329
15. Jabbour P, Fehlings M, Vaccaro AR, Harrop JS. Traumatic spine injuries in the geriatric population. Neurosurg Focus 2008;25(5):E16
16. Atkinson PP, Atkinson JL. Spinal shock. Mayo Clin Proc 1996;71(4):384–389

17. Hanigan WC, Anderson RJ. Commentary on NASCIS-2. J Spinal Disord 1992;5(1):125–131, discussion 132–133
18. Hugenholtz H. Methylprednisolone for acute spinal cord injury: not a standard of care. CMAJ 2003;168(9):1145–1146
19. Nesathurai S. Steroids and spinal cord injury: revisiting the NASCIS 2 and NASCIS 3 trials. J Trauma 1998;45(6):1088–1093
20. Dvorak MF, Fisher CG, Hoekema J, et al. Factors predicting motor recovery and functional outcome after traumatic central cord syndrome: a long-term follow-up. Spine 2005;30(20): 2303–2311
21. Bosch A, Stauffer ES, Nickel VL. Incomplete traumatic quadriplegia. A ten-year review. JAMA 1971;216(3):473–478
22. Tow AM, Kong KH. Central cord syndrome: functional outcome after rehabilitation. Spinal Cord 1998;36(3):156–160
23. Aito S, D'Andrea M, Werhagen L, et al. Neurological and functional outcome in traumatic central cord syndrome. Spinal Cord 2007;45(4 292–297
24. Perkash I. Management of neurogenic bladder dysfunctions following acute traumatic cervical central cord syndrome (incomplete tetraplegia) [proceedings]. Paraplegia 1977;15(1):21–37
25. Fehlings MG, Vaccaro A, Wilson JR, Singh A, Cadotte DW, et al. Early versus delayed decompression for traumatice cervical spinal cord injury: results of the Surgical Timing in Acute Spinal Cord Injury Study (STASCIS). PLoS ONE 2012; 7(2):e32037
26. Papadopoulos SM, Selden NR, Quint DJ, Patel N, Gillespie B, Grube S. Immediate spinal cord decompression for cervical spinal cord injury: feasibility and outcome. J Trauma 2002;52(2): 323–332
27. Furlan JC, Fehlings MG. The impact of age on mortality, impairment, and disability among adults with acute traumatic spinal cord injury. J Neurotrauma 2009;26(10):1707–1717
28. Chen TY, Dickman CA, Eleraky M, Sonntag VK. The role of decompression for acute incomplete cervical spinal cord injury in cervical spondylosis. Spine 1998;23(22):2398–2403
29. Duh MS, Shepard MJ, Wilberger JE, Bracken MB. The effectiveness of surgery on the treatment of acute spinal cord injury and its relation to pharmacological treatment. Neurosurgery 1994;35(2):240–248, discussion 248–249
30. Fehlings MG, Perrin RG. The timing of surgical intervention in the treatment of spinal cord injury: a systematic review of recent clinical evidence. Spine 2006;31(11, Suppl):S28–S35, discussion S36
31. Maroon JC, Abla AA, Wilberger JI, Bailes JE, Sternau LL. Central cord syndrome. Clin Neurosurg 1991;37:612–621
32. Chen L, Yang H, Yang T, Xu Y, Bao Z, Tang T. Effectiveness of surgical treatment for traumatic central cord syndrome. J Neurosurg Spine 2009;10(1):3–8
33. Ng WP, Fehlings MG, Cuddy B, et al. Surgical Treatment for Acute Spinal Cord Injury Study pilot study #2: evaluation of protocol for decompressive surgery within 8 hours of injury. Neurosurg Focus 1999;6(1):e3
34. Baptiste DC, Tighe A, Fehlings MG. Spinal cord injury and neural repair: focus on neuroregenerative approaches for spinal cord injury. Expert Opin Investig Drugs 2009;18(5):663–673

III

Neuroprotective and Neuroregenerative Approaches

28

Research in Spinal Cord Injury: Building an Effective Translational Research Program

W. Dalton Dietrich

Key Points

1. Spinal cord injury is a complex clinical problem.
2. Translational studies provide a solid basis for clinical investigations.
3. A multidisciplinary approach brings together required expertise to target this condition.
4. Core facilities can provide the capability to conduct difficult procedures.
5. Discovery research generates new knowledge on which to base future questions.
6. A bench to bedside approach in translating new discoveries is required to advance this field.

Traumatic injuries to the central nervous system represent a complex insult to the most complicated organ in the human body. Injuries to the spinal cord produced by primary insults initiate a series of secondary injury mechanisms that each by itself can participate in the eventual destruction of tissues and long-term neurological disorders. Although significant progress has been made in understanding the pathogenesis of spinal cord injury (SCI) and the identification of novel targets for therapeutic interventions, today there are no treatments that have been shown to be effective when tested in phase 3 clinical trials in SCI patients.[1] Although the use of methylprednisolone is recommended following SCI in specific cases, its use has declined over the last several years due to emerging information regarding the harmful side effects of this steroid. Thus, continued investigations into injury mechanisms initiated by SCI as well as the development of novel therapeutic interventions to protect and promote reparative strategies are critical. Because of the complexity of SCI, including a wide range of cellular, molecular, and biochemical responses, it is clear that more work is required to help identify novel treatments to target this patient population in well-designed clinical trials.

Because of the complex nature of SCI and the multifactorial nature of its immediate and later-occurring consequences, it is critical that research programs addressing this clinical problem are multidisciplinary and include expertise from different research areas (**Fig. 28.1**). Such a multidisciplinary approach allows for a wide range of expertise to tackle different aspects of the injury and treatment process.[2] To this end, various SCI centers have been established that attract a range of scientists and clinicians interested in making a difference in these patients' lives. As we move closer to testing our basic science discoveries in translational models of SCI and ultimately to initiate clinical trials (**Fig. 28.2**), it is clear that there are specific steps that need to be included in the investigative process to make such a translational program successful (**Fig. 28.3**). This chapter reviews several of the prerequisites that are felt to be critical as we attempt to move new therapies to the clinic.

Spinal Cord Models

As already mentioned, SCI is a complex clinical problem that is relatively difficult to replicate in the laboratory. Over the past 25 years, various models of SCI have been developed that mimic many of the aspects of human SCI.[3] Although no one model exactly mimics all aspects of human SCI, various models do reproduce in a consistent manner many of the biomechanical aspects and cellular response characteristics that occur in an injured patient. These injury models include spinal cord transection, clip compression, and contusive injury. Using other approaches, SCI is produced by occluding feeding blood vessels, producing a focal ischemic insult leading to long-term paralysis. The importance of having multiple

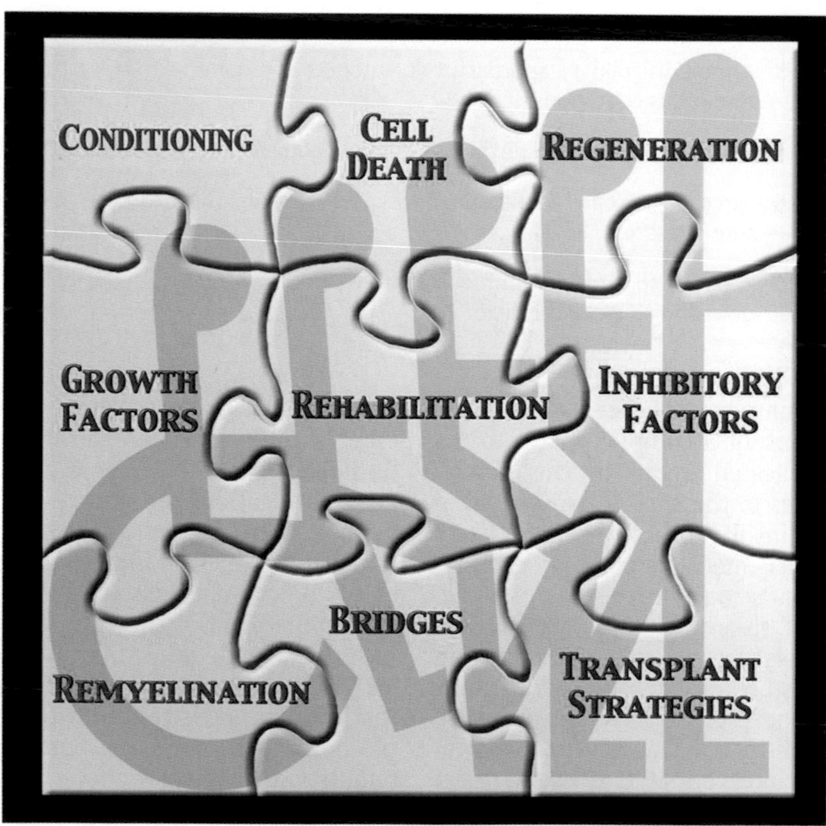

Fig. 28.1 The puzzle diagram indicates different research disciplines that are required for the successful development of therapies to promote protection and recovery after spinal cord injury and emphasizes major components of a multidisciplinary research program needed to achieve this objective.

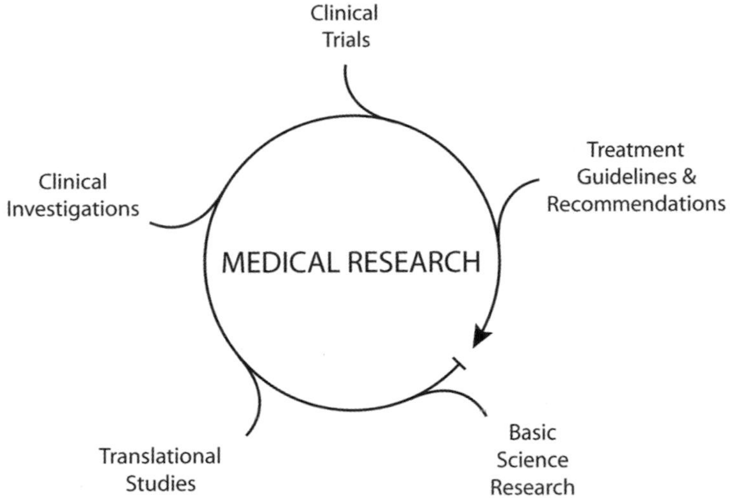

Fig. 28.2 Various steps for moving a discovery from the bench to the bedside are necessary. It is advantageous for translational research programs to incorporate each of these steps.

models in a translational laboratory is that the heterogeneous nature of SCI can be replicated with the various approaches. Also, it is anticipated that, if a particular therapy works in one type of SCI model, it might be advantageous to test that promising therapy in another model that may mimic another subpopulation of individuals with SCI.[4]

Another consideration regarding SCI is the level of injury. Recent models have allowed reproducible injuries to be produced at specific levels, including the most common cervical and thoracic levels. Currently, a high frequency of SCI patients sustain cervical SCI.[5] Thus, although in the past more conventional thoracic injuries were frequently produced and evaluated for motor assessment, more recent studies have concentrated on cervical injury, lead ing to reproducible histopathological and behavioral deficits. Importantly, clinically relevant behavioral consequences, including forelimb function and decreased hand function, can be evaluated.[6,7] In a successful translational research program in SCI, it is important to consider evaluating new therapies in both cervical and thoracic models.

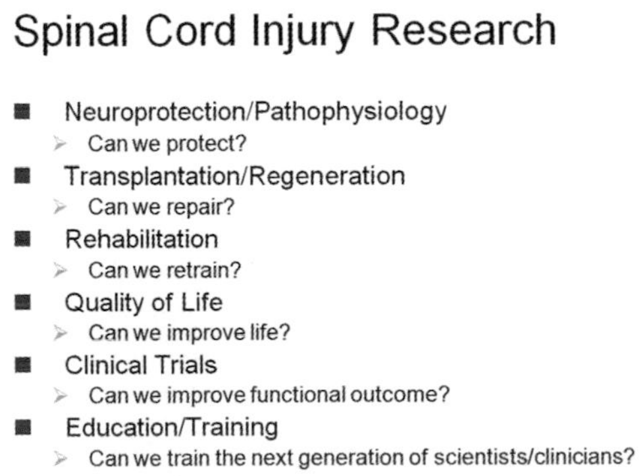

Spinal Cord Injury Research

- Neuroprotection/Pathophysiology
  - Can we protect?
- Transplantation/Regeneration
  - Can we repair?
- Rehabilitation
  - Can we retrain?
- Quality of Life
  - Can we improve life?
- Clinical Trials
  - Can we improve functional outcome?
- Education/Training
  - Can we train the next generation of scientists/clinicians?

Fig. 28.3 Multidisciplinary research programs targeting SCI may include several key elements.

Another variable regarding injury models is whether the model mimics mild, moderate, or severe injury. As previously mentioned, the SCI population includes a range of injury severities that can be replicated in a controlled laboratory environment. In contrast to severe injury, mildly and moderately injured animals show more robust evidence for spontaneous patterns of functional recovery that sometimes can make the assessment of therapeutic interventions challenging. Thus the use of SCI models that take into consideration injury severity and the heterogeneity of human SCI will maximize the chances of finding effective therapies that protect and promote recovery in the clinic.

Functional Outcome Measures

A variety of functional outcome measures are used to assess injury severity and therapeutic interventions in animal models of SCI. The Basso, Beattie, Bresnahan (BBB) Locomotive Assessment Scale is routinely used to evaluate locomotive function in rodents following thoracic SCI.[8] This 21-point scale is an advantageous method to assess different aspects of walking over a repetitive testing period. Other motor tests, including the inclined plane, number of foot faults, and beam walking, can provide important information regarding deficits in motor function that are so critical to the human population with SCI. In terms of cervical injury, new testing strategies are now being conducted to evaluate forelimb function, including hand grip and strength. The ability of animals to remove pellets from a cylinder allows investigators to more critically evaluate fine motor hand skills after SCI.[9]

Over the last several years, abnormal sensation following SCI has become an important quality of life issue in terms of modeling SCI in the laboratory.[10] A significant number of patients show abnormal sensations, including neuropathic pain, that seriously affect their ability to carry out normal daily functions. Thus more emphasis is being placed on assessing sensory function through a variety of approaches after SCI. Because some treatment strategies may have the potential to reduce or aggravate neuropathic pain, these types of sensory outcomes are critical in preclinical work.

Structural Outcome Measures

In the majority of SCI preclinical studies, histopathological approaches are used to evaluate contusion size as well as percentages of gray and white matter sparing following various treatment strategies.[11] Nonbiased stereological approaches can be recommended to quantitate numbers of cells either by routine histological stains or by immunofluorescent approaches. These types of morphological strategies allow for the characterization of neuropathological changes at the injury site or occurring in spinal cord levels rostral or caudal at specific times after injury. Because different treatments may selectively affect gray or white matter pathology, the assessment of both gray and white matter vulnerability and sparing after treatments is critical as we attempt to move our discoveries forward.

Confocal microscopy is also being used to identify endogenous and migrating cell types in spinal cord tissues after injury and to evaluate treatment effects on cell survival and other cellular responses to injury.[12] With immunofluorescent approaches, cells can be labeled with one or more specific antibodies that allow critical questions to be asked concerning the phenotype or function of a particular cell. These imaging approaches are becoming very useful to investigate spinal cord regeneration,[13] endogenous reparative responses to trauma and cellular transplantation strategies to promote reparative processes and recovery.[14]

Electron microscopy continues to be an important tool in the area of SCI where evidence for axonal demyelination and remyelination is frequently seen. Ultrathin sections are examined with a transmission electron microscope to clarify the ultrastructural characteristics of various cell types and complement the evaluation procedures using other microscopic approaches that have been discussed. The availability of these different morphological outcome measures provides important information regarding the structural integrity of the tissue as well as the effects of various treatment strategies.

Core Facilities

In many instances, established core facilities can facilitate the successful steps necessary for an effective translational program. Core facilities that involve animal surgery, for example, can recruit personnel with expertise in producing SCI. Core facilities can maintain expensive instruments, including SCI devices, that therefore do not have to be replicated in multiple principle investigator laboratories. This approach helps maximize the consistency of lesion production and reduces potential drift in injury severity that can be seen over time.

The increased use of transgenic mice has emphasized the need for well-maintained transgenic facilities within research programs. These facilities are built especially to house and breed these expensive animals for research programs. Special needs, including environmental filters and care of the animals to enhance breeding, are all important for these types of facilities.

An important component of translational programs is critical animal care after SCI. SCI animals are highly susceptible to infection and require special attention to maximize good outcome and long-term survival. These animals can become infected and require care to reduce discomfort and other consequences of the injury. Personnel experienced in caring for these animals, including bladder expression and conducting other steps that ensure the health of the animals, are critical.

As discussed, behavioral testing is an extremely important clinical outcome measure that is commonly used in SCI investigations. Several different behavioral tasks are often utilized, and expertise is required to ensure that the behavioral tasks are conducted and scored properly. Testing must be done in a blinded fashion so no information is given to the evaluators regarding the various treatment groups. Thus, randomization and blind assessment strategies are necessary as interventions are assessed. Because behavioral testing apparatuses are expensive, a behavioral core facility allows for the maximization of the equipment and alleviates the need for similar devices to be purchased in multiple principal investigator laboratories.

A histopathology/immunocytochemistry core also allows investigators to have tissues processed for routine histopathological approaches, including paraffin, frozen, or vibratome sectioning. This core ensures the quality and consistency of the product in terms of embedding, sectioning, and specimen staining. Automatic processing machines allow for the tissue to be embedded by the core, again with the appropriate expertise to minimize damage to the tissue. Once the tissue is embedded, technicians qualified to cut the tissue allow consistency of cutting and staining and maximizing tissue availability.

Imaging cores can contain and maintain expensive microscopes and other equipment that are used by multiple investigators using a sign-up sheet approach. Confocal microscopes, transmission electron microscopes, fluorescent microscopes, and double-head scopes are made available to the investigators in such a core environment. Recently, the critical need for nonbiased stereological approaches for evaluating histopathological outcome has been emphasized in the scientific literature. Thus various approaches, including multiple imaging stations that allow for the use of nonbiased approaches for the evaluation of tissue responses to injury, are best located in these core facilities.

One of the exciting areas of SCI research is the use of cell therapies to protect and promote recovery.[14] Various cells, including adult human cells, stem cells, or engineered cells, are transplanted to enhance protection and repair after SCI. Thus it is important that core cell culture facilities also be considered in a successful translational program. These cores are set up and run with the appropriate technical staff to maintain healthy cultured cells as well as to prepare cells for transplantation. Other specialty cores, including viral vector or high content screening, are now being added to the list of core programs to emphasize the cutting-edge nature of our research field.

Replication Studies

One question that scientists commonly debate at traumatic brain injury and SCI conferences is what specific information should be required by the scientific community prior to moving a new treatment into the clinic. It would be helpful if there were a defined road map to follow in testing a particular drug or other agent in preclinical models prior to human testing. Many agree that some type of replication studies would be very advantageous prior to moving new therapies to the clinic.[11] Using this approach, published data from peer-reviewed manuscripts that are clinically relevant are considered for replication by independent laboratories. Fortunately, the National Institutes of Health/ National Institute of Neurological Disorders and Stroke over the last several years has funded several laboratories to conduct these replication studies for this particular reason.[11,15–17] It is felt that, if studies can be successfully replicated and published, it may provide a strong rationale for moving the studied therapy to the clinic. Similar strategies are also being considered in other clinical fields, such as traumatic injury and stroke, to enhance the successful translation of preclinical findings. In these cases, multiple laboratories using different models of central nervous system (CNS) injury will test similar therapeutic strategies to document efficacy. It is felt that if multiple laboratories show efficacy of a particular agent using their own established injury models and outcome measures, it is strong evidence that these treatments may prove efficacious in a heterogeneous patient population. Because of the large number of failures that have been reported in clinical trials targeting CNS injury, it is suggested that established translational research SCI programs be involved in replication studies supported by the scientific community.

Research Team Approach

As previously discussed, the complexity of human SCI demands the involvement of many types of scientists and clinicians who can provide specific expertise as we think about this clinical problem. For example, cell biologists are required to understand the normal function of cells and what surface or intracellular mechanisms might be appropriate for targeting therapies to stop destructive mechanisms.[12] Developmental neuroscientists have become very important because of their expertise in brain and spinal cord development, including complex cellular maturation processes and the role of guidance and inhibitory molecules in circuit formation and target recognition during development. These concepts, which were first described in the developmental literature, now are being evaluated and discussed in the acute CNS injury field. Systems neuroscientists bring critical expertise in terms of circuit and synaptic function underlying the behavioral consequences of SCI. Because of the complexity of the spinal cord, including injury severity and potential for circuit dysfunction and plasticity that may occur after injury, it is important that these investigators be included in the investigations.

As already emphasized, functional testing involving behavioral and electrophysiological studies is critical as we evaluate therapies and the consequences of injury. Scientists trained in the fields of psychology and animal behavior are critical as we develop clinically relevant outcome measures that may help predict successful clinical trials. Electrophysiological expertise continues to be important as we assess cellular responses to injury and evaluate circuit function and plasticity.

A critical component of a translational spinal cord research program is the involvement of clinicians at all steps of the investigative and discovery process. Clinicians who treat SCI patients regularly can bring to the laboratory useful information regarding clinical questions that merit investigation. While moving bench findings to the clinic, it is also clear that clinical problems or questions that require attention be introduced into the preclinical setting for the basic scientists to work on. Therapeutic approaches that are being anticipated for clinical testing need to be discussed with treating physicians to determine their clinical relevance as well as potential risk factors. Because of the emergence of bioengineering in the area of restorative strategies to improve function in the disabled population, the communication between laboratories doing medical research and biomedical engineering should also be enhanced.[18,19] This research team approach invites many different types of experts to focus on the problem of SCI and allows for a holistic approach to be concentrated on this complex clinical problem.

Federal Regulations Involving Clinical Trials

The regulatory guidelines for moving new discoveries to the clinic include multiple steps and approaches.[20] Many of these steps are not routinely used in laboratories where animal models of injury are being produced and novel treatments are tested. Therefore, expertise in US Food and Drug Administration (FDA) regulations and guidelines is critical as one attempts to obtain approval for new treatments. Preclinical studies assessing efficacy, risk factors, toxicity, or other factors that could influence or alter a drug's effect on a patient have to be fully characterized prior to initiation of a trial. In effective translational research programs, that type of regulatory expertise can be found within the university setting or through consultant agreements that allow a successful stepwise approach to moving things forward for FDA approval.

In addition to FDA guidelines, specialized facilities are also required to obtain FDA approval for a new treatment.[21] Good laboratory practice (GLP) is required on some aspects of the preclinical studies to ensure quality control of the various experiments. GLP facilities can be partnered with companies that have expertise in these approaches. Good manufacturing practices (GMP) are also critical as one processes cells or drugs for clinical use. Again, expertise is required to ensure that these procedures are done properly with appropriate reagents and paperwork requirements.

Translational Clinical Programs in Spinal Cord Injury

As one attempts to move discoveries forward, it is clear that various clinical programs are required to make such a program successful. In traumatic SCI, for example, departments of emergency medicine, neurosurgery, clinical care units, neuroradiology, and rehabilitation all are critical components of the patient treatment programs. Thus it is important that these various departments and programs be integrated into the translational research program so that clinical expertise at different levels can be incorporated into the overall treatment strategy. It is clear that an SCI patient goes through various phases of treatment, evaluation, and care, and a smooth transition from one treatment phase to the next is required for optimal benefit of the various treatment modalities. In the acute setting, stabilization of the patient with attention to physiological variables is of critical importance to limiting secondary insults and injury mechanisms.[22,23] In the critical care unit, management of the patient for days after injury necessitates expertise in these areas. Surgical strategies, including decompression procedures as well as stabilization of the spinal column, also offer the patient the best opportunity to recover from the injuries. When appropriate, rehabilitation strategies need to be introduced that will maximize recovery patterns and improve the ability of the individual to have a good quality of life.[24]

Technology Transfer

In today's world, the importance of intellectual property and patent applications is becoming ever more important. Research discoveries that have the potential for translation into the clinic require significant amounts of funding to support clinical studies and trials. Thus the ability to obtain intellectual property rights or patents for these particular discoveries will help investigators move their science to the clinic. Alternatively, funding for investigations can be obtained through federal grants and various SCI foundations. The ability to have intellectual property expertise in a university setting to support translational research greatly enhances the ability to move discoveries into the clinic.

Education, Training, and Awareness Programs

Another important function of an integrated SCI center is to train the next generation of scientists to conduct spinal cord research. Many center faculty are associated with basic science, clinical departments, and various graduate programs. Thus there is the opportunity to recruit young trainees, including high school, medical, and graduate students and postdoctoral fellows into the laboratory. Also, visiting scientists from universities and hospitals can spend dedicated research time on conducting SCI studies. These training experiences establish lifelong relationships between the scientists and institutions.

As new information regarding recent advancements in SCI become available, it is critical that consumers be introduced to existing support groups and have a place to be educated and informed regarding progress. Established research centers and programs can take a lead role in providing SCI awareness and in directing individuals to appropriate surgical and rehabilitation programs. Thus education, training, and the promotion of awareness of SCI programs and discoveries are important functions of translational research programs. Through tours, presentations, and information placed on SCI program Web sites, all of these strategies can be efficiently communicated to the public.

Fundraising and Philanthropy

Most scientists rely on research funds to support their programs through grant applications to the federal government as well as other SCI funding agencies. Grant applications usually require a significant amount of preliminary data and remain extremely competitive. Another complementary strategy that is used to obtain research funding is through philanthropy and fundraising efforts. Grateful patients as well as individuals interested in neuroscience are introduced to the subject matter and progress being made in the field. Funds available through philanthropy can allow for the purchase of expensive pieces of equipment, provide startup funds for new collaborations, as well as support studies that, although high risk, may have significant implications for the field. Scientists and laboratories thus need to consider multiple sources of funding to support their research programs.

Conclusion

An effective translational research program targeting the area of SCI today is multidisciplinary and involves different types of scientists and clinicians. SCI is an extremely complicated problem and therefore requires a concentrated effort from various investigators bringing time and effort into this exciting but difficult field. These are truly exciting times in the area of SCI, with new treatments on the horizon and clinical trials being proposed and conducted. Only with the continued support of the private and research communities will the successful translation of our basic science discoveries be moved into treatment of patients with paralysis.

Pearls

- Published studies are being replicated by independent groups.
- These are exciting times in SCI research.
- Some treatments are being translated to the clinic.
- Public awareness regarding SCI has been emphasized.
- Large SCI research groups are working together.

Pitfalls

- SCI is a complicated injury.
- SCI affects many organ systems, not just the spinal cord.
- Clinical trials are expensive and difficult to conduct.
- There is a need for clinical trial networks to recruit patients.

References

1. Hawryluk GW, Rowland J, Kwon BK, Fehlings MG. Protection and repair of the injured spinal cord: a review of completed, ongoing, and planned clinical trials for acute spinal cord injury. Neurosurg Focus 2008;25(5):E14
2. Kleitman N. Under one roof: the Miami Project to Cure Paralysis model for spinal cord injury research. Neuroscientist 2001;7(3):192–201
3. Akhtar AZ, Pippin JJ, Sandusky CB. Animal models in spinal cord injury: a review. Rev Neurosci 2008;19(1):47–60
4. Dietrich WD. Confirming an experimental therapy prior to transfer to humans: what is the ideal? J Rehabil Res Dev 2003;40(4, Suppl 1):63–69
5. Anderson KD, Sharp KG, Hofstadter M, Irvine KA, Murray M, Steward O. Forelimb locomotor assessment scale (FLAS): novel assessment of forelimb dysfunction after cervical spinal cord injury. Exp Neurol 2009;220(1):23–33
6. Pearse DD, Lo TP Jr, Cho KS, et al. Histopathological and behavioral characterization of a novel cervical spinal cord displacement contusion injury in the rat. J Neurotrauma 2005;22(6):680–702
7. Montoya CP, Campbell-Hope LJ, Pemberton KD, Dunnett SB. The "staircase test": a measure of independent forelimb reaching and grasping abilities in rats. J Neurosci Methods 1991;36(2-3):219–228
8. Basso DM, Beattie MS, Bresnahan JC. A sensitive and reliable locomotor rating scale for open field testing in rats. J Neurotrauma 1995;12(1):1–21
9. Whishaw IQ, Pellis SM. The structure of skilled forelimb reaching in the rat: a proximally driven movement with a single distal rotatory component. Behav Brain Res 1990;41(1):49–59
10. Gris D, Marsh DR, Oatway MA, et al. Transient blockade of the CD11d/CD18 integrin reduces secondary damage after spinal cord injury, improving sensory, autonomic, and motor function. J Neurosci 2004;24(16):4043–4051
11. Pinzon A, Marcillo A, Pabon D, Bramlett HM, Bunge MB, Dietrich WD. A re-assessment of erythropoietin as a neuroprotective agent following rat spinal cord compression or contusion injury. Exp Neurol 2008;213(1):129–136
12. Kwon BK, Tetzlaff W, Grauer JN, Beiner J, Vaccaro AR. Pathophysiology and pharmacologic treatment of acute spinal cord injury. Spine J 2004; 4(4):451–464
13. Verma P, Fawcett J. Spinal cord regeneration. Adv Biochem Eng Biotechnol 2005;94:43–66
14. Eftekharpour E, Karimi-Abdolrezaee S, Fehlings MG. Current status of experimental cell replacement approaches to spinal cord injury. Neurosurg Focus 2008;24(3-4):E19
15. Pinzon A, Marcillo A, Quintana A, et al. A re-assessment of minocycline as a neuroprotective agent in a rat spinal cord contusion model. Brain Res 2008;1243:146–151
16. Steward O, Sharp K, Selvan G, et al. A re-assessment of the consequences of delayed transplantation of olfactory lamina propria following complete spinal cord transection in rats. Exp Neurol 2006;198(2):483–499
17. Steward O, Sharp K, Yee KM, Hofstadter M. A re-assessment of the effects of a Nogo-66 receptor antagonist on regenerative growth of axons and locomotor recovery after spinal cord injury in mice. Exp Neurol 2008;209(2):446–468
18. Grill WM, Norman SE, Bellamkonda RV. Implanted neural interfaces: biochallenges and engineered solutions. Annu Rev Biomed Eng 2009;11:1–24
19. Willerth SM, Sakiyama-Elbert SE. Approaches to neural tissue engineering using scaffolds for drug delivery. Adv Drug Deliv Rev 2007;59(4-5): 325–338
20. Sagen J. Cellular therapies for spinal cord injury: what will the FDA need to approve moving from the laboratory to the human? J Rehabil Res Dev 2003;40(4, Suppl 1):71–79
21. Laurencot CM, Ruppel S. Regulatory aspects for translating gene therapy research into the clinic. Methods Mol Biol 2009;542:397–421
22. Deletis V, Sala F. Intraoperative neurophysiological monitoring of the spinal cord during spinal cord and spine surgery: a review focus on the corticospinal tracts. Clin Neurophysiol 2008;119(2):248–264
23. Schinkel C, Anastasiadis AP. The timing of spinal stabilization in polytrauma and in patients with spinal cord injury. Curr Opin Crit Care 2008;14(6):685–689
24. Sadowsky CL, McDonald JW. Activity-based restorative therapies: concepts and applications in spinal cord injury-related neurorehabilitation. Dev Disabil Res Rev 2009;15(2):112–116

29

North American Clinical Trials Network: Building a Clinical Trials Network for Spinal Cord Injury

Robert G. Grossman, Elizabeth G. Toups, Ralph F. Frankowski, Keith D. Burau, Susan P. Howley for the NACTN Investigators

Key Points

1. Organizational, regulatory and financial barriers must be overcome to bring new basic scientific discoveries that have the promise of improving the outcome of spinal cord injury to clinical trials. The present chapter describes the steps taken to overcome these barriers and to develop a clinical trials network for new treatments for spinal cord injury.

The rapid advance of knowledge of the cellular and molecular responses of the spinal cord to injury has led to therapies that have improved functional recovery after spinal cord injury (SCI) in laboratory studies.[1] Some of these therapies have been used in small numbers of SCI patients.[2] However, most of these promising developments have not been brought to phase 2 or 3 clinical trials that have the design and statistical power to demonstrate efficacy because of the formidable organizational, regulatory, and financial barriers that must be overcome to conduct such trials. This chapter describes the steps in building the North American Clinical Trials Network (NACTN) for Treatment of Spinal Cord Injury. NACTN was created in 2004 with the support of the Christopher Reeve Foundation with the goal of overcoming these barriers. The Telemedicine and Advanced Technology Research Center (TATRC) United States Army Medical Research and Materiel Command (USAMRMC) of the Department of Defense has supported NACTN since 2006. Since 2007, Walter Reed Army Medical Center (WRAMC) has been part of NACTN with the goal of comparing the natural history of military and civilian injuries. NACTN's mission is to carry out clinical trials of the comparative effectiveness of new therapies for SCI using a consortium of neurosurgery departments at university-affiliated medical center hospitals with medical, nursing, and rehabilitation personnel who are skilled in the evaluation and management of SCI. NACTN is the only standing network for clinical trials for SCI in North America. NACTN is composed of clinical, data management, and pharmacological centers.

NACTN Centers and Investigators

Clinical Centers (Fig. 29.1)

- The Methodist Hospital, Houston–Coordinating Center
  - Principal Investigator, Robert G. Grossman, MD
  - Clinical Trials Manager, Elizabeth Toups, MS, RN, CCRP
- The University of Texas–Memorial Hermann Hospital, Houston
  - Investigator, Michele Johnson, MD
- The University of Virginia Hospital, Charlottesville
  - Investigators, Christopher I. Shaffrey, MD, John Jane, Sr., MD, PhD
- The University of Toronto, Toronto
  - Investigators, Michael Fehlings, MD, PhD, Charles Tator, MD, PhD
- The University of Louisville, Louisville
  - Investigators, Susan Harkema, PhD, Jonathan Hodes, MD
- University of Maryland, Baltimore
  - Investigator, Bizhan Aarabi, MD
- Walter Reed Army Medical Center
  - Investigator, Michael Rosner, MD
- University of Miami, Miami
  - Investigator, James Guest, MD, PhD
- Thomas Jefferson University, Philadelphia
  - Investigator, James Harrop, MD

Data Management Center

- The University of Texas School of Public Health, Houston
  - Investigators, Ralph Frankowski, PhD, Keith Burau, PhD

Pharmacological Center

- University of Houston, College of Pharmacy, Houston
  - Investigator, Diana Chow, PhD

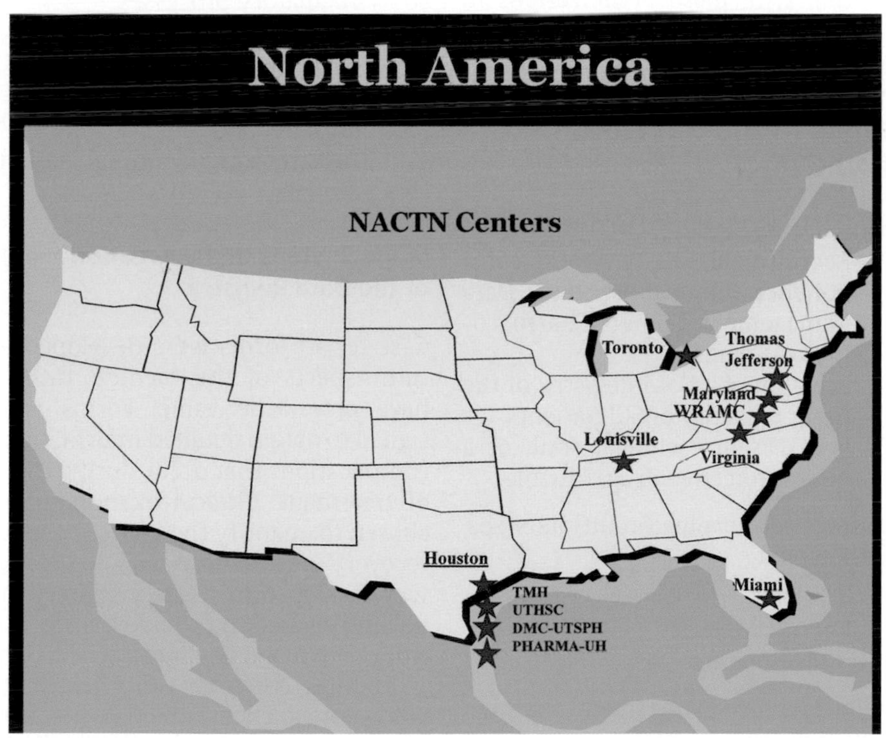

Fig. 29.1 NACTN clinical centers.

Background

An increasing number of clinical trial networks have been formed to study a wide variety of diseases.[3] This growth has been encouraged by the National Institutes of Health (NIH)[4] and the Institute of Medicine,[5] and it has been facilitated by Internet communication and the formation of societies and journals devoted to clinical trials.[6] The prototype of a clinical trial network for SCI was the National Acute Spinal Cord Injury Study (NASCIS) supported by the NIH, which published its first trial of corticosteroid therapy for SCI in 1984.[7] NASCIS did not continue as a clinical trial organization for testing new therapies after the publication of its third corticosteroid trial in 1997.[8] In the past decade, SCI clinical trial networks have been organized in Europe—the European Multicenter Study about Spinal Cord Injury (EMSCI)[9]—and in Canada and the United States—the Surgical Treatment in Acute Spinal Cord Injury Study (STASCIS),[10] which was formed to study early surgical decompression of cord injuries. NACTN is collaborating with these organizations in studies of outcome after SCI.

Stages in the Development of NACTN

- NACTN has developed in three stages:
  1. Recruitment of network components: Clinical Centers, Data Management Center, Pharmacological Center
  2. Creation of a Data Registry of the natural history of SCI patients
  3. NACTN's first clinical trial, of a neuroprotective drug, riluzole

Each stage has involved multiple steps, as described next.

Stage 1: Recruitment of Network Components

- *Clinical centers* were sought that met the following criteria:
  1. Emergency transport systems providing rapid transport of SCI patients to a level 1 emergency department at the clinical center
  2. An intensive care unit with neurointensivists
  3. Neurosurgical, orthopedic, critical care, and physiatry staff with research and clinical expertise in neurotraumatology
  4. A closely affiliated rehabilitation hospital
  5. Mutual trust of the centers in each other based upon previous joint experience in research

The initial five clinical centers were expanded to nine centers between 2006 and 2008. Each center is led by a principal investigator and at some centers a co-principal investigator. Each clinical center has a study coordinator, usually a nurse-clinician, and two clinical research assistants.

- *A Data Management and Statistical Center (DMC)* was sought that had experience with large clinical trials, experimental design, and familiarity with medical and governmental regulatory processes.
- *A Pharmacological Center* was sought that had experience in pharmacokinetic and pharmacodynamic measurements of medications, including metabolism in animal and human studies.

Stage 2: Steps in the Creation of the Data Registry

Case report forms were developed to capture aspects of the medical history that have prognostic value. Forms were designed to obtain detailed information about complications that occur during the course of treatment. Clinical examinations were chosen to quantify the course of functional recovery in patients. A data archival system was developed to create a registry that can be interrogated to provide a historical control group to aid in clinical trial design.

Multiple meetings were held by the investigators to choose the data elements that would be collected and to design the case report forms. The investigators had the benefit of consulting existing SCI registries, including those of the Model Spinal Cord Injury Systems,[11] the International Spinal Cord Injury Data Set Elements that are currently being incorporated into the NIH–National Institute of Neurological Disorders and Stroke (NINDS) Common Data Elements[12] and those of STASCIS and EMSCI. Developing prognostic algorithms required collecting comprehensive data that included a medical history, medications, the radiology of the injury, medical and surgical treatment, the physiological response to injury and complications, as well as neurological examinations from the earliest feasible time to examinations during rehabilitation and for a year after injury.

The case report forms are divided between measures obtained during the acute hospitalization following injury and functional outcome measures obtained during rehabilitation. The case report forms are available from the coordinating center to investigators who are developing clinical trials.

Acute Hospitalization Forms

Data are collected under 12 headings:

- Contact Sheet: Hospital Name, ID Number, Patient and Family Contact
- Page 1 Demographic Data; Medical History
- Page 2 Circumstances of Injury, Evacuation Details
- Page 3 Initial Clinical Status; Glasgow Coma Scale (GCS) score; Abbreviated Injury Score (AIS)
- Page 4A,B ASIA (American Spinal Injury Association) Motor, Sensory Scales at < 72 h and 2 wk
- Page 5 Type of Neurological Injury; Type of Bony Injury
- Page 6 Imaging Cord and Canal Diameters: CT; MRI; CT/Myelogram
- Page 7A,B Nonoperative Treatment: Medical; Traction–Reduction
- Page 8A,B Posterior Surgical Treatment: Procedural Details; Levels
- Page 9A,B Anterior Surgical Treatment: Procedural Details; Levels
- Page 10A–D Complications: Cardiac; Pulmonary; Hematological; GI/GU; Infection; Skin; Psychiatric
- Page 11 Acute Hospitalization Outcome Summary

Rehabilitation and Long-Term Follow-Up Forms

Functional outcomes are measured at specified times:

- ASIA Scale (American Spinal Injury Association) at 3, 6, and 12 months after injury
- FIM (Functional Independence Measure) at Acute Discharge, Rehabilitation Discharge, 3, 6, 12 months
- SCIM (Spinal Cord Independence Measure) at Acute Discharge, Rehabilitation Discharge, 3, 6, 12 months
- WISCI-II (Walking Index for Spinal Cord Injury) at Acute Discharge, Rehabilitation Discharge, 3, 6, 12 months

Data Quality Control: The NACTN Manual of Operations

The Manual of Operations (MOO) was written to serve as a guide for completing the data forms. It is a 55-page document that summarizes the research protocol and inclusion/exclusion criteria, and gives explicit instructions about each form. The center study coordinators are also in frequent telephone and e-mail communication with the Clinical Coordinating Center and the Data Management and Statistical Center (DMC) to clarify questions that arise.

Data Form Design and Transmission of Data from the Centers to the Data Management and Statistical Center

A multipart paper/optical scanning system was judged to be the best initial system for data collection because it would allow for multiple protocol iterations and adjustments required as experience was gained in data collection. The data collection system is a high-security system. Data from patients that are submitted to the DMC are identified only by a code number for the center and a number for the patient. Each data collection form was designed in Verity TeleForm software that uses an optical recognition system to digitally capture paper-based images and their content by scanner and allows customized field-by-field data verification. The data processing activities are managed by an integrated data system that uses TeleForm for data entry and verification and then uploads data to a secure Structured Query Language (SQL) server, which simultaneously generates Microsoft (MS) Access files and tables. This integrated system is augmented by a parallel data quality control system.

The NACTN registry receives completed paper forms via mail from the clinical centers. Data forms are reviewed for completeness before being sent to the optical scanner. Forms are held by the electronic data processing system until they are audited by a verification program that allows field-by-field data verification. Each scanned form is maintained in the system as a TIF file, allowing computerized images of the data forms to be stored electronically. Once the data forms have been verified, the data go to a secure password-protected SQL server database. This server is backed up nightly with archival storage maintained at two alternate off-site locations. Once data have been committed to the data tables, the data are subjected to logic and edit checks as well as cross-checks between different form types. A separate file tracks each batch of data entered through the scanning system. Additionally, a correction database has been developed to document data change or data transactions that result from logic/error checks or updates received from clinical centers. Computer programs have also been written to generate one-page patient narrative reports. Export procedures were developed to convert data to Statistical Analysis System (SAS) and State formats to facilitate statistical analyses. Programs have been developed to tabulate summary statistics and generate reports. All steps from data logging, entry, committing to SQL and MS Access, editing, reporting, and summary analysis have been closely documented and are known by multiple members at the DMC. This redundancy and shared responsibility reduces the turnaround time from receipt of forms to generation of data-editing reports sent back to the clinics. As patients are enrolled in the registry, the quality of data on key measures is evaluated and, when necessary, measures are refined or clarified in the DMC Manual of Operations.

Steps in the Initiation of the Data Registry

Protocol Development

A protocol was written that stated the goals of the registry, the inclusion/exclusion enrollment criteria, the process of data collection, and the precautions to ensure patient protection and the security of the data.

An Informed Consent Form and an Explanatory Brochure

An Informed Consent Form (ICF) and an Explanatory Brochure for patients were written.

Institutional Review Board Approval of the Protocol and the Informed Consent Form

Institutional review board (IRB) Approval of the Protocol and the ICF was obtained from the institutional review boards of the centers, and from the Human Research Protection Office (HRPO), Department of Defense (DOD).

Training in Data Collection

Two workshops were held for the investigators, nurse clinicians, physiatrists, and coordinators at which they received training in the ASIA examination and in the data collection methodologies.

Data in the Registry

The registry has enrolled 414 patients with ASIA grades A to E, from October 2005 to October 2010.

Stage 3: NACTN's Initial Clinical Trial

A Phase 1 Study of the Safety and Pharmacokinetics of Riluzole in Patients with Traumatic Acute Spinal Cord Injury was undertaken to investigate its therapeutic effect in SCI.

Riluzole is a neuroprotective drug that blocks glutamate-mediated sodium and calcium ion entry into neurons and glia and blocks glutamate release from presynaptic terminals. It has been shown to be effective in limiting traumatic damage to the spinal cord in laboratory studies.[13] Riluzole presented several advantages as a therapy in NACTN's first trial, in which the working of the network was being tested. Riluzole is used clinically in the treatment of amyotrophic lateral sclerosis (ALS).[14] It is relatively inexpensive, it can be given orally, it has a favorable safety profile in ALS patients, it can be measured in blood and cerebrospinal fluid, and costs are reasonable for laboratory studies that are necessary for monitoring its use.

Research Design and Methods

The initial phase of the study is a multisite, single-arm active treatment pilot study involving 36 subjects. If the rate of adverse effects in the initial trial group is no greater than that in the NACTN database, a phase 2 study of a larger number of patients will be undertaken as a comparative efficacy trial. Features of the riluzole protocol are the detail in which possible adverse effects of the therapy are being studied, and the use of pharmacokinetic and pharmacodynamic data and its correlation with adverse effects and efficacy. Previous studies of drug therapy for SCI have not measured blood and cerebrospinal fluid levels of the therapeutic drugs to see if effective or toxic levels of drug were reaching the spinal cord and brain.

Multiple steps were involved in planning and in implementing the riluzole trial, which enrolled its first patient on April 12, 2010.

Selection of a Therapy and Development of the Protocol

1. Selection of riluzole after discussion by the investigators of candidate therapies
2. Writing the research protocol
3. Creation of a schedule of events, a day-by-day hourly schedule of tests, procedures, laboratory work, rules for drug administration
4. Modifying elements of the registry case report forms for the requirements of the trial
5. Designing case report forms (CRFs)
6. Writing a Manual of Operations and patient brochure
7. Writing the Informed Consent Form
8. Setting up the study database at the DMC
9. Developing new methods of measuring riluzole in plasma and cerebrospinal fluid

Trial Initiation: Compliance with Regulatory Requirements

1. Approval of the research protocol by the HRPO, DOD
2. Harmonization of the IRB requirements of each center with requirements of the HRPO; final approval of harmonized protocol and ICF by each IRB
3. Appointment of a central trial monitor, a distinguished physiatrist at a university not affiliated with any of the centers. For a phase 2 study, a data monitoring and safety committee will be established.
4. Appointment of a local trial monitor at each clinical center
5. Trial initiation meeting of all investigators and coordinators; intensive 2 day review of the protocol, the schedule of events, the rules and procedures for reporting adverse events, interim analysis, and stopping rules
6. Writing and signing of site agreements between the trial sponsor and the network centers. The site agreements are a contract setting forth the statement of work, the responsibilities of the center, and deadlines for completion of work.

Trial Conduct at Each Center

1. Creation of patient data binders
2. Creation of regulatory binders
3. At the Coordinating Center, files of all regulatory documents and files of adverse events

Appointment of a Site Monitor

An individual trained in monitoring clinical trials who has been conducting onsite monitoring at each clinical center and reviewing CRFs, regulatory documents, source documentation, adherence to protocol, and drug accountability in accordance with federal regulations and Good Clinical Practices (GCPs)

Ensuring Communication between Network Centers

1. Writing a Governance Manual
2. Forming committees: Executive; Selection of Therapies; Publications; Data Management
3. Forming Neurological Outcomes Assessment Task Force, led by Dr. Susan Harkema, to develop improved quantitative outcome measures
4. Conducting monthly conference calls by the investigators and coordinators, the committees, and the Neurological Outcome Assessment (NOA) Task Force
5. Posting of NACTN documents and communications on an FTP Web site

Acknowledgments

- Dr. Branko Kopjar, Associate Professor, Department of Health Services, University of Washington, contributed to the development of the riluzole protocol.
- The study sponsor was the Christopher Reeve Foundation, Short Hills, New Jersey.
- Support was provided by the Telemedicine and Advanced Technology Research Center (TATRC) US Army Medical Research and Materiel Command.
- Additional support was provided by Mission Connect, a project of the TIRR Foundation.

Pearls

- Clinical trial organization and implementation require a fusion of many disparate elements in our complex, nonintegrated medical system.
- The most important elements in building a clinical trials network is the dedication of the investigators and the clinical and scientific staff and the willing participation of patients, to whom we owe our gratitude.
- Current thinking is that a trial of a new therapy for SCI will require a cohort of 200 to 250 patients to achieve statistical significance. Depending on the therapy, the cost of such a study can be in the millions of dollars. An urgent question is how to apportion these costs between governmental and private funding agencies, pharmaceutical companies, voluntary health organizations, not-for-profit hospitals, philanthropy, and health insurers. NACTN has combined support from multiple sources to develop a clinical trial network. We believe that a parallel effort to develop a consortium of funding sources is required to support clinical trials of new therapy to improve the outcome of SCI.

Pitfalls

- Randomized, multicenter, clinical trials require extensive planning that frequently takes 1 to 2 years to complete. Additional time is required for harmonization of the protocol with specific requirements that individual IRBs request, and which must be acceptable to all of the other IRBs, requiring frequent protocol revisions and IRB filings.
- The complexity of planning and initiating multicenter clinical trials and the cost of such trials have been major factors in preventing new therapies from being brought from the laboratory into clinical practice.

References

1. Rossignol S, Schwab M, Schwartz M, Fehlings MG. Spinal cord injury: time to move? J Neurosci 2007;27(44):11782–11792
2. Human Spinal Cord Injury: New and Emerging Therapies. http://www.sci-therapies.info, 2006. Accessed May 22, 2012
3. Cobb JP, Cairns CB, Bulger E, et al. The United States critical illness and injury trials group: an introduction. J Trauma 2009;67(2, Suppl): S159–S160
4. National Institutes of Health. NIH Roadmap for Medical Research. NIH Common Fund Web site. 2006. http://nihroadmap.nih.gov. Accessed May 11, 2012
5. Institute of Medicine. Spinal Cord Injury: Progress, Promise and Priorities. Committee on Spinal Cord Injury, Board on Neuroscience and Behavioral Health; Liverman CT, et al, eds. Washington, DC: National Academies Press; 2005
6. Society for Clinical Trials. http://sctweb.org
7. Bracken MB, Collins WF, Freeman DF, et al. Efficacy of methylprednisolone in acute spinal cord injury. JAMA 1984;251(1):45–52
8. Bracken MB, Shepard MJ, Holford TR, et al. Administration of methylprednisolone for 24 or 48 hours or tirilazad mesylate for 48 hours in the treatment of acute spinal cord injury. Results of the Third National Acute Spinal Cord Injury Randomized Controlled Trial. National Acute Spinal Cord Injury Study. JAMA 1997;277(20):1597–1604
9. European Multicenter Study about Spinal Cord Injury. http://www.emsci.org, 2006. Accessed May 11, 2012
10. Fehlings M, Vaccaro A, Aarabi B, et al. A prospective, multicenter trial to evaluate the role and timing of decompression in patients with cervical spinal cord injury: One year results of the STASCIS study. Can J Surg 2009;52(Suppl):10
11. Marino RJ, Ditunno JF Jr, Donovan WH, Maynard F Jr. Neurologic recovery after traumatic spinal cord injury: data from the Model Spinal Cord Injury Systems. Arch Phys Med Rehabil 1999;80(11):1391–1396
12. Biering-Sørensen F, Charlifue S, Devivo MJ, et al. Incorporation of the International Spinal Cord Injury Data Set elements into the National Institute of Neurological Disorders and Stroke Common Data Elements. Spinal Cord 2011;49(1):60–64
13. Schwartz G, Fehlings MG. Evaluation of the neuroprotective effects of sodium channel blockers after spinal cord injury: improved behavioral and neuroanatomical recovery with riluzole. J Neurosurg 2001;94(2, Suppl):245–256
14. Bensimon G, Lacomblez L, Meininger V; ALS/Riluzole Study Group. A controlled trial of riluzole in amyotrophic lateral sclerosis. N Engl J Med 1994;330(9):585–591

30

Considerations for the Initiation and Conduct of Spinal Cord Injury Clinical Trials

John D. Steeves

Key Points

1. Overall therapeutic goals are discussed, including neuroprotection, neural repair, and functional recovery.
2. Necessary steps in the preclinical translation of a discovery to human application are outlined.
3. The differences between clinical trial phases are highlighted.
4. Potential confounding factors that can alter the outcomes of a clinical trial are described.
5. The guiding principles for the development of clinical trial protocols are listed.

Over the past few years there has been increasing interest in the translation of experimental therapeutic interventions to improve functional outcomes after spinal cord injury (SCI). The number of reported successes using preclinical animal models have been substantial and encouraged the development of several clinical trial programs.

The overall goals for the treatment of SCI might be summarized as a series of temporally overlapping targets or goals to preserve or improve functional capacity (**Table 30.1**). At this time there is limited human efficacy data; thus, the timelines for effective neuroprotective, reparative, regenerative, and recovery treatments are necessarily vague. It is not the intent of this chapter to review the mechanisms underlying experimental treatment strategies. Instead, the focus is on the principled pathway for translation of discoveries, as well as the factors that may influence outcomes or confound the accurate interpretation of clinical trial results.

Therapeutic Goals after Spinal Cord Injury

Protection strategies are directed against the mechanical, pathological, and inflammatory effects on spinal cord tissues immediately following the primary injury

Table 30.1 Overall Goals for Improving Functional Capacity after Spinal Cord Injury

Therapeutic targets or clinical goals	Timeline for human application after SCI	Selected underlying biological mechanisms
Protection	Within first few weeks	Edema Secondary cell death Inflammation Immune system responses
Repair (endogenous)	Weeks to months	Angiogenesis Myelination Astrocyte responses
Regeneration (exogenous)	Weeks to years	Cell transplants Axonal outgrowth Biocompatible substrates
Recovery	Weeks to years	Activity-dependent training Axonal sprouting Synaptic plasticity Neuronal circuit rewiring

and throughout the first few weeks when secondary cell death processes are most active. Surgical decompression of the cord and mechanical stabilization of the spine constitute standard acute care to ensure the spinal column does not impinge on the cord and cause further damage. The maintenance of adequate vascular perfusion of the spinal cord is also a current standard of care, whereas the reduction of spinal edema and minimization of secondary cell death (e.g., apoptosis) are research goals for acute treatments.[1,2]

Repair includes endogenous cellular and tissue responses that are spontaneously activated after injury or need appropriate stimulation to provide a benefit. For example, stimulation of appropriate angiogenesis or decreasing widespread demyelination is likely to be beneficial.[3,4] Current thinking also suggests astrogliosis after SCI is maladaptive to functional recovery, and limiting such responses by astrocytes may be a worthy therapeutic target.[5–7] Interventions that enhance the expression of required growth factors, stimulate the proliferation and differentiation of resident neural progenitors, or activate endogenous “developmental programs” to facilitate intrinsic neuronal outgrowth are also areas of active preclinical investigation.[1,8]

Regeneration is often used as a synonym for repair, but here the emphasis is on *exogenous* interventions that specifically stimulate or facilitate outgrowth from severed axons, as well as strategies, such as cell and biocompatible material transplants, that replace lost tissue or provide scaffolds for neural growth.[9] Obvious approaches include transplantation of autologous or allograft neural stem cells or neural progenitors.[10] Although cell transplantation is a most promising therapeutic intervention, at this time there is little scientific consensus as to what are the most appropriate cellular candidates for transplantation after SCI. In addition, different therapeutic goals may require different cell transplant phenotypes. Further preclinical studies are essential before this approach will have a meaningful and widespread clinical application.

Recovery of a clinically meaningful functional capacity is the ultimate goal and may necessarily involve all the above approaches, but activity-dependent rehabilitation alone can provide benefit. The underlying basis is collectively referred to as neuroplasticity, which includes a variety of mechanisms, such as the formation of novel synaptic connections by axonal sprouts from existing (i.e., preserved) fibers, to alterations in synaptic strength, or the rewiring of functional circuits within intact (uninjured) spinal and brain regions.[11] Treatments, such as bodyweight-supported walking, robot-assisted training, and functional electric stimulation, capitalize on and facilitate plasticity.[12,13] Activity-dependent efforts are also important to consolidate any functional anatomical repair induced by a biological intervention that protects, repairs, or regenerates the injured cord.

SCI is a complex disorder, and functional recovery will undoubtedly require more than one type of intervention. Many preclinical investigations are examining the combined or sequential manipulations of promoters, inhibitors, intracellular modulators of axonal growth, cell transplants, and activity-dependent training.[14,15] The steps for the clinical translation of combinatorial therapies are necessarily more involved because each individual component, as well as the proposed combination, must be examined for safety at both the preclinical and the clinical level before any evaluation for efficacy can begin.

Preclinical Translation of Discoveries

A disconnect between preclinical and clinical results is undesirable, especially considering the extensive investment of time and money in a translation process. Thus, the adoption of high-quality preclinical protocols, with blinded assessments, adequate power, and the incorporation of "functional" outcome measures similar to those used in a human study, provide increased confidence. Likewise, most scientists would agree that the optimal preclinical translation process would include independent replication of promising preclinical strategies.[16] Furthermore, in the case of SCI, independent replication efforts might involve the use of different SCI models (e.g., severe vs moderate injury, lacerating vs contusive SCI) or variations of the treatment paradigms. This would establish both the relevance and the robustness of the initial discovery. In addition, finding similar beneficial outcomes of the experimental intervention after SCI in different species would demonstrate the fundamental nature of the therapeutic target and increase the likelihood that the treatment would benefit humans. Finally, if a therapy purports to be a useful acute treatment, it should be demonstrated to have benefit in animals when administered within a clinically relevant time frame (in most circumstances, at least several hours after the initial spinal injury). If an intervention is suggested to benefit people living with chronic SCI, then it should be shown to be effective in a chronic animal model.

As outlined in **Table 30.2**, there are several characteristics of an experimental treatment that should be established prior to beginning a human study. Nevertheless, some experimental interventions enter into clinical trials without being directly studied in a preclinical animal model of the human disorder. This may occur, for example, if the treatment has a previous clinical use for a different disorder but involves a related clinical therapeutic target. The advantages for such a translational path include a prior understanding of the safety and toxicology of the treatment in humans. Thus, when translated to SCI, there is reduced risk that the intervention might deteriorate neurological function or have other adverse effects (**Fig. 30.1**).

Spinal Cord Injury Clinical Trial Process

Initial guidelines for the conduct of valid SCI clinical trials have become progressively more important. The development of basic cell culture and surgical transplant technologies is relatively inexpensive and requires only modest biological or surgical expertise. Thus there has been a rapid expansion of "for-profit" clinics offering such treatments. The increasing attractiveness of these transplantation practices has understandable appeal to patients when presented as a "cure," but patients' desperation can be exploited. The claims of beneficial outcomes are often based on media

Table 30.2 Necessary Characterization and Development of an Experimental Treatment Prior to Human Study

Therapeutic trait	Approach	Outcome
Temporal "window of opportunity"	Test different time limits for therapeutic strategy after SCI	Determine early and late time points for the therapeutic benefit
Formulation	Examine different forms of drug, types of cells, or rehabilitation training programs	Identify which formulation provides best actions with minimal adverse effects
Route of administration	Investigate the most effective route to achieve therapeutic benefit (e.g., intravenous, intrathecal, intraparenchymal)	Determine best potential route for administering intervention in human patients
Dosage	Test different levels (dose response) of therapy (e.g., drug doses, cell numbers, or length and number of rehabilitation sessions) (also see adverse effects)	Define the optimal dosage that will potentially achieve a meaningful benefit, without unwanted side effects or adverse events
Adverse effects	Determine doses that cause unwanted side effects or adverse events	Identify tolerable and maximal dosages of therapeutic intervention
Fate of drug, transplanted cells, or rehabilitation strategy	Drugs: pharmacodynamics (action of drug on body) and pharmacokinetics (actions of body on drug—absorption, diffusion, metabolism, excretion) Cells: integration with host tissue, distribution, survival, tumorigenicity Rehabilitation: discover persistence of rehabilitative benefit	Outline the expected duration (length) of benefit that may be achieved through the therapy Gain better understanding of how the body interacts with the therapeutic intervention
Mechanism of action	Identify target or biological action of the intervention (e.g., altered biochemical pathway)	Provides information for development of subsequent (next-generation) therapeutics

Note: Rehabilitation strategies (activity-dependent training programs) should undergo similar characterization.

reports that are powerfully emotive, but unsubstantiated, and usually rely on anecdotal testimonials from hopeful patients or biased practitioners who stand to profit.

To ensure public safety, most countries in the developed world have regulatory agencies that have established criteria for an experimental therapy to enter a clinical trial program. Unfortunately, regulatory requirements are only as good as their enforcement, and this has not been uniform across the globe. To provide some objective assistance to a complex series of decisions weighing the possible risks and benefits for a human study, an initial set of SCI clinical trial guidelines was recently developed and published by an international panel of scientists and clinicians. This series of papers detailed the degree of spontaneous recovery after SCI,[17] outlined approaches for trial outcome measures,[18] discussed inclusion/exclusion criteria and ethics,[19] and outlined various trial designs and protocols.[20] In addition, the same authors created a document written for the general public and allied health care professionals (www.icord.org).

Each phase of a clinical trial program has distinct goals and thus different parameters, protocols, outcome measures, and end points that can govern the conduct for each stage of investigation. The over-

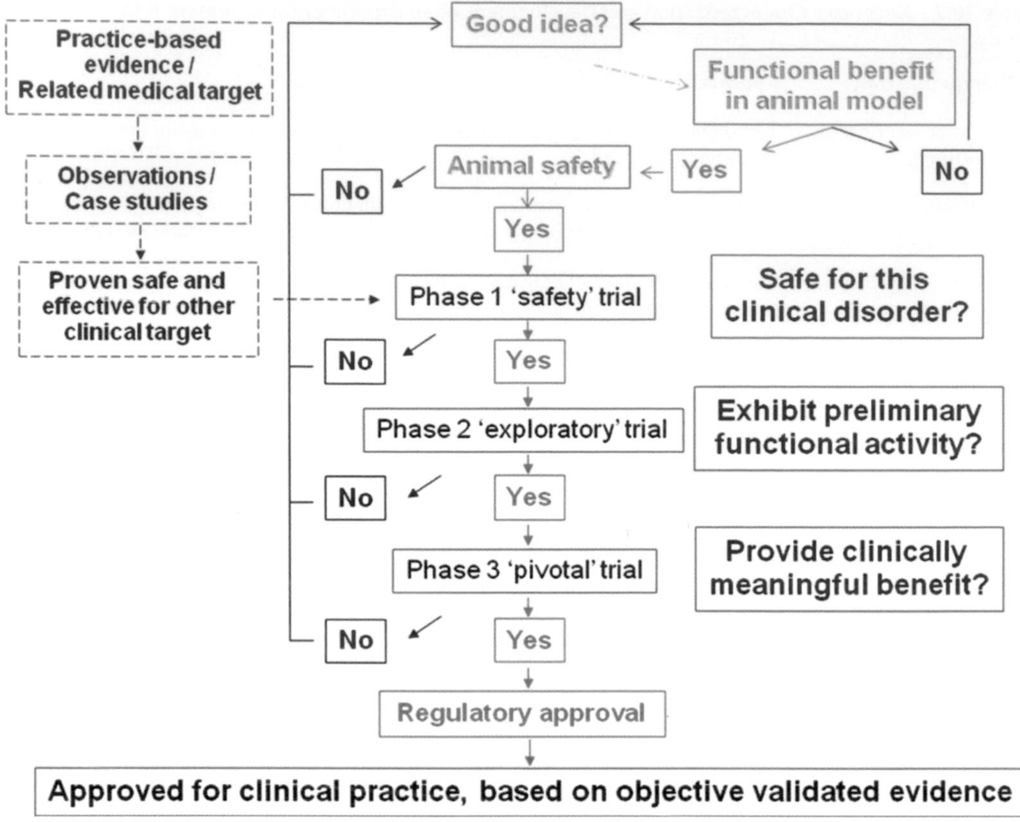

Fig. 30.1 Summary chart of a translational path for a therapeutic intervention from discovery to approval for clinical use.

all translational path for an experimental intervention through the various stages of preclinical and clinical study might be summarized as shown in **Fig. 30.1**.

Phase 1 trials are centered on the initial exploration of safety, and in the case of a drug, often include an evaluation of the responses to different therapeutic doses. Of course, safety is continuously monitored throughout all subsequent trial phases. Phase 1 trials will sometimes attempt to collect pilot data on functional outcomes, primarily to justify the continued funding of the trial program.

Phase 2 trials are still exploratory, with a focus on the preliminary demonstration of functional biological activity and functional benefit of the intervention. They will usually measure several different clinical or functional outcomes to determine which end point is likely to measure a reliable, clinically meaningful outcome in a sensitive and accurate manner.

Phase 3 trials are the pivotal studies, where an intervention must demonstrate benefit in a clinically meaningful manner, which is then weighed against the associated risks before it can be approved by the relevant regulatory body. A clinically meaningful benefit for a therapeutic can be difficult to define when examining a disorder like SCI. At present, there are no clearly established benchmarks for demonstrating a "subtle" change in efficacy or relating a small but statistically significant improvement to an enhanced functional capacity (e.g., activities of daily living) or quality of life.

After regulatory approval and adoption of the intervention as standard clinical practice, most interventions enter a surveillance period where the greatly increased exposure of a more heterogeneous array of patients allows potential detection of less frequent adverse events and may provide additional information on efficacy. At this stage, it is also possible to perform phase 4 clinical studies that continue to examine additional questions of efficacy, optimal treatment approaches, and safety in a more controlled way.

Characteristics of Human Spinal Cord Injury and Confounding Factors Influencing Clinical Trials

It is also not the intent of this chapter to review specific SCI clinical trials; please see other chapters in this volume and recent review articles.[21–24]

In the transition from preclinical animal experiments to human studies there are several considerations to contemplate. As already mentioned, human SCI is not the relatively homogeneous situation created in an experimental laboratory. Although the design of special impact devices has allowed scientists to create animal injuries within the same relative time frame of most human spinal injuries (< 10 msec sec), human SCI often involves mechanical damage that simultaneously compresses, dislocates, and distracts the spinal cord (i.e., disruption along three different axes). Human SCI can also be acquired from a variety of nontraumatic incidents, including: infection, vertebral stenosis, or spinal tumors. Thus SCI is heterogeneous in terms of the following:

- Spinal levels of injury (from ventilator-dependent, high cervical SCI to ambulatory, cauda equina injury)
- Severity of injury (from incomplete spinal damage to complete sensory and motor loss below the level of injury)
- Temporal differences (from the acute stage, through subacute, to more chronic time points after SCI)

Therefore, from a clinical study perspective, it is wise to minimize the variability between study subjects. If the enrolled subjects range from incomplete to sensorimotor complete, the potentially different outcomes (including the differing rates of spontaneous recovery) may obscure, offset, or cancel each other in the statistical analysis, leading an investigator to erroneously conclude there is no treatment effect. Finally, the greater the variability of SCI types allowed within a study, the higher the requirement for stratification and thus the lower the statistical power (significance) of any analyses. The primary way to overcome subject heterogeneity in a study is to increase the number of enrolled participants or start again; either choice will mean more time and money. In every possible respect, the (placebo) control group should be matched to the composition of the experimental study group.

A list of potential confounding factors that could jeopardize the accurate interpretation of the outcomes in a clinical trial is provided in **Table 30.3**. More detailed discussions of SCI subject inclusion/exclusion criteria and ethics[10] or SCI clinical trial design[20] can also be consulted.

General Principles for the Conduct of Valid Clinical Trials

Past SCI clinical trial programs have provided valuable lessons and knowledge, which will be instructive to future trials.[25–35] Many of the lessons are not unique to SCI studies and emphasize fundamental truths in the translation of any therapeutic intervention.[36] The most prominent past acute SCI trials (e.g., the National Acute Spinal Cord Injury Study [NASCIS], Sygen, and GK-11) were well-conducted protocols that incorporated appropriate controls and utilized blinded assessments over an adequate recovery period. Unfortunately, none of these trials was successful in demonstrating unequivocal efficacy based on prospectively defined primary end points.

Thus the field of SCI research does not currently have the clearly validated clinical end points that must be achieved in a

Table 30.3 Confounding Factors That Could Alter the Accurate Interpretation of Clinical Trial Outcomes

Possible confounding factor(s)	Can this confounder always be controlled by study investigator (Y/N)
Prior emergency or primary care, intensive care treatment and management	N
Surgical decompression and spine stabilization (and timing of surgery after SCI)	N
Damage to other organs or subsequent medical complications after SCI	N
Onset, type, and extent of rehabilitation activity in which subject engages during trial	N
Unsuitable study protocol design or statistical analysis of trial results	Y
Inappropriate inclusion and exclusion criteria for subject to participate in trial (e.g., different: spinal segmental levels of SCI, severities of SCI, time since SCI)	Y
Lack of "blinded" randomization of subjects and randomization of treatment allocation sequence	Y
Lack of appropriate control subjects who match criteria of experimental treatment group	Y
Investigator or subject expectations and bias because they know the type of treatment provided to the subject	Y
Inappropriate, insensitive, or unreliable clinical outcome tools or primary outcome measure (clinical trial end point)	Y
Lack of independent "blinded" assessments of trial outcome measures	Y
Poor intra- and interrater reliability of outcome assessments (lack of ongoing training of trial assessors)	Y
Lack of sufficient follow-up assessments (often at least 6 to 12 months after trial completion)	Y

Note: These factors may or may not be controlled by the study investigator, but should be carefully noted prior to analysis of data.

study (i.e., outcome measures of efficacy or clinically meaningful benefit). It is possible to interpret the past clinical end points as overly ambitious or insensitive to detect a subtle change, but this may also be because the treatment effects (if any) were of insufficient magnitude. It is easy to blame the measurement tool when the measurement does not provide the desired conclusion. The validation of an accurate, sensitive clinical end point that can reliably detect a significant but subtle treatment effect is difficult until such an effect is accurately defined and distinct from what might be achieved via spontaneous recovery. There is currently no consensus on what are the most appropriate outcome tools to discern *subtle*, but *clinically meaningful*, benefits for the variety of clinical SCI targets. Understanding the natural history of spontaneous recovery after SCI can facilitate the determination of a reasonable threshold that might be exceeded to demonstrate a valid therapeutic effect.[17,18,37,38] Recent reviews of SCI outcome measures and tools provide additional information and discussion.[18,39]

The optimal foundations for an ideal clinical trial program are difficult to guarantee, but planning how to achieve some of these is instructive. The considerations may include the following:

- Compelling preclinical data and an understanding of the mechanism of therapeutic action that will allow enthusiasm and financial support to withstand any setbacks in the clinic during the early trial phases. (Financing clinical programs is difficult and usually limits the opportunities for trial and error learning.)
- Sensitive and reliable outcome measures to show an objectively measurable effect of the treatment
- Prospectively designed criteria for establishing clinically meaningful effects (clinical end points) sufficient to convince *others* that there is a real benefit to balance against the costs and risks of the intervention
- A plan for dealing with partial success (e.g., small therapeutic benefit), with an understanding that there may be no practical way back or forward from a partial success
- An understanding that randomized studies and appropriate placebo controls are essential for validating any clinical intervention
- A clear understanding of the natural history of the conditions, including the spontaneous (untreated) recovery to be expected
- Enrollment criteria that can be set to provide a pool of participants sufficiently homogeneous to show a treatment effect with the chosen end points

Conclusion

The independent replication of any preclinical discovery, using good laboratory practices, elevates confidence in the initial findings and facilitates the translation of experimental treatments to human study. It is difficult to develop the optimal trial design and protocol for a disorder, like SCI, which has yet to achieve a treatment that has been shown to have a clear clinical benefit. As outlined in this chapter, there are several factors that need to be considered prospectively to increase the potential for a successful outcome.

To achieve a successful outcome by the end of the pivotal phase 3 trial, an investigator should be able to demonstrate an improved *functional capacity* that affects a relevant activity of daily living. However, the performance of any activity of daily living is subject to the influence of a variety of factors (e.g., motivation) that are often independent of the particular experimental treatment being examined. In short, *capacity* and *performance* are not synonymous; whether a person makes use of any improved capacity is up to the individual and beyond the control of any clinical study. The pace of preclinical discovery and translation in SCI means it is timely to consider how to best conduct human studies in a logical, objective, and efficient manner.

Pearls

- Studies without appropriate control data and blinded assessments are *not* valid clinical trials. Payment (by a subject) for an experimental treatment automatically means it is *not* a clinical trial because the investigator has a financial incentive (i.e., bias).
- Valid clinical trial programs require the following:
  - Suitable preclinical (or prior clinical) evidence for potential benefit of therapeutic intervention
  - Randomization of an appropriate number of participants to experimental and control groups
  - Blinded assessments over a sufficient recovery period (often up to 1 year posttreatment)
  - An appropriate outcome tool (with a sensitive detection threshold) to accurately detect a significant difference between experimental and control groups for a meaningful functional clinical end point

Pitfalls

- Fundamental preclinical (animal study) translational requirements that should be completed or understood before moving forward to a clinical trial include the following:
  - Independent validation of discovery by another laboratory
  - Therapeutic target (population most likely to benefit)
  - Possible toxic side effects or adverse events (as determined in multiple animal species)
  - Effective time and duration for therapeutic application ("window of opportunity")
  - Amount of treatment (dosage)
- Common pitfalls during a clinical trial include the factors listed in **Table 30.3** of this chapter.

References

1. Ramer LM, Ramer MS, Steeves JD. Setting the stage for functional repair of spinal cord injuries: a cast of thousands. Spinal Cord 2005;43(3): 134–161
2. Onose G, Anghelescu A, Muresanu DF, et al. A review of published reports on neuroprotection in spinal cord injury. Spinal Cord 2009;47(10): 716–726
3. Karimi-Abdolrezaee S, Eftekharpour E, Wang J, Morshead CM, Fehlings MG. Delayed transplantation of adult neural precursor cells promotes remyelination and functional neurological recovery after spinal cord injury. J Neurosci 2006;26(13): 3377–3389
4. Biernaskie J, Sparling JS, Liu J, et al. Skin-derived precursors generate myelinating Schwann cells that promote remyelination and functional recovery after contusion spinal cord injury. J Neurosci 2007;27(36):9545–9559
5. McGraw J, Hiebert GW, Steeves JD. Modulating astrogliosis after neurotrauma. J Neurosci Res 2001; 63(2):109–115
6. Galtrey CM, Fawcett JW. The role of chondroitin sulfate proteoglycans in regeneration and plasticity in the central nervous system. Brain Res Brain Res Rev 2007;54(1):1–18
7. Fitch MT, Silver J. CNS injury, glial scars, and inflammation: inhibitory extracellular matrices and regeneration failure. Exp Neurol 2008;209(2): 294–301
8. Lu P, Jones LL, Tuszynski MH. Axon regeneration through scars and into sites of chronic spinal cord injury. Exp Neurol 2007;203(1):8–21
9. Nomura H, Tator CH, Shoichet MS. Bioengineered strategies for spinal cord repair. J Neurotrauma 2006;23(3-4):496–507
10. Mackay-Sim A, Féron F, Cochrane J, et al. Autologous olfactory ensheathing cell transplantation in human paraplegia: a 3-year clinical trial. Brain 2008;131(Pt 9):2376–2386
11. Dunlop SA. Activity-dependent plasticity: implications for recovery after spinal cord injury. Trends Neurosci 2008;31(8):410–418
12. Dunlop SA, Steeves JD. Neural activity and facilitated recovery by training after CNS injury: implications for rehabilitation. Top Spinal Cord Inj Rehabil 2003;8:92–103
13. Lynskey JV, Belanger A, Jung R. Activity-dependent plasticity in spinal cord injury. J Rehabil Res Dev 2008;45(2):229–240
14. Blesch A, Tuszynski MH. Spinal cord injury: plasticity, regeneration and the challenge of translational drug development. Trends Neurosci 2009;32(1):41–47
15. Benowitz LI, Yin Y. Combinatorial treatments for promoting axon regeneration in the CNS: strategies for overcoming inhibitory signals and activating neurons' intrinsic growth state. Dev Neurobiol 2007;67(9):1148–1165
16. Kwon BK, Okon EB, Tsai E, et al. A grading system to evaluate objectively the strength of pre-clinical data of acute neuroprotective therapies for clini-

cal translation in spinal cord injury. J Neurotrauma 2011;28(8):1525–1543

17. Fawcett JW, Curt A, Steeves JD, et al. Guidelines for the conduct of clinical trials for spinal cord injury as developed by the ICCP panel: spontaneous recovery after spinal cord injury and statistical power needed for therapeutic clinical trials. Spinal Cord 2007;45(3):190–205

18. Steeves JD, Lammertse D, Curt A, et al; International Campaign for Cures of Spinal Cord Injury Paralysis. Guidelines for the conduct of clinical trials for spinal cord injury (SCI) as developed by the ICCP panel: clinical trial outcome measures. Spinal Cord 2007;45(3):206–221

19. Tuszynski MH, Steeves JD, Fawcett JW, et al; International Campaign for Cures of Spinal Cord Injury Paralysis. Guidelines for the conduct of clinical trials for spinal cord injury as developed by the ICCP Panel: clinical trial inclusion/exclusion criteria and ethics. Spinal Cord 2007;45(3):222–231

20. Lammertse D, Tuszynski MH, Steeves JD, et al; International Campaign for Cures of Spinal Cord Injury Paralysis. Guidelines for the conduct of clinical trials for spinal cord injury as developed by the ICCP panel: clinical trial design. Spinal Cord 2007; 45(3):232–242

21. Amador MJ, Guest JD. An appraisal of ongoing experimental procedures in human spinal cord injury. J Neurol Phys Ther 2005;29(2):70–86

22. Baptiste DC, Fehlings MG. Update on the treatment of spinal cord injury. Prog Brain Res 2007; 161;217–233

23. Knafo S, Choi D. Clinical studies in spinal cord injury: moving towards successful trials. Br J Neurosurg 2008;22(1):3–12

24. Hawryluk GW, Rowland J, Kwon BK, Fehlings MG. Protection and repair of the injured spinal cord: a review of completed, ongoing, and planned clinical trials for acute spinal cord injury. Neurosurg Focus 2008;25(5):E14

25. Bracken MB, Collins WF, Freeman DF, et al. Efficacy of methylprednisolone in acute spinal cord injury. JAMA 1984;251(1):45–52

26. Bracken MB, Shepard MJ, Hellenbrand KG, et al. Methylprednisolone and neurological function 1 year after spinal cord injury. Results of the National Acute Spinal Cord Injury Study. J Neurosurg 1985;63(5):704–713

27. Bracken MB, Shepard MJ, Collins WF, et al. A randomized, controlled trial of methylprednisolone or naloxone in the treatment of acute spinal-cord injury. Results of the Second National Acute Spinal Cord Injury Study. N Engl J Med 1990;322(20):1405–1411

28. Bracken MB, Shepard MJ, Collins WF Jr, et al. Methylprednisolone or naloxone treatment after acute spinal cord injury: 1-year follow-up data. Results of the Second National Acute Spinal Cord Injury Study. J Neurosurg 1992;76(1):23–31

29. Bracken MB, Shepard MJ, Holford TR, et al. Administration of methylprednisolone for 24 or 48 hours or tirilazad mesylate for 48 hours in the treatment of acute spinal cord injury. Results of the Third National Acute Spinal Cord Injury Randomized Controlled Trial. National Acute Spinal Cord Injury Study. JAMA 1997;277(20):1597–1604

30. Bracken MB, Shepard MJ, Holford TR, et al. Methylprednisolone or tirilazad mesylate administration after acute spinal cord injury: 1-year follow up. Results of the Third National Acute Spinal Cord Injury Randomized Controlled Trial. J Neurosurg 1998;89(5):699–706

31. Otani K, Abe H, Kadoya S, et al. Beneficial effects of methylprednisolone sodium succinate in the treatment of acute spinal cord injury. Sekitsy Sekizu.i 1994;7:633–647

32. Geisler FH, Dorsey FC, Coleman WP. Recovery of motor function after spinal-cord injury—a randomized, placebo-controlled trial with GM-1 ganglioside. N Engl J Med 1991;324(26):1829–1838

33. Geisler FH, Coleman WP, Grieco G, Poonian D; Sygen Study Group. The Sygen multicenter acute spinal cord injury study. Spine 2001;26(24, Suppl): S87–S98

34. Tadié M, Gaviria J-F, Mathé P, et al. Early care and treatment with the neuroprotective drug gacyclidine in patients with acute spinal cord injury. RACHIS 2003;15:363–376 (translation)

35. Cardenas DD, Ditunno J, Graziani V, et al. Phase 2 trial of sustained-release fampridine in chronic spinal cord injury. Spinal Cord 2007;45(2): 158–168

36. Steeves JD, Zariffa J, Kramer JL. Are you "tilting at windmills" or undertaking a valid clinical trial? Yonsei Med J 2011;52(5):701–716

37. Steeves JD, Kramer JK, Fawcett JW, et al; EMSCI Study Group. Extent of spontaneous motor recovery after traumatic cervical sensorimotor complete spinal cord injury. Spinal Cord 2011; 49(2):257–265

38. Zariffa J, Kramer JL, Fawcett JW, et al. Characterization of neurological recovery following traumatic sensorimotor complete thoracic spinal cord injury. Spinal Cord 2011;49(3):463–471

39. Alexander MS, Anderson KD, Biering-Sorensen F, et al. Outcome measures in spinal cord injury: recent assessments and recommendations for future directions. Spinal Cord 2009;47(8): 582–591

31

Animal Models of Spinal Cord Injury

Aileen J. Anderson, Sheri L. Peterson, and Christopher J. Sontag

Key Points

1. SCI researchers utilize a wide range of animal models that incorporate various aspects of injury progression and inform on pathophysiological progression, mechanisms, and potential treatments for SCI.
2. Different animal models have different strengths and weaknesses; understanding these characteristics, along with any underlying assumptions, is essential in drawing the proper conclusions from a given model.
3. Animal models of SCI can focus on recapitulating clinical correlates or testing proof-of-concept variables that are applicable to SCI, and each has its importance to advancing the field.
4. SCI researchers have a variety of tools to assess animal models of SCI, including histology, motor and sensory behavioral tasks, and electrophysiology.

The goal of all spinal cord injury (SCI) models is to create a reproducible, standardized, and consistent method of assessing damage and recovery of the spinal cord. Animal models of SCI are an important tool for understanding the pathophysiological progression, mechanisms, and potential therapeutic intervention points for SCI. This chapter reviews the principal animal models of SCI and their clinical correlates. Additionally, the text addresses proof-of-concept models for remyelination, ischemia, and regeneration, as well as histological and behavioral assessment issues in these models (**Table 31.1**).

A variety of species have been utilized in SCI research (**Table 31.2**). The majority of work in recent years has been done in rats, mainly due to the low cost and established methods of functional behavioral analysis; however, the mouse has seen increased use, primarily due to the advantage of genetic manipulations and the development of new injury devices. Although these species fulfill an extremely useful role for research purposes, larger-scale animal models may have a role in clinical translation for some therapies,[1] particularly in the context of scaling from mouse, to rat, to human spinal cord (**Fig. 31.1**). Nonhuman primate

Table 31.1 A Summary of Injury Models Used in Spinal Cord Injury Research

	Model	Features	Limitations
Blunt force trauma	Contusion	Most common clinically Real-time injury feedback Well characterized in literature Reproducible Graded	Difficult to assess regeneration due to spared fibers
	Compression	Ischemic component of injury similar to clinical Reproducible Graded	Difficult to assess regeneration due to spared fibers
	Crush	Simplest of the blunt force trauma models Graded, forceps-dependent Reproducible	Difficult to assess regeneration due to spared fibers
Transection	Full transection	Tissue engineering and bridge compatible Optimal for study of axonal regeneration of descending motor tracts	Difficult animal care Careful validation of lesion required for interpretation
	Partial transection	Can provide a platform to study tract-specific regeneration May provide a contralateral control	Careful validation of lesion required for interpretation Spared axon sprouting and behavioral compensation
	Root avulsion	Strength of clinical parallel; functional improvement with root reimplantation in patients Optimal for study of regeneration across the PNS/CNS interface	Does not model the full spectrum of combined avulsion/traumatic SCI
Proof of concept	Chemical demyelination	Useful for the study of endogenous remyelination factors and treatments	Reductionist model, no traumatic component
	Photochemical lesion	Isolate ischemic component of injury, useful for the study of ischemia treatments	Reductionist model, no traumatic component
	Peripheral conditioning	Useful for studying the regeneration inhibitory environment of the injured CNS, and strategies to promote PNS/CNS axonal growth	Reductionist model, no traumatic component
	Optic nerve crush	Useful for studying the regeneration inhibitory environment of the injured CNS, and strategies to promote PNS/CNS axonal growth Well characterized and clearly identified anatomical system	Reductionist model, no traumatic component CNS but not spinal cord

Abbreviations: CNS, central nervous system; PNS, peripheral nervous system.

Table 31.2 Summary of Animals Used in Spinal Cord Injury Research

Animal	Features	Limitations
Rodents	Larger N possible (lower cost and technical hurdles) Reproducible injuries Well-defined behavioral assessments Clinically similar respiratory neuroanatomy Clinically similar cellular immune response	Small size and shorter lifespan Strain differences add complexity Some differences in vasculature and tract locations and features from humans Some differences in humoral immune response from humans Lack paw and digit dexterity Quadrupedal locomotion: different musculoskeletal anatomy; strong role for forelimbs in locomotion
Mouse	High potential for gene manipulation Immunodeficient models for assessment of human cell therapies in absence of rejection confounds	Smallest size Lesion epicenter forms fibronectin-filled scar, unlike many clinical cases
Rat	Best-characterized injury and behavioral assessments Some immunodeficient models Lesion epicenter cavitation	Reduced potential for gene manipulation
Larger mammals	Larger size provides scaling information for regeneration, transplanted cell migration and procedural safety Similar vasculature and tract organization to humans Hindlimbs drive locomotion	Smaller N possible (higher cost and technical hurdles) Lack of standardized injury models and established behavioral assessments Very limited potential for gene manipulation
Cat	Historically important model Some standardization of injury and behavioral assessment	
Dog	Potential for assessment of naturally injured domestic dogs via veterinary clinics	
Mini pig	Closely mimics human vasculature	
Nonhuman primates	Larger size provides scaling information for regeneration, transplanted cell migration, and procedural safety Highly similar vasculature and tract locations and features to humans Genetic similarity to humans (good for pharmacological interventions) Bipedal locomotion assessments Physical therapy interventions Assessment of hand dexterity Complex cortical circuits for simple motor tasks mimic human plasticity potential Motivational aspects can be evaluated	Very low N possible (highest cost, technically difficult, not available to all researchers) Increased ethical considerations Difficult, although sensitive, behavioral measures Very limited potential for genetic manipulation High hurdle to achieve adequate long-term immunosuppression for xenograft transplantation studies
Marmoset	Established contusion model	Small primate (rodent equivalent)
Macaque	Large primate	Injury limited to partial transection, while contusion is most common clinically

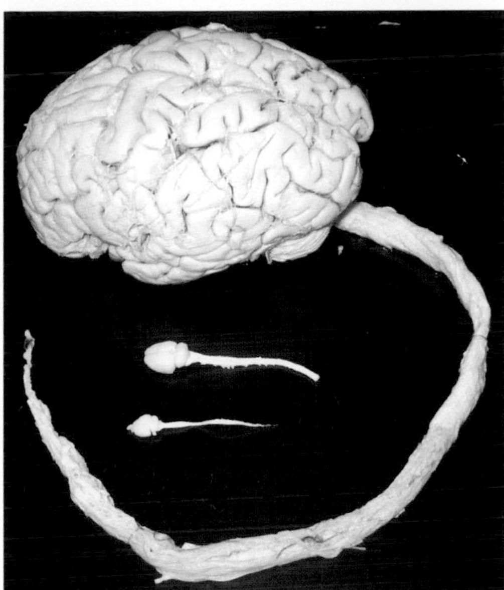

Fig. 31.1 Size comparison of mouse, rat, and human spinal cords. Note the much larger human spinal cord and the possible challenges that this difference may create for translation from rodents to humans, especially with regard to cell transplantation, lesion dynamics, and distance traversed by regenerating fibers.

models of SCI are rare in comparison to rodent models, mainly due to the high cost, specialized care required, and difficulty of producing reproducible lesions.[2] In parallel, smaller animal species have been critical to advancing the identification of new molecules and pathways in central nervous system (CNS) regeneration.

The critical criterion required of an animal model is how well it addresses or can be applied to human SCI. Injuries in humans are a heterogeneous mix of types and severities at different levels, accompanied by differing degrees of functional deficits. Consequently, animal models need to be capable of incorporating these factors.

The first factor a model must address is the injury type and severity. Injury types in humans have been classified into four broad categories: solid cord injury (10% of cases), contusion/cavity (49% of cases), laceration (21% of cases), and massive compression (20% of cases), with the majority of these injuries being anatomically incomplete.[3] Consequently, animal models have been focused on mimicking these types of injuries and are discussed based on their method of injury here. Additionally, the ability to create graded injuries of varying severities and to detect these differences in a behavioral and histological manner is critical for translatable success to the varied human SCI population and has been a chief criterion for the development of these models.

Another important factor to address is injury level. Many animal models have utilized midthoracic injuries, resulting in various degrees of hindlimb paralysis and trunk instability. Since the species used are predominantly quadrupeds, this level of injury has significantly different behavioral outcomes than what can occur in bipeds, like humans. The majority of human injuries are in the cervical region,[3] and a recent survey of individuals with SCI has shown that regaining the ability to walk is lower in priority than other functions, such as arm movement, bladder and bowel control, and sexual function.[4] Thus it is critical that animal models be designed to address these needs, and there has been a recent surge in efforts to develop cervical injury and assessment models. The biggest obstacle to the implementation of consistently reproducible cervical SCI models has been with regard to gaining access to the spinal cord due to the more complex musculature and neuroanatomy at that level. Regardless, the majority of injury paradigms and models discussed throughout this chapter can be applied at any desired vertebral level, given the proper training and reproducibility.

Furthermore, induction of SCI in animal models is performed under anesthesia in the absence of other conflicting variables. In contrast, many human SCI cases are accompanied by comorbidities and secondary trauma (e.g., in the case of automobile accidents, one of the leading causes of SCI).[3,5] These situations lead to quite different conditions between clinical reality and animal models.

Finally, some consideration should be given to what has been learned about differences in SCI among different species. First, despite a great deal of conservation of neuroanatomy and function across species, there are distinct differences in the transition from rodent to primate to human.[6] Furthermore, even rodents have their differences: rats and mice have been shown to have different inflammatory reactions following SCI,[7] and different strains of mice have been shown to have different levels of complement activity,[8] excitotoxicity, secondary degeneration, and wound healing following SCI.[9] Finally, age has been shown to be a critical factor in humans[10] as well as rats,[11,12] with increased age being correlated to higher mortality and greater locomotor and histological deficits. This is particularly critical because the vast majority of rodent SCI models are conducted in young adult animals, 8 to 12 weeks of age, whereas the average age of human clinical SCI is currently 40.[5]

Ultimately, it is important to be aware of the strengths and weaknesses of a model and the assumptions being made regarding it as well. Although some models are more clinically translatable, all of the animal models presented here have strongly shaped what is known about SCI and have influenced where treatments are headed in the future.

Animal Spinal Cord Injury Models with Clinical Correlates

Many commonly used animal models of SCI mimic the injury, pathology, and behavior observed in human patients. This section focuses on contusion, compression, transection, and root avulsion models and their individual contributions to the understanding of the underlying mechanisms and treatment of SCI in humans.

Laminectomies

Laminectomies are frequently performed as the first step of most animal injury models. Care should be taken to ensure that extensive damage to the musculature or inadvertent damage to the spinal cord is avoided when exposing and removing the vertebrae. Additionally, the musculature and skin need to be sutured properly to avoid the development of kyphosis in animals. Ultimately, with training and practice, laminectomies can be incident-free and a reliable and reproducible way of exposing the spinal cord for further experimentation.

Compression and Contusion Models of Spinal Cord Injury

Contusion models are widely used in an effort to mimic what occurs in the majority of human injuries.[3] These models all utilize some form of blunt trauma, followed by compression of the spinal cord, which results in the development of a progressive lesion that is very similar to that seen in human SCI.[13] It should also be noted that the dura is not disrupted in these injuries, and none include stretching or shearing, which is sure to be a clinical factor. The focus presented here is on the blunt injury models that have the highest prevalence within the scientific literature.

The clip compression model utilizes a modified aneurysm clip to produce consistent and reproducible injuries. Compression time can be varied to alter injury severity, or clips with different compressive force can be used while keeping time consistent.[14] Alternatively, the use of graded forceps has also been described as a way to create a range of injuries in mice that can be visualized both behaviorally and histologically.[15] When used properly, either of these models is a cost-effective method of creating reproducible injuries across a variety of species. However, they lack some of the more advanced features and data output of recently developed computer-controlled devices.

Computer-assisted contusion devices are advantageous due to their consistency and the amount of data they report, which can be used to determine injury reliability, efficacy, and animal exclusions at the time of surgery. The OSU impactor[16] was first used in rats, and was later modified to improve consistency and accommodate the use of mice.[17] It utilizes the amount of cord displacement as a variable for injury and reports the total amount of displacement and force transmitted to the spinal cord. The NYU impactor[18] is a weight-drop method of inducing contusion injuries in rats. Height is varied to affect injury severity and a variety of parameters are reported, including rod impact velocity, compression rate and distance, and the total force applied to the cord. The Infinite Horizon Impactor (Precision Systems and Instrumentation, Fairfax Station, VA)[19] utilizes a computer-controlled probe to vary the amount of user-defined force that is applied to the spinal cord of a variety of species. The device reports a wealth of parameters, including the actual force applied, the velocity at maximum force, and the displacement of the cord, and it also generates a graph that plots changes in force and displacement as a function of time.

As noted in the introduction, age, like strain and species variations, is likely an important variable in both the initial injury and recovery from SCI. Contusion injury models have shown greater deficits in functional recovery in aged animals after SCI, but, due to the complex nature of these models, the biological rationale behind this difference is difficult to determine.[11,12]

Complete and Partial Transection Models of Spinal Cord Injury

Complete transection models involve the severing of the spinal cord, resulting in a complete injury, often called a "spinalized" animal. Clinically, this model mimics a complete laceration of the spinal cord, which can occur from stabbing or bullet wounds, but these injuries are often incomplete and are rare.[3] However, the complete nature of the injury provides a clean way for researchers to judge axonal regeneration and behavioral recovery. Care must be taken to ensure that the injury is complete or spared axons can be mistakenly counted as regenerating axons.[20] Retrograde and anterograde tracers are utilized to visualize the presence of regenerating versus spared axons. The distinct, localized trauma can also be advantageous for studies looking at less complex injuries and interested in a specific scientific question regarding axonal regeneration, but the model does not show the same extent of pathophysiological changes seen in contusion injuries.[21] Finally, it should be noted that behavioral recovery due to intervention after complete transection should be confirmed by retransection to avoid the possibility of native locomotion reported in fully transected animals.[22]

Partial transections are generally utilized to examine specific tracts or regions of the spinal cord. Clinically, this model is comparable to incomplete lacerations of the human spinal cord, albeit in a much more clean and precise fashion. Although these models carry some of the same limitations as complete transection, they do have some advantages. A partial lateral transection allows for comparison with the uninjured contralateral side in the same animal. Furthermore, specific tracts and pathways can be targeted depending on the scientific question or clinical relevance. Due to the incomplete nature of the injury, it is important to distinguish between spared axons and potential regenerating axons even more so than with a complete transection. Retrograde and anterograde tracers can aid in this determination. One important confound with regard to behavior for these animals is that recovery can sometimes be accomplished through the use of compensation and plasticity of spared regions.[23]

Root Avulsion Models of Spinal Cord Injury

Another animal model of SCI is root avulsion, in which motoneurons, parasympathetic neurons, and dorsal root ganglia (DRG) cells are axotomized at the interface between CNS and peripheral nervous system (PNS).[24] Because of the increased regenerative capacity of the PNS versus the CNS, the location of the injury in this model poses a unique scientific question. Following laminectomy, the injury is performed using forceps to deliver longitudinal traction to either dorsal[25] or ventral roots[26] of the brachial plexus,[27] lumbosacral plexus,[28] or cauda equina.[26]

The clinical correlate of this model is often a complex injury involving rupture and avulsion of both dorsal and ventral roots resulting from motor vehicle accidents or complications during birth. Lumbosacral plexus avulsions are much less common clinically than brachial plexus avulsions, due to the anatomy of the spinal column.[29] The animal model shares the clinically described deficits in motor, sensory, autonomic, bladder, and bowel function.[30,31] The emergence of pain and the dramatic loss of neurons after avulsion is also evident in these animals, similar to the human condition.[29] The root avulsion injury model has been used to characterize the inflammatory response and the number of motoneurons remaining after progressive loss following axotomy.[26]

Clinically, this SCI animal model was pivotal in developing root reimplantation surgery, which is today the only successful treatment for not only brachial plexus injuries but also any SCI in humans. Reimplantation of the avulsed ventral root (or PNS graft) into the lateral white matter of the spinal cord (or into the ventral root exit zone) has been demonstrated to lead to recovery of motor and bladder function accompanied by pain reduction within 1 year in both animals and humans.[29,32] A combinatorial approach including neurotrophin treatment to reduce motoneuron death may prove to be most beneficial clinically.[33]

Proof of Concept for Myelination, Ischemia, and Regeneration in Spinal Cord Injury

In addition to traditional animal models with clinical SCI correlates, several other commonly employed models include chemical demyelination, photochemical lesions, and peripheral conditioning injuries. These proof-of-concept models allow researchers to isolate a process of interest in SCI and to study this process in a system with relatively few variables before moving to a more complex, clinically translatable model. Thus, studies using these paradigms are integral to our understanding of the molecular mechanisms of processes associated with SCI or recovery from injury, including myelination, ischemia, and regeneration.

Chemical Demyelination Models of Spinal Cord Injury

The myelination component of SCI has been studied using ethidium bromide (EB) or lysolecithin (LL) to create focal demyelination lesions in animals in the absence of mechanical SCI.[34] These models induce the synchronous and rapid demyelination of axons as a result of oligodendrocyte death, with little direct axonal damage. In addition, there is evidence for depletion of the endogenous oligoprecursor population within the lesion site, and spontaneous, essentially complete, host-mediated remyelination takes place over a period of 2 to 3 weeks in animals lesioned at a young age (8 to 10 weeks). Further, transplantation of a variety of oligodendrocyte precursor cell (OPC) populations results in spinal lesion remyelination.[34]

A significant variable that has emerged is the role of age at time of lesion, with age-related deficits in remyelination seen in rodents over 5 months in comparison with those under 3 months of age.[34,35] As mentioned previously, a reduction in functional recovery and myelination with age has also been demonstrated in the contusion model, demonstrating that proof-of-concept models can yield valuable mechanistic insight to the more complex clinical models.

Photochemical Lesion Model of Spinal Cord Injury

One method of initiating an ischemic lesion is through the use of rose bengal, a photosensitive dye. The dye is injected into animals intravenously and activated by irradiation of the spinal cord with a 560 nm laser beam.[36] This ischemic lesion differs from surgical occlusion models in that platelet aggregation is the primary initiator of the ischemic event. Numerous groups have characterized the morphological and electrophysiological aspects of the lesion and have shown that lesion size, severity, and location can be controlled.[37] Furthermore, the surgery requires no laminectomy, due to the translucent properties of rodent bone. Finally, the injury model lacks the complications of hemorrhaging seen in mechanical trauma models. However, the model does not mimic the type of injury commonly seen in human patients, the contusion injury. Nonetheless, it is a useful tool for focusing on the ischemic component of SCI.

Peripheral Conditioning Lesion Model of Spinal Cord Regeneration

Peripheral and central branches of sensory neurons are known to respond differently to injury, with marked regeneration of the peripheral axons and no regeneration of the central axons contained within the dorsal column of the spinal cord.[38,39] This lack of central regeneration is due to a reduced intrinsic growth state of CNS neurons combined with inhibitory cues from CNS myelin and the glial scar. CNS axons have been demonstrated to grow into a PNS tissue graft after injury in rodents and humans, which points to the importance of the microenvironment in nervous system regeneration.[29,38,40] However, conditioning peripheral nerve lesions in rats and mice have recently been demonstrated to increase axonal regeneration through the injured tissue and rostral to the site of dorsal column transection without the aid of a PNS graft.[41,42]

This central regeneration was originally demonstrated with sciatic nerve transection 1 week prior to dorsal column injury[42] ("prepriming"), and more recently with sciatic nerve transection at the time of dorsal column injury and again 1 week after dorsal column injury[41] ("priming plus postpriming"). Although the latter paradigm is more clinically relevant with regard to timing, a peripheral nerve lesion cannot be conducted on human patients for ethical reasons. In addition, motor regeneration and functional motor recovery would not be expected to result from sensory regrowth. Therefore, the usefulness of this animal model lies in the elucidation of the mechanism of a rare instance of CNS regeneration, and the use of that knowledge to augment regeneration after diverse spinal cord insults.

Considering the difference in PNS versus CNS regenerative capacity, and the elongation of central DRG axons after axotomy to both branches (but not to the central axon alone), the mechanism of central regeneration in this model likely involves changes in protein expression at the level of the DRG cell soma. Indeed, many signaling proteins and transcription factors appear to be involved in regeneration of sensory afferents in the spinal cord.[43–45] Interestingly, the conditioning lesion effect on central axon regeneration is mimicked by intraganglionic injection of a cyclic adenosine monophosphate (cAMP) analogue.[46]

It is important to note that, although central sensory axons from conditioned DRGs regenerate through a spinal cord lesion, many axons also adopt tortuous trajectories within the injured tissue and do not emerge rostrally.[42] Also, the functional capacity of the regenerated sensory afferents is questionable because they appear to remain in a chronic pathological state according to electrophysiological measures, such as conduction velocity.[47] Nevertheless, the DRG conditioning lesion is a powerful model of CNS regeneration, allowing for the exploration of regenerative mechanisms and of the impact of environmental and intrinsic factors on spinal cord regeneration, possibly leading to future SCI treatments.

A parallel and widely used model of CNS regeneration is the optic nerve crush model, in which lens puncture combined with forcep crush of the optic nerve induces axonal elongation into the optic nerve.[48] This model has the advantages of being completely contained within the CNS, and the relative simplicity of the optic nerve compared with the spinal cord. Many of the same proteins and processes, including cAMP, are involved in both models of regeneration.[49]

Assessments for Animal Models of Spinal Cord Injury

The assessment of recovery after SCI may involve histology, motor and sensory behavioral tasks, and occasionally electrophysiology.

Histology

Common histological considerations include lesion volume and tissue sparing, but neuroanatomical tracing of regenerating fibers and quantification of inflammatory cells are also used, depending on the model and hypothesis being addressed. It is important to note that variations in total spinal cord volume can accompany injury, and the recovery from injury.[11] Importantly, unbiased stereological quantification is equipped to account for these changes in volume, and therefore provides a more accurate evaluation of histopathological parameters.

Behavior

Many behavioral tasks are available for the evaluation of deficit and recovery after SCI.[50] Behavioral measures should be chosen on the basis of sensitivity to injury level, type, and severity. Therefore, appropriate tasks are chosen based on the outcome variable of interest, and constrained by the methods of the study. A particularly useful tool for screening of hindlimb function in rats is the Basso, Beattie, Bresnahan scale (BBB), in which gross assessment of locomotor recovery is evaluated in an open field, resulting in a score of 0 to 21, with 21 as normal and 0 as completely paralyzed.[51] An open-field rating scale has also been developed for mice—the Basso Mouse Scale (BMS).[52] Although these open-field measures are an important first step, both suffer from nonlinearity and differences in sensitivity across the broad spectrum of recovery. Accordingly, linearly valid secondary measures, such as gait analysis (e.g., CatWalk, Noldus, Wageningen, The Netherlands),[53] kinematic analysis,[54] horizontal ladder beam,[55] inclined plane,[56] grid walking,[57] ground reaction force measurement,[58] and swim testing,[59] can be used to tease apart more subtle differences in recovery. In addition, common behavioral assessments of forelimb function after cervical SCIs include limb hanging,[60] grip strength,[61] rope climbing,[62] paw preference,[63] and pellet reaching[64] tasks. In addition, Von Frey's testing[65] evaluates mechanical allodynia, whereas Hargreaves, or hot plate, testing[66] evaluates temperature sensitivity. Improvement in bladder/bowel and sexual function is of paramount importance to the SCI patient population,[4] and hurdles to clinical translation may not be as high for autonomic function as for locomotion, but these outcome measures are widely underassessed in SCI models. Methods for evaluation of micturition,[67] erection,[68] and autonomic dysreflexia[69] do exist and should therefore be assessed in all SCI animal models.

Conclusion

Studies employing animal models of SCI are essential for driving the understanding of the underlying mechanisms of the injured or diseased CNS and human clinical functional and pathological deficits. Much of what is known about the human condition is derived from animals, because more stringent controls as well as more potential treatment approaches and exploratory experiments are available to the animal researcher than to the clinician. With little or no scientifically sound treatment options currently available for the majority of SCIs in humans, translation from animal studies, including current and planned clinical trials,[70] will prove to be integral in alleviating the functional deficits and pain suffered by spinal cord injured patients in the future.

Pearls

- Human SCI is heterogeneous, and animal models allow researchers to control injury-associated variables.
- Animal models provide a means for acquiring graded, reproducible injuries from which pathological and behavioral comparisons between treatment groups can be made.
- Proof-of-concept animal models of SCI allow for isolation of specific aspects of the clinical picture for treatment proof-of-concept and mechanism questions.
- Some animal models of SCI mimic most aspects of the clinical picture, allowing for the evaluation of potential human therapies in a complex environment.
- The overall number of human SCI patients and the ability of researchers to acquire histological and electrophysiological data from these patients are very limited, emphasizing the need for animal models.

Pitfalls

- Most patients with an SCI have other injuries or diseases requiring surgical or pharmacological intervention, which may interact with therapies developed in animal models.
- Many patients with an SCI also undergo physical therapy, which is not usually modeled in combination with developed therapies in animals.
- Most SCI experiments are conducted using young adult animals, whereas it is common for human SCI to occur later in life.
- Most animal SCI experiments focus on the acute phase of injury, whereas the vast majority of current SCI patients have lived with the injury for years.
- Most SCI experiments are conducted using female animals due to bladder complications, and there is some evidence for increased neuroprotection in females in response to trauma.
- In animal models but not in most human SCI, anesthesia is present at the time of injury.
- There are limitations of each animal and injury method as it applies to the specific research question.

References

1. Blesch A, Tuszynski MH. Spinal cord injury: plasticity, regeneration and the challenge of translational drug development. Trends Neurosci 2009; 32(1):41–47
2. Robins SL, Fehlings MG. Models of experimental spinal cord injury: translational relevance and impact. Drug Discov Today Dis Models 2008; 5(1):5–11
3. Norenberg MD, Smith J, Marcillo A. The pathology of human spinal cord injury: defining the problems. J Neurotrauma 2004;21(4):429–440
4. Anderson KD. Targeting recovery: priorities of the spinal cord-injured population. J Neurotrauma 2004;21(10):1371–1383
5. CDRF. Prevalence of Paralysis Including Spinal Cord Injuries in the United States. 2009. http://www.christopherreeve.org/atf/cf/%7B3d83418f-b967-4c18-8ada-adc2e5355071%7D/8112REPTFINAL.PDF
6. Courtine GBM, Bunge MB, Fawcett JW, et al. Can experiments in nonhuman primates expedite the translation of treatments for spinal cord injury in humans? Nat Med 2007;13(5):561–566
7. Sroga JM, Jones TB, Kigerl KA, McGaughy VM, Popovich PG. Rats and mice exhibit distinct inflammatory reactions after spinal cord injury. J Comp Neurol 2003;462(2):223–240
8. Galvan MD, Luchetti S, Burgos AM, et al. Deficiency in complement C1q improves histological and functional locomotor outcome after spinal cord injury. J Neurosci 2008;28(51):13876–13888
9. Inman D, Guth L, Steward O. Genetic influences on secondary degeneration and wound healing following spinal cord injury in various strains of mice. J Comp Neurol 2002;451(3):225–235
10. Irwin ZN, Arthur M, Mullins RJ, Hart RA. Variations in injury patterns, treatment, and outcome for spinal fracture and paralysis in adult versus geriatric patients. Spine 2004;29(7):796–802
11. Galvan MDPE, Anderson AJ. The effects of age after a moderate contusion spinal cord injury in female rats. Neurobiol Aging, Submitted
12. Siegenthaler MM, Ammon DL, Keirstead HS. Myelin pathogenesis and functional deficits following SCI are age-associated. Exp Neurol 2008;213(2): 363–371
13. Metz GA, Curt A, van de Meent H, Klusman I, Schwab ME, Dietz V. Validation of the weight-drop contusion model in rats: a comparative study of human spinal cord injury. J Neurotrauma 2000; 17(1):1–17
14. Fehlings MG, Tator CH. The relationships among the severity of spinal cord injury, residual neurological function, axon counts, and counts of retrogradely labeled neurons after experimental spinal cord injury. Exp Neurol 1995;132(2):220–228

15. Plemel JR, Duncan G, Chen KW, et al. A graded forceps crush spinal cord injury model in mice. J Neurotrauma 2008;25(4):350–370
16. Bresnahan JC, Beattie MS, Todd FD III, Noyes DH. A behavioral and anatomical analysis of spinal cord injury produced by a feedback-controlled impaction device. Exp Neurol 1987;95(3):548–570
17. Jakeman LB, Guan Z, Wei P, et al. Traumatic spinal cord injury produced by controlled contusion in mouse. J Neurotrauma 2000;17(4):299–319
18. Gruner JA. A monitored contusion model of spinal cord injury in the rat. J Neurotrauma 1992;9(2):123–126, discussion 126–128
19. Scheff SW, Rabchevsky AG, Fugaccia I, Main JA, Lumpp JE Jr. Experimental modeling of spinal cord injury: characterization of a force-defined injury device. J Neurotrauma 2003;20(2):179–193
20. Steward O, Zheng B, Tessier-Lavigne M. False resurrections: distinguishing regenerated from spared axons in the injured central nervous system. J Comp Neurol 2003;459(1):1–8
21. Siegenthaler MM, Tu MK, Keirstead HS. The extent of myelin pathology differs following contusion and transection spinal cord injury. J Neurotrauma 2007;24(10):1631–1646
22. Edgerton VR, Leon RD, Harkema SJ, et al. Retraining the injured spinal cord. J Physiol 2001;533(Pt 1):15–22
23. Loy DN, Magnuson DS, Zhang YP, et al. Functional redundancy of ventral spinal locomotor pathways. J Neurosci 2002;22(1):315–323
24. Carlstedt T. Root repair review: basic science background and clinical outcome. Restor Neurol Neurosci 2008;26(2-3):225–241
25. Carlstedt T, Cullheim S, Risling M, Ulfhake B. Nerve fibre regeneration across the PNS-CNS interface at the root-spinal cord junction. Brain Res Bull 1989;22(1):93–102
26. Hoang TX, Nieto JH, Tillakaratne NJ, Havton LA. Autonomic and motor neuron death is progressive and parallel in a lumbosacral ventral root avulsion model of cauda equina injury. J Comp Neurol 2003;467(4):477–486
27. Carlstedt T, Aldskogius H, Hallin RG, Nilsson-Remahl I. Novel surgical strategies to correct neural deficits following experimental spinal nerve root lesions. Brain Res Bull 1993;30(3-4):447–451
28. Risling M, Cullheim S, Hildebrand C. Reinnervation of the ventral root L7 from ventral horn neurons following intramedullary axotomy in adult cats. Brain Res 1983;280(1):15–23
29. Lang EM, Borges J, Carlstedt T. Surgical treatment of lumbosacral plexus injuries. J Neurosurg Spine 2004;1(1):64–71
30. Carlstedt T, Anand P, Hallin R, Misra PV, Norén G, Seferlis T. Spinal nerve root repair and reimplantation of avulsed ventral roots into the spinal cord after brachial plexus injury. J Neurosurg 2000;93(2, Suppl):237–247
31. Hoang TX, Pikov V, Havton LA. Functional reinnervation of the rat lower urinary tract after cauda equina injury and repair. J Neurosci 2006;26(34):8672–8679
32. Carlstedt T, Lindå H, Cullheim S, Risling M. Reinnervation of hind limb muscles after ventral root avulsion and implantation in the lumbar spinal cord of the adult rat. Acta Physiol Scand 1986;128(4):645–646
33. Bergerot A, Shortland PJ, Anand P, Hunt SP, Carlstedt T. Co-treatment with riluzole and GDNF is necessary for functional recovery after ventral root avulsion injury. Exp Neurol 2004;187(2):359–366
34. Blakemore WF, Franklin RJ. Remyelination in experimental models of toxin-induced demyelination. Curr Top Microbiol Immunol 2008;318:193–212
35. Chari DM, Crang AJ, Blakemore WF. Decline in rate of colonization of oligodendrocyte progenitor cell (OPC)-depleted tissue by adult OPCs with age. J Neuropathol Exp Neurol 2003;62(9):908–916
36. Watson BD, Prado R, Dietrich WD, Ginsberg MD, Green BA. Photochemically induced spinal cord injury in the rat. Brain Res 1986;367(1-2):296–300
37. Verdú E, García-Alías G, Forés J, et al. Morphological characterization of photochemical graded spinal cord injury in the rat. J Neurotrauma 2003;20(5):483–499
38. Ramon y Cajal S. Degeneration and Regeneration of the Nervous System. New York: Oxford University Press; 1991
39. Schwab ME, Bartholdi D. Degeneration and regeneration of axons in the lesioned spinal cord. Physiol Rev 1996;76(2):319–370
40. Richardson PM, McGuinness UM, Aguayo AJ. Axons from CNS neurons regenerate into PNS grafts. Nature 1980;284(5753):264–265
41. Neumann S, Skinner K, Basbaum AI. Sustaining intrinsic growth capacity of adult neurons promotes spinal cord regeneration. Proc Natl Acad Sci U S A 2005;102(46):16848–16852
42. Neumann S, Woolf CJ. Regeneration of dorsal column fibers into and beyond the lesion site following adult spinal cord injury. Neuron 1999;23(1):83–91
43. Lu P, Yang H, Jones LL, Filbin MT, Tuszynski MH. Combinatorial therapy with neurotrophins and cAMP promotes axonal regeneration beyond sites of spinal cord injury. J Neurosci 2004;24(28):6402–6409
44. Mills CD, Allchorne AJ, Griffin RS, Woolf CJ, Costigan M. GDNF selectively promotes regeneration of injury-primed sensory neurons in the lesioned spinal cord. Mol Cell Neurosci 2007;36(2):185–194
45. Seijffers R, Mills CD, Woolf CJ. ATF3 increases the intrinsic growth state of DRG neurons to enhance peripheral nerve regeneration. J Neurosci 2007;27(30):7911–7920
46. Neumann S, Bradke F, Tessier-Lavigne M, Basbaum AI. Regeneration of sensory axons within the injured spinal cord induced by intraganglionic cAMP elevation. Neuron 2002;34(6):885–893
47. Tan AM, Petruska JC, Mendell LM, Levine JM. Sensory afferents regenerated into dorsal columns after spinal cord injury remain in a chronic pathophysiological state. Exp Neurol 2007;206(2):257–268
48. Leon S, Yin Y, Nguyen J, Irwin N, Benowitz LI. Lens injury stimulates axon regeneration in the mature rat optic nerve. J Neurosci 2000;20(12):4615–4626
49. Monsul NT, Geisendorfer AR, Han PJ, et al. Intraocular injection of dibutyryl cyclic AMP pro-

motes axon regeneration in rat optic nerve. Exp Neurol 2004;186(2):124–133

50. Sedý J, Urdzíková L, Jendelová P, Syková E. Methods for behavioral testing of spinal cord injured rats. Neurosci Biobehav Rev 2008;32(3):550–580
51. Basso DM, Beattie MS, Bresnahan JC. A sensitive and reliable locomotor rating scale for open field testing in rats. J Neurotrauma 1995;12(1):1–21
52. Basso DM, Fisher LC, Anderson AJ, Jakeman LB, McTigue DM, Popovich PG. Basso Mouse Scale for locomotion detects differences in recovery after spinal cord injury in five common mouse strains. J Neurotrauma 2006;23(5):635–659
53. Hamers FP, Lankhorst AJ, van Laar TJ, Veldhuis WB, Gispen WH. Automated quantitative gait analysis during overground locomotion in the rat: its application to spinal cord contusion and transection injuries. J Neurotrauma 2001;18(2):187–201
54. Gimenez y Ribotta M, Orsal D, Feraboli-Lohnherr D, Privat A, Provencher J, Rossignol S. Kinematic analysis of recovered locomotor movements of the hindlimbs in paraplegic rats transplanted with monoaminergic embryonic neurons. Ann N Y Acad Sci 1998;860:521–523
55. Cummings BJ, Engesser-Cesar C, Cadena G, Anderson AJ. Adaptation of a ladder beam walking task to assess locomotor recovery in mice following spinal cord injury. Behav Brain Res 2007;177(2): 232–241
56. Rivlin AS, Tator CH. Objective clinical assessment of motor function after experimental spinal cord injury in the rat. J Neurosurg 1977;47(4): 577–581
57. Metz GA, Merkler D, Dietz V, Schwab ME, Fouad K. Efficient testing of motor function in spinal cord injured rats. Brain Res 2000;883(2):165–177
58. Webb AA, Muir GD. Unilateral dorsal column and rubrospinal tract injuries affect overground locomotion in the unrestrained rat. Eur J Neurosci 2003;18(2):412–422
59. Smith RR, Burke DA, Baldini AD, et al. The Louisville Swim Scale: a novel assessment of hindlimb function following spinal cord injury in adult rats. J Neurotrauma 2006;23(11):1654–1670
60. Pearse DD, Lo TP Jr, Cho KS, et al. Histopathological and behavioral characterization of a novel cervical spinal cord displacement contusion injury in the rat. J Neurotrauma 2005;22(6):680–702
61. Meyer OA, Tilson HA, Byrd WC, Riley MT. A method for the routine assessment of fore- and hindlimb grip strength of rats and mice. Neurobehav Toxicol 1979;1(3):233–236
62. Hendriks WT, Eggers R, Ruitenberg MJ, et al. Profound differences in spontaneous long-term functional recovery after defined spinal tract lesions in the rat. J Neurotrauma 2006;23(1):18–35
63. Gensel JC, Tovar CA, Hamers FP, Deibert RJ, Beattie MS, Bresnahan JC. Behavioral and histological characterization of unilateral cervical spinal cord contusion injury in rats. J Neurotrauma 2006; 23(1):36–54
64. Whishaw IQ, Whishaw P, Gorny B. The structure of skilled forelimb reaching in the rat: a movement rating scale. J Vis Exp 2008;18(18):e816
65. Lambert GA, Mallos G, Zagami AS. Von Frey's hairs—a review of their technology and use—a novel automated von Frey device for improved testing for hyperalgesia. J Neurosci Methods 2009;177(2): 420–426
66. Hargreaves K, Dubner R, Brown F, Flores C, Joris J. A new and sensitive method for measuring thermal nociception in cutaneous hyperalgesia. Pain 1988;32(1):77–88
67. Chang HY, Havton LA. Re-established micturition reflexes show differential activation patterns after lumbosacral ventral root avulsion injury and repair in rats. Exp Neurol 2008;212(2):291–297
68. Allard J, Edmunds NJ. Reflex penile erection in anesthetized mice: an exploratory study. Neuroscience 2008;155(1):283–290
69. Inskip JA, Ramer LM, Ramer MS, Krassioukov AV. Autonomic assessment of animals with spinal cord injury: tools, techniques and translation. Spinal Cord 2009;47(1):2–35
70. Rowland JW, Hawryluk GW, Kwon B, Fehlings MG. Current status of acute spinal cord injury pathophysiology and emerging therapies: promise on the horizon. Neurosurg Focus 2008;25(5):E2

32

Glial Scar and Monocyte-Derived Macrophages Are Needed for Spinal Cord Repair: Timing, Location, and Level as Critical Factors

Michal Schwartz and Ravid Shechter

Key Points

1. Chondroitin sulfate proteoglycan, the major glial scar–associated matrix protein, is essential for repair at the hyperacute phase following injury and becomes a barrier to regeneration at the chronic stage.
2. Monocyte-derived macrophages, acting as immunoregulatory cells, are pivotal for spinal cord repair and display a distinct role from that of activated resident microglia.
3. An active dialogue takes place between the glial scar and monocyte-derived macrophages, which synchronizes the repair process.
4. Circulating CNS-specific recognizing T lymphocytes orchestrate monocyte recruitment to the injured spinal cord (this function of T cells is referred to as protective autoimmunity).

The poor recovery following central nervous system (CNS) insults has been a major issue of research over the last 3 decades; numerous studies have attempted to resolve why such an indispensible, precious, and pivotal organ has such a poor potential for recovery. Several factors have been suggested in attempts to resolve this puzzle, but no fully satisfactory explanation has been found. The changes induced following injury have been collectively assumed to create a hostile microenvironment, which not only is nonpermissive for regeneration but also leads to further damage through a process known as secondary degeneration.[1,2] Among such factors are the activation of local immune cells, often referred to as inflammation, and the formation of glial scar tissue following CNS injuries, which are generally considered to be major obstacles for survival, repair, and regeneration[3–6] (**Fig. 32.1**-I_{1-4}). Yet, these two processes are not unique characteristics of the CNS and are in fact pivotal components of the wound healing response in the peripheral nervous system, as well. Yet these two processes are not unique characteristics of the CNS and are, in fact, also pivotal components of the wound healing response in the peripheral nervous system.

The perception of the CNS, an immune-privileged site, as a "tissue behind walls," led to the general belief that any immune response at the injured CNS is destructive, and thus should be suppressed or eliminated. In addition, the well-documented growth-inhibitory nature of the glial scar led to the widespread conception of the glial scar as an obstacle to regeneration and, therefore, as an additional factor contributing to impaired CNS repair. Moreover, the observed spatial and temporal association between glial scar deposition and the local immune response was thought to support the negative roles of both these elements in recovery from CNS

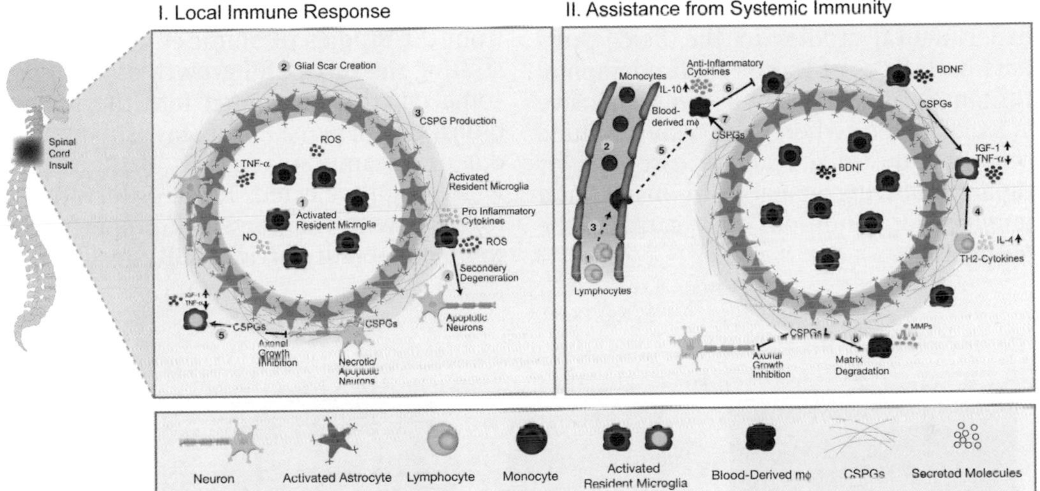

Fig. 32.1 The immunological scenario following spinal cord injury; assistance from systemic immunity is essential. (I) The local immediate response to the insult. Central nervous system insult results in the immediate activation of the local resident microglia (1) and the astrocytes. This activation leads to the creation of a dense structure, termed the glial scar (2). The major matrix component at the glial scar is chondroitin sulfate proteoglycan (CSPG), which is secreted mainly by the reactive astrocytes, and thus accumulates at the lesion margin (3). At this early stage of recovery, CSPG is required to limit the spread of damage by creating a physical barrier. The activated microglia are professional phagocytes, a function that is essential for clearance of debris; however, these cells are also associated with secretion of toxic compounds, including proinflammatory cytokines, such as interleukin (IL)-1, tumor necrosis factor-α (TNF-α), and IL-6, reactive oxygen species (ROS), and nitric oxide (NO). Thus, if the microglial response is uncontrolled or prolonged, this leads to the death of surrounding neurons, a process termed secondary degeneration (4). CSPG contributes to the limitation of this vicious cycle by activating microglia to a beneficial phenotype, which is associated with high levels of insulin-like growth factor (IGF-1) and low levels of TNF-α (5). (II) The assistance from systemic immunity. Both the adaptive (lymphocytes; 1) and the innate (monocytes; 2) arms participate in the immunological response to the insults. The lymphocytes, and more specifically helper T cells, contribute to this scenario by augmenting the recruitment of blood monocytes to the CNS (3) and by regulating the phenotype of microglia via the secretion of Th-2 cytokines (4). Blood monocytes infiltrate the damaged parenchyma and locally differentiate to macrophages (5). These blood-derived macrophages locally acquire an antiinflammatory function, which is associated with the secretion of IL-10, and thereby regulate the microglial response (6). This essential regulatory role of blood-derived macrophages is critically dependent on their interaction with CSPG (7). In turn, the blood-derived macrophages contribute to the timely degradation of this matrix (8) with well-known growth-inhibitory properties, thereby contributing to regeneration.

injury. Accordingly, research efforts were directed at attempts to block or even circumvent these two presumably hostile processes.[7–12]

However, more recent studies, pioneered by our group, questioned this blanket view and further revisited the contribution of the local inflammatory response and the scar tissue to the repair of the injured CNS. Essentially, we found that both inflammation[13–15] and scar tissue formation[16,17] are required for healing following cord insults (**Fig. 32.2**), and it is their location, level, and timing that determine whether their effect is beneficial or detrimental to the recovering neuronal tissue. This chapter, by summarizing the current experimental studies in the field, presents both faces of these two fundamental responses and suggests a comprehensive view of when, where, and why immune cells and the glial scar are essential for repair following spinal cord insult, and under what conditions they can become obstacles.

The History of the Understanding of Inflammation in the Context of CNS Repair

Although the immune system represents the defense mechanism of the body's tissues against internal or external threats, irrespective of whether the potential or actual assailants are mechanical, chemical, or biological in nature, the effects of this system on CNS repair are still elusive. From an immunological point of view, the CNS enjoys a privileged status. One of the first lines of evidence for the immune-privileged status of the brain emerged from the studies of Shirai et al.[18] demonstrating the successful growth of a rat sarcoma when transplanted into the mouse brain parenchyma, whereas subcutaneous or intramuscular grafts of the tumor were rapidly rejected. These observations, together with the perceived properties of the blood–brain barrier (BBB), resulted in

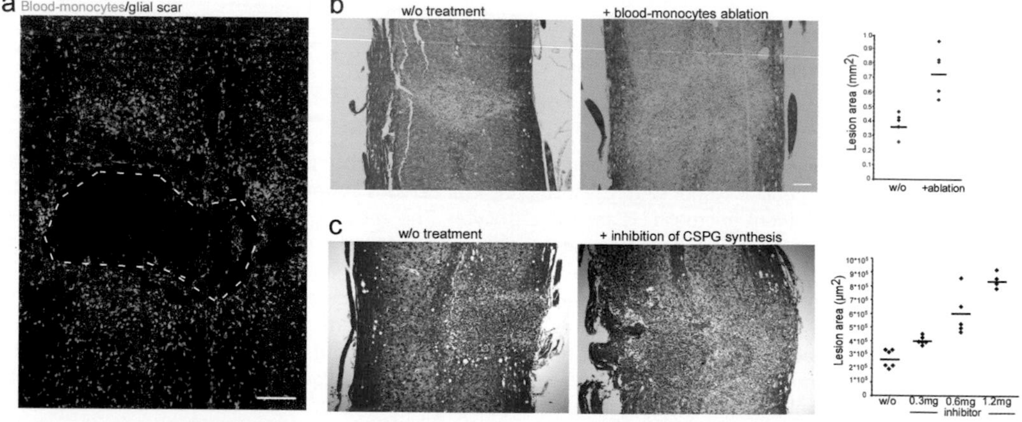

Fig. 32.2 The glial scar and blood-derived macrophages are essential for recovery from acute spinal cord injury. **(A)** Spatial association between the glial scar, represented by reactive astrocytes (*red*) and the blood-derived macrophages, shown in [Cx3cr1^{GFP} > wt]BM chimeric mice carrying the green fluorescent protein (GFP) label under the control of a myeloid-specific promoter (*green*). **(B)** The spread of damage following either conditional ablation of blood-derived macrophages or **(C)** prevention of the glial scar matrix (CSPG) formation. (From Shechter R, London A, Varol C, et al. Infiltrating blood-derived macrophages are vital cells playing an anti-inflammatory role in recovery from spinal cord injury in mice. PLoS Med 2009;6(7):e1000113; Rolls A, Shechter R, London A, et al. Faces of chondroitin sulfate proteoglycan in spinal cord repair: a role in microglia/macrophage activation. PLoS Med 2008;5(8):e171. Reprinted with permission.)

the commonly accepted view of the brain as a sealed organ, deprived of immune interactions.[19] Yet the understanding of this "privileged" status had been taken to an extreme as if no immune cell is allowed to enter the CNS from the circulation. We now know that this simplistic view is inaccurate because the degree of immune privilege is not uniform within the CNS, with some areas of the brain known to be quite active immunologically.[20] In fact, it is now well established that continuous immunosurveillance occurs in unique compartments of the CNS.

Partly because of the common view of the CNS as an immune-privileged site, the traditional belief was that any immune activity in the damaged CNS is harmful and must therefore be eliminated or suppressed.[21–23] In support of this view, mounting evidence indicated that the local inflammatory response is associated with production of toxic substances, known to be produced by various leukocytes, such as reactive oxygen species (ROS) and proinflammatory cytokines. Moreover, possibly due to erroneous projections from inflammatory diseases like multiple sclerosis to other neurodegenerative conditions, it was commonly assumed that local inflammation represents a systemic inflammatory process[24] that should be suppressed; therefore, it was persuasively suggested that the therapy of choice following injury should comprise systemic immunosuppressive drugs.[23] These drugs were thought to have great promise as a potential therapy for spinal cord injuries. Disappointingly, anti-inflammatory drugs have a narrow therapeutic window, and only a modest effect in the best of cases. Furthermore, because in some cases such treatment even accelerated damage,[25–28] a spirited debate has ensued, questioning the significance and efficiency of these sorts of systemic anti-inflammatory treatments. Moreover, potent immunosuppressive treatments were found to be accompanied by increased risk of infectious diseases, the leading cause of morbidity and mortality in patients following acute CNS injury.[29] Therefore, the utility of steroids following acute CNS insults is generally limited, and steroids are no longer automatically administered.[30] As will be discussed next, over the last few years, additional pieces were added to the puzzle by studies recognizing that the immune response to injury is not uniform in terms of the place, time, and identity of the responding cells.

The Immunological Response to Injury: A Pivotal Friend If Well Controlled

The Innate Component: The Microglial/Macrophage Response

A decade ago, we reported that "alternatively activated" blood macrophages, when locally transplanted at the margin of a spinal cord lesion, resulted in improved recovery.[13] The success of such macrophage transplantation was found to be dependent on the site of injection (no effect was found when cells were administered at the center of the lesion or far from its margins), the number of injected cells, and the time elapsed between the injury and the injection.[31] The success of this manipulation was received with a high degree of skepticism, primarily due to the lack of appreciation of macrophage heterogeneity within the CNS, a well-established phenomenon in peripheral tissues,[32,33] and due to the mistaken view of the entire local immune response as destructive within any immune-privileged site.[21,22,34] Moreover, because the site of injury is spontaneously overwhelmed with locally activated microglia, the idea of deriving therapeutic benefit by adding macrophages seemed puzzling.

A recent study in a mouse model of spinal cord injury suggested that the missing link lies in the distinction between the contribution of local versus systemic macrophages to both the widely accepted detrimental local inflammatory response and, more crucially, to its resolution.[15] The basis of this perception is our discovery of a functional distinction between the

CNS-resident macrophages, the so-called microglia, and their peripheral counterparts, the blood-derived macrophages. We found that the blood-derived macrophages, which are recruited to the site of the injury only following the insult (**Fig. 32.1**-II_5), rather than contributing to the ongoing inflammation, terminate the local immune response by displaying an antiinflammatory function required for the regulation of the activated microglia whose activity is apparently poorly controlled[15] (**Fig. 32.1**-II_6). Accordingly, recovery from CNS insults is likely to involve similar phases to those occurring in wound repair, in which the first line of defense involves a local inflammatory response needed to clean the site of injury and to create optimal conditions for the repair process. Following this phase, there is an active process of immune termination. Suppressing the immune response at any of these stages is counterproductive and is likely to result in a chronic wound with no repair. However, according to our model, if timely termination does not occur, the blessing of the first phase becomes a curse; the bright side of the local immune response is eclipsed by its negative outcomes, as a prolonged proinflammatory response becomes neurotoxic to the surrounding intact tissue. Outside the CNS, these two phases involve recruitment of naive monocytes from the blood, which locally acquire inflammatory, followed by antiinflammatory, functions, during the first and second phase, respectively.[35,36] According to our view, in the CNS, the first phase is mediated by the resident microglia without the need for assistance from circulating monocytes. Yet the termination phase critically depends on the timely and efficient recruitment of blood-derived monocytes. This does not negate the beneficial role of a "classically" activated microglial response at the early posttraumatic phase of the recovery. Rather, we argue that the mere presence of activated microglia/macrophages does not predict whether they will promote inflammation or induce its termination. This distinction calls for a careful definition of *inflammation*, which should be identified based on the activity of the relevant immune cell populations at specific time points, and not only based on their mere presence or number. These findings not only support the heterogeneity of the macrophage population at the lesion site but also indicate the essential function of blood-derived macrophages for CNS repair. This model requires an entirely different understanding of the role of macrophages in the resolution of CNS damage, versus that suggested previously. The lack of a clear distinction between the origins and functions of various macrophage subpopulations, and disregarding the need for blood-derived monocytes to mitigate damage that the microglia can no longer contain, can, in part, explain the failure of the systemic antiinflammatory drugs. Importantly and unexpectedly, we discovered that as much as these blood monocytes are needed for repair, their spontaneous recruitment is limited, unlike that of the activated resident microglia. Although the reason for the limited recruitment is not completely understood, systemic CD4+ T cells were found to be beneficial in boosting the levels of these cells[15,37] (**Fig. 32.1**-II_3).

The Role of Adaptive Immunity: CD4+ T Lymphocytes

Although the specific distinction between the CNS-resident and blood-derived subpopulations is relevant only to macrophages, many other reports indicated the necessity of additional systemic immune cells of other lineages to enable repair. It was demonstrated almost a decade ago that adaptive immune elements, and more particularly T cells, have a neuroprotective role as part of the physiological response to the CNS trauma, perhaps insufficient in its natural state but amenable to boosting.[14,38–42] It was further shown that T cells specific for CNS self-antigens, though not those reactive with irrelevant peptides, are responsible for such CNS protection. Based on these results, we have termed this phenomenon protective autoimmunity.[43] Recently, it was shown that beneficial roles of adaptive immunity are not restricted to acute traumas because these cells were found to be essential players for resolution of chronic neurodegenerative diseases, as well.[44,45] Intense research in this field revealed that these beneficial autoreactive T cells are responsible, at least in part, for the modulation of the microglial/macrophage phenotype[46–48] (**Fig. 32.1**-II_4). T cell–based vaccination results in shifting of the microglial/macrophage phenotype to a noncytotoxic beneficial one, which is mainly associated with low production of TNF-α and high levels of IGF-1.[48] Using in vitro experimental systems, it was further demonstrated that the profile of the cytokines secreted from T cells can directly affect the characteristics of the microglia. Moreover, both following acute insult and in chronic degenerative conditions, it was shown that these autoreactive T cells are involved in boosting the spontaneous infiltration of blood monocytes to the injured nervous tissue (**Fig. 32.1**-II_3), which, as described earlier, is essential for the regulation or termination of the local microglial response.[15,37]

The involvement of adaptive immunity as well as circulating monocytes in the process of repair calls for a reinterpretation of the assumption that destructive local inflammation derives from systemic inflammation. As already discussed, many studies reached opposing conclusions regarding the effects of the immune response, and thus of its inhibition, on repair. We suggest that, although CNS traumas are associated with detrimental local inflammation, this does not imply that the systemic immune system shares such an inflammatory state. Rather, we propose that the systemic immune response must be boosted/recruited to locally mitigate the inflammation and thereby reduce the damage.[49] Accordingly, blocking the systemic immune response, as is often tested in the treatment of many neurodegenerative conditions, may be counterproductive by eliminating the capacity of the systemic immune cells to introduce essential regulating and restorative factors into the inflamed area.

The Common Wisdom Regarding the Glial Scar

The glial scar consists predominantly of reactive astrocytes and microglia/macrophages embedded in extracellular matrix molecules, especially chondroitin sulfate proteoglycans (CSPGs).[50,51] The glial scar tissue is mainly known for its inhibitory effect on axonal growth.[52] Numerous studies attributed the negative aspects of the scar to the growth-inhibitory nature of some of its components. For example, CSPGs have been shown to induce neurite retraction and growth cone collapse in vitro.[53] Similarly, studies that compared the effects of different types of astrocytes on neurons revealed that reactive astrocytes, which produce NG2 (also known as CSPG4), inhibit axonal growth.[54] Moreover, the developmental role of CSPGs in the CNS is associated with the formation of boundaries because they prevent growing neurons from spreading to sites that are rich in these molecules.[55] Other studies indicated that inducing the degradation of CSPGs using specific enzymes, or inhibiting their formation, results in a dramatic increase in axonal growth and regeneration.[8,9,56] In light of its well-known activity in limiting axonal growth, the intensive secretion of CSPGs reported to follow CNS traumas has been largely blamed for the lack of axonal regeneration and detrimental outcomes.[52] These findings led to general support for therapeutic approaches targeted at scar modulation and resolution. Various approaches have attempted to eliminate and reorganize the chemical components of the glial scar, or to regulate its purportedly negative effects. Such treatments include using degrading enzymes to eliminate scar components (especially CSPGs),[8,57] blocking the activity of the growth-inhibitory components,[58] regulating intracellular signals induced by the growth-inhibitory compounds,[59,60] inhibiting astrocyte proliferation to attenuate scar formation,[61] application of growth-inducing agents,[62] and others. Obviously, all of these approaches have been based on the perception that the glial scar is an obstacle to recovery that should be modified, eliminated, suppressed, or circumvented. Yet recovery following injury has additional steps that precede regrowth, and the constructive role of the scar in these steps may have been overlooked, probably due to nonoptimal regulation of its resolution in the subsequent stage.

Although the growth-inhibitory effect of the scar and of the matrix-bound proteoglycans is the most widely studied phenomenon associated with this issue, other studies have revealed that proteoglycans actually vary in their activities. Studies of developmental processes revealed that the structure of proteoglycans and their availability in the tissue are crucial determinants of their function. Thus, for example, growth-promoting features were demonstrated for oversulfated CSPGs,[63,64] and trophic effects were attributed to several CSPGs in their soluble form.[65,66] Moreover, as will be discussed in the next sections, accumulating evidence indicates that the scar tissue and its components might have an important role in the immediate response to CNS injury.

The Glial Scar: A Pivotal Friend for Protection and a Foe for Regrowth

Despite extensive characterization of the glial scar, there is still no uniform view of its properties and function in CNS recovery. As already discussed, although the scar is mainly recognized as a major growth inhibitor, recent evidence suggests that its participation in CNS repair is much more complex than previously appreciated. In a comprehensive review,[17] which was based on our recent studies[16] and other accumulating data,[67] we proposed that the general view of the scar merely as a barrier for regeneration ignores its positive and protective effects during the acute phase of recovery. The following text summarizes the newly identified beneficial functions of this tissue and suggests how these can be reconciled with its well established growth-inhibitory role.

A Protective Mechanical Barrier

In the acute phase after the injury, the scar tissue is required for sealing the site of injury and to enable tissue remodeling. Astrocytes form a dense scar tissue that has been suggested to demarcate the lesion area and to separate the injured toxic tissue from its still-healthy surroundings.[68–70] This impermeable barrier also actively functions to restore homeostasis; astrocytes have an important scavenging activity, which is crucial for regulating excessive levels of glutamate and ions released as a result of injury.[71,72] CSPGs, secreted at the lesion margins, create a diffusion barrier for molecules that are potentially harmful to the spared tissue, thereby attenuating the spread of neurotoxicity.[68,73] Moreover, astrocytes supply tropic and metabolic support at the injury site.[74–76] Owing to their adhesiveness to growth factors, proteoglycans—and more specifically CSPGs—capture these factors, increasing their focal concentration. An additional aspect of the glial scar that may be crucial for neuronal survival following injury relates to its interim activity in filling gaps in the lesion area, creating a scaffold for the vascularization network, and regulating the intensity of blood flow.[77] Taken together, these finding indicate that the glial scar has an important role in the immediate response to insult.

An Immunoregulatory Function

A series of recent studies indicated that the scar tissue has an additional role in regulating the immunological response at the lesion site boundaries. As mentioned earlier, the phenotype acquired by immune cells and their regulation are both crucial determinants of the functional outcomes of their activity. We recently showed that the scar tissue can control the functional, temporal, and spatial immune activity at the sites of axonal injury.[16] Evidence supporting the notion that the glial scar affects immune activity has emerged from recent studies indicating that the scar is required to maintain a balanced inflammatory response. Using various techniques, including conditional ablation of predetermined cell types and specific knockdown transgenic mice, it was demonstrated that reduction of astrocyte migration/activation results in marked and widespread infiltration of inflammatory cells, emphasizing the role of astrocytes in immune regulation.[67,69,70,78] Astrocytes can further contribute to immune regulation through the secretion of relevant immune-modulating molecules, such as cytokines[79] and proteoglycans. By analogy to the elimination of astrocytes, inhibition of CSPG production using xyloside immediately after acute spinal cord injury results in an alteration of the immune response, manifested by decreased insulin-like growth factor (IGF-1) production by microglia/macrophages, and increased tumor necrosis factor-α (TNF-α) levels[16] (**Fig. 32.1**-I_5). Moreover, CSPG spatially and temporally controls the activity of infiltrating blood-derived macrophages[16] because it is required for their compartmentalization around the lesion site and for their acquisition of an inhibitory phenotype (Shechter et al., unpublished data; **Fig. 32.1**-II_7). These findings are in agreement with other reports indicating that, in the periphery, CSPGs regulate the motility and activation of macrophages,[80] dendritic cells,[81] and other immune cell types.[82] By virtue of their adhesiveness to chemoattractive agents that are needed for recruiting and activating immune cells,[83] proteoglycans capture these factors, increasing their focal concentration, and thereby target the circulating immune cells to the damaged area. This is especially important in the context of the injured CNS, which has low tolerance for immune activity; immune cells that are not confined to the injury site can cause further damage. According to this view, the glial scar, and more specifically CSPG, is needed for neuroprotection; but what about regrowth?

When Does the Scar Tissue Become an Obstacle?

As already discussed, although the glial scar participates in sealing the lesion site and modulating immune activity, it is also a major growth inhibitor. Thus many studies have reached opposing conclusions regarding the effects of this tissue and its components on repair. In our opinion, the timing of the scar generation and degradation are crucial in determining its effects.[17] In the acute phase after the injury, the scar tissue is required for wound sealing and restoring homeostasis, thereby promoting neuroprotection, whereas in the subsequent phase, further recovery requires axonal regrowth, and thus in these stages, the tissue can benefit from scar degradation. Consistent with this time-dependent view of the scar, application of inhibitors of CSPG production immediately following the insult is counterproductive, whereas their delayed administration has beneficial effects.[16] Similarly, it was shown that astrocyte ablation at different time points after injury has distinct effects on the outcome; astrocytes in the acute phase are crucial for recovery, whereas their presence in the chronic phase is inhibitory.[67] Interestingly, recent lines of evidence suggest a mutual relationship between infiltrating blood-borne macrophages and the glial scar matrix as a self-contained regulatory mechanism essential for CNS repair. The recruited macrophages, which are activated by CSPG to their essential antiinflammatory phenotype (**Fig. 32.1**-II_7), are induced by this matrix to produce proteases, such as MMP-13, that eventually degrade the matrix, resulting in the temporal restriction of the expression of this matrix molecule.[84] Thus the bidirectional relationship between the glial scar and the immune response allows the temporal, spatial, and quantitative regulation of both elements, as required for repair. However, this regulatory process does not always work optimally—the recruitment of systemic immune cells is often insufficient and thus the feedback loop does not optimally operate in the absence of intervention.

Conclusion

Although intensive efforts have been directed in attempts to reveal the individual roles of each of the participants in the local response to the insult, there is still no uniform view regarding their contribution to the repair process. Based on our recent studies and other publications over the last few years, we suggest that the debate, dilemma, and conflict all result from ignoring the fact that the response to any insult is a multistep dynamic process in which the needs of the tissue differ at each step (**Fig. 32.3**). Another source of confusion emerges from the fact that, in many studies, activation of the immune system was based on the use of bacteria or yeast-derived cell-wall components, assuming that these would induce strong immune activation. However, one should bear in mind that those activators, although they induce a strong response, do not mimic endogenous response to trauma but rather induce a different mode of activation suitable for coping with external threats. Undoubtedly, as mentioned earlier, an acute response to injury that is not terminated can turn into a chronic proinflammatory response that is destructive and shares many features with microorganism-induced activities. However, one should not attempt to make inferences from this to the participation of specific immune components in the early steps following the insult.

Similarly, we do not argue against the deleterious effects of overwhelming accumulation of CSPG or of specific immune cells, but rather suggest that the timing of both phenomena should be carefully controlled according to the changing requirements of the ongoing dynamic repair process (**Fig. 32.3**).

Over all, the "pearls" and the "pitfalls" of both phenomena, the immune response and glial scar, lie in the timing of their appearance and resolution, as well as the extent of their coordination with the tissue's needs. Although in the immediate acute phase, the tissue can benefit from neuroprotection and from rescue of the surrounding cells from the toxic environment, in the subsequent phases, regeneration must be supported. Because CSPG and proinflammatory cells share opposing effects at these two stages, their timely regulation is essential. CSPG is required at the early stages of recovery to recruit and activate microglia/blood macrophages and to limit the spread of damage by creating a physical barrier, whereas in the chronic postinjury phase, or when present in excessive amounts, its presence inhibits axonal growth. Similarly, proinflammatory cells are needed as part of the initial response for engulfment of toxic components and

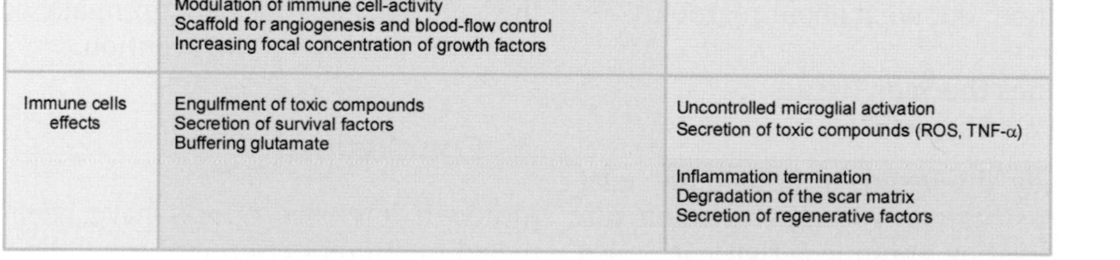

Injury → Time	Acute/sub-acute phase (hours/days – days/weeks)	Chronic phase (weeks/years)
Tissue needs	Neuroprotection Rescue of surrounding cells Removal of debris and toxic compounds Revascularization	Regeneration
Glial scar effects	Sealing the toxic site; physical barrier Compartmentalization Buffering toxicity and supply of metabolic factors by astrocytes Accumulation of chemokines, cytokines and tropic factors Modulation of immune cell-activity Scaffold for angiogenesis and blood-flow control Increasing focal concentration of growth factors	Axonal growth inhibition
Immune cells effects	Engulfment of toxic compounds Secretion of survival factors Buffering glutamate	Uncontrolled microglial activation Secretion of toxic compounds (ROS, TNF-α) Inflammation termination Degradation of the scar matrix Secretion of regenerative factors

Fig. 32.3 The dynamic repair process as a function of the tissue's needs, and the effects of both the scar and the immune response on these requirements. The main requirements for the rescue and repair at each phase are plotted as "tissue needs" (*gray*). The effects of the glial scar and the immune response are indicated. The blue box indicates potential beneficial effects, whereas the red box indicates a potentially harmful contribution. As discussed in the text, in the acute/immediate phase, both phenomena are essential for protection and for tissue sparing, whereas their uncontrolled levels and timing in the subsequent phases turn them into obstacles for repair and regeneration.

the recruitment of other essential immune cells; however, their uncontrolled response can lead to neuronal death because their phenotype is associated with the secretion of neurotoxic compounds. Such temporal and spatial regulation is achieved, for example, by the mutual relationship between these two components; CSPG is needed to promote the termination of the proinflammatory response by activating the blood-derived macrophages to an antiinflammatory phenotype, whereas these monocyte-derived cells contribute to CSPG degradation in the subsequent phase (Shechter et al., unpublished data). Because these two phenomena are so closely interrelated, it seems that optimizing one would be sufficient to ensure that the other is synchronized. One such approach is boosting levels of recruited monocytes at the optimal timeframe after the insult.[15]

Although we do not negate the potentially destructive functions of the glial scar and of the local immune response if they are not optimally controlled, we argue that viewing them as wholly detrimental is an inaccurate generalization. Thus we suggest that, rather than altogether suppressing the inflammatory response and eliminating buildup of the matrix that is associated with the glial scar, as has been attempted in the treatment of many neurodegenerative conditions, controlling their levels and timing should enable the injured neurons to benefit from their essential roles without the risk of an overwhelming and destructive response. A better understanding of the regulation of each of these phenomena, and of their mutual relationship following CNS insults, might enable the development of novel approaches or even more timely tuning of the existing approaches as ways of refining the endogenous repair mechanism, thereby improving currently available therapies for CNS insults.

Pearls

- The microglia are the first cell type to be activated following injury; they clean the injured site and signal for help. Blood-derived macrophages are essential for resolution of the microglial response and for activating the healing process; enzyme production is needed for scar resolution and to induce axonal growth, while growth factors are required for cell renewal.
- Recruitment of antiinflammatory/alternatively activated (M-2) blood macrophages cannot be replaced by administration of antiinflammatory cytokines or drugs; these "antiinflammatory" cells bring to the site not only terminating factors but also neuroprotective compounds, healing factors, such as cytokines and growth factors, and scar-degrading enzymes that promote axonal regeneration.
- The development of glial scar tissue, including formation of extracellular matrix CSPG, is not in itself a negative process. Scar formation represents an interim stage in the healing process. The scar is required first for delineating the lesion site and protecting the spared tissue, and, additionally, for controlling macrophage location and activity.

Pitfalls

- If microglial response is not resolved in a timely manner, an ongoing microglial response continues and becomes chronically cytotoxic.
- Classically activated (proinflammatory) macrophages, if not resolved on time, impair both axonal growth and cell renewal.
- The scar tissue often lacks temporal and spatial control. As with the inflammatory response, if not resolved in a timely fashion, the scar becomes a major barrier to regeneration.

References

1. Crowe MJ, Bresnahan JC, Shuman SL, Masters JN, Beattie MS. Apoptosis and delayed degeneration after spinal cord injury in rats and monkeys. Nat Med 1997;3(1):73–76
2. Park E, Velumian AA, Fehlings MG. The role of excitotoxicity in secondary mechanisms of spinal cord injury: a review with an emphasis on the implications for white matter degeneration. J Neurotrauma 2004;21(6):754–774
3. Pan JZ, Ni L, Sodhi A, Aguanno A, Young W, Hart RP. Cytokine activity contributes to induction of inflammatory cytokine mRNAs in spinal cord following contusion. J Neurosci Res 2002;68(3): 315–322
4. Young W, Kume-Kick J, Constantini S. Glucocorticoid therapy of spinal cord injury. Ann N Y Acad Sci 1994;743:241–263, discussion 263–265
5. Donnelly DJ, Popovich PG. Inflammation and its role in neuroprotection, axonal regeneration and functional recovery after spinal cord injury. Exp Neurol 2008;209(2):378–388
6. Weaver LC, Marsh DR, Gris D, Brown A, Dekaban GA. Autonomic dysreflexia after spinal cord injury: central mechanisms and strategies for prevention. Prog Brain Res 2006;152:245–263
7. Fawcett JW. Overcoming inhibition in the damaged spinal cord. J Neurotrauma 2006;23(3-4): 371–383
8. Bradbury EJ, Moon LD, Popat RJ, et al. Chondroitinase ABC promotes functional recovery after spinal cord injury. Nature 2002;416(6881): 636–640
9. Moon LD, Asher RA, Rhodes KE, Fawcett JW. Regeneration of CNS axons back to their target following treatment of adult rat brain with chondroitinase ABC. Nat Neurosci 2001;4(5):465–466
10. Nesathurai S. The role of methylprednisolone in acute spinal cord injuries. J Trauma 2001;51(2): 421–423
11. Gris D, Marsh DR, Oatway MA, et al. Transient blockade of the CD11d/CD18 integrin reduces secondary damage after spinal cord injury, improving sensory, autonomic, and motor function. J Neurosci 2004;24(16):4043–4051
12. Yong VW, Wells J, Giuliani F, Casha S, Power C, Metz LM. The promise of minocycline in neurology. Lancet Neurol 2004;3(12):744–751
13. Rapalino O, Lazarov-Spiegler O, Agranov E, et al. Implantation of stimulated homologous macrophages results in partial recovery of paraplegic rats. Nat Med 1998;4(7):814–821
14. Hauben E, Agranov E, Gothilf A, et al. Posttraumatic therapeutic vaccination with modified myelin self-antigen prevents complete paralysis while avoiding autoimmune disease. J Clin Invest 2001;108(4):591–599
15. Shechter R, London A, Varol C, et al. Infiltrating blood-derived macrophages are vital cells playing an anti-inflammatory role in recovery from spinal cord injury in mice. PLoS Med 2009;6(7): e1000113
16. Rolls A, Shechter R, London A, et al. Two faces of chondroitin sulfate proteoglycan in spinal cord repair: a role in microglia/macrophage activation. PLoS Med 2008;5(8):e171
17. Rolls A, Shechter R, Schwartz M. The bright side of the glial scar in CNS repair. Nat Rev Neurosci 2009;10(3):235–241
18. Shirai M, Izumi H, Yamagami T. Experimental transplantation models of mouse sarcoma 180 in ICR mice for evaluation of anti-tumor drugs. J Vet Med Sci 1991;53(4):707–713
19. de Micco C, Toga M. [The immune status of the central nervous system]. Rev Neurol (Paris) 1988;144(12):776–788
20. Schwartz M, Shechter R. Protective autoimmunity functions by intracranial immunosurveillance to support the mind: the missing link between health and disease. Mol Psychiatry 2010; 15(4):342–354
21. Block ML, Zecca L, Hong JS. Microglia-mediated neurotoxicity: uncovering the molecular mechanisms. Nat Rev Neurosci 2007;8(1):57–69
22. Popovich PG, Guan Z, Wei P, Huitinga I, van Rooijen N, Stokes BT. Depletion of hematogenous macrophages promotes partial hindlimb recovery and neuroanatomical repair after experimental spinal cord injury. Exp Neurol 1999;158(2):351–365
23. Nesathurai S. Steroids and spinal cord injury: revisiting the NASCIS 2 and NASCIS 3 trials. J Trauma 1998;45(6):1088–1093
24. Ankeny DP, Lucin KM, Sanders VM, McGaughy VM, Popovich PG. Spinal cord injury triggers systemic autoimmunity: evidence for chronic B lymphocyte activation and lupus-like autoantibody synthesis. J Neurochem 2006;99(4):1073–1087
25. Suberviola B, González-Castro A, Llorca J, Ortiz-Melón F, Miñambres E. Early complications of high-dose methylprednisolone in acute spinal cord injury patients. Injury 2008;39(7):748–752
26. George ER, Scholten DJ, Buechler CM, Jordan-Tibbs J, Mattice C, Albrecht RM. Failure of methylprednisolone to improve the outcome of spinal cord injuries. Am Surg 1995;61(8):659–663, discussion 663–664
27. Prendergast MR, Saxe JM, Ledgerwood AM, Lucas CE, Lucas WF. Massive steroids do not reduce the zone of injury after penetrating spinal cord injury. J Trauma 1994;37(4):576–579, discussion 579–580
28. Guízar-Sahagún G, Rodríguez-Balderas CA, Franco-Bourland RE, et al. Lack of neuroprotection with pharmacological pretreatment in a paradigm for anticipated spinal cord lesions. Spinal Cord 2009; 47(2):156–160
29. Meisel C, Schwab JM, Prass K, Meisel A, Dirnagl U. Central nervous system injury-induced immune deficiency syndrome. Nat Rev Neurosci 2005;6(10):775–786
30. Rozet I. Methylprednisolone in acute spinal cord injury: is there any other ethical choice? J Neurosurg Anesthesiol 2008;20(2):137–139
31. Schwartz M, Yoles E. Immune-based therapy for spinal cord repair: autologous macrophages and beyond. J Neurotrauma 2006;23(3-4):360–370
32. Gordon S, Taylor PR. Monocyte and macrophage heterogeneity. Nat Rev Immunol 2005;5(12):953–964
33. Gordon S. Alternative activation of macrophages. Nat Rev Immunol 2003;3(1):23–35
34. Mabon PJ, Weaver LC, Dekaban GA. Inhibition of monocyte/macrophage migration to a spinal cord

injury site by an antibody to the integrin alphaD: a potential new anti-inflammatory treatment. Exp Neurol 2000;166(1):52–64

35. Nahrendorf M, Swirski FK, Aikawa E, et al. The healing myocardium sequentially mobilizes two monocyte subsets with divergent and complementary functions. J Exp Med 2007;204(12): 3037–3047
36. Arnold L, Henry A, Poron F, et al. Inflammatory monocytes recruited after skeletal muscle injury switch into antiinflammatory macrophages to support myogenesis. J Exp Med 2007;204(5): 1057–1069
37. Butovsky O, Kunis G, Koronyo-Hamaoui M, Schwartz M. Selective ablation of bone marrow-derived dendritic cells increases amyloid plaques in a mouse Alzheimer's disease model. Eur J Neurosci 2007;26(2):413–416
38. Moalem G, Leibowitz-Amit R, Yoles E, Mor F, Cohen IR, Schwartz M. Autoimmune T cells protect neurons from secondary degeneration after central nervous system axotomy. Nat Med 1999;5(1):49–55
39. Hofstetter HH, Sewell DL, Liu F, et al. Autoreactive T cells promote post-traumatic healing in the central nervous system. J Neuroimmunol 2003;134(1-2):25–34
40. Lobell A, Weissert R, Eltayeb S, et al. Suppressive DNA vaccination in myelin oligodendrocyte glycoprotein peptide-induced experimental autoimmune encephalomyelitis involves a T1-biased immune response. J Immunol 2003;170(4): 1806–1813
41. Ibarra A, Avendaño H, Cruz Y. Copolymer-1 (Cop-1) improves neurological recovery after middle cerebral artery occlusion in rats. Neurosci Lett 2007;425(2):110–113
42. Ibarra A, Hauben E, Butovsky O, Schwartz M. The therapeutic window after spinal cord injury can accommodate T cell-based vaccination and methylprednisolone in rats. Eur J Neurosci 2004;19(11):2984–2990
43. Schwartz M, Shaked I, Fisher J, Mizrahi T, Schori H. Protective autoimmunity against the enemy within: fighting glutamate toxicity. Trends Neurosci 2003;26(6):297–302
44. Banerjee R, Mosley RL, Reynolds AD, et al. Adaptive immune neuroprotection in G93A-SOD1 amyotrophic lateral sclerosis mice. PLoS ONE 2008; 3(7):e2740
45. Beers DR, Henkel JS, Zhao W, Wang J, Appel SH. CD4+ T cells support glial neuroprotection, slow disease progression, and modify glial morphology in an animal model of inherited ALS. Proc Natl Acad Sci U S A 2008;105(40):15558–15563
46. Butovsky O, Hauben E, Schwartz M. Morphological aspects of spinal cord autoimmune neuroprotection: colocalization of T cells with B7-2 (CD86) and prevention of cyst formation. FASEB J 2001;15(6):1065–1067
47. Butovsky O, Koronyo-Hamaoui M, Kunis G, et al. Glatiramer acetate fights against Alzheimer's disease by inducing dendritic-like microglia expressing insulin-like growth factor 1. Proc Natl Acad Sci USA 2006;103(31):11784–11789
48. Butovsky O, Ziv Y, Schwartz A, et al. Microglia activated by IL-4 or IFN-gamma differentially induce neurogenesis and oligodendrogenesis from adult stem/progenitor cells. Mol Cell Neurosci 2006;31(1):149–160
49. Schwartz M, Shechter R. Systemic inflammatory cells fight off neurodegenerative disease. Nat Rev Neurol 2010;6(7):405–410
50. Jones LL, Margolis RU, Tuszynski MH. The chondroitin sulfate proteoglycans neurocan, brevican, phosphacan, and versican are differentially regulated following spinal cord injury. Exp Neurol 2003;182(2):399–411
51. McKeon RJ, Jurynec MJ, Buck CR. The chondroitin sulfate proteoglycans neurocan and phosphacan are expressed by reactive astrocytes in the chronic CNS glial scar. J Neurosci 1999;19(24): 10778–10788
52. Silver J, Miller JH. Regeneration beyond the glial scar. Nat Rev Neurosci 2004;5(2):146–156
53. McKeon RJ, Schreiber RC, Rudge JS, Silver J. Reduction of neurite outgrowth in a model of glial scarring following CNS injury is correlated with the expression of inhibitory molecules on reactive astrocytes. J Neurosci 1991;11(11):3398–3411
54. Fidler PS, Schuette K, Asher RA, et al. Comparing astrocytic cell lines that are inhibitory or permissive for axon growth: the major axon-inhibitory proteoglycan is NG2. J Neurosci 1999; 19(20):8778–8788
55. Snow DM, Steindler DA, Silver J. Molecular and cellular characterization of the glial roof plate of the spinal cord and optic tectum: a possible role for a proteoglycan in the development of an axon barrier. Dev Biol 1990;138(2):359–376
56. Smith-Thomas LC, Stevens J, Fok-Seang J, Faissner A, Rogers JH, Fawcett JW. Increased axon regeneration in astrocytes grown in the presence of proteoglycan synthesis inhibitors. J Cell Sci 1995; 108(Pt 3):1307–1315
57. Moon LD, Fawcett JW. Reduction in CNS scar formation without concomitant increase in axon regeneration following treatment of adult rat brain with a combination of antibodies to TGFbeta1 and beta2. Eur J Neurosci 2001;14(10):1667–1677
58. Tan AM, Colletti M, Rorai AT, Skene JH, Levine JM. Antibodies against the NG2 proteoglycan promote the regeneration of sensory axons within the dorsal columns of the spinal cord. J Neurosci 2006;26(18):4729–4739
59. Neumann S, Bradke F, Tessier-Lavigne M, Basbaum AI. Regeneration of sensory axons within the injured spinal cord induced by intraganglionic cAMP elevation. Neuron 2002;34(6):885–893
60. Dergham P, Ellezam B, Essagian C, Avedissian H, Lubell WD, McKerracher L. Rho signaling pathway targeted to promote spinal cord repair. J Neurosci 2002;22(15):6570–6577
61. Tian DS, Dong Q, Pan DJ, et al. Attenuation of astrogliosis by suppressing of microglial proliferation with the cell cycle inhibitor olomoucine in rat spinal cord injury model. Brain Res 2007; 1154:206–214
62. Romero MI, Rangappa N, Garry MG, Smith GM. Functional regeneration of chronically injured sensory afferents into adult spinal cord after neurotrophin gene therapy. J Neurosci 2001; 21(21):8408–8416
63. Hikino M, Mikami T, Faissner A, Vilela-Silva AC, Pavão MS, Sugahara K. Oversulfated dermatan sulfate exhibits neurite outgrowth-promoting

activity toward embryonic mouse hippocampal neurons: implications of dermatan sulfate in neuritogenesis in the brain. J Biol Chem 2003; 278(44):43744–43754

64. Bicknese AR, Sheppard AM, O'Leary DD, Pearlman AL. Thalamocortical axons extend along a chondroitin sulfate proteoglycan-enriched pathway coincident with the neocortical subplate and distinct from the efferent path. J Neurosci 1994;14(6):3500–3510
65. Sato Y, Nakanishi K, Tokita Y, et al. A highly sulfated chondroitin sulfate preparation, CS-E, prevents excitatory amino acid-induced neuronal cell death. J Neurochem 2008;104(6):1565–1576
66. Brittis PA, Silver J. Exogenous glycosaminoglycans induce complete inversion of retinal ganglion cell bodies and their axons within the retinal neuroepithelium. Proc Natl Acad Sci U S A 1994;91(16):7539–7542
67. Okada S, Nakamura M, Katoh H, et al. Conditional ablation of Stat3 or Socs3 discloses a dual role for reactive astrocytes after spinal cord injury. Nat Med 2006;12(7):829–834
68. Roitbak T, Syková E. Diffusion barriers evoked in the rat cortex by reactive astrogliosis. Glia 1999;28(1):40–48
69. Faulkner JR, Herrmann JE, Woo MJ, Tansey KE, Doan NB, Sofroniew MV. Reactive astrocytes protect tissue and preserve function after spinal cord injury. J Neurosci 2004;24(9):2143–2155
70. Bush TG, Puvanachandra N, Horner CH, et al. Leukocyte infiltration, neuronal degeneration, and neurite outgrowth after ablation of scar-forming, reactive astrocytes in adult transgenic mice. Neuron 1999;23(2):297–308
71. Cui W, Allen ND, Skynner M, Gusterson B, Clark AJ. Inducible ablation of astrocytes shows that these cells are required for neuronal survival in the adult brain. Glia 2001;34(4):272–282
72. Chen Y, Vartiainen NE, Ying W, Chan PH, Koistinaho J, Swanson RA. Astrocytes protect neurons from nitric oxide toxicity by a glutathione-dependent mechanism. J Neurochem 2001;77(6): 1601–1610
73. Vorísek I, Hájek M, Tintera J, Nicolay K, Syková E. Water ADC, extracellular space volume, and tortuosity in the rat cortex after traumatic injury. Magn Reson Med 2002;48(6):994–1003
74. do Carmo Cunha J, de Freitas Azevedo Levy B, de Luca BA, de Andrade MS, Gomide VC, Chadi G. Responses of reactive astrocytes containing S100beta protein and fibroblast growth factor-2 in the border and in the adjacent preserved tissue after a contusion injury of the spinal cord in rats: implications for wound repair and neuroregeneration. Wound Repair Regen 2007;15(1):134–146
75. Schwartz JP, Nishiyama N. Neurotrophic factor gene expression in astrocytes during development and following injury. Brain Res Bull 1994;35(5-6):403–407
76. Wu VW, Nishiyama N, Schwartz JP. A culture model of reactive astrocytes: increased nerve growth factor synthesis and reexpression of cytokine responsiveness. J Neurochem 1998;71(2):749–756
77. Parri R, Crunelli V. An astrocyte bridge from synapse to blood flow. Nat Neurosci 2003;6(1):5–6
78. Herrmann JE, Imura T, Song B, et al. STAT3 is a critical regulator of astrogliosis and scar formation after spinal cord injury. J Neurosci 2008;28(28): 7231–7243
79. Chung IY, Benveniste EN. Tumor necrosis factor-alpha production by astrocytes: induction by lipopolysaccharide, IFN-gamma, and IL-1 beta. J Immunol 1990;144(8):2999–3007
80. Hayashi K, Kadomatsu K, Muramatsu T. Requirement of chondroitin sulfate/dermatan sulfate recognition in midkine-dependent migration of macrophages. Glycoconj J 2001;18(5):401–406
81. Kodaira Y, Nair SK, Wrenshall LE, Gilboa E, Platt JL. Phenotypic and functional maturation of dendritic cells mediated by heparan sulfate. J Immunol 2000;165(3):1599–1604
82. Rolls A, Cahalon L, Bakalash S, Avidan H, Lider O, Schwartz M. A sulfated disaccharide derived from chondroitin sulfate proteoglycan protects against inflammation-associated neurodegeneration. FASEB J 2006;20(3):547–549
83. Nandini CD, Sugahara K. Role of the sulfation pattern of chondroitin sulfate in its biological activities and in the binding of growth factors. Adv Pharmacol 2006;53:253–279
84. Shechter R, Raposo C, London A, Sagi I, Schwartz M. The glial scar-monocyte interplay: a pivotal resolution phase in spinal cord repair. PLoS ONE 2011;6:e27979

33

Promising Preclinical Pharmacological Approaches to Spinal Cord Injury

Michael S. Beattie and Jacqueline C. Bresnahan

Key Points

1. CNS injury induces a cascade of overlapping degradative and reparative processes that interact to determine the final functional outcome.
2. Targeting these processes for therapeutic purposes will be complicated by differential responses of individual cell types and the time course over which they respond.
3. Sensitive and reliable preclinical models are critical for translation of therapies.
4. Several promising pharmacological treatments are now available based on preclinical studies.

Edema and excitotoxic cell death have long been targets for therapies aimed at reducing secondary damage after central nervous system (CNS) injury.[1–3] Recently, it has become clear that acute inflammatory reactions to injury interact with, and may drive, some aspects of secondary injury.[4] The concept of secondary injury is key to the search for acute therapies, although details of the complex cascade of secondary events in spinal cord injury (SCI) and other acute neural damage are lacking. It is generally thought that, in SCI, a frank mechanical disruption of cellular membranes, including breakage of endothelial cells and the release of peripheral blood products into the cord, is followed by the centripetal spread of injury mediated by the biochemical and biological consequences of this initial damage[1,3,5] (**Fig. 33.1**). But the relative roles of extracellular glutamate, blood products released from the injury site, inflammation, and oxidative stress are really not well understood, although each has been the target of intensive investigations. In addition, injury initiates reparative processes as well as degradation, and it is often difficult to differentiate the "positive" from the "negative" biological events after injury. One way to conceptualize this complexity is to view secondary injury and repair in terms of the cell–cell interactions that occur between the multiple cellular constituents of the injured spinal cord or brain

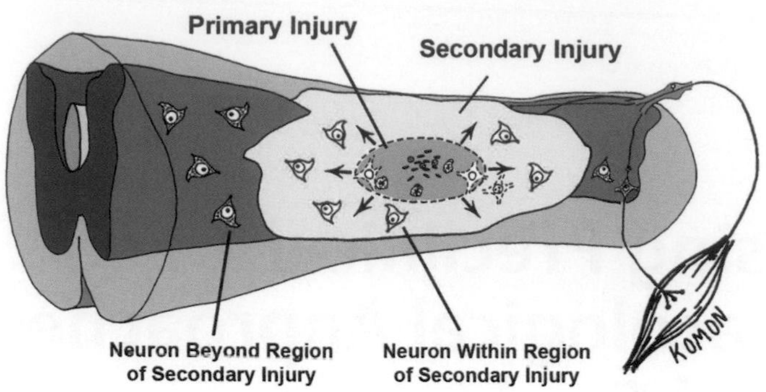

Fig. 33.1 Schematic of the secondary injury process after spinal cord injury. Mechanical impact to the cord concentrates energy in the central region where blood vessels and cell membranes are disrupted immediately. Products of that destruction include glutamate and cytosolic contents that are thought to produce a wave of cell death moving outward from the primary lesion. Cells on the periphery of the expanding lesion are in danger of excitotoxic cell death due to the effects of cytokines and reactive oxygen (see **Fig 33.2** and legend), and are the targets for pharmacological treatments aimed at increasing sparing.

(**Fig. 33.2**). Although each of the cellular constituents of the cord can be identified as a group of phenotypically related cells (e.g., glia, neurons, endothelia), they share many biological response elements, including common neurotransmitter and cytokine receptors, protective mechanisms aimed at reducing cellular stress, and effectors (e.g., glutamate and cytokine release) that make targeting isolated aspects of the injury process problematic.

This chapter discusses several new, promising therapeutic strategies aimed at secondary injury in the context of the interaction between neurons, astrocytes, oligodendrocytes, and their precursor cells (OPCs), microglia and vascular elements, and how those effects may be translated into alterations in the response to injury characterized by edema, excitoxicity, and acute inflammation.

Therapies Aimed at One Target May Affect Multiple Aspects of Secondary Injury

The classic example of this is, of course, methylprednisolone (MP), which is a steroid with high activity at glucocorticoid receptors. Its multiple mechanisms of action, however, are thought to include reduction of both edema and lipid peroxidation.[6–8] Further, there is evidence that MP reduces endothelial cell damage, thus promoting vascular stability and blood flow,[9,10] that MP is antiinflammatory,[8] and that MP can reduce axonal retraction after SCI.[10] Because there are extensive cell–cell interactions between the multiple cell types affected by SCI, and because many of the potential targets of therapies are shared between multiple elements of secondary injury, it is useful to consider how promising therapies may interact with multiple targets. This is the strategy behind looking for "dirty drugs" that might be most useful in reducing secondary injury.[1] It is also worth noting that the drugs that might reduce secondary injury might also affect the endogenous reparative responses of the cord to injury. For example, reduction of the acute inflammatory response to injury by MP has also been associated with a reduction in the production of neurotrophic factors or progenitor cell proliferation that might aid in repair.[11–13] Although MP meets many of the criteria of a promising dirty drug, and there is some evidence supporting its promise in rodent models,[14] there have been continued failures in attempts to show consistent effects in rodent contusion models of SCI.[15] Indeed, it has been difficult to find any treatments aimed at secondary injury that show consistently

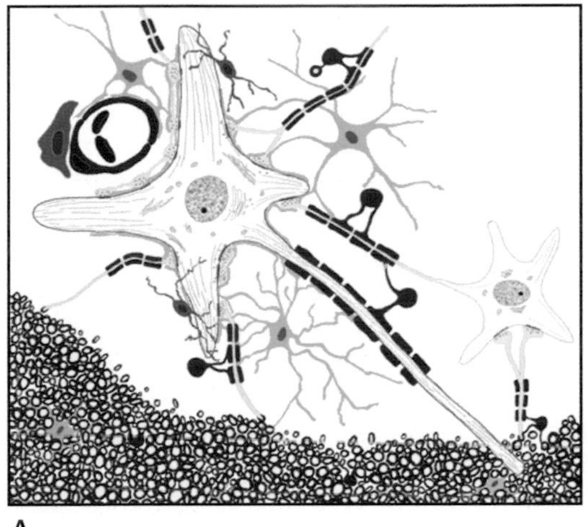

A

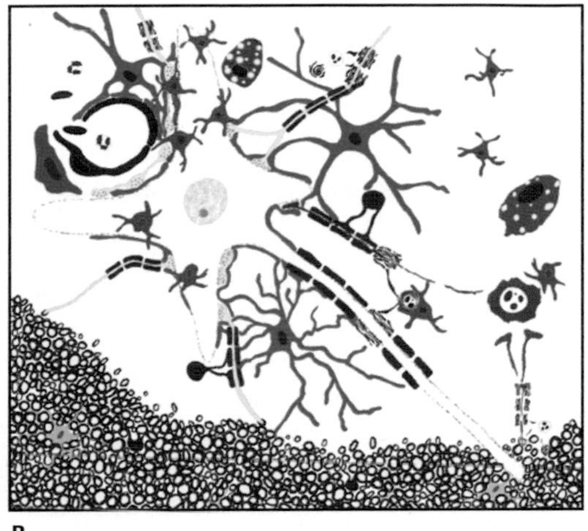

B

Fig. 33.2 A cartoon of the cellular constituents **(A)** before and **(B)** after injury. The central importance of the "neurovascular unit" (NVU) in the secondary injury response should be emphasized. Endothelial cell breakdown leads to extravasation of blood and plasma, which contain fibrin, and which can result in vasogenic and cytotoxic edema, leading to swelling of astrocytes, vascular stasis, and continued blood-brain barrier disruption. These events can induce microglial activation, which releases a host of cytokines, including the proinflammatory cytokine tumor necrosis factor-α (TNF-α). TNF can induce the release of glutamate from astrocytes as well. This, in combination with release of glutamate from damaged axons and neurons, can depolarize intact neurons, leading to excess Ca^{2+} influx via *N*-methyl-D-aspartate (NMDA) receptors. Excess TNF can move Ca^{2+} permeable α-amino-3-hydroxy-5-methyl-4-isoxazoleproprionic acid (AMPA) receptor to the neuronal surface, thus increasing the CA^{2+} load on surviving neurons. All of the resulting cellular death releases intracellular molecules that can in turn activate microglial cells and astrocytes further through, for example, the activation of purinergic receptors and Toll-like receptor 4 signaling. The resultant reactive oxygen species (ROS), along with cytokines, can attack nearby oligodendrocytes, which also respond to glutamate through AMPA receptors, resulting in acute or delayed oligodendrocyte death and demyelination of intact axons. At the same time, glial responses to injury can be protective, including the rapid removal of glutamate from the extracellular space by astrocytic glutamate transporters, and the production of neurotrophic and neuroprotective molecules by both astrocytes and microglia. In addition, injury induces the proliferation and differentiation of endogenous progenitor cells, including those characterized by surface expression of the proteoglycan NG2. In more chronic phases after injury, the result of all these interactions may be the deposition of glial scar and extracellular matrix molecules that retard axonal growth. Even this rather long list of events is really just a snapshot of the complexity inherent in the response of the spinal cord parenchyma to injury. Each of these events represents a target for therapies. (Astrocytes, turquoise; apoptotic neuron and degenerating axons and terminals, brown; normal axons and terminals, yellow; endothelial and red blood cells, red; microglia and macrophages, orange; pericyte, orange; neurons, gray; oligodendrocytes, blue with magenta nuclei and myelin, blue; polymorphonuclear leukocytes,– white with blue nuclei.)

positive effects in multiple laboratories.[16,17] This is likely due, at least in part, to the complicated multiple and redundant pathways leading to tissue damage after injury.

Blood Vessel Injury Is a Point of First Defense

Figure 33.1 shows the central hemorrhagic injury due to breakage of blood vessels by trauma. However, vascular damage appears not to be a single mechanical event, but rather is part of the injury cascade can also proceed over time. This has been appreciated in earlier studies of blood flow and vascular status,[18,19] but recent attention has been placed on a dynamic expansion of secondary hemorrhage. Progressive hemorrhagic necrosis appears to be related to active breakdown of vascular endothelial cells through a process of endothelial cell swelling and oncosis that is mediated by sulfonylurea receptor 1 (SUR1)-regulated NC(Ca-ATP) channels and transient potential cation channel subfamily M member 4 (TRPM4) channels expressed in response to injury and hypoxia.[20,21] SCI induces upregulation of both SUR1-regulated channels and Trpm4. Blockade of SUR1-regulated channel expression, or receptor blockade using glibenclamide or other drugs, produces remarkable reduction in progressive hemorrhagic necrosis. Trpm4 -/- mice have much attenuated vascular breakdown after a cervical contusion injury.[20] Reductions of channel expression or activity have marked effects on injury progression and appear to improve outcome substantially.[20,21] The prevention of progressive vascular disruption and protection of endothelial cells presumably blunts all of the downstream complex sequelae, including glutamate and adenosine triphosphate (ATP) production, microglial activation, and cytokine production, and the progression of cell death that ensues, including the longer-term effects on oligodendrocyte apoptosis.[22,23] It is less clear how this endothelial cell progression of damage may affect injuries that are less mechanical and more ischemic in origin, but SUR1-regulated channels are also implicated in the progression of hemorrhagic necrosis seen in ischemic stroke models.[24] Disruption of the blood–brain barrier is therefore linked to endothelial cell edema, and the critical importance of the "neurovascular unit" in secondary injury is emphasized.[25] In this regard, it is interesting that hypertonic saline, which is thought to provide protection for endothelial cells by reducing cellular swelling,[26] has been shown in our laboratory to reduce magnetic resonance imaging indices of edema and hemorrhage[27] in the first 8 hours after a cervical contusion injury model similar to that used to demonstrate the positive effects of endothelial cell protection by blocking SUR1-regulated NC-Ca-ATP channels or Trpm4 already described.

Cellular Energy Loss and Depletion of ATP Appear to Be Important in Cellular Dysregulation after Injury

For example, dysregulation of the Trpm4 channels results in unchecked Na^+ influx, swelling, and oncosis of endothelial cells, as well as astrocytes and neurons.[20] In turn, release of ATP by dying cells can play a role in the production of secondary injury. This has been highlighted by recent work in which blockade of ATP activation of P2X7 receptors has been shown to improve outcomes after experimental SCI in rats.[28,29] Wang et al.[28] provided an elegant demonstration of the release of extracellular ATP after SCI using luciferase-mediated breakdown of luciferin in the presence of ATP to image ATP release in vivo after a mechanical injury to the dorsal spinal cord. After laminectomy, a charge coupled device (CCD) camera and in vivo microscopy were used to show the spread of luciferase-mediated fluorescence after a mechanical injury to the surface of the exposed cord. Concentrations of ATP were estimated qualitatively, but the experiment clearly showed a progression of ATP release over time, yielding another confirmation of the concept of secondary injury spread. When ATP activation of P2X7 receptors was blocked by OxATP, cell death was reduced and recovery was enhanced. Treatments reduced apoptosis after a thoracic contusion injury in rats, as measured in a TUNEL assay, and also dramatically improved Basso, Beattie, Bresnahan (BBB) locomotor scores[30] at 6 weeks postinjury from ~9 to 14, corresponding to a difference between weight support and no or little stepping, to consistent plantar stepping and consistently coordinated locomotion in the treatment group.

In a follow-up study,[29] P2X7 receptor blockade was obtained using a novel antagonist, brilliant blue G (BBG), a Coomasie dye analogue of the food coloring additive FD&C blue dye no. 1. Even large doses of this dye are not toxic, and indeed, the authors point out that humans consume massive quantities of this food coloring every day. Thus it was particularly intriguing that this treatment also had significant effects on outcomes from thoracic contusion injuries in rats. BBB locomotor scores were improved from an average of 9.4 to 11.9 at 6 weeks, corresponding to a difference between weight support and no or little plantar stepping in untreated subjects and consistent plantar stepping with some coordinated locomotion in the treatment groups. BBG treatments of 10 or 50 mg/kg were also found to improve tissue sparing at the lesion site, and, importantly, to reduce microglial activation at early times after injury (as measured by immunocytochemistry and microglial morphology). In addition, BBG treatment reduced the infiltration of macrophages, neutrophils, and CD8-positive T-cells. All of these results are consistent with a powerful antiinflammatory effect mediated by blockade of microglial activation through the P2X7 receptor. But, in addition, neurons (and to a lesser extent astrocytes) also have P2X7 receptors. Because ATP can induce activity and excitotoxicity in neurons as well, the BBG treatment also represents a multiple-cell targeted therapy. If this work can be replicated, it should serve as an important stimulus for more secondary injury treatments aimed at early stages in the inflammatory cascade. This work supports the use of antiinflammatory strategies, even though the reports of efficacy of antiinflammatory drugs like minocycline have shown mixed positive and negative effects.[17,31,32]

ATP Activation of Microglia and Neurons, As Well As Cell Death–Induced Release of Intracellular Stores of Glutamate, Contribute to Excitotoxicity

Glutamate reaches toxic levels minutes after SCI,[33] and drugs that reduce the activity of glutamate receptors, allowing Ca^{2+} influx, have been used for many studies of secondary neuroprotection. However, the most effective agents, including MK-801, tetrodotoxin (TTX), and others,[34–36] are not suitable for clinical use. Recently, increased attention has been given to neuroprotective drugs that are used as antiepileptic agents, including phenytoin and riluzole. These drugs also share multiple mechanisms of action, including reduction of Na^+ influx to ligand and voltage-gated channels,[37] and reduction of glutamate release. Studies in models of epilepsy also show reduced cellular damage and excitotoxicity.[38] In addition, riluzole has been tested in human clinical trials for amyotrophic lateral sclerosis (ALS), with some efficacy demonstrated.[39,40] In rat SCI models, antagonists of glutamate receptors, including the AMPA/kainate receptor antagonists NBQX[34] and GYKI 52466,[41] have shown some positive effects on behavioral recovery (BBB score outcomes of ~2 points difference). Riluzole, typically used as an anticonvulsant, has shown rather impressive neuroprotection and amelioration of neurological deficits in a rat clip-compression model of SCI.[37] Interestingly, several other compounds that are thought to share the Na^+ channel blocking properties of riluzole (e.g., phenytoin) failed to show efficacy in the same study. Another study using a more rapid contusion injury model, also in rats, showed efficacy only when riluzole was given in combination with MP.[42] Riluzole's actions might also be due to its apparent reduction of glutamate release by astrocytes.[43] Riluzole is currently in clinical trials for SCI and has also shown efficacy in trials for ALS.[39,40] Riluzole also has activity in reducing glutamate release[43] and thus affects multiple mechanisms of action against secondary injury. Again, multiple targets are better, but it is difficult to predict efficacy in rodent models based on mechanisms of action alone.

Importantly, the actions of glutamate on oligodendrocytes and oligodendrocyte progenitor cells via AMPA-receptor-mediated cell death and apoptosis are also critical in secondary injury.[3] Indeed, many of the drugs that show some efficacy against neuronal excitotoxicity also have been shown to inhibit secondary oligodendrocyte cell death and demyelination.[32]

Proinflammatory Cytokines Play an Important Role in the Secondary Injury Cascade

Finally, we turn to the role of proinflammatory cytokines in secondary injury. The tetracycline derivative minocycline has antiinflammatory properties and has been used to reduce microglial activation in an attempt to reduce the production and release of proinflammatory tumor necrosis factor-α (TNF-α), for example, which rise precipitously after SCI.[44] Proinflammatory cytokines in turn can activate microglia as well as increase glutamate release from astrocytes.[45] Although a direct "bystander effect" has been postulated for both neurons and oligodendrocytes,[46] recent work in our laboratory and others has highlighted an interactive effect between cytokine actions and glutamate-induced excitotoxicity. Thus, TNF-α greatly exacerbates the excitotoxic effects of kainic acid nano-injected into the spinal cord gray matter.[47] This effect is completely blocked by the AMPA/kainic acid receptor antagonist 6-cyano-7-nitroquinoxaline-2,3-drone (CNQX). Thus TNF has an amplifying effect on glutamate signaling through AMPARs. This amplifying effect was shown in vitro to be due to a specific TNF-α effect on the trafficking of AMPARs to the surface of the neuronal membrane.[48] This increased the effects of AMPAR-mediated cell death, and the death was blocked by drugs that reduced PI3K activity and thereby the TNF-induced increases in trafficking.[49] Contusion SCI also could be shown to increase the surface localization of AMPARs that lacked GluR2.[50] Such AMPARs allow passage of Ca^{2+} ions, which are normally blocked by the presence of the GluR2 subunit. Thus more GluR1-containing and fewer Glur2-containing receptors on the surface would lead to increased excitotoxic effects of the same amount of extracellular glutamate. This was confirmed by using a soluble TNF receptor protein 1 (sTNFr1) to sequester injury-induced TNF. This treatment reduced surface expression of GluR2-lacking AMPARs and also reduced neuronal cell death after SCI.[50]

Conclusion

Despite the frustrations of numerous failures to show consistent positive outcomes using drugs aimed at secondary injury in CNS trauma and stroke,[1] the exciting results of the selected positive outcomes reviewed in this chapter suggest that the prospects for better therapies for secondary injury after SCI seem promising indeed. Growing understanding of the roles of multiple destructive and reparative pathways under the control of complex cell–cell interactions is providing more insight into how drugs targeted to "nodal" mechanisms might be effective. Further, it is clear that combinatorial therapies are likely to be needed, as has been the case in pharmacological approaches to multiple treatment targets in cancer therapeutics.[1] It does seem clear that the concept of an evolving secondary injury after SCI is holding up to continued scrutiny, and that these events evolve over a long enough time to provide a window of therapeutic opportunity. The results of human trials under way, for example riluzole,[51] will hopefully pave the way for continued efforts aimed at this elusive target.

Pearls

- The complex interactions between the multiple cellular constituents of the nervous system (glia, neurons, endothelial cells) present in the neuropil determine the outcome of injury, and the cascade of events that ensues includes both degradative and reparative processes.
- The proinflammatory cytokine, TNF, rapidly released in response to injury, exacerbates the excitotoxic effect of injury-induced release of glutamate by increasing the surface expression of AMPA-type glutamate receptors. This same process is involved in the physiological regulation of synaptic strength. Thus injury hijacks a normal physiological process to produce an injury cascade.

Pitfalls

- Because multiple cell types can all respond differently to individual aspects of the secondary injury cascade (e.g., inflammation), and because the processes of degradation and repair change over time, targeting secondary injury is fraught with pitfalls.

References

1. Faden AI, Stoica B. Neuroprotection: challenges and opportunities. Arch Neurol 2007;64(6):794–800
2. Kwon BK, Tetzlaff W, Grauer JN, Beiner J, Vaccaro AR. Pathophysiology and pharmacologic treatment of acute spinal cord injury. Spine J 2004;4(4):451–464
3. Park E, Velumian AA, Fehlings MG. The role of excitotoxicity in secondary mechanisms of spinal cord injury: a review with an emphasis on the implications for white matter degeneration. J Neurotrauma 2004;21(6):754–774
4. Beattie MS. Inflammation and apoptosis: linked therapeutic targets in spinal cord injury. Trends Mol Med 2004;10(12):580–583
5. Beattie MS, Bresnahan JC. Cell death, repair and recovery of function after spinal cord contusion injuries in rats. In: Kalb R, Strittmatter S, eds. Neurobiology of Spinal Cord Injury. Totowa, NJ: Humana Press; 2000:1–21
6. Bracken MB, Shepard MJ, Collins WF, et al. A randomized, controlled trial of methylprednisolone or naloxone in the treatment of acute spinal-cord injury. Results of the Second National Acute Spinal Cord Injury Study. N Engl J Med 1990;322(20):1405–1411
7. Braughler JM. Lipid peroxidation-induced inhibition of gamma-aminobutyric acid uptake in rat brain synaptosomes: protection by glucocorticoids. J Neurochem 1985;44(4):1282–1288
8. Hall ED. Neuroprotective actions of glucocorticoid and nonglucocorticoid steroids in acute neuronal injury. Cell Mol Neurobiol 1993;13(4):415–432
9. Young W, Flamm ES. Effect of high-dose corticosteroid therapy on blood flow, evoked potentials, and extracellular calcium in experimental spinal injury. J Neurosurg 1982;57(5):667–673
10. Oudega M, Vargas CG, Weber AB, Kleitman N, Bunge MB. Long-term effects of methylprednisolone following transection of adult rat spinal cord. Eur J Neurosci 1999;11(7):2453–2464
11. Chari DM, Zhao C, Kotter MR, Blakemore WF, Franklin RJM. Corticosteroids delay remyelination of experimental demyelination in the rodent central nervous system. J Neurosci Res 2006;83(4):594–605
12. Fumagalli F, Madaschi L, Brenna P, et al. Single exposure to erythropoietin modulates Nerve Growth Factor expression in the spinal cord following traumatic injury: comparison with methylprednisolone. Eur J Pharmacol 2008;578(1):19–27
13. Schröter A, Lustenberger RM, Obermair FJ, Thallmair M. High-dose corticosteroids after spinal cord injury reduce neural progenitor cell proliferation. Neuroscience 2009;161(3):753–763
14. Behrmann DL, Bresnahan JC, Beattie MS. Modeling of acute spinal cord injury in the rat: neuroprotection and enhanced recovery with methylprednisolone, U-74006F and YM-14673. Exp Neurol 1994;126(1):61–75
15. Pereira JE, Costa LM, Cabrita AM, et al. Methylprednisolone fails to improve functional and histological outcome following spinal cord injury in rats. Exp Neurol 2009;220(1):71–81
16. Pinzon A, Marcillo A, Pabon D, Bramlett HM, Bunge MB, Dietrich WD. A re-assessment of erythropoietin as a neuroprotective agent following rat spinal cord compression or contusion injury. Exp Neurol 2008;213(1):129–136
17. Pinzon A, Marcillo A, Quintana A, et al. A reassessment of minocycline as a neuroprotective agent in a rat spinal cord contusion model. Brain Res 2008;1243:146–151
18. Tator CH, Fehlings MG. Review of the secondary injury theory of acute spinal cord trauma with emphasis on vascular mechanisms. J Neurosurg 1991;75(1):15–26
19. Tator CH, Koyanagi I. Vascular mechanisms in the pathophysiology of human spinal cord injury. J Neurosurg 1997;86(3):483–492
20. Gerzanich V, Woo SK, Vennekens R, et al. De novo expression of Trpm4 initiates secondary hemorrhage in spinal cord injury. Nat Med 2009;15(2):185–191
21. Simard JM, Tsymbalyuk O, Ivanov A, et al. Endothelial sulfonylurea receptor 1-regulated NC Ca-ATP channels mediate progressive hemorrhagic necrosis following spinal cord injury. J Clin Invest 2007;117(8):2105–2113
22. Beattie MS, Farooqui AA, Bresnahan JC. Apoptosis and secondary damage after experimental spinal cord injury. Top Spinal Cord Inj Rehabil 2000;6:14–26
23. Beattie MS, Harrington AW, Lee R, et al. ProNGF induces p75-mediated death of oligodendrocytes following spinal cord injury. Neuron 2002;36(3):375–386
24. Simard JM, Chen M, Tarasov KV, et al. Newly expressed SUR1-regulated NC(Ca-ATP) channel mediates cerebral edema after ischemic stroke. Nat Med 2006;12(4):433–440
25. Iadecola C, Nedergaard M. Glial regulation of the cerebral microvasculature. Nat Neurosci 2007;10(11):1369–1376
26. Ziai WC, Toung TJ, Bhardwaj A. Hypertonic saline: first-line therapy for cerebral edema? J Neurol Sci 2007;261(1-2):157–166
27. Nout YS, Mihai G, Tovar CA, Schmalbrock P, Bresnahan JC, Beattie MS. Hypertonic saline attenuates cord swelling and edema in experimental spinal cord injury: a study utilizing magnetic resonance imaging. Crit Care Med 2009;37(7):2160–2166
28. Wang X, Arcuino G, Takano T, et al. P2X7 receptor inhibition improves recovery after spinal cord injury. Nat Med 2004;10(8):821–827
29. Peng W, Cotrina ML, Han X, et al. Systemic administration of an antagonist of the ATP-sensitive receptor P2X7 improves recovery after spinal cord injury. Proc Natl Acad Sci USA 2009;106(30):12489–12493
30. Basso DM, Beattie MS, Bresnahan JC. A sensitive and reliable locomotor rating scale for open field testing in rats. J Neurotrauma 1995;12(1):1–21
31. Teng YD, Choi H, Onario RC, et al. Minocycline inhibits contusion-triggered mictochondrial cytochrome c release and mitigates functional deficits after spinal cord injury. Proc Natl Acad Sci U S A 2004;101(9):3071–3076
32. Stirling DP, Khodarahmi K, Liu J, et al. Minocycline treatment reduces delayed oligodendrocyte death, attenuates axonal dieback, and improves

functional outcome after spinal cord injury. J Neurosci 2004;24(9):2182–2190

33. Panter SS, Yum SW, Faden AI. Alteration in extracellular amino acids after traumatic spinal cord injury. Ann Neurol 1990;27(1):96–99

34. Wrathall JR, Teng YD, Choiniere D. Amelioration of functional deficits from spinal cord trauma with systemically administered NBQX, an antagonist of non-N-methyl-D-aspartate receptors. Exp Neurol 1996;137(1):119–126

35. Rosenberg LJ, Wrathall JR. Time course studies on the effectiveness of tetrodotoxin in reducing consequences of spinal cord contusion. J Neurosci Res 2001;66(2):191–202

36. Rosenberg LJ, Teng YD, Wrathall JR. Effects of the sodium channel blocker tetrodotoxin on acute white matter pathology after experimental contusive spinal cord injury. J Neurosci 1999;19(14): 6122–6133

37. Schwartz G, Fehlings MG. Evaluation of the neuroprotective effects of sodium channel blockers after spinal cord injury: improved behavioral and neuroanatomical recovery with riluzole. J Neurosurg 2001;94(2, Suppl):245–256

38. Farber NB, Jiang XP, Heinkel C, Nemmers B. Antiepileptic drugs and agents that inhibit voltage-gated sodium channels prevent NMDA antagonist neurotoxicity. Mol Psychiatry 2002;7(7):726–733

39. Wagner ML, Landis BE. Riluzole: a new agent for amyotrophic lateral sclerosis. Ann Pharmacother 1997;31(6):738–744

40. Zoccolella S, Santamato A, Lamberti P. Current and emerging treatments for amyotrophic lateral sclerosis. Neuropsychiatr Dis Treat 2009;5: 577–595

41. Colak A, Soy O, Uzun H, et al. Neuroprotective effects of GYKI 52466 on experimental spinal cord injury in rats. J Neurosurg 2003;98(3, Suppl):275–281

42. Mu X, Azbill RD, Springer JE. Riluzole and methylprednisolone combined treatment improves functional recovery in traumatic spinal cord injury. J Neurotrauma 2000;17(9):773–780

43. Estevez AG, Stutzmann JM, Barbeito L. Protective effect of riluzole on excitatory amino acid-mediated neurotoxicity in motoneuron-enriched cultures. Eur J Pharmacol 1995;280(1):47–53

44. Wang CX, Nuttin B, Heremans H, Dom R, Gybels J. Production of tumor necrosis factor in spinal cord following traumatic injury in rats. J Neuroimmunol 1996;69(1-2):151–156

45. Santello M, Volterra A. Synaptic modulation by astrocytes via Ca2+-dependent glutamate release. Neuroscience 2009;158(1):253–259

46. Miller BA, Crum JM, Tovar CA, Ferguson AR, Bresnahan JC, Beattie MS. Activated microglia reduce oligodendrocyte progenitor cell viability but protect mature oligodendrocytes from apoptotic cell death. J Neuroinflammation 2007;4:27

47. Hermann GE, Rogers RC, Bresnahan JC, Beattie MS. Tumor necrosis factor-alpha induces cFOS and strongly potentiates glutamate-mediated cell death in the rat spinal cord. Neurobiol Dis 2001; 8(4):590–599

48. Beattie EC, Stellwagen D, Morishita W, et al. Control of synaptic strength by glial TNFalpha. Science 2002;295(5563):2282–2285

49. Leonoudakis D, Zhao P, Beattie EC. Rapid tumor necrosis factor alpha-induced exocytosis of glutamate receptor 2-lacking AMPA receptors to extrasynaptic plasma membrane potentiates excitotoxicity. J Neurosci 2008;28(9):2119–2130

50. Ferguson AR, Christensen RN, Gensel JC, et al. Cell death after spinal cord injury is exacerbated by rapid TNF alpha-induced trafficking of GluR2-lacking AMPARs to the plasma membrane. J Neurosci 2008;28(44):11391–11400

51. Hawryluk GWJ, Rowland J, Kwon BK, Fehlings MG. Protection and repair of the injured spinal cord: a review of completed, ongoing, and planned clinical trials for acute spinal cord injury. Neurosurg Focus 2008;25(5):E14

34

Cellular Transplantation in Spinal Cord Injury

Wolfram Tetzlaff

Key Points

1. Although many cellular transplantation studies have shown very encouraging results, the application of these approaches to truly repair the chronically injured spinal cord (vs protecting the acutely injured cord) is still a huge challenge. The survival and integration of transplanted cells are still far from optimal and conceivably could be optimized in conjunction with better substrates (e.g., engineered biomaterials and trophic factors). Few preclinical studies have used blunt cervical injuries, and few studies had been performed in the chronic state.
2. The actual mechanisms for how the transplanted cells exert their beneficial effects are poorly understood. Behavioral improvements are likely due to protection, modulation of host plasticity, remyelination of denuded axons, and short-distance axonal regeneration—and these contributions vary among cell types.
3. There is a need for standardization of how to generate and control the quality of cells to minimize variability, especially in autotransplantation settings where the cells are not "off the shelf."

Cell transplantation strategies are extensively investigated for their potential to treat humans with spinal cord injury (SCI). The rationale for studying a particular cell type is based on the availability of the cells as well as the ability of these cells to integrate into the injured spinal cord, where they may myelinate denuded axons or bridge the SCI site and promote axonal sprouting/regeneration. In addition, it has become apparent that many cells used also modify inflammation, provide neuroprotection, and enhance plasticity of the spared host spinal cord, and some cells are doing just that without integration or long-term survival. Given the large number of cell candidates that are reportedly found to be beneficial in animal models of SCI, it is impossible for this chapter to cover the field comprehensively. In addition, the reader has to keep in mind when analyzing preclinical data that even the best-studied cell types can vary considerably among laboratories due to differences in source materials (age, gender, and species from which the cells are taken or progenitors from which the cells are generated), cell purity and contamination with other cell types, culture conditions (such as number of passages), and variability of media used. Hence the focus here is on the cell types best studied in animal models, each followed by a brief outlook on clinical treatment attempts in many parts of the world despite the fact that such interventions have not been validated in controlled clinical trials. **Table 34.1** summarizes previous studies in cellular transplantation (**Fig. 34.1**). **Table 34.2** presents the pros and cons of the different cell types.

Schwann Cells

Schwann cells (SCs) are the myelin-forming cells of the peripheral nervous system. Their ability to form cellular bands (of von Buengner) and to support axonal regeneration after nerve injury was recognized almost a century ago.[1] This and the ability of SCs to remyelinate central nervous system (CNS) axons sparked the exploration of SCs for the treatment of SCI.[2] Over 30 preclinical studies employed either blunt contusion/compression type lesions or full/partial transection injuries of rat spinal cords to treat them with SCs isolated from peripheral nerves of rodents.[3] In the sharp injury

Table 34.1 Summary of Cellular Transplantation Studies in Spinal Cord Injury

Cell type	Animal species and number of studies	Type of injury tested	Studies with human cells	Behavioral outcomes
Schwann cells	Rats 41, mice 1	Thoracic: contusion/blunt 14 Partial and full Tx 26 Cervical partial Tx 1 Cervical contusion 1	2 in rat	10 positive; 7 needed cotreatment 5 no improvement
OECs	Rats 26	Thoracic: contusion/blunt 5 Th. Partial and full TX 15 Cervical partial Tx 6	1 with questionable human OECs (from abortions)	12 positive; needed cotreatment 5 no improvement
NS/PCs	Rats 22, mice 8, dogs 1, cats 1, marmosets 1	Thoracic contusions 18 Thoracic partial and full Tx 8 Cervical partial Tx 5 Cervical contusion blunt 2	5 with human cell lines (immortalized) 1 from primary human embryo 10 passages	17 positive outcomes 5 needed cotreatment 3 no improvement
GRP/NRPs OPCs ES-OPCs*	Rats 11 Rats 3	Thoracic contusion 10 Cervical partial Tx 3 Thoracic contusions 2 Cervical contusion 1	0 3 human ESC (H7) derived OPCs	5 positive studies 1 needed cotreatment 2 positive studies
BMSC	Rats 38, mice 2; pig 1 monkey 1	Thoracic blunt 31 Thoracic full Tx 3 Partial Tx 1 Cervical partial Tx 7	8 studies with human BMSCs all rat 6 with contusions 4/2	20 positive studies 2 needed cotreatment 11 no improvements

Abbreviations: BMSCs, bone marrow–derived stromal cells; ESC, embryonic stem cell; OECs, olfactory ensheathing cells; OPCs, oligodendrocyte precursor cells; Tx, transection.

Table 34.2 Pros and Cons of Different Cell Types

Schwann cells

PROS:
- Extensively studied cell type that guides axons, remyelinates, and provides neuroprotection (subacute)
- Behavioral effects demonstrated by numerous investigators, including efficacy in "chronic" rodent contusion model
- Can be harvested from patients for an autologous transplantation approach, which circumvents rejection problems, ethical concerns, and tumor risks

CONS:
- In many cases, appear to require adjuvant treatment to increase efficacy (e.g., Matrigel [BD Biosciences], Rolipram [Tocris Bioscience], cAMP, neurotrophic factors)
- Somewhat limited integration into the host compared with neural stem cells
- Optimal source for Schwann cells has yet to be determined, and cell quality in autotransplantation setting may be variable

OECs

PROS:
- Demonstrate good integration into host spinal cord; repeated claims of axonal sprouting and regeneration in partial- or full-transection SCI models, possible myelination and trophic effects
- Behavioral improvements have been frequently reported
- Offer the possibility of autologous transplantation

CONS:
- No robust behavioral benefits after transplantation into moderate or severe thoracic contusion injuries
- Human protocols for OEC cultures still need refinement and cell quality in autotransplantation setting may be variable
- In many cases, OECs require cotreatments to increase efficacy (e.g., Schwann cells, Matrigel, Rolipram, cAMP, neurotrophic factors)

NSPC

PROS:
- Good integration into the host spinal cord
- Can differentiate into oligodendroglial cells and myelinate, but likely act by other beneficial mechanisms as well
- The majority of studies reported behavioral benefits, including with humans cells

CONS:
- NSPCs do not provide optimal bridges for axonal regeneration
- Sourcing of the cells is challenging. Harvesting NSPCs from human fetuses or adult brain material is met with ethical and safety issues and will likely result in variable quality and will require suppression; this difficulty might be overcome by using iPCs

Human embryonic stem cell–eerived oligodendrocytes

PROS:
- Provide myelin, are neuroprotective, and modify the host endogenous myelination response
- Off-the-shelf preparation in production by Geron Pharmaceuticals
- FDA-approved phase 1 trials were approved in 2010

CONS:
- Embryonic stem cell–derived OPCs bear a tumor risk due to possible contamination with pluripotent stem cells
- Published preclinical data all from one group; independent replication desirable

(Continued on page 402)

Table 34.2 **Pros and Cons of Different Cell Types** *(Continued)*

BMSC
PROS: • Easily harvested for autotransplantations, which circumvents rejection issues • Both human and rodent BMSCs effective in rodent SCI models • Large animal and primate studies successful, as well as studies in chronic contusion injuries (although not independently confirmed)
CONS: • BMSCs are a somewhat ill-defined populations of cells, hence cell quality hard to assess and likely variable • Integration in the injured spinal cord is limited, mainly neuroprotective and trophic effects • No convincing differentiation into neural cells despite claims to the contrary

Abbreviations: BMSCs, bone marrow–derived stromal cells; cAMP, cyclic adenosine monophosphate; FDA, US Food and Drug Administration; IPCs, induced pluripotent cells; NSPCs, neural stem/progenitor cells; OECs, olfactory ensheathing cells; OPCs, oligodendrocyte precursor cells; SCI, spinal cord injury.

models, SCs were used in combination with Matrigel (BD Biosciences, Franklin Lakes, NJ) and/or guidance channels providing some scaffold; such models allowed investigation of SCs' abilities to promote axonal regeneration. There is convincing evidence that SCs enhance the regeneration of sensory axons from the dorsal root ganglia, as well as propriospinal axons adjacent to the injury site.[2] However, SCs alone have only limited capacity to promote regeneration of long brain-to-spinal cord projection axons. In any case, those axons regenerating into SC bridges typically fail to reenter the host spinal cord at the other side of the bridge (referred to as off-ramp phenomenon) unless additional treatment strategies are used. In the most prominent study that also achieved behavioral benefits after full spinal cord transections, the SCs were used in combination with a Matrigel-filled polyacrylonitrile/polyvinylchloride channel plus olfactory ensheathing cell (OEC) injections into the stumps plus chondroitinase ABC and mouse immunoglobulin G (IgG).[4] Some of the treated rats regained weight-

Transplanted cells may secrete factors that provide NEUROPROTECTION and enhance host PLASTICITY; replace lost myelin-forming cells to promote REMYELINATION; integrate and form BRIDGES across the lesion site to promote axonal REGENERATION; and may replace lost NEURONS

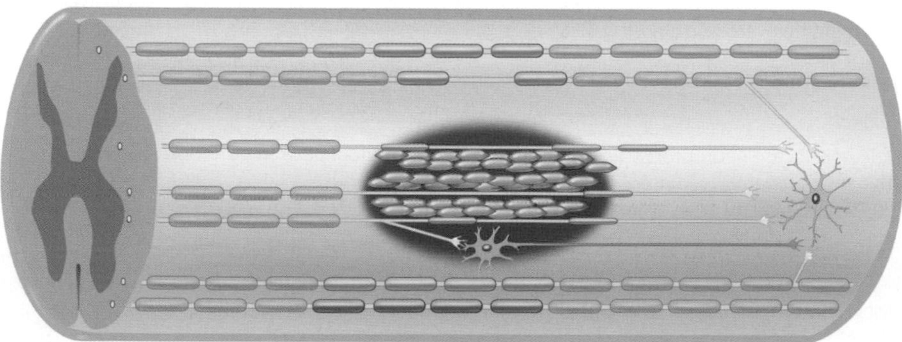

Fig. 34.1 Cellular transplantation for spinal cord injury. Transplanted cells (green) may remyelinate denuded axons and/or bridge the lesion site (red) where they promote axonal regeneration and/or differentiate into relay neurons that in turn connect onto neurons in the caudal spinal cord (in blue). In addition, transplanted cells may stimulate plasticity in the host spinal cord, e.g., sprouting of spared axons (yellow).

supported stepping, which is arguably the most convincing example of restoration of function after complete spinal cord transection in the preclinical literature.

However, the majority of clinical injuries are incomplete and best modeled by blunt contusion injuries. Significant behavioral benefits in open-field locomotion after SC transplantation alone were reported by Takami et al.[5] after injecting the SC 7 days after contusion injury and in a study by Barakat et al.[6] transplanting into an 8-week chronic contusion injury (the only chronic study in the SC literature). The three other studies saw benefits when SCs were used in combination with either Rolipram (Tocris Bioscience, Minneapolis, MN) plus cyclic adenosine monophosphate (cAMP), or in combinations of methylprednisolone, interleukin (IL)-10, and OECs.[7] But even without cotreatments, nerve-derived rodent SCs improved forelimb grip strength and function after transplantation into a cervical contusion injury.[8] In light of the fact that a large number of SCIs occur at the cervical level, this is very encouraging.

Human SCs were evaluated in only two studies with thoracic full transections of rats, yielding a small but significant behavioral benefit on the Basso, Beattie, Bresnahan (BBB) scale and the inclined plane test.[9] More preclinical experiments with human SCs in cervical and thoracic contusion models are highly desirable. Taken together, the results of SC transplantation into the injured spinal cord show some promise, and the possibility to obtain autologous SCs for transplantation eliminates concerns regarding ethics, contamination, and immune rejection. However, the use of autologous transplants necessitates an additional peripheral nerve injury (e.g., sural nerve excision), which results in additional minor sensory deficits. Recently, alternative sources for SCs from postnatal skin or adult bone marrow have been pursued and tested after thoracic transection[10] or contusion[11] injuries. Both studies reported modest (but significant) improvements in open-field locomotion, suggesting that other sources that circumvent peripheral nerve biopsies may be an alternative source for autologous SCs. Intriguingly, the SCs from skin-derived progenitors formed bridges across the injury site, migrated into the host parenchyma, and formed myelin with minimal astrocyte hypertrophy.[11]

Clinical trials with autologous human SCs are moving ahead. Saberi and colleagues[12] in Iran recently published the first results from four of 33 patients who underwent autologous transplantation of human SCs into thoracic SCIs of 2 to 6.5 years. No detrimental (nor beneficial) effect of SC transplants was reported in the first four patients; however, magnetic resonance imaging (MRI) failed to detect the SC transplants in the study by Saberi et al.[12] This trial, following the International Campaign for Cures of Spinal Cord Injury Paralysis (ICCP) guidelines, is a promising first step in the move toward human clinical trials of SCs for SCI.

Olfactory Ensheathing Cells

OECs are found in the nerve fiber layer of the olfactory bulb and in the nasal olfactory mucosa. OECs have attracted considerable interest because of their ability to facilitate the lifelong growth of olfactory receptor axons from the peripheral nervous system (PNS) environment of the nasal olfactory mucosa to the central nervous system (CNS) environment of the olfactory bulb.[13] This sparked the evaluation of OECs in axonal regeneration studies, such as complete thoracic spinal cord transactions, based on the rationale that OECs may promote axonal regeneration across a spinal cord lesion site and facilitate the reentry of axons into the host at the distal host–graft interface, in analogy to the PNS–CNS interface at the olfactory bulb. The study by Ramón-Cueto et al.[14] gained great attention due to the apparent regeneration of corticospinal axons and improvements of motor behavior in a grid-climbing test at 3 and 7 months postinjury. When combining this OEC treatment after full transection injury with treadmill step training, the ability of rats to perform plantar stepping was further improved.[15] Similarly, in an independent study, Cao et al.[16] injected OECs as well as OECs modified to overexpress glial-derived neurotrophic factor into the stumps of the fully transected spinal cord and reported significant motor improvements. However, a study similar to that by Ramón-Cueto et al.,[14] this time using primate OECs in nude rats, failed to reveal any corticospinal tract (CST) regeneration and saw only modest regeneration of 5-HT fibers and only transient improvement in behavior.[17] Retransection of those animals that demonstrated some improved behavior did not change function, supporting the notion that the improved behavior was not due to long axonal regeneration but to plasticity in the caudal spinal cord.

Studies of axonal regeneration in incomplete transection models were even more equivocal. Although some authors claimed spectacular successes after dorsal column injury or small electrolytic lesions,[18] other authors could not confirm axonal growth through and beyond the site of injury.[3,19] The reasons for these discrepancies are not fully understood, and sparing of tissue, experimental bias, and variability of the cell culture conditions and sources and animal or injury model systems are likely playing a role.

Human SCIs are typically incomplete and contusive in nature, but none of the studies with OEC transplantation into contusion sites (n = 3) reported that OECs alone conferred any behavioral benefits in either the subacute[5] or the chronic setting at 8 weeks postinjury.[6] The combination of OECs with SCs, however, seemed to convey significant behavioral benefits, yet in direct comparisons SCs were more effective.[5]

Only one preclinical study to date has reported benefits with human OECs harvested from the outer layers of the olfactory bulbs from human fetuses of 5 to 7 months' gestation.[20] Although these are p75-positive "OEC-like" cells at best, protocols to harvest OECs from the nasal mucosa of humans are under development to pursue the possibility for autotransplantations. Even in the absence of convincing data with human cells in animals, OECs are already used in some form or another in humans using autotransplantation of mucosal pieces in which OECs are mixed with other cells or in crude cell mixes from the olfactory bulb of aborted fetuses. These reports are uncontrolled and not blinded. Nevertheless, an improvement in 11 of 20 individuals with chronic SCI (> 18 months) and six of 20 persons showing an American Spinal Injury Association Impairment Scale (AIS) score increase from A to C is intriguing,[21] although it must not be overlooked that this was in combination with an aggressive physiotherapy regimen. Hence, more basic and clinical studies are needed to understand the biology of human OECs, including these mixed-cell preparations, to improve on the preclinical findings and to design better-controlled clinical trials with better-understood cell preparations.

Neural Stem/Progenitor Cells

Neural stem/progenitor cells (NPCs) are typically harvested from the subventricular zone of the brain or the spinal cord of rodent embryos or adult rodents and amplified as neurospheres in epidermal growth factor (EGF) and/or basic fibroblast growth factor (bFGF) for several rounds of passages. They contain precursors for neurons, astroglia, and oligodendrocytes, and likely some stemlike cells with capacity for self-renewal.

Adult rodent NPCs have been applied to thoracic contusion or compression injuries in rats and mice and to cervical dorsal column transections in rat studies.[3] A subacute regimen was chosen in most cases except in the study by Karimi-Abdolrezaee et al.[22] Although some authors reported mainly astrocytic differentiation of the transplanted aNPCs,[23] many authors observed in addition the expression of up to 60% oligodendroglial markers,[3] yet the expression of neuron markers was generally rare (0 to 1%). There is some inconsistency in the extent to which these oligodendrocytes can mature and generate compact myelin in the injured spinal cord.[24,25] The majority of the studies using contusion injuries found significant improvements of open-field locomotion scores after transplantation of aNPCs in rats[24–26] and in mice.[27] However, it needs to be pointed out that cotreatments were used in some of these studies like vaccination with myelin or a cocktail of trophic factors infused intrathecally for 1 week.[25] Similarly, only the combination of aNPCs with trophic factors and chondroitinase ABC promoted recovery when administered 8 weeks after a chronic clip compression injury—the first successful chronic treatment with this cell type.[22] However, the logistics of obtaining adult NPCs routinely and with consistent quality for treatments of SCI appear difficult; hence embryonic NPCs are also pursued.

Embryonic NPCs (eNPCs) have been assessed in almost a dozen compression/contusion injuries as well as in several full transection or partial transection models of rodents.[3] Expression of astrocyte, oligodendrocyte, and neuronal markers was observed to a variable degree. Of interest, eNPC transplantation into cervical weight-compression lesions revealed improvements on a skilled reaching task in rats. In thoracic contusion models, significant effects in open-field locomotion were observed in several studies, and the effects were further enhanced if pretreatments with noggin, which antagonizes bone morphogenic proteins (BMPs), or bFGF-expressing rat amniotic epithelial cells were given. In addition, eNPCs yielded functional benefits in (4/5) sharp lesion models of SCI, including full transections, and the effects where enhanced with various cotreatments.[3]

Interesting from a translational perspective is the transplantation of eNPCs from human fetuses (8 weeks of gestation) into cervical contusion sites of marmoset monkeys.[28] Behaviorally, bar grip power and spontaneous motor activity were improved, which is promising. Given the ethical controversy around the use of human abortion material to harvest human eNPCs as well as the technical variability and logistical problems involved, several authors have pursued human immortalized neural stem cell lines (HB1.F3 clone; line K048 and line c17.2[3]) or long-term human neurosphere cultures[29] and transplanted them to rodents. Although some studies were met with behavioral success,[29] others reported "pain without gain" with the c17.2 line studied.[30] It remains to be seen whether these approaches will yield viable sources of human cells for clinical translation.

A new alternative route for the generation of NPCs was recently opened by the discovery of inducible pluripotent cells from skin fibroblasts[31,32] or more recently from peripheral blood.[33] As few as four transcription factors (Oct4, Sox2, Klf4, and c-Myc) suffice to convert human skin fibroblast cells into pluripotent cells, which in turn may be induced to differentiate into a wide variety of cells, including NPCs, oligodendrocytes, neurons, or SCs. Hence a patient's own cells could be used, or more standardized human leukocyte antigen (HLA)-compatible lines could be generated for transplantation into the injured spinal cord. Although the risk of tumors from undifferentiated cells (i.e., teratomas) cannot yet be well assessed, it is hoped that the fast technological advancements in this area will allow for the elimination of undesired pluripotent cells.

Neural and Glial Restricted Precursors, Including Embryonic Stem Cell Derived Oligodendrocyte Precursors

Neural restricted precursors (NRPs) and/or glial restricted precursors (GRPs) are more restricted versions of eNPCs also harvested from embryos. Although transplantation of NRPs alone into uninjured spinal cords resulted in neural differentiation, such neuronal differentiation is far less complete in the environment of the SCI site, underlining that the SCI environment inhibits neuronal differentiation.[34] Similarly, GRPs differentiate mainly into astroglial cells in the lesion center, whereas some express oligodendrocyte markers, usually after migration into the spared host spinal cord.[35–37] Still, the degree to form myelinating oligodendrocytes by GRPs in the contused spinal cord is somewhat limited, and it appears that behavioral recovery requires the transduction with the neurotrophin D14A[38] that has brain-derived neurotrophic factor (BDNF) and neurotrophin-3 (NT-3) activities and also enhances oligodendrocyte differentiation. As with many other transplantation strategies, it can only be speculated to what extent the observed benefits are due to increased myelination, neuroprotection, or neural plasticity.

From a translational perspective, harvesting human GRPs and NRPs from abortion materials is met with logistic and ethical concerns in many countries. Hence alternative sources for oligodendrocyte precursors have been pursued. Most prominent is the differentiation of oligodendrocyte precursor cells (OPCs) from a human embryonic stem cell line, which was recently approved for a phase 1 clinical trial (Geron Inc. www.geron.com/grnopc1 clearance). In essence, these ESC-derived OPCs enhance myelination, are neuroprotective, and mediate moderate improvement of locomotor function when transplanted after acute, but not chronic, SCI.[39] This study has not been independently replicated by other laboratories, although Geron performed extensive "in house" safety and efficacy studies on over 2000 rats prior to US Food and Drug Administration (FDA) approval, which has yet to be released to the SCI academic community. Efficacy in blunt cervical models would be desirable if that will be a major human target for translation. Similarly, no larger animal models with OPC transplants exist so far. Concerns regarding the risk of teratoma formation have been voiced due to possible contamination with undifferentiated stem cells.

Bone Marrow–Derived Stromal Cells

Bone marrow cells are a mixture of stromal cells and hematopoietic stem cells. The mesenchymal bone marrow stromal cells (BMSCs) can be isolated and separated from the hematopoietic cell fraction of the bone marrow by their property of adhering to plastic culture dishes. For a systematic review of BMSC transplantation, see Tetzlaff et al.[3] BMSCs can differentiate into chondrocytes, osteoblasts, and adipocytes and are thus multipotent precursors; however, the claims of neural differentiation after transplantation into the injured spinal cord have been debated. There is considerable heterogeneity among BMSCs isolated by plastic adhesion, which partly explains the highly variable results among different laboratories regarding the ability of these cells to survive, integrate, and differentiate as neural cells in the injured spinal cord. In addition, there is evidence that rather nonspecific treatments can induce the expression of neuronal markers without truly specifying these cells as neurons or glial cells.[40]

The majority of the over 20 studies transplanting rodent BMSCs into blunt SCIs (mainly contusions of the rat thoracic spinal cords) reported positive behavioral effects, whereas four failed to see any benefits.[3,41–43] In most studies the cells were injected directly into or next to the SCI site, yet, in some hands, intrathecal and even intravenous (IV) delivery is claimed to be successful; although some researchers did not have success with IV delivery. As for most cell transplantations, most studies used a subacute or acute timing for the transplantation, except for Zurita and Vaquero,[44] who delayed the treatment to 3 months after spinal cord contusion by weight drop at T6–8. These authors allowed the rats to survive for up to 12 months and claimed significant locomotor improvements. Independent replications are eagerly awaited.

In the light of the widely observed behavioral benefits, it is somewhat surprising that the histological data are very divergent and range from good survival and differentiation of BMSC into neural cells, to poor survival and no differentiation into neural cells. Claims of differentiation are often not credible when in vitro dyes have been used to prelabel the transplanted cells (e.g., the chromatin stain Hoechst[17]). Still the heterogeneity of histological results once more underlines that beneficial behavioral effects can be brought about by multiple factors, ranging from neuroprotection (via secretion of trophic factors and modification of inflammation) to recruitment of endogenous cells, including stem cells and remyelinating cells and vascular endothelial cells, which enhance endogenous repair, and, last but not least, differentiation and integration as neurons (which is highly debated). Indeed several studies reported more preserved white matter or less cell death, indicative of neuroprotection.[3,43] The claims of axonal regeneration in contusion studies can only be interpreted within the site of lesion but not the host spinal cord itself, where spared axons and regenerated axons are not easily distinguishable. Such questions are better addressed in sharp models of SCI, and a few studies with full transections reported mild behavioral benefits.[45] Although this may be due to some axonal regeneration, other mechanisms like trophic effects on spinal circuits below the level of the injury site cannot be ruled out. BMSCs do promote axonal growth, and these effects may be attributed to invading SCs (see earlier discussion), and axon growth can be greatly enhanced with co-expression of trophic factors by the transplanted BMSCs.[46]

Given the fairly easy access to human bone marrow, it does not surprise that almost a dozen studies have been performed with human BMSC, and about two thirds of them reported transplant-related behavioral improvements. Deng and colleagues[20] claimed impressive BBB scores of 13 (weight-supported stepping with frequent coordination) versus BBB of 6 in their controls; however, Kim et al.[47] found less dramatic benefits (13 vs 10) in a milder contusion model when combining these cells with FGF. Similarly, Cízková et al.[48] reported benefits with human BMSC using a balloon compression model. However, Neuhuber et al.[49] tested human BMSC from four different donors and found highly variable outcomes in a rat hemisection model using various tests, which underlines the possible heterogeneity of these cells. Hence, it appears that we need a better understanding of the types of cells in the BMSC fraction that are mediating these benefits.

Nevertheless, from a translational perspective, BMSCs are the most widely studied human cells using rodents, large mammals, and primates. This and the easy access to bone marrow for autotransplantation have fueled several unproven human treatment attempts. However, most of these human treatments are using crude mixtures of mesenchymal and hematopoietic cells[50–53] and not the cultured plastic-adherent BMSC fractions. Several centers are routinely administering these autologous cell mixes to individuals with chronic SCI, at considerable costs and surgical risks (e.g., www.xcell-center.com). Unfortunately, the assessments are thus far based on small patient cohorts only and are mostly uncontrolled; hence it is difficult to discern any possible BMSC-related benefits from placebo effects or from untethering of the cord and removing scar tissue during surgery. In light of a booming interest in cell transplantation, a systematic preclinical and clinical validation of this approach is overdue.

Other Cells

Several other cell types are claimed to hold promise for the treatment of SCI and could not be dealt with here. These include radial glial cells, amnion epithelial cells, umbilical cord cells (mesenchymal and hematopoietic), adipose-derived mesenchymal cells, hair follicle–derived progenitor cells, skin-derived progenitor cells, and more. Some of these cell types are still not well defined, and there is little independent confirmation regarding their benefits for the injured spinal cord. Nevertheless, uncontrolled clinical treatments with some of these cells are ongoing, as many of these cells are easily obtained without destroying human embryos. More preclinical data are needed before we can judge their true potential for repairing the injured spinal cord.

Outlook

We are seeing very encouraging results with many of the cells discussed in this chapter, yet it is remarkably surprising how few preclinical studies have used blunt cervical injuries (the most frequent clinical injury type), how few studies had been performed in the chronic state, and how little we understand the actual mechanisms whereby the transplanted cells exert their beneficial effects. Behavioral improvements are likely due to protection, modulation of host plasticity, remyelination of denuded axons, and short-distance axonal regeneration—and these contributions vary among cell types. The survival and integration are still far from optimal and conceivably could be optimized in conjunction with better substrates (e.g., engineered biomaterials and trophic factors). In addition, there is the need for standardization of how to generate and control the quality of cells so as to minimize variability, especially in autotransplantation settings where the cells are not "off the shelf." And, last but not least, the application of these approaches to truly repair the chronically injured spinal cord (vs protecting the acutely injured cord) is still a huge challenge. In the meantime, thousands of patients are traveling around the world to buy unproven cell treatments for their injured spinal cord, reminding us that cell transplantation as such is feasible and that we need to close the gaps in our preclinical data and work effectively toward FDA-approved controlled trials of these promising treatments. The clinical trial by GERON Corporation with human ESC-OPCs was suspended in Fall 2011 due to financial reasons; a clinical safety and feasibility trial of human NSPCs sponsored by STEM CELL INC. was initiated in 2012 in Switzerland.

Pearls

- "Stem cells" hold great promise to enhance recovery from SCI by providing cell replacement and thus enhancing multiple mechanisms, including neuroprotection, plasticity in the injured spinal cord, remyelination, and axonal regeneration.
- Hence the therapeutic spectrum is broad.

Pitfalls

- Cell transplantation is invasive and expensive.
- There is no agreement upon which cell type is optimal to use, and the understanding of the mechanisms is limited.
- Cell transplantation may pose ethical, logistic, and safety problems.

References

1. Ramon y Cajal S. Degeneration and Regeneration of the Nervous System. May RM, trans. Oxford: Oxford University Press; 1928
2. Oudega M. Schwann cell and olfactory ensheathing cell implantation for repair of the contused spinal cord. Acta Physiol (Oxf) 2007;189(2):181–189
3. Tetzlaff W, Okon EB, Karimi-Abdolrezaee S, et al. A systematic review of cellular transplantation therapies for spinal cord injury. J Neurotrauma 2011;28(8):1611–1682
4. Fouad K, Schnell L, Bunge MB, Schwab ME, Liebscher T, Pearse DD. Combining Schwann cell bridges and olfactory-ensheathing glia grafts with chondroitinase promotes locomotor recovery after complete transection of the spinal cord. J Neurosci 2005;25(5):1169–1178
5. Takami T, Oudega M, Bates ML, Wood PM, Kleitman N, Bunge MB. Schwann cell but not olfactory ensheathing glia transplants improve hindlimb locomotor performance in the moderately contused adult rat thoracic spinal cord. J Neurosci 2002;22(15):6670–6681
6. Barakat DJ, Gaglani SM, Neravetla SR, et al. Survival, integration, and axon growth support of glia transplanted into the chronically contused spinal cord. Cell Transplant 2005;14(4):225–240
7. Pearse DD, Pereira FC, Marcillo AE, et al. cAMP and Schwann cells promote axonal growth and functional recovery after spinal cord injury. Nat Med 2004;10(6):610–616
8. Schaal SM, Kitay BM, Cho KS, et al. Schwann cell transplantation improves reticulospinal axon growth and forelimb strength after severe cervical spinal cord contusion. Cell Transplant 2007;16(3):207–228
9. Guest JD, Rao A, Olson L, Bunge MB, Bunge RP. The ability of human Schwann cell grafts to promote regeneration in the transected nude rat spinal cord. Exp Neurol 1997b;148(2):502–522
10. Kamada T, Koda M, Dezawa M, et al. Transplantation of bone marrow stromal cell-derived Schwann cells promotes axonal regeneration and functional recovery after complete transection of adult rat spinal cord. J Neuropathol Exp Neurol 2005;64(1):37–45
11. Biernaskie J, Sparling JS, Liu J, et al. Skin-derived precursors generate myelinating Schwann cells that promote remyelination and functional recovery after contusion spinal cord injury. J Neurosci 2007;27(36):9545–9559
12. Saberi H, Moshayedi P, Aghayan HR, et al. Treatment of chronic thoracic spinal cord injury patients with autologous Schwann cell transplantation: an interim report on safety considerations and possible outcomes. Neurosci Lett 2008;443(1):46–50

13. Doucette R. PNS-CNS transitional zone of the first cranial nerve. J Comp Neurol 1991;312(3): 451–466
14. Ramón-Cueto A, Cordero MI, Santos-Benito FF, Avila J. Functional recovery of paraplegic rats and motor axon regeneration in their spinal cords by olfactory ensheathing glia. Neuron 2000; 25(2):425–435
15. Kubasak MD, Jindrich DL, Zhong H, et al. OEG implantation and step training enhance hindlimb-stepping ability in adult spinal transected rats. Brain 2008;131(Pt 1):264–276
16. Cao L, Liu L, Chen ZY, et al. Olfactory ensheathing cells genetically modified to secrete GDNF to promote spinal cord repair. Brain 2004;127(Pt 3):535–549
17. Guest JD, Herrera L, Margitich I, Oliveria M, Marcillo A, Casas CE. Xenografts of expanded primate olfactory ensheathing glia support transient behavioral recovery that is independent of serotonergic or corticospinal axonal regeneration in nude rats following spinal cord transection. Exp Neurol 2008;212(2):261–274
18. Li Y, Field PM, Raisman G. Repair of adult rat corticospinal tract by transplants of olfactory ensheathing cells. Science 1997;277(5334): 2000–2002
19. Bretzner F, Liu J, Currie E, Roskams AJ, Tetzlaff W. Undesired effects of a combinatorial treatment for spinal cord injury—transplantation of olfactory ensheathing cells and BDNF infusion to the red nucleus. Eur J Neurosci 2008;28(9):1795–1807
20. Deng YB, Liu Y, Zhu WB, et al. The co-transplantation of human bone marrow stromal cells and embryo olfactory ensheathing cells as a new approach to treat spinal cord injury in a rat model. Cytotherapy 2008;10(6):551–564
21. Lima C, Escada P, Pratas-Vital J, et al. Olfactory mucosal autografts and rehabilitation for chronic traumatic spinal cord injury. Neurorehabil Neural Repair 2010;24(1):10–22
22. Karimi-Abdolrezaee S, Eftekharpour E, Wang J, Schut D, Fehlings MG. Synergistic effects of transplanted adult neural stem/progenitor cells, chondroitinase, and growth factors promote functional repair and plasticity of the chronically injured spinal cord. J Neurosci 2010;30(5):1657–1676
23. Cao QL, Zhang YP, Howard RM, Walters WM, Tsoulfas P, Whittemore SR. Pluripotent stem cells engrafted into the normal or lesioned adult rat spinal cord are restricted to a glial lineage. Exp Neurol 2001;167(1):48–58
24. Parr AM, Kulbatski I, Zahir T, et al. Transplanted adult spinal cord-derived neural stem/progenitor cells promote early functional recovery after rat spinal cord injury. Neuroscience 2008;155(3): 760–770
25. Karimi-Abdolrezaee S, Eftekharpour E, Wang J, Morshead CM, Fehlings MG. Delayed transplantation of adult neural precursor cells promotes remyelination and functional neurological recovery after spinal cord injury. J Neurosci 2006; 26(13):3377–3389
26. Hofstetter CP, Holmström NA, Lilja JA, et al. Allodynia limits the usefulness of intraspinal neural stem cell grafts; directed differentiation improves outcome. Nat Neurosci 2005;8(3): 346–353
27. Ziv Y, Avidan H, Pluchino S, Martino G, Schwartz M. Synergy between immune cells and adult neural stem/progenitor cells promotes functional recovery from spinal cord injury. Proc Natl Acad Sci U S A 2006;103(35):13174–13179
28. Iwanami A, Kaneko S, Nakamura M, et al. Transplantation of human neural stem cells for spinal cord injury in primates. J Neurosci Res 2005;80(2):182–190
29. Cummings BJ, Uchida N, Tamaki SJ, et al. Human neural stem cells differentiate and promote locomotor recovery in spinal cord-injured mice. Proc Natl Acad Sci USA 2005;102(39):14069–14074
30. Macias MY, Syring MB, Pizzi MA, Crowe MJ, Alexanian AR, Kurpad SN. Pain with no gain: allodynia following neural stem cell transplantation in spinal cord injury. Exp Neurol 2006;201(2): 335–348
31. Takahashi K, Yamanaka S. Induction of pluripotent stem cells from mouse embryonic and adult fibroblast cultures by defined factors. Cell 2006;126(4):663–676
32. Takahashi K, Tanabe K, Ohnuki M, et al. Induction of pluripotent stem cells from adult human fibroblasts by defined factors. Cell 2007;131(5): 861–872
33. Yamanaka S. Patient-specific pluripotent stem cells become even more accessible. Cell Stem Cell 2010;7(1):1–2
34. Cao QL, Howard RM, Dennison JB, Whittemore SR. Differentiation of engrafted neuronal-restricted precursor cells is inhibited in the traumatically injured spinal cord. Exp Neurol 2002;177(2): 349–359
35. Hill CE, Proschel C, Noble M, et al. Acute transplantation of glial-restricted precursor cells into spinal cord contusion injuries: survival, differentiation, and effects on lesion environment and axonal regeneration. Exp Neurol 2004; 190(2):289–310
36. Enzmann GU, Benton RL, Woock JP, Howard RM, Tsoulfas P, Whittemore SR. Consequences of noggin expression by neural stem, glial, and neuronal precursor cells engrafted into the injured spinal cord. Exp Neurol 2005;195(2):293–304
37. Han SS, Liu Y, Tyler-Polsz C, Rao MS, Fischer I. Transplantation of glial-restricted precursor cells into the adult spinal cord: survival, glial-specific differentiation, and preferential migration in white matter. Glia 2004;45(1):1–16
38. Cao QL, Xu XM, Devries WH, et al. Functional recovery in traumatic spinal cord injury after transplantation of multineurotrophin-expressing glial-restricted precursor cells. J Neurosci 2005;25(30):6947–6957
39. Keirstead HS, Nistor G, Bernal G, et al. Human embryonic stem cell-derived oligodendrocyte progenitor cell transplants remyelinate and restore locomotion after spinal cord injury. J Neurosci 2005;25(19):4694–4705
40. Lu P, Blesch A, Tuszynski MH. Induction of bone marrow stromal cells to neurons: differentiation, transdifferentiation, or artifact? J Neurosci Res 2004;77(2):174–191

41. Chopp M, Zhang XH, Li Y, et al. Spinal cord injury in rat: treatment with bone marrow stromal cell transplantation. Neuroreport 2000;11(13):3001–3005
42. Hofstetter CP, Schwarz EJ, Hess D, et al. Marrow stromal cells form guiding strands in the injured spinal cord and promote recovery. Proc Natl Acad Sci U S A 2002;99(4):2199–2204
43. Ankeny DP, McTigue DM, Jakeman LB. Bone marrow transplants provide tissue protection and directional guidance for axons after contusive spinal cord injury in rats. Exp Neurol 2004;190(1):17–31
44. Zurita M, Vaquero J. Bone marrow stromal cells can achieve cure of chronic paraplegic rats: functional and morphological outcome one year after transplantation. Neurosci Lett 2006;402(1-2):51–56
45. Koda M, Kamada T, Hashimoto M, et al. Adenovirus vector-mediated ex vivo gene transfer of brain-derived neurotrophic factor to bone marrow stromal cells promotes axonal regeneration after transplantation in completely transected adult rat spinal cord. Eur Spine J 2007;16(12):2206–2214
46. Lu P, Jones LL, Tuszynski MH. Axon regeneration through scars and into sites of chronic spinal cord injury. Exp Neurol 2007;203(1):8–21
47. Kim KN, Oh SH, Lee KH, Yoon DH. Effect of human mesenchymal stem cell transplantation combined with growth factor infusion in the repair of injured spinal cord. Acta Neurochir Suppl (Wien) 2006;99:133–136
48. Cízková D, Rosocha J, Vanický I, Jergová S, Cízek M. Transplants of human mesenchymal stem cells improve functional recovery after spinal cord injury in the rat. Cell Mol Neurobiol 2006;26(7-8):1167–1180
49. Neuhuber B, Timothy Himes B, Shumsky JS, Gallo G, Fischer I. Axon growth and recovery of function supported by human bone marrow stromal cells in the injured spinal cord exhibit donor variations. Brain Res 2005;1035(1):73–85
50. Yoon SH, Shim YS, Park YH, et al. Complete spinal cord injury treatment using autologous bone marrow cell transplantation and bone marrow stimulation with granulocyte macrophage-colony stimulating factor: phase I/II clinical trial. Stem Cells 2007;25(8):2066–2073
51. Chernykh ER, Stupak VV, Muradov GM, et al. Application of autologous bone marrow stem cells in the therapy of spinal cord injury patients. Bull Exp Biol Med 2007;143(4):543–547
52. Geffner LF, Santacruz P, Izurieta M, et al. Administration of autologous bone marrow stem cells into spinal cord injury patients via multiple routes is safe and improves their quality of life: comprehensive case studies. Cell Transplant 2008;17(12):1277–1293
53. Saito F, Nakatani T, Iwase M, et al. Spinal cord injury treatment with intrathecal autologous bone marrow stromal cell transplantation: the first clinical trial case report. J Trauma 2008;64(1):53–59

35

Neuroregeneration Approaches

Lisa McKerracher, Michael G. Fehlings, Alyson Fournier, and Stephan Ong Tone

Key Points

1. After CNS injury, many growth inhibitors are released that block repair and regeneration.
2. Many of these inhibitors use the Nogo and Rho pathways, so blocking these pathways could lead to improved functional repair and recovery.
3. Animal models support the targeting of this pathway for drug development, and preclinical studies of the drugs that act on this pathway are providing promising results.

Over the past 30 years, the major molecular components and signaling cascades that block axon regeneration in the adult spinal cord have been elucidated. Multiple lines of evidence have validated the Rho pathway as important in controlling both regeneration and neuroprotection after central nervous system (CNS) injury. Of the several different strategies that promote repair that have now been translated toward clinical trials, the drug called BA-210 (trademarked as Cethrin, Alseres Pharmaceuticals, Inc., Hopkinton, MA) is the first to target the multiple inhibitory proteins that block inhibition signaling to neurons by blocking activation of Rho. This chapter reviews growth inhibition in the central nervous system (CNS) and the evidence that multiple inhibitory pathways signal to Rho, then describes the steps used to translate this discovery toward an Investigational New Drug (IND) application for clinical trial approval by the US Food and Drug Administration (FDA) and by Health Canada.

Growth Inhibition in the Central Nervous System

The failure of axon regeneration in the injured spinal cord is largely caused by the growth-inhibitory environment of the adult CNS that is especially prominent in white matter. The inhibitors of CNS regeneration can be classified into three main categories: (1) inhibitors associated with the glial scar that forms after injury, (2) myelin-associated inhibitors, and (3) inhibitors of the "guidance type." There are many types of ligands and receptor complexes that convey signals from the multiple growth-inhibitory proteins (**Fig. 35.1**). However, despite this diversity, inside neuronal cells, most if not all inhibitory signaling complexes converge on the Rho pathway.

Inhibitors Associated with the Glial Scar

The glial reaction to CNS injury occurs almost immediately as a mechanism to protect healthy CNS tissue from inflammatory damage and to repair the blood–brain barrier.[1] The glial scar forms both a physical and a chemical barrier that is composed of astrocytes, microglia, macrophages, oligodendrocyte precursor cells, and an extracellular matrix of secreted basal membrane components.[1,2] Astrocytes undergo reactive gliosis and are a major contributor to the inhibitory nature of the glial scar by releasing chondroitin sulfate proteoglycans (CSPGs), which are potent inhibitors of axon growth.[1] Recently, the receptor for CSPG inhibitory signaling has been identified as protein tyrosine phosphatase (PTPs), and PTPs gene disruption promotes axon regeneration.[3,4] It is known that inactivating Rho will overcome growth inhibition on CSPG substrates,[5] but the full signaling cascades still need to be elaborated.

Myelin-Associated Inhibitors

Myelin Inhibitors

Many potent growth-inhibitory proteins exist in myelin, and the myelin debris in the environment of the injured CNS is a formidable barrier to regeneration The best-characterized myelin-derived growth-inhibitory proteins are myelin-associated glycoprotein (MAG), Nogo, and oligodendrocyte myelin glycoprotein (OMgp),[6] although other inhibitors, such

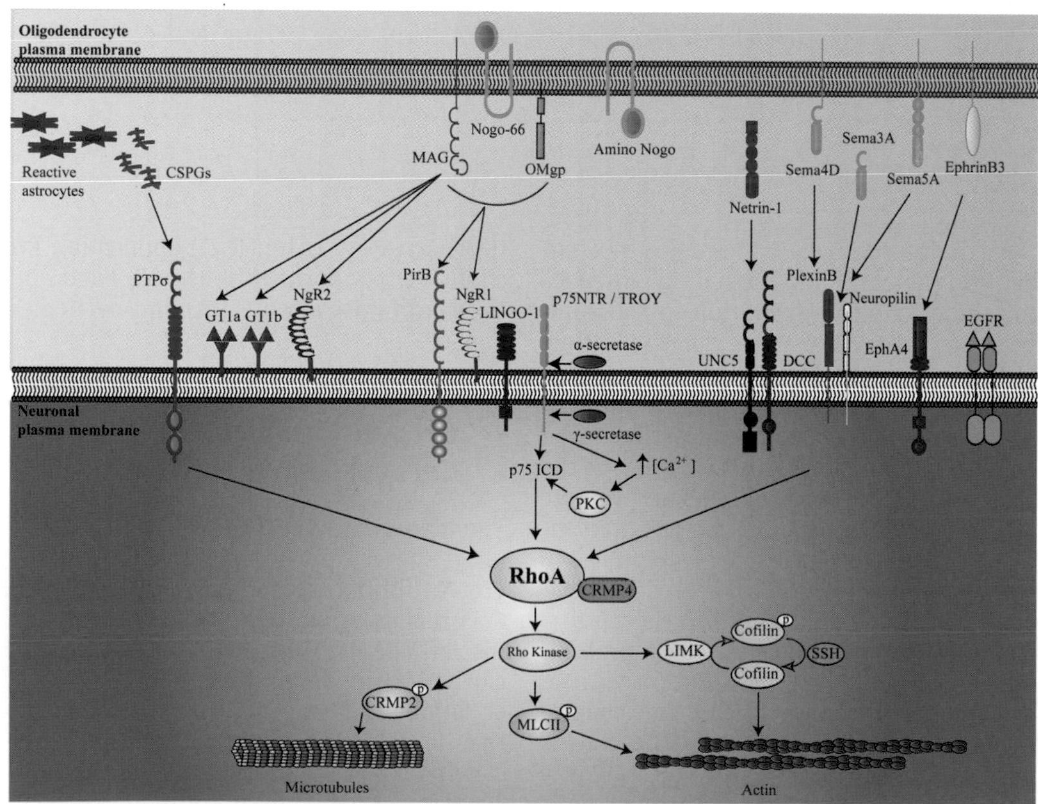

Fig. 35.1 A schematic diagram that shows the ligands and receptors that participate in central nervous system growth-inhibitory signaling. Inside neurons, the growth-inhibitory signals converge to Rho, a master switch that regulates the growth cone cytoskeleton in motility.

as versican,[7] are also present in myelin. MAG was the first myelin inhibitor identified[8,9] after the Schwab group first characterized CNS inhibitory activity.[10] Nogo was next identified through the use of IN-1 antibody to identify the antigen peptide sequence.[11–13] OMgp is another myelin-derived inhibitor identified[14,15] and may play a role in preventing collateral sprouting and determining the spacing of the nodes of Ranvier.[16] MAG, Nogo, and OMgp all have in common the ability to share interaction with the Nogo receptor complex.[6]

Nogo Receptors

The receptors for the various myelin-derived growth-inhibitory proteins have taken longer to identify and new receptors are still being added to the list. The difficulty in identifying receptors is that MAG, Nogo, and OMgp all signal to receptor complexes on the neuronal membrane that may have different components on different types of neuronal cells. MAG, Nogo, and OMgp signal through a receptor complex composed of Nogo-66 receptor (NgR1)[17] or paired immunoglobulin-like receptor B (PirB),[18] leucine rich repeat and Ig domain containing 1 (LINGO1),[19] and either p75 neurotrophin receptor (p75 NTR)[20] or tumor necrosis factor receptor superfamily, member 19 (TROY/TNSRF19).[21,22]

NgR1 is localized to the axolemma in many classes of CNS neurons, and because it lacks an intracellular domain, additional co-receptors transduce the signal following ligand binding.[17] The p75NTR co-receptor can physically interact with NgR1 to mediate intracellular signaling,[20] although in many neurons TROY takes the place of p75 NTR. The p75NTR is known to signal directly to Rho,[20] and TROY also signals to Rho.[21,22] The other components of the NgR receptor complex are LINGO1, a transmembrane protein,[19] and PirB.[18] PirB is expressed in a subset of neurons in the brain, and interfering with PirB activity, either genetically or with a function-blocking antibody, reduces neurite outgrowth inhibition in response to Nogo-66, MAG, OMgp, and myelin.[18]

Gangliosides and NgR2

Other receptors may be involved in mediating some of the extracellular inhibitory signals by myelin-derived inhibitors. Two additional human homologues for NgR1 have been identified: NgR2 and NgR3.[23,24] NgR2 mRNA levels have been detected in neurons in the adult mouse brain that project to the spinal cord.[25] Neither NgR2 nor NgR3 can bind Nogo-66, but NgR2 has been demonstrated to bind MAG.[26] The gangliosides GT1b and GD1a act as receptors for MAG that signal to Rho.[20,26,27] However, although MAG is not thought to be a very important growth-inhibitory protein, it may have an important role in promoting resistance to axonal injury and disease.[28]

Guidance-Type Growth Inhibitors: Eph/Ephrins, Netrins, and Semaphorins

Chemorepulsive axon guidance molecules are known to be important in the development of the nervous system, and now it is clear that many of the developmentally expressed proteins act as inhibitors in CNS injury by signaling to Rho. Three classes of proteins have been implicated in inhibiting nerve regeneration: Ephrins/Eph receptors, netrins, and semaphorins.

Ephrins and Eph proteins are part of the large receptor tyrosine kinase family capable of bidirectional signaling between neurons and oligodendrocytes (**Fig. 35.1**). Both Ephs and Ephrins have been localized to CNS tissue following a spinal cord injury (SCI),[29,30] and Ephrin-B3 is persistently expressed in oligodendrocytes, where it has strong axon growth-inhibitory activity.[31] Studies with knockout mice show that Ephrin-B3 and Eph4 play a role in limiting axonal regeneration and functional recovery following SCI,[31] and Rho is activated by inhibitory Ephrin signaling.[32]

Netrins are a family of proteins that play an important role in development of spinal cord, and Netrin-1 is expressed in the neurons and oligodendrocytes of the adult spinal cord.[33] Netrin-1 is a bifunctional ligand that can function as a chemoattractant or chemorepellent depending on the receptor type it interacts with. Netrin-1 inhibits axon growth,[34] and netrins affect Rho signaling.[35]

The semaphorin family has both soluble and transmembrane-bound members that mediate repulsion in development, and these proteins are re-expressed in CNS injury.[36,37] Sema4D is an oligodendrocyte transmembrane protein that inhibits axon growth and is transiently up-regulated following CNS injury,[38] as is Sema3A, which is a soluble inhibitory protein.[39] Sema5A induces growth cone collapse, and blocking Sema5A with a function-blocking antibody neutralizes these effects.[40] Semaphorins inhibit axon growth via the activation of Rho.[41,42] Therefore, inactivation of Rho should be effective to overcome many of the guidance-type of axon growth inhibitors.

Growth Inhibition: All Roads Lead to Rho

The challenge for translational medicine to treat SCI is to find a strategy that blocks all the CNS growth-inhibitory activity. The growing body of evidence indicates that Rho regulates the neuronal response to diverse growth-inhibitory proteins. Therefore, Rho is a potentially very powerful target to promote repair after SCI.

Rho guanidine triphosphate (GTPases) are a family of highly related proteins that are present in all cells as important signaling switches. GTPases have two conformations: a guanidine diphosphate (GDP)-bound inactive state and a GTP-bound active state. Treating neurons with C3 transferase to inactivate Rho was first demonstrated by us as an effective way to overcome growth inhibition on myelin.[43] C3 transferase is a bacterial protein that adenosine diphosphate (ADP) ribosylates Rho to keep it in its inactive state. Rho kinase interacts with Rho, and inhibition of Rho kinase with Y-27632 has similar effects—both C3 and Rho kinase inhibitors promote growth on inhibitory substrates in vitro and in vivo.[43–57] Moreover, both compounds override growth inhibition by myelin as well as by the CSPGs.[5] Newer evidence also indicates that many of the guidance-type inhibitors signal to Rho. The in vitro studies have been followed by a wealth of studies on animal models of SCI and regeneration (**Table 35.1**). The general finding is that inactivating Rho after SCI has beneficial effects on tissue sparing and functional recovery, and anatomical studies indicate that inactivation of Rho stimulates axon regeneration and prevents apoptotic cell death (**Table 35.1**).

We are now beginning to understand the molecular mechanisms that explain why Rho is such an important target to block growth inhibition and promote regeneration. Rho activation signals through downstream effectors to modulate the cytoskeleton and influence growth cone behavior. Rho kinase is activated in response to Rho activation, leading to phosphorylation of myosin light chain II[58,59] that in turn regulates myosin in motility. The actin depolymerizing factor/cofilin family is also important in cytoskeleton rearrangements in the growth cone, and these proteins are also regulated by Rho.[60] Collapsing response mediator protein (CRMP) is implicated in the signaling cascade activated in response to myelin-associated inhibitors and CSPGs and can physically interact with Rho to mediate growth inhibition.[61,62] The current findings suggest that inhibitory signaling from myelin inhibitors and CSPGs converge on Rho-CRMP4 to cause cytoskeletal rearrangements.

Translational Medicine

The in vitro and in vivo demonstration that C3 transferase could specifically inactivate Rho to overcome growth inhibition suggested it could be a good drug candidate. As a biologic drug, breakdown products are amino acids, so there is less risk of a phase 3 failure due to toxicity. With a view to translating early preclinical findings on Rho inactivation to clinical testing, it was necessary to (1) develop a method to obtain highly purified active protein and standardize the enzymatic activity of different purification batches, (2) develop a suitable delivery method and determine effective dose, and (3) complete proof-of-concept and confirm delivery method. We have developed a drug candidate, called BA-210, by modifying the properties of C3 transferase to enhance its ability to penetrate cells. BA-210 has been given the trademark name of Cethrin (Alseres Phar-

Table 35.1 Summary of Preclinical Studies on Rho as a Target for Treatment of Spinal Cord Injury

Drug	Method of delivery	Injury model	Anatomical observations	Functional outcome	Reference
Rho inhibitors					
C3	Lesion (Gel-foam, Baxter, Deerfield, IL)	Rat ON	Regeneration	N/A	Lehmann et al., 1999[43]
C3	Lesion site (in fibrin)	Mouse SC	Regeneration	↑ Locomotion	Dergham et al., 2002[5]
C3–05*	Lesion site (in fibrin)	Rat SC Mouse SC	Neuroprotective	N/A	Dubreuil et al., 2003[50]
C3-TAT	N/A	In vitro on injured SC	N/A	N/A	Monnier et al., 2003[51]
C3	Intrathecal	Rat SC	Less scar formation	↓ Locomotion	Fournier et al., 2003[46]
C3	Adeno-assoc. virus	Rat ON	Regeneration Neuroprotective	N/A	Fischer et al., 2004[52]
C3–05 C3–07*	Intraocular (delayed)	Rat ON	Regeneration Neuroprotective	N/A	Bertrand et al., 2005[47]
C3–07	Intraocular (multiple)	Rat ON	Regeneration Neuroprotective	N/A	Bertrand et al., 2007[48]
C3–11* + CNTF/cAMP	Intraocular (multiple)	Rat ON	Regeneration Neuroprotective	N/A	Hu et al., 2007[53]
BA-210	Extradural (in fibrin)	Rat SC/ Mouse SC	Tissue sparing	↑ Locomotion NC allodynia	Lord-Fontaine et al., 2008[15]
Rho kinase inhibitors					
HA1077	Intraperitoneal	Rat SC	Tissue sparing	↑ Locomotion	Hara et al., 2000[49]
Y-27632	Lesion site (fibrin)	Mouse SC	Regeneration	↑ Locomotion	Dergham et al., 2002[5]
Y-27632/ HA1077	Oral/ Intraperitoneal	Rat SC	Decreased SC damage	↑ Locomotion	Sung et al., 2003[54]
Y-27632	Intrathecal	Rat SC	Regeneration	↑ Locomotion	Fournier et al., 2003[46]
Y-27632	N/A	Mouse SC	Regeneration	N/A	Borisoff et al., 2003[55]
Y-27632	Intrathecal	Rat SC	Regeneration	↑ Locomotion	Chan et al., 2005[56]
Rho kinase mutant mice	N/A	Mouse SC	Regeneration	NC locomotion	Duffy et al., 2009[57]

*C3–05, C3–07, and C3–11 are different versions of C3 created during the drug development process.
Abbreviations: cAMP, cyclic adenosine monophosphate; N/A, not applicable; NC, no change; ON, optic nerve; SC, spinal cord.

maceuticals). The steps that were needed to bring BA-210 to clinical trial are shown in **Fig. 35.2**.

Chemistry, Manufacturing, and Control

With any drug, and especially with a protein drug, a critical component is to scale up production and purification procedures and develop assays to characterize purity, potency, and reproducibility. Before this step, we ensured that we had the best drug candidate possible by engineering several cell-permeable versions of C3 and comparing their biological activity.[44] We also optimized expression systems for synthesis and the method of purification.[45]

To use a drug in a clinical trial, chemistry, manufacturing and control (CMC) must be performed according to good manufacturing practices (GMPs) (**Fig. 35.2**). Although a discussion of GMPs is beyond this chapter, it is important to state that the earlier the procedures needed for GMPs are developed, the better, and the importance of rigorous characterization of a drug candidate as early as possible cannot be overstated. There are many reasons for putting an early effort into quality control: (1) Impurities can have unwanted biological effects and influence preclinical findings. For example, endotoxins in protein drugs are likely to cause variability in SCI experiments because of their effect on inflammation. (2) Assays required to monitor potency, purity, and reproducibility are not trivial and may require a significant development effort. (3) Thinking about formulation is a critical component with respect to drug delivery and drug stability in storage.

In the development of BA-210, we made different variants along the way[44,45] (**Table 35.1**). BA-210 manufactured at large scale is functionally interchangeable with its predecessors, having the same or better enzymatic and biological activities but

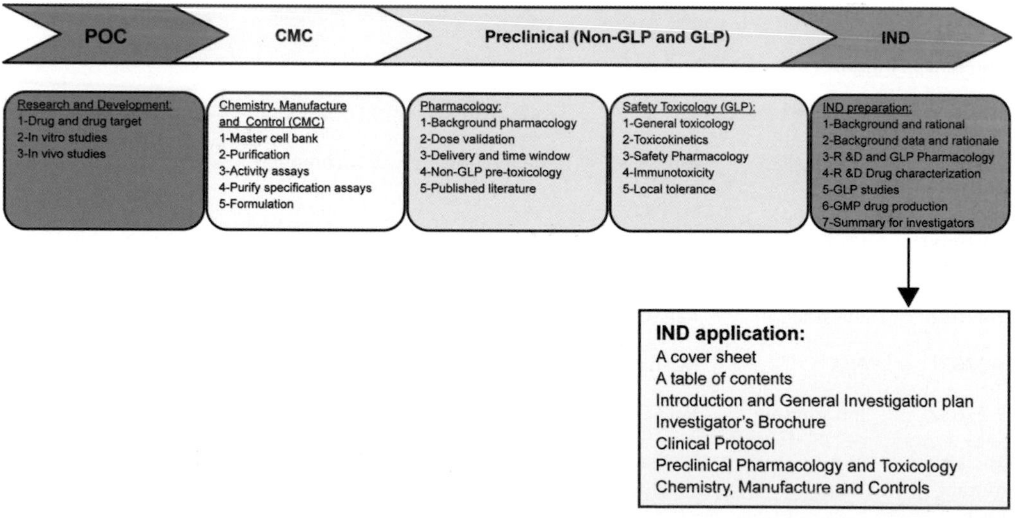

Fig. 35.2 Diagram to illustrate the development path for BA-210 from proof-of-concept (POC) research to investigational new drug (IND) application. After the decision to go forward from POC data, BA-210 was synthesized following chemistry, manufacture, and control (CMC) guidelines. This well-characterized drug was used for further dose-validation and delivery studies, for good laboratory practice (GLP)-compliant safety studies, and to finalize GLP-compliant drug purity and activity assays. A good manufacturing practice (GMP) compliant batch of drug was synthesized for the clinical trials.

fewer impurities, and a standardized enzymatic activity. An example of a change made during the CMC development process can be seen in the removal of a single cysteine that was located in a nonfunctional region of the protein. This was done after it was noted that the C3 variants had a tendency to aggregate during scale-up purification.[63]

Preclinical Proof of Concept and the Preclinical Package

The preclinical package for an IND application has two major components: (1) the preclinical data that support the clinical plan, and (2) the safety and toxicology package, which must be completed according to GLPs. Due to the rigors of GLP studies, safety and toxicology studies were outsourced to a contract research organization specializing in drug development, and these will not be discussed here. However, it is important to emphasize that the safety and toxicology studies are a key element to deciding if a drug should go into clinical trial; data from these studies will help determine the starting dose based on a no-observed-adverse-effect level from the panel of studies. In the case of BA-210, a panel of safety studies with different delivery methods was completed; the delivery methods included intravenous (single and repeated dose), extradural, and subcutaneous.

Drug Delivery

To choose a delivery method for clinical trial, we sought a noninvasive delivery that did not require the insertion of needles or catheters into the spinal cord or cerebrospinal fluid. Fibrin-mediated delivery was chosen because local delivery would minimize systemic exposure, and fibrin formulations have been approved for use in humans and are routinely used during decompression and stabilization surgeries after SCI. Fibrin had already been used as a delivery vehicle for SCI in rats, and it acts as a slow-release matrix[64] (**Table 35.1**). Other studies in monkeys showed the safety of fibrin sealant application onto the spinal cord with respect to the inflammatory and neurophysiological responses.[65] In a rat SCI model, dural closure with a fibrin matrix reduced the lesion gap and scar formation.[66] Therefore, fibrin as a delivery method for clinical trial had many advantages in terms of safety.

The biochemical mechanism of action of C3 compounds has been well studied in the literature, as already discussed, but we wished to understand more fully the possible mechanism of action on the spinal cord. We showed that the penetration of BA-210 in the spinal cord after extradural delivery was superior to C3 lacking a transport sequence and superior to mutated C3 lacking enzymatic activity.[45] We and others documented that, after SCI injury, Rho is activated in both white matter and gray matter, and activated Rho is present in both cell bodies of neurons and glia, and in axonal fibers.[67–69] We went on to show that BA-210 penetrated into the area of the spinal cord with abnormal Rho activation, and delayed delivery was effective. Studies using rats with SCI demonstrated tissue sparing and improved locomotion after treatment with BA-210.[45] Therefore, results of studies with BA-210 were consistent with the wealth of preclinical experiments in animals supporting Rho as a target for regeneration (**Table 35.1**).

Therapeutic Dose

Of critical importance for drug development is determining a potential therapeutic dose for testing in patients. Rho activation in vivo can be quantified by a biochemical method known as a pull-down assay. Studies on injured rat spinal cord demonstrated that Rho activation is sustained after SCI, and that application of BA-210 to the injured spinal cord could reverse Rho activation. These findings were important to translate the discovery of Rho as a potential target for SCI repair because it allowed a quantitative read-out for determination of an effective dose in rodent spinal cord. In rats, a low dose of 15 µg BA-210 completely abolished SCI-induced Rho activation.[45] To further study dosage, we examined penetration of BA-210 into pig spinal cord because it approximates the size of the human spinal cord. By comparing effective doses in rats with penetration in pigs and rats, we determined that 0.5 mg might be expected to be an effective dose in humans, but likely the optimal dose would be 1 to 3 mg. The clinical protocol was designed to ensure the safety of the patients, and thus, a starting dose of 0.3 mg was chosen, which was well below the no-observed-effect level. Dose escalation to 6 mg was planned.

Clinical Studies with Cethrin to Treat Spinal Cord Injury

The primary goal of the clinical study was to determine the safety and tolerability of BA-210 when administered in conjunction with fibrin sealant to the dura mater of the spinal cord. The secondary objectives were to evaluate (1) the pharmacokinetic profile of BA-210, (2) the neurological status of patients as measured by the American Spinal Injury Association (ASIA) assessment, and (3) the appropriate dose range for BA-210 in humans.

The planned clinical trial was an open-label study using five dose levels of BA-210. There were two patient groups in the study. Group 1 consisted of patients with acute thoracic (T2–12) SCI. Group 2 consisted of patients with acute cervical (C4–T1) SCI. The first patients were enrolled in group 1, and cumulative safety data were assessed before the decision to enroll patients in group 2. This stratification of enrollment was followed until all doses had been tested in first thoracic then cervical patients. Patient enrollment is now complete, and the data are being analyzed. The results will be reported in a full publication (Fehlings et al., in preparation).

Pearls

- Many of the growth inhibitory proteins that block regeneration and repair after CNS injury use the Rho pathway.
- Preclinical and clinical research supports using a Rho inhibitor to improve outcomes after spinal cord injury.
- Animal models of SCI support the selection of Rho as the target for drug development and clinical testing; preclinical studies have been undertaken to determine the safety of BA-210, delivery and mechanism of action, time window of activity, and therapeutic dose. Finishing the current clinical study and further clinical studies will be needed to determine the effectiveness of BA-210 (Cethrin); thus far, the outlook is promising.

Pitfalls

- Following CNS injury, many growth inhibitory proteins block regeneration and repair. These inhibitors include proteins associated with the glial scar myelin-associated inhibitors, and guidance-type inhibitors.
- Blocking just one of these proteins would likely have limited success in improving outcomes so broader approaches, such as targeting the Rho pathway, are needed.

References

1. Fitch MT, Silver J. CNS injury, glial scars, and inflammation: inhibitory extracellular matrices and regeneration failure. Exp Neurol 2008;209(2): 294–301
2. Fawcett JW, Asher RA. The glial scar and central nervous system repair. Brain Res Bull 1999; 49(6):377–391
3. Fry EJ, Chagnon MJ, López-Vales R, Tremblay ML, David S. Corticospinal tract regeneration after spinal cord injury in receptor protein tyrosine phosphatase sigma deficient mice. Glia 2010;58(4): 423–433
4. Shen Y, Tenney AP, Busch SA, et al. PTPsigma is a receptor for chondroitin sulfate proteoglycan, an inhibitor of neural regeneration. Science 2009; 326(5952):592–596
5. Dergham P, Ellezam B, Essagian C, Avedissian H, Lubell WD, McKerracher L. Rho signaling pathway targeted to promote spinal cord repair. J Neurosci 2002;22(15):6570–6577
6. Nash M, Pribiag H, Fournier AE, Jacobson C. Central nervous system regeneration inhibitors and their intracellular substrates. Mol Neurobiol 2009; 40(3):224–235
7. Schweigreiter R, Walmsley AR, Niederöst B, et al. Versican V2 and the central inhibitory domain of

Nogo-A inhibit neurite growth via p75NTR/NgR-independent pathways that converge at RhoA. Mol Cell Neurosci 2004;27(2):163–174
8. McKerracher L, David S, Jackson DL, Kottis V, Dunn RJ, Braun PE. Identification of myelin-associated glycoprotein as a major myelin-derived inhibitor of neurite growth. Neuron 1994;13(4): 805–811
9. Mukhopadhyay G, Doherty P, Walsh FS, Crocker PR, Filbin MT. A novel role for myelin-associated glycoprotein as an inhibitor of axonal regeneration. Neuron 1994;13(3):757–767
10. Caroni P, Schwab ME. Two membrane protein fractions from rat central myelin with inhibitory properties for neurite growth and fibroblast spreading. J Cell Biol 1988;106(4):1281–1288
11. Chen MS, Huber AB, van der Haar ME, et al. Nogo-A is a myelin-associated neurite outgrowth inhibitor and an antigen for monoclonal antibody IN-1. Nature 2000;403(6768):434–439
12. GrandPré T, Nakamura F, Vartanian T, Strittmatter SM. Identification of the Nogo inhibitor of axon regeneration as a Reticulon protein. Nature 2000;403(6768):439–444
13. Prinjha R, Moore SE, Vinson M, et al. Inhibitor of neurite outgrowth in humans. Nature 2000; 403(6768):383–384
14. Kottis V, Thibault P, Mikol D, et al. Oligodendrocyte-myelin glycoprotein (OMgp) is an inhibitor of neurite outgrowth. J Neurochem 2002; 82(6):1566–1569
15. Wang KC, Koprivica V, Kim JA, et al. Oligodendrocyte-myelin glycoprotein is a Nogo receptor ligand that inhibits neurite outgrowth. Nature 2002;417(6892):941–944
16. Huang JK, Phillips GR, Roth AD, et al. Glial membranes at the node of Ranvier prevent neurite outgrowth. Science 2005;310(5755):1813–1817
17. Fournier AE, GrandPre T, Strittmatter SM. Identification of a receptor mediating Nogo-66 inhibition of axonal regeneration. Nature 2001; 409(6818):341–346
18. Atwal JK, Pinkston-Gosse J, Syken J, et al. PirB is a functional receptor for myelin inhibitors of axonal regeneration. Science 2008;322(5903): 967–970
19. Mi S, Lee X, Shao Z, et al. LINGO-1 is a component of the Nogo-66 receptor/p75 signaling complex. Nat Neurosci 2004;7(3):221–228
20. Yamashita T, Higuchi H, Tohyama M. The p75 receptor transduces the signal from myelin-associated glycoprotein to Rho. J Cell Biol 2002;157(4): 565–570
21. Park JB, Yiu G, Kaneko S, et al. A TNF receptor family member, TROY, is a coreceptor with Nogo receptor in mediating the inhibitory activity of myelin inhibitors. Neuron 2005;45(3):345–351
22. Shao Z, Browning JL, Lee X, et al. TAJ/TROY, an orphan TNF receptor family member, binds Nogo-66 receptor 1 and regulates axonal regeneration. Neuron 2005;45(3):353–359
23. Laurén J, Airaksinen MS, Saarma M, Timmusk T. Two novel mammalian Nogo receptor homologs differentially expressed in the central and peripheral nervous systems. Mol Cell Neurosci 2003; 24(3):581–594
24. Pignot V, Hein AE, Barske C, et al. Characterization of two novel proteins, NgRH1 and NgRH2, structurally and biochemically homologous to the Nogo-66 receptor. J Neurochem 2003;85(3): 717–728
25. Barrette B, Vallières N, Dubé M, Lacroix S. Expression profile of receptors for myelin-associated inhibitors of axonal regeneration in the intact and injured mouse central nervous system. Mol Cell Neurosci 2007;34(4):519–538
26. Venkatesh K, Chivatakarn O, Lee H, et al. The Nogo-66 receptor homolog NgR2 is a sialic acid-dependent receptor selective for myelin-associated glycoprotein. J Neurosci 2005;25(4):808–822
27. Mehta NR, Lopez PH, Vyas AA, Schnaar RL. Gangliosides and Nogo receptors independently mediate myelin-associated glycoprotein inhibition of neurite outgrowth in different nerve cells. J Biol Chem 2007;282(38):27875–27886
28. Nguyen T, Mehta NR, Conant K, et al. Axonal protective effects of the myelin-associated glycoprotein. J Neurosci 2009;29(3):630–637
29. Miranda JD, White LA, Marcillo AE, Willson CA, Jagid J, Whittemore SR. Induction of Eph B3 after spinal cord injury. Exp Neurol 1999;156(1): 218–222
30. Bundesen LQ, Scheel TA, Bregman BS, Kromer LF. Ephrin-B2 and EphB2 regulation of astrocyte-meningeal fibroblast interactions in response to spinal cord lesions in adult rats. J Neurosci 2003;23(21): 7789–7800
31. Benson MD, Romero MI, Lush ME, Lu QR, Henkemeyer M, Parada LF. Ephrin-B3 is a myelin-based inhibitor of neurite outgrowth. Proc Natl Acad Sci U S A 2005;102(30):10694–10699
32. Wahl S, Barth H, Ciossek T, Aktories K, Mueller BK. Ephrin-A5 induces collapse of growth cones by activating Rho and Rho kinase. J Cell Biol 2000;149(2):263–270
33. Manitt C, Colicos MA, Thompson KM, Rousselle E, Peterson AC, Kennedy TE. Widespread expression of netrin-1 by neurons and oligodendrocytes in the adult mammalian spinal cord. J Neurosci 2001;21(11):3911–3922
34. Löw K, Culbertson M, Bradke F, Tessier-Lavigne M, Tuszynski MH. Netrin-1 is a novel myelin-associated inhibitor to axon growth. J Neurosci 2008; 28(5):1099–1108
35. Moore SW, Correia JP, Lai Wing Sun K, Pool M, Fournier AE, Kennedy TE. Rho inhibition recruits DCC to the neuronal plasma membrane and enhances axon chemoattraction to netrin 1. Development 2008;135(17):2855–2864
36. Luo Y, Raible D, Raper JA. Collapsin: a protein in brain that induces the collapse and paralysis of neuronal growth cones. Cell 1993;75(2):217–227
37. Pasterkamp RJ, Verhaagen J. Semaphorins in axon regeneration: developmental guidance molecules gone wrong? Philos Trans R Soc Lond B Biol Sci 2006;361(1473):1499–1511
38. Moreau-Fauvarque C, Kumanogoh A, Camand E, et al. The transmembrane semaphorin Sema4D/CD100, an inhibitor of axonal growth, is expressed on oligodendrocytes and upregulated after CNS lesion. J Neurosci 2003;23(27): 9229–9239
39. Pasterkamp RJ, Giger RJ, Ruitenberg MJ, et al. Expression of the gene encoding the chemorepellent semaphorin III is induced in the fibroblast component of neural scar tissue formed following injuries of adult but not neonatal CNS. Mol Cell Neurosci 1999;13(2):143–166

40. Goldberg JL, Vargas ME, Wang JT, et al. An oligodendrocyte lineage-specific semaphorin, Sema5A, inhibits axon growth by retinal ganglion cells. J Neurosci 2004;24(21):4989–4999

41. Aurandt J, Vikis HG, Gutkind JS, Ahn N, Guan K-L. The semaphorin receptor plexin-B1 signals through a direct interaction with the Rho-specific nucleotide exchange factor, LARG. Proc Natl Acad Sci U S A 2002;99(19):12085–12090

42. Swiercz JM, Kuner R, Behrens J, Offermanns S. Plexin-B1 directly interacts with PDZ-RhoGEF/LARG to regulate RhoA and growth cone morphology. Neuron 2002;35(1):51–63

43. Lehmann M, Fournier A, Selles-Navarro I, et al. Inactivation of Rho signaling pathway promotes CNS axon regeneration. J Neurosci 1999;19(17):7537–7547

44. Winton MJ, Dubreuil CI, Lasko D, Leclerc N, McKerracher L. Characterization of new cell permeable C3-like proteins that inactivate Rho and stimulate neurite outgrowth on inhibitory substrates. J Biol Chem 2002;277(36):32820–32829

45. Lord-Fontaine S, Yang F, Diep Q, et al. Local inhibition of Rho signaling by cell-permeable recombinant protein BA-210 prevents secondary damage and promotes functional recovery following acute spinal cord injury. J Neurotrauma 2008;25(11):1309–1322

46. Fournier AE, Takizawa BT, Strittmatter SM. Rho kinase inhibition enhances axonal regeneration in the injured CNS. J Neurosci 2003;23(4):1416–1423

47. Bertrand J, Winton MJ, Rodriguez-Hernandez N, Campenot RB, McKerracher L. Application of Rho antagonist to neuronal cell bodies promotes neurite growth in compartmented cultures and regeneration of retinal ganglion cell axons in the optic nerve of adult rats. J Neurosci 2005;25(5):1113–1121

48. Bertrand J, Di Polo A, McKerracher L. Enhanced survival and regeneration of axotomized retinal neurons by repeated delivery of cell-permeable C3-like Rho antagonists. Neurobiol Dis 2007;25(1):65–72

49. Hara M, Takayasu M, Watanabe K, et al. Protein kinase inhibition by fasudil hydrochloride promotes neurological recovery after spinal cord injury in rats. J Neurosurg 2000;93(1, Suppl):94–101

50. Dubreuil CI, Winton MJ, McKerracher L. Rho activation patterns after spinal cord injury and the role of activated Rho in apoptosis in the central nervous system. J Cell Biol 2003;162(2):233–243

51. Monnier PP, Sierra A, Schwab JM, Henke-Fahle S, Mueller BK. The Rho/ROCK pathway mediates neurite growth-inhibitory activity associated with the chondroitin sulfate proteoglycans of the CNS glial scar. Mol Cell Neurosci 2003;22(3):319–330

52. Fischer D, Petkova V, Thanos S, Benowitz LI. Switching mature retinal ganglion cells to a robust growth state in vivo: gene expression and synergy with RhoA inactivation. J Neurosci 2004;24(40):8726–8740

53. Hu Y, Cui Q, Harvey AR. Interactive effects of C3, cyclic AMP and ciliary neurotrophic factor on adult retinal ganglion cell survival and axonal regeneration. Mol Cell Neurosci 2007;34(1):88–98

54. Sung JK, Miao L, Calvert JW, Huang L, Louis Harkey H, Zhang JH. A possible role of RhoA/Rho-kinase in experimental spinal cord injury in rat. Brain Res 2003;959(1):29–38

55. Borisoff JF, Chan CCM, Hiebert GW, et al. Suppression of Rho-kinase activity promotes axonal growth on inhibitory CNS substrates. Mol Cell Neurosci 2003;22(3):405–416

56. Chan CCM, Khodarahmi K, Liu J, et al. Dose-dependent beneficial and detrimental effects of ROCK inhibitor Y27632 on axonal sprouting and functional recovery after rat spinal cord injury. Exp Neurol 2005;196(2):352–364

57. Duffy P, Schmandke A, Schmandke A, et al. Rho-associated kinase II (ROCKII) limits axonal growth after trauma within the adult mouse spinal cord. J Neurosci 2009;29(48):15266–15276

58. Alabed YZ, Grados-Munro E, Ferraro GB, Hsieh SH-K, Fournier AE. Neuronal responses to myelin are mediated by rho kinase. J Neurochem 2006;96(6):1616–1625

59. Kubo T, Endo M, Hata K, et al. Myosin IIA is required for neurite outgrowth inhibition produced by repulsive guidance molecule. J Neurochem 2008;105(1):113–126

60. Hsieh SH-K, Ferraro GB, Fournier AE. Myelin-associated inhibitors regulate cofilin phosphorylation and neuronal inhibition through LIM kinase and Slingshot phosphatase. J Neurosci 2006;26(3):1006–1015

61. Mimura F, Yamagishi S, Arimura N, et al. Myelin-associated glycoprotein inhibits microtubule assembly by a Rho-kinase-dependent mechanism. J Biol Chem 2006;281(23):15970–15979

62. Alabed YZ, Pool M, Ong Tone S, Fournier AE. Identification of CRMP4 as a convergent regulator of axon outgrowth inhibition. J Neurosci 2007;27(7):1702–1711

63. Lasko D, McKerracher L. Fluorescent assay of cell-permeable C3 transferase activity. Methods Enzymol 2006;406:512–520

64. Guest JD, Hesse D, Schnell L, Schwab ME, Bunge MB, Bunge RP. Influence of IN-1 antibody and acidic FGF-fibrin glue on the response of injured corticospinal tract axons to human Schwann cell grafts. J Neurosci Res 1997;50(5):888–905

65. Kassam A, Nemoto E, Balzer J, et al. Effects of Tisseel fibrin glue on the central nervous system of nonhuman primates. Ear Nose Throat J 2004;83(4):246–248, 250, 252 passim

66. Zhang YP, Iannotti C, Shields LBE, et al. Dural closure, cord approximation, and clot removal: enhancement of tissue sparing in a novel laceration spinal cord injury model. J Neurosurg 2004;100(4, Suppl Spine):343–352

67. McKerracher L, Higuchi H. Targeting Rho to stimulate repair after spinal cord injury. J Neurotrauma 2006;23(3-4):309–317

68. Madura T, Yamashita T, Kubo T, Fujitani M, Hosokawa K, Tohyama M. Activation of Rho in the injured axons following spinal cord injury. EMBO Rep 2004;5(4):412–417

69. Schwab JM, Conrad S, Elbert T, Trautmann K, Meyermann R, Schluesener HJ. Lesional RhoA+ cell numbers are suppressed by anti-inflammatory, cyclooxygenase-inhibiting treatment following subacute spinal cord injury. Glia 2004;47(4):377–386

36

Neuroprotective Trials in Spinal Cord Injury

Shelly Wang, Gregory W. J. Hawryluk, and Michael G. Fehlings

Key Points

1. Despite numerous drugs having been trialed for neuroprotection after SCI in the past, only MPSS has been translated to the clinic.
2. Despite not producing clinically used strategies, the trials from the past have informed research.
3. Current promising trials are being conducted on riluzole, minocycline, early surgical decompression and therapeutic hypothermia.
4. In the future, these strategies may be used in combination with neuroregenerative methods.

Over the past 25 years, therapeutic strategies to protect neural tissue have emerged as a promising approach for improving outcome from spinal cord injury (SCI). Central to this approach has been the acceptance of *secondary injury*, which involves a period of progressive and prolonged tissue damage following the initial *primary injury* (**Fig. 36.1**). This delayed damage results from interrelated pathological cellular events, which include ischemia, excitotoxicity, electrolyte dysregulation, free radical production, mitochondrial dysfunction, and vasogenic edema leading to cell death, which are often exacerbated by systemic hypotension and hypoxia, which can accompany SCI.[1–3]

Following successful preclinical trials in animal models, many neuroprotective agents have been tested in human clinical trials. Recent decades have seen the trial process advance as much as the agents being tested. Thus, ongoing studies that combine promising new agents with more appropriate and sensitive outcome measurements have strong potential for human translation.

Completed Neuroprotective Trials in Spinal Cord Injury

Pharmacological Agents

Numerous pharmacological agents have been shown to have the potential to reduce secondary injury and improve functional outcomes in animal studies. However, human trials of most agents have had disappointing results, and to date, only methylprednisolone sodium succinate (MPSS) has been

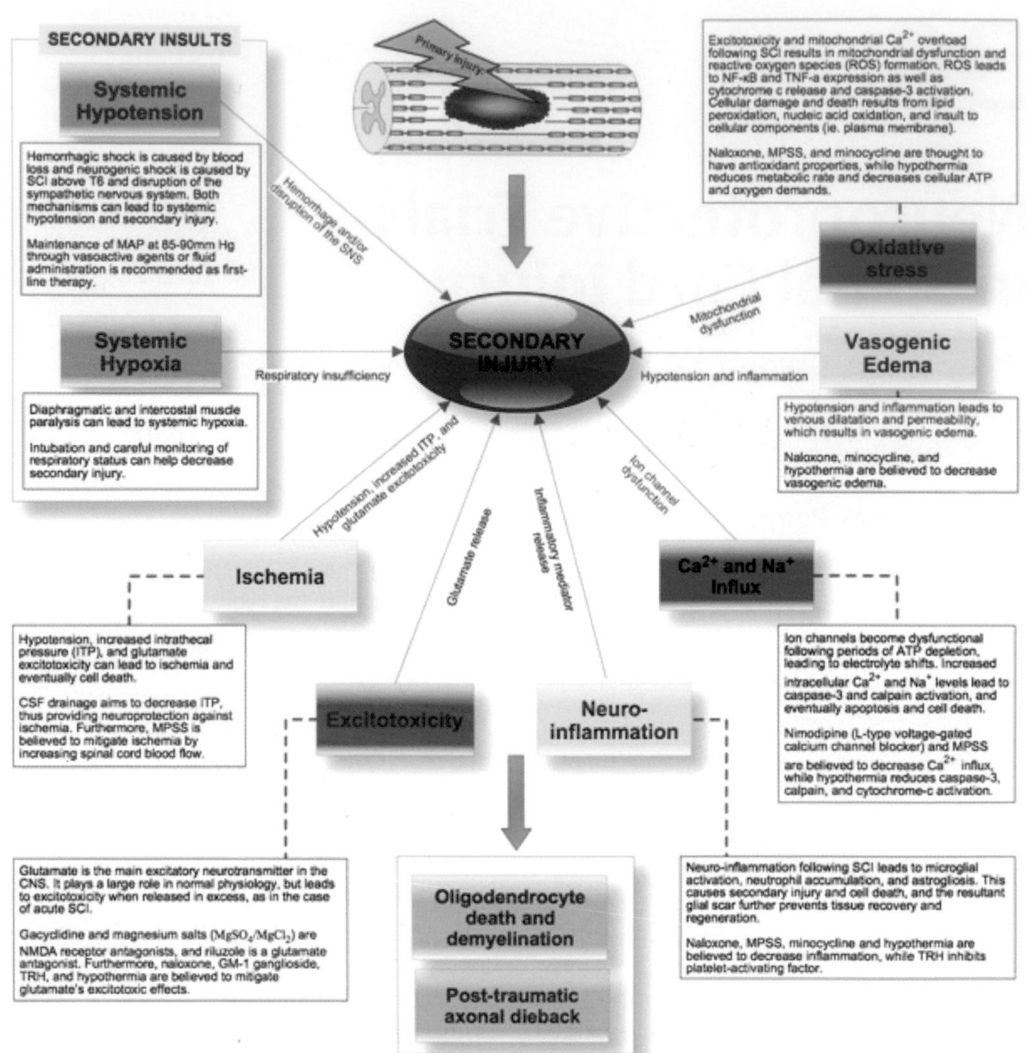

Fig. 36.1 Secondary injury mechanisms following acute spinal cord injury (SCI), and the proposed neuroprotective agents that have been studied or are planned for clinical trials in SCI to attempt to mitigate these processes. The complex secondary injury mediator interactions that follow acute SCI are only shown in part by this simplified figure. ATP, adenosine triphosphate; CNS, central nervous system; CSF, cerebrospinal fluid; ITP, intrathecal pressure; MAP, mean arterial pressure; MPSS, methylprednisolone sodium succinate; NF-kB, nuclear factor kappaB, NMDA, *N*-methyl-D-aspartate; ROS, reactive oxygen species; SCI, spinal cord injury; SNS, sympathetic nervous system; TNF-α, tumor necrosis factor-α; TRH, thyrotropin-releasing hormone.

translated to the clinic. Nonetheless, it is important to understand current trials in the context of those that preceded them, and key trials are reviewed here.

Gacyclidine is a noncompetitive, *N*-methyl-d-aspartate (NMDA) receptor antagonist that mitigates secondary injury by reducing glutamate-dependent excitotoxicity. In 1999, three escalating gacyclidine doses were tested against placebo in a phase 2 clinical trial in France.[4] The study involved 280 patients with complete and incomplete SCI. A nonsignificant increase in motor function in incomplete cervical injury patients was observed. Because the overall results of the trial were negative, this line of clinical investigation was discontinued. Gacyclidine is now being investigated for the treatment of traumatic brain injury (TBI), organophosphate poisoning, and tinnitus, but it is no longer being explored for use in SCI.[3]

Naloxone is a competitive opioid antagonist that is believed to reduce secondary injury by antagonizing dynorphin A, a harmful endogenous opioid released following SCI.[5] It also reduces edema, free-radical generation, excitotoxic amino acid release, and superoxide production by microglia.[6] Following preclinical studies that suggested benefit, naloxone underwent a phase 1 human clinical trial in 1985.[7] Benefit was suggested in this small trial, and in 1990, the more definitive National Acute Spinal Cord Injury Study II (NASCIS II) trial included naloxone as one of its treatment arms (alongside MPSS and placebo).[8] Unlike MPSS, naloxone failed to show an improvement in motor or sensory function.

Nimodipine is a dihydropyridine L-type voltage-gated calcium channel blocker that decreases intracellular calcium levels, thus inhibiting the activation of calpains and other destructive enzymes.[3] A 1996 phase 3 randomized, controlled trial (RCT) involving 100 patients with complete and incomplete SCI failed to demonstrate benefit.[9]

Thyrotropin-releasing hormone (TRH) is a neurohormone that mitigates secondary injury by antagonizing the actions of excitotoxic amino acids, peptidoleukotrienes, endogenous opioids, and platelet-activating factor.[2,10] TRH demonstrated efficacy in treating brain injury and SCI in preclinical animal studies and in 1995 was studied in a small phase 2 human SCI trial.[11] Although statistically significant functional improvement was seen in incomplete (but not complete) SCI patients, patient attrition and the limited sample size necessitate cautious interpretation.[3] No further trials with this agent are on the horizon despite this suggestion of benefit.

GM-1 ganglioside (Sygen, Fidia Pharma USA, Inc., Parsipanny, NJ) is a member of a heterogeneous family of complex glycosphingolipids, which are abundant in neurons. GM-1 mimics endogenous neurotrophic factors, which stimulate nerve-fiber growth and repair, and it has been explored as a therapy for multiple neurodegenerative diseases.[12] GM-1 may also reduce glutamate-mediated excitoxicity and subsequent apoptosis.[13] A small phase 2 trial of GM-1 in SCI in 1991 suggested improved neurological recovery,[14] and the following year, a larger phase 3 RCT (the Sygen Multi-Center Acute Spinal Cord Injury Study) was initiated.[15] GM-1 failed to show a significant benefit, although a nonsignificant trend toward greater motility on the Modified Benzel Walking Scale was noted. A low dose of GM-1 ganglioside (300 mg loading dose and then 100 mg/d for 56 d) is recommended as an option by the American Association of Neurological Surgeons/ Congress of Neurological Surgeons (AANS/ CNS),[16] although it is not used in clinical practice due to the lack of availability of this compound.

Methylprednisolone sodium succinate (MPSS) is by far the most extensively researched pharmacotherapy for SCI, having been investigated in five large, human clinical trials over the past 25 years. Despite controversy surrounding its side effects, MPSS is also the most widely used pharmacotherapy in the treatment of acute SCI.

As a synthetic glucocorticoid, MPSS has antiinflammatory and antioxidant properties that mitigate oxidative stress, calcium influx, and lipid peroxidation, leading to increased oligodendrocyte survival and decreased posttraumatic axonal dieback following acute SCI.[3,17] Subsequent to promising preclinical study results, a series of five human clinical trials (**Table 36.1**) was launched to study the efficacy, safety, and dosage of MPSS. The most influential were the three NASCIS trials, which set the foundation for current SCI treatment protocols.

Despite extensive human clinical trials involving multiple centers and more than 1500 patients, expert opinions on MPSS administration remain divided. Neurological benefits were modest, inconsistent, and only apparent in post hoc analyses. Fur-

Table 36.1 Human Clinical Trials of Neuroprotective Approaches

Agent	Trial name	Authors/ organization	Year	Size
Pharmacotherapy, historical				
Thyrotropin-releasing hormone (TRH)	TRH	Pitts et al.[11]	1995 *(completed)*	20
Naloxone	Naloxone	Flamm et al.[7]	1985 *(completed)*	29
	NASCIS II (*against MPSS*)	Bracken et al.[8]	1990 *(completed)*	487
Nimodipine (against MPSS)	Pointillart et al.	Pointillart et al.[9]	2000 *(completed)*	100
Gacyclidine	Gacyclidine	Tadie et al.[4]	1999 *(completed)*	280
Pharmacotherapy, in clinical use				
GM-1 ganglioside	Maryland	Geisler et al.[14]	1991 *(completed)*	34
	Sygen Multi-Center Acute Spinal Cord Injury Study	Geisler et al.[15]	2001 *(completed)*	797
Methylprednisolone sodium succinate (MPSS)	NASCIS I	Bracken et al.[18]	1984 *(completed)*	330
	NASCIS II	Bracken et al.[8]	1990 *(completed)*	487
	NASCIS III	Bracken et al.[19]	1997 *(completed)*	499
	Otani et al.	Otani et al.[20]	1994 *(completed)*	158
	Pointillart et al.	Pointillart et al.[9]	1996 *(completed)*	100
Pharmacotherapy, ongoing and future trials				
Minocycline	Minocycline	University of Calgary[21]	2009 *(completed)*	52
Riluzole	Riluzole	University of Toronto, North American Clinical Trials Network[22]	2009 *(initiated)*	36
$MgSO_4$ and $MgCl_2$ in polyethylene glycol (PEG)				

Study design	Assessment tool(s)	Conclusions
Phase 2 RC—pilot study	NASCIS Sunnybrook	Suggested improvement in neurological function
Phase 1 RCT	NASCIS	Suggested improvement in neurological function
Phase 3 RCT	NASCIS	Unlike MPSS, no benefit was noted in naloxone
Phase 3 RCT	ASIA	Negative No benefit could be ascribed to MPSS or nimodipine
Phase 2 RCT	ASIA	Negative Non–statistically significant improvement of motor recovery with incomplete cervical injuries
Phase 2 RCT—pilot study	ASIA	Improved neurological outcome
Phase 3 RCT	ASIA Modified Benzel Classification System	Nonsignificant trend toward improvement in neurological outcome
Phase 3 RCT	NASCIS	No difference between high- and low-dose groups
Phase 3 RCT	NASCIS	Negative primary analysis Improved motor recovery if treated with MPSS within 8 hours of injury
Phase 3 RCT	NASCIS FIM	Improved neurological outcome with 48 h MPSS regimen if SCI is 3–8 h
Nonblinded RCT	?	Sensory improvement, no motor differences
Phase 3 RCT	ASIA	Negative No benefit could be ascribed to MPSS or nimodipine
Phase 1/2 RCT—pilot study	?	Recently reported as negative, unpublished data
Phase 2 RCT	ASIA SCIM Brief Pain Inventory	Ongoing trial, promising preliminary data
		Future trial Preclinical studies suggest benefit

(Continued on page 426)

Table 36.1 Human Clinical Trials of Neuroprotective Approaches *(Continued)*

Agent	Trial name	Author/ organization	Year	Size
Nonpharmacological strategies				
Cerebrospinal Fluid (CSF) Drainage	CSF Drainage	Kwon et al.[23]	2009 *(completed)*	22
Therapeutic hypothermia	The Miami Project to Cure Paralysis	University of Miami Levi et al.[24]	2009 *(completed)*	14
		Neurological Emergencies Treatment Trials (NETT) Group		100 *(proposed)*
Timing of surgical decompression	STASCIS	Spine Trauma Study Group[25]	2012	313

Abbreviations: ASIA, America Spinal Injury Association; FIM, Functional Independence Measure; n/a, not available; NASCIS, National American Spinal Cord Injury Study; RCT, randomized, controlled trial; SCIM, Spinal Cord Independence Measure; STASCIS, Surgical Treatment for Acute Spinal Cord Injury Study.

thermore, important side effects of MPSS have been consistently seen and include pulmonary complications, gastrointestinal complications, infections, delayed wound healing, and death. Many physicians now choose not to administer MPSS,[26–29] although the senior author (MGF) and many other clinicians support its use when confronted with severe neurological consequences and the lack of alternatives.[3] The AANS/CNS guidelines recommend MPSS at an optional level because its modest benefits are balanced by important side effects.[30]

Ongoing and Future Trials of Neuroprotective Approaches in Acute Spinal Cord Injury

New trials combine a greater understanding of SCI with improved clinical trial methodology. Minocycline and riluzole are currently being investigated in human clinical trials, whereas magnesium salts in polyethylene glycol (PEG) showed successful preclinical results and promise for future human translation. Nonpharmacological neuroprotective strategies, including cerebrospinal fluid (CSF) drainage, early surgical decompression, and therapeutic hypothermia, are also undergoing human clinical trials.

Pharmacological Agents

Minocycline is a synthetic tetracycline antibiotic. In addition to its bacteriostatic properties, it has antiinflammatory and antiapoptotic properties, acting to suppress cytokine production by inflammatory cells, microglial activation, and neuronal death.[31,32] In animal models, it has shown efficacy in numerous neurological conditions,[33] and in particular, it has decreased oligodendrocyte loss, motor axon dieback, and lesion size in SCI.[34] In 2004, a phase 1/2 human clinical trial was initiated by the University of Calgary to test the efficacy of minocycline against placebo. The results of this trial have recently been published. The authors report that minocyline treatment was safe and feasible, but did not

Study design	Assessment tool(s)	Conclusions
Phase 1/2 RCT	ASIA	Negative; study was underpowered to show neurological improvement No adverse effects associated with CSF drainage
Phase 1 RCT—pilot study	n/a	Hypothermia shows safety and feasibility
Phase 2 RCT		Future trial Pending approval
Nonrandomized prospective observational	ASIA	Ongoing trial, preliminary data suggests neurological improvement and decreased complications associated with early decompression

result in statistically significant improvement in patient outcomes. However, there were tendencies toward an improvement in some outcome measures and the authors conclude that a phase 3 clinical trial is warranted.

Riluzole is a US Food and Drug Administration (FDA)-approved benzothiazole anticonvulsant traditionally used in the treatment of amyotrophic lateral sclerosis (ALS).[35] Recently it has been applied in the treatment of other neurological conditions, including acute SCI. Riluzole antagonizes glutamate excitotoxicity by inhibiting presynaptic glutamate release and increasing high-affinity glutamate uptake, mitigating its neurotoxic mechanisms.[36] Animal studies have revealed favorable results and synergy with MPSS,[37] demonstrating decreased neuronal death and enhanced outgrowth of sensory neurons.[38] In August 2009, a human trial investigating riluzole was initiated under the leadership of Dr. Michael Fehlings and the North American Clinical Trial Network (NACTN).[22] Patients are randomized to receive riluzole (by mouth 50 mg every 12 hours) or placebo within 12 hours of injury. The study will employ the American Spinal Injury Association (ASIA) scale, the Spinal Cord Independence Measure (SCIM), and the Brief Pain Inventory in patient assessments.

Magnesium sulfate and chloride recovers endogenous Mg^{2+} ion levels, which are presumably depleted following SCI, and leads to improved neurological functioning. Magnesium is also believed to block NMDA receptors and attenuate glutamate excitotoxicity, radical generation, and apoptosis.[23] Its coadministration within PEG, a hydrophilic polymer and pharmacological excipient with independent neuroprotective properties, has led to improved neurological outcome in a rodent SCI model.[39] A recent preclinical study suggests that $MgSO_4$ and $MgCl_2$ in PEG are equally as effective in treating acute SCI (although $MgCl_2$ showed improved early recovery), and if administered within 4 hours, lead to a statistically significant decrease in SCI lesion size and improvement in neurological function.[23] Further investigation into the efficacy of $MgSO_4$ and $MgCl_2$ in PEG may be achieved through human clinical trials.

Nonpharmacological Neuroprotective Strategies

Surgical decompression is typically performed following SCI to relieve pressure on the damaged spinal cord and to stabilize the spine. There is debate surrounding the timing of this intervention, however. Although animal studies have strongly suggested neurological benefit from early surgical decompression, many physicians prefer to delay surgery for unstable trauma patients.[40] In 1999, a multicenter retrospective study found little agreement on the optimal timing of surgical treatment and identified the need for a prospective human trial to address this issue.[41] In 2003, the Surgical Treatment of Acute Spinal Cord Injury Study (STASCIS) was initiated by Drs. Michael Fehlings (University of Toronto) and Alex Vaccaro (Thomas Jefferson University). This prospective observational study analyzed neurological and functional outcomes in 313 patients receiving either early (<24 hours postinjury) or late surgical decompression. Of the 222 patients with follow-up available at 6 months postinjury, 19.8% of patients undergoing early surgery showed a ≥2 grade imporvement in AIS compared to 8.8% in the late decompression group.[25] Following the early promising results from the STASCIS study in support of early surgical decompression, the University of Toronto has established the practice of performing decompression by traction or open surgery immediately following SCI.[3]

Cerebrospinal fluid (CSF) drainage lowers intrathecal pressure (ITP) and is routinely performed in thoracoabdominal aortic aneurysm surgery to prevent spinal cord ischemia and paraplegia.[42] In SCI, it is believed to increase spinal cord perfusion pressure, attenuate ischemia, and provide neuroprotection.[43] A human clinical trial was recently completed to study intrathecal pressure changes before and after surgical decompression, as well as to evaluate the safety, feasibility, and efficacy of CSF drainage.[43] Completed in 2009, this phase 1/2 RCT randomized 22 patients with acute SCI to receive CSF drainage versus no drainage within 72 hours of injury. CSF drainage was not associated with adverse effects, but it did not show improved neurological outcome, though this is not unexpected in a small, underpowered pilot study such as this.

Therapeutic hypothermia (28°C to 32°C) has been studied for various conditions since the 1970s and has become the treatment guideline for comatose and out-of-hospital cardiac arrest patients.[44] Hypothermia mitigates secondary injury by decreasing metabolic rate and the neuroinflammatory response to injury.[45] It has also been shown to stabilize cell membranes and to prevent caspase-3 and calpain activation.

In 2008, the Miami Project to Cure Paralysis began a prospective clinical trial exploring the role of systemic hypothermia (as opposed to localized cooling investigated in historic studies). Immediately following SCI, patients undergo systemic cooling with chilled intravenous saline to decrease the core body temperature to ~34°C. A phase 1 pilot study, involving 14 patients with complete SCI, was completed in 2009 to assess the safety and efficacy of systemic modest hypothermia (33°C) using an intravascular cooling catheter.[24] Although respiratory complications and arrhythmias were noted, systemic hypothermia showed promise as a potential neuroprotective intervention. A larger, multicenter phase 2/3 RCT involving the Neurological Emergencies Treatment Trials (NETT) group is pending approval. The larger RCT hopes to better delineate the potential efficacy as well as the risks associated with systemic hypothermia.

Conclusion

Many putative neuroprotective treatments for acute SCI have been investigated in human clinical trials. Though only MPSS has reached the clinical realm, we have learned much from the trials completed in the past. Ongoing human clinical trials in early surgical decompression, therapeutic hypothermia, and riluzole hold great promise and may also see clinical use alone or in combination with strategies that enhance regeneration or replace lost cells.

Pearl

- Subsequent to the NASCIS trials, it has been recommended that MPSS prescribed for blunt SCI less than 3 hours old should be administered as a 30 mg/kg bolus followed by a 5.4 mg/kg/h infusion for 24 hours. For injuries treated within 3 to 8 hours, a 48 hour infusion following the bolus has been recommended. It is the senior author's (MGF) preference to use the 24 hour NASCIS II protocol to minimize the adverse side effects of MPSS on wound healing and infectious complications. MPSS is not recommended for use in SCI beyond 8 hours after injury or for penetrating SCI.

Pitfall

- At this time, therapeutic hypothermia remains insufficiently studied in human SCI, and it carries life-threatening risks, such as cardiac dysrhythmias and coagulopathy. It is also associated with increased susceptibility to infection, pancreatitis, and longer hospital stay.[38]

References

1. Dumont RJ, Okonkwo DO, Verma S, et al. Acute spinal cord injury, I: Pathophysiologic mechanisms. Clin Neuropharmacol 2001;24(5):254–264
2. Dumont RJ, Verma S, Okonkwo DO, et al. Acute spinal cord injury, II: Contemporary pharmacotherapy. Clin Neuropharmacol 2001;24(5):265–279
3. Hawryluk GW, Rowland J, Kwon BK, Fehlings MG. Protection and repair of the injured spinal cord: a review of completed, ongoing, and planned clinical trials for acute spinal cord injury. Neurosurg Focus 2008;25(5):E14
4. Tadie M, D'Arbigny P, Mathé J, et al. Acute spinal cord injury: early care and treatment in a multicenter study with gacyclidine. Soc Neurosci 1999;25:1090
5. Long JB, Kinney RC, Malcolm DS, Graeber GM, Holaday JW. Intrathecal dynorphin A1-13 and dynorphin A3-13 reduce rat spinal cord blood flow by non-opioid mechanisms. Brain Res 1987;436(2):374–379
6. Chang RC, Rota C, Glover RE, Mason RP, Hong JS. A novel effect of an opioid receptor antagonist, naloxone, on the production of reactive oxygen species by microglia: a study by electron paramagnetic resonance spectroscopy. Brain Res 2000;854(1-2):224–229
7. Flamm ES, Young W, Collins WF, Piepmeier J, Clifton GL, Fischer B. A phase I trial of naloxone treatment in acute spinal cord injury. J Neurosurg 1985;63(3):390–397
8. Bracken MB, Shepard MJ, Collins WF, et al. A randomized, controlled trial of methylprednisolone or naloxone in the treatment of acute spinal-cord injury. Results of the Second National Acute Spinal Cord Injury Study. N Engl J Med 1990;322(20):1405–1411
9. Pointillart V, Petitjean ME, Wiart L, et al. Pharmacological therapy of spinal cord injury during the acute phase. Spinal Cord 2000;38(2):71–76
10. Hashimoto T, Fukuda N. Effect of thyrotropin-releasing hormone on the neurologic impairment in rats with spinal cord injury: treatment starting 24 h and 7 days after injury. Eur J Pharmacol 1991;203(1):25–32
11. Pitts LH, Ross A, Chase GA, Faden AI. Treatment with thyrotropin-releasing hormone (TRH) in patients with traumatic spinal cord injuries. J Neurotrauma 1995;12(3):235–243
12. Rabin SJ, Bachis A, Mocchetti I. Gangliosides activate Trk receptors by inducing the release of neurotrophins. J Biol Chem 2002;277(51):49466–49472
13. Vorwerk CK, Bonheur J, Kreutz MR, Dreyer EB, Laev H. GM1 ganglioside administration protects spinal neurons after glutamate excitotoxicity. Restor Neurol Neurosci 1999;14(1):47–51
14. Geisler FH, Dorsey FC, Coleman WP. Recovery of motor function after spinal-cord injury—a randomized, placebo-controlled trial with GM-1 ganglioside. N Engl J Med 1991;324(26):1829–1838
15. Geisler FH, Coleman WP, Grieco G, Poonian D; Sygen Study Group. The Sygen multicenter acute spinal cord injury study. Spine 2001;26(24, Suppl):S87–S98
16. Hadley MN, Walters BC, Grabb PA, et al. Guidelines for the management of acute cervical spine and spinal cord injuries. Clin Neurosurg 2002;49:407–498
17. Oudega M, Vargas CG, Weber AB, Kleitman N, Bunge MB. Long-term effects of methylprednisolone following transection of adult rat spinal cord. Eur J Neurosci 1999;11(7):2453–2464
18. Bracken MB, Collins WF, Freeman DF, Shepard MJ, Wagner FW, Silten RM, et al. Efficacy of methylprednisolone in acute spinal cord injury. JAMA 1984;251(1):45–52
19. Bracken MB, Shepard MJ, Holford TR, Leo-Summers L, Aldrich EF, Fazl M, et al. Administration of methylprednisolone for 24 or 48 hours or tirilazad mesylate for 48 hours in the treatment of acute spinal cord injury. Results of the Third National Acute Spinal Cord Injury Randomized Controlled Trial. JAMA 1997;277(20):1597–1604
20. Otani K, et al. Beneficial effect of methylprednisolone sodium succinate in the treatment of acute spinal cord injury. Sekitsui Sekizui 1994;7:633–647
21. Casha S, Zygun D, McGowan MD, Bains I, Yong VW, John HR. Results of a phase II placebo-controlled randomized trial of mincycline in acute spinal cord injury. Brain 2012;135(4):1224–1236

22. Fehlings MG, Wilson JR, Frankowski RF, Toups EG, Aarabi B, Harrop JS, et al. Riluzole for the treatment of acute traumatic spinal cord injury: rationale for and design of the NACTN Phase I Clinical Trial. Clinical Journal of Neurosurgery: Spine AO Spine Supplement 2012
23. Kwon BK, Roy J, Lee JH, et al. Magnesium chloride in a polyethylene glycol formulation as a neuroprotective therapy for acute spinal cord injury: preclinical refinement and optimization. J Neurotrauma 2009;26(8):1379–1393
24. Levi AD, Green BA, Wang MY, et al. Clinical application of modest hypothermia after spinal cord injury. J Neurotrauma 2009;26(3):407–415
25. Fehlings MG, Vaccaro A, Wilson JR, Singh AW, Cadotte D, Harrop JS, et al. Early versus delayed decompression for traumatic cervical spinal cord injury: results of the Surgical Timing in Acute Spinal Cord Injury Study (STASCIS). PLoS ONE 2012;7(2):e32037
26. Coleman WP, Benzel D, Cahill DW, et al. A critical appraisal of the reporting of the National Acute Spinal Cord Injury Studies (II and III) of methylprednisolone in acute spinal cord injury. J Spinal Disord 2000;13(3):185–199
27. Hurlbert RJ. The role of steroids in acute spinal cord injury: an evidence-based analysis. Spine 2001;26(24, Suppl):S39–S46
28. Hurlbert RJ, Moulton R. Why do you prescribe methylprednisolone for acute spinal cord injury? A Canadian perspective and a position statement. Can J Neurol Sci 2002;29(3):236–239
29. Nesathurai S. Steroids and spinal cord injury: revisiting the NASCIS 2 and NASCIS 3 trials. J Trauma 1998;45(6):1088–1093
30. AANS/CNS. Pharmacological therapy after acute cervical spinal cord injury. Neurosurgery 2002; 50(3, Suppl):S63–S72
31. Festoff BW, Ameenuddin S, Arnold PM, Wong A, Santacruz KS, Citron BA. Minocycline neuroprotects, reduces microgliosis, and inhibits caspase protease expression early after spinal cord injury. J Neurochem 2006;97(5):1314–1326
32. Tikka TM, Koistinaho JE. Minocycline provides neuroprotection against N-methyl-D-aspartate neurotoxicity by inhibiting microglia. J Immunol 2001;166(12):7527–7533
33. Yong VW, Wells J, Giuliani F, Casha S, Power C, Metz LM. The promise of minocycline in neurology. Lancet Neurol 2004;3(12):744–751
34. Stirling DP, Khodarahmi K, Liu J, et al. Minocycline treatment reduces delayed oligodendrocyte death, attenuates axonal dieback, and improves functional outcome after spinal cord injury. J Neurosci 2004;24(9):2182–2190
35. Bhatt JM, Gordon PH. Current clinical trials in amyotrophic lateral sclerosis. Expert Opin Investig Drugs 2007;16(8):1197–1207
36. Azbill RD, Mu X, Springer JE. Riluzole increases high-affinity glutamate uptake in rat spinal cord synaptosomes. Brain Res 2000;871(2):175–180
37. Mu X, Azbill RD, Springer JE. Riluzole and methylprednisolone combined treatment improves functional recovery in traumatic spinal cord injury. J Neurotrauma 2000;17(9):773–780
38. Shortland PJ, Leinster VH, White W, Robson LG. Riluzole promotes cell survival and neurite outgrowth in rat sensory neurones in vitro. Eur J Neurosci 2006;24(12):3343–3353
39. Ditor DS, John SM, Roy J, Marx JC, Kittmer C, Weaver LC. Effects of polyethylene glycol and magnesium sulfate administration on clinically relevant neurological outcomes after spinal cord injury in the rat. J Neurosci Res 2007;85(7):1458–1467
40. Fehlings MG, Perrin RG. The timing of surgical intervention in the treatment of spinal cord injury: a systematic review of recent clinical evidence. Spine 2006;31(11, Suppl):S28–S35, discussion S36
41. Tator CH, Fehlings MG, Thorpe K, Taylor W. Current use and timing of spinal surgery for management of acute spinal surgery for management of acute spinal cord injury in North America: results of a retrospective multicenter study. J Neurosurg 1999;91(1, Suppl):12–18
42. Estrera AL, Sheinbaum R, Miller CC, et al. Cerebrospinal fluid drainage during thoracic aortic repair: safety and current management. Ann Thorac Surg 2009;88(1):9–15, discussion 15
43. Kwon BK, Curt A, Belanger LM, et al. Intrathecal pressure monitoring and cerebrospinal fluid drainage in acute spinal cord injury: a prospective randomized trial. J Neurosurg Spine 2009; 10(3):181–193
44. Nolan JP, Morley PT, Vanden Hoek TL, et al; International Liaison Committee on Resuscitation. Therapeutic hypothermia after cardiac arrest: an advisory statement by the advanced life support task force of the International Liaison Committee on Resuscitation. Circulation 2003;108(1):118–121
45. Kwon BK, Mann C, Sohn HM, et al; NASS Section on Biologics. Hypothermia for spinal cord injury. Spine J 2008;8(6):859–874

37

Approaches Using Biomaterials for Tissue Engineering

Catherine E. Kang, Howard Kim, Violeta Talpag, and Molly Sandra Shoichet

Key Points

1. Biomaterials are designed in accordance with the type of injury.
2. Biomaterials are either synthesized or derived from natural sources.
3. Biomaterial scaffolds can be designed to promote host tissue regeneration and/or support cell transplantation.
4. Local delivery strategies provide a minimally invasive way to release biomolecules directly to CNS tissue.

Biomaterials in Neural Tissue Engineering

The complexity of the secondary injury after traumatic spinal cord injury (SCI) has limited the success of clinical treatment regimes with respect to restoring neurobehavioral function. For this reason, much research has been devoted to investigating experimental strategies utilizing a variety of materials to enhance tissue sparing and regeneration following an injury. Tissue engineering involves the improvement, restoration, or replacement of tissue or organs in the human body by manipulating three basic constituents of biological tissues: cells, molecular signals, and extracellular matrices (ECMs). Materials that interface with biological tissues to evaluate, treat, or replace these basic constituents or their function in the body are termed biomaterials.[1] Biomaterials comprise a diversity of natural and synthetic materials that are often designed to be biomimetic. The primary requirement for any biomaterial is biocompatibility—that is "the ability of a material to perform with an appropriate response in a specific application."[2] A biomaterial should not cause a significant immune response locally or systemically and must not be appreciably cytotoxic. The safety of a material for in vivo applications is highly dependent on these properties but is also impacted by its size, shape, mechanical properties, and degradation products. Other properties that are important for the choice of a biomaterial are degradation rate, cell adhesion, ease of chemical manipulation for protein or peptide attachment, as well as the ability to process materials into desired shapes with the porosity required for cellular infiltration and macromolecular diffusion.

Injury-Specific Biomaterial Design

In SCI, the lack of ECM at the lesion site presents a challenge to cell migration and formation of tissue bridges across cavities or gaps that can form in the cord after injury. Biomaterial scaffolds provide a physical substrate on which cells attach and grow, serving as a replacement for the natural ECM during the regenerative process. The type of SCI sustained dictates the type of biomaterial that would be suitable for a given tissue-engineering strategy, and reviews by Nomura et al.,[3] Hejcl et al.,[4] and Samadikuchaksaraei[5] discuss these at length.

Full transection and hemisection injury models in which the spinal cord is completely or partially severed are often used in preclinical research because these injuries provide a clear delineation of the injury site, are highly reproducible, and can easily accommodate scaffold implantation. Full transection injuries require a physical support to reconnect the two stumps of the spinal cord; thus biomaterial strategies that have been employed in these models include guidance channels and fiber networks, both of which provide directional cues to enhance tissue regeneration. Hemisection models often have scaffolds implanted[6–8] to promote repair, or they combine scaffolds with drug delivery to achieve greater efficacy.[9]

Compression injuries are the most common type of SCI in humans, and they represent the most clinically relevant model for treatment. However, the injury model does not allow facile implantation of preformed scaffolds because there is not a clear implantation site, thereby necessitating the use of injectable tissue engineering strategies. Most of the research with cavity-forming injuries has been focused on drug delivery and neuroprotective strategies.

Biomaterial Sources

Polymeric hydrogels are the most commonly used biomaterials for tissue engineering in the central nervous system (CNS) due to their high water content (similar to tissues in vivo) and because the properties of these materials are highly tunable to meet biological requirements. Natural polymers, including polysaccharides and native ECM proteins, are prominent in neural tissue applications. These materials are generally biodegradable and well tolerated in vivo. Because synthetic materials are often easier to manipulate chemically and mechanically, they too have been used extensively for various applications in CNS regeneration. **Table 37.1** summarizes commonly used biomaterials for spinal cord repair strategies.

Natural biomaterials are derived and purified from biological sources, mammalian or otherwise, and are appealing because they are often found in native mammalian tissue and include collagen, hyaluronan, laminin, and fibronectin. Collagen is a fibrillar protein and the main structural component of most connective tissues in the body. Glycosaminoglycans, such as hyaluronan, chondroitin sulfates, and heparin sulfates, are highly hydrated molecules and ubiquitous in the CNS.[10] Other natural biomaterials are derived from plant and nonmammalian sources. Chitosan, a deacetylated form of the polysaccharide chitin (a major component of fungi and arthropod exoskeletons), has been used extensively in the development of guidance channels for spinal cord regeneration.[11,12] The degree of deacetylation of chitosan allows degradation rate, cell adhesion, and amount of neurite extension to be tailored.[13] Other polysaccharides, including agarose, alginate, methylcellulose, and dextran, have also been investigated as biomaterials in neural tissue engineering (**Table 37.1**).

Synthetic polymeric hydrogels are also of interest because they can be uniformly produced, and their properties easily tuned. Examples of synthetic biomaterials include derivatives of both poly(acrylate) and poly(acrylamide), and notably poly(2-hydroxyethyl methacrylate) (PHEMA) and poly(2-hydroxypropyl methacrylate) (pHPMA), which have been studied as nerve-guidance-channel materials with controlled structure and wall porosity.[14] Because surgical removal of nondegradable materials is undesirable, several re-

Table 37.1 Common Biomaterials Used in SCI Research

Material	Description	Device designs
Natural materials		
Agarose	Thermogelling polysaccharide that is non-cell-adhesive and nondegradable	Hydrogel[27]
Alginate	Polysaccharide that undergoes ionic crosslinking in the presence of calcium	Hydrogel[57]
Collagen	Fibrillar cell-adhesive ECM protein	Hydrogel,[58] fibers[22]
Chitosan	Polysaccharide derived from chitin degradation and cell adhesion properties can be tuned[13]	Channel,[17] Hydrogel[59]
Fibrin	Enzymatically polymerized fibrinogen; can potentially be derived from autologous sources; non-cell-adhesive	Hydrogel[29]
Hyaluronic acid	ECM glycosaminoglycan that is injectable and non-cell-adhesive	Hydrogel[26,56,60]
Matrigel	Derived from mouse tumor cells, limited clinical relevance; highly cell adhesive	Hydrogel[18]
Methylcellulose	Reverse thermogelling, degradable polysaccharide that is non-cell-adhesive	Hydrogel[26,56]
Synthetic materials (degradable)		
PLA/PGA/PLGA	Poly α-hydroxyacids of lactic and glycolic acids; degradation occurs via hydrolysis and can be tuned based on composition	Channel,[43] scaffold,[21] fibers[61]
PCL	A degradable polyester of ε-caprolactone; degrades by hydrolysis, but more slowly than PLA	Channel,[62] fibers[63]
PHB	Polyhydroxybutyrate is a biocompatible polyester that degrades by surface erosion but more slowly than PLA	Channel,[58] fibers[64]
Amphiphilic peptides	Can be made to express cell-adhesive peptide sequences, and can self-assemble into nanofibers	Fibers[65,66]
Synthetic materials (nondegradable)		
PHEMA/PHEMA-MMA	Poly(2-hydroxyethyl methacrylate) and copolymers are synthetic hydrogels whose mechanical properties can be matched to the spinal cord	Channel,[67] scaffold[68]
PHEMA (NeuroGel, Aqua Gel Technologies)	Porous crosslinked hydrogel used in spinal cord and brain applications	Hydrogel[69]
PAN/PVC	Copolymer of polyacrylonitrile and polyvinylchloride can be used to form stable and nontoxic channels	Channel[70]

Abbreviations: ECM, extracellular matrix; PAN/PVC, poly(acrylonitrile-*co*-vinyl chloride); PGA, poly(glycolide); PHEMA/PHEMA-MMA, poly(2-hydroxyethyl methacrylate)/poly(2-hydroxyethyl methacrylate-*co*-methyl methacrylate); PHPMA, poly[N-(2-hydroxypropyl)methacrylamide]; PLA, polylactic acid; PLGA, polylactic-co-glycolic acid.

sorbable synthetic polymers have been investigated for nerve-guidance materials, including polyesters, polycarbonates, and polyurethanes. Most of the synthetic polyesters used in these applications are based on only a few monomer units, used alone or in combination, including poly(glycolide) (PGA), poly(L-lactide) (PLLA), poly(D,L-lactide) (PDLLA), and poly(ε-caprolactone) (PCL). The mechanical and biological properties of these materials can vary widely based on changes in the copolymer composition and fabrication method. For example, scaffolds consisting of PGA or its copolymers with PDLLA or PLLA generally show much shorter degradation times (2 to 12 months) than those composed of PLLA alone or in combination with PCL (up to 2 years). Newer generations of biomaterials incorporate several elements and mechanisms that govern axonal extension and guidance, including physical guidance cues of scaffolds and fiber networks, chemical guidance molecules of cell-signaling molecules, and cell–cell interactions. The following sections describe some of the in vitro and in vivo published literature in these areas and their application to translational neural tissue engineering strategies.

Scaffolds for Neural Tissue Engineering

Physical Guidance Systems for Regeneration

Popularized by their clinical success in treating peripheral nerve injuries,[15] guidance channels have been widely investigated in SCI repair. The channel provides a substrate for directed growth while shielding the local area from the surrounding environment, which is inhibitory to regeneration. Guidance channels can be made from synthetic or naturally occurring polymers and can be degradable or nondegradable. Early studies with guidance channels focused on the use of nondegradable materials, such as silicone, poly(acrylonitrile-*co*-vinyl chloride) PAN/PVC, and poly(2-hydroxyethyl methacrylate-*co*-methyl methacrylate) (PHEMA-MMA), to ensure stability of the channels; however, biodegradable materials, such as polylactic-co-glycolic acid (PLGA) and chitosan, have become more popular for clinical translation. These materials can be tuned to degrade on the order of months to years, allowing for the relatively long time thought to be required for neural regeneration. Animal studies conducted in rats have used chitosan guidance channels to promote the formation of a tissue bridge between the rostral and caudal stumps as early as 5 weeks after injury,[16] whereas animals receiving no treatment fail to form a distinct tissue bridge after 14 weeks.[17] Tissue bridges formed inside guidance channels contain numerous axons, indicating that a host neural regenerative response is being stimulated. When combined with cellular therapy, these channels were shown to greatly enhance transplant survival.[17]

Several groups have incorporated intricate engineering designs to provide greater surface area for tissue ingrowth. This includes matrix-filled channels,[18,19] channels within scaffolds,[20,21] and aligned fiber networks.[22] Moreover, immobilized growth factor patterning[23,24] and electrically active materials[20] are also being investigated as potential methods for guiding regeneration.

Hydrogel Networks

Hydrogels are crosslinked hydrophilic polymer networks that contain high water content, making them highly attractive for implantation in soft tissue. Hydrogels generally have open porous networks ideal for cell migration and free nutrient exchange between surrounding tissue. However, the most appealing property of hydrogels is that many are injectable or can undergo scaffold formation in situ, facilitating space-filling of irregularly shaped gaps or cavities while minimizing the invasiveness of implantation. A hydrogel strategy for filling a spinal cord cavity is illustrated in **Fig. 37.1**. The most common biomedical

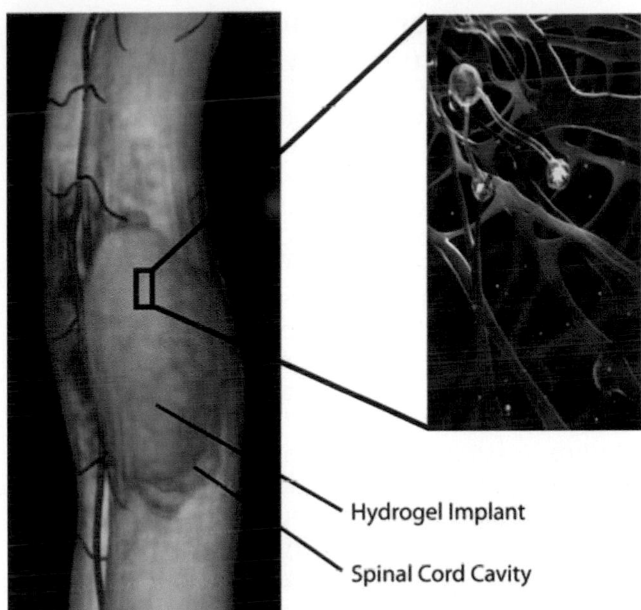

Fig. 37.1 Illustration of a hydrogel implant into a spinal cord cavity showing neurite extension into the scaffold. (Permission courtesy of Hyun-Joo Lee).

hydrogels include those that are derived from natural polymers, such as chitosan, methylcellulose, collagen, hyaluronan, agarose, alginate, dextran, and fibrin, and those that are synthetic, such as poly[N-(2-hydroxypropyl)methacrylamide] (PHPMA or NeuroGel™, Aqua Gel Technologies, Inc., Quebec City, Quebec, CA),[25] PHEMA, poly(N-isopropyl acrylamide) (pNiPAAm), and polyethylene glycol (PEG).

Hydrogel networks are formed by physical or chemical crosslinks. Physically crosslinked gels have hydrogen bonds or hydrophobic interactions, whereas chemically crosslinked gels have ionic or covalent bonds. Bioengineers take advantage of the thermodynamics and kinetics of bond formation in these systems to optimize implantation techniques. For example, physically crosslinked hydrogels are generally held together by weaker forces that are easily broken and readily reform, making them injectable,[26] whereas others are environmentally responsive and can be tuned to gel based on changes in temperature[27] or pH.[28] Chemically crosslinked hydrogels can be formed in situ through chemical or photochemical crosslinking at or just prior to the time of implantation. For example, soluble fibrinogen solution rapidly forms a scaffold when reacted with the enzyme thrombin,[29,30] and photocrosslinkable polyethylene glycol-co-lactic acid diacrylate can be crosslinked in situ by exposure to UV light and a photoinitiator to form hydrogel scaffolds in situ.[31]

Hydrogels allow facile modification with proteins or peptides that modulate cellular functions, such as proliferation, differentiation, and morphogenesis. Adhesion proteins or peptides derived from laminin or fibronectin are routinely immobilized to the scaffold's surface to improve cell adhesion.[32] Likewise, growth factor immobilization can direct cell proliferation or differentiation.[33,34] All of these properties suggest that hydrogels may provide an ideal delivery vehicle for cell transplantation and local and sustained release of therapeutically relevant molecules, both of which are discussed in more detail next.

Biomaterials for Cell Transplantation Therapies

Cell-based therapies for SCI offer a promising means of replacing lost or damaged tissue. Many cell types have been transplanted into SCI models with successful outcomes,[35,36] and human clinical trials are under way with oligodendrocyte-enriched progenitors.[37] Typically, in these studies, cells are delivered as a suspension in culture media and injected directly into the spinal cord, often resulting in poor survival rates.[38–40] It is believed that providing an adherent substrate for cells prior to introducing them into the hostile environment of the injured spinal cord will greatly enhance their ability to survive.

When designing hydrogel systems as cell-delivery vehicles, it is important to consider the optimal microenvironment for the cell type of interest, because mechanical and chemical properties of the material significantly affect cell behavior. Moreover, properties like porosity and cell adhesiveness have profound effects on cell seeding efficiency and distribution. It is possible to encapsulate cells during scaffold formation, provided the mechanism used to crosslink the scaffold (e.g., heat, ultraviolet exposure, chemical initiators) does not significantly affect cell viability.

Several studies have highlighted the benefit of transplanting cells within a biomaterial carrier. For example, bone marrow stromal cells transplanted within a fibrin matrix survived and migrated better after SCI compared with controls without a matrix.[41] Similarly, PLGA scaffolds preseeded with neural stem cells prior to implantation resulted in better functional recovery in SCI rats relative to implanted scaffolds or cells alone.[6] Several guidance-channel strategies have also demonstrated the ability to successfully promote cell-transplant survival and subsequent integration with host tissue.[17,42–45] Biomaterial support for cell delivery not only improves cell survival but, through functional design, allows researchers to better control other cell outcomes, such as migration and differentiation.

Biomaterials for Localized Drug Delivery

Drug-delivery strategies encompass both neuroregenerative and neuroprotective approaches following traumatic injury to the CNS. The main goal in limiting degeneration after SCI has been to preserve functional behavior through axonal sparing and reduced lesion volumes. Currently, the only drug used clinically is intravenously administered methylprednisolone, an antiinflammatory steroid, despite its limited efficacy.[46,47] Several clinical trials of systemically administered drugs have been performed in the last 2 decades; however, none has been successful in improving functional recovery. Additionally, systemic delivery is not suitable for many therapeutic agents because the blood–spinal cord barrier limits their diffusion into the spinal cord, requiring extremely high doses and resulting in undesirable systemic side effects. This has led to a recent surge of research utilizing biomaterials for localized and sustained delivery strategies in the treatment of SCI.

Epidural delivery is more localized than systemic delivery and relatively minimally invasive yet requires the therapeutic molecule to cross the dura mater, arachnoid mater, fluid-filled intrathecal space, and pia mater before penetrating the spinal cord, likely resulting in the loss of most of the dosage.[48] This delivery route has been exploited using a poloxamer gel[49] and through liposomes for analgesic delivery.[50] Notwithstanding these limitations, the Rho inhibitor Cethrin (Alseres Pharmaceuticals, Inc., Hopkinton, MA) administered to the intact dura in a fibrin glue is currently being tested in clinical trials.[51]

Intrathecal delivery requires the dura and arachnoid maters to be punctured but achieves localized release at the injury site, requiring the therapeutic molecules to diffuse only across the pia mater and into the spinal cord.[52] Mini-pump/catheter systems have been investigated most commonly for this route, but long-term use of catheters is undesirable due to the possibility of infection, chronic in-

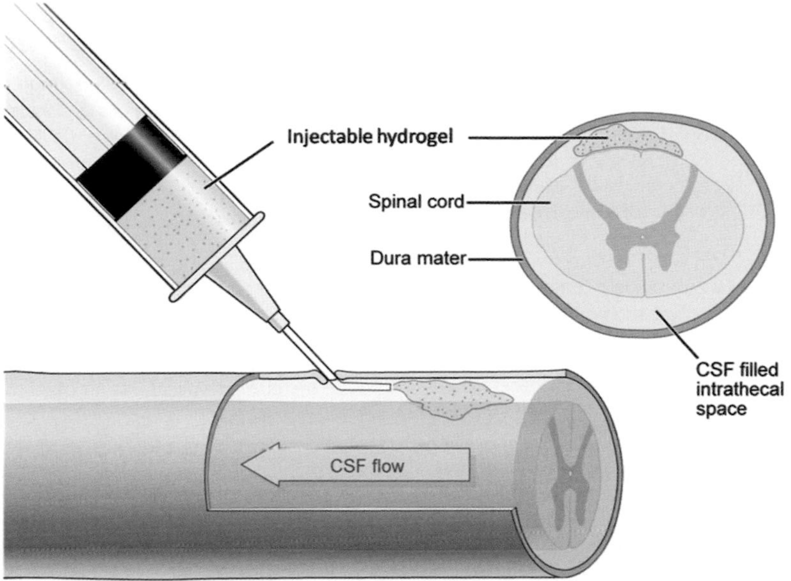

Fig. 37.2 Illustration of a hydrogel that can be injected into the intrathecal space to achieve localized drug delivery at the site of spinal cord injury. (Permission courtesy of Michael Corrin).

flammation, scarring, and compression of the spinal cord.[53] Intrathecal delivery of injectable hydrogels, illustrated in **Fig. 37.2**, avoids these concerns and was first tested with a fast-gelling collagen for local delivery of epidermal growth factor and basic fibroblast factor and was shown to be safe in vivo.[54,55] Methylcellulose is an inverse thermal gelling polymer that solidifies upon a temperature increase and has been combined with hyaluronan to form a gel at physiological temperatures.[26] When injected intrathecally, this biopolymer blend alone showed reduced inflammation compared with injection of an artificial cerebrospinal fluid (aCSF) in compression models of SCI[26] and demonstrated reduced cavity areas and moderate neuronal sparing when used to locally deliver the neuroprotective protein, erythropoietin.[56] These studies demonstrate the promise of a local delivery system for clinically relevant SCI models and are easily translatable to SCI treatment.

Conclusion

A broad range of polymeric biomaterial strategies have been tested for SCI repair. They encompass scaffold strategies that have been utilized in transection and hemisection models of SCI as well as injectable strategies that have been used for drug delivery in compression and/or contusive injuries. Although the strategies are different and each has demonstrated some success in neuroprotection and/or neuroregeneration, the biomaterials are always designed to be biocompatible and cytocompatible, eliciting the desired cellular response. Thus the biomaterials themselves have an active role in tissue regeneration and sparing, including axonal guidance provided by fibers, or the release of therapeutic factors from polymeric hydrogels injected at the injury site. These bioengineering strategies provide significant promise and require rigorous preclinical testing for translation to the clinic.

Pearls

- Biomaterials are highly versatile and can be tailored with respect to their biological, chemical, and mechanical properties.
- Modifications of biomaterials are used to tune their strength, porosity, adhesiveness, and degradability.
- Biomaterial implants provide a temporary scaffold to aid cell transplant survival.
- Biomaterials can act synergistically with native tissue to enhance cellular integration for tissue regeneration.
- Tissue-engineered constructs can combine physical cellular support and drug delivery to overcome the complexities of SCI and achieve a meaningful improvement in tissue function.

Pitfalls

- Regulatory approval for tissue-engineered constructs that comprise cells and biomaterials is slower than that for medical devices to ensure consistency in manufacturing and safety prior to clinical trials.
- Cellular transplantation strategies have to overcome the following challenges to be successful:
  - Immunosuppression required for nonautologous cell sources
  - Insufficient vascularity in many biomaterial constructs
- Potential difficulties in translating biomaterial strategies from bench to bedside include the following:
  - Variability of SCI in humans; SCI is more controlled in animal studies

References

1. Williams DF. On the nature of biomaterials. Biomaterials 2009;30(30):5897–5909
2. Williams DF. The Williams' Dictionary of Biomaterials. Liverpool, UK: Liverpool University Press; 1999
3. Nomura H, Tator CH, Shoichet MS. Bioengineered strategies for spinal cord repair. J Neurotrauma 2006;23(3-4):496–507
4. Hejcl A, Lesný P, Prádný M, et al. Biocompatible hydrogels in spinal cord injury repair. Physiol Res 2008;57(Suppl 3):S121–S132
5. Samadikuchaksaraei A. An overview of tissue engineering approaches for management of spinal cord injuries. J Neuroeng Rehabil 2007;4:15
6. Teng YD, Lavik EB, Qu X, et al. Functional recovery following traumatic spinal cord injury mediated by a unique polymer scaffold seeded with neural stem cells. Proc Natl Acad Sci USA 2002; 99(5):3024–3029
7. Xu XM, Zhang SX, Li H, Aebischer P, Bunge MB. Regrowth of axons into the distal spinal cord through a Schwann-cell-seeded mini-channel implanted into hemisected adult rat spinal cord. Eur J Neurosci 1999;11(5):1723–1740
8. Stokols S, Tuszynski MH. Freeze-dried agarose scaffolds with uniaxial channels stimulate and guide linear axonal growth following spinal cord injury. Biomaterials 2006;27(3):443–451
9. Kim YT, Caldwell JM, Bellamkonda RV. Nanoparticle-mediated local delivery of Methylprednisolone after spinal cord injury. Biomaterials 2009; 30(13):2582–2590
10. Novak U, Kaye AH. Extracellular matrix and the brain: components and function. J Clin Neurosci 2000;7(4):280–290
11. Archibald SJ, Shefner J, Krarup C, Madison RD. Monkey median nerve repaired by nerve graft or collagen nerve guide tube. J Neurosci 1995;15(5 Pt 2):4109–4123
12. Liu S, Bodjarian N, Langlois O, et al. Axonal regrowth through a collagen guidance channel bridging spinal cord to the avulsed C6 roots: functional recovery in primates with brachial plexus injury. J Neurosci Res 1998;51(6):723–734
13. Freier T, Koh HS, Kazazian K, Shoichet MS. Controlling cell adhesion and degradation of chitosan films by N-acetylation. Biomaterials 2005;26(29): 5872–5878
14. Dalton PD, Flynn L, Shoichet MS. Manufacture of poly(2-hydroxyethyl methacrylate-co-methyl methacrylate) hydrogel tubes for use as nerve guidance channels. Biomaterials 2002;23(18): 3843–3851
15. Ichihara S, Inada Y, Nakamura T. Artificial nerve tubes and their application for repair of peripheral nerve injury: an update of current concepts. Injury 2008;39(Suppl 4):29–39
16. Zahir T, Nomura H, Guo XD, et al. Bioengineering neural stem/progenitor cell-coated tubes for spinal cord injury repair. Cell Transplant 2008; 17(3):245–254
17. Nomura H, Zahir T, Kim H, et al. Extramedullary chitosan channels promote survival of transplanted neural stem and progenitor cells and create a tissue bridge after complete spinal cord transection. Tissue Eng Part A 2008;14(5):649–665
18. Tsai EC, Dalton PD, Shoichet MS, Tator CH. Matrix inclusion within synthetic hydrogel guidance channels improves specific supraspinal and local axonal regeneration after complete spinal cord transection. Biomaterials 2006;27(3): 519–533

19. Li X, Yang Z, Zhang A, Wang T, Chen W. Repair of thoracic spinal cord injury by chitosan tube implantation in adult rats. Biomaterials 2009; 30(6):1121–1132
20. Li GN, Hoffman-Kim D. Tissue-engineered platforms of axon guidance. Tissue Eng Part B Rev. 2008;14(1):33–51
21. Moore MJ, Friedman JA, Lewellyn EB, et al. Multiple-channel scaffolds to promote spinal cord axon regeneration. Biomaterials 2006;27(3): 419–429
22. Yoshii S, Ito S, Shima M, Taniguchi A, Akagi M. Functional restoration of rabbit spinal cord using collagen-filament scaffold. J Tissue Eng Regen Med 2009;3(1):19–25
23. Luo Y, Shoichet MS. A photolabile hydrogel for guided three-dimensional cell growth and migration. Nat Mater 2004;3(4):249–253
24. Yu LM, Wosnick JH, Shoichet MS. Miniaturized system of neurotrophin patterning for guided regeneration. J Neurosci Methods 2008; 171(2):253–263
25. Woerly S, Pinet E, de Robertis L, Van Diep D, Bousmina M. Spinal cord repair with PHPMA hydrogel containing RGD peptides (NeuroGel). Biomaterials 2001;22(10):1095–1111
26. Gupta D, Tator CH, Shoichet MS. Fast-gelling injectable blend of hyaluronan and methylcellulose for intrathecal, localized delivery to the injured spinal cord. Biomaterials 2006;27(11): 2370–2379
27. Jain A, Kim YT, McKeon RJ, Bellamkonda RV. In situ gelling hydrogels for conformal repair of spinal cord defects, and local delivery of BDNF after spinal cord injury. Biomaterials 2006;27(3): 497–504
28. Chiu YL, Chen SC, Su CJ, et al. pH-triggered injectable hydrogels prepared from aqueous N-palmitoyl chitosan: in vitro characteristics and in vivo biocompatibility. Biomaterials 2009;30(28): 4877–4888
29. Taylor SJ, Rosenzweig ES, McDonald JW III, Sakiyama-Elbert SE. Delivery of neurotrophin-3 from fibrin enhances neuronal fiber sprouting after spinal cord injury. J Control Release 2006; 113(3):226–235
30. Petter-Puchner AH, Froetscher W, Krametter-Froetscher R, Lorinson D, Redl H, van Griensven M. The long-term neurocompatibility of human fibrin sealant and equine collagen as biomatrices in experimental spinal cord injury. Exp Toxicol Pathol 2007;58(4):237–245
31. Piantino J, Burdick JA, Goldberg D, Langer R, Benowitz LI. An injectable, biodegradable hydrogel for trophic factor delivery enhances axonal rewiring and improves performance after spinal cord injury. Exp Neurol 2006;201(2):359–367
32. Lévesque SG, Shoichet MS. Synthesis of cell-adhesive dextran hydrogels and macroporous scaffolds. Biomaterials 2006;27(30):5277–5285
33. Shen YH, Shoichet MS, Radisic M. Vascular endothelial growth factor immobilized in collagen scaffold promotes penetration and proliferation of endothelial cells. Acta Biomater 2008;4(3): 477–489
34. Leipzig ND, Xu C, Zahir T, Shoichet MS. Functional immobilization of interferon-gamma induces neuronal differentiation of neural stem cells. J Biomed Mater Res A 2010;93(2):625–633
35. Louro J, Pearse DD. Stem and progenitor cell therapies: recent progress for spinal cord injury repair. Neurol Res 2008;30(1):5–16
36. Eftekharpour E, Karimi-Abdolrezaee S, Fehlings MG. Current status of experimental cell replacement approaches to spinal cord injury. Neurosurg Focus 2008;24(3-4):E19
37. Alper J. Geron gets green light for human trial of ES cell-derived product. Nat Biotechnol 2009;27(3):213–214
38. Parr AM, Kulbatski I, Tator CH. Transplantation of adult rat spinal cord stem/progenitor cells for spinal cord injury. J Neurotrauma 2007;24(5): 835–845
39. Himes BT, Neuhuber B, Coleman C, et al. Recovery of function following grafting of human bone marrow-derived stromal cells into the injured spinal cord. Neurorehabil Neural Repair 2006;20(2):278–296
40. Mothe AJ, Kulbatski I, Parr A, Mohareb M, Tator CH. Adult spinal cord stem/progenitor cells transplanted as neurospheres preferentially differentiate into oligodendrocytes in the adult rat spinal cord. Cell Transplant 2008;17(7):735–751
41. Itosaka H, Kuroda S, Shichinohe H, et al. Fibrin matrix provides a suitable scaffold for bone marrow stromal cells transplanted into injured spinal cord: a novel material for CNS tissue engineering. Neuropathology 2009;29(3):248–257
42. Nomura H, Baladie B, Katayama Y, Morshead CM, Shoichet MS, Tator CH. Delayed implantation of intramedullary chitosan channels containing nerve grafts promotes extensive axonal regeneration after spinal cord injury. Neurosurgery 2008;63(1):127–141, discussion 141–143
43. Oudega M, Gautier SE, Chapon P, et al. Axonal regeneration into Schwann cell grafts within resorbable poly(alpha-hydroxyacid) guidance channels in the adult rat spinal cord. Biomaterials 2001;22(10):1125–1136
44. Fouad K, Schnell L, Bunge MB, Schwab ME, Liebscher T, Pearse DD. Combining Schwann cell bridges and olfactory-ensheathing glia grafts with chondroitinase promotes locomotor recovery after complete transection of the spinal cord. J Neurosci 2005;25(5):1169–1178
45. Olson HE, Rooney GE, Gross L, et al. Neural stem cell- and Schwann cell-loaded biodegradable polymer scaffolds support axonal regeneration in the transected spinal cord. Tissue Eng Part A 2009; 15(7):1797–1805
46. Bracken MB, Shepard MJ, Collins WF Jr, et al. Methylprednisolone or naloxone treatment after acute spinal cord injury: 1-year follow-up data. Results of the second National Acute Spinal Cord Injury Study. J Neurosurg 1992;76(1): 23–31
47. Bracken MB, Shepard MJ, Holford TR, et al. Methylprednisolone or tirilazad mesylate administration after acute spinal cord injury: 1-year follow up. Results of the third National Acute Spinal Cord Injury randomized controlled trial. J Neurosurg 1998;89(5):699–706
48. Dergham P, Ellezam B, Essagian C, Avedissian H, Lubell WD, McKerracher L. Rho signaling path-

way targeted to promote spinal cord repair. J Neurosci 2002;22(15):6570–6577

49. Paavola A, Tarkkila P, Xu M, Wahlström T, Yliruusi J, Rosenberg P. Controlled release gel of ibuprofen and lidocaine in epidural use—analgesia and systemic absorption in pigs. Pharm Res 1998; 15(3):482–487

50. Paavola A, Kilpeläinen I, Yliruusi J, Rosenberg P. Controlled release injectable liposomal gel of ibuprofen for epidural analgesia. Int J Pharm 2000;199(1):85–93

51. Baptiste DC, Tighe A, Fehlings MG. Spinal cord injury and neural repair: focus on neuroregenerative approaches for spinal cord injury. Expert Opin Investig Drugs 2009;18(5):663–673

52. Ethans KD, Schryvers OI, Nance PW, Casey AR. Intrathecal drug therapy using the Codman Model 3000 Constant Flow Implantable Infusion Pumps: experience with 17 cases. Spinal Cord 2005;43(4):214–218

53. Jones LL, Tuszynski MH. Chronic intrathecal infusions after spinal cord injury cause scarring and compression. Microsc Res Tech 2001;54(5): 317–324

54. Jimenez Hamann MC, Tator CH, Shoichet MS. Injectable intrathecal delivery system for localized administration of EGF and FGF-2 to the injured rat spinal cord. Exp Neurol 2005;194(1): 106–119

55. Jimenez Hamann MC, Tsai EC, Tator CH, Shoichet MS. Novel intrathecal delivery system for treatment of spinal cord injury. Exp Neurol 2003; 182(2):300–309

56. Kang CE, Poon PC, Tator CH, Shoichet MS. A new paradigm for local and sustained release of therapeutic molecules to the injured spinal cord for neuroprotection and tissue repair. Tissue Eng Part A 2009;15(3):595–604

57. Prang P, Müller R, Eljaouhari A, et al. The promotion of oriented axonal regrowth in the injured spinal cord by alginate-based anisotropic capillary hydrogels. Biomaterials 2006;27(19): 3560–3569

58. Mitsui T, Shumsky JS, Lepore AC, Murray M, Fischer I. Transplantation of neuronal and glial restricted precursors into contused spinal cord improves bladder and motor functions, decreases thermal hypersensitivity, and modifies intraspinal circuitry. J Neurosci 2005;25(42):9624–9636

59. Crompton KE, Goud JD, Bellamkonda RV, et al. Polylysine-functionalised thermoresponsive chitosan hydrogel for neural tissue engineering. Biomaterials 2007;28(3):441–449

60. Baumann MD, Kang CE, Stanwick JC, et al. An injectable drug delivery platform for sustained combination therapy. J Control Release 2009;138(3):205–213

61. Bini TB, Gao S, Wang S, Ramakrishna S. Development of fibrous biodegradable polymer conduits for guided nerve regeneration. J Mater Sci Mater Med 2005;16(4):367–375

62. Wong DY, Leveque JC, Brumblay H, Krebsbach PH, Hollister SJ, Lamarca F. Macro-architectures in spinal cord scaffold implants influence regeneration. J Neurotrauma 2008;25(8):1027–1037

63. Nisbet DR, Yu LM, Zahir T, Forsythe JS, Shoichet MS. Characterization of neural stem cells on electrospun poly(epsilon-caprolactone) submicron scaffolds: evaluating their potential in neural tissue engineering. J Biomater Sci Polym Ed 2008;19(5):623–634

64. Novikov LN, Novikova LN, Mosahebi A, Wiberg M, Terenghi G, Kellerth JO. A novel biodegradable implant for neuronal rescue and regeneration after spinal cord injury. Biomaterials 2002;23(16):3369–3376

65. Tysseling-Mattiace VM, Sahni V, Niece KL, et al. Self-assembling nanofibers inhibit glial scar formation and promote axon elongation after spinal cord injury. J Neurosci 2008;28(14): 3814–3823

66. Guo J, Su H, Zeng Y, et al. Reknitting the injured spinal cord by self-assembling peptide nanofiber scaffold. Nanomedicine 2007;3(4):311–321

67. Tsai EC, Dalton PD, Shoichet MS, Tator CH. Synthetic hydrogel guidance channels facilitate regeneration of adult rat brainstem motor axons after complete spinal cord transection. J Neurotrauma 2004;21(6):789–804

68. Hejcl A, Lesný P, Prádný M, et al. Macroporous hydrogels based on 2-hydroxyethyl methacrylate. Part 6: 3D hydrogels with positive and negative surface charges and polyelectrolyte complexes in spinal cord injury repair. J Mater Sci Mater Med 2009;20(7):1571–1577

69. Woerly S, Doan VD, Evans-Martin F, Paramore CG, Peduzzi JD. Spinal cord reconstruction using NeuroGel implants and functional recovery after chronic injury. J Neurosci Res 2001;66(6): 1187–1197

70. Guest JD, Rao A, Olson L, Bunge MB, Bunge RP. The ability of human Schwann cell grafts to promote regeneration in the transected nude rat spinal cord. Exp Neurol 1997;148(2):502–522

IV

Neurophysiology and Imaging

38

Electrophysiological Measures after Spinal Cord Injury

James Xie and Maxwell Boakye

Key Points

1. MEPS and SSEPs are predictive of hand and ambulatory capacity. MEP amplitudes and latencies do not appear to correlate with recovery in longitudinal studies
2. The sympathetic skin response can indirectly assess supraspinal pathways and reflects the integrity of the autonomic pathways. SSRs are absent below the level of the spinal lesion and should be used to identify populations at risk for autonomic hyperreflexia (AH).
3. The electrical perceptual test may be a better test to assess sensory physiology and recovery after SCI. Used in conjunction with dSSEPs, the two tests provide better results than traditional SSEP tests.

There is an increasing interest in the use of clinical electrophysiological assessments in the evaluation of severity and outcomes after spinal cord injury (SCI). Electrophysiological measures offer several advantages over qualitative clinical measures. First, electrophysiological recordings provide quantitative, objective data that can be analyzed by blinded researchers.[1] This is particularly relevant in designing appropriate clinical trials that aim to compare functional outcome measures. For example, the reliability of measurements between assessments and between investigators is increased relative to traditional clinical tests, which are dependent on human evaluation. Second, the measures are more flexible and environmentally independent, thus allowing researchers to perform recordings on unresponsive, uncooperative, or comatose patients.[2] The greater feasibility and flexibility that electrophysiological measures provide give clinicians and investigators freedom to assess previously unexaminable patients. Third, measures of evoked potentials complement existing SCI recovery assessments, such as the American Spinal Injury Association (ASIA) sensory and motor scores, because they are able to assess specific parts of the spinal segments and peripheral nerve tracts and autonomic nervous system. In particular, measures can target specific spinal segments below the level of injury.[3] Finally, combinations of recording techniques can provide detailed quantitative information about a patient's condition that cannot be determined through other clinical means. There is much promise in using these measures to assess SCI, predict functional outcomes, and inform clinicians about the planning and results of therapeutic interventions.

This chapter provides an overview of the most common electrophysiological tests: motor evoked potential (MEP), somatosensory evoked potential (SSEP or SEP), dermatomal somatosensory evoked potential (dSSEP), electromyography (EMG), nerve conduction studies and F waves, sympathetic skin response (SSR), H-reflex recordings, and electrical perceptual threshold (EPT) recordings. A summary of these techniques is provided in **Tables 38.1** and **38.2**.

■ Motor Evoked Potentials

MEPs are produced by transcranial magnetic stimulation (TMS). Developed in 1985,[4] TMS generates a magnetic field, which, in turn, induces an electrical current that elicits descending corticospinal volleys, which are recorded as MEPs using surface electrodes on muscles of interest. Measurable MEP parameters (**Table 38.1**) include the stimulation intensity that elicits MEPs (MEP threshold), amplitude and latency of MEPs, and the slope of plots of amplitude against intensity (input–output or recruitment curve)[5] (**Fig. 38.1**). These parameters provide information about the state of cortical excitability after injury. The slope of the steep portion of the curve increases with increasing cortical excitability, such as following treadmill training (**Fig. 38.2**).[6]

Additional information about sensorimotor physiology can be obtained by performing paired pulse TMS studies. In paired pulse studies, a conditioning subthreshold or suprathreshold stimulus is followed by a second test pulse to determine the effect of the conditioning pulse on the size of MEP response generated by the test pulse alone. At interstimulus intervals between 1 and 5 msec, subthreshold conditioning pulses inhibit suprathreshold test pulses and are referred to as short-interval intracortical inhibition (SICI). Intracortical facilitation (ICF) is at interstimulus intervals between 10 and 25 msec. By varying parameters

Table 38.1 Parameters That Can Be Measured in Transcranial Magnetic Stimulation Studies in SCI Patients[32]

TMS parameter	Function	Main findings in SCI
MEP amplitude	Measure of cortical excitability and corticospinal tract integrity	↓↓
MEP threshold	Measure of cortical excitability	↑↑
MEP latency	Measure of total conduction time	↑↑
CCT	Measure of conduction time to motor neurons	↑↑
Cortical silent period	Measure of cortical and spinal inhibition	↑↑
SAI	Measure of sensorimotor integration	Not studied
SICI	Measure of intracortical inhibition	Not studied
Slope of input–output curve	Measure of cortical excitability and corticospinal tract integrity	Not studied
MEP facilitation		↓↓

Abbreviations: CCT, central conduction time; MEP, motor evoked potential; SAI, short-latency afferent inhibition; SCI, spinal cord injury; SICI, short-interval intracortical inhibition; TMS, transcranial magnetic stimulation.

Table 38.2 A Summary of Electrophysiological Tests for Assessment of Spinal Cord Injury

Test	Key features	Key findings and potential use in SCI
Motor evoked potentials (MEPs)	Assess descending corticospinal tract function via signals induced by transcranial magnetic stimulation (TMS) of the motor cortex	MEP latencies remain unchanged over time, suggesting that recovery in SCI patients is not related to improvements in spinal conductivity Correlated to recovery of hand and ambulatory capacity Can be used to predict level of injury Absence is indicative of poorer prognosis Increase in amplitude may correlate to functional recovery
Somatosensory evoked potentials (SSEPs)	Assess ascending spinal tract function via stimulation of peripheral nerves Record response in the somatosensory cortex using an electrode on the subject's scalp	Signal amplitudes have been shown to correlate with functional outcomes SSEPs can be used to determine injury level in unexaminable patients
Dermatomal somatosensory evoked potentials (dSSEPs)	Similar to SSEPs but are obtained by cutaneous electrical stimulation of dermatomal points Appear to correlate with EPT results	When paired with electrical perceptual threshold tests and electrical pain perception, dSSEPs reliably measure segmental integrity
Electromyography (EMG) and F-waves and compound muscle action potentials	Assess peripheral nerve injury and anterior horn damage; F-waves are elicited by supramaximal stimulation of peripheral nerves and test the integrity of the efferent peripheral motor pathway and may test excitability of the motor neuron pool	Analysis of surface EMG patterns may be able to identify patients with discomplete injuries
Sympathetic skin response (SSR)	Assesses spinal cord autonomic integrity using electric or magnetic stimulation from above the spinal lesion Records response on the palmar, plantar skin surface or perineum using surface electromyographic (EMG) electrodes	SSR is absent below the level of complete lesion Loss of palmar SSR was associated with development of AH in 93% of patients Useful in assessing injury level and injury completeness
Hoffmann reflex (H-reflex)	H-reflex is a measure of spinal cord excitability elicited by submaximal stimulation of a mixed peripheral nerve and caused by activation of a motor neuron Records response with surface EMG electrodes	Amplitude of H-reflex increases over time post-SCI The H-reflex test may be useful as a marker of spinal cord excitability and plasticity
Electrical perceptual thresholds (EPTs)	Assess the level and degree of sensory impairment of SCI by cutaneous electrical stimulation of American Spinal Injury Association (ASIA) sensory points Record subject's perceived response at minimal ascending and descending stimulation intensities	Provide a more objective test of sensory function that is as accurate as clinical assessment according to ASIA classifications

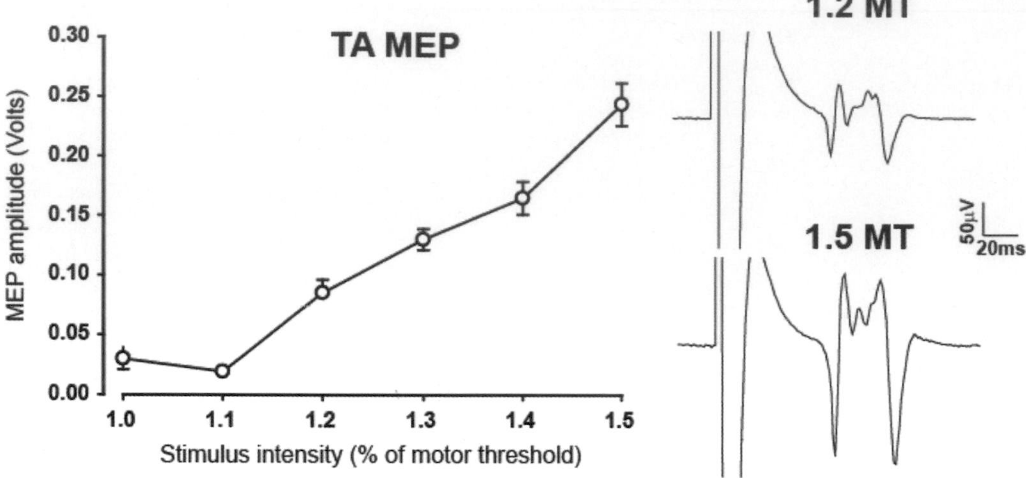

Fig. 38.1 Input–output recruitment curve of the resting tibialis anterior muscle. On the right are examples of motor evoked potentials at intensities of 1.2 and 1.5 times motor threshold.

other types of inhibition have been described. Suprathreshold conditioning pulses paired with suprathreshold test pulses at interstimulus intervals of 50 to 200 msec cause long-interval intracortical inhibition (LICI). Conditioning median nerve stimulation inhibits test MEP responses at ISIs between 20 and 30 msec or at ISIs between 100 and 200 msec. These are referred to as short-latency afferent inhibition (SAI) and long-latency afferent inhibition (LAI), respectively (**Fig. 38.3**). The central conduction time (CCT) measures the conduction time between the cortex and motor neuron pool. The silent period refers to a period of EMG silence following the MEP when TMS is performed during a sustained muscle contraction.

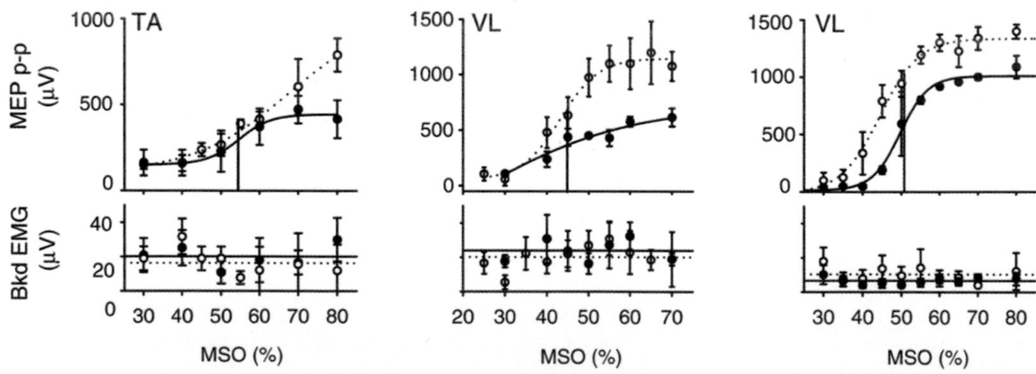

Fig. 38.2 Representative recruitment curves from three different subjects before (—) and after (- - -) treadmill training. (*Top*) Recruitment curves from the tibialis anterior (TA) and vastus lateralis (VL) muscles (middle; right). In all three examples, the recruitment curves after training rested above the recruitment curves before training, especially at intermediate- and high-stimulation intensities. The slope of the steep portion of the sigmoid line fit to the recruitment curve also increased after training. (*Bottom*) The mean background electromyography (EMG) results after training (· · ·) were similar to the background EMG results before training (—). Data points represent trial means ± standard deviation. (From Thomas SL, Gorassini MA. Increases in corticospinal tract function by treadmill training after incomplete spinal cord injury. J Neurophysiol 2005;94:2844–2855. Reprinted with permission.)

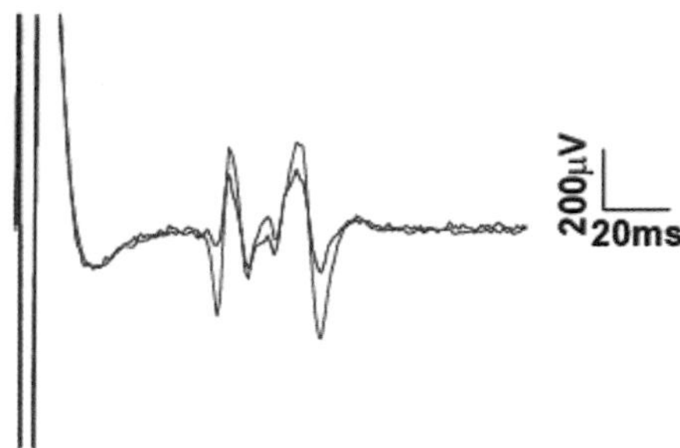

Fig. 38.3 Motor evoked potentials of the tibialis anterior showing short afferent inhibition (*red*) of the conditioning response (*black*) at an interstimulus interval of 42 msec. The latency of the somatosensory evoked potentials was at 43 msec.[6]

■ Motor Evoked Potentials in Spinal Cord Injury

MEPs are frequently pathological in SCI patients, with abnormal amplitude or latency.[7] In addition, the facilitation of MEPs with voluntary contraction is significantly reduced in SCI patients.[8] In one study,[9] MEPs were predictive of the level of injury, although they are not used routinely for that purpose. The clinical exam is presently the standard way of determining injury level and injury severity in addition to neuroimaging. As a prognostic tool, MEPs are predictive of hand and ambulatory function. Abductor digiti minimi MEPs were significantly correlated to hand function outcome, with very poor prognosis in patients with absent MEPs.[10] Similarly, tibialis anterior MEPs were predictive of ambulatory capacity with sensitivity similar to ASIA scores. Tibialis anterior MEPs were present in 70% of patients who recovered ambulatory capacity. Most SCI patients who achieve full ambulatory capacity had normal MEP latencies, and only 20% with initial loss of MEPs achieved functional ambulatory capacity.[10,11]

In a large, multicenter study, the functional recovery mechanisms of compensation, neural plasticity, and repair of the central nervous system were tracked over a 1-year period.[12] Other than a small increase in MEP amplitudes in ASIA D tetraplegic patients, evoked potential latencies remained unchanged over time, thus indicating that functional recovery in SCI patients was not related to improvements in spinal conductivity. Over all, improvements in function as assessed by the Walking Index for Spinal Cord Injury (WISCI) and Spinal Cord Independence Measure (SCIM) scores did not correlate with reductions in evoked potential latencies. The findings strongly supported the idea that recovery mainly occurs through compensation in complete spinal cord injury (cSCI) and through facilitation by neural plasticity in incomplete spinal cord injury (iSCI) rather than physical repair. In another longitudinal study over a 6-month period, MEP latencies and thresholds did not change despite improvements in clinical scores.[13] To date there have not been any longitudinal studies using other indices, such as MEP recruitment curve slopes.

Electromyography and Nerve Conductance Studies

EMG is often used in conjunction with motor nerve conduction studies to evaluate the motor neuron pool and peripheral nervous system. Compound nerve action potentials can be used to distinguish between peripheral and cord lesions and to assess the extent of anterior horn damage.[10] F-waves are elicited following supramaximal stimulation of a peripheral nerve and can be used to assess the efferent peripheral motor pathway. F-waves have been used to assess the excitability of the spinal motor neuron pool.[14,15] The voluntary response index (VRI)[16] is a measure derived from surface EMG recordings and compares the pattern of EMG activation in patients to a prototypical pattern generated from a group of neurologically intact individuals. It has two components, a magnitude scale that measures excitability and a similarity index that measures the balance of excitation and inhibition. There is a moderate correlation between both scales and the ASIA score. Thus far, there have been limited studies in SCI, and more studies are needed to determine utility in longitudinal evaluations of recovery or therapeutic interventions. The term *discomplete injuries* has been used to describe patients who have clinically complete injuries but who have residual connectivity. It is hoped that analysis of surface EMG patterns measures may also be able to identify such patients, who would be most suitable for therapeutic interventions.[17]

Somatosensory Evoked Potentials

SSEPs are recorded after an electrical stimulus is applied to Ia afferents of a peripheral nerve. SSEPs are typically recorded using surface electrodes after median or tibial nerve stimulation but can also be recorded after ulnar and peroneal nerve stimulation. Measureable SSEP parameters include the amplitude and latency of the peak activation along the pathway from the dorsal columns to the somatosensory cortex. For median nerve stimulation, the most important parameters are the amplitude and latencies of the N_9, N_{13}, N_{18}, N_{20}, and P_{14} waveforms, where N is a negative deflection on the tracing, P is a positive deflection, and the subscript refers to latency. N_{20} is thought to originate from thalamocortical radiations to the somatosensory cortex, N_{18} from the upper brain stem, N_{13} from the dorsal horn neurons, and P_{14} from the caudal medial lemniscus. Typical waveforms of interest after tibial nerve stimulation are the P_{37}, which is from the sensory cortex, and N_{34} from the brain stem.

Somatosensory evoked potentials are frequently pathological in SCI.[18] As a prognostic tool, they have been found to have predictive value in overall outcomes[18,19] and in determining ambulatory outcomes, although not to a degree more accurate than conventional clinical examination.[20] A positive relationship has been shown between median and ulnar nerve SSEP amplitudes and the outcome of hand function, with sensitivity similar to ASIA scores. Tibial SSEPs are also predictive of ambulatory function. At least 80% of patients with initial tibial SSEPs do regain some ambulatory capacity at 1-year follow-up,[10] whereas the absence of median, ulnar, and tibial SSEPs early after injury usually indicates a poor prognosis.[10,18] In one longitudinal study, ~20% of patients showed an improvement of SSEP parameters over time; however, a direct correlation with neurological recovery is unlikely.[18] Another large longitudinal study showed no significant change in SSEPs over time.[12]

Dermatomal Somatosensory Evoked Potentials

Dermatomal SSEPs are elicited with cutaneous electrical stimulation of ASIA sensory points. Previously, dSSEPs were considered to be of limited value in determining the level of cervical SCI when compared with MEPs.[9] However, it has been shown that dSSEPs in conjunction with electrical perceptual threshold and electrical pain perception tests provide reliable data to assess the segmental integrity of the spinal cord.[21] By combining these tests, improved sensitivity in the monitoring of changes in function post-SCI becomes possible.

Sympathetic Skin Response

SSR is another noninvasive electrophysiological assessment using EMG electrodes on the skin's surface to record signals from electric or magnetic stimulation above the spinal lesion.[10] Physiological (auditory and inspiratory gasp) stimulation can also be used to elicit SSR.[22] These recordings can be used to assess damage to the spinal sympathetic nervous system and the respective peripheral sympathetic nerve fibers connecting to the areas of the skin from which the signal is being recorded. The palmar (**Fig. 38.4**) (testing the pathway from spinal cord to the sweat glands of the hands), plantar (pathway from spinal cord to feet), and perineal (from spinal cord to pre- and postganglionic sympathetic nerve fibers) pathways are tested most often.[23]

In general, SSRs are absent below the level of a complete injury.[10,23] In general, palmar, plantar and perineal SSRs are absent in complete injuries above T4. Plantar and perineal SSRs are absent in complete injuries between T4 and T10. Only perineal SSRs are absent in injuries between T10 and

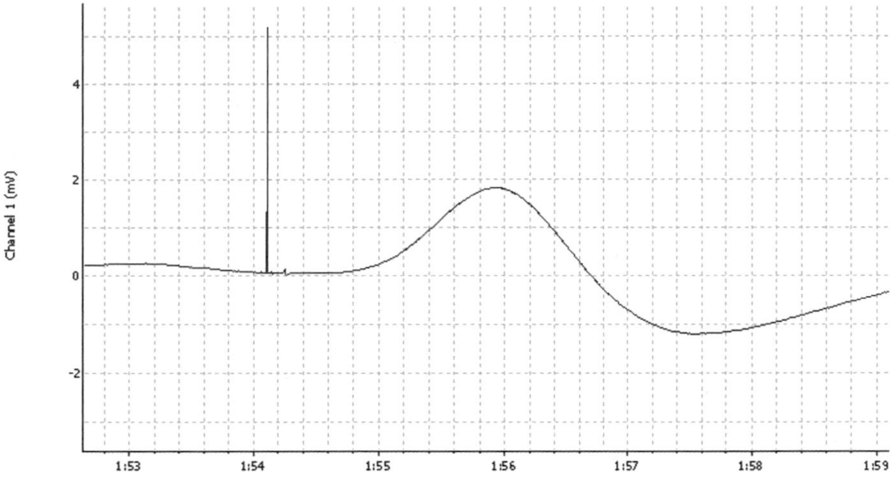

Fig. 38.4 Upper extremity palmer sympathetic skin response in a healthy subject elicited by median nerve stimulation.

L2. Injuries of the conus or cauda do not affect plantar, palmar, or perineal SSR. SSR is also helpful in the evaluation of patients at risk for autonomic dysreflexia. A study performed in 1999 demonstrated that the loss of palmar SSR was associated with development of autonomic hyperreflexia in 93% of patients.[10] In other studies, a clinical exam alone was not adequately sensitive to identify complete autonomic injury in 27% of patients.[23,24] In iSCI subjects, the presence of SSRs are dependent on the preservation of supraspinal connections. Whereas SSR has not traditionally been used to provide an assessment of the completeness of an SCI lesion to the same extent as somatic tests, such as MEPs and SSEPs, the addition of sympathetic nervous system tests may provide a more complete picture for studying SCI.[10,22] Furthermore, ASIA scores alone are not predictive of severity of autonomic injury or autonomic injury completeness.[25]

Hoffmann Reflex

The Hoffmann reflex (H-reflex) test is the electrical analogue of the monosynaptic stretch reflex. It can be elicited by low-intensity (submaximal) electrical stimulation of the afferent fibers (Ia) of a mixed peripheral nerve, such as the tibial nerve or the common peroneal nerve. Afferent nerve stimulation leads to the activation of the α-motor neuron, which is recorded using a surface EMG electrode. Unlike F-waves, H-reflexes are present during spinal shock despite the loss of tendon reflexes. The presence of H-reflexes in spinal shock confirms a normal reflex arc, with the absence of peripheral nerve lesions below the lesion. H-reflex amplitudes increase over time after SCI.[26] Typical parameters measured in H-reflex studies include the H_{max}:M_{max} ratio, the H_{mean}, and the slope of the H-reflex recovery curve.[27] With regard to the H_{max}:M_{max} ratio, M_{max} is the maximal motor response of the motor neuron pool and H_{max} is the maximal response of the motor pool reflexively activated by the stimulus. This ratio is increased in the case of spasticity. H_{mean} is the mean H-reflex amplitude within a specified range of M-wave amplitudes. For the H-reflex recovery curve, the H-reflex amplitude of a test stimulus as a percentage of the H-reflex amplitude to a conditioning stimulus of equal intensity is plotted as a function of interstimulus interval between the conditioning and test stimuli. There is typically a bimodal pattern of inhibition between 30 and 75 msec and also between 300 and 900 msec. This curve can be used to evaluate spinal inhibitory circuits, such as recurrent inhibition and presynaptic inhibition.[27] The H-reflex recruitment curve is a plot of the H-reflex amplitude (usually with the M-wave amplitude) at increasing intensities (*x*-axis) (**Fig. 38.5**). Over all, the H-reflex is a measure of motor neuron excitability. Changes in H-reflex parameters as a result of an intervention or a conditioning stimulus can be used to probe spinal cord excitability, pathophysiology, and plasticity.[28]

Electrical Perceptual Thresholds

The EPT test is a noninvasive quantitative sensory test developed to assess the level and degree of impairment in patients with SCI. The test mimics light touch/pinprick tests with cutaneous electrical stimulation of ASIA sensory points along spinal dermatomes.[29] The use of this test has been validated as a simple and reproducible means of testing in SCI subjects.[30] The level of SCI as determined by EPT was found to be as accurate as clinical assessment according to ASIA classifications. Moreover, the use of EPT was concluded to perhaps be able to provide greater sensitivity and resolution to clinical testing that could be used in monitoring SCI subjects in clinical investigations.

Assessment of Bowel and Bladder Function

Bladder function can be evaluated using pudendal SSEPs.[10] This test monitors the somatic fibers of the external urethral sphincter. Similar to upper extremity and lower extremity SSEPs, a complete loss of pudendal SSEP indicates a poor prognosis, with no patient with complete loss achieving normal function. For full evaluation of bladder function, urodynamic studies are required to evaluate detrusor function in addition to pudendal SSEPs. The detrusor is innervated by parasympathetic fibers that travel through the pelvic nerve. For evaluation of bowel incontinence, rectal EMGs can be used to assess the function of the external anal sphincter and are routinely used in urodynamic studies.

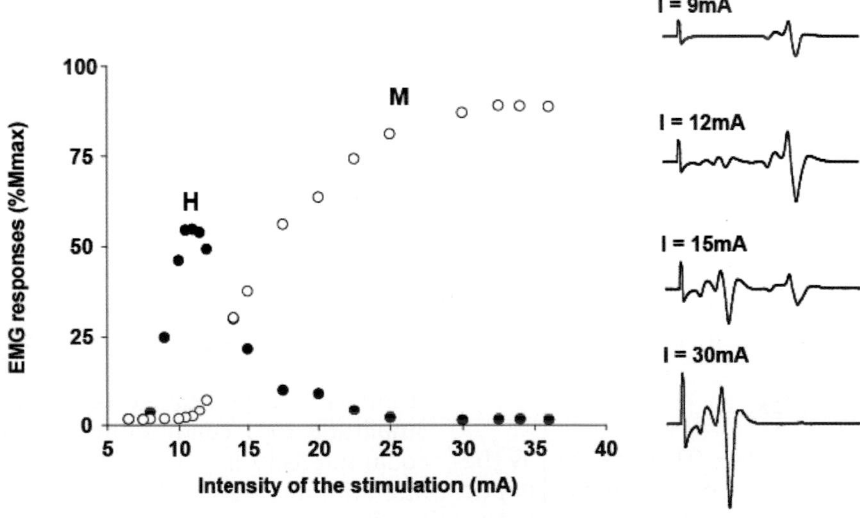

Fig. 38.5 H-reflex input–output recruitment curve of the soleus H-reflex (H) and M-wave (M) expressed as a percentage of M_{max}. Illustrated on the right are the corresponding H-reflex waveforms at intensities of 9 mA, 12 mA, 15 mA, and 30 mA.

■ Conclusion

Electrophysiological measures are increasingly being used to provide objective measures for SCI assessment. They are able to provide predictive value with a similar degree of significance as clinical examinations by ASIA scoring and provide informative, quantitative data on the changes that occur in neural circuitry. Used in conjunction with conventional clinical examinations, electrophysiological exams have come to be a good complement to assessing function after SCI. Furthermore, the tests themselves also complement each other in providing a broader picture of the condition. Ultimately, finding out the underlying significance of these measures may provide a better understanding of the way in which neural plasticity, repair, compensation, and improvement interrelate in regard to SCI.

However, despite the benefits of these measures, they have yet to be completely standardized and validated in the clinic, thus prompting the push for further research and detailed guidelines.[1] The relationship between changes in electrophysiological measures and different quantifiers of recovery has not yet been fully explored, and the mechanisms of recovery from incomplete and complete SCI are still in need of further investigation. Although there have been efforts to do so, much is still unknown about how these electrophysiological measures correlate to recovery. Continuing research using these methodologies should yield a better understanding of the mechanisms behind SCI recovery and thus provide potentially greater predictive and evaluative power.

Pearls

- Electrophysiological methods must be included in overall initial assessment of SCI injury severity and completeness.
- Electrophysiological studies show evidence of significant plasticity after SCI.
- There is a need for longitudinal studies of SCI patients using additional electrophysiological parameters, such as slopes of MEP recruitment curves and SSR and EPT.

Pitfalls

- There is significant variability of MEPs and SSEPs within and across sessions. This must be taken into account when interpreting longitudinal MEP and SEP studies to avoid attributing a treatment or therapy effect when none exists.
- SCIs may be accompanied by traumatic brain injuries. Transcranial magnetic stimulation may cause seizures in patients with brain injuries and MEP parameters may be altered by undiscovered brain injuries. So brain injuries and brain lesions should be ruled out prior to performing MEP studies.
- Electrophysiological factors may be affected by several parameters, including age, so studies should be performed with age-matched controls. It is also important to control for temperature when performing SSR studies because they are affected by room temperature.

References

1. Steeves JD, Lammertse D, Curt A, et al; International Campaign for Cures of Spinal Cord Injury Paralysis. Guidelines for the conduct of clinical trials for spinal cord injury (SCI) as developed by the ICCP panel: clinical trial outcome measures. Spinal Cord 2007;45(3):206–221
2. Houlden DA, Schwartz ML, Klettke KA. Neurophysiologic diagnosis in uncooperative trauma patients: confounding factors. J Trauma 1992; 33(2):244–251
3. Fawcett JW, Curt A, Steeves JD, et al. Guidelines for the conduct of clinical trials for spinal cord injury as developed by the ICCP panel: spontaneous recovery after spinal cord injury and statistical power needed for therapeutic clinical trials. Spinal Cord 2007;45(3):190–205
4. Barker AT, Jalinous R, Freeston IL. Non-invasive magnetic stimulation of human motor cortex. Lancet 1985;1(8437):1106–1107
5. Thomas SL, Gorassini MA. Increases in corticospinal tract function by treadmill training after in-

complete spinal cord injury. J Neurophysiol 2005; 94(4):2844–2855

6. Sandbrink F. The MEP in clinical neurodiagnosis. In: Wassermann EM, Epstein CM, Ziemann U, Walsh V, Paus T, Lisanby SH, eds. The Oxford Handbook of Transcranial Magnetic Stimulation. Oxford, England: Oxford University Press; 2008:237–283
7. Davey NJ, Smith HC, Savic G, Maskill DW, Ellaway PH, Frankel HL. Comparison of input-output patterns in the corticospinal system of normal subjects and incomplete spinal cord injured patients. Exp Brain Res 1999;127(4):382–390
8. Diehl P, Kliesch U, Dietz V, Curt A. Impaired facilitation of motor evoked potentials in incomplete spinal cord injury. J Neurol 2006;253(1):51–57
9. Shields CB, Ping Zhang Y, Shields LB, Burke DA, Glassman SD. Objective assessment of cervical spinal cord injury levels by transcranial magnetic motor-evoked potentials. Surg Neurol 2006; 66(5):475–483, discussion 483
10. Curt A, Dietz V. Electrophysiological recordings in patients with spinal cord injury: significance for predicting outcome. Spinal Cord 1999; 37(3):157–165
11. Curt A, Keck ME, Dietz V. Functional outcome following spinal cord injury: significance of motor-evoked potentials and ASIA scores. Arch Phys Med Rehabil 1998;79(1):81–86
12. Curt A, Van Hedel HJ, Klaus D, Dietz V; EM-SCI Study Group. Recovery from a spinal cord injury: significance of compensation, neural plasticity, and repair. J Neurotrauma 2008;25(6):677–685
13. Smith HC, Savic G, Frankel HL, et al. Corticospinal function studied over time following incomplete spinal cord injury. Spinal Cord 2000;38(5): 292–300
14. Inghilleri M, Lorenzano C, Conte A, Frasca V, Manfredi M, Berardelli A. Effects of transcranial magnetic stimulation on the H reflex and F wave in the hand muscles. Clin Neurophysiol 2003; 114(6):1096–1101
15. Lin JZ, Floeter MK. Do F-wave measurements detect changes in motor neuron excitability? Muscle Nerve 2004;30(3):289–294
16. Lee DC, Lim HK, McKay WB, Priebe MM, Holmes SA, Sherwood AM. Toward an objective interpretation of surface EMG patterns: a voluntary response index (VRI). J Electromyogr Kinesiol 2004; 14(3):379–388
17. McKay WB, Lim HK, Priebe MM, Stokic DS, Sherwood AM. Clinical neurophysiological assessment of residual motor control in post-spinal cord injury paralysis. Neurorehabil Neural Repair 2004;18(3):144–153
18. Spiess M, Schubert M, Kliesch U, Halder P; EM-SCI Study group. Evolution of tibial SSEP after traumatic spinal cord injury: baseline for clinical trials. Clin Neurophysiol 2008;119(5):1051–1061
19. Li C, Houlden DA, Rowed DW. Somatosensory evoked potentials and neurological grades as predictors of outcome in acute spinal cord injury. J Neurosurg 1990;72(4):600–609
20. Jacobs SR, Yeaney NK, Herbison GJ, Ditunno JF Jr. Future ambulation prognosis as predicted by somatosensory evoked potentials in motor complete and incomplete quadriplegia. Arch Phys Med Rehabil 1995;76(7):635–641
21. Kramer JL, Moss AJ, Taylor P, Curt A. Assessment of posterior spinal cord function with electrical perception threshold in spinal cord injury. J Neurotrauma 2008;25(8):1019–1026
22. Nicotra A, Catley M, Ellaway PH, Mathias CJ. The ability of physiological stimuli to generate the sympathetic skin response in human chronic spinal cord injury. Restor Neurol Neurosci 2005; 23(5-6):331–339
23. Curt A, Weinhardt C, Dietz V. Significance of sympathetic skin response in the assessment of autonomic failure in patients with spinal cord injury. J Auton Nerv Syst 1996;61(2):175–180
24. Curt A, Nitsche B, Rodic B, Schurch B, Dietz V. Assessment of autonomic dysreflexia in patients with spinal cord injury. J Neurol Neurosurg Psychiatry 1997;62(5):473–477
25. Claydon VE, Krassioukov AV. Orthostatic hypotension and autonomic pathways after spinal cord injury. J Neurotrauma 2006;23(12):1713–1725
26. Hiersemenzel LP, Curt A, Dietz V. From spinal shock to spasticity: neuronal adaptations to a spinal cord injury. Neurology 2000;54(8):1574–1582
27. Mazzini L, Balzarini C. An overview of H-reflex studies in amyotrophic lateral sclerosis. Amyotroph Lateral Scler Other Motor Neuron Disord 2000; 1(5):313–318
28. Knikou M, Taglianetti C. On the methods employed to record and measure the human soleus H-reflex. Somatosens Mot Res 2006;23(1-2): 55–62
29. Davey NJ, Nowicky AV, Zaman R. Somatopy of perceptual threshold to cutaneous electrical stimulation in man. Exp Physiol 2001;86(1):127–130
30. Savic G, Bergström EM, Frankel HL, Jamous MA, Ellaway PH, Davey NJ. Perceptual threshold to cutaneous electrical stimulation in patients with spinal cord injury. Spinal Cord 2006;44(9): 560–566

39

Quantitative Tests of Sensory, Motor, and Autonomic Function

Peter H. Ellaway

Key Points

1. Quantitative and objective electrophysiological tests of sensory, motor, and autonomic function are reviewed as adjuncts to the International Standards for Neurological Classification of Spinal Cord Injury (ISNSCI) and the American Spinal Injury Association Impairment Scale (AIS) neurological assessment.
2. The merits of the electrical perceptual test of cutaneous sensibility and the use of dermatomal sensory evoked potentials are assessed and compared.
3. The use of noninvasive electromyographic recording of muscle function and the ability to test the patency of the corticospinal tract with transcranial magnetic stimulation is reviewed.
4. The use of a specific test of autonomic function in SCI, the sympathetic skin response, is described as having the potential to provide insight into the supraspinal access to the sympathetic chain.

A limited number of clinical trials for the repair of spinal cord injury (SCI) are under way, with additional trials based on novel therapies being widely anticipated from successful preclinical studies. One integral aspect of the design of clinical trials for SCI is identifying the type and breadth of the primary and secondary outcome measures.[1] This chapter is devoted to discussing several novel and improved techniques for ascertaining the level and completeness of an SCI. Although the general goal of a clinical trial will have been an improvement in functional outcome, and hence anticipated, the actual outcome will inevitably be uncertain and may even be adverse. Outcome measures for physiological systems should therefore be based on methods that allow both for improvements and for worsening of the condition. Additionally, the methods employed as outcome measures should be capable of detecting small physiological changes that could be limited to change at a single vertebral level of the spinal cord. Preclinical studies of novel therapies designed to promote regeneration of spinal cord axons indicate that regenerating axons may descend or ascend the cord for only a few centimeters.[2] Translated to humans, this amount of potential reinnervation would result in renewed or new functional connections restricted to one or two vertebral levels. The current gold standard for clinical assessment of SCI is the American Spinal Injury Association (ASIA) Impairment Scale (AIS), a set of standard neurological classifications that comprises tests of sensory and motor function. There are several limitations to the AIS assessment. First, sensory cutaneous evaluation of each dermatome is scored simply as either normal, absent, or abnormal sensation. Abnormal sensation currently includes both heightened and lowered sensitivity as well as allodynia. Second, motor assessment is confined to the myotomes of the four limbs and ignores the trunk. A recent improvement has been the recommendation to score the upper and lower limbs separately.[3] Furthermore, the minimal clinically important difference is generally regarded as not having been established for either sensory or motor AIS assessments.[4] There is no component of autonomic assessment in the ASIA standard neurological classification of spinal injury. The only references to visceral function are questions on voluntary anal contraction and anal sensation. It is currently recognized that bladder and bowel require functional testing and that sexual, cardiac, vasomotor, and sudomotor function should be addressed.[5]

The following sections represent physiological tests that have been developed or improved upon in the Clinical Initiative funded by the International Spinal Research Trust (ISRT) (http://www.spinal-research.org).[6]

■ Cutaneous Sensory Function

At the time of an assessment, subjects may have lived for months or years with a disability caused by their SCI. Their impression of what constitutes normal sensibility for a dermatome may well have changed with time. Any test that is objective, quantitative, and does not rely on reporting the quality of sensation would augment the limited AIS sensory grading. Methods that fit this description are frequently bracketed under the description of quantitative sensory testing (QST).[7] Two electrophysiological techniques that also provide quantitative and objective measures of somatosensory function are the electrical perceptual threshold (EPT) test and somatosensory evoked potentials.

Electrical Perceptual Threshold

The EPT was developed for the assessment of cutaneous sensibility[8] and later validated against the AIS sensory grading.[9] EPT measures the threshold, or minimally detectable sensory appreciation, of constant-current square-wave pulses applied to the AIS test point of a dermatome. EPT determinations for subjects with SCI may be superimposed on a normal template constructed from the results of up to 40 neurologically normal individuals (**Fig. 39.1**). EPT values were found to lie outside the normal range below the level of injury defined clinically by the AIS sensory grading.[9] However, Savic et al. also reported a large number of abnormal EPT readings at the level of injury (i.e., the most caudal clinically normal dermatome), and even up to two or three dermatomes higher (**Fig. 39.1**), indicating that the ASIA clinical assessment had placed the level of injury too low.[9] The discrepancy was tentatively attributed to adaptation over time to sensations elicited by cutaneous stimulation of dermatomes affected by the injury. The EPT has since undergone repeatability evaluation for both inter- and intrarater trials in SCI[10] and compared different stimulators. Good intra- and interrater reliability for the EPT has now been confirmed[11] in control subjects for the C3, T1, L3, and S2 dermatomes.

The EPT is most likely testing the state of the posterior (dorsal) column pathway. In support of this, it is generally accepted that low-amplitude and short-duration current pulses applied to the skin will preferentially excite nerve endings or axons of large Aαβ myelinated fibers that convey innocuous modalities of cutaneous sensation, which agrees with reports of subjects that EPT test pulses are perceived as a light tapping sensation. Also supporting the as-

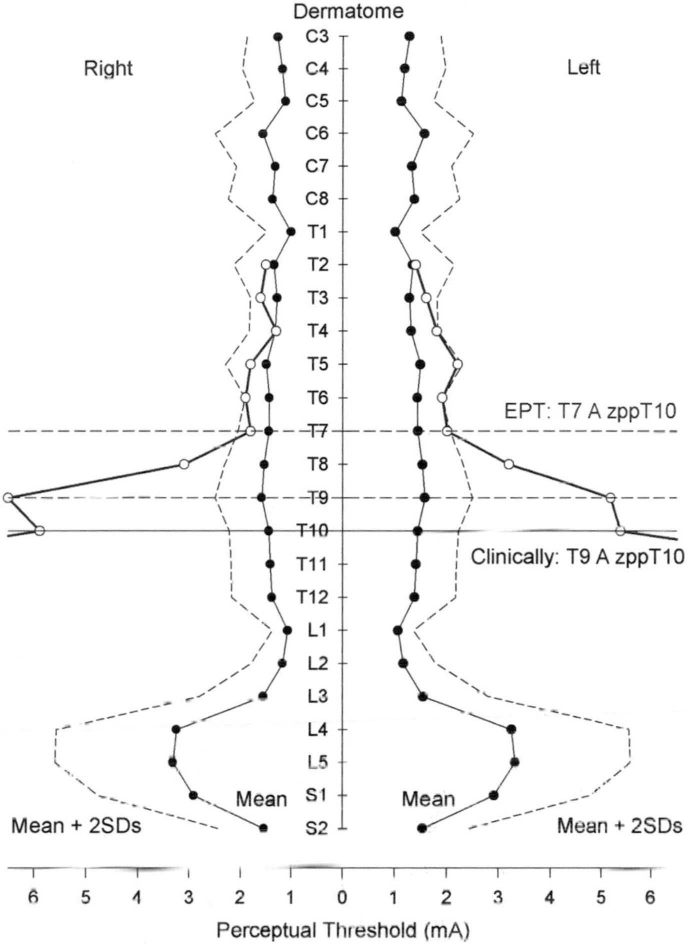

Fig. 39.1 Electrical perceptual threshold (EPT) results from a subject with complete spinal cord injury (*open circles, red line*) superimposed on the normal template (*solid circles, black line*). The clinical level of injury (American Spinal Injury Association Impairment Scale sensory) was T9 with a zone of partial preservation to T10. The EPT reveals the most caudal normal dermatome to be T7. (From Savic G, Bergstrom EMK, Frankel HL, Jamous MA, Ellaway PH, Davey NJ. Perceptual threshold to cutaneous electrical stimulation in patients with spinal cord injury. Spinal Cord 2006;44:560–566. Reprinted with permission.)

sociation is the observation that some individuals with incomplete SCI lack any pain perception to large current pulses (>10 mA) but have normal EPT values for certain dermatomes below the level of the lesion.[12] Similarly, a patient (T2 AIS D) with anterior spinal artery infarction has been reported with preserved light touch sensation and proprioception but abnormal pinprick discrimination consistent with an anterior cord syndrome, and EPT values within the normal range.[11]

In summary, EPT provides an adjunct to the AIS for sensory function by being a more quantitative and more objective measure. The method has good inter- and intrarater reliability. It is likely that EPT tests the posterior (dorsal) column pathway for light touch and proprioception rather than the anterolateral spinothalamic tract.

Somatosensory Evoked Potentials

The clinical neurological assessment of SCI may be augmented by employing somatosensory evoked potentials (SSEPs). Such neurophysiological evaluation of the sensory pathways from the skin has provided greater accuracy in determining the level and extent of an injury and has been correlated with functional outcomes.[13] The technique assesses the posterior (dorsal) column pathways of the spinal cord. A refinement of the technique is the dermatomal somatosensory evoked potential (dSSEP), which relates to a specific spinal segment. Rather than place the peripheral stimulating electrodes over a large nerve, electrodes are applied to the skin of a specific dermatome. The resulting evoked potentials are usually smaller in amplitude and lack the definition of SSEPs evoked by stimulation of a large nerve. However, the advantage is that dSSEPs may determine the level and extent of a spinal cord lesion with greater accuracy.

Validation of the EPT has been provided against dSSEPs.[12] Above the level of a spinal cord lesion, the dSSEP and EPT were comparable to those of control subjects. Close to the level of lesion, the dSSEP appeared abnormal and was of longer latency, and the EPT was raised above control values. Below the lesion, when the dSSEP was abolished, the EPT was raised further or unobtainable.

In conclusion, the requirement to improve on the insufficient sensitivity of the AIS sensory assessment[1] may be met by either the EPT or dSSEP methods. Either or both appear sufficiently sensitive as an adjunct to the AIS sensory assessment to detect change over individual segments and so provide assurance in terms of both safety and quantitative evidence that an intervention is working in a beneficial manner in early phase 1 or 2 clinical trials. Applying these techniques to measure cutaneous sensibility above and below the level of a lesion during trials could also point to the neurophysiological basis of the mechanism of change. An intervention may well induce changes in spinal cord circuitry as a result of sprouting or regeneration but additionally induce secondary plastic changes. These may occur above as well as at and below the lesion. EPT and dSSEPs have the potential to identify such change and, by indicating the basis of recovery, assist the refinement of any physical, pharmacological, or cell-based intervention designed to effect recovery of function.[14]

■ Motor Function

The current clinical gold standard for determining voluntary control of human motor function is the AIS assessment. This is limited to five key muscle groups of the upper limbs and five for the lower limbs. The trunk is not currently assessed. Moreover, the scores for the upper and lower limbs tend to be combined, presenting an overall score that, by itself, cannot provide a clear picture of the nature and extent of the injury. Electromyographic (EMG) investigation provides direct, quantitative, and objective insight into the integrity of the principal pathway involved in executing voluntary skeletal muscle activity, the corticospinal tract. The EMG approach that directly addresses the function of the corticospinal pathway is the use of transcranial magnetic stimulation (TMS) of the motor cortex.

Transcranial Magnetic Stimulation

There are numerous reviews of the TMS technique and applications to the investigation of several neurological conditions,[15] and TMS has frequently been used to provide motor outcome for SCI.[16–19] Measures of the threshold, latency, and size of motor evoked potentials (MEPs) to TMS have been made longitudinally during natural recovery in SCI. These studies have failed to show a direct link between MEP parameters and functional or clinical recovery.[20,21] In contrast, recovery of MEPs has been closely linked with functional recovery in response to weight-assisted treadmill training in SCI.[22] The observations of impaired facilitation of MEPs to voluntary effort in subjects with incomplete SCI are likely to be of significance in developing the TMS technique as an outcome measure for recovery of corticospinal tract function.[23] A further application that would contribute greatly to motor assessment is the potential for TMS to be used with trunk muscles (**Fig. 39.2**). MEPs may be recorded from abdominal muscles, paravertebral muscles,[24] and respiratory muscles.[19,25] Moreover, the technique is able to provide insight into the ipsilateral projections of the corticospinal tract.[26,27]

The brain motor control assessment (BMCA)[28] provides a quantitative analysis of surface EMG recordings during voluntary movement based on a voluntary response index (VRI). The method also has the potential to extend the limited range of muscles included in the AIS assessment, in addition to meeting the criteria for a more quantitative and objective measure. Usefully, the facility for TMS to demonstrate connection between the motor cortex and spinal motor neurons in persons with SCI has been related to the quality of postinjury voluntary motor control as assessed by the VRI.[29]

Finally, the inclusion of TMS for provision of quantitative outcome measures in SCI is supported by its being a noninvasive technique that is well tolerated by subjects. A recent review of risks associated with conventional TMS protocols reports few side effects and provides guidelines with respect to safety.[30]

■ Autonomic Function

The autonomic nervous system controls disparate body functions and also interacts closely with somatosensory systems and the central nervous control of voluntary movement. Apart from the innervation provided by cranial nerves, autonomic control is potentially affected by SCI at cervical,

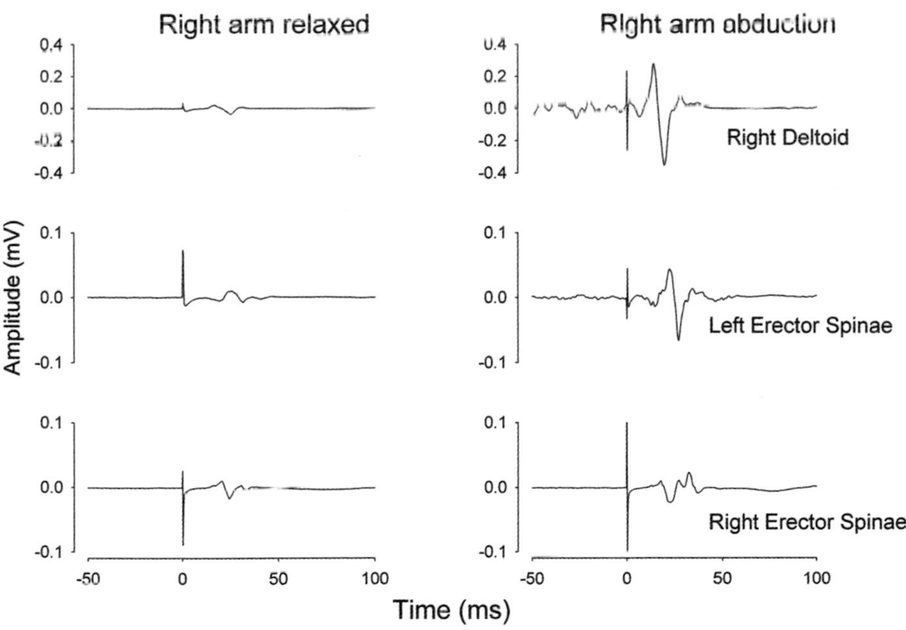

Fig. 39.2 Motor evoked potentials (MEPs) recorded from deltoid and erector spinae muscles of a control subject in response to transcranial magnetic stimulation (time zero) of the motor cortex. (*Left*) MEPs recorded with both arms relaxed and (*right*) with the right arm abducted. Note the greater facilitation of the left compared with the right erector spinae MEP during arm abduction. Unaveraged, single recordings. (Unpublished records)

thoracic, lumbar, and sacral levels. Routine measurements of blood pressure and heart rate and questionnaires relating to bladder, bowel, and sexual function are important in determining the impact of an SCI on the autonomic nervous system. Detailed assessment, however, may require elaborate functional and physiological tests. Those tests may be impractical when repeated, and quantitative estimates are required for monitoring change in response to treatment on a clinical trial. A test that could be considered when cost, time, and patient acceptability are of concern is the sympathetic skin response (SSR).

The Sympathetic Skin Response

The SSR is an electrodermal recording of the activation of palmar and plantar sweat glands in response to an arousal stimulus. The ability to control sweat is not high on the list of priorities for regaining function voiced by either tetraplegic or paraplegic sufferers.[31] The SSR does, however, provide insight into the supraspinal access to the sympathetic chain. In complete SCI, sweating is reduced or absent (anhidrosis) below the level of injury,[32] and the SSR is absent for complete injuries above T1.[33] The spinal cord when isolated from the brain stem appears also to be incapable of generating an SSR even when a normally adequate arousal stimulus (e.g., electrical nerve stimulation) is applied below the level of a lesion[34]; pudendal nerve stimulation may be an exception.[35] The integrity of central sympathetic descending tracts to the upper thoracic segments (T2-6) is required to elicit the palmar SSR, and all thoracic segments appear to be required for the plantar SSR, although the output is restricted to T8 to T10.[36]

The SSR in normal subjects is usually biphasic, with an initial negative wave (volar surface with respect to dorsal surface of the hand, plantar to the dorsum of the foot) followed by a positive-going wave. However, adaptation to repeated stimuli, which is a common feature of the SSR, can result in a decline in amplitude of the SSR[37] and a tendency to revert simply to an initial negative wave. Of functional interest, the presence of the second positive wave appears to be necessary for actual sweat secretion to be recorded.[38] The SSR records from a subject with a complete SCI at T7 would typically have preserved SSR of the hands in response to median nerve stimulation at 1.5 times motor threshold but no SSR recordable for the feet (**Fig. 39.3**), which is consonant with the level of the lesion. Such consistency is not always observed when the diagnosis of completeness of SCI has been determined clinically based solely on sensory and motor AIS assessments. In a study of 20 subjects with chronic SCI, preserved palmar and plantar SSRs were found in a complete C7 subject and a further case of preserved plantar (and palmar) SSRs in a complete T6 subject.[33] The study's conclusion was that the SCI was incomplete with regard to descending sympathetic neural control.

Therefore, SSR has the potential to assess a major element of autonomic function (descending sympathetic drive) in SCI, with regard to both the level and the completeness of the injury. The test is a relatively well-tolerated, straightforward, noninvasive, electrophysiological investigation that is not time consuming. It is currently being considered for inclusion in the revised battery of tests as a supplement to the ASIA clinical assessment of SCI in clinical trials.[39]

■ Conclusion

This chapter reports largely on novel and improved physiological methods of assessment for monitoring recovery (or deterioration) in SCI. The methods were developed in the ISRT Clinical Initiative. The raison d'être of the Clinical Initiative was that existing methods lacked the sensitivity that might be required to detect change following novel interventional measures designed to promote recovery of function in SCI. Among the battery of tests reported here, it is unlikely that

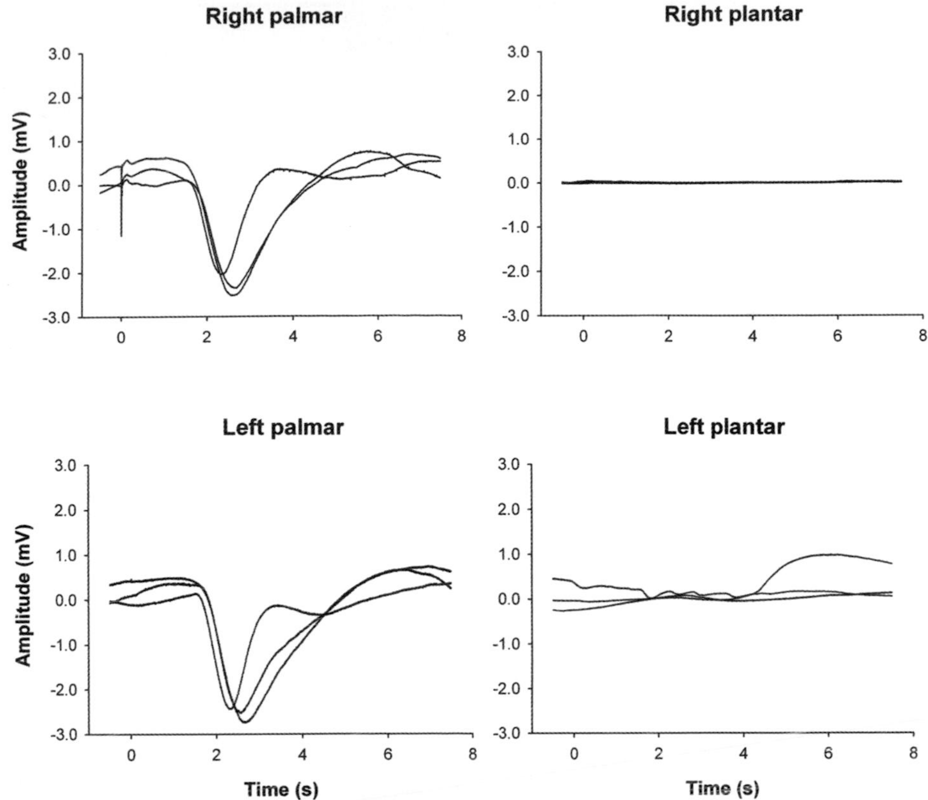

Fig. 39.3 Palmar and plantar sympathetic skin responses to electrical stimulation of the median nerve at 1.5 times motor threshold in a subject with a complete T7 spinal cord injury. Three sequential responses superimposed. Stimulation at time zero. Note the absence of plantar responses. (Unpublished records)

limiting assessment to any single procedure would be appropriate. The choice of test(s) to supplement AIS assessments will depend on several factors. An intervention may target specifically sensory, motor, or autonomic systems. The level and completeness of the spinal cord lesion will constitute further factors in the choice of test, as will the anticipated degree of improvement in function. Factors unrelated to the type of injury include tolerance by the subjects, health and safety issues, and the time and cost of administering the test. Tests that come closest to satisfying the foregoing considerations are the EPT as a test for innocuous cutaneous sensation and the SSR for sympathetic nervous system function. TMS and recording of MEPs have the potential for revealing connectivity of corticospinal function to voluntary muscle but currently are less acceptable measures in terms of sensitivity and practicality than is the EPT test for sensory input. These emerging tools, despite their shortcomings, do target specific systems and should not be ignored if they can provide significant clinically meaningful changes in physiology. The data that they provide are likely to be essential for the refinement of novel strategies to promote recovery of function in SCI.

Pearls

- The EPT test of cutaneous function has low cost, is quick to administer, and requires little training. It provides increased sensitivity to supplement the AIS measure of sensory function in SCI.
- Latencies of TMS evoked MEPs within the normal range for specific muscles are currently the most reliable indication of preserved corticospinal transmission in the injured spinal cord.
- The sympathetic skin response provides a convenient test with the potential to reveal an incomplete SCI with regard to autonomic function in subjects with cervical ASIA A (motor and sensory complete) or B (motor complete, sensory incomplete) clinical diagnosis.

Pitfalls

- The EPT technique requires cooperation and alertness on the part of the subject to report on the minimal sensation evoked by electrical stimulation at the threshold for perception.
- With TMS, crosstalk from electromyographic activity, generated in muscles innervated from a level above the level of SCI, may erroneously indicate a lower level of lesion when testing muscles residing in close anatomical proximity in a limb.
- The sensory stimulus required to elicit a sympathetic skin response must be applied via innervation above the level of an SCI or by voluntary gasp. The sympathetic skin response requires integration in supraspinal structures and cannot be generated by sensory input to the spinal cord isolated below a complete injury.

References

1. Steeves JD, Lammertse D, Curt A, et al; International Campaign for Cures of Spinal Cord Injury Paralysis. Guidelines for the conduct of clinical trials for spinal cord injury (SCI) as developed by the ICCP panel: clinical trial outcome measures. Spinal Cord 2007;45(3):206–221
2. Verma P, Fawcett J. Spinal cord regeneration. Adv Biochem Eng Biotechnol 2005;94:43–66
3. Graves DE, Frankiewicz RG, Donovan WH. Construct validity and dimensional structure of the ASIA motor scale. J Spinal Cord Med 2006;29(1): 39–45
4. Furlan JC, Fehlings MG. The impact of age on mortality, impairment, and disability among adults with acute traumatic spinal cord injury. J Neurotrauma 2009;26(10):1707–1717
5. Krassioukov AV, Karlsson AK, Wecht JM, Wuermser LA, Mathias CJ, Marino RJ; Joint Committee of American Spinal Injury Association and International Spinal Cord Society. Assessment of autonomic dysfunction following spinal cord injury: rationale for additions to International Standards for Neurological Assessment. J Rehabil Res Dev 2007;44(1):103–112
6. Ellaway PH, Anand P, Bergstrom EM, et al. Towards improved clinical and physiological assessments of recovery in spinal cord injury: a clinical initiative. Spinal Cord 2004;42(6):325–337
7. Savic G, Bergström EM, Davey NJ, et al. Quantitative sensory tests (perceptual thresholds) in patients with spinal cord injury. J Rehabil Res Dev 2007;44(1):77–82
8. Davey NJ, Nowicky AV, Zaman R. Somatopy of perceptual threshold to cutaneous electrical stimulation in man. Exp Physiol 2001;86(1):127–130
9. Savic G, Bergström EM, Frankel HL, Jamous MA, Ellaway PH, Davey NJ. Perceptual threshold to cutaneous electrical stimulation in patients with spinal cord injury. Spinal Cord 2006;44(9):560–566
10. King NK, Savic G, Frankel H, Jamous A, Ellaway PH. Reliability of cutaneous electrical perceptual threshold in the assessment of sensory perception in patients with spinal cord injury. J Neurotrauma 2009;26(7):1061–1068
11. Kramer JK, Taylor P, Steeves JD, Curt A. Dermatomal somatosensory evoked potentials and electrical perception thresholds during recovery from cervical spinal cord injury. Neurorehabil Neural Repair 2010;24(4):309–317
12. Curt A, Dietz V. Electrophysiological recordings in patients with spinal cord injury: significance for predicting outcome. Spinal Cord 1999;37(3): 157–165
13. Leong GW, Gorrie CA, Ng K, Rutkowski S, Waite PM. Electrical perceptual threshold testing: a validation study. J Spinal Cord Med 2009;32(2): 140–146
14. Fawcett JW, Curt A, Steeves JD, et al. Guidelines for the conduct of clinical trials for spinal cord injury as developed by the ICCP panel: spontaneous recovery after spinal cord injury and statistical power needed for therapeutic clinical trials. Spinal Cord 2007;45(3):190–205
15. Pascual-Leone A, Davey NJ, Rothwell J, Wasserman EM, Puri BK. Handbook of Transcranial Magnetic Stimulation. London: Arnold; 2002
16. Davey NJ, Smith HC, Wells E, et al. Responses of thenar muscles to transcranial magnetic stimulation of the motor cortex in patients with incomplete spinal cord injury. J Neurol Neurosurg Psychiatry 1998;65(1):80–87
17. Calancie B, Alexeeva N, Broton JG, Suys S, Hall A, Klose KJ. Distribution and latency of muscle responses to transcranial magnetic stimulation of motor cortex after spinal cord injury in humans. J Neurotrauma 1999;16(1):49–67

18. Davey NJ, Smith HC, Savic G, Maskill DW, Ellaway PH, Frankel HL. Comparison of input-output patterns in the corticospinal system of normal subjects and incomplete spinal cord injured patients. Exp Brain Res 1999;127(4):382–390

19. Ellaway PH, Catley M, Davey NJ, et al. Review of physiological motor outcome measures in spinal cord injury using transcranial magnetic stimulation and spinal reflexes. J Rehabil Res Dev 2007;44(1):69–76

20. Smith HC, Savic G, Frankel HL, et al. Corticospinal function studied over time following incomplete spinal cord injury. Spinal Cord 2000;38(5): 292–300

21. Curt A, Van Hedel HJ, Klaus D, Dietz V; EM-SCI Study Group. Recovery from a spinal cord injury: significance of compensation, neural plasticity, and repair. J Neurotrauma 2008;25(6):677–685

22. Thomas SL, Gorassini MA. Increases in corticospinal tract function by treadmill training after incomplete spinal cord injury. J Neurophysiol 2005;94(4):2844–2855

23. Diehl P, Kliesch U, Dietz V, Curt A. Impaired facilitation of motor evoked potentials in incomplete spinal cord injury. J Neurol 2006;253(1):51–57

24. Cariga P, Catley M, Nowicky AV, Savic G, Ellaway PH, Davey NJ. Segmental recording of cortical motor evoked potentials from thoracic paravertebral myotomes in complete spinal cord injury. Spine 2002;27(13):1438–1443

25. Lissens MA, Vanderstraeten GG. Motor evoked potentials of the respiratory muscles in tetraplegic patients. Spinal Cord 1996;34(11):673–678

26. Ferbert A, Caramia D, Priori A, Bertolasi L, Rothwell JC. Cortical projection to erector spinae muscles in man as assessed by focal transcranial magnetic stimulation. Electroencephalogr Clin Neurophysiol 1992;85(6):382–387

27. Kuppuswamy A, Catley M, King NK, Strutton PH, Davey NJ, Ellaway PH. Cortical control of erector spinae muscles during arm abduction in humans. Gait Posture 2008;27(3):478–484

28. Lee DC, Lim HK, McKay WB, Priebe MM, Holmes SA, Sherwood AM. Toward an objective interpretation of surface EMG patterns: a voluntary response index (VRI). J Electromyogr Kinesiol 2004; 14(3):379–388

29. McKay WB, Lee DC, Lim HK, Holmes SA, Sherwood AM. Neurophysiological examination of the corticospinal system and voluntary motor control in motor-incomplete human spinal cord injury. Exp Brain Res 2005;163(3):379–387

30. Rossi S, Hallett M, Rossini PM, Pascual-Leone A; Safety of TMS Consensus Group. Safety, ethical considerations, and application guidelines for the use of transcranial magnetic stimulation in clinical practice and research. Clin Neurophysiol 2009;120(12):2008–2039

31. Anderson KD. Targeting recovery: priorities of the spinal cord-injured population. J Neurotrauma 2004;21(10):1371–1383

32. Mathias CJ, Frankel HL. Autonomic disturbances in spinal cord lesions. In: Mathias CJ, Bannister R, eds. Autonomic Failure. New York: Oxford University Press; 2002:494–513

33. Nicotra A, Catley M, Ellaway PH, Mathias CJ. The ability of physiological stimuli to generate the sympathetic skin response in human chronic spinal cord injury. Restor Neurol Neurosci 2005;23(5-6):331–339

34. Cariga P, Catley M, Mathias CJ, Savic G, Frankel HL, Ellaway PH. Organisation of the sympathetic skin response in spinal cord injury. J Neurol Neurosurg Psychiatry 2002;72(3):356–360

35. Reitz A, Schmid DM, Curt A, Knapp PA, Schurch B. Sympathetic sudomotor skin activity in human after complete spinal cord injury. Auton Neurosci 2002;102(1-2):78–84

36. Schurch B, Curt A, Rossier AB. The value of sympathetic skin response recordings in the assessment of the vesicourethral autonomic nervous dysfunction in spinal cord injured patients. J Urol 1997;157(6):2230–2233

37. Cariga P, Catley M, Mathias CJ, Ellaway PH. Characteristics of habituation of the sympathetic skin response to repeated electrical stimuli in man. Clin Neurophysiol 2001;112(10):1875–1880

38. Ellaway PH, Kuppuswamy A, Nicotra A, Mathias CJ. Sweat production and the sympathetic skin response: improving the clinical assessment of autonomic function. Auton Neurosci 2010;155(1-2):109–114

39. Alexander MS, Biering-Sorensen F, Bodner D, et al. International standards to document remaining autonomic function after spinal cord injury. Spinal Cord 2009;47(1):36–43

40

Basic Neurophysiological Approaches to Probing Spinal Circuits

Rose Katz and Jean-Charles Lamy

Key Points

1. Monosynaptic reflexes, ongoing EMG modulation, and post-stimulus time histogram are indirect techniques that allow probing of spinal circuitries in humans.
2. Recurrent inhibition of motoneurons, reciprocal to inhibition, and presynaptic mechanisms are described in healthy subjects and spinal cord injury (SCI) patients, both at rest and during motor activities.

Noninvasive studies of central nervous system (CNS) networks in humans have been considerably improved by the progress in imaging techniques, including functional magnetic resonance imaging (fMRI), positron emission tomographic (PET) scanning, magnetoencephalography (MEG), and electroencephalography (EEG). However, up to now, these techniques have been suitable mainly for probing cerebral activities. At the spinal cord level, the small size of networks and motoneuron (MN) pools prevents their functional study with imaging techniques. Fortunately, the activity of muscle fibers is easily recorded with electrodes placed on the skin over a muscle belly. Because muscle fiber activity (except in rare pathological cases) relies only on MN activity, EMG is a "window" through which to explore MN excitability (**Fig. 40.1**).

The knowledge of motor control in animals has emerged from experiments performed with monosynaptic reflexes (i.e., with techniques whose underlying principles are similar to those currently used in humans). Their validities have been fully confirmed with direct recordings from MNs.

Even though methods used in humans cannot be controlled as those in animals, congruent results obtained with methods relying on different principles as well as control experiments performed in cats ensure their reliability. Moreover, it is likely that the effects of therapeutics aimed at facilitating CNS plasticity or regeneration in spinal cord injured (SCI) patients will first be detected with electrophysiological techniques, with clinical or MRI modifications being delayed.

■ Methodological Overview

The Monosynaptic Reflex: H- and T-Reflexes

The pathway of the monosynaptic reflex arc is sketched in **Fig. 40.2A**: Ia afferents from muscle-spindle primary endings have monosynaptic connections to a MN innervating the muscle from which Ia afferents originate. This pathway underlies both the Hoffmann reflex (H-reflex) and the tendon jerk (T-reflex).

In humans, at rest, percutaneous electrical stimulation of peripheral nerves usually evokes H-reflexes in the soleus, quadriceps, and flexor carpi radialis (FCR) muscles and, to a lesser extent, in hamstrings. A typical example of soleus H-reflex recordings and recruitment curves is illustrated in **Fig. 40.2**: when the intensity of the electrical stimulus is progressively augmented, a monosynaptic response (~30 msec latency) appears on electromyography (EMG) and gradually increases in amplitude. When the threshold for motor activation is reached, a direct motor response (~10 msec latency) appears on EMG, increases with the intensity of the electrical stimulus before reaching a maximum: the maximal motor response (M_{max}) reflecting the discharge of the totality of α motor axons contained in the nerve. In proximal muscles (i.e., biceps or triceps brachii), motor and reflex responses are evoked together and overlapped.

The T-reflex can also be used to assess the excitability of the MN pool via monosynaptic reflex amplitude: transient mechanical tap, elicited by an electromagnetic hammer, results in a tendon jerk in a wide range of muscles. However, the mechanical percussion is not as stable as the electrical shock applied on the peripheral nerve. Both H- and T-reflexes are simple, painless, and do not require the cooperation of the subject, only that the subject remain quiet. An excitatory input to the MN pool (i.e., induced by a conditioning stimulation) will increase the amplitude of unconditioned monosynaptic reflexes, whereas an inhibitory input will suppress it. There are some limitations to the use of changes in monosynaptic reflex amplitude to assess changes in MN excitability: (1) monosynaptic reflexes are mediated by Ia afferents, so the mechanisms controlling the Ia afferent volleys, including presynaptic Ia inhibition and postactivation depression (see later discussion), have to be taken into consideration; and (2) there are some limitations due to both properties of the MN pool and inhomogeneous distribution of afferent inputs within the MN pool.[1]

On the whole, the H-reflex technique remains the most valuable method for investigating spinal pathways in healthy subjects and patients with CNS lesions, whether at rest or during motor activities, when the following rules are taken into account: (1) the amplitude of the unconditioned H-reflex amplitude must be within the ascending part of the recruitment curve (**Fig. 40.2**); (2) the H-reflex size has to be expressed as a percentage of the M_{max}; (3) the unconditioned H-reflex size has to be the same in all the situations (rest, motor activities, etc.); and (4) conditioned and unconditioned reflexes have to be randomly alternated.

Ongoing Electromyographic Modulations

In this method, the ongoing EMG is rectified to sum both positive and negative deflections in the raw EMG and is therefore averaged. The ongoing unconditioned EMG is compared with that following a conditioning stimulus (conditioned EMG). An excitatory input to the MN pool will augment ongoing EMG activity, whereas an inhibitory input will suppress it (**Fig. 40.1**). Although this method is simple, it comes with certain limitations: (1) it can be used

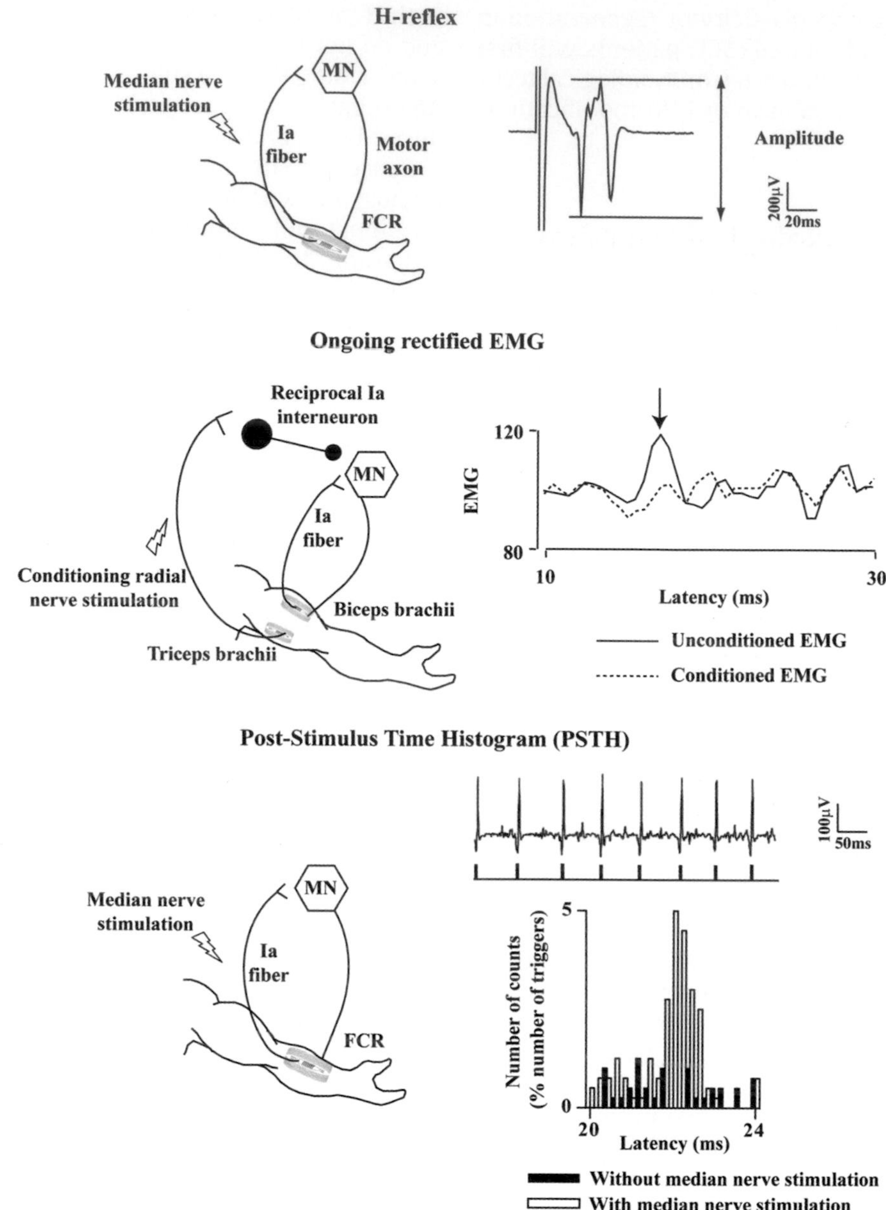

Fig. 40.1 Common methods used to probe spinal circuitry in humans. From top to bottom: Y-shaped bars represent excitatory connections and small filled circles represent inhibitory connections. H-reflex: percutaneous electrical stimulation of a peripheral nerve, such as the median nerve innervating the flexor carpi radialis (FCR) muscle, results in an H-reflex on electromyography (EMG). The peak-to-peak amplitude of this response reflects the excitability of the myotatic arc (see **Fig.40.2** legend for more details). Ongoing rectified EMG: during a voluntary contraction of a target muscle (e.g., the biceps brachii muscle), the ongoing EMG activity is rectified and averaged (*continuous line*—unconditioned EMG). A conditioning electrical stimulation applied to the nerve supplying the antagonist muscle (e.g., the radial nerve innervating the triceps brachii muscle) results in a depression (*arrow*) in the EMG (*dashed lines*—conditioned EMG) due to reciprocal inhibition (see **Fig. 40.3**). Poststimulus time histogram (PSTH): changes in firing probability of a voluntary repetitively activated motor unit during a weak contraction of a target muscle (e.g., the FCR muscle) are determined by comparing the histogram of occurrence of motoneuronal (MN) discharges without homonymous nerve (e.g., median nerve) stimulation (*filled histograms*) and with homonymous nerve stimulation (*opened histograms*). The electrical stimulation induces a peak of occurrence of MN discharges due to the monosynaptic activation of a MN.

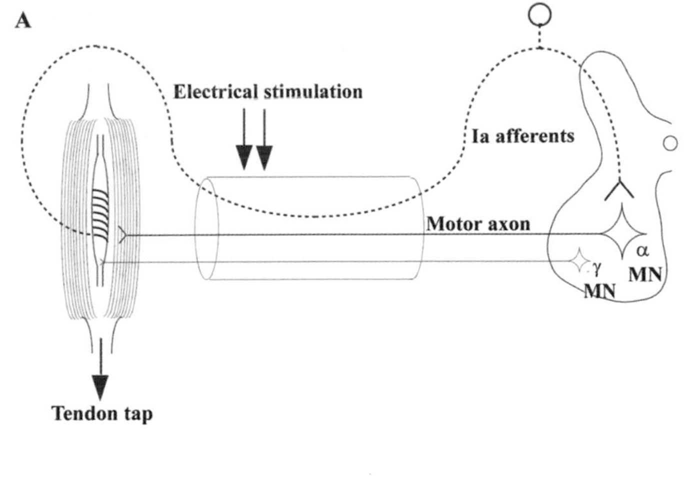

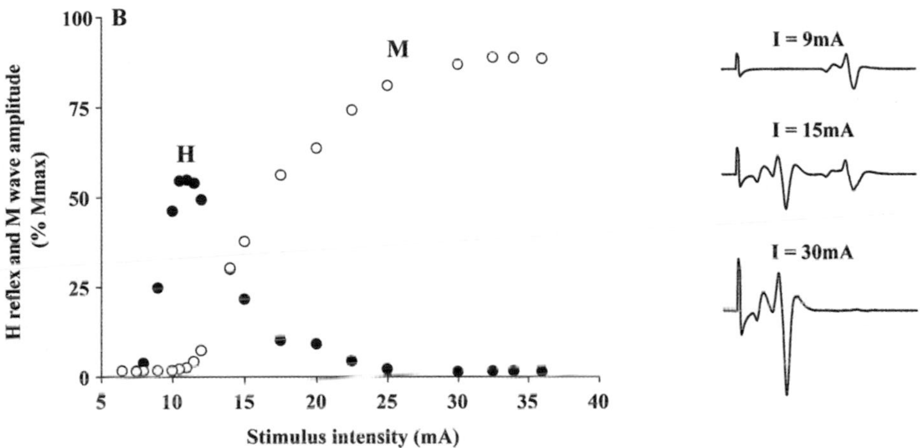

Fig. 40.2 Monosynaptic reflexes and M wave. **(A)** Sketch of the pathway of the monosynaptic reflexes. Ia afferents from muscle spindle primary endings have monosynaptic connections to a motoneurons (MNs) innervating the muscle from which Ia afferents originate. The H-reflex is produced by electrical stimulation of Ia afferents that bypasses the muscle spindle, whereas the T-reflex stretches the muscle spindle and therefore also depends on the gamma drive. The M wave reflects the direct activation of the motor axon. Y-shaped bars represent excitatory connections. **(B)** Recruitment curve of H reflex and M wave in soleus muscle. A weak stimulation activating Ia afferents only (9 mA) results in the electromyogram (EMG) in an H-reflex (*filled circles*), which progressively augments in amplitude with the intensity of the stimulus. A moderate stimulus (15 mA) results in decreased H-reflex amplitude and an M wave (*opened circles*) appears because the threshold for motor axon activation is reached. A strong stimulus (30 mA) produces the maximal motor response (M_{max}) and suppresses the H-reflex because of the collision between the reflex volley and the antidromic motor volley in the motor axons.

only on subjects able to perform a voluntary contraction for ~1 to 2 minutes and, and (2) it suffers from a poor temporal resolution, and the changes in ongoing EMG following the early facilitation are difficult to interpret.[1]

Poststimulus Time Histograms of the Discharge of Single Motor Units

Poststimulus time histograms (PSTHs) (**Fig. 40.1**) rely on the recording of a single isolated motor unit potential during a very weak voluntary contraction. In this technique, changes in firing probability of a voluntary repetitively activated motor unit are determined by constructing a histogram of occurrence of MN discharges, following repeated presentation of a conditioning stimulus. The main advantage of this method is that it allows for investigating single MNs and thus eliminates problems that are linked to the study of an MN pool (see earlier discussion). However, because this method is contingent upon the activation, by the subject, of an isolated motor unit at a rather stable frequency, it is challenging to use it in patients with motor control disorders.

Changes in excitability of human MNs can also be investigated using F-waves, cortical stimulation, and coherence analysis between EMG/EMG or EMG/EEG signals (see Chapters 38 and 42).

To summarize, each technique comes with its advantages and its limitations, given that these noninvasive methods are indirect and explore the excitability of spinal MNs through the "window" of EMG. To probe spinal circuits in healthy subjects, at rest and during various motor activities, the combined use of different methods allows for overcoming their specific drawbacks. In SCI patients, activation of MNs via peripheral inputs (H- or T-reflexes, F-waves) can be used regardless of the impairment of the motor command, whereas methods based on voluntary activation of MNs will be related to the latent motor command capabilities.

Recurrent Inhibition of a Motoneurons

In 1941, Renshaw[2] showed in the cat that antidromic impulses flowing along motor axons inhibit homonymous and synergistic monosynaptic reflexes. This inhibition is due to interneurons (termed Renshaw cells), activated by axon recurrent collaterals, which project back to inhibit MNs (**Fig. 40.3**).

Recurrent inhibition of a MN is the first feedback system described in the CNS and has been extensively studied in the cat.[3] Renshaw cells have projections to (1) both α and γ MNs, even though finger and toe MNs have no recurrent inhibition, (2) Ia inhibitory interneurons, (3) other Renshaw cells, and (4) cells originating in the ventral spinocerebellar tract.

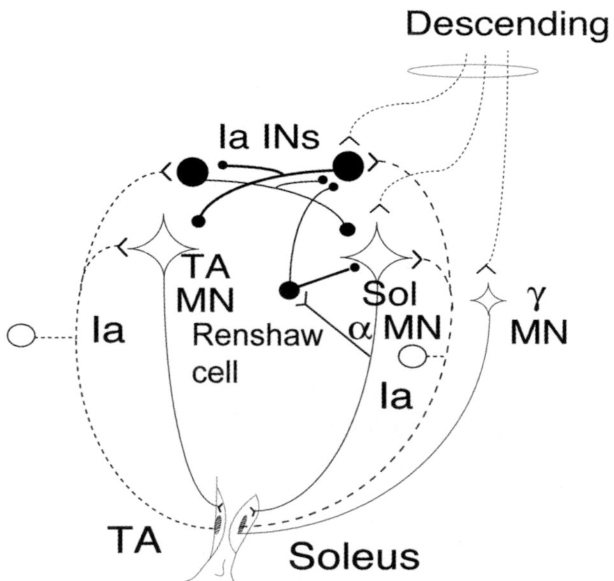

Fig. 40.3 Diagram of reciprocal Ia inhibition at the ankle joint. Y-shaped bars represent excitatory connections and small filled circles represent inhibitory connections. Ia afferents from the soleus (Sol) muscle-spindle primary endings have monosynaptic connections to α motoneurons (MNs) and activate Ia interneurons (Ia INs), inhibiting MNs of the antagonist TA, and vice versa. Ia INs are inhibited by Renshaw cells and by "opposite" Ia INs (i.e., Sol-coupled Ia INs inhibit TA-coupled Ia INs and vice versa). The α (and γ) MNs and their corresponding Ia INs receive a parallel descending input from a higher center.

Study of Homonymous Recurrent Inhibition in Humans: The Paired H-Reflex Technique

The method used in animals to selectively activate Renshaw cells, based on a section of the dorsal roots, is obviously not suitable for human experiments. In the paired H-reflex, Renshaw cells are activated by a conditioning monosynaptic reflex discharge and, for conditioning-test intervals larger than 10 msec, the inhibition of the test reflex is due to recurrent inhibition.[4]

Physiological Changes of Recurrent Inhibition During Voluntary Contractions and Active Maintenance of Posture in Healthy Subjects

During homonymous voluntary tonic contractions of graduated forces, recurrent inhibition is increased during weak contractions, whereas it is decreased during strong ones. This unexpected result has led to the reconsideration of the role of recurrent inhibition, and it has been proposed that it acts as a variable gain regulator at the motor pool level. During antagonistic voluntary contraction, recurrent inhibition is increased and likely contributes to preventing the appearance of a stretch reflex in the noncontracting muscle. During cocontractions or active maintenance of posture, recurrent inhibition is enhanced.[5]

Changes in Recurrent Inhibition in Spinal Cord Injured Patients

Before the development of methods for studying recurrent inhibition in humans, decreased recurrent inhibition had been proposed as a possible mechanism underlying spasticity. In fact, at rest, there is evidence for reinforced recurrent inhibition in SCI patients. Decreased recurrent inhibition was only reported in patients with amyotrophic lateral sclerosis and in patients with hereditary spastic paraparesis. During voluntary agonistic or antagonistic contractions and active maintenance of posture in paraparetic patients, modulations observed in healthy subjects are mostly absent.[5]

■ Reciprocal Ia Inhibition

The relaxation of the muscle antagonistic to that undergoing the contractions is among the mechanisms that have been the most studied in both animals and humans. The pathway of reciprocal Ia inhibition is mediated by a single interneuron (**Fig. 40.3**).[6] In humans, reciprocal inhibition was first described from the tibialis anterior (TA) to the soleus[3] and was then extended to other agonistic/antagonistic muscles acting at the knee, elbow, and wrist joints. The experimental design is simple: a conditioning electrical stimulus is applied to the nerve innervating the antagonistic muscle to that involved in the unconditioned reflex. At both ankle and elbow joints, the pathways of reciprocal inhibition exhibit all the features described in the cat, whereas at the wrist level, the early radial-induced inhibition of the FCR H-reflex is not depressed by activation of extensor carpi radialis (ECR)-coupled Renshaw cells, suggestive of a nonreciprocal group I inhibition.[1]

Physiological Changes of Reciprocal Ia Inhibition During Voluntary Contractions and Maintenance of Posture in Healthy Subjects

During a voluntary contraction, reciprocal Ia inhibition directed to the contracting muscle is decreased, and the stronger the contraction, the weaker the reciprocal inhibition. Results obtained during voluntary contractions of the antagonistic muscle led to controversial results. To sum up, an increase in reciprocal inhibition is revealed when the possible interaction between the "natural" TA Ia volleys generated by the TA contractions and the "artificial" TA Ia volleys generated by the electrical stimulus applied to the CPN is discarded.[1]

Changes in Reciprocal Ia Inhibition in Spinal Cord Injured Patients

Reciprocal Ia inhibition directed from the TA to the soleus has been studied in patients both at rest and during voluntary contractions. At rest, in SCI patients, controversial results have been obtained that may be partly due to methodological issues. Indeed, a weak decreased reciprocal Ia inhibition,[7] a correlation with motor impairment and spasticity,[8] a reinforcement in patients with good recovery,[9] or an early facilitation substituting the inhibition[10] have all been reported. In multiple sclerosis patients, the reciprocal Ia inhibition is reduced.[11,12]

To our knowledge, reciprocal inhibition at the wrist joint has not been investigated in SCI patients.

During voluntary contractions, changes in reciprocal Ia inhibition induced in the soleus H-reflex have been explored in multiple sclerosis patients[13]; the main finding is the absence of reinforced reciprocal Ia inhibition at the onset of antagonistic contractions.

Presynaptic Inhibition of Ia Fibers

In 1957, Frank and Fuortes[14] described in the cat a long-lasting inhibition (~300 msec) without any change in MN membrane potential. Subsequent studies revealed that this inhibition, termed presynaptic Ia inhibition, is due to primary afferent depolarization (PAD) that controls the efficacy of the Ia afferent volley, before its target in the spinal cord. PAD interneurons receive many peripheral and descending controls. The main descending control decreases PAD interneuron excitability and thus reduces presynaptic inhibition even though there is also a weak facilitatory control.[15]

Several techniques have been set up to study presynaptic Ia inhibition in humans. Two commonly used techniques are described here.

D1 Inhibition

D1 inhibition is the long-lasting inhibition that follows reciprocal inhibition (**Fig. 40.4**). This inhibition can be induced in both the soleus[3] and the FCR H-reflexes.[16,17] For specific conditioning-test intervals, the antagonistic nerve stimulation decreases the H-reflex amplitude but not the motor evoked potential (**Fig. 40.4**), suggesting that this inhibition is presynaptic in origin.

Heteronymous Monosynaptic Ia Facilitation of the H-Reflex

This method relies on the fact that a constant conditioning stimulus eliciting a given monosynaptic excitatory postsynaptic potential in MN should induce a constant reflex facilitation, except if the presynaptic Ia inhibition changes.[18] The amount of monosynaptic facilitation can be used to assess the presynaptic inhibition of the Ia fibers: the greater the facilitation, the smaller the presynaptic Ia inhibition.

Physiological Changes of Presynaptic Ia Inhibition During Voluntary Contractions and Maintenance of Posture in Healthy Subjects

The main finding of the experiments performed in the lower limb is that, contrary to what was hypothesized from earlier animal experiments, presynaptic Ia inhibition is accurately adjusted with respect to the motor task. For example, in the lower limb, at the onset of a phasic voluntary contraction of a given muscle, presynaptic inhibition directed to the MNs of the contracting muscle is decreased, whereas presynaptic inhibition of Ia fibers projecting to the synergist noncontracting or antagonistic motor pools is increased. In active maintenance of posture, presynaptic inhibition of Ia fibers projecting to the soleus and quadriceps MNs is increased and unchanged to TA.[1]

Changes in Presynaptic Ia Inhibition in Spinal Cord Injured Patients

Since the findings that a long-lasting vibration depressed the monosynaptic reflex in healthy subjects but not in spastic patients,[19] many studies have been devoted to the possible changes in presynaptic Ia inhibition in spastic patients. The ideas have evolved with the development of selective methods to access presynaptic inhibition. In SCI patients, at ankle level, presynaptic Ia inhibition is decreased whatever the origin of the lesion: traumatic spinal cord lesions, multiple sclerosis, or amyotrophic lateral sclerosis. In the upper limb, presynaptic Ia inhibition projecting to FCR Ia afferents was found to

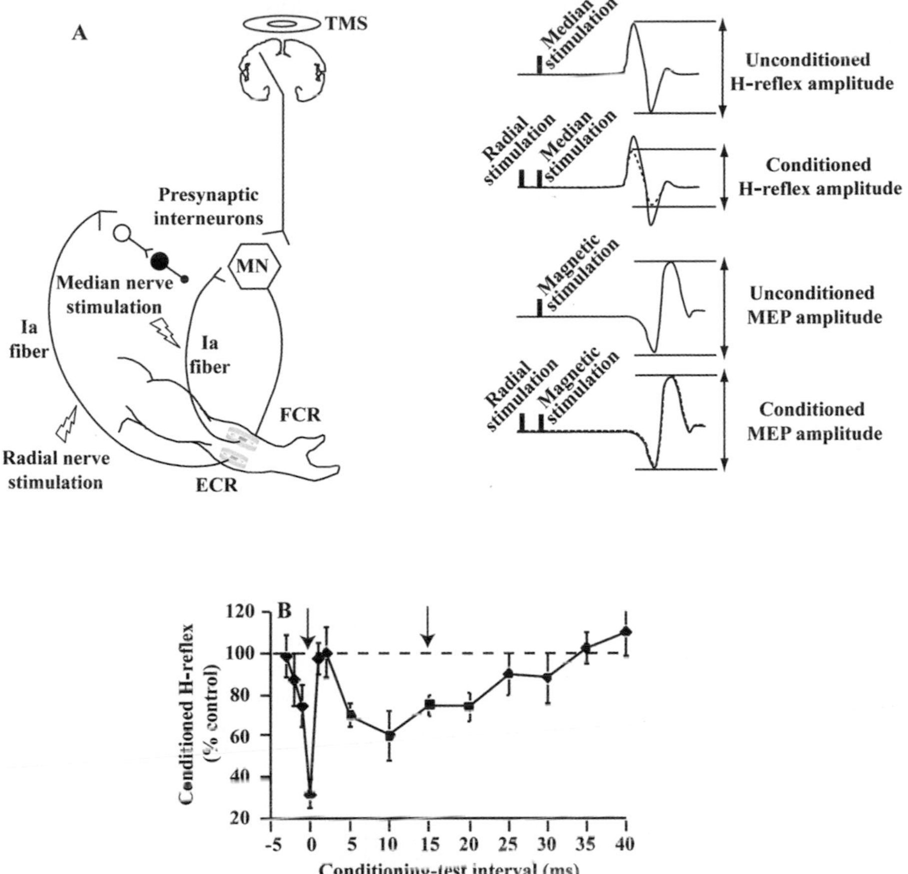

Fig. 40.4 Method of D1 inhibition to assess presynaptic Ia inhibition in humans. **(A)** General methodological arrangement. In this example, unconditioned H-reflex (*continuous line*) is evoked in the flexor carpi radialis (FCR) muscle by stimulation of the median nerve. A conditioning stimulus applied to the radial nerve supplying the antagonist muscle (i.e., radial nerve innervating the extensor carpi radialis—ECR) depresses the H-reflex amplitude (*dashed line*—conditioned H-reflex). However, motor evoked potentials (MEPs), evoked by transcranial magnetic stimulation (TMS) targeting the motor representation of the FCR muscle, is not affected by the radial nerve stimulation (compare unconditioned and conditioned MEPs). This strongly suggests that radial-induced inhibition of the FCR H-reflex occurs before the Ia afferent volley reaches α MN at a presynaptic level. **(B)** Time course of radial-induced depression of the FCR H-reflex. The time interval between conditioned (radial stimulation) and unconditioned (median stimulation) was progressively varied between −5 and +40 msec. Positive intervals mean that the conditioning stimulation is delivered before the unconditioned one, and reciprocally. At a short interval (i.e., ~ 0 msec—*left arrow*), radial-induced depression of the FCR H-reflex is due to reciprocal Ia inhibition, whereas at a longer interval (i.e., ranging from ~ 4 to +35 msec—*right arrow*) it is due to presynaptic Ia inhibition.

be suppressed in two tetraplegic patients. In multiple sclerosis patients, presynaptic inhibition of the soleus Ia terminals is not reinforced at the onset of voluntary ankle dorsiflexion.[1]

Even though most of the studies reported decreased presynaptic inhibition in spastic patients, it is likely that this pathway does not play a key role in the pathophysiology of spasticity: (1) no correlation was found between the severity of spasticity and the extent of decreased presynaptic inhibition, and (2) presynaptic inhibition is also reduced on the unaffected side of stroke patients[20] or in patients with movement disorders other than spasticity, such as dystonia.[21]

Postactivation Depression at the Ia Afferent-α Motoneuron Synapses

The fact that repetitive stimulation of Ia fibers dramatically decreases the size of monosynaptic reflexes was described in both cats and humans in the 1950s. Kuno[22] revealed that in cats this phenomenon is likely due to changes in the probability of transmitter release. Hultborn and Nielsen[23] provided arguments that in humans this phenomenon is presynaptic in origin. In humans, postactivation depression can be easily investigated by measuring changes in H-reflex amplitude following previous activation of Ia fiber muscle, induced either by a stretch reflex or an electrical nerve stimulus adjusted below the motor threshold. The ratio of the size of the H-reflex elicited every 2 seconds to the size of the H-reflex elicited every 8 seconds can be used to quantify the amount of postactivation depression.[20]

Postactivation Depression in Spinal Cord Injured Patients

Postactivation depression has been found to be regularly decreased in spastic SCI patients whatever the origin of the lesion. However, until recently, no significant correlation had been found between the degree of abnormality of a spinal mechanism and the severity of spasticity.[1] Although usually well linked (but not significantly, likely due to the relatively small sample of patients enrolled) to the severity of spasticity in SCI patients, impaired postactivation depression has been shown to be correlated with the intensity of spasticity in a large sample of stroke patients.[20] Even though a correlation cannot be used as a proof of causality, this suggests that decreased postactivation depression may be a contributing factor to the expression of spasticity. In this view, diminished postactivation depression has been suggested to be involved in the transition between flaccid and spastic paralysis, even though it occurred before displaying clinically observable signs of spasticity.[24]

Pearls

- The noninvasive but selective methods developed in the past 40 years in humans to probe spinal circuits rely on recordings of EMG activity and electrical or magnetic stimulation of the nervous system. On the whole, these methods present the following advantages:
  - In uninjured subjects, the combination of the different methods (ongoing EMG, monosynaptic reflexes, motor evoked potentials, poststimulus time histogram) overcomes the drawbacks of each specific method.
  - In injured patients, most of these techniques can be used regardless of the impairment of motor capabilities (with the exception of patients with complete SCI).
  - In injured patients, changes in network excitability implied in motor control are likely to appear before clinical changes; therefore, their study will be a major tool with which to (1) follow-up during the course of recovery, or (2) reveal the effects of new therapeutics before any clinical evidence.

Pitfalls

- In contrast, these techniques are also associated with some inconveniences:
  - Each method available in humans is indirect and has its own specific drawbacks.
  - Both ongoing EMG and poststimulus time histogram rely on the voluntary activation of a target muscle and cannot be used in patients with complete SCI; similarly, changes in network excitability implied in motor control occurring during movement can only be explored in patients who are able to maintain an appreciable contraction.
  - In injured patients, it must be kept in mind that, even if a strong correlation is found between a clinical symptom and the dysfunction of a given network, it is not a definitive proof of causality.

References

1. Pierrot-Deseilligny E, Burke D. The Circuitry of the Human Spinal Cord: Its Role in Motor Control and Movement Disorders. Cambridge: Cambridge University Press; 2005
2. Renshaw B. Influence of discharge of motoneurones upon excitation of neighboring motoneurons. J Neurophysiol 1941;4:167–183
3. Mizuno Y, Tanaka R, Yanagisawa N. Reciprocal group I inhibition on triceps surae motoneurons in man. J Neurophysiol 1971;34(6):1010–1017
4. Bussel B, Pierrot-Deseilligny E. Inhibition of human motoneurons, probably of Renshaw origin, elicited by an orthodromic motor discharge. J Physiol 1977;269(2):319–339
5. Katz R, Pierrot-Deseilligny E. Recurrent inhibition in humans. Prog Neurobiol 1999;57(3): 325–355
6. Baldissera F, Hultborn H, Illert M. Integration in spinal neuronal systems. In: Brook VB, ed. Handbook of Physiology, Sect. I, The Nervous System, Vol. II Motor Control. Bethesda, MD: American Physiological Society 1981:509–595
7. Perez MA, Field-Fote EC. Impaired posture-dependent modulation of disynaptic reciprocal Ia inhibition in individuals with incomplete spinal cord injury. Neurosci Lett 2003;341(3):225–228
8. Okuma Y, Mizuno Y, Lee RG. Reciprocal Ia inhibition in patients with asymmetric spinal spasticity. Clin Neurophysiol 2002;113(2):292–297
9. Boorman G, Hulliger M, Lee RG, Tako K, Tanaka R. Reciprocal Ia inhibition in patients with spinal spasticity. Neurosci Lett 1991;127(1):57–60
10. Crone C, Johnsen LL, Biering-Sørensen F, Nielsen JB. Appearance of reciprocal facilitation of ankle extensors from ankle flexors in patients with stroke or spinal cord injury. Brain 2003;126(Pt 2):495–507
11. Crone C, Nielsen J, Petersen N, Ballegaard M, Hultborn H. Disynaptic reciprocal inhibition of ankle extensors in spastic patients. Brain 1994;117(Pt 5):1161–1168
12. Ørsnes G, Crone C, Krarup C, Petersen N, Nielsen J. The effect of baclofen on the transmission in spinal pathways in spastic multiple sclerosis patients. Clin Neurophysiol 2000;111(8):1372–1379
13. Morita H, Crone C, Christenhuis D, Petersen NT, Nielsen JB. Modulation of presynaptic inhibition and disynaptic reciprocal Ia inhibition during voluntary movement in spasticity. Brain 2001; 124(Pt 4):826–837
14. Frank K, Fuortes M. Presynaptic and postsynaptic inhibition of monosynaptic reflexes. Fed Proc 1957;16:39–40
15. Rudomin P, Schmidt RF. Presynaptic inhibition in the vertebrate spinal cord revisited. Exp Brain Res 1999;129(1):1–37
16. Day BL, Marsden CD, Obeso JA, Rothwell JC. Reciprocal inhibition between the muscles of the human forearm. J Physiol 1984;349:519–534
17. Berardelli A, Day BL, Marsden CD, Rothwell JC. Evidence favouring presynaptic inhibition between antagonist muscle afferents in the human forearm. J Physiol 1987;391:71–83
18. Hultborn H, Meunier S, Morin C, Pierrot-Deseilligny E. Assessing changes in presynaptic inhibition of I a fibres: a study in man and the cat. J Physiol 1987;389:729–756
19. Delwaide PJ. Human monosynaptic reflexes and presynaptic inhibition. In: Desmedt, JE, ed. New Developments in Electromyography and Clinical Neurophysiology, Vol. 3. Munchen: Karger-Basel 1973:508–522
20. Lamy JC, Wargon I, Mazevet D, Ghanim Z, Pradat-Diehl P, Katz R. Impaired efficacy of spinal presynaptic mechanisms in spastic stroke patients. Brain 2009;132(Pt 3):734–748
21. Nakashima K, Rothwell JC, Day BL, Thompson PD, Shannon K, Marsden CD. Reciprocal inhibition between forearm muscles in patients with writer's cramp and other occupational cramps, symptomatic hemidystonia and hemiparesis due to stroke. Brain 1989;112(Pt 3):681–697
22. Kuno M. Mechanism of Facilitation and Depression of the Excitatory Synaptic Potential in Spinal Motoneurones. J Physiol 1964;175:100–112
23. Hultborn H, Nielsen JB. Modulation of transmitter release from Ia afferents by their preceding activity: a "post-activation depression." In: Rudomin P, Romo R, Mendell L, eds. Presynaptic Inhibition and Neural Control. New York: Oxford University Press; 1998:178–191
24. Schindler-Ivens S, Shields RK. Low frequency depression of H-reflexes in humans with acute and chronic spinal-cord injury. Exp Brain Res 2000; 133(2):233–241

41

Neuroimaging after Spinal Cord Injury: Evaluating Injury Severity and Prognosis Using Magnetic Resonance Imaging

Maxwell Boakye

Key Points

1. The presence of hematoma at injury level on MRI is generally associated with the worst outcomes.
2. Significantly decreased fractional anisotropy (FA) values occur at injury levels in patients with acute cervical spine cord injury compared with normal volunteers. Tractography may be used to visualize residual tracts after injury in the near future.
3. Functional MRI studies of the brain show significant reorganizational changes in the sensorimotor cortex after spinal cord injury.

Magnetic resonance imaging (MRI) is essential in the evaluation and management of spinal cord injury (SCI) and is considered the imaging modality of choice for identification of ligamentous injury, hematoma, disk compression, spinal cord edema, and myelomalacia. This chapter reviews the role of MRI in the evaluation of injury severity and prediction of recovery, with a focus on identification of parameters that have been found to be useful markers of injury severity. Chapter 3 discusses the clinical use of MRI in the determination of injury characteristics and classification and for the initial treatment planning for patients in the emergency room. This chapter focuses on identifying findings on conventional MRI that can be helpful in predicting outcome. It also describes emerging MRI technologies not currently routinely used in clinical care but likely to find utility in the near future.

■ Conventional Magnetic Resonance Imaging for Spinal Cord Injury

The pattern of MRI findings has been of great interest for assessment of injury severity and prognosis. **Table 41.1** lists the most common qualitative MRI findings shown in

Table 41.1 Potential Predictive Markers in Spinal Cord Injury

Qualitative MRI predictors
• Presence of hematoma • Edema or signal change on T2-weighted images • Cord compression • Cord transection
Quantitative MRI predictors
• Maximal canal compromise • Maximal spinal cord compression • Length of edema • Length of hematoma
Other potential predictors
• Fractional anisotropy in diffusion tensor imaging studies • Tractography • N-acetylaspartate and N-acetylaspartate:creatine ratios on magnetic resonance spectroscopy studies

peer-reviewed studies to correlate with injury severity and recovery.[1–4] Lammertse et al.[5] provide a systematic review. The presence of hematoma is generally associated with the worst outcomes.[1,6–9] Traumatic spinal cord hematoma is best identified as focal decreased signal on T2-weighted (**Fig. 41.1**) or gradient echo images. Quantitative parameters shown to adversely impact recovery are the length of cord edema or signal change,[2,3] extent or size of hematoma,[1,4] and degree of spinal cord compression.[3] The degree of spinal cord compression can be calculated in two ways[10]: The maximal canal compromise (MCC) and maximal spinal cord compression (MSCC) are defined by the following equations[3,10]:

$$MSCC\,(\%) = [1 - (\frac{di}{(da + db)/2})] \times 100\%$$

$$MCC\,(\%) = [1 - (\frac{Di}{(Da + Db)/2})] \times 100\%$$

Di represents the anteroposterior canal diameter at the level of maximum injury, Da is the anteroposterior canal diameter at the nearest normal level above the site of injury, and Db is the anteroposterior canal diameter at the nearest normal level below the site of injury; di is the anteroposterior spinal cord diameter at the level of maximum injury, da is the anteroposterior spinal cord diameter at the nearest normal level above the site of injury, and db is the anteroposterior spinal cord diameter at the nearest normal level below the site of injury. The use of the MCC and MSCC has

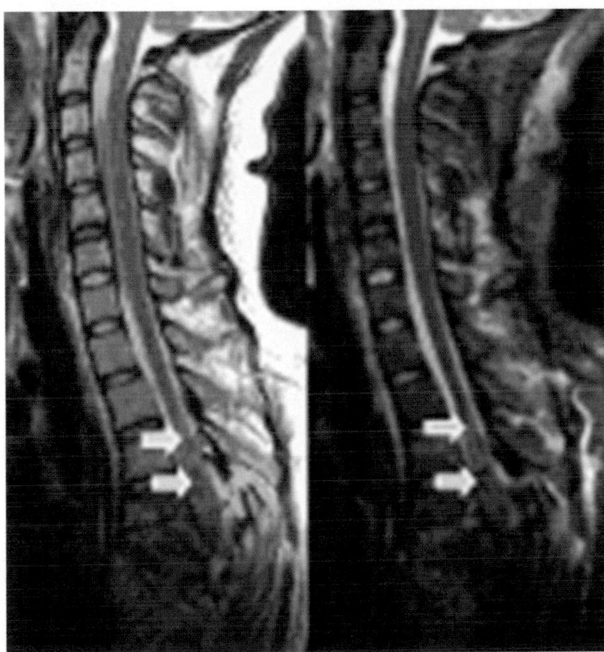

Fig. 41.1 A 23-year-old female status post–motor vehicle accident with T3–5 spinal cord injury. Sagittal fast spin echo T2-weighted image (*left*) and sagittal short T1-weighted inversion recovery (STIR) images. The low signal in the middle of the cord (*orange arrow*) is hematoma. There is also significant edema (*blue arrows*).

been shown to have good interrater reliability and to be predictive of severity of injury.[3,10] **Figure 41.2** is an MRI scan of a 41-year-old patient with a C6-7 fracture dislocation SCI and illustrates severe spinal cord compression and canal compromise at the injury level.

Over all, MRI appears to be of tremendous value in augmenting the clinical exam and American Spinal Injury Association (ASIA) scale and motor scores, which are considered to be the best predictors of neurological recovery.[7,11] Attention to details on the MRI will provide further information on prognostication in patients with the same ASIA grade or motor score. The main limitation of MRI in SCI prognostication is its inability to identify spared white matter tracts. This disadvantage may be overcome with the development of diffusion tensor imaging (DTI) technology.

■ Diffusion Tensor Imaging

DTI is a relatively new imaging modality that can permit the imaging of directional asymmetry in the diffusion of water protons to make maps of white matter fiber bundles. This is an established technique in the brain, and early reports suggest that it is likely to be of significant use in the evaluation of SCI and diseases. DTI has potentially two main uses in SCI. The first is tractography, which is a technique to visualize the white matter tracts and therefore is of interest in identifying residual pathways after injury.[12] A second area of interest is generation of quantitative parameters with prognostication value. The fractional anisotropy is one of several quantitative parameters that are mathematically derived from the eigenvalues of the diffusion tensor. The role of quantitative parameters like the fractional anisotropy in predicting injury severity and prognosis is the subject of intense research. The fractional anisotropy is a value between 0 (isotropic or unrestricted diffusion along all axes) and 1 (restricted diffusion along a single axis). It is a measure of white matter axonal diameter, myelination, and fiber density. It can be calculated using the following formulas:

$$FA = \frac{\sqrt{3\{(\lambda_1 - \lambda)^2 + (\lambda_2 - \lambda)^2 + (\lambda_3 - \lambda)^2\}}}{\sqrt{2(\lambda_1^2 + \lambda_2^2 + \lambda_3^2)}}$$

where $\lambda = \frac{\lambda_1 + \lambda_2 + \lambda_3}{3}$ and $(\lambda_1, \lambda_2, \lambda_3)$ are the eigenvalues of the diffusion tensor.

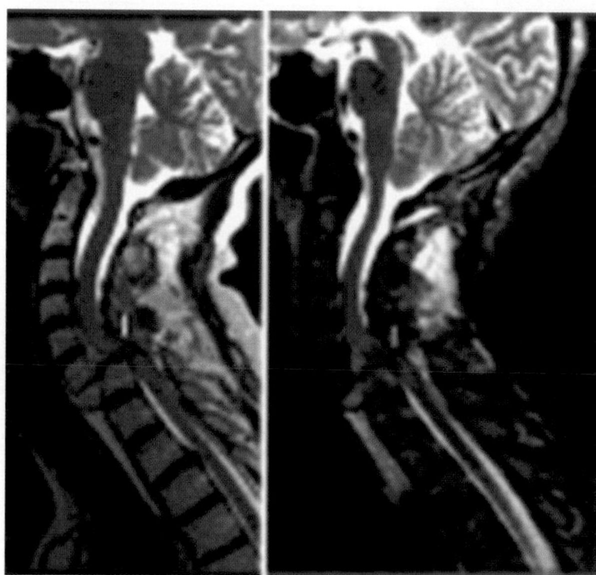

Fig. 41.2 A 41-year-old patient status post–motor vehicle accident with a C6–7 fracture dislocation injury. Sagittal fast spin echo T2 (*left image*) and sagittal short T1-weighted inversion recovery (STIR) showing significant dislocation, cord compression, and severe canal compromise at C6–7 (*white bars*).

Ellingson et al.[13] performed DTI in 13 neurologically intact subjects and 10 subjects with chronic SCI (> 4 years postinjury). They found that the fractional anisotropy was significantly lower at the chronic lesion site, and the extent of reduction in FA appeared dependent on the completeness of the injury. Similarly, Shanmuganathan et al.[14] reported significantly decreased lesional FA values in 20 symptomatic patients with acute cervical spine trauma compared with normal volunteers. To date there have been no studies of correlations between FA values and clinical scores in acute SCI patients, and a central role of DTI for injury prognostication is premature at the present time. **Figure 41.3** illustrates a DTI study in a patient with a 9 year history of C7 ASIA B chronic SCI showing significantly reduced fractional anisotropy at the injury site. The corresponding tractography images illustrate few fibers below the injury site. There was no recovery of lower extremity motor function.

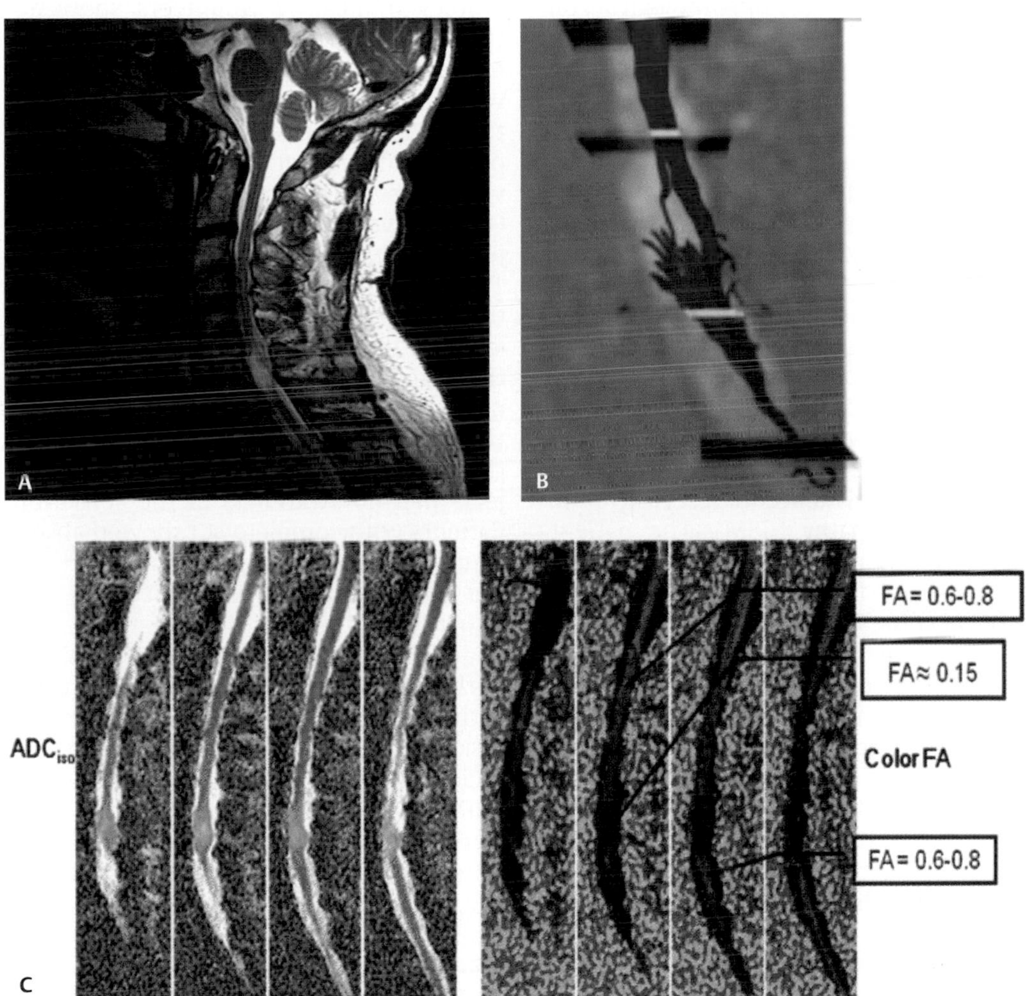

Fig. 41.3 A 61-year-old patient with a C7 American Spinal Injury Association (ASIA) B injury from a motor vehicle accident in 2000. **(A)** Sagittal T2-weighted image showing focal C7 signal change and myelomalacia. **(B)** Tractography images show few fibers (*red and blue*) below the lesion site. Diffusion tensor images are shown: ADC (**C**, *left*) and fractional anisotropy (**C**, *right*) are shown. There is significantly reduced fractional anisotropy at the C7 injury site.

Magnetic Resonance Spectroscopy

Magnetic resonance spectroscopy is commonly used to provide cellular and metabolic information in the brain and has proven useful in the differential diagnosis of intracranial pathology. Typical spectral peaks of interest are the N-acetylaspartate (NAA), choline (Cho), creatine (Cr), and lactate.[15] NAA is considered a marker of neuronal density and loss. Decreases in NAA are reflective of axonal loss. Creatine is a marker of energy metabolism. Its peak is stable under a variety of pathological conditions and is therefore used as an internal control for calculating metabolite ratios, such as Cho:Cr and NAA:Cr ratios. Cho is a metabolic marker of membrane density and integrity and is influenced by phospholipid synthesis and degradation and cellular turnover. Lactate levels increase significantly under conditions of anaerobic metabolism, as in failure of aerobic oxidation during ischemia.

Recently, the technique has been applied in the evaluation of cervical spondylotic myelopathy by Holly et al.[16] They performed magnetic resonance spectroscopy (MRS) in 21 patients with clinical and radiographic evidence of cervical spondylotic myelopathy (CSM). The patients underwent preoperative neurological examination, functional assessment, and cervical spine MRS. MRS spectra peaks for NAA, Cho, lactate (Lac), and Cr were measured using voxels placed at the C2 level. Thirteen age-matched healthy volunteers served as controls. The NAA:Cr ratio was significantly lower in patients with CSM than in controls. The Cho:Cr ratio was not significantly different between the two groups. Seven of the patients with CSM had a Lac peak, whereas no peaks were noted in the control group ($p < 0.05$). The authors concluded that the reduced NAA:Cr was likely due to axonal and neuronal loss, whereas the presence of Lac peaks in a third of the patients was supportive of the role of ischemia. Other studies have documented reduced NAA concentrations in multiple sclerosis patients.[17] Further studies are needed to establish a prognostic role for MRS in acute SCI.

Functional Magnetic Resonance Imaging

Functional magnetic resonance imaging (fMRI) techniques can be used to measure the pattern and extent of activation in brain regions in response to motor and sensory tasks. Recently, several groups have performed fMRI of the spinal cord. Studies in healthy volunteers show activation patterns corresponding to anatomical location of the activated myotome, with a signal intensity proportional to the intensity of effort.[18–20] Stroman et al.[18] performed fMRI of the spinal cord in 27 volunteers with cervical or thoracic SCIs. Of these volunteers, 18 had complete injuries, and nine had incomplete injuries. Thermal stimulation at 10°C was applied to the fourth lumbar dermatome on each leg, and images were obtained of the entire lumbar spinal cord. Areas of neuronal activity were consistently observed in the lumbar spinal cord in response to the thermal stimulation, even when the subjects had no awareness of the sensation. Patients with complete SCI showed absent or diminished dorsal gray matter activity but had enhanced ventral activity, particularly contralateral to the stimulation. In another study, Kornelsen and Stroman[21] performed fMRI of the spinal cord using active and passive lower limb movement tasks in 12 volunteers with cervical or thoracic SCIs. Activity was detected in all volunteers regardless of the extent of injury. During both active and passive participation, activity was seen caudal to the injury site, although the number of active voxels detected with passive movement was less than with the active movement task. Over all, there are limited clinical studies of spinal cord fMRI, but the technique has the potential for monitoring and anatomically localizing functional areas of intact cord within injured spinal cord.

■ Brain fMRI and Plasticity after Spinal Cord Injury

Functional MRI studies of the brain show significant reorganizational changes in the sensorimotor cortex (**Table 41.2**). Kokotilo et al. provide a systematic review.[22] Two patterns of activation are generally observed. The first pattern involves alteration of volumes of activation in the motor and associated motor cortices and/or creation of new areas of activation. In the systematic review,[22] five studies showed increased activation in several motor cortical areas. Areas of activation common to the five studies included bilateral primary motor cortex (M1), supplementary motor area (SMA), premotor area, cingulate motor area, and contralateral primary somatosensory cortex (S1). In addition, there were new areas of activation in bilateral cerebellum, thalamus, and basal ganglia compared with controls. Three studies reported activation patterns similar to controls, and two studies reported reduced activation in these areas.

The second reorganizational pattern involves changes in somatotopy. This generally takes two forms: posterior displacements of motor activation maxima into the primary somatosensory cortex[23,24] and displacement of cortical representations of rostral muscles into areas previously represented by the deafferented area. Examples of the latter include activation of the leg area by hand movements[25] or superior and medial shift of activation foci for tongue movements into the hand area.[26] In a recent study of six patients with chronic SCI, Lotze et al. demonstrated a displacement of 11.9 mm of biceps brachii cortical maps into the

Table 41.2 Some fMRI Studies of Sensorimotor Cortical Plasticity in Spinal Cord Injury (SCI) Patients

Author and date	Study description	Results
Curt et al., 2002[29]	fMRI study of nine patients with chronic SCI injuries, L1–4	No change in somatotopy of upper limb representations; increased activation in M1, SMA, S1, cerebellum, parietal lobe
Lotze et al., 1999[30]	fMRI study of four patients with subacute and chronic injuries	Change in somatotopy with cranial shift of elbow representation
Turner et al., 2003[24]	fMRI study of 13 patients with chronic SCI injuries between T2 and L1	Posterior shift of hand motor representation in SCI group
Mikulis et al., 2002[26]	fMRI study of nine patients with chronic SCI, C4–7	Superior and medial shift of tongue movement representations
Alkadhi et al., 2005[31]	fMRI study of eight chronic SCI patients, T3–L1	Greater activation in SCI patients on imagined foot movements
Cramer et al., 2005[23]	fMRI study of 12 patients with chronic SCI, C5–T6	Reduced activation on leg movement; posterior shift of sensorimotor activation during imagined movement
Lotze et al., 2006[27]	fMRI study of six patients with chronic SCI T3–T11	Displacement of elbow cortical maps into deafferented thoracic area
Jurkiewicz et al., 2007[32]	Longitudinal fMRI study of six patients with acute C5–8 cervical injury	Initial injury associated with decreased contralateral M1 activation and increased secondary motor activations after injury; increased contralateral M1 activation and decreased secondary motor activation during recovery
Jurkiewicz et al., 2009[33]	fMRI study of four patients with persistent paralysis after injury	Progressive decrease in M1 activation and decrease in activation in associated motor areas

thoracic deafferented area.[27] The finding of posterior shifts in motor cortical activity in SCI patients compared with controls is in agreement with an electroencephalographic (EEG) study.[28] Increased posterior displacement of motor activity may be related to increased somatomasensory activation due to neuropathic pain or increased contribution of S1 to the corticospinal tract deprived of M1 input.[22] In general, mechanisms of reorganization are poorly understood.

There are a significant number of contradictory results reported by brain fMRI studies in SCI patients. For example, although some studies reported increased motor cortical activation, others found no increases. In patients with thoracic injury, some studies reported that movements of unaffected upper extremity muscles generate greater activation volumes.[25,29] Other studies failed to find increases in activation volumes of unaffected upper extremity muscles.[30] Imaginary movements of lower extremity affected muscles seem to show increased activation in some studies[31] but decreased activation in another study.[23] The discrepancies in the literature may be due to differing age groups, injury types, injury levels, and rehabilitation regimens between studies.[22]

The amount and pattern of activation can be influenced by the completeness of the lesion, the level of injury, the use of rehabilitative interventions, and the time after injury. Kokotilo et al.[22] found in their systematic review that 24/25 patients with posterior shifts in activation had complete injuries and suggested that posterior displacements may be more common than anterior displacements in complete SCI. They also noted that posterior shifts of activation maxima may be more common in thoracic injury level and higher lesions (70/83 patients), whereas medial shifts of activation foci tended to occur in lower lesions (24/36 patients). Using positron emission tomography ([15O]-H_2O-PET), Bruehlmeier et al.[25] studied paraplegics performing hand movements. The extent of activation of contralateral sensorimotor cortex, supplementary motor area, and ipsilateral cerebellum correlated with the number of disconnected spinal segments (i.e., patients with higher thoracic injuries had greater changes in cerebral activation). Curt[29] showed greater activation in paraplegic patients compared with tetraplegic patients in response to movements of the wrist and concluded that differences were likely related to differential impairment of wrist movements in tetraplegic patients.

The amount of reorganizational plasticity is a dynamic process that evolves over time. Jurkiewicz et al. performed a longitudinal study of six patients with C5–8 SCI.[32] Three patients were studied at 1, 3, 6, and 12 months after injury. Two patients were studied at 0.25, 1, 3, and 12 months and at 0.25, 3, and 6 months. The last patient was studied at 6, 9, and 12 months. Three patients had ASIA A injuries, and three had ASIA B injuries. During a right wrist extension task, fMRI was performed. The outcome was evaluated using ASIA motor scores. The authors reported greater activation of secondary sensorimotor cortical activity and minimal contralateral primary motor cortical (M1) activity at the initial scanning. During recovery, they found increased task-related activation in M1 activation and decreased activation in the secondary motor areas. Although the number of patients was small, the study demonstrated for the first time the evolution of sensorimotor cortical plasticity during recovery from traumatic cervical SCI. In a subsequent study in four tetraplegic patients with persistent paralysis, they found significantly decreased activation in M1 and progressive decrease in activation in the associated sensorimotor areas.[33]

■ Brain fMRI Changes after Training

The amount of cortical plasticity can also be influenced by training and rehabilitation. Winchester et al.[34] performed fMRI studies before and after 12 weeks of robotic body weight-supported treadmill training in four subjects with chronic SCI. All four subjects showed increased activation of the sensorimotor cortex after training. Substantial improvement in locomotor ability was present in two subjects who showed significant increase in cerebellum. Although the number of subjects was small, it illustrates the potential of fMRI to identify brain areas where activation correlates with training effects.

Conclusion

A variety of neuroimaging tools discussed in this chapter have become available for assessment of SCI. Research using these tools is necessary to assess their value beyond the ASIA clinical exam. The availability of these neuroimaging technologies promises to significantly increase our ability to evaluate SCIs, predict recovery, and assess plasticity after injury.

Pearls

- The presence of hematoma or extensive signal change on T2-weighted MRI is generally associated with poor outcomes.
- Complete injuries do not disrupt ability of the brain activation with imaginary movements of the impaired muscle. Future technology may be able to harness the preservation of motor cortical activity for activation of a brain neuroprosthesis.
- Complete injuries as determined by the ASIA clinical exam do not necessarily mean a complete loss of anatomical continuity of white matter tracts.

Pitfalls

- Ignoring the pattern of MRI findings may miss potentially important injury prognostication data.
- Longitudinal SCI studies should control for injury timing, type of rehabilitation, completeness, and injury-level factors that affect amount of plasticity after injury.

References

1. Boldin C, Raith J, Fankhauser F, Haunschmid C, Schwantzer G, Schweighofer F. Predicting neurologic recovery in cervical spinal cord injury with postoperative MR imaging. Spine 2006; 31(5):554–559
2. Flanders AE, Spettell CM, Friedman DP, Marino RJ, Herbison GJ. The relationship between the functional abilities of patients with cervical spinal cord injury and the severity of damage revealed by MR imaging. AJNR Am J Neuroradiol 1999;20(5):926–934
3. Miyanji F, Furlan JC, Aarabi B, Arnold PM, Fehlings MG. Acute cervical traumatic spinal cord injury: MR imaging findings correlated with neurologic outcome—prospective study with 100 consecutive patients. Radiology 2007;243(3):820–827
4. Selden NR, Quint DJ, Patel N, d'Arcy HS, Papadopoulos SM. Emergency magnetic resonance imaging of cervical spinal cord injuries: clinical correlation and prognosis. Neurosurgery 1999;44(4): 785–792, discussion 792–793
5. Lammertse D, Dungan D, Dreisbach J, et al; National Institute on Disability and Rehabilitation. Neuroimaging in traumatic spinal cord injury: an evidence-based review for clinical practice and research. J Spinal Cord Med 2007;30(3):205–214
6. Flanders AE, Spettell CM, Tartaglino LM, Friedman DP, Herbison GJ. Forecasting motor recovery after cervical spinal cord injury: value of MR imaging. Radiology 1996;201(3):649–655
7. Kirshblum SC, O'Connor KC. Predicting neurologic recovery in traumatic cervical spinal cord injury. Arch Phys Med Rehabil 1998;79(11): 1456–1466
8. Marciello MA, Flanders AE, Herbison GJ, Schaefer DM, Friedman DP, Lane JI. Magnetic resonance imaging related to neurologic outcome in cervical spinal cord injury. Arch Phys Med Rehabil 1993;74(9):940–946
9. Ramón S, Domínguez R, Ramírez L, et al. Clinical and magnetic resonance imaging correlation in acute spinal cord injury. Spinal Cord 1997; 35(10):664–673
10. Furlan JC, Fehlings MG, Massicotte EM, et al. A quantitative and reproducible method to assess cord compression and canal stenosis after cervical spine trauma: a study of interrater and intrarater reliability. Spine 2007;32(19):2083–2091
11. Maynard FM Jr, Bracken MB, Creasey G, et al; American Spinal Injury Association. International Standards for Neurological and Functional Classification of Spinal Cord Injury. Spinal Cord 1997;35(5):266–274

12. Thurnher MM, Law M. Diffusion-weighted imaging, diffusion-tensor imaging, and fiber tractography of the spinal cord. Magn Reson Imaging Clin N Am 2009;17(2):225–244
13. Ellingson BM, Ulmer JL, Kurpad SN, Schmit BD. Diffusion tensor MR imaging in chronic spinal cord injury. AJNR Am J Neuroradiol 2008; 29(10):1976–1982
14. Shanmuganathan K, Gullapalli RP, Zhuo J, Mirvis SE. Diffusion tensor MR imaging in cervical spine trauma. AJNR Am J Neuroradiol 2008;29(4): 655–659
15. Soares DP, Law M. Magnetic resonance spectroscopy of the brain: review of metabolites and clinical applications. Clin Radiol 2009;64(1): 12–21
16. Holly LT, Freitas B, McArthur DL, Salamon N. Proton magnetic resonance spectroscopy to evaluate spinal cord axonal injury in cervical spondylotic myelopathy. J Neurosurg Spine 2009;10(3): 194–200
17. Ciccarelli O, Wheeler-Kingshott CA, McLean MA, et al. Spinal cord spectroscopy and diffusion-based tractography to assess acute disability in multiple sclerosis. Brain 2007;130(Pt 8):2220–2231
18. Stroman PW, Kornelsen J, Bergman A, et al. Noninvasive assessment of the injured human spinal cord by means of functional magnetic resonance imaging. Spinal Cord 2004;42(2):59–66
19. Stroman PW. Magnetic resonance imaging of neuronal function in the spinal cord: spinal FMRI. Clin Med Res 2005;3(3):146–156
20. Xie CH, Kong KM, Guan JT, et al. SSFSE sequence functional MRI of the human cervical spinal cord with complex finger tapping. Eur J Radiol 2009; 70(1):1–6
21. Kornelsen J, Stroman PW. fMRI of the lumbar spinal cord during a lower limb motor task. Magn Reson Med 2004;52(2):411–414
22. Kokotilo KJ, Eng JJ, Curt A. Reorganization and preservation of motor control of the brain in spinal cord injury: a systematic review. J Neurotrauma 2009;26(11):2113–2126
23. Cramer SC, Lastra L, Lacourse MG, Cohen MJ. Brain motor system function after chronic, complete spinal cord injury. Brain 2005;128(Pt 12): 2941–2950
24. Turner JA, Lee JS, Schandler SL, Cohen MJ. An fMRI investigation of hand representation in paraplegic humans. Neurorehabil Neural Repair 2003; 17(1):37–47
25. Bruehlmeier M, Dietz V, Leenders KL, Roelcke U, Missimer J, Curt A. How does the human brain deal with a spinal cord injury? Eur J Neurosci 1998;10(12):3918–3922
26. Mikulis DJ, Jurkiewicz MT, McIlroy WE, et al. Adaptation in the motor cortex following cervical spinal cord injury. Neurology 2002;58(5): 794–801
27. Lotze M, Laubis-Herrmann U, Topka H. Combination of TMS and fMRI reveals a specific pattern of reorganization in M1 in patients after complete spinal cord injury. Restor Neurol Neurosci 2006; 24(2):97–107
28. Green JB, Sora E, Bialy Y, Ricamato A, Thatcher RW. Cortical sensorimotor reorganization after spinal cord injury: an electroencephalographic study. Neurology 1998;50(4):1115–1121
29. Curt A, Alkadhi H, Crelier GR, Boendermaker SH, Hepp-Reymond MC, Kollias SS. Changes of non-affected upper limb cortical representation in paraplegic patients as assessed by fMRI. Brain 2002;125(Pt 11):2567–2578
30. Lotze M, Laubis-Herrmann U, Topka H, Erb M, Grodd W. Reorganization in the primary motor cortex after spinal cord injury: a functional magnetic resonance (fMRI) study. Restor Neurol Neurosci 1999;14(2-3):183–187
31. Alkadhi H, Brugger P, Boendermaker SH, et al. What disconnection tells about motor imagery: evidence from paraplegic patients. Cereb Cortex 2005;15(2):131–140
32. Jurkiewicz MT, Mikulis DJ, McIlroy WE, Fehlings MG, Verrier MC. Sensorimotor cortical plasticity during recovery following spinal cord injury: a longitudinal fMRI study. Neurorehabil Neural Repair 2007;21(6):527–538
33. Jurkiewicz MT, Mikulis DJ, Fehlings MG, Verrier MC. Sensorimotor cortical activation in patients with cervical spinal cord injury with persisting paralysis. Neurorehabil Neural Repair 2010; 24(2):136–140
34. Winchester P, McColl R, Querry R, et al. Changes in supraspinal activation patterns following robotic locomotor therapy in motor-incomplete spinal cord injury. Neurorehabil Neural Repair 2005; 19(4):313–324

42

The Role of Neurophysiology in the Study of Recovery and Spasticity

Jens Bo Nielsen

Key Points

1. Transcranial magnetic stimulation
2. Corticomuscular coherence
3. Galvanic stimulation
4. Auditory startle reactions
5. Treatment of spasticity

Optimal individualized intervention following lesions in the central nervous system requires a detailed understanding of the structures and pathways that have been damaged in the individual patient. Furthermore, plastic changes occurring spontaneously or in response to intervention must be monitored to evaluate the efficiency of treatment. These plastic changes involve structures above the lesion, the spinal neuronal circuitries below the lesion, and the interaction between supraspinal and spinal circuitries. Most of these plastic changes are not apparent anatomically and are therefore out of reach for imaging techniques. The anatomical extent of a spinal lesion is also often not well correlated to the functional deficit.[1] Physiological techniques by which transmission in specific spinal and supraspinal pathways may be evaluated are therefore of paramount importance for the evaluation of the underlying mechanisms of plastic changes and recovery of function following spinal cord lesions. This chapter reviews the present state of these techniques and sketches their use in evaluation of plastic changes in the nervous system in relation to (1) recovery of function following spinal cord lesion and (2) the development of spasticity.

■ Evaluation of Transmission in the Corticospinal Tract

The use of transcranial magnetic stimulation (TMS) to evaluate transmission in surviving corticospinal tract fibers following spinal cord lesion is reviewed in other chapters. Here, it should only be added that the latency and amplitude of motor evoked potentials (MEPs) recorded at rest or during weak static voluntary activation of the target muscle, which is the normal standardized procedure, may not provide a fully functionally relevant measure of the subject's ability to use the remaining corticospinal connectivity to control the full range of voluntary movements. It should therefore be noted that techniques are now available that allow the use of TMS during functional motor tasks, such as standing,[2] walking,[3,4] and even jumping and hopping.[5] TMS may also be used during these motor tasks to condition Hoffmann reflexes (H-reflexes) (**Fig. 42.1A**) and in this way obtain specific information of task-related changes in activity of specific corticospinal pathways to the spinal motoneurons.[4] This kind of information has the potential to provide a more specific and more functionally relevant indication of plastic changes in the recruitment of corticospinal pathways for control of specific tasks following spinal cord lesions and may turn out to be more optimal physiological outcome measures than the routine MEP measurements in sitting subjects.

However, such measurements are not easy to do, especially in a routine clinical setting, and TMS also has the drawback that it involves an external stimulation of the corticospinal system and thus does not necessarily reflect the (unperturbed) normal neural activity in the pathway. Coherence and cross-correlation of electroencephalographic (EEG) and electromyographic (EMG) signals therefore provide attractive alternative techniques for evaluation of corticospinal transmission.[6,7] With these techniques, events in different biological signals (such as EEG or EMG) that are time- or phase-locked to each other may be revealed. Activity in the motor cortex measured by EEG and in a voluntarily activated muscle measured by EMG thus show coupling in both the time and frequency domain reflecting the corticospinal activation of the muscle and the resulting sensory feedback.[8] This corticomuscular coupling has also been shown to be greatly reduced or absent following lesion of both descending and ascending pathways in patients with stroke.[9] The appearance of corticomuscular coupling also coincides closely with the development of the corticospinal tract and the acquisition of an adult-like control of fine finger movements during childhood.[10] Different motor unit populations within the same muscle or in synergistic muscles show central short-term (lasting 10 to 20 msec) coupling in the time domain and characteristic peaks of coherence around 10 Hz and 15 to 35 Hz during voluntary movements.[11] There is good evidence to believe that shared synaptic drive from corticospinal tract neurons is responsible for these features.[6,11] Both the central short-term peaks of synchronization in the time domain and the 15 to 25 Hz coherence peaks have been shown to be reduced or absent in patients with stroke as well as patients with spinal cord injury (SCI).[12,13]

Cross-correlation and coherence techniques have the disadvantage that they require collaboration of the subject and cannot be used if the subject has no remaining voluntary effort. However, the techniques are simple and may easily be performed in a routine clinical setting because they require only a couple of minutes of paired surface EEG or EMG recordings. Furthermore, new analysis techniques allow measurements during functional motor tasks like walking[14] and reaching[15] to also be obtained. It has thus been demonstrated that healthy subjects show a characteristic modulation of coupling of populations of motor units during gait, which likely reflects the contribution of descending drive to the activation of the muscles.[14] This coupling is greatly reduced or absent during gait in SCI patients and on the injured side in stroke patients.[16,17] It shows a very good correlation to the functional deficit in the patients, and it appears to be a good marker of functional recovery in relation to gait training in SCI patients.[18] These features and the ease of its use make this an optimal method for physiological outcome evaluation in relation to assessment of interventions in SCI patients.

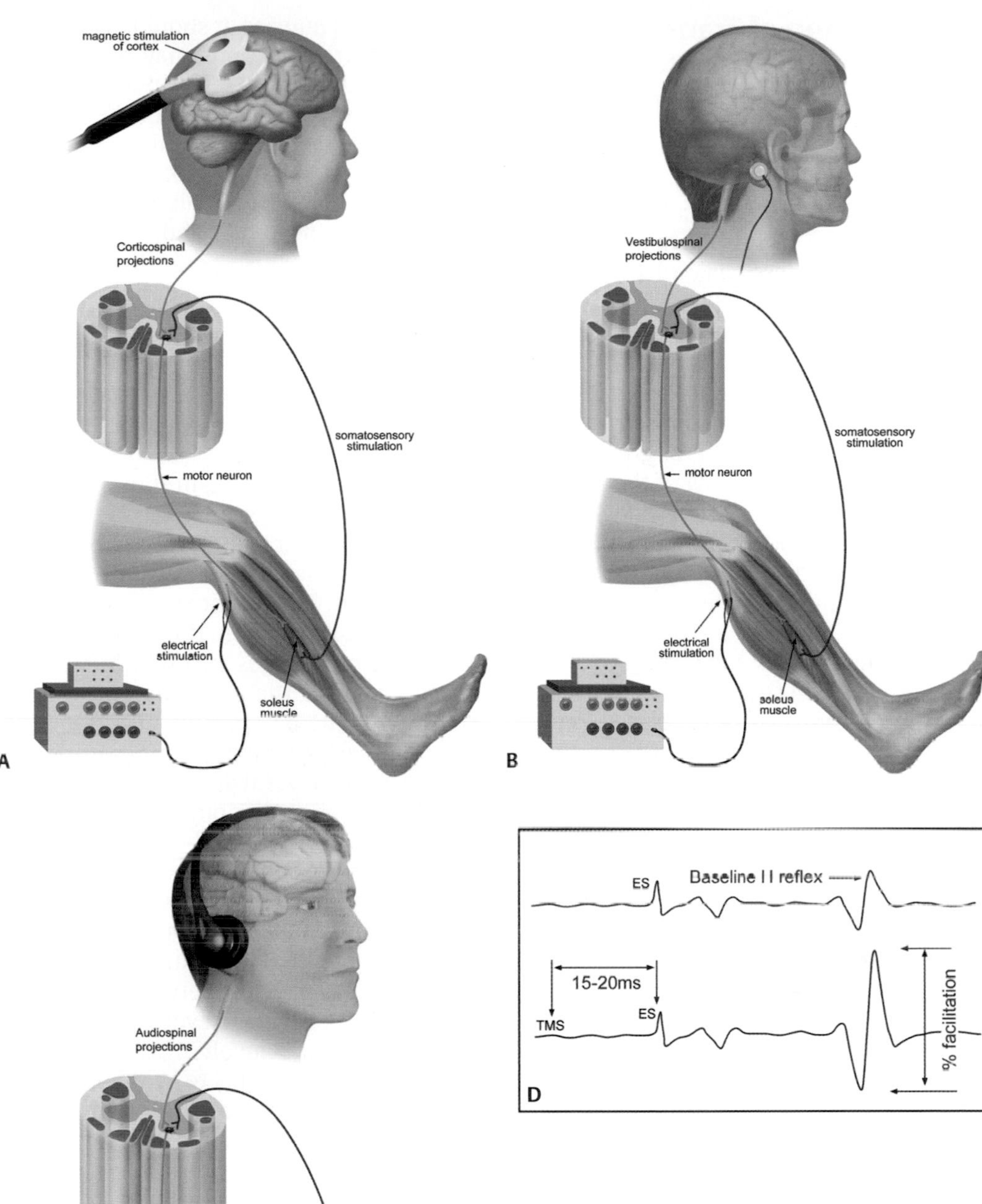

Fig. 42.1 **(A)** Transcranial magnetic stimulation, **(B)** galvanic stimulation, and **(C)** audiospinal stimulation can be used to modulate soleus H-reflex **(D)** to investigate corticospinal, vestibulospinal, and reticulospinal tracts, respectively.

Evaluation of Transmission in Descending Motor Tracts from the Brain Stem

The role of descending motor tracts other than the corticospinal tract for functional recovery following SCI has been somewhat neglected, probably mainly due to the relative inaccessibility of these tracts for electrophysiological testing. However, in recent years techniques have been developed that appear to provide some information of the conduction in the vestibulospinal and reticulospinal tracts. This information is likely to be of great importance for an understanding of the recovery of posture, balance, and gait following SCI. Galvanic stimulation (**Fig. 42.1B**) involves application of a small constant electric current (around 1 mA) between electrodes placed behind the ears on the mastoid processes, which elicits enhanced body sway in the direction of the ear behind which the anode is placed.[19] The muscular responses evoked by the stimulation in leg muscles are in all likelihood mediated by transmission in the vestibulospinal tract[20] and appear to provide valuable information about altered transmission in the tract following stroke[21] and SCI.[22]

Auditory stimulation or startle reactions (**Fig. 42.1C**) are in all likelihood generated by reticulospinal tracts from the brain stem.[23] They have been shown to be hyperactive in muscles rostral to a spinal cord lesion, possibly as a plastic adaptation to the impaired control of muscles below the lesion.[24] Startle reactions are also exaggerated in cortical stroke patients.[25] There is evidence in rats that assessment of auditory startle reactions may be useful in evaluating the extent of lesion of reticulospinal tracts,[23] but this is of limited use in human subjects, where startle responses are seldom seen in most distal arm and leg muscles. However, startle stimuli have been shown to trigger patterned movements in various muscles, including leg muscles during standing.[26] In all likelihood these responses are also mediated by reticulospinal projections and may therefore possibly be used to assess reticulospinal transmission across spinal injuries. It should also be noted that startle reactions may be observed in leg muscles also in relation to functional motor tasks.[27] Modification of the H-reflex (**Fig. 42.1D**) by TMS, galvanic stimulation, and audiospinal stimulation thus provides a way of studying transmission in corticospinal, vestibulospinal, and reticulospinal tracts, respectively.

Evaluation of Transmission in Spinal Neuronal Pathways in Relation to Spasticity

Changes in transmission in spinal neuronal pathways have been investigated following lesion of descending motor pathways in numerous studies since the beginning of the 1970s.[28,29] The focus of most of this research has been on the possible contribution of changes in inhibitory spinal mechanisms to the development of spasticity with the perspective of finding target points for therapeutic interventions.[30] Alteration in several spinal control mechanisms has been demonstrated, including presynaptic inhibition,[31,32] postactivation depression,[32] disynaptic reciprocal inhibition,[33,34] and persistent inward currents in the motoneurons.[35] From this research it appears clear that no single mechanism explains the development of spasticity, but that alteration in several interdependent mechanisms involving different neuronal pathways is likely to be involved. The relative changes in these different mechanisms have been shown to depend on several factors, which vary between subjects and determine the severity of spasticity relative to the subject´s functional ability. Spasticity should thus be seen as a plastic adaptation to the altered activity in the spinal neuronal circuitry secondary to the lesion of the descending pathways *and* secondary to the altered activity pattern in surviving descending motor tracts and sensory afferents. Short- and long-lasting plastic changes in the mechanisms that are involved in spasticity have thus been demonstrated in relation to immobilization[36] and the extent and type of exercise.[37] With this degree of modifiability of the mechanisms involved in spasticity, it seems within reach to find interventions that may help the surviving descending motor tracts to make more optimal use of the altered spinal neuronal circuitries and thus promote functional recovery. There is indeed an increasing understanding that weak to moderate spasticity may not be a "bad" thing and that spasticity may often be used by the patient to perform voluntary movements.[38] Rather than to simply remove spasticity, the goal of "antispastic" treatment should therefore in many cases be to find ways to help the patient—and the surviving descending tracts—to make new use of the altered settings in the spinal circuitries. Research into how the altered spinal circuitries may contribute to spontaneous recovery of function and how different interventions may make use of the altered spinal circuitries and induce changes in them and their descending control has already been conducted in relation to gait training,[39,40] and more research will undoubtedly appear when the full potential of this approach is generally realized.

Pearls

- Electrophysiological techniques provide information about functional transmission, adaptation, and reorganization of specific supraspinal and spinal neural pathways that is inaccessible with other techniques.
- Coherence and cross-correlation analysis of biological signals provides information about the functional organization and reorganization of unperturbed neural networks during natural movements.

Pitfalls

- Most neurophysiological techniques require somewhat sophisticated equipment and considerable expertise. They may therefore be difficult to implement in a routine setting.
- There is still insufficient knowledge regarding the relation between electrophysiological parameters and functional outcome measures. The value of many of the parameters for evaluation of functional recovery following lesion is therefore still unclear, and more research is required.

References

1. Nidecker A, Kocher M, Maeder M, et al. MR-imaging of chronic spinal cord injury. Association with neurologic function. Neurosurg Rev 1991; 14(3):169–179
2. Petersen TH, Rosenberg K, Petersen NC, Nielsen JB. Cortical involvement in anticipatory postural reactions in man. Exp Brain Res 2009;193(2): 161–171
3. Schubert M, Curt A, Jensen L, Dietz V. Corticospinal input in human gait: modulation of magnetically evoked motor responses. Exp Brain Res 1997;115(2):234–246
4. Petersen N, Christensen LO, Nielsen J. The effect of transcranial magnetic stimulation on the soleus H reflex during human walking. J Physiol 1998; 513(Pt 2):599–610
5. Taube W, Leukel C, Schubert M, Gruber M, Rantalainen T, Gollhofer A. Differential modulation of spinal and corticospinal excitability during drop jumps. J Neurophysiol 2008;99(3):1243–1252
6. Farmer SF. Rhythmicity, synchronization and binding in human and primate motor systems. J Physiol 1998;509(Pt 1):3–14
7. Halliday DM, Rosenberg JR, Amjad AM, Breeze P, Conway BA, Farmer SF. A framework for the analysis of mixed time series/point process data—theory and application to the study of physiological tremor, single motor unit discharges and electromyograms. Prog Biophys Mol Biol 1995;64(2-3): 237–278
8. Conway BA, Halliday DM, Farmer SF, et al. Synchronization between motor cortex and spinal motoneuronal pool during the performance of a maintained motor task in man. J Physiol 1995; 489(Pt 3):917–924
9. Mima T, Toma K, Koshy B, Hallett M. Coherence between cortical and muscular activities after subcortical stroke. Stroke 2001;32(11):2597–2601
10. James LM, Halliday DM, Stephens JA, Farmer SF. On the development of human corticospinal oscillations: age-related changes in EEG-EMG coherence and cumulant. Eur J Neurosci 2008;27(12): 3369–3379
11. Datta AK, Farmer SF, Stephens JA. Central nervous pathways underlying synchronization of human motor unit firing studied during voluntary contractions. J Physiol 1991;432:401–425

12. Farmer SF, Swash M, Ingram DA, Stephens JA. Changes in motor unit synchronization following central nervous lesions in man. J Physiol 1993; 463:83–105
13. Davey NJ, Ellaway PH, Friedland CL, Short DJ. Motor unit discharge characteristics and short term synchrony in paraplegic humans. J Neurol Neurosurg Psychiatry 1990;53(9):764–769
14. Halliday DM, Conway BA, Christensen LO, Hansen NL, Petersen NP, Nielsen JB. Functional coupling of motor units is modulated during walking in human subjects. J Neurophysiol 2003;89(2): 960–968
15. Fang Y, Daly JJ, Sun J, et al. Functional corticomuscular connection during reaching is weakened following stroke. Clin Neurophysiol 2009; 120(5):994–1002
16. Hansen NL, Conway BA, Halliday DM, et al. Reduction of common synaptic drive to ankle dorsiflexor motoneurons during walking in patients with spinal cord lesion. J Neurophysiol 2005;94(2): 934–942
17. Nielsen JB, Brittain JS, Halliday DM, Marchand-Pauvert V, Mazevet D, Conway BA. Reduction of common motoneuronal drive on the affected side during walking in hemiplegic stroke patients. Clin Neurophysiol 2008;119(12):2813–2818
18. Norton JA, Gorassini MA. Changes in cortically related intermuscular coherence accompanying improvements in locomotor skills in incomplete spinal cord injury. J Neurophysiol 2006; 95(4):2580–2589
19. Britton TC, Day BL, Brown P, Rothwell JC, Thompson PD, Marsden CD. Postural electromyographic responses in the arm and leg following galvanic vestibular stimulation in man. Exp Brain Res 1993; 94(1):143–151
20. Fitzpatrick RC, Day BL. Probing the human vestibular system with galvanic stimulation. J Appl Physiol 2004;96(6):2301–2316
21. Marsden JF, Playford DE, Day BL. The vestibular control of balance after stroke. J Neurol Neurosurg Psychiatry 2005;76(5):670–678
22. Iles JF, Ali AS, Savic G. Vestibular-evoked muscle responses in patients with spinal cord injury. Brain 2004;127(Pt 7):1584–1592
23. Gruner JA, Kersun JM. Assessment of functional recovery after spinal cord injury in rats by reticulospinal-mediated motor evoked responses. Electroencephalogr Clin Neurophysiol Suppl 1991; 43:297–311
24. Kumru H, Vidal J, Kofler M, Benito J, Garcia A, Valls-Solé J. Exaggerated auditory startle responses in patients with spinal cord injury. J Neurol 2008;255(5):703–709
25. Jankelowitz SK, Colebatch JG. The acoustic startle reflex in ischemic stroke. Neurology 2004;62(1): 114–116
26. Valls-Solé J, Rothwell JC, Goulart F, Cossu G, Muñoz E. Patterned ballistic movements triggered by a startle in healthy humans. J Physiol 1999; 516(Pt 3):931–938
27. Nieuwenhuijzen PH, Horstink MW, Bloem BR, Duysens J. Startle responses in Parkinson patients during human gait. Exp Brain Res 2006;171(2): 215–224
28. Ashby P, Verrier M. Neurophysiological changes following spinal cord lesions in man. Can J Neurol Sci 1975;2(2):91–100
29. Morin C, Pierrot-Deseilligny E, Bussel B. Role of muscular afferents in the inhibition of the antagonist motor nucleus during a voluntary contraction in man. Brain Res 1976;103(2):373–376
30. Nielsen JB, Crone C, Hultborn H. The spinal pathophysiology of spasticity—from a basic science point of view. Acta Physiol (Oxf) 2007; 189(2):171–180
31. Faist M, Mazevet D, Dietz V, Pierrot-Deseilligny E. A quantitative assessment of presynaptic inhibition of Ia afferents in spastics: differences in hemiplegics and paraplegics. Brain 1994;117(Pt 6):1449–1455
32. Nielsen J, Petersen N, Crone C. Changes in transmission across synapses of Ia afferents in spastic patients. Brain 1995;118(Pt 4):995–1004
33. Yanagisawa N, Tanaka R, Ito Z. Reciprocal Ia inhibition in spastic hemiplegia of man. Brain 1976;99(3):555–574
34. Crone C, Nielsen J, Petersen N, Ballegaard M, Hultborn H. Disynaptic reciprocal inhibition of ankle extensors in spastic patients. Brain 1994;117(Pt 5):1161–1168
35. Gorassini MA, Knash ME, Harvey PJ, Bennett DJ, Yang JF. Role of motoneurons in the generation of muscle spasms after spinal cord injury. Brain 2004;127(Pt 10):2247–2258
36. Lundbye-Jensen J, Nielsen JB. Immobilization induces changes in presynaptic control of group Ia afferents in healthy humans. J Physiol 2008; 586(Pt 17):4121–4135
37. Perez MA, Lundbye-Jensen J, Nielsen JB. Task-specific depression of the soleus H-reflex after cocontraction training of antagonistic ankle muscles. J Neurophysiol 2007;98(6):3677–3687
38. Dietz V, Sinkjaer T. Spastic movement disorder: impaired reflex function and altered muscle mechanics. Lancet Neurol 2007;6(8):725–733
39. Dietz V, Wirz M, Curt A, Colombo G. Locomotor pattern in paraplegic patients: training effects and recovery of spinal cord function. Spinal Cord 1998; 36(6):380–390
40. Barbeau H, Ladouceur M, Mirbagheri MM, Kearney RE. The effect of locomotor training combined with functional electrical stimulation in chronic spinal cord injured subjects: walking and reflex studies. Brain Res Brain Res Rev 2002;40(1-3):274–291

V

Plasticity and Recovery

43

Spinal and Supraspinal Plasticity after Spinal Cord Injury

Serge Rossignol and Alain Frigon

Key Points

1. The recovery of motor functions after spinal cord injuries depends on neuroplastic changes occurring at various levels of the central nervous system, including the spinal cord itself.
2. There is abundant evidence in the animal literature of recovery of motor functions like locomotion after complete spinal section. There is also evidence that, after partial spinal lesions, the spinal cord is changed and participates in the recovery of locomotion.
3. There are multiple sites in reflex pathways where transmission can be altered. Spinal lesions may for instance remove important descending inputs that control alternative spinal pathways.
4. Neuroplastic changes may include regeneration of damaged descending pathways as well as changes in various membrane properties of cells in the spinal cord.
5. The evidence of neuroplastic changes as a major component of the recovery of function may justify the use of enhanced sensory inputs to foster the recovery.

This chapter discusses various observations and possible mechanisms of neural plasticity following spinal cord injury (SCI). Although plasticity is an underlying theme of several chapters of this book, it is important to integrate some of the neural plastic changes with the known anatomy and physiology as presented in Chapter 1. Although several observations are made in animals, the aim is to highlight some mechanisms (proofs of principle) that should be considered in clinical conditions. It is indeed likely that the underlying mechanisms involved in the recovery of sensorimotor functions are conserved in several animal species, including humans. The expression *translational research* can imply that concepts developed in one animal species are simply transposed in another species more or less as a physical object is translated in the physical space. In the linguistic sense, translation implies that a concept expressed in one language is expressed in another language using the symbols of that second language. Some of the concepts exposed here must be translated from animals to humans, taking into consideration the specificity of the various species (bipedality, etc.).

■ Spinal Plasticity after a Complete Spinal Cord Section

Recovery of Locomotion

Although initially well studied in kittens,[1,2] the recovery of hindlimb locomotion after complete SCI is just as impressive in the adult cat,[3] adult mouse,[4] and adult rat,[5,6] provided an adequate stimulation is applied (e.g., locomotor training, pharmacology). In cats, a few days after a complete SCI at low thoracic levels, perineal stimulation evokes small alternate movements of the hindlimbs, especially at the hip, on a treadmill belt while the cat stands with its forelimbs on a fixed platform. At this stage the cat inadequately places the paw on the foot dorsum and weight bearing is absent. After 2 to 3 weeks of daily treadmill training (15 to 30 minutes), cats can regain hindlimb walking with some hindquarter weight support while making plantar foot contacts and generating much larger steps. **Figure 43.1** compares the hindlimb locomotor pattern of a cat before and 40 days after spinalization. Although there are some differences between the two patterns, the similarities are striking, considering that all connections to and from the brain have been lost. It must then be concluded that the spinal cord can by itself generate the basic locomotor pattern of the hindlimbs. As mentioned in Chapter 1, spinal circuits exist within the cord that are capable of expressing such rhythmicity, even in very primitive vertebrates such as the lamprey.[7] The neuronal elements essential for the generation of such locomotor patterns are largely unknown in mammals, but the fact that locomotion can be expressed after a complete SCI is proof of their existence.

Among the most prominent deficits in spinal locomotion are the absence of voluntary movements, severe equilibrium deficits, a reduced weight support of the hindquarters, reduced step length, and a variable amount of foot drag at the onset of swing. Diminished weight support probably results from the loss of reticulospinal and vestibulospinal pathways because similar deficits are observed with partial spinal lesions of ventral and ventrolateral spinal pathways. Similarly, the simultaneous activation of hip and ankle flexors may lead to foot drag, which could be seen as the equivalent of a foot drop in humans. Such specific deficits in the timing of hindlimb flexors may result from damage to corticospinal pathways because they are also observed after dorsolateral spinal lesions in the cat.[8]

The notion of a spinal central pattern generator (CPG) is important in a clinical context because these spinal circuits may contribute to the recovery of locomotion (see Chapters 44 and 45). The existence of a spinal CPG, capable of generating autonomous rhythmic activity in humans, has often been debated. However, there are reports[9–11] of patients with complete or incomplete lesions who present involuntary rhythmic movements of the legs (often called myoclonus). In a patient with a complete SCI, it was shown that, despite synchronous discharges in some muscles (even in some antagonists), others may contract out-of-phase,[12] as is usually the case between flexors and extensors during locomotion. Such observations should not be too surprising because there are striking descriptions of involuntary movements in the lower limbs of war-injured patients with complete SCI.[12] As reviewed in Chapter 12, the lower limbs of some patients with complete spinal thoracic cord lesions had to be strapped to the bed because of uncontrollable large amplitude rhythmic movements involving all the joints of the leg.

The importance of the spinal CPG will become even more obvious later, when we give evidence that, in cats, the CPG may have a role in locomotion not only after complete SCI but also after partial spinal lesions. Chapters 44 and 45 provide a more detailed view of this subject.

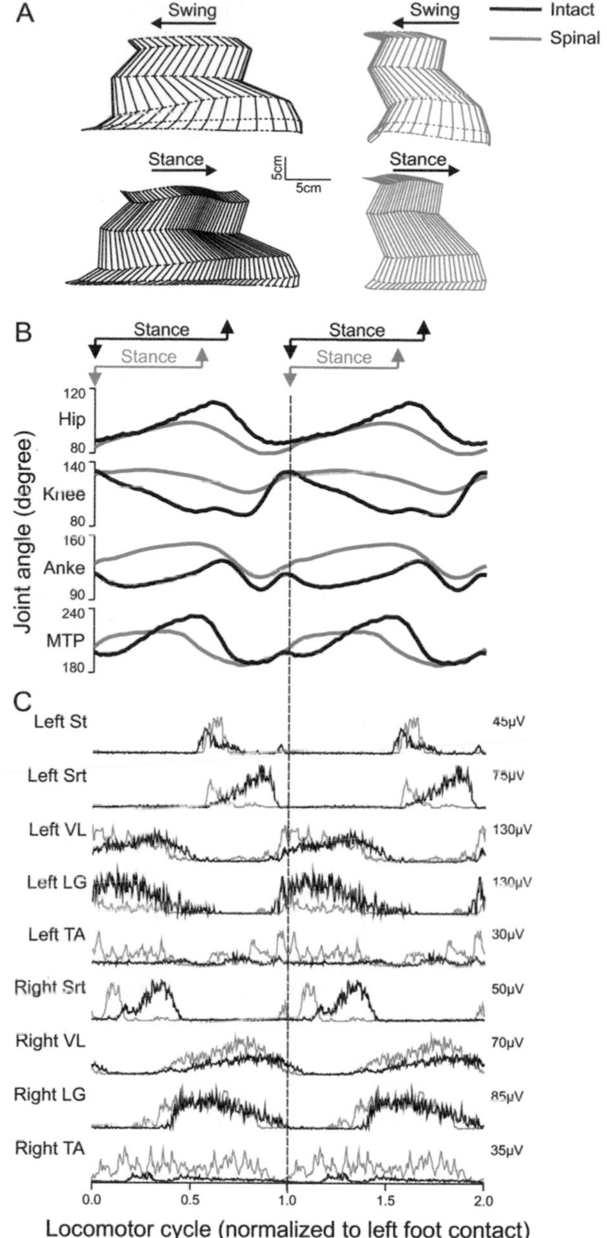

Fig. 43.1 Kinematics and muscle activity in a cat during locomotion before and 40 days after a complete spinal transection. **(A)** Stick diagrams of swing and stance phases before (*black*) and after (*blue*) spinalization in one cat. The stick diagrams are reconstructed from reflective markers positioned over prominent bony landmarks, including the iliac crest, greater trochanter, lateral epicondyle, lateral malleolus, metatarsophalangeal (MTP) joint, and tip of the fourth toe. **(B)** Angular excursions relative to left foot contact of the hip, knee, ankle, and MTP joints during locomotion. Each line is the average of ~ 20 locomotor cycles. **(C)** Single rectified bursts of electromyography obtained with intramuscular wire electrodes during locomotion before and after spinalization in the same cat. Each waveform is the average of ~ 20 locomotor cycles. St, semitendinosus (knee flexor/hip extensor); Srt, anterior sartorius (hip flexor/knee extensor); VL, vastus lateralis (knee extensor); LG, lateral gastrocnemius (ankle extensor/knee flexor); TA, tibialis anterior (ankle flexor). The cycle time was 1079 msec and 684 msec before and after spinalization, respectively.

Recovery of Reflexes

As discussed in Chapter 1, spinal reflexes are evoked by stimulating peripheral receptors or afferents and by recording the activity within or over a given muscle, which provides a means to evaluate changes in the excitability of sensorimotor pathways following SCI, at rest and during motor behaviors. Reflex excitability is governed by many factors, and it is important to consider all components of the pathway that may be altered after SCI, including peripheral receptors, primary afferents, synapse(s), motoneurons, and properties of the muscle (see Fig. 1.4 in Chapter 1).

It does not appear that morphological or functional properties of sensory receptors and axons are greatly affected by SCI.[13] On the other hand, once the input reaches the spinal cord, there can be considerable changes in how this input is processed and hence in reflex excitability.[14,15] Reflex excitability depends on the baseline activity of the target motoneuron pool, and in the case of di-, tri- and polysynaptic pathways, on the activity of interposed interneurons. It is known that motoneuron excitability is reduced for a time following SCI due to the loss of persistent inward currents (PICs), sustained depolarizing currents that greatly amplify the excitability of motoneurons to a given input.[16] Motoneuron excitability and PICs are largely regulated by descending monoaminergic pathways from the brain stem, which are disrupted or completely abolished after SCI. It is probable that interneuronal activity is also depressed due to a similar phenomenon. As a result, spinal reflex excitability is diminished for some time after SCI. Over time, however, PICs return, and as motoneuronal excitability recovers, spinal reflexes return. However, because descending pathways are important in turning off PICs, some reflexes become exaggerated due to abnormal control of neuronal excitability. In other words, a given input produces large sustained responses because the excitability within the spinal circuitry is not as tightly regulated as before SCI.[16] Due in part to changes in motoneuron excitability, the muscle can also undergo considerable alterations following SCI in humans and in animal models.[17] For instance, after SCI, hindlimb muscle fibers can substantially atrophy and there can be fiber type transformations over time. Changes in the size, number, and composition of muscle fibers can, in turn, influence not only the biomechanical responses of muscles but also the signal recorded over or within the muscle (i.e., electromyography), which can affect reflex excitability measurements.

The excitability within spinal reflex pathways is also controlled by direct and indirect interactions between various sources. For instance, supraspinal structures exert a powerful influence on several reflex pathways, as do other reflex pathways at a segmental level[18] (see Fig. 1.4 in Chapter 1). Thus it is important to consider how these interactions are modified to gain a better understanding of the pathophysiology of SCI. For instance, some pathways appear much more affected than others after SCI, such as reciprocal inhibition. As described in Chapter 1, in neurologically intact human subjects, stretching a muscle evokes a contraction of the agonist via a monosynaptic excitatory reflex pathway and relaxation of the antagonist via a disynaptic inhibitory reflex pathway (i.e., reciprocal inhibition). However, after SCI, reciprocal inhibition, assessed by conditioning the soleus Hoffmann reflex (H-reflex) with stimulation of the common peroneal nerve, is reduced in human subjects, and in some cases there is a reciprocal facilitation, instead of inhibition, which produces coactivation of agonists and antagonists at a particular joint.[19] **Figure 43.2**, derived from Fig. 1.4 in Chapter 1, explains how changes in reciprocal interactions can occur after SCI.

The coupling between agonists and antagonists, such as ankle dorsiflexors and plantarflexors, is important for the control of movement, and disrupting this coordination can impair motor control. The H-reflex itself is reduced after SCI, but it recovers with time and can be used as a tool to probe the excitability of other pathways, such as presynaptic, recurrent, and reciprocal inhibition, which are also influenced by SCI.[14]

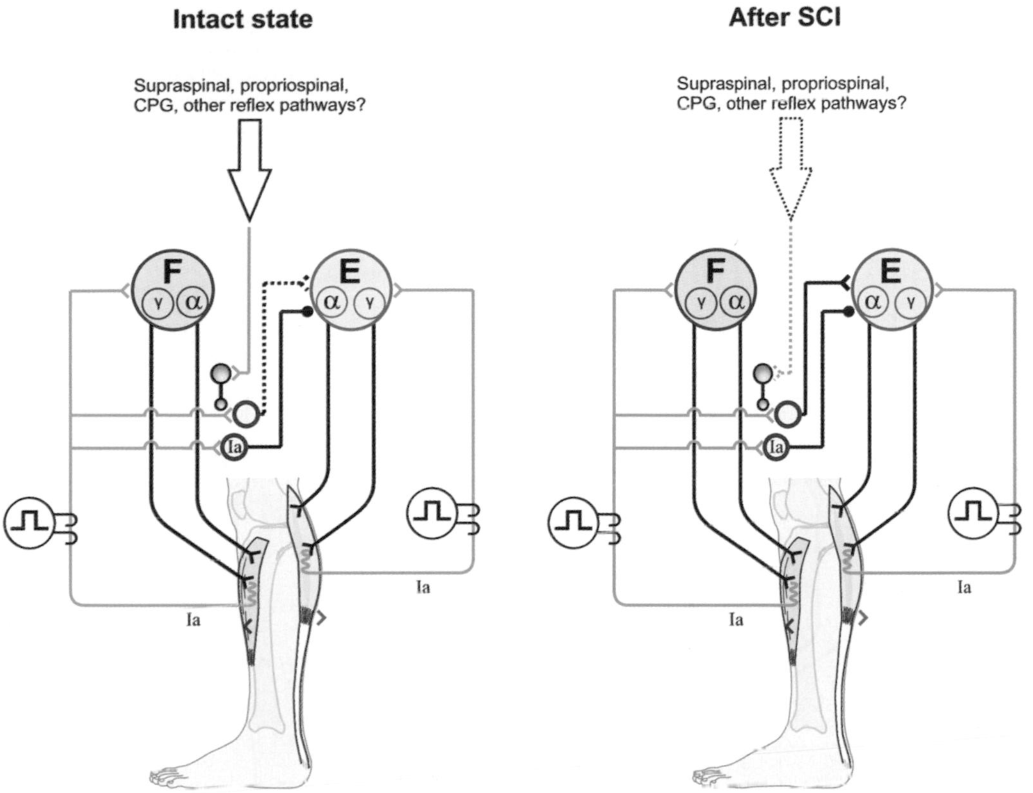

Fig. 43.2 Appearance of reciprocal facilitation following spinal cord injury (SCI). In humans with SCI, the normal reciprocal inhibition between antagonists mediated by the stretch or H-reflex pathway is disrupted, and instead there can be a reciprocal facilitation producing co-contraction at a given joint.[19,56] The figure illustrates the putative activation of an alternate reflex pathway following SCI due to a change in the balance between excitatory and inhibitory connections within the injured spinal cord. In the intact state (*left panel*), the pathway that mediates reciprocal facilitation is normally inhibited due to mechanisms that are unclear, but after SCI (*right panel*), the pathway can become active and produce reciprocal facilitation. The dotted lines indicate changes within descending pathways.

Cutaneous reflexes, evoked by stimulating the skin or cutaneous nerves, are also modified following SCI.[14] For example, a useful clinical tool is the Babinski sign or plantar reflex, which is evoked by slowly passing a blunt instrument on the lateral plantar aspect of the foot.[20] After damage to the central nervous system, such as SCI, or in infants in whom the corticospinal tract is immature, the Babinski sign is characterized by dorsiflexion of the big toe and fanning of the other toes. It should be emphasized that SCI most likely does not alter the circuitry of the spinal pathway but produces biases within one of several possible alternate pathways. What is modified is the supraspinal control of this pathway and of other spinal pathways that converge on interneurons interposed in the plantar reflex pathway. Thus the reflex itself after SCI is not pathological, but its control is; a phenomenon that probably extends to most tested reflex pathways. **Figure 43.3** explains how a cutaneous pathway may give rise to an inhibitory response or else an excitatory response after SCI.

Evaluating changes in reflex pathways after SCI is important because treadmill training in SCI patients is based on the principle that providing sensory cues con-

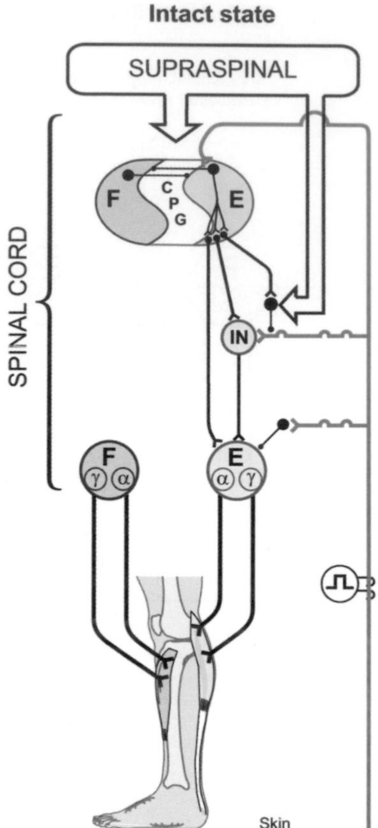

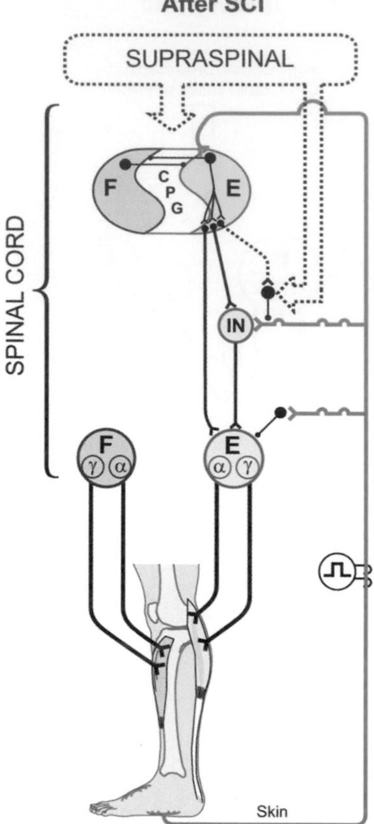

Fig. 43.3 Appearance of short-latency excitation after incomplete or complete spinal cord injury (SCI). In the cat, stimulating cutaneous afferents evokes a short-latency inhibition in ankle extensors (E) during the stance phase of locomotion. After complete[57] or incomplete SCI, short-latency excitatory responses can be observed following the same afferent stimulation. The most likely explanation is that an alternate reflex pathway becomes activated due to changes within the balance between excitatory and inhibitory connections within the injured spinal cord. The appearance of short-latency excitation can be due to mechanisms acting via the spinal locomotor central pattern generator (CPG) or more directly due to disrupted connections from supraspinal inputs to interneurons interposed in the excitatory cutaneous pathway. The dotted lines indicate changes within descending pathways or from the spinal CPG.

sistent with walking will induce beneficial plastic changes within the spinal locomotor circuitry.[21] Therefore, as the patient "relearns" to walk, activity-dependent processes induce changes within the spinal circuitry and in how it interacts with spared descending pathways and peripheral sensory feedback. Changes in these interactions are thought to be critical in optimizing remnant locomotor functions after SCI. Changes in reflex pathways could also be forerunners for locomotor recovery because some studies have shown that the appearance of long-latency reflex responses, evoked at rest, was associated with the development of walking in humans and adult rats.[22,23] These long-latency responses are thought to be components of the spinal locomotor circuitry.[11] An alternative explanation is that sensory feedback from the periphery regains the ability to activate key components of the spinal CPG due to the return of excitability within the neuronal locomotor circuitry.

Pharmacological Intervention to Trigger or Modulate Locomotor Functions

As discussed in other chapters, pharmacological interventions may become more and more important in the context of rehabilitation after SCI. The basic approach here may be (1) to replace neurotransmitters, such as noradrenaline and serotonin, that are normally synthesized in the brain stem, which largely disappear after SCI; (2) to offset changes in the excitability of neurotransmitter receptors (i.e., upregulation) caused by the reduction of neurotransmitters; (3) to create a new equilibrium between neurotransmitters released by spared descending inputs and those produced locally in the SC. Pharmacological interventions could be used temporarily to increase the excitability of spinal circuits (i.e., to offset paralysis) or to decrease the excitability of others (i.e., to reduce spasticity), which may interfere with the expression of basic motor patterns.[24]

The concept of a CPG for locomotion evolved from early work showing that the noradrenaline precursor L-dopa evoked a rhythmic discharge pattern in hindlimb nerves of acute spinal cats paralyzed with curare.[25] This "fictive" locomotion resembles normal locomotion with an alternation between flexors and extensors as well as bilateral alternation of both hindlimbs. Noradrenergic agonists, such as clonidine (α-2 noradrenergic receptor agonist), also evoked hindlimb locomotion in spinal cats.[26] It is important to mention that the effects of noradrenergic agonists (clonidine) or antagonists (yohimbine) differ whether the cats have an intact spinal cord or a complete or partial SCI. In cats with a large ventral and ventrolateral lesion, intrathecal clonidine injection can altogether stop voluntary quadrupedal locomotion.[27] Therefore, the sensitivity of receptors as well as the presence of pre- and postsynaptic receptors in various neural circuits may differ with different spinal lesions, which influences the effectiveness of various drugs. This is an important concept when evaluating a particular drug treatment in humans because the extent of the lesion is hard to quantify and the state of the receptors is completely unknown.[28]

Although serotoninergic (5-HT) agonists (e.g., quipazine, 5-O-DMT)[29] do not initiate locomotion in spinal cats, they strengthen the activity of hindlimb muscles (especially extensors) and paraxial muscles. In cats with ventrolateral spinal lesions, 5-HT agonists increased weight support as well as the ability of cats to walk uninterrupted for prolonged periods.[27] 5-HT may, however, initiate locomotion in rats when embryonic raphe cells are grafted below a complete SCI[5] or when agonists are administered.[6] 5-HT antagonists, such as cyproheptadine, can also block locomotion or reduce spasticity that may prevent locomotion in humans.[30] The importance of better understanding neurochemical changes in the spinal cord after injury is well exemplified by the recent work in spinal rats showing that some serotoninergic receptors can become constitutively active (i.e., their activity then does not require stimulation by an agonist). This could be the basis for the development of spasticity and even be part of the recovery of locomotion.[31]

Space limitations preclude discussing in detail other neurotransmitter systems, such as amino acids acting on excitatory glutamate receptors or inhibitory receptors acting on gamma-aminobutyric acid (GABA)ergic receptors, which might play a role after SCI. In the latter case, GABAergic agonists like baclofen may be used through intrathecal pumps to relieve spasticity

Supraspinal and Spinal Plasticity after Partial Spinal Cord Lesions in Animal Models

In humans, the majority of SCIs resulting from car accidents or falls are incomplete and may damage several ascending and descending pathways to varying extents. It is therefore important to look at the deficits that result from more circumscribed surgical lesions in animal models as well as other models that approximate human SCI, such as those resulting from spinal compressions produced by clips or weight drops.

Severance of Ventral or Dorsal Tracts

In cats, none of the spinal quadrants, and therefore none of the descending pathways, plays an indispensable role in the basic generation of locomotion, although severe and specific deficits may be observed as a result of disrupted supraspinal controls.[26]

Ventrolateral Pathways

Locomotion is generally considered to be initiated via activation of the mesencephalic locomotor region (MLR),[32] which activates reticulospinal cells projecting down to the SC and thus the CPG. The reticular formation also plays a major role in the control of locomotion and associated posture.[33] Consequently, it would be expected that lesioning reticulospinal pathways would greatly impact locomotion.[27,34] Although it is difficult to completely section reticulospinal pathways, the consequences of major damage to these pathways can be observed using ventral and ventrolateral spinal lesions. Cats with such lesions could eventually regain voluntary quadrupedal locomotion but retained diminished weight support and lack of normal coordination between the fore- and hindlimbs. Similarly, humans who had a surgical section of ventral pathways for intractable pain retained walking ability.[35]

Dorsolateral Pathways

After large lesions of the dorsolateral quadrant,[3] cats can walk over ground. Contrary to ventral lesions, after which cats maintained a well organized intralimb walking cycle, cats with dorsolateral lesions had deficits in the temporal recruitment of flexor muscles, leading to a significant foot drag at the initiation of swing, akin to a foot drop in humans.

How is this recovery of locomotion achieved? The remaining reticulospinal and rubrospinal cells may participate in the recovery of locomotion (i.e., functional substitution). Propriospinal neurons could be strategically placed to participate in such compensation, as suggested by others.[36,37] However, corticospinal pathways may contribute to locomotor recovery, as shown in other chapters.

Hemisections

A spinal hemisection implies surgically sectioning half of the spinal cord at a specific segment, and can be grouped into one of three categories (dorsal, ventral, and lateral). In humans, a lateral spinal hemisection is also referred to as the Brown-Séquard syndrome. It is characterized by the loss of sensorimotor functions on the side ipsilateral to the lesion and the loss of temperature sensation on the contralateral side. Brown-Séquard syndrome is most often caused by spinal tumors, piercing trauma (e.g., gunshot or stabbing wounds), ischemia, or vertebral disk herniation. It is a relatively less common form of SCI in humans compared with compressive injuries (see next section).

The extent of the lesion and locomotor training are important factors in the recovery of walking following lateral hemisection. In humans, complete paralysis can occur if the secondary injury leads to a large final lesion. In most cases, patients will recover some sensorimotor functions below the injury. In experimental models, a lateral hemisection implies surgically sectioning the left or right side of the spinal cord, which abolishes all ventral and dorsal descending and ascending pathways on one side of the spinal cord. After such lesions in various animal species, treadmill and normal walking recovers within a few days or weeks, depending on the severity of the injury.[3]

It is very difficult to perform a "perfect" hemisection, but in all cases animals respond well to training regardless of whether the lesion is large or small. Animals with smaller lesions generally recover faster and maintain better locomotor performance over time.[38,39] In cats, in the first few days following the hemisection, the limb ipsilateral to the lesion usually exhibits flaccid paresis and drags on the treadmill while the animal adopts a "tripod" gait. Over time the affected limb recovers adequate locomotion with weight support and proper foot placement. Although voluntary quadrupedal locomotion recovers, some deficits can persist over time. For example, large lesions can permanently impair the coupling between the fore- and hindlimbs (i.e., interlimb coordination), with the forelimbs adopting a faster rhythm than the hindlimbs. This might be a strategy to provide more excitability to the hindlimbs via spared propriospinal connections between cervical and lumbosacral CPGs.

Lateral hemisections also provide a useful model to evaluate spinal and supraspinal plasticity. For instance, after hemisection, the stance phase of the hindlimb contralateral to the lesion usually occupies a greater percentage of the locomotor cycle in cats,[40] which minimizes the amount of time that the affected limb contacts the ground until it recovers sufficient excitability. Over time the asymmetry is reduced or disappears. However, if the hemisection is followed by a complete spinal transection, the asymmetry can reverse, with the stance phase of the ipsilateral hindlimb occupying a greater percentage of the locomotor cycle. More importantly, animals can walk within 24 hours of complete spinal transection, a process normally requiring 2 to 3 weeks of treadmill training. This near immediate expression of locomotion following spinalization indicates that considerable plasticity occurred at the spinal level, whereas the reversal suggests that the return toward symmetry before spinalization was accomplished by supraspinal pathways.

Descending motor pathways are also very important for skilled motor tasks, such as reaching/grasping and skilled walking (e.g., horizontal ladder or rope walking), compared with treadmill or normal locomotion. Indeed, marked deficits in reaching and grasping are observed in the ipsilateral forelimb following a lateral spinal hemisection at C5 in adult rats.[41] Rats that showed some functional recovery in skilled motor tasks had greater sparing of the corticospinal tract. Moreover, there is evidence that spared descending pathways, such as the reticulospinal tract, are morphologically altered (e.g., collateral sprouting) after lateral hemisection of the spinal cord, and that this plasticity is associated with locomotor recovery.[42] Therefore, after lateral spinal hemisection, motor adaptation is a distributed process involving spinal and supraspinal structures. The extent of this plasticity, both functional and morphological, and the relative contribution of specific structures in the recovery of locomotion largely remain to be determined.

Compressive Lesions

Experimental compressive lesions are usually made in one of two ways. The first method involves using a calibrated clip to compress the spinal cord for a specific amount of time, whereas the second method involves dropping a weight on the exposed spinal cord from specific heights. In both methods the extent of injury can be graded by changing the amount of time that the clip is applied, or by varying the height of the weight-drop. Contrary to surgical sections of the spinal cord, compressive injuries produce more diffuse damage with a central cavitation surrounded by spared white matter (i.e., the secondary injury). The secondary injury is important because it can account for a substantial proportion of the final lesion. In general, the cavitation volume and lesion extent play a large role in determining locomotor recovery. In addition, following a compressive SCI in adult rats, the extent of spared white matter is more closely associated with locomotor recovery than spared gray matter,[43] indicating that the integrity of descending motor and ascending sensory pathways is critical for locomotor adaptation. In the adult rat, the same type of compressive injury at T13–L2 causes more severe locomotor deficits than at L3–4.[43] Damage at T13–L2 might damage key elements of the spinal CPG, which in the rat are thought to be located at upper lumbar levels.[44]

The locomotor deficits and extent of recovery following compressive SCI are comparable to those for other types of lesions. Hindlimb locomotion generally recovers over time, and locomotor training is effective in facilitating the recovery of walking. More severe compressive injuries can permanently disrupt the coordination between the fore- and hindlimbs. Inputs from peripheral afferents also appear to be involved in locomotor recovery following compressive SCI. For instance, following a compressive injury at T9, swimming in adult rats is effective in enhancing normal walking.[45] Moreover, providing cutaneous feedback to the feet during swim training further enhances locomotor recovery, as is also found following a lateral spinal hemisection in the chick.[46] It is likely that the processes involved in locomotor recovery are very similar in different types of SCI. That is, spared pathways/structures and the extent of injury largely dictate residual sensorimotor functions, whereas the amount/quality of training and pharmacological interventions promote functional recovery by modifying interactions between different control levels of the neuraxis.

However, even mild compressive SCIs can completely abolish the corticospinal tract, which can have profound consequences on skilled motor tasks.[47,48] On the other hand, rubrospinal and vestibulospinal pathways are only partially damaged. Recovery of motor skills after compressive SCI might be accomplished by functional substitution, where other descending pathways take over the function normally accomplished by other structures. If some corticospinal axons are spared, locomotor training can enhance their effectiveness. For example, using transcranial magnetic stimulation, it was shown that motor-evoked potentials in some leg muscles were greater following several weeks of treadmill training in human SCI subjects.[49] Recently, it was shown that treadmill locomotion induced considerable cortical plasticity after complete SCI in neonatal rats.[50] Cortical plasticity also occurs after incomplete SCI, and it is possible that spared descending corticospinal axons are more effective in activating spinal neurons.

Studies in Humans

Although animal models of SCI cannot be directly extrapolated to humans with SCI, the framework provided by animal work has been useful in conceptualizing therapeutic interventions in humans. Some reviews are particularly useful in relating animal work and clinical conditions.[21,24,51,52]

The first question to raise is whether humans also have a CPG. Although there is no direct evidence, several studies indicate that it might be the case. For instance, patients with complete spinal section after a war injury can develop autonomous rhythmic movements of the legs.[12] Patients with SCI may also develop such spontaneous movements, and rhythmic movements can be triggered by electrical epidural stimulation.[53]

Patients with partial spinal cord lesions can walk, albeit with some deficits.[54,55] Animal and human experiments suggesting a potential for an involuntary rhythmogenesis at the spinal cord/brain stem level have encouraged the promotion of locomotor training on a treadmill with body weight support, robotics, or muscle stimulation, with remarkable results (see Chapter 45).

Pearls

- The existence of spinal circuits capable of generating a well-organized locomotor pattern (central pattern generator) in several animal species after complete spinal lesions may indicate similar capabilities in humans.
- Reflex studies show that physiological and pathophysiological conditions can bias reflexes toward one or the other alternative pathways. These reflex pathways may participate in the recovery of function.
- After lesion, plastic changes occur in the spinal cord. These may include changes in circuitry as well as cellular membrane properties.
- Pharmacological interventions could promote or decrease these intrinsic changes in the spinal cord.
- Studies with partial spinal lesions reveal that the CPG probably also participates in the recovery of locomotor functions after SCI and would justify basic locomotor training after SCI.

Pitfalls

- Neuroplasticity may also be maladaptive, so that hyper-/hyponeuronal excitability may interfere with recovery of function. For instance, hypersensitivity or hyperactivity of some receptors of neurotransmitters can lead to an increase of muscle tone but also to an unwarranted hypertonicity, such as in spasticity, that is in part maladaptive.
- Although "abnormal or pathological" reflexes may be convenient clinical signs, they do not necessarily reflect the development of abnormal reflex circuits but rather biases in existing alternative reflex pathways.
- Neuroplasticity is often considered to be the result of morphological changes in circuitry. Although some anatomical changes may indeed occur, physiological changes in the efficacy of transmission within existing circuits (spinal or supraspinal) may also be prominent.
- After a spinal lesion, it is often thought that the main neuroplastic mechanisms occur in supraspinal structures. However, important neurologic changes also occur below the lesion within the spinal cord itself.

References

1. Forssberg H, Grillner S, Halbertsma J, Rossignol S. The locomotion of the low spinal cat, II: Interlimb coordination. Acta Physiol Scand 1980; 108(3):283–295
2. Forssberg H, Grillner S, Halbertsma J. The locomotion of the low spinal cat, I: Coordination within a hindlimb. Acta Physiol Scand 1980;108(3): 269–281
3. Rossignol S, Barrière G, Alluin O, Frigon A. Re-expression of locomotor function after partial spinal cord injury. Physiology (Bethesda) 2009;24: 127–139
4. Leblond H, L'Esperance M, Orsal D, Rossignol S. Treadmill locomotion in the intact and spinal mouse. J Neurosci 2003;23(36):11411–11419
5. Ribotta MG, Provencher J, Feraboli-Lohnherr D, Rossignol S, Privat A, Orsal D. Activation of locomotion in adult chronic spinal rats is achieved by transplantation of embryonic raphe cells reinnervating a precise lumbar level. J Neurosci 2000;20(13):5144–5152
6. Courtine G, Gerasimenko Y, van den Brand R, et al. Transformation of nonfunctional spinal circuits into functional states after the loss of brain input. Nat Neurosci 2009;12(10):1333–1342
7. Grillner S, Wallén P, Saitoh K, Kozlov A, Robertson B. Neural bases of goal-directed locomotion in vertebrates—an overview. Brain Res Brain Res Rev 2008;57(1):2–12
8. Jiang W, Drew T. Effects of bilateral lesions of the dorsolateral funiculi and dorsal columns at the level of the low thoracic spinal cord on the control of locomotion in the adult cat, I: Treadmill walking. J Neurophysiol 1996;76(2):849–866
9. Calancie B. Spinal myoclonus after spinal cord injury. J Spinal Cord Med 2006;29(4):413–424
10. Calancie B, Needham-Shropshire B, Jacobs P, Willer K, Zych G, Green BA. Involuntary stepping after chronic spinal cord injury: evidence for a central rhythm generator for locomotion in man. Brain 1994;117(Pt 5):1143–1159
11. Bussel B, Roby-Brami A, Azouvi P. Organization of reflexes elicited by flexor reflex afferents in paraplegic man: evidence for a stepping generator.

In: Jami L, Pierrot-Deseilligny E, Zytnicki D, eds. Muscle Afferents and Spinal Control of Movement. Oxford: Pergamon; 1992:427–432

12. Nadeau S, Jacquemin G, Fournier C, Lamarre Y, Rossignol S. Spontaneous motor rhythms of the back and legs in a patient with a complete spinal cord transection. Neurorehabil Neural Repair 2010;24(4):377–383
13. Thomas CK, Westling G. Tactile unit properties after human cervical spinal cord injury. Brain 1995;118(Pt 6):1547–1556
14. Frigon A, Rossignol S. Functional plasticity following spinal cord lesions. Prog Brain Res 2006; 157(16):231–260
15. Rossignol S, Frigon A. Recovery of locomotion after spinal cord injury: some facts and mechanisms. Annu Rev Neurosci 2011;34:413–440
16. Heckmann CJ, Gorassini MA, Bennett DJ. Persistent inward currents in motoneuron dendrites: implications for motor output. Muscle Nerve 2005; 31(2):135–156
17. Biering-Sørensen B, Kristensen IB, Kjaer M, Biering-Sørensen F. Muscle after spinal cord injury. Muscle Nerve 2009;40(4):499–519
18. Nielsen JB, Crone C, Hultborn H. The spinal pathophysiology of spasticity—from a basic science point of view. Acta Physiol (Oxf) 2007;189(2): 171–180
19. Crone C, Johnsen LL, Biering-Sørensen F, Nielsen JB. Appearance of reciprocal facilitation of ankle extensors from ankle flexors in patients with stroke or spinal cord injury. Brain 2003;126(Pt 2): 495–507
20. Babinski J. Sur le reflexe cutané plantaire dans certaines affections organiques du système nerveux central. C R Soc Biol 1896;48:207–208
21. Harkema SJ. Neural plasticity after human spinal cord injury: application of locomotor training to the rehabilitation of walking. Neuroscientist 2001;7(5):455–468
22. Dietz V, Grillner S, Trepp A, Hubli M, Bolliger M. Changes in spinal reflex and locomotor activity after a complete spinal cord injury: a common mechanism? Brain 2009;132(Pt 8):2196–2205
23. Lavrov I, Gerasimenko YP, Ichiyama RM, et al. Plasticity of spinal cord reflexes after a complete transection in adult rats: relationship to stepping ability. J Neurophysiol 2006;96(4):1699–1710
24. Barbeau H, Rossignol S. Enhancement of locomotor recovery following spinal cord injury. Curr Opin Neurol 1994;7(6):517–524
25. Rossignol S. Neural control of stereotypic limb movements. In: Rowell LB, Sheperd JT, eds. Handbook of Physiology, Section 12. Exercise: Regulation and Integration of Multiple Systems. New York: Oxford University Press; 1996:173–216
26. Rossignol S. Plasticity of connections underlying locomotor recovery after central and/or peripheral lesions in the adult mammals. Philos Trans R Soc Lond B Biol Sci 2006;361(1473):1647–1671
27. Brustein E, Rossignol S. Recovery of locomotion after ventral and ventrolateral spinal lesions in the cat. II. Effects of noradrenergic and serotoninergic drugs. J Neurophysiol 1999;81(4): 1513–1530
28. Giroux N, Rossignol S, Reader TA. Autoradiographic study of alpha1- and alpha2-noradrenergic and serotonin1A receptors in the spinal cord of normal and chronically transected cats. J Comp Neurol 1999;406(3):402–414
29. Barbeau H, Rossignol S. The effects of serotonergic drugs on the locomotor pattern and on cutaneous reflexes of the adult chronic spinal cat. Brain Res 1990;514(1):55–67
30. Norman KE, Barbeau H. Comparison of cyproheptadine, clonidine and baclofen on the modulation of gait pattern in subjects with spinal cord injury. In: Thilmann A, Burke D, Rymer Z, eds. Spasticity. New York: Springer-Verlag; 1992:410–425
31. Murray KC, Nakae A, Stephens MJ, et al. Recovery of motoneuron and locomotor function after spinal cord injury depends on constitutive activity in 5-HT2C receptors. Nat Med 2010;16(6): 694–700
32. Orlovsky GN, Shik ML. Control of locomotion: a neurophysiological analysis of the cat locomotor system. In: Porter R, ed. International Review of Physiology. Neurophysiology II. Baltimore, MD: University Park Press; 1976:281–309
33. Drew T, Prentice S, Schepens B. Cortical and brainstem control of locomotion. Prog Brain Res 2004;143:251–261
34. Brustein E, Rossignol S. Recovery of locomotion after ventral and ventrolateral spinal lesions in the cat, I: Deficits and adaptive mechanisms. J Neurophysiol 1998;80(3):1245–1267
35. Nathan PW. Effects on movement of surgical incisions into the human spinal cord. Brain 1994;117(Pt 2):337–346
36. Jordan LM, Schmidt BJ. Propriospinal neurons involved in the control of locomotion: potential targets for repair strategies? Prog Brain Res 2002; 137:125–139
37. Bareyre FM, Kerschensteiner M, Raineteau O, Mettenleiter TC, Weinmann O, Schwab ME. The injured spinal cord spontaneously forms a new intraspinal circuit in adult rats. Nat Neurosci 2004; 7(3):269–277
38. Barrière G, Leblond H, Provencher J, Rossignol S. Prominent role of the spinal central pattern generator in the recovery of locomotion after partial spinal cord injuries. J Neurosci 2008;28(15): 3976–3987
39. Barrière G, Frigon A, Leblond H, Provencher J, Rossignol S. Dual spinal lesion paradigm in the cat: evolution of the kinematic locomotor pattern. J Neurophysiol 2010;104(2):1119–1133
40. Frigon A, Barrière G, Leblond H, Rossignol S. Asymmetric changes in cutaneous reflexes after a partial spinal lesion and retention following spinalization during locomotion in the cat. J Neurophysiol 2009;102(5):2667–2680
41. Anderson KD, Gunawan A, Steward O. Quantitative assessment of forelimb motor function after cervical spinal cord injury in rats: relationship to the corticospinal tract. Exp Neurol 2005;194(1): 161–174
42. Ballermann M, Fouad K. Spontaneous locomotor recovery in spinal cord injured rats is accompa-

nied by anatomical plasticity of reticulospinal fibers. Eur J Neurosci 2006;23(8):1988–1996

43. Magnuson DS, Lovett R, Coffee C, et al. Functional consequences of lumbar spinal cord contusion injuries in the adult rat. J Neurotrauma 2005;22(5):529–543

44. Bertrand S, Cazalets JR. The respective contribution of lumbar segments to the generation of locomotion in the isolated spinal cord of newborn rat. Eur J Neurosci 2002;16(9):1741–1750

45. Smith RR, Shum-Siu A, Baltzley R, et al. Effects of swimming on functional recovery after incomplete spinal cord injury in rats. J Neurotrauma 2006;23(6):908–919

46. Muir GD, Steeves JD. Phasic cutaneous input facilitates locomotor recovery after incomplete spinal injury in the chick. J Neurophysiol 1995;74(1):358–368 PubMed

47. Conta AC, Stelzner DJ. Differential vulnerability of propriospinal tract neurons to spinal cord contusion injury. J Comp Neurol 2004;479(4): 347–359

48. Anderson KD, Sharp KG, Steward O. Bilateral cervical contusion spinal cord injury in rats. Exp Neurol 2009;220(1):9–22

49. Thomas SL, Gorassini MA. Increases in corticospinal tract function by treadmill training after incomplete spinal cord injury. J Neurophysiol 2005; 94(4):2844–2855

50. Kao T, Shumsky JS, Murray M, Moxon KA. Exercise induces cortical plasticity after neonatal spinal cord injury in the rat. J Neurosci 2009;29(23): 7549–7557

51. Dietz V, Harkema SJ. Locomotor activity in spinal cord-injured persons. J Appl Physiol 2004;96(5): 1954–1960

52. Rossignol S. Locomotion and its recovery after spinal injury. Curr Opin Neurobiol 2000;10(6): 708–716

53. Dimitrijevic MR, Gerasimenko Y, Pinter MM. Evidence for a spinal central pattern generator in humans. Ann N Y Acad Sci 1998;860:360–376

54. Pépin A, Ladouceur M, Barbeau H. Treadmill walking in incomplete spinal-cord-injured subjects: 2. Factors limiting the maximal speed. Spinal Cord 2003;41(5):271–279

55. Pépin A, Norman KE, Barbeau H. Treadmill walking in incomplete spinal-cord-injured subjects, I: Adaptation to changes in speed. Spinal Cord 2003;41(5):257–270

56. Xia R, Rymer WZ. Reflex reciprocal facilitation of antagonist muscles in spinal cord injury. Spinal Cord 2005;43(1):14–21

57. Frigon A, Rossignol S. Adaptive changes of the locomotor pattern and cutaneous reflexes during locomotion studied in the same cats before and after spinalization. J Physiol 2008;586(Pt 12): 2927–2945

44

The Human Central Pattern Generator and Its Role in Spinal Cord Injury Recovery

Volker Dietz

Key Points

1. There is evidence for a spinal central pattern generator for locomotion in humans.
2. Human bipedal locomotion uses a quadrupedal limb coordination.
3. A locomotor pattern can be induced and can be trained in complete human SCI when an appropriate afferent input is provided.

Locomotion in mammals is largely dependent upon the central pattern generator (CPG); that is to say, neuronal circuits (networks of interneurons) within the spinal cord. The CPG is defined as a neural circuit that can produce self-sustained patterns of behavior, independent of sensory input.[1] The understanding of basic principles of CPG function is based on research in invertebrates and primitive fish like the lamprey.[2] There is no comparable research in mammals, especially human beings, where our understanding is only based on indirect evidence.

Knowledge about the neuronal control of human locomotion is also of broad interest for clinical reasons. Characteristic disorders of locomotion are often the first sign of a central lesion of the motor system. Advances in our understanding of movement control allow us to define more precisely the requirements for the rehabilitation of patients with movement disorders. This chapter focuses on the role of the CPG and its interaction with proprioception during human locomotion. In a more general sense, locomotion is representative of movement control. It is a subconsciously performed, everyday movement that is highly reproducible. It is adapted automatically to existing conditions, such as ground irregularities, within a large safety margin.

The selection of, and interaction between, different sources of afferent input is task dependent. Simple stretch reflexes are thought to be involved primarily in the control of focal movements. For more complex motor behaviors, such as locomotion, afferent input related to load and hip-joint position probably has an important role in the proprioceptive contribution to the activation pattern of the leg muscles. There is increasing evidence that the movement disorder after a spinal cord injury (SCI) involves the defective use of afferent input in combination with secondary compensatory processes. This has implications for therapy, which should be directed to take advantage of the plasticity of the central nervous system.

Central Pattern Generation

Spinal Locomotor Pattern Generation: Evidence in Animals

For most quadruped mammals, it is assumed that the neural control of locomotion is based on CPGs within the spinal cord.[3] This network generates the rhythm and shapes the pattern of bursts of motoneurons.[4] For the cat, it is assumed that there is at least one such CPG for each limb and that these CPGs are mainly located within the thoracolumbar region.[3] The rhythmogenic capacity of the hindlimb innervating segments of the spinal cord decreases substantially in the rostrocaudal direction, so that the caudal lumbar segments are incapable of producing the rhythm.[5,6]

Neuronal circuits (networks of interneurons) within the spinal cord that interact with specific sensory information are responsible for locomotion in nonprimate mammals.[1] These spinal neuronal circuits are defined as CPGs and were identified as being able to generate self-sustained patterns of locomotor-like neural activity independently of supraspinal and peripheral afferent input.[7]

Further evidence that neuronal networks in the spinal cord are able to produce rhythmic output was obtained by experiments in which such output was generated even though movement-related afferent input was eliminated through pharmacological blocking of the movements.[8] By recording the output at muscle nerves, rhythmic periods of activity, which are reciprocally organized between agonists and antagonists (fictive locomotion), were demonstrated in hindlimbs[9] and forelimbs[10] of the spinal cat. The CPG model is not restricted to the cat; fictive locomotion has also been demonstrated in a wide variety of invertebrates and vertebrates.[11]

Spinal Locomotor Pattern Generation: Evidence in Humans

In contrast to the abundance of data gained from invertebrates, rats, and cats, leading to the general assumption of a CPG underlying the central control of locomotion, there is relatively little known about spinal networks acting like CPGs in humans. Nevertheless, there are observations indicating that the neural control of human locomotion is based on the activity of spinal CPGs.[3]

The existence of CPGs in humans is difficult to demonstrate because it requires observations of oscillating neural networks after anatomically complete spinal lesions and deafferentation. Nevertheless, several human studies have provided evidence of oscillatory neural networks that interact with afferent input with limited or no detectable functional supraspinal input. Electrical stimulation of flexor reflex afferents show characteristics of neuronal networks in humans[12] that are similar to those identified as CPGs in animals. Furthermore, rhythmic contractions of the trunk and lower limb extensor muscles were described in an individual with clinically complete SCI.[13] This rhythmic activity could be induced, stopped, and modulated by peripheral stimulation of flexor reflex afferents.[14] Also, involuntary steplike movements that were modulated by sensory input were observed in an individual with chronic incomplete cervical SCI several years after injury.[15]

Interaction between Pattern Generation and Afferent Input

Pattern generation is basically innate. In humans, steplike movements are present at birth; they are spontaneously initiated or triggered by peripheral stimuli. A central origin of these movements is implied because an electromyographic (EMG) burst precedes the actual mechanical events.[16] Central programming can be influenced by sensory input.[17] This again is illustrated by infant-stepping. Although rhythmic alternating leg movements are coordinated by a CPG, the infant is unable to maintain body equilibrium. Infants lack an integration of the appropriate afferent input into the programmed leg muscle EMG pattern. To achieve body equilibrium, afferent information from a variety of sources within the visual, vestibular, and proprioceptive systems is utilized by the CPG for adaptation to actual needs (**Fig. 44.1**).

The convergence of spinal reflex pathways and descending pathways on common spinal interneurons seems to play an integrative role[18] similar to that in the cat.[19] For example, visual feedforward information reduces the activity that arises from the length sensors of muscles (the muscle spindles). Furthermore, the amount of proprioceptive feedback from the legs during various locomotor activities determines the influence of vestibulospinal input on the stabilization of body movement.[20] Conversely, somatosensory loss increases vestibulospinal sensitivity.[21]

The selection of an appropriate locomotor pattern determines the mode of organization of muscle synergies that are designed to meet multiple conditions of stance and gait.[22,23] Afferent information influences the central (spinal) pattern and, conversely, the CPG selects the appropriate afferent information according to the external requirements.[1,24] Both the CPG and the reflexes that mediate afferent input to the spinal cord are under the control of the brainstem.[25] The actual weighting of proprioceptive, vestibular, and visual inputs to the equilibrium control is context dependent and can profoundly modify the central program.[23]

In addition, proprioceptive information provides the basis for a conscious representation of the body in space, which becomes disturbed in deafferented individuals.[26] Furthermore, there is phase-linked corticospinal control of locomotion in humans[27] and other mammals.[28] Voluntary commands have to interact with the spinal locomotor generator to change, for example, the direction of gait or to avoid an obstacle.[29]

Spinal reflexes adapt the preprogrammed motor patterns of leg muscles to the terrain.[30] Whereas this neuronal mechanism explains quick, unilateral reflex activity in leg extensor muscles, more complex bilateral coordination of leg muscle activation is needed to maintain body equilibrium when gait is disturbed by an obstacle. Irrespective of the conditions under which stance

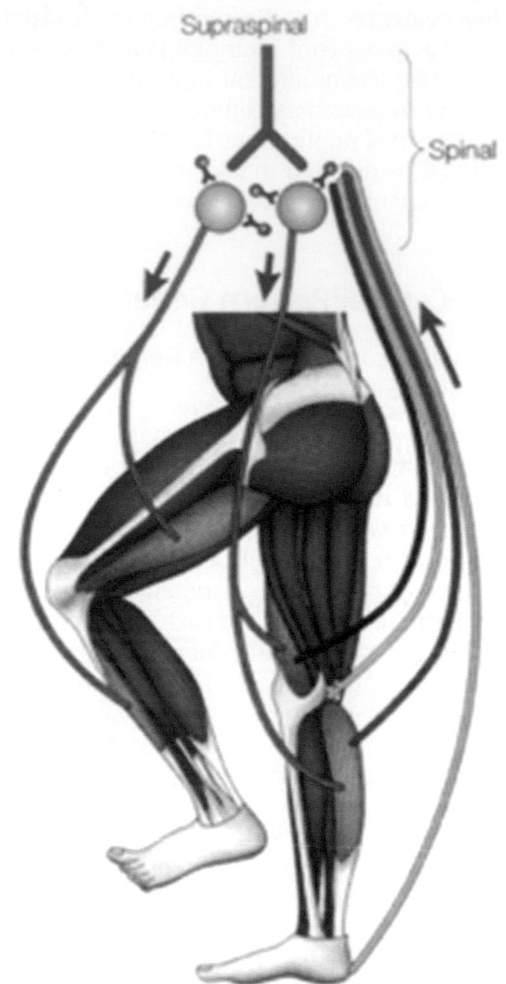

Fig. 44.1 Schematic drawing of the neuronal mechanisms involved in human gait. Leg muscles become activated by a programmed pattern that is generated in spinal neuronal circuits (*turquoise pathway*). This pattern is modulated by multisensory afferent input, which adapts the pattern to meet existing requirements. Both the programmed pattern and the reflex mechanisms are under supraspinal control. In addition, there is differential neuronal control of leg extensor and flexor muscles. Whereas extensors are mainly activated by proprioceptive feedback, the flexors are predominantly under central control.[65]

and gait are investigated, the neuronal pattern that is evoked during a particular task is always directed to hold the body's center of mass over the base of support. Consequently, the selection of afferent input by central mechanisms must correspond to the requirements for body stabilization.

Quadrupedal versus Bipedal Coordination of Locomotion

The coordination of forelimb and hindlimb rhythmic activities is a main characteristic feature of quadrupedal locomotion.[31] Specialized neural circuits located in the caudal spinal cord (the CPG) organize hindlimb locomotor activity, whereas specialized circuits in the rostral spinal cord control forelimb movements.[3] The coordination of both circuits is mediated by propriospinal neurons with long axons, which couple the cervical and lumbar enlargements of the spinal cord.[32]

According to observations made in humans during the last years, bipedal and quadrupedal locomotion share common spinal neuronal control mechanisms. As in quadrupeds, long projecting propriospinal neurons couple the cervical and lumbar enlargements in humans.[33] Furthermore, the coordination of limb movements during walking is similar in human infants,[34] adults,[29] and quadrupeds.[1]

Nevertheless, there are also distinct differences because the upper limb in primates has become specialized to perform skilled hand movements. The evolution of upright stance and gait, in association with a differentiation of hand movements, represents a basic requirement for human cultural development.[35] The phylogenetic development does not, however, exclude that human bipeds still use quadrupedal coordination for their locomotor activities.[20] Recent research indicates that interlimb coordination during human locomotion is organized in a similar way to that in the cat.[18] Hence, during locomotion, corticospinal excitation of upper limb motoneurons is mediated indirectly, via propriospinal neurons in the cervical spinal cord. This allows a task-dependent neuronal linkage of cervical and thoracolumbar propriospinal circuits controlling leg and arm movements during human locomotor activities (**Fig. 44.2**).

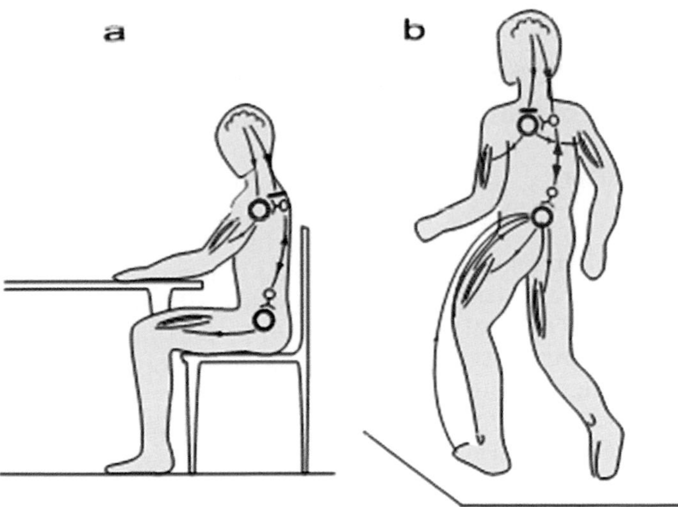

Fig. 44.2 Movement control during different motor tasks. According to the research cited in this review, neuronal control of arm movement is task dependent. **(A)** During skilled hand movements, strong direct cortical-motoneuronal excitation is predominant (*red lines*) and the cervical propriospinal neuronal system is inhibited. **(B)** During locomotion, it is assumed that the brain commands are predominantly mediated by interneurons. Cervical and thoracolumbar propriospinal systems become coupled and coordinate arm and leg movements (*red lines*). (From Dietz V. Do human bipeds use quadrupedal coordination? Trends in neurosciences 2002;25(9):462–467. Reprinted with permission.)

According to recent studies using functional magnetic resonance imaging,[36] the supplementary motor area might be involved in the supraspinal control of this coupling between upper and lower limb movements.

There is a neuronal coupling of upper and lower limb muscles during various human locomotor activities.[37] In such conditions, arm and leg movements are locked with a fixed frequency relationship. The frequency relationship characterizing this coordination corresponds to that observed in well-defined biological systems consisting of coupled oscillators.[38] Also during gait, swinging of the arms serves to regulate the rotation of the body (i.e., it counteracts torsion-related movements of the trunk).

These observations indicate a flexible task-dependent neuronal coupling between upper and lower limbs. The pathway that couples upper and lower limb movements seems to become gated by the activity of the CPG during walking. The stronger impact of leg flexors in interlimb coordination is in line with the increasing evidence that leg flexor and leg extensor muscles are differentially controlled in both animals[39] and humans.[22,27]

Central Pattern Generation after a Spinal Cord Injury

Interlimb Coupling after a Spinal Cord Injury

Evidence for neuronal coupling between upper and lower limbs also comes from studies in patients with cervical SCI. So-called interlimb reflex responses can be evoked with short latency in distal muscles of upper limbs by electrical stimulation of the tibial nerve at the ankle.[40] These reflex connections might reflect a loss of supraspinal inhibition or, alternatively, a sprouting of ascending propriospinal systems occupying synaptic locations vacated by degenerating descending connections.

Furthermore, it has been shown that the more rostral the spinal cord lesion, the more "normal" the locomotor pattern induced in patients with complete paraplegia or tetraplegia.[5] This observation indicates that neuronal circuits underlying locomotor "pattern generation" in humans are not restricted to any specific level of the spinal cord but, rather, that an intricate neuronal network contributing to bipedal locomotion extends from thoracolumbar to cervical levels.

Neuronal Plasticity after a Spinal Cord Injury: Animal Models

There is convincing evidence in spinal animals that use-dependent plasticity of spinal neuronal circuits modifies the sensorimotor function of the adult mammalian lumbosacral spinal cord.[41] Regular training after complete spinal cord transection in adult cats improves the recovery of hindlimb function. For example, the lumbosacral spinal cord of the cat could function to execute stepping or standing more successfully if that particular task was specifically practiced. When stand training alone was practiced, stepping ability was compromised.[41] Observations in spinal cats also indicated that, if the training of a motor task was discontinued, the performance of that task deteriorated.[42] These results show that repetitive motor training provides sufficient stimulation of specific neural pathways to facilitate functional reorganization within the spinal cord and to improve motor output. Furthermore, appropriate sensory input during training is of critical importance to achieve an optimal motor output of the spinal neuronal circuitry.[43] Consequently, a much greater level of functional recovery might be possible if the concept of use dependence is applied.

Locomotor Capacity of the Isolated Human Spinal Cord

The notion that "locomotor-like patterns" can be released also in humans and that there is a basic similarity between the spinal locomotor circuitry of cats and humans is supported by observations made in patients with complete spinal cord transection. In these patients, electrical stimulation of flexor reflex afferents (FRAs) shows characteristics of the neuronal networks similar to those seen in the cat.[12,44] Early descriptions of involuntary stepping movements generated by the spinal cord in human subjects with complete paraplegia date back to the work of Lhermitte[45] and Kuhn.[46] Later on, in a patient with a complete spinal cord lesion, rhythmic contractions of the trunk and lower limb extensor muscles were described.[13,47] Furthermore, in persons with complete spinal lesion, spinal cord stimulation is followed by "stepping movements" with reciprocally organized EMG activity of symmetric muscles of both sides.[48] Evidence for a spinal CPG for locomotion in humans after SCI has also come from locomotor movements induced on a treadmill with body-weight support in people with incomplete and complete paraplegia.[49]

Further indirect evidence for the capacity of the spinal CPG has been suggested from recordings of locomotor activity induced in patients with complete paraplegia standing on a moving treadmill with body-weight support.[49–51] According to these experiments, it appears that the strength of the locomotor pattern depends on the level of the lesion (i.e., the higher the lesion, the more "normal" is the pattern).[5] This would imply that neuronal circuits up to a cervical level contribute to the locomotor activity, as it was suggested for the mudpuppy.[39] The pattern of leg muscle activation during such locomotion resembles in many aspects the pattern observed in an intact cat or a healthy individual. However, the amplitude of leg muscle EMG activity in the individuals with clinically complete SCI is lower than that of healthy subjects, and no independent leg movements resulted from this leg muscle activation.[52]

Neuronal Plasticity after a Human Spinal Cord Injury

After an SCI of the cat, rat, or human, neuronal centers below the level of lesion exhibit plasticity that can be exploited by specific training paradigms. The coordination of human gait seems to be controlled in much the same way as that in other mammals.[18] Therefore, it is not surprising that in persons with complete or incomplete paraplegia, locomotor EMG activity can be both elicited and trained, as in the cat. This is achieved by partially unloading (up to 80%) the patients, who are standing on a moving treadmill.[29,50,52–54] In severely affected patients, the leg movements usually have to be externally assisted, especially during the transition from stance to swing. It is supposed that by moving the limbs through trajectories under close physiological conditions, providing an appropriate afferent input (i.e., loading, hip joint), spinal neuronal circuits become activated. The timing of the pattern of leg muscle EMG activity recorded in such a condition is similar to that seen in healthy subjects. However, the amplitude of leg muscle EMG is considerably reduced and is less well modulated. This makes the body unloading necessary for the locomotor training.

The analysis of the locomotor pattern in completely paraplegic patients indicates that it is unlikely to be due to rhythmic stretches of the leg muscle because leg muscle EMG activity is, as in healthy subjects, equally distributed during muscle lengthening and shortening.[50] In addition, recent observations indicate that locomotor movements induced in patients who are completely unloaded do not lead to leg muscle activation.[43] This implies that the generation of the leg muscle EMG pattern in these patients is programmed at a spinal level rather than being generated by stretch reflexes.

Individuals with an incomplete SCI benefit from locomotor training such that they improve their ability to walk over ground. Load- or hip joint-related afferent input seems to be of crucial importance for both the generation of a locomotor pattern and the effectiveness of the training. However, a critical combination of afferent signals may be needed to generate a locomotor pattern after severe SCI. Several neurotransmitter systems within the spinal cord are suggested to be involved in the generation of locomotor patterns and their adaptation to repetitive use. In spinal cats, serotonin agonists modulate established locomotor patterns, whereas antagonists worsen the locomotor pattern.[55]

Using a driven gait orthosis (DGO), the effects of locomotor movements restricted to hip joints were studied in people with complete paraplegia.[43] An important observation was that the pattern of leg muscle activation was almost unchanged after knee-joint movements were blocked in these patients. Furthermore, isolated joint movements of the foot evoked only local responses. This indicates that afferent input related to hip-joint position also has an important influence on leg muscle activation by the isolated spinal cord.

During the course of daily locomotor training, the amplitude of the EMG in the leg extensor muscles increases during the stance phase, and inappropriate leg flexor activity decreases. Such training effects are seen in both complete and incomplete paraplegic patients.[50,52] These training effects lead to a greater weight-bearing function of the extensors. This indicates that the isolated human spinal cord has the capacity not only to generate a locomotor pattern but also to show some plasticity. However, only persons with incomplete paraplegia benefit from the training program insofar as they can learn to perform unsupported stepping movements on solid ground.[50,52] In complete paraplegic patients, the training effects on leg muscle activation become lost after the training has been stopped.[56]

There are several reports about the beneficial effect of locomotor training in incomplete paraplegic patients,[55,57] and patients who undergo locomotor training have a greater mobility compared with a control group without training.[58] Afferent input from receptors signaling contact forces during the stance phase of gait is essential for the activation of spinal locomotor centers[43,51] and is important to achieve training effects in paraplegic patients.[50,52] Furthermore, hip-joint-related afferent input seems to be essential to generate a locomotor pattern.[43]

The improvement of locomotor activity could also be attributed to spontaneous recovery of spinal cord function.[59] However, recent observations indicate that in both incomplete and complete paraplegic patients, the increase of leg extensor EMG activity occurs independently of the spontaneous recovery of spinal cord function.[53,54,59]

In severely affected chronic (in-) complete SCI subjects, an exhaustion of leg muscle activity during assisted locomotion was observed.[60] It was assumed that a degradation of spinal neuronal circuits deprived of their supraspinal input occurs that could not be reversed by training. This exhaustion of locomotor activity was associated with a decrease of the early component and an increase of the late component of spinal reflex activity.[61]

Significance of Load Receptor Input for Training Effects in Spinal Cord Injury Subjects

The significance of loading for the regulation of stance and gait has previously been established in healthy human subjects.[22] Proprioceptive inputs from the extensor muscles, and probably also from mechanoreceptors in the sole of the foot, provide load-related afferent information. The signals arising from the afferent input are likely to be integrated into the polysynaptic spinal reflex pathway, which adapts the programmed locomotor pattern to the actual ground conditions. The role of afferent activity for the rhythmic locomotor pattern is to shape the pattern, control phase-transitions, and reinforce ongoing activity.[62]

Load-related input has an important role in inducing and training the locomotor pattern in SCI subjects. However, the effects of training are lost over time in people with complete paraplegia.[56] These results indicate that there is training-induced plasticity of neuronal centers in the isolated spinal cord that is dependent on specific afferent input. This might be of relevance to future interventional therapies (by combining training with regeneration-inducing agents). When locomotor movements were assisted by a DGO that allows stepping movements to be induced, even with 100% body unloading, physiological locomotor-like movements alone did not lead to leg muscle activation.[43] This occurs only in combination with loading of the legs in both healthy subjects and people with complete paraplegia or tetraplegia.

The amplitude of muscle activation in the legs is directly related to the level of loading on the legs during stepping of healthy and SCI subjects.[51] Therefore, it is not surprising that body unloading and reloading play an essential role in the success of locomotor training in paraplegic patients. However, an appropriate rhythmic loading of one extended leg alone while stepping movements are performed by the contralateral leg is not always sufficient for the activation of the static leg.[43] This indicates that a combination of different afferent inputs is required to achieve locomotor-like leg muscle activation.

Significance of Hip-Joint Afferents for Training Effects in Spinal Cord Injury Subjects

Afferent input from hip joints is important for muscle activation during locomotion in mammals, mainly because it initiates the transition from stance to swing. Hip kinematics have been shown to modulate muscle activation during locomotion in humans.[43] The pattern of leg muscle activation was shown to be similar when the knee joint movements are blocked while physiological hip movements are induced. Furthermore, isolated foot joint movements (simulated stepping with or without loading the sole of the foot) evoke only local responses, which is in line with earlier reports.[22,63] These results suggest that hip-joint afferents play a role in the leg muscle activation in the functionally isolated human spinal cord.

■ Conclusion

There is increasing evidence that in typical movement disorders, such as spasticity after an incomplete SCI, a defective utilization of afferent input, in combination with secondary compensatory processes, is involved. Furthermore, it becomes evident from cat experiments that neuronal networks underlying the generation of motor patterns are quite flexible after central neural lesions.[64] This has implications for therapy. The aim of rehabilitation should be the improvement of function by taking advantage of the plasticity of neuronal centers, and should be less directed to the correction of isolated clinical signs, such as the reflex excitability. To monitor outcome and to assess the effectiveness of any interventional therapy, standardized functional tests should be applied.

Locomotor training is an effective method for improving the recovery of walking in many individuals with incomplete SCI. However, at this point, complete recovery of walking is not routinely attained with severe injury. Looking ahead, it may be important to discover combination strategies to further enhance the locomotor output, such as the application of pharmacological interventions, spinal electrical stimulation, and functional electrical stimulation. Furthermore, rehabilitation approaches should be refined and directed to take advantage of the plasticity of the central nervous system and the intrinsic neuronal properties of the human spinal cord.[65] However, the most promising approach may be to induce some regeneration of corticospinal axons within the spinal cord.[66] In the future, individuals with complete or almost complete SCI may profit from a combination of regeneration approaches and exploitation of neuronal plasticity driven by appropriate retraining of the nervous system, taking advantage of spinal neural networks and critical sensory cues.

Pearls

- For the exploitation of neuronal plasticity after SCI, the provision of an appropriate afferent input is required.
- Hip-joint-related and load receptor afferent inputs are essential to induce locomotor activity and to achieve training effects.
- Locomotor activity can be trained in complete paraplegic subjects, without profit for locomotor ability.
- In immobilized, severely affected SCI subjects, a neuronal dysfunction develops over time after injury, which limits the success of any regeneration-inducing therapy.

Pitfalls

- Problems in translational medicine include the fact that regeneration-inducing therapy in human SCI (e.g., olfactory ensheathing cells) is not yet successfully applied.
- Adequacy of animal SCI models is not yet fully established for translational studies.
- Mechanisms of neuronal dysfunction in chronic severe human SCI are not yet fully understood.
- An adequate chronic SCI model is not yet available.

References

1. Grillner S. Interaction between sensory signals and the central networks controlling locomotion in lamprey, dogfish and cat. In: Grillner S, Stein PSG, Stuart DG, Fossberg F, Herman RM, eds. Neurobiology of Vertebrate Locomotion. Wenner Gren International Symposium Series, Vol. 45. London: Macmillan; 1986:505–512
2. Marder E. From biophysics to models of network function. Annu Rev Neurosci 1998;21: 25–45
3. Duysens J. Neural control of locomotion: the central pattern generator from cats to humans. Gait Posture 1998;7(2):131–141
4. Grillner S, Deliagina T, Ekeberg O, et al. Neural networks that co-ordinate locomotion and body orientation in lamprey. Trends Neurosci 1995; 18(6):270–279
5. Dietz V, Nakazawa K, Wirz M, Erni T. Level of spinal cord lesion determines locomotor activity in spinal man. Exp Brain Res 1999;128(3):405–409
6. Lev-Tov A, Delvolvé I. Pattern generation in non-limb moving segments of the mammalian spinal cord. Brain Res Bull 2000;53(5):671–675
7. Grillner S, Zangger P. How detailed is the central pattern generation for locomotion? Brain Res 1975; 88(2):367–371
8. Perret C, Cabelguen JM. Main characteristics of the hindlimb locomotor cycle in the decorticate cat with special reference to bifunctional muscles. Brain Res 1980;187(2):333–352
9. Floeter MK, Sholomenko GN, Gossard JP, Burke RE. Disynaptic excitation from the medial longitudinal fasciculus to lumbosacral motoneurons: modulation by repetitive activation, descending pathways, and locomotion. Exp Brain Res 1993;92(3): 407–419
10. Yamaguchi T. Muscle activity during forelimb stepping in decerebrate cats. Jpn J Physiol 1992; 42(3):489–499
11. Rossignol S. Neuronal control of stereotypic limb movements. In: Rowell LB, Sheperd JT, eds. Exercise: Regulation and Integration of Multiple Systems. Handbook of Physiology, section 112. Bethesda, MD: American Physiological Society; 1996:173–216
12. Roby-Brami A, Bussel B. Long-latency spinal reflex in man after flexor reflex afferent stimulation. Brain 1987;110(Pt 3):707–725
13. Bussel B, Roby-Brami A, Azouvi P, Biraben A, Yakovleff A, Held JP. Myoclonus in a patient with spinal cord transection: possible involvement of the spinal stepping generator. Brain 1988;111(Pt 5):1235–1245
14. Bussel B, Roby-Brami A, Yakovleff A, Bennis N. Late flexion reflex in paraplegic patients: evidence for a spinal stepping generator. Brain Res Bull 1989;22(1):53–56
15. Calancie B, Needham-Shropshire B, Jacobs P, Willer K, Zych G, Green BA. Involuntary stepping after chronic spinal cord injury: evidence for a central rhythm generator for locomotion in man. Brain 1994;117(Pt 5):1143–1159
16. Forssberg H. A developmental model of human locomotion. In: Grillner S, Stein PSG, Stuart DG, Fossberg F, Herman RM, eds. Neurobiology of Vertebrate Locomotion. Wenner Gren International Symposium Series, 45. London: Macmillan; 1986;485–501
17. Brooks V. Motor programs revisited. In: Talbott RE, Humphrey DR, eds. Posture and Movement. New York, NY: Raven Press; 1979:13–49
18. Dietz V. Do human bipeds use quadrupedal coordination? Trends Neurosci 2002;25(9): 462–467
19. Schomburg ED. Spinal sensorimotor systems and their supraspinal control. Neurosci Res 1990;7(4):265–340
20. Dietz V, Fouad K, Bastiaanse CM. Neuronal coordination of arm and leg movements during human locomotion. Eur J Neurosci 2001;14(11): 1906–1914

21. Horak FB, Hlavacka F. Somatosensory loss increases vestibulospinal sensitivity. J Neurophysiol 2001;86(2):575–585
22. Dietz V. Human neuronal control of automatic functional movements: interaction between central programs and afferent input. Physiol Rev 1992; 72(1):33–69
23. MacKay-Lyons M. Central pattern generation of locomotion: a review of the evidence. Phys Ther 2002;82(1):69–83
24. Mulder T, Duysens J. Neural control of locomotion: sensory control of the central pattern generator and its relation to treadmill training. Gait Posture 1998;7(3):251–263
25. Jankowska E, Lundberg A. Interneurones in the spinal cord. Trends Neurosci 1981;(4):230–233
26. Sanes JN, Mauritz KH, Dalakas MC, Evarts EV. Motor control in humans with large-fiber sensory neuropathy. Hum Neurobiol 1985;4(2): 101–114
27. Schubert M, Curt A, Jensen L, Dietz V. Corticospinal input in human gait: modulation of magnetically evoked motor responses. Exp Brain Res 1997;115(2):234–246
28. Leblond H, Ménard A, Gossard JP. Corticospinal control of locomotor pathways generating extensor activities in the cat. Exp Brain Res 2001;138(2): 173–184
29. Dietz V. Neurophysiology of gait disorders: present and future applications. Electroencephalogr Clin Neurophysiol 1997;103(3):333–355
30. Dietz V, Quintern J, Sillem M. Stumbling reactions in man: significance of proprioceptive and pre-programmed mechanisms. J Physiol 1987; 386:149–163
31. Gans C, Gaunt AS, Webb PS, et al. Vertebrate locomotion. In: Terjung R, ed. Handbook of Physiology, Vol. 13: Comparative Physiology. New York: Wiley-Blackwell; 1997:55–213
32. Cazalets JR, Bertrand S. Coupling between lumbar and sacral motor networks in the neonatal rat spinal cord. Eur J Neurosci 2000;12(8): 2993–3002
33. Nathan PW, Smith M, Deacon P. Vestibulospinal, reticulospinal and descending propriospinal nerve fibres in man. Brain 1996;119(Pt 6): 1809–1833
34. Pang MY, Yang JF. The initiation of the swing phase in human infant stepping: importance of hip position and leg loading. J Physiol 2000;528(Pt 2):389–404
35. Herder J. Ideen zur Philosophie der Geschichte der Menschheit. Hartknoch, Bd 1. Leipzig: 1785
36. Debaere F, Swinnen SP, Béatse E, Sunaert S, Van Hecke P, Duysens J. Brain areas involved in interlimb coordination: a distributed network. Neuroimage 2001;14(5):947–958
37. Wannier T, Bastiaanse C, Colombo G, Dietz V. Arm to leg coordination in humans during walking, creeping and swimming activities. Exp Brain Res 2001;141(3):375–379
38. Bartos M, Manor Y, Nadim F, Marder E, Nusbaum MP. Coordination of fast and slow rhythmic neuronal circuits. J Neurosci 1999;19(15): 6650–6660
39. Cheng J, Stein RB, Jovanović K, Yoshida K, Bennett DJ, Han Y. Identification, localization, and modulation of neural networks for walking in the mudpuppy (Necturus maculatus) spinal cord. J Neurosci 1998;18(11):4295–4304
40. Calancie B, Lutton S, Broton JG. Central nervous system plasticity after spinal cord injury in man: interlimb reflexes and the influence of cutaneous stimulation. Electroencephalogr Clin Neurophysiol 1996;101(4):304–315
41. De Leon RD, Hodgson JA, Roy RR, Edgerton VR. Retention of hindlimb stepping ability in adult spinal cats after the cessation of step training. J Neurophysiol 1999;81(1):85–94
42. Edgerton VR, de Leon RD, Tillakaratne N, Recktenwald MR, Hodgson JA, Roy RR. Use-dependent plasticity in spinal stepping and standing. Adv Neurol 1997;72:233–247
43. Dietz V, Müller R, Colombo G. Locomotor activity in spinal man: significance of afferent input from joint and load receptors. Brain 2002;125(Pt 12):2626–2634
44. Roby-Brami A, Bussel B. Effects of flexor reflex afferent stimulation on the soleus H reflex in patients with a complete spinal cord lesion: evidence for presynaptic inhibition of Ia transmission. Exp Brain Res 1990;81(3):593–601
45. L'Hermite J. La section totale de la moelle dorsal. Bourges, Tardy-Pigelet; 1919
46. Kuhn RA. Functional capacity of the isolated human spinal cord. Brain 1950;73(1):1–51
47. Bussel B, Roby-Brami A, Néris OR, Yakovleff A. Evidence for a spinal stepping generator in man: electrophysiological study. Acta Neurobiol Exp (Warsz) 1996;56(1):465–468
48. Rosenfeld J, Sherwood A, Halter J, Dimitrijevic M. Evidence of a pattern generator in paralyzed subjects with spinal cord stimulation. Soc Neurosci 1995;21:688
49. Dobkin BH, Harkema S, Requejo P, Edgerton VR. Modulation of locomotor-like EMG activity in subjects with complete and incomplete spinal cord injury. J Neurol Rehabil 1995;9(4):183–190
50. Dietz V, Colombo G, Jensen L, Baumgartner L. Locomotor capacity of spinal cord in paraplegic patients. Ann Neurol 1995;37(5):574–582
51. Harkema SJ, Hurley SL, Patel UK, Requejo PS, Dobkin BH, Edgerton VR. Human lumbosacral spinal cord interprets loading during stepping. J Neurophysiol 1997;77(2):797–811
52. Dietz V, Colombo G, Jensen L. Locomotor activity in spinal man. Lancet 1994;344(8932): 1260–1263
53. Dietz V, Wirz M, Colombo G, Curt A. Locomotor capacity and recovery of spinal cord function in paraplegic patients: a clinical and electrophysiological evaluation. Electroencephalogr Clin Neurophysiol 1998;109(2):140–153
54. Dietz V, Wirz M, Curt A, Colombo G. Locomotor pattern in paraplegic patients: training effects and recovery of spinal cord function. Spinal Cord 1998;36(6):380–390
55. Barbeau H, Rossignol S. Enhancement of locomotor recovery following spinal cord injury. Curr Opin Neurol 1994;7(6):517–524

56. Wirz M, Colombo G, Dietz V. Long term effects of locomotor training in spinal humans. J Neurol Neurosurg Psychiatry 2001;71(1):93–96
57. Wernig A, Müller S. Laufband locomotion with body weight support improved walking in persons with severe spinal cord injuries. Paraplegia 1992;30(4):229–238
58. Wernig A, Müller S, Nanassy A, Cagol E. Laufband therapy based on 'rules of spinal locomotion' is effective in spinal cord injured persons. Eur J Neurosci 1995;7(4):823–829
59. Curt A, Keck ME, Dietz V. Functional outcome following spinal cord injury: significance of motor-evoked potentials and ASIA scores. Arch Phys Med Rehabil 1998;79(1):81–86
60. Dietz V, Müller R. Degradation of neuronal function following a spinal cord injury: mechanisms and countermeasures. Brain 2004;127(Pt 10):2221–2231
61. Dietz V, Grillner S, Trepp A, Hubli M, Bolliger M. Changes in spinal reflex and locomotor activity after a complete spinal cord injury: a common mechanism? Brain 2009;132(Pt 8):2196–2205
62. Whelan PJ, Pearson KG. Plasticity in reflex pathways controlling stepping in the cat. J Neurophysiol 1997;78(3):1643–1650
63. Sinkjaer T, Andersen JB, Larsen B. Soleus stretch reflex modulation during gait in humans. J Neurophysiol 1996;76(2):1112–1120
64. Pearson KG. Neural adaptation in the generation of rhythmic behavior. Annu Rev Physiol 2000;62:723–753
65. Dietz V. Proprioception and locomotor disorders. Nat Rev Neurosci 2002;3(10):781–790
66. Schwab ME, Bartholdi D. Degeneration and regeneration of axons in the lesioned spinal cord. Physiol Rev 1996;76(2):319–370

45

Electrophysiological Predictors of Lower Limb Motor Recovery: The Rehabilitation Perspective

Jessica Hillyer and Susan Harkema

Key Points

1. Optimal outcome assessment for SCI clinical trials is widely debated. Although much of the SCI literature focuses on neurological status, motor and sensory function, and functional capacity, electrophysiological assessments offer the potential to detect subclinical changes in neurological functioning objectively and sensitively.
2. Two electrophysiological assessment tools are highlighted in this review. Electrical perceptual threshold testing measures minimally detectable sensations, and the method is well tolerated by individuals, can be performed in less time than the American Spinal Injury Association Impairment Scale (AIS) sensory exam, and provides a simple, reproducible, quantitative sensory assessment of the level and degree of impairment in SCI. The brain motor control assessment analyzes suprasegmental control of segmental motor activity using EMG. The protocol response is quantitative and objective, and it provides measurable parameters of the neural components of each assessed motor task.
3. The SCI literature reflects a growing consensus that current outcome measures for recovery after SCI are insufficient. Most researchers agree that electrophysiological tests offer the best opportunity for enhancing assessments, especially as a complement to AIS; however, until there is more work done on the standardization of the acquisition and analysis of data, clinical applicability of these tests will be limited.

Awareness of spinal cord injury (SCI) and its consequences is becoming more widespread. Recently, the prevalence of SCI in the United States was estimated to be ~1.27 million, with 11,000 new cases reported annually.[1] Resultant impairments can include motor and sensory deficits, ranging from complete paralysis to mildly disturbed gait or balance; autonomic dysfunction, including cardiovascular and respiratory disturbances; bowel, bladder, and sexual dysfunction; and a significant number of secondary complications, such as pressure sores, osteoporosis, and depression.[2] Fortunately, advances in the treatment of experimental SCI are being made at an accelerated pace.[3,4] Developments in neuroprotection, regeneration, and rehabilitation support the field's general optimism and provide realistic hope that a cure is imminent. Although effectively treating experimental SCI in animals is an enormously important task, translating this research into clinically feasible interventions for humans will not necessarily follow.

■ Translation of Spinal Cord Injury Research

Translation of medical research into the clinical sector is a difficult task for any field. First, anatomical, physiological, and sheer size differences between experimental animal models and humans can lead to vastly distinct outcomes when a treatment is translated.[5] To account for this expected variation, the medical community requires rigorous testing and infallible findings from preliminary research before an intervention can be successfully translated. As such, most clinical treatments are safe, reliable, and effective, but innovation is tremendously challenging. The issue of running clinical trials for SCI therapies has been well documented.[2,5–7] Briefly, to translate a therapy from bench to bedside, researchers must (1) establish its efficacy in animal models, (2) overcome general model-to-model obstacles like size and anatomy, (3) verify safety and potential benefit despite confounding variables, (4) recruit an appropriate sample of human participants to minimize injury variability without creating a group so specific that results won't be generalizable to the SCI population at large, and (5) demonstrate that the treatment is efficacious.[5,7] This chapter addresses only the final step of this demanding process by outlining the issue of outcomes measures, explaining how currently available measures for SCI are insufficient, and providing suggestions for their improvement, specifically, encouraging the refinement and expanded use of electrophysiological measures, such as the electrical perceptual threshold (EPT) test and the brain motor control assessment (BMCA) protocol.

Outcome Measures

The objective and valid conduct of successful clinical studies, and, eventually, the effective choice of therapeutic approach and rehabilitation planning, requires the development of appropriate tools and measures.[6,8] However, validly and reliably measuring any type of behavior is difficult because variation in baseline, recovery, and confounding factors produces unique patterns of activity.[9] Evaluating neuronal function presents additional challenges; the intricacy, organization, and widespread involvement of the nervous system make it nearly impossible to directly map anatomy to function.[2,6] Assessing the capacity of the spinal cord usually involves analyzing locomotor behavior, which adds yet another layer of complexity because it is a multifaceted behavior involving several distinct functions and physiological systems.[10] Particularly challenging is the establishment of reliable baseline measures immediately following SCI because it usually results from trauma, and patients initially present with comorbid injuries and are often unconscious or unresponsive for considerable periods immediately following the insult, which allows only subjective assessments. Initial assessments, then, can often be misleading or simply erroneous if they can be obtained at all after accounting for limitations in sensation and voluntary behavior.

Accordingly, the nature of optimal outcomes for clinical trials investigating therapies for SCI remains a controversial and uncertain issue.[7] Researchers and clinicians often disagree about what types of behaviors are important, or at least which are most relevant for analytical focus. SCI includes a complicated interplay of impairments, including neurological insult, autonomic dysfunction, changes in quality of life and community integration, pain, spasticity, and sensorimotor deficits, which do not necessarily recover along the same trajectories.[2,6,11] Ideally, individual outcomes that have been standardized and have demonstrated statistical efficacy would be assessed at cellular, physiological, and behavioral levels for all of these behaviors[6,7,10]; however, this ideal is constrained by the reality of confirming the usefulness of the suite of assessments and of the clinical impossibility of administering them all to patients.[12]

Another divisive issue surrounding the outcomes debate is the definition of clinically meaningful change.[6,13] Most researchers agree that subtle neurological changes should not be underestimated because subclinical function may indicate where recovery is more feasible,[14] but small effect sizes in highly variable subject pools lead to nonsignificant results and trial "failures."[15] Although there are accepted thresholds for clinically meaningful change in most of the widely used outcome measures for SCI, these blanketing guidelines add little to the field in terms of recognizing therapeutic benefit for all patients. For example, most researchers acknowledge that the Berg Balance Scale (BBS) has the capacity to demonstrate change over time and that increases of 5 to 7 points (out of a total of 56 points given for 14 different actions) represent clinically meaningful improvement.[16] Tests of ambulation speed and endurance, like the ten meter walk test (10MWT) and the six minute walk test (6MWT), are also recognized for their capacity to detect change over time, as well as their profound floor and ceiling effects and their disregard for assistive devices.[10] Ditunno et al. report that only 14/124 participants were actually able to complete the 6MWT due to the severity of their paralysis.[16] Participants are deemed "slow" walkers if their speed is < 0.8 m/s, and individuals ambulating faster than this are often fully functional.[17] Another suggestion is that neither of these tests is relevant to real life situations, nor do they reflect the individual's true capacity. To summarize, agreeing upon an all-encompassing guideline for clinical relevance may be completely unnecessary, if not obstructive. Gains of even 0.01 m/s, or doing so with a less invasive assistive device, could be of great personal relevance to an individual who was not able to walk at all before, whereas gains > 0.5 m/s could mean little to individuals who can already walk faster than the "fully functional" 0.8 m/s. Clinical significance, then, is a concept that must be carefully considered, especially when considering groups of SCI patients with wide-ranging skill levels and functional capacities. Over all, researchers recognize that a battery of powerfully sensitive instruments, focusing on several domains of function, is most desirable. Standardizing excellent outcome measures will lead to decreases in necessary sample size, increased positive findings, and more accurate prediction of when and which candidates are likely to benefit from interventions, ultimately decreasing cost.[5]

Commonly Used Outcome Measures for Spinal Cord Injury

Outcome measures that are commonly used to document deficit and recovery after SCI are as varied as the typical sequelae of impairments they attempt to analyze. In a recent review, Alexander outlines several categories of popular assessments for SCI, including neurological—assessing behavior to understand the severity and prognosis of the injury; neuroimaging using magnetic resonance imaging to access neurological information; sensorimotor function using a variety of techniques to document motor and sensory capacity; functional potential using self-report and objective tests to monitor overall activities of daily living; extremity function using generic tests of hand or foot function to assess motor and sensory impairment of complex tasks; ambulation tests to monitor speed, endurance, and functionality; autonomic function using general measures for blood pressure, heart rate, and orthostatic regulation; colon and rectal function, typically documenting either physiology or subjective reports of activity; lower urinary tract function, mainly urodynamics;

sexual function; pain; spasticity, typically assessed with electromyography (EMG); depression, quality of life; and participation.[6] Devices for many of these categories were initially developed for other disorders and, thus, are currently not standardized or statistically tested for use in the SCI population.[6,18] Much of the SCI literature focuses on just three of these categories: neurological status, motor and sensory function, and functional capacity. Rather than outlining the shortcomings of this limited focus (e.g., many have noted that there are few outcome measures that assess autonomic function, especially sweating, temperature regulation, and respiration,[6,8,12] despite the fact that autonomic dysfunction is related to a majority of the most common causes of death for individuals with SCI[19]), this chapter addresses shortcomings within this focus, demonstrating how currently available outcome measures used within the popular categories are insufficient (**Table 45.1**).

Clinical Neurological Assessment

As soon as possible (i.e., when the patient is stable and conscious), patients diagnosed with SCI are assessed on the American Spinal Injury Association's (ASIA) Impairment Scale (AIS).[5,6] The AIS is an index based on a clinical neurological examination from which several measures of neurological damage are generated (neurological, sensory, and motor injury level).[20] Reliability and validity of the AIS have been shown time and again, but although it is accepted and used as the gold standard outcome measure for SCI, most researchers and clinicians acknowledge that the AIS has limitations, specifically in sensitivity.[6,12] Two of the most obvious contributions to the insensitivity of the AIS are its exclusion of tests for thoracic motor function, muscles that are innervated by the thoracic segments where most of the limited recovery is anticipated to occur, and its classification of sensory function into "normal," "absent," or "abnormal" categories.[12] Simply put, AIS is valid as a tool for classification of injuries but not as an outcome measure,[21] and, accordingly, many of the other outcome measures we will discuss demonstrate validity by correlating with AIS classifications.

Functional, Motor, and Sensory Assessments

A plethora of devices have been either developed for SCI or modified from use for other disorders to assess either functional, motor, or sensory impairments, or some combination of the three. These outcome measures are typically considered either functional (i.e., they monitor an individual's capacity to perform various tasks) or electrophysiological (referring mostly to the method by which neurological functioning is assessed).

Functional Assessment of Neurological Functioning

Functional Independence Measure

Probably the most commonly used outcome measure for neurological disorders worldwide, the Functional Independence Measure (FIM) monitors functional ability in daily activities, focusing on the amount of assistance, or burden of care, required.[5,10,13] Although the FIM requires extensive training to administer correctly, research has shown that the test is reliable and has good predictive validity, especially for life satisfaction and burden of care.[13] The FIM was not originally developed for SCI, and although this allows the score to include all levels of disability, its broadness creates several issues for use in SCI.[10,13] First, some SCI patients simply cannot perform FIM tasks within 72 hours of their injury, due to the unstable nature of their condition, lack of consciousness, or other injuries.[13] Most importantly, the FIM suffers from profound insensitivity to impairments in individuals with less severe SCI who do not require assistance.[10] In short, the FIM simply has no real utility for SCI recovery assessment.[13]

Spinal Cord Independence Measure

After encountering the aforementioned issues with the FIM, researchers specifically designed the Spinal Cord Independence

Table 45.1 Advantages and Limitations of Commonly Used Outcomes Assessments

Outcomes assessments: electrophysiological measures	Advantages	Limitations
Reflex testing	• Statistically valid and reliable • Sensitive and applicable for individuals with SCI at all levels and severities • Provides objective, quantitative data • Correlated with spasticity • Indicative of both short- and long-term plasticity in the nervous system	• Assessment requires time, training, and equipment • Need standardization of protocol and data management • Data can be affected by extraneous factors that produce noise that can lead to misinterpretation
Sensory evoked potential	• Statistically valid and reliable • Sensitive and applicable for individuals with SCI at all levels and severities, conscious patient involvement is limited • Provides objective, quantitative data	• Assessment requires time, training, and equipment • Need standardization of protocol and data management • Assessment is restricted to fast conducting tracts • Monitors specific pathways only
Motor evoked potential	• Statistically valid and reliable • Sensitive and applicable for individuals with SCI at all levels and severities, conscious patient involvement is limited • Provides objective, quantitative data	• Assessment requires time, training, and equipment • Need standardization of protocol and data management • Assessment is restricted to fast conducting tracts • Monitors specific pathways only
Electrical perceptual threshold (EPT)	• Statistically valid and reliable • Sensitive and applicable for individuals with SCI at all levels and severities • Provides objective, quantitative data • Assessment of both fast and slow conducting tracts • Can be integrated to provide a complete sensorimotor analysis	• Assessment requires time, training, and equipment • Need standardization of protocol and data management • Conscious patient involvement is required
Brain motor control assessment (BMCA)	• Statistically valid and reliable • Sensitive and applicable for individuals with SCI at all levels and severities • Provides objective, quantitative data • Assessment of both fast and slow conducting tracts • Can be integrated to provide a complete sensorimotor analysis	• Assessment requires time, training, and equipment • Need standardization of protocol and data management • Conscious patient involvement is required

Measure (SCIM) to comprehensively test functionality in SCI.[6,13] The SCIM is made up of three subscales that test individuals with SCI on their ability to perform relevant daily tasks and their corresponding assistance needs.[5,13] The tool is growing in popularity and usage, especially as a complement to AIS assessments, and is more sensitive than both the AIS and the FIM, particularly for mobility, bladder, bowel, and respiratory functioning.[13] Psychometric analyses demonstrate that the SCIM is valid and reliable and has good predictive validity, and can, therefore, be used to plan rehabilitation programs.[13] Still, even as the SCIM is much more sensitive than other measures of global disability, it also fails to detect either subclinical changes, improvements on either end of the disability spectrum, or nuances of motor behavior, such as quality of gait, balance, and real-life mobility (like ambulation over uneven surfaces).[13]

Walking Index for Spinal Cord Injury

The Walking Index for SCI (WISCI) is an outcome measure that evaluates walking in a standard environment while accounting for bracing, ambulation aids, and assistance.[5,10] The score depends on the participant's device requirements and is therefore widely inclusive, but it does not account for speed, gait quality, or sit-to-stand capacity.[10] Psychometric analyses have shown the test's reliability and validity by correlating scores with the lower extremity motor score of the AIS, the FIM, and measures of balance, speed, and distance.[6,10,16] Once again, however, this outcome measure lacks sensitivity at both ends of the disability spectrum, in chronic injuries, and for subclinical changes.[10]

Ten Meter and Six Minute Walk Tests

Outcome measures that assess walking speed over a given distance or within a specified time frame are considered overall measures of walking ability and provide some predictive value for independent ambulation.[10,17] The 10MW and 6MW tests were originally developed and standardized to detect functional capacity in other neurological disorders because it is assumed that gait mechanics, strength, and proprioception all have a direct effect on ambulation speed.[10,22] Psychometric analyses have shown that both timed measures are more reliable, valid, and sensitive than qualitative functional measures, at least in individuals with incomplete SCI who already have the capacity to ambulate.[10,23] Both tests produce substantial floor and ceiling effects, given that some individuals are unable to perform the tests at all and others can perform them without any real effort.[10] Additional methodological issues include decreased reliability with repeated testing, environmental effects (like the number of turns on a course), examiner effects (such as type and amount of encouragement given),[10] and use of compensation, such as assistive devices.

Electrophysiological Assessment of Neurological Functioning

Another method for assessing outcomes after SCI includes electrophysiological measures (see Chapter 38 for a thorough review). These noninvasive and precise tests have the potential to fill the field's need for a tool that can predict outcome early after injury.[8,24–27] Sensory and motor evoked potentials and reflex testing can provide information beyond the clinical exam, be completed in impaired patients, help more completely characterize the injury, and detect changes, allowing prompt responses in treatment plans.[8,26,28] Electrophysiological assessments offer the potential to detect subclinical changes in neurological functioning because they are objective and much more sensitive than the AIS or functional tests.[6,8,12,14,15,27,29–31] The tests are sensitive not only for monitoring recovery of motor and sensory capacity as well as spasticity but also for establishing baseline measures of impairment.[32,33] One study reported that an electrophysiological assessment of sensory capacity placed 41% of subjects into less severe categories of injury than suggested by their AIS scores.[31] Therefore, most researchers agree that electrophysiological tests will increase the clinician's ability to determine the level and "completeness" of an SCI in addition to monitoring outcomes and suggest administering them alongside the AIS to complement and enhance evaluations.[8,15] Psychometric analyses have shown that, in general, they are sensitive, reliable, and valid because they closely correspond to actual neurological functioning,[29,33] and over all these measures are quickly becoming viewed as the best tools for detecting functional capacity of neurons after injury.[6,30,31]

The rationale behind electrophysiological testing is that retention or recovery of voluntary control or reflexive activation of a muscle or conscious perception of a sensation is indicative of intact, uninjured, or recovered neurological processes. Sensory evoked potentials demonstrate the integrity of sensory impulse transmission, are not affected by spinal shock, and can be conducted in unconscious patients, whereas motor evoked potentials demonstrate the integrity of motoneuron pathways, can be conducted painlessly in conscious patients, and can be used to supplement the clinical exam in characterizing the injury and assessing its extent.[8,26] Peripheral testing, such as EMGs and reflex assessments, can be used to distinguish peripheral lesions, assess motoneuron functioning, and detect the development of neuropathologies, such as spasticity.[8,26,34] There are many different protocols for electrophysiological tests, but they all share the same basic principles. An electrical stimulation is given to a sensory dermatome (usually mimicking key AIS evaluation points) or muscle, and the pattern of output response is noted either by patient report or EMG.[27,31] Decreased latency of response indicates improved neurological conduction and, accordingly, some degree of neurological recovery.[12,35,36] These measures have already been successfully used to demonstrate improved conduction following pharmaceutical intervention,[36] the reestablishment of synaptic activity after transplant therapy (despite the failure of these grafts to regenerate),[37,38] and a distinction between the capacity for patients with sexual impairments to achieve or maintain erections.[39] Some studies also tout the prognostic value of these assessments, especially for sympathetic failure and autonomic hyperreflexia,[8,39] bladder functioning, and future ambulatory capacity.[8]

Electrical Perceptual Threshold

A method for quantitative sensory testing, the EPT test, was developed by Belci et al.[40] for the assessment of cutaneous sensibility and has been validated against the AIS[12] (see Chapter 39 for a thorough review). The EPT has also demonstrated repeatability for both inter- and intrarater trials.[29] In brief, the EPT measures the threshold, or minimally detectable sensory appreciation, of constant current square wave pulses (0.5 msec) applied at a frequency of 3 Hz to an adhesive, disposable cathodal electrode applied to the AIS test point of a dermatome. A larger indifferent anode is attached to the skin at a remote location. The method of limits is then used to determine threshold, increasing the strength of stimulation until a participant just reports sensation at the location of the cathode, and subsequently reducing it until sensation is reported as lost. The test is repeated three times for each dermatome, and the average of the descending thresholds is taken as the EPT. The method is well tolerated by individuals and can be performed in less time than the AIS sensory exam, with relatively modest increases in total cost.

The technique of perceptual threshold to cutaneous electrical stimulation (EPT) was developed on persons with intact neurological systems. Thresholds differed according to the dermatome tested (n = 7 C3-L5), but a correlation was established for equivalent dermatomes on the left and right sides. Women had slightly lower EPTs than men, but the difference was significant only for the lumbar (L3, L5) dermatomes and not elsewhere (C3, C4, C5, C6, and T8). The technique has been adapted to assess individuals with SCI at any level and of any impairment grade.[31] First, a thorough evaluation of normal EPT values was established for 30 control subjects for all dermatomes (C3 through S2). The results confirmed and extended the earlier study with regard to variation in EPT between dermatomes and the good correlation between left and right sides. The data provided a template against which to evaluate subjects with SCI. EPT was measured in 45 patients at AIS key sensory points for selected dermatomes at, above, and below the clinically defined level of lesion. The level of lesion determined by AIS was compared with the EPT readings and was the same in 48% of tests. In 41%, the EPT was actually more cranial than the clinical level, and in only 11% of tests was it lower. The EPT also revealed asymmetries in sensory perception that were not evident from the AIS grading, particularly in the zone of partial preservation. For dermatomes with preserved but impaired light touch (AIS grade 1) and absent pinprick sensation (AIS grade 0), EPT was measurable but elevated above control values. This provided preliminary evidence that EPT reflects conduction in the posterior column pathways rather than the anterolateral spinothalamic tract. A more recent unpublished study has produced further evidence to support this association (**Fig. 45.1**). The conclusion was that EPT provides a simple, reproducible quantitative sensory assessment of the level and degree of impairment in SCI. EPT adds to the sensitivity and resolution of the AIS clinical grading by (1) increasing objectivity through machine- rather than human-applied stimulation; (2) providing a continuous numerical scale of sensitivity, rather than a discontinuous ordinal scale, that is able to reveal asymmetries (left, right) and subtle changes with time/recovery not indicated by AIS testing; and (3) revealing deficits in sensory perception not

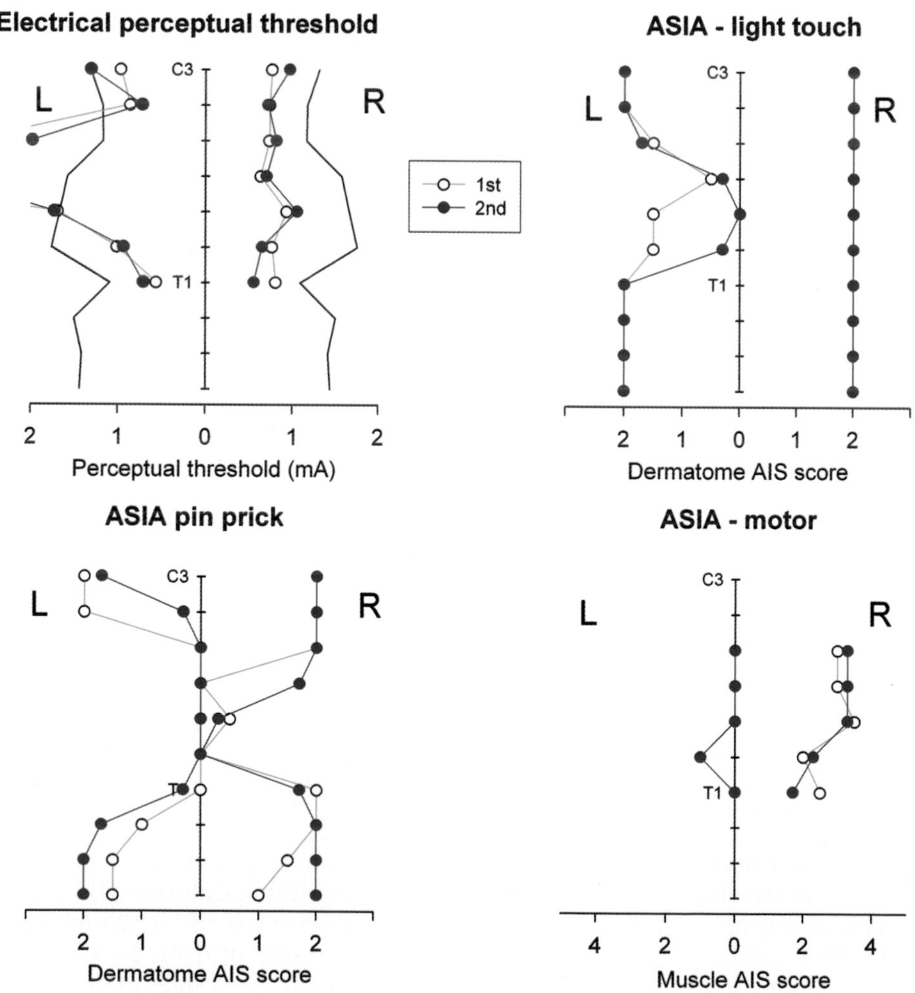

Fig. 45.1 Results of electrical perceptual threshold (EPT) and American Spinal Injury Association (ASIA) Impairment Scale testing on an individual with an ASIA D spinal cord injury at C4.

detected by AIS sensory ratings (i.e., raised EPT for AIS light touch and pinprick scores of 2 (normal).[29]

A recently published study on the reliability of cutaneous EPT for the assessment of sensory perception in individuals with clinically incomplete SCI ($n = 2$, chronic, >20 months; $n = 10$, subacute, <9 months postinjury) and noninjured individuals ($n = 12$) showed no significant differences in mean intra- or interrater EPT values at, above, or below the level of lesion (AIS sensory level) for participants with clinically incomplete SCI.[29] The intraclass correlation coefficient (ICC) ranged from 0.56 to 0.80 for intrarater and 0.52 to 0.91 for interrater classes, depending on the neurological level tested. Additionally, there was a significant correlation (Pearson's $r = 0.93$) between EPTs for four different dermatomes of noninjured (NI) individuals assessed using two different types of stimulators. Therefore, EPT provides an objective and quantitative measure of threshold for cutaneous sensory function with good inter- and intrarater reliability and can be assessed using different stimulators. This conclusion has now been independently confirmed in a repeatability study by Leong et al.,[41] and a further study has validated EPT against dermatomal somatosensory evoked potentials in persons with SCI.[42]

Brain Motor Control Assessment

A well-researched electrophysiological protocol for assessment of motor functioning is the BMCA, a neurophysiological method for characterizing impaired neurological motor function in persons with neurological dysfunction.[30,32,43] The test was designed to objectively and reproducibly assess suprasegmental control of segmental motor activity using EMG.[14,30] In the BMCA, composite motor unit activity recorded from multiple muscles is used to indicate the state of spinal motor excitability relative to a motor task requested or required by the protocol.[30,44] Thus the BMCA measures the amplitude, duration, and time to peak of EMG activity of multiple muscles during standardized voluntary, passive, and reflexive maneuvers.

The BMCA was originally designed to identify and characterize residual supraspinal central nervous system influence on motor output following a severe SCI, but it has since been validated in persons with motor complete SCI (AIS A and B).[32,43,45] Using the BMCA, Sherwood et al.[43] reported the presence of supralesional influence over reinforcement maneuvers, vibration response, and/or withdrawal reflex suppression in 84% of 88 participants with motor-complete SCI. Recently repeated, these neurophysiological markers were found in 64% of a convenience sample of 67 participants with motor-complete SCI.[32,45] These markers allow researchers to classify participants distinct from AIS groups.[14] Neurophysiological distinctions of motor complete (indicating limited reflex activation and the absence of contralateral and tonic activation), discomplete (indicating segmental function in the absence of voluntary movement), and incomplete (preservation of segmental and voluntary control), injuries are more sensitive than AIS classification and provide a more accurate representation of the person's functional capacity.[14]

To develop the protocol for assessing EMG during standard movements and to determine the appropriate stimulation pattern, the voluntary control maneuvers of the BMCA profile were evaluated in neurologically intact individuals.[30,45] From this preliminary study, a baseline was generated for each movement, so that future assessments could focus on the change in activation per movement, rather than the variation of amplitudes between participants.[30] The resultant voluntary response index (VRI) is a comparison of EMG responses in individuals with SCI with the collected measures from intact participants, providing a profile for comparison of recovery of function.[30,44,46] The VRI is related to the condition of the corticospinal system and allows the quantification of the quality of voluntary control relative to corticospinal patency.[45] It consists of two components, the magnitude of the EMG response and the similarity index (SI). VRI has been shown to be constant for intact neurological systems and reliably distinguished among SCI groups and between individuals with SCI and those without.[46]

Lee et al. examined the VRI reliability using three repetitions of each of 10 volitional motor tasks in 69 participants with SCI (34 AIS-C, 35 AIS-D).[30] In six of the 69 participants (3 AIS-C, 3 AIS-D), the study was repeated 1 week later. Reliability and validity were assessed by intraclass correlation coefficient (ICC), analysis of variance, coefficient of variance, and Pearson's correlation. Good reliability was found for magnitude (ICC = 0.71 to 0.99, Pearson's r = 0.77 to 0.99) and for SI (ICC = 0.65 to 0.96, Pearson's r = 0.72 to 0.93) for three repeated tests (within-day). The SI showed less variation than magnitude (p <0.001). No significant difference of magnitude and SI was observed between tasks. Further, the index was used to differentiate weak voluntary motor function from spasm activation in those with clinically motor complete SCI and showed a strong relationship to motor evoked potentials elicited by transcranial magnetic motor cortex stimulation.[36]

The BMCA maintains the advantage realized in the AIS exam of targeting the essential motor movements that represent specific neurological segments. The exceptional advantage of the BMCA is that the response is quantitative, does not rely on the subjectivity of the examiner, and provides measurable parameters of the neural components of the motor task. The limitation of the currently validated BMCA protocol is that it is limited to the lumbosacral segments. Thus our current objective is to expand the BMCA to cervical and thoracic segments (**Fig. 45.2**). We will include muscles innervated by the cranial nerve to primarily serve as control muscles above the lesion of SCI regardless of level. The protocol will include 17 neurological segments, adding an additional sensitivity of four cervical motor segments and four thoracic motor segments beyond that currently available with AIS examination. The maneuvers associated with the muscles innervated by the segments are also outlined in **Fig. 45.2**. By extending the BMCA to include these segments, we will be able to

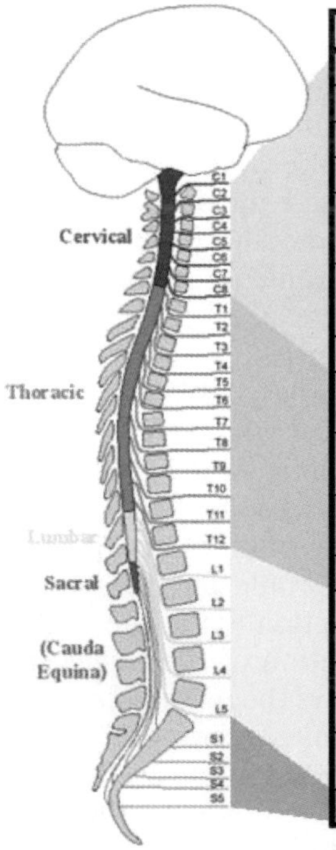

Spinal roots	Muscle	Maneuver	AIS Maneuver
CN XI, C1-C2	Sternocleidomastoid(C1-3)	Shoulder elevation	
C3	Upper Trapezius(C3-4)	Shoulder elevation	
C4	Scalene(C4-8)	Forced inspiration	
C5	Biceps Brachii	Elbow flexion	Elbow flexion
C6	Extensor Carpi Radialis(C6-7)	Wrist Extension	Wrist extension
	Flexor Carpi Radialis(C6-7)	Wrist Flexion	
C7	Extensor Digitorum Communis(C7-8)	Finger extension	
	Triceps Brachii(C7-8)	Elbow extension	Elbow extension
C8	Flexor Digitorum Profundus(C8-T1)	Finger flexion	Finger flexion
T1	Abductor Pollicis Brevis(C8-T1) Abductor Digiti Quinti(C8-T1)	Finger abduction	Finger abduction
T2-T5	Intercostals(C6-T10)	Trunk flexion Forced inspiration & expiration	
T6-9	Rectus Abdominus(T6-12)	Trunk flexion Forced inspiration & expiration	
T10-12	Erector Spinae	Trunk extension	
L1	Paraspinal, lumbosacral (L1-S1)	Hip extension	
L2	Rectus Femoris(L2-4)	Hip flexion	Hip flexion
L3	Vastus Lateralis(L2-4)	Knee extension	Knee extension
L4	Tibialis Anterior(L4-5)	Ankle dorsiflexion	Ankle dorsiflexion
L5	Extensor Digitorum Longus(L5-S1), Extensor Hallucis Longus(L5-S1)	Long toe extension	Long toe extension
S1	Soleus(L5-S2)	Ankle plantarflexion	Ankle plantarflexion

Fig. 45.2 Protocol for the expanded version of the brain motor control assessment (BMCA).

provide motor assessments that are more precise, sensitive, and reliable measures of motor recovery in persons with SCI. We have begun to collect and analyze data from noninjured individuals and individuals with SCI who have participated in pilot protocols for the cervical segments and thoracic segments showing the feasibility of these protocols.[47] Hence we can see that the BMCA provides a more precise analysis of function than the AIS. We recorded EMG bursting from an individual with C4 traumatic SCI at days, weeks, and months after injury (**Fig. 45.3**). Further studies are warranted to standardize the assessment and analyses, conduct reliability and validity studies, and develop a protocol that is clinically feasible within the first week of injury. In addition, combining the ETP and BMCA would provide a more comprehensive assessment of neurological function.

The SCI literature reflects a growing consensus that current outcome measures for recovery after SCI are insufficient. Most researchers agree that electrophysiological tests offer the best opportunity for enhancing assessments, especially as a complement to AIS.[15] Moreover, whereas sensorimotor integration is essential for successful movement, it is not tested by any available measures. Studies show that, in addition to the special senses, balanced standing is achieved by the integration of proprioceptive and cutaneous feedback from limbs with voluntary drive to the leg and trunk muscles.[48] The ability to judge muscle power required to lift a weight depends on somatosensory input,[49] as does controlled locomotion.[50] Fine motor movements necessary for manipulating objects require sensorimotor integration (e.g., if motor function scores are high); however, sensation is severely impaired and the individual will not be able to effectively perform the motor task and ultimately be limited in activities of daily living. Adopting a sensorimotor neurological method of evaluation using tools such as the BMCA *and* EPT would present several advantages: (1) quantification of the neuromuscular activation and sensation response during standardized and controlled conditions; (2) examination of many different motor spinal segments and dermatomes, including some that are not currently assessed; (3) early and late recovery assessment, including the first day of injury through follow-up years later; (4) reproducibility and reliability across multiple clinical sites; and (5) a more sensitive assessment of neurological motor and sensory level and function than is now available.

Although the tests themselves are relatively simple, electrophysiological assessment and interpretation require specialized equipment, trained staff, and time for acquisition and analyses.[25,26,51] Until there is more work done on the standardization of the acquisition and analysis of data, clinical availability of these tests will be limited. Moreover, when all three protocols are combined (upper limb, lower limb, and trunk) the number of muscles tested and the time to conduct the protocol may not be clinically feasible, so targeted protocols for specific injury levels need to be developed. Based on analyses from preliminary data in our laboratory of the three protocols, we suggest that the critical information regarding neurophysiological function can be obtained by specifying the protocol to include the motor tasks associated with the level of injury, three segments above, three segments below, and the most rostral and distal muscles. This protocol also is comparable to the EPT protocol.

Over all, these measures are accepted as objective, reliable, and precise; however, there are reports of some issues with variable electrode placement, differences in scoring based on patient subjectivity, and confounding electrical noise from abnormal activations (spasms).[6,30,31] For BMCA, there are some modest floor effects as validity decreases in AIS A participants, due to the very low EMG activation.[44] The most notable limitation is that some measures (like the latencies of evoked potentials) do not correlate with observed functional improvements,[24] whereas others (like H-reflex sensitivity) continue to recover despite behavioral plateaus.[52] Although reports like these seem to limit the applicability of electrophysiological methods, the argument could be made that discrepancies like these are exactly why further development

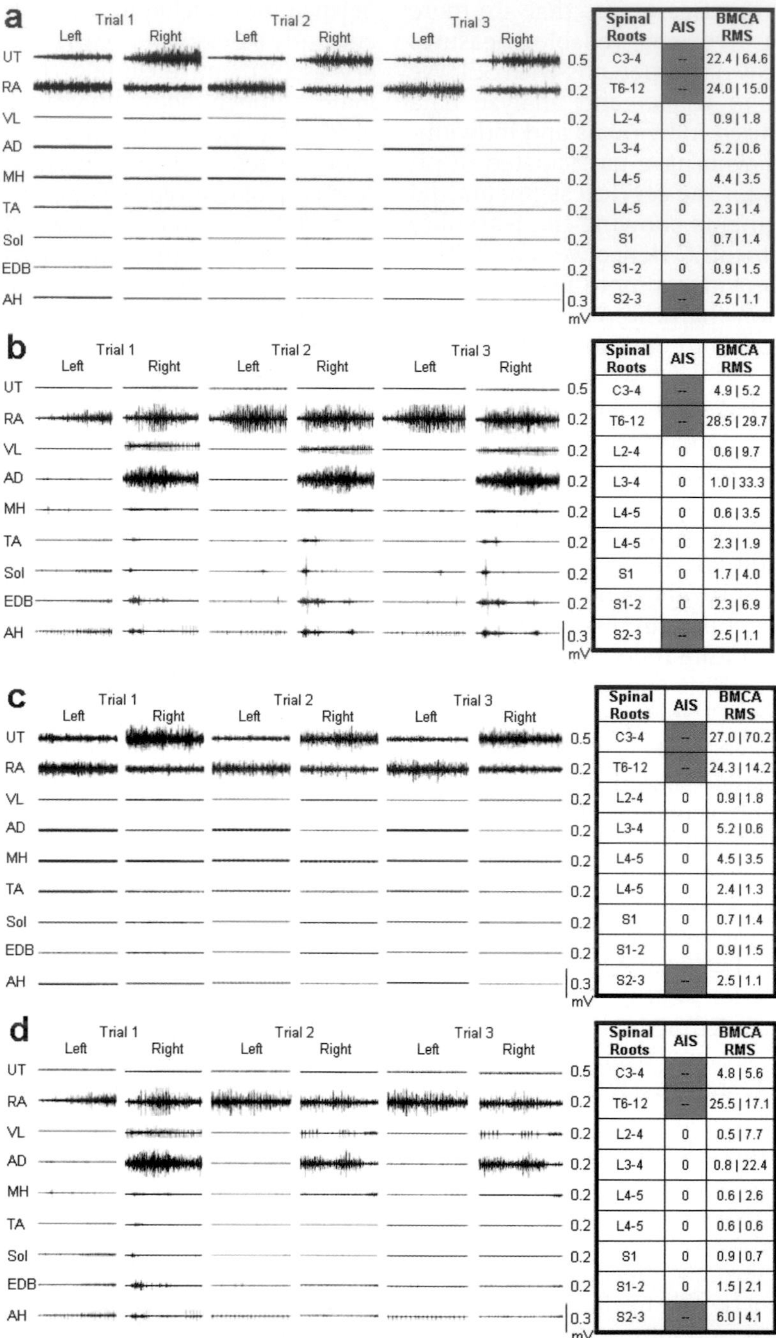

Fig. 45.3 Electromyographic bursting recorded from an individual with a traumatic C4 spinal cord injury, assessed days, weeks, and months postinjury.

is warranted. Varied protocols combining neurological, functional, and conductivity outcomes are crucial for distinguishing between processes of compensation, plasticity, and repair.[24] Functional recovery after SCI is a multifaceted problem and will require multidisciplinary approaches and outcomes that assess multiple, and quite possibly, independent, aspects of recovery.

Conclusion

We are continuing work aimed at integrating the BMCA and EPT, including the (1) standardization of the hardware, software, and protocols needed to produce reliable and valid results in multiple clinical centers; (2) assessment of these tools in persons with SCI within 1 week after injury up to 1 year postinjury and before and after activity-based therapy; and (3) relation of the quantitative measures to each individuals' functional outcomes. Standardization of the protocol and administration of the test will allow for its utilization in multicenter clinical trials.

Generating a powerful treatment for neurological disorders is an extremely difficult task. First, the nervous system is intricate, delicate, and not fully understood. Second, the implications of neurological injury are so widespread and interrelated that addressing any one of them requires multisystem evaluations and multitargeted interventions. Third, even our best experimental models are failing to translate clinically, indicating some disconnect between bench and bedside methods. To make this task even more arduous, designing sensitive, valid, reliable outcome measures for complicated behaviors, such as autonomic function and locomotion, and their successful standardization and implementation are challenging. However, funding for clinical trials depends on the researcher's ability to demonstrate the efficacy of a given intervention, which, in turn, is reliant on the efficacy of the outcome measure used. A combinatorial approach will be needed, so it is essential that we have available outcome measures that can detect incremental improvements in neurological levels in the early stages after SCI. Therefore, while it is obvious that in the quest for a cure for SCI there are urgent and addressable issues regarding continued basic research needs, inadequate experimental models, and improper clinical trial design, the lack of powerful outcome measures will undermine all of these efforts. Future efforts need to focus on developing, assessing for reliability and validity, and standardizing quantitative, sensitive outcome measures for utilization in clinical trials. Expansion of electrophysiological methods, like the BMCA and EPT, will further the field not only in terms of improving assessment but also toward the ultimate goal of a cure.

Pearls

- Electrophysiological measures, like the BMCA and EPT, provide objective, quantitative data and are useful for all individuals with SCI at any time point after their injury.
- Integration of the BMCA and EPT will provide a measure of sensorimotor function, which is currently unavailable, thereby enhancing current assessments by monitoring a variety of motor spinal segments and dermatomes with higher sensitivity.
- These tests are statistically valid, reliable, and sensitive and can provide insight into the neurological mechanisms of injury.

Pitfalls

- The BMCA and EPT assessments require a significant time commitment, extensive training, and specialized equipment to be conducted properly.
- Acquisition and analysis of the resultant data must be standardized to increase clinical availability. Additionally, the development of targeted protocols may be necessary because combining all three protocols (upper limb, lower limb, and trunk) may not be clinically feasible.
- Confounds such as variable electrode placement, electrical noise from spasms, and floor effects in participants diagnosed as AIS A will limit the functionality of the tests until more work can be done to advance their use.

References

1. Gibson C, Turner S, Donnelly M. One Degree of Separation: Paralysis and Spinal Cord Injury in the United States. Short Hills, NJ: Christopher and Dana Reeve Foundation; 2009
2. Alexander MS, Biering-Sorensen F, Bodner D, et al. International standards to document remaining autonomic function after spinal cord injury. Spinal Cord 2009;47(1):36–43
3. Courtine G, Gerasimenko Y, van den Brand R, et al. Transformation of nonfunctional spinal circuits into functional states after the loss of brain input. Nat Neurosci 2009;12(10):1333–1342
4. Onose G, Anghelescu A, Muresanu DF, et al. A review of published reports on neuroprotection in spinal cord injury. Spinal Cord 2009;47(10): 716–726
5. Steeves JD, Lammertse D, Curt A, et al; International Campaign for Cures of Spinal Cord Injury Paralysis. Guidelines for the conduct of clinical trials for spinal cord injury (SCI) as developed by the ICCP panel: clinical trial outcome measures. Spinal Cord 2007;45(3):206–221
6. Alexander MS, Anderson KD, Biering-Sorensen F, et al. Outcome measures in spinal cord injury: recent assessments and recommendations for future directions. Spinal Cord 2009;47(8):582–591
7. Anderson DK, Beattie M, Blesch A, et al. Recommended guidelines for studies of human subjects with spinal cord injury. Spinal Cord 2005;43(8): 453–458
8. Curt A, Dietz V. Electrophysiological recordings in patients with spinal cord injury: significance for predicting outcome. Spinal Cord 1999; 37(3):157–165
9. Dobkin B, Barbeau H, Deforge D, et al; Spinal Cord Injury Locomotor Trial Group. The evolution of walking-related outcomes over the first 12 weeks of rehabilitation for incomplete traumatic spinal cord injury: the multicenter randomized Spinal Cord Injury Locomotor Trial. Neurorehabil Neural Repair 2007;21(1):25–35
10. Jackson AB, Carnel CT, Ditunno JF, et al; Gait and Ambulation Subcommittee. Outcome measures for gait and ambulation in the spinal cord injury population. J Spinal Cord Med 2008;31(5): 487–499
11. Bowden MG, Hannold EM, Nair PM, Fuller LB, Behrman AL. Beyond gait speed: a case report of a multidimensional approach to locomotor rehabilitation outcomes in incomplete spinal cord injury. J Neurol Phys Ther 2008;32(3):129–138
12. Ellaway PH, Anand P, Bergstrom EM, et al. Towards improved clinical and physiological assessments of recovery in spinal cord injury: a clinical initiative. Spinal Cord 2004;42(6):325–337
13. Anderson K, Aito S, Atkins M, et al; Functional Recovery Outcome Measures Work Group. Functional recovery measures for spinal cord injury: an evidence-based review for clinical practice and research. J Spinal Cord Med 2008;31(2):133–144
14. Dimitrijevic MR, Hsu CY, McKay WB. Neurophysiological assessment of spinal cord and head injury. J Neurotrauma 1992;9(Suppl 1):S293–S300
15. Kramer JK, Taylor P, Steeves JD, Curt A. Dermatomal somatosensory evoked potentials and electrical perception thresholds during recovery from cervical spinal cord injury. Neurorehabil Neural Repair 2010;24(4):309–317
16. Ditunno JF Jr, Barbeau H, Dobkin BH, et al; Spinal Cord Injury Locomotor Trial Group. Validity of the walking scale for spinal cord injury and other domains of function in a multicenter clinical trial. Neurorehabil Neural Repair 2007;21(6): 539–550
17. Barbeau H, Elashoff R, Deforge D, Ditunno J, Saulino M, Dobkin BH. Comparison of speeds used for the 15.2-meter and 6-minute walks over the year after an incomplete spinal cord injury: the SCILT Trial. Neurorehabil Neural Repair 2007;21(4): 302–306
18. Dawson J, Shamley D, Jamous MA. A structured review of outcome measures used for the assessment of rehabilitation interventions for spinal cord injury. Spinal Cord 2008;46(12):768–780
19. Krassioukov A. Autonomic function following cervical spinal cord injury. Respir Physiol Neurobiol 2009;169(2):157–164
20. Marino RJ, Barros T, Biering-Sorensen F, et al; ASIA Neurological Standards Committee 2002. International standards for neurological classification of spinal cord injury. J Spinal Cord Med 2003;26(Suppl 1):S50–S56
21. Graves DE, Frankiewicz RG, Donovan WH. Construct validity and dimensional structure of the ASIA motor scale. J Spinal Cord Med 2006;29(1):39–45
22. Winchester P, Smith P, Foreman N, et al. A prediction model for determining over ground walking speed after locomotor training in persons with motor incomplete spinal cord injury. J Spinal Cord Med 2009;32(1):63–71
23. van Hedel HJ, Wirz M, Curt A. Improving walking assessment in subjects with an incomplete spinal cord injury: responsiveness. Spinal Cord 2006;44(6):352–356
24. Curt A, Van Hedel HJ, Klaus D, Dietz V; EM-SCI Study Group. Recovery from a spinal cord injury: significance of compensation, neural plasticity, and repair. J Neurotrauma 2008;25(6):677–685
25. Ellaway PH, Kuppuswamy A, Balasubramaniam AV, et al. Development of quantitative and sensitive assessments of physiological and functional outcome during recovery from spinal cord injury: a clinical initiative. Brain Res Bull 2011;84(4-5): 343–357
26. Grundy BL, Friedman W. Electrophysiological evaluation of the patient with acute spinal cord injury. Crit Care Clin 1987;3(3):519–548
27. Xie J, Boakye M. Electrophysiological outcomes after spinal cord injury. Neurosurg Focus 2008;25(5):E11
28. Phadke CP, Flynn SM, Thompson FJ, Behrman AL, Trimble MH, Kukulka CG. Comparison of single bout effects of bicycle training versus locomotor training on paired reflex depression of the soleus H-reflex after motor incomplete spinal cord injury. Arch Phys Med Rehabil 2009;90(7):1218–1228
29. King NK, Savic G, Frankel H, Jamous A, Ellaway PH. Reliability of cutaneous electrical perceptual threshold in the assessment of sensory perception in patients with spinal cord injury. J Neurotrauma 2009;26(7):1061–1068

30. Lee DC, Lim HK, McKay WB, Priebe MM, Holmes SA, Sherwood AM. Toward an objective interpretation of surface EMG patterns: a voluntary response index (VRI). J Electromyogr Kinesiol 2004; 14(3):379–388
31. Savic G, Bergström EM, Frankel HL, Jamous MA, Ellaway PH, Davey NJ. Perceptual threshold to cutaneous electrical stimulation in patients with spinal cord injury. Spinal Cord 2006;44(9):560–566
32. McKay WB, Lim HK, Priebe MM, Stokic DS, Sherwood AM. Clinical neurophysiological assessment of residual motor control in post-spinal cord injury paralysis. Neurorehabil Neural Repair 2004;18(3):144–153
33. Sherwood AM, Graves DE, Priebe MM. Altered motor control and spasticity after spinal cord injury: subjective and objective assessment. J Rehabil Res Dev 2000;37(1):41–52
34. Benito Penalva J, Opisso E, Medina J, et al. H reflex modulation by transcranial magnetic stimulation in spinal cord injury subjects after gait training with electromechanical systems. Spinal Cord 2010;48(5):400–406
35. Ellaway PH, Catley M, Davey NJ, et al. Review of physiological motor outcome measures in spinal cord injury using transcranial magnetic stimulation and spinal reflexes. J Rehabil Res Dev 2007;44(1):69–76
36. McKay WB, Stokic DS, Dimitrijevic MR. Assessment of corticospinal function in spinal cord injury using transcranial motor cortex stimulation: a review. J Neurotrauma 1997;14(8):539–548
37. Skinner RD, Houle JD, Reese NB, Garcia-Rill EE. Electrophysiological investigations of neurotransplant-mediated recovery after spinal cord injury. Adv Neurol 1997;72:277–290
38. Toft A, Scott DT, Barnett SC, Riddell JS. Electrophysiological evidence that olfactory cell transplants improve function after spinal cord injury. Brain 2007;130(Pt 4):970–984
39. Schmid DM, Curt A, Hauri D, Schurch B. Clinical value of combined electrophysiological and urodynamic recordings to assess sexual disorders in spinal cord injured men. Neurourol Urodyn 2003;22(4):314–321
40. Belci M, Catley M, Husain M, Frankel HL, Davey NJ. Magnetic brain stimulation can improve clinical outcome in incomplete spinal cord injured patients. Spinal Cord 2004;42(7):417–419
41. Leong GW, Gorrie CA, Ng K, Rutkowski S, Waite PM. Electrical perceptual threshold testing: a validation study. J Spinal Cord Med 2009;32(2): 140–146
42. Kramer JL, Moss AJ, Taylor P, Curt A. Assessment of posterior spinal cord function with electrical perception threshold in spinal cord injury. J Neurotrauma 2008;25(8):1019–1026
43. Sherwood AM, McKay WB, Dimitrijević MR. Motor control after spinal cord injury: assessment using surface EMG. Muscle Nerve 1996;19(8): 966–979
44. Lim HK, Sherwood AM. Reliability of surface electromyographic measurements from subjects with spinal cord injury during voluntary motor tasks. J Rehabil Res Dev 2005;42(4):413–422
45. McKay WB, Lee DC, Lim HK, Holmes SA, Sherwood AM. Neurophysiological examination of the corticospinal system and voluntary motor control in motor-incomplete human spinal cord injury. Exp Brain Res 2005;163(3):379–387
46. Lim HK, Lee DC, McKay WB, et al. Analysis of sEMG during voluntary movement, II: Voluntary response index sensitivity. IEEE Trans Neural Syst Rehabil Eng 2004;12(4):416–421
47. McKay WB, Ovechkin AV, Vitaz TW, Terson de Paleville DG, Harkema SJ. Long-lasting involuntary motor activity after spinal cord injury. Spinal Cord 2011;49(1):87–93
48. Maurer C, Mergner T, Peterka RJ. Multisensory control of human upright stance. Exp Brain Res 2006;171(2):231–250
49. Miall RC, Ingram HA, Cole JD, Gauthier GM. Weight estimation in a "deafferented" man and in control subjects: are judgements influenced by peripheral or central signals? Exp Brain Res 2000; 133(4):491–500
50. Pearson KG, Misiaszek JE, Hulliger M. Chemical ablation of sensory afferents in the walking system of the cat abolishes the capacity for functional recovery after peripheral nerve lesions. Exp Brain Res 2003;150(1):50–60
51. Savic G, Bergström EM, Davey NJ, et al. Quantitative sensory tests (perceptual thresholds) in patients with spinal cord injury. J Rehabil Res Dev 2007;44(1):77–82
52. Lee JK, Emch GS, Johnson CS, Wrathall JR. Effect of spinal cord injury severity on alterations of the H-reflex. Exp Neurol 2005;196(2):430–440

46

Somatosensory Function and Recovery after Spinal Cord Injury: Advanced Assessment of Segmental Sensory Function

John L. Kipling Kramer, John D. Steeves, and Armin Curt

Key Points

1. Clinical light touch and pinprick testing disclose changes in the perception of sensation with limited insight into the physiology of sensory pathways.
2. Quantitative sensory testing complements sensory testing due to increased sensitivity and responsiveness in the assessment of sensory pathways.
3. Segmental sensory evoked potentials may indicate changes in the conduction of large- and small-diameter pathways that are missed by clinical testing.

The assessment of somatosensory deficits after spinal cord injury (SCI) is an important component of the clinical examination. Impairments to different sensory modalities (e.g., proprioception, touch, and temperature) may vary depending on the disruption of ascending fibers in the spinal cord, range from diminished or absent sensation to complex hypersensitivity or hyperalgesia, and change during the course of spontaneous neurological recovery or secondary neurological deterioration (i.e., syringomyelia). The preservation of sensation after SCI is also considered a requisite for achieving desirable motor outcomes during rehabilitation and is related to the prediction of future performance of activities of daily living (ADLs), quality of life (QoL), and functional independence. Additionally, the plasticity of the somatosensory system may be a neural target for rehabilitation and therapeutic strategies that promote repair and regeneration, but which may also result in detrimental aberrant sprouting underlying neuropathic pain. Given the importance of closely monitoring sensory function after SCI for diagnosis, prognosis, and recovery (spontaneous or therapeutically derived), developing and implementing valid and reliable sensory measures that are responsive to subtle changes in afferent neurophysiology and related to functional outcomes are priorities of clinicians and researchers.

This chapter focuses on the three main pillars of the clinical assessment of somatosensory function after SCI: (1) the American Spinal Injury Association (ASIA) Impairment Scale (AIS), (2) quantitative sensory testing (QST), and (3) electrophysiological recordings. The validity, reliability, and responsiveness of these measures to detect deficits in the spinothalamic tract and dorsal column are discussed in relation to the stable neurological condition (chronic SCI) and during spontaneous neurological recovery (transition from acute to chronic SCI). Also discussed is the utility of the outcomes measured during the course of a clinical trial in SCI to assess the effectiveness and potential side-effects of intervention.

Sensory Examination According to the ASIA Impairment Scale

The classification of SCI by the AIS has undergone years of intensive study to examine psychometric properties[1–11] and the responsiveness to spontaneous neurological recovery.[12–17] Adopted by both the clinical and the research communities worldwide as a relatively undemanding test of basic motor and sensory function after SCI, the AIS has served as a stratification tool and primary outcome measure in all of the randomized clinical trials in SCI to date.[18,19] The sensory component of the AIS is based on the theoretical framework that dermatomes with defined boundaries in the periphery represent individual spinal segments anatomically organized into large- (light touch) and small-diameter (pinprick) fiber functions, which ascend in the dorsal column and spinothalamic tract, respectively (**Fig. 46.1**). The decussation points of these afferent fibers into the ventrolateral spinothalamic tract (i.e., small-diameter fibers, on entry into the spinal cord segment), and dorsal column (i.e., large-diameter, dorsal column nuclei in the brain stem) represent the key anatomical difference accounting for the dissociation of light touch and pinprick sensory impairments after SCI. The outcomes of sensory examination are at first integral in diagnosing and predicting long term the severity (i.e., sensory preservation at S4–5), neurological level, and functional deficits associated with SCI, and later, the planning of an appropriate rehabilitation program.

The reliability of AIS sensory outcomes is well supported in the literature by several large and statistically powerful studies. In general, studies examining the test–retest (i.e., intrarater) and interrater reliability of light touch and pinprick scores in the chronic, stable SCI condition demonstrate intraclass correlations that exceed the minimal requirements of clinical standards and strong interrater agreement. However, the reliability of light touch and pinprick may be influenced by several factors, including when the examination is performed after SCI, characteristics of the individual being examined (i.e., age), severity of SCI, and formal training of the examiner.

The two primary outcomes of the sensory component of the AIS (completeness of injury and cumulative light touch and pinprick sensory scores) are both subject to change during the course of spontaneous neurological recovery. First, the return of anal sensation (fourth and fifth sacral spinal cord segment) marks an important clinical event by which an individual spontaneously converts from a complete (AIS A) SCI to an incomplete (AIS B–D) SCI. So termed "AIS grade conversion" can be observed most prominently within the first year of SCI,[13,15,19,20] but it has been reported infrequently between 1 and 5 years after injury.[21] Recovering sensation in dermatomes near the level of lesion may also shift the neurological level of SCI caudally, thereby improving function in a segmental fashion. Unfortunately, conversion from complete to incomplete SCI occurs rather infrequently spontaneously or due to therapeutic intervention, and the spontaneous recovery of sensory scores (light touch and pinprick) is also

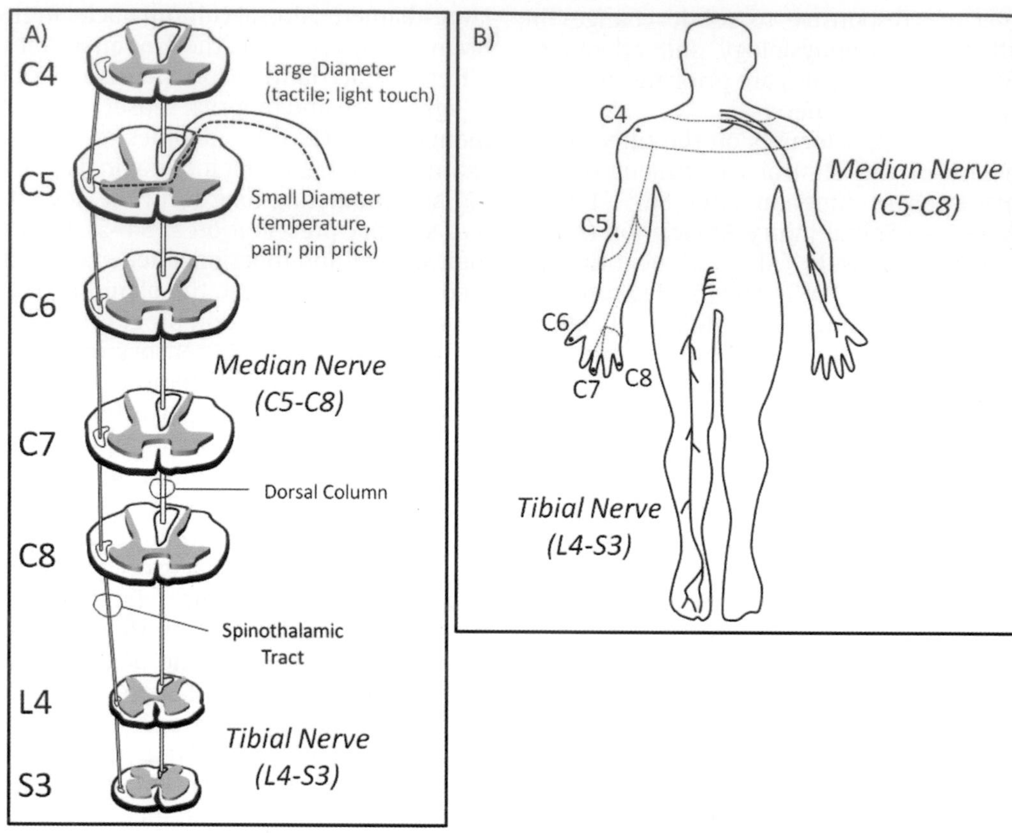

Fig. 46.1 **(A)** The segmental and longitudinal anatomical organization of ascending pathways in the spinal cord. **(B)** The distribution of key American Spinal Injury Association (ASIA) Impairment Scale (AIS) dermatomes in the upper limbs examined for light touch and pinprick sensation after spinal cord injury. The median (upper limb) and tibial (lower limb) nerves examined by conventional sensory evoked potentials are also shown.

quite small. These findings should be interpreted with caution, to illustrate the insensitivity of an ordinal measurement scale incapable of tracking changes within "impaired" dermatomes (i.e., hyper- and hyposensitive) rather than unchanging sensory deficits after SCI.

Quantitative Sensory Testing

The primary goal of implementing QST as an adjunct to the standard examination of sensory function is to improve the overall sensitivity and clinical meaningfulness of sensory outcomes after SCI. Specifically, QST methods aim to (1) detect underlying deficits in dermatomes with "normal" sensation, and (2) distinguish differences in dermatomes with "impaired" sensation. QST methods still require that the individual being tested report the sensation to an examiner but differ from the AIS by allowing a continuous scaled outcome to mark distinct sensory thresholds (i.e., perception and pain).

Several different QST modalities have been tested in individuals with SCI (**Table 46.1**).[22–28] Typically, thresholds are achieved by increasing the intensity of stimulation at a set rate from baseline until the individual verbally reports a change in sensation (i.e., method of limits). QST outcomes have generally been found to correlate with electrophysiological outcomes and the AIS examination and

Table 46.1 The Reported Reliability of QST Modalities in Individuals with SCI

Study author (date)	Study description	QST modality	ICC results	Interpretation
Krassioukov et al., 1999[26]	• Incomplete SCI subjects ($n = 21$), examined dermatomes below the level of SCI at chronic (mean, 6 years) time points • Intrarater (range)	Warm Cold Cold pain Vibration	.23–69 .45–81 .65–89 .76–90	• Depended on the dermatome and modality tested • Day-to-day variability higher in SCI subjects than uninjured controls • Repeated examination on separate days required to establish a baseline
Felix and Widerström-Noga, 2009[22]	• Complete and incomplete SCI subjects, examined dermatomes at and below the level of SCI with chronic (mean, 6 years) neuropathic pain ($n = 10$) • Intrarater (95% confidence)	*Mechanical Vibration Cool Warm Cold pain Hot pain	.84(0.75–90) .90(0.84–94) .90(0.83–94) .95(0.91–97) .50(0.28–67) .50(0.28–66)	• Moderate to fair reliability, comparable to uninjured controls • Innocuous modalities can be measured in one test session (do not require repeated examinations)
King et al., 2009[24]	• Incomplete SCI subjects ($n = 12$); examined all ASIA sensory points at chronic (>20 months) and subacute (<9 months) time points • Intra- and interrater (range)	Electrical *Intra-* *Inter-*	 .56–80 .52–91	• Good intra- and interrater reliability to measure cutaneous sensory function • Depended on the dermatome tested
Kramer et al., 2009[25]	• Incomplete SCI subjects ($n = 18$), examined *unaffected* dermatomes (according to dSSEP interpretation), during first year of spontaneous recovery • Intrarater (overall ICC from all dermatomes)	Electrical	.24	• Reliably recorded from dermatomes unaffected by SCI during recovery (no significant change in threshold over time) • Acquiring from the very acute phase after SCI (9 days) may account for lower ICC than previously reported (King et al., 2009[24]) • Most suitable when combined with electrophysiological readouts (i.e., dSSEPs)

* Monofilaments

Abbreviations: ASIA, American Spinal Injury Association; dSSEP, dermatomal somatosensory evoked potential; ICC, intraclass correlation coefficient; QST, quantitative sensory testing; SCI, spinal cord injury.

appear more sensitive to sensory impairments rostral to the neurological level of SCI. However, most QST measures have not been employed by clinicians due in part to practical limitations (i.e., time-consuming procedure and expensive equipment), but also a lack of sufficient data regarding their utility to reliably distinguish differences in dermatomes with clearly impaired sensation (i.e., hypersensitive vs hyposensitive) and track changing sensory deficits during spontaneous recovery.[29]

To address many of the concerns about existing QST measures, electrical perception threshold (EPT) testing was introduced to SCI in 2006[28] and has been well studied regarding psychometric properties in both control subjects and individuals with chronic SCI. This assessment technique, which requires a subject to report perception of an increasing electrical stimulation from self-adhesive surface electrodes positioned on key areas of each dermatome, requires minimal technical experience, uses relatively inexpensive equipment, and appears sensitive to varying degrees of sensory deficits after SCI. Independent groups have shown the reliability of this measure in chronic SCI, and responsiveness studies in acute SCI are under way. Proposed as a measure of dorsal column function,[29] the major drawback of EPT at present is that stimulation is not physiologically specific; rather, it may broadly activate both small- and large-diameter fibers in the periphery.

Neurophysiological Recordings of Sensory Function

Largely considered a complementary assessment to the AIS examination of SCI severity, the inclusion of electrophysiology as a standard outcome measure intends to provide a more sensitive and objective index of spinal cord function. Conventional somatosensory evoked potential (SSEP) outcomes (i.e., amplitude and latency) are most commonly examined by upper- and lower-limb stimulation of mixed nerves in the periphery using square-wave electrical pulses to record the function of the dorsal column. The characteristic waveforms of SSEPs recorded from scalp electrodes following peripheral electrical stimulation of the median and tibial nerves (upper/lower panel) are shown in **Fig. 46.2A**. After incomplete SCI (black line), prominent negative and positive peak potentials (N20, median nerve; P40, tibial nerve) are marked at increased latencies and decreased amplitudes compared with neurologically intact subjects (gray line). In general, the outcomes of electrophysiological assessment improve the prediction of long-term functional outcomes based on AIS preservation of sensation in S4-5 alone[30] and are clinically very useful to detect SCI in unconscious individuals.

In theory, implementing electrophysiology during the first year after SCI also allows a greater understanding of the mechanisms involved in spontaneous recovery (i.e., remyelination and/or regeneration). However, the responsiveness of conventional SSEPs during spontaneous recovery has only recently been studied in a large and statistically powerful cohort of individuals with SCI.[13,17] In general, it seems that, although severely deteriorated SSEPs may undergo minor recovery of delayed latency and reduced amplitude, these changes do not correspond with the extent of the functional improvement typically achieved during spontaneous recovery.

Electrical stimulation of individual dermatomes using the same electroencephalographic (EEG) methodological principles and protocol as for conventional SSEPs provides a more precise segmental neurophysiological assessment of posterior spinal cord innervation (dorsal root entry and ascending dorsal column conduction). Termed dermatomal SSEPs (dSSEPs), this approach shares the advantages of the AIS examination to record segment-by-segment sensory outcomes above, at, and below the level of lesion, and conventional electrophysiological outcomes to assess sensory function relatively independent of examiner or examinee interpretation and bias (**Fig. 46.2B**). In the example shown in **Fig. 46.2B**, a dSSEP is recorded in both an individual with SCI (i.e., above the level of the lesion) and a neurologically healthy control subject at normal N1/onset latencies. As the stimulation site moves caudally (from C4 to C8), the dSSEP recording latency of the prominent N1 component is increased greater than two standard deviations of normal control

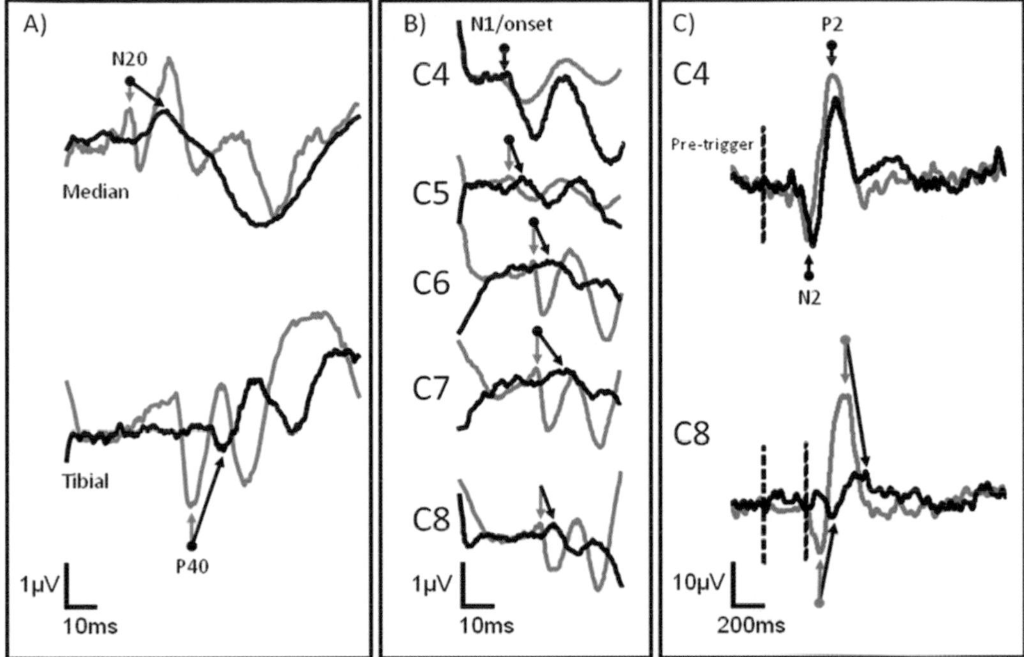

Fig. 46.2 **(A)** Conventional mixed nerve somatosensory evoked potentials (SSEPs), **(B)** cervical (C4-8) dermatomal SSEPs (dSSEPs), and **(C)** cervical contact heat evoked potentials (CHEPs) recorded from neurologically intact control subjects (*gray*), and after incomplete spinal cord injury (SCI) (*black*). Arrows indicate the marking of the most prominent and reliable component of the waveforms. The increased latency and decreased amplitude of sensory evoked potentials are characteristic of spinal conductive deficits after SCI; however, only a segmental approach is useful to track changes within different levels above, at, and below the injury.

values in the individual with SCI, indicating impaired spinal conduction at and below the level of SCI. The reliability of this technique recorded from cervical dSSEPs has been demonstrated in neurologically healthy control subjects and recently in individuals with chronic-stable SCI.[25,29]

The electrophysiological readouts discussed so far provide information only regarding conduction in large-diameter fibers that ascend in the dorsal column. To address sensory impairments due to lesion in the spinothalamic tract, another small-diameter fiber stimulation modality must be employed. To date, most studies that attain measures of conduction in the spinothalamic tract have used supramaximal CO_2 laser pulses to irradiate specific areas of skin within a dermatome affected by a small-diameter fiber neuropathy.[31] The painful response and long latency of the laser evoked potentials (LEPs) correspond with the known properties of activation and conduction in small-diameter and unmyelinated fibers (A-delta and C-fibers, respectively) ascending in the spinothalamic tract.

To address the practical limitations of acquiring LEPs (i.e., skin burns and safety precautions) in a clinical setting, contact heat has reemerged as a modality for the electrophysiological assessment of conduction in small-diameter fibers, with recent technological advances that permit safe, continuous surface contact and rapid warming (70°C/s) and cooling of the skin's surface up to 55°C. An additional advantage of contact heat is the physiological relevancy of stimulation, from which large-amplitude, long-latency evoked potentials can be built based on a small number of stimulation repetitions (i.e., fewer than 20). So-called contact heat evoked potentials (CHEPs, **Fig. 46.2C**) have demonstrated promising intrarater reliability in neurologically uninjured control subjects measured from the surface of cervical and thoracic dermatomes, and can be recorded at increased latencies and decreased amplitudes after SCI in dermatomes with impaired temperature sensation at and below the level of the lesion.[32,33]

There is preliminary evidence that dermatomal evoked potentials measured during the course of the first year after SCI are more sensitive to the period of spontaneous recovery than are conventional, longitudinal approaches (i.e., median or tibial nerve, **Fig. 46.3**). In a study that reviewed initial and follow-up dSSEP findings from individuals with complete and incomplete cervical SCI, the latency

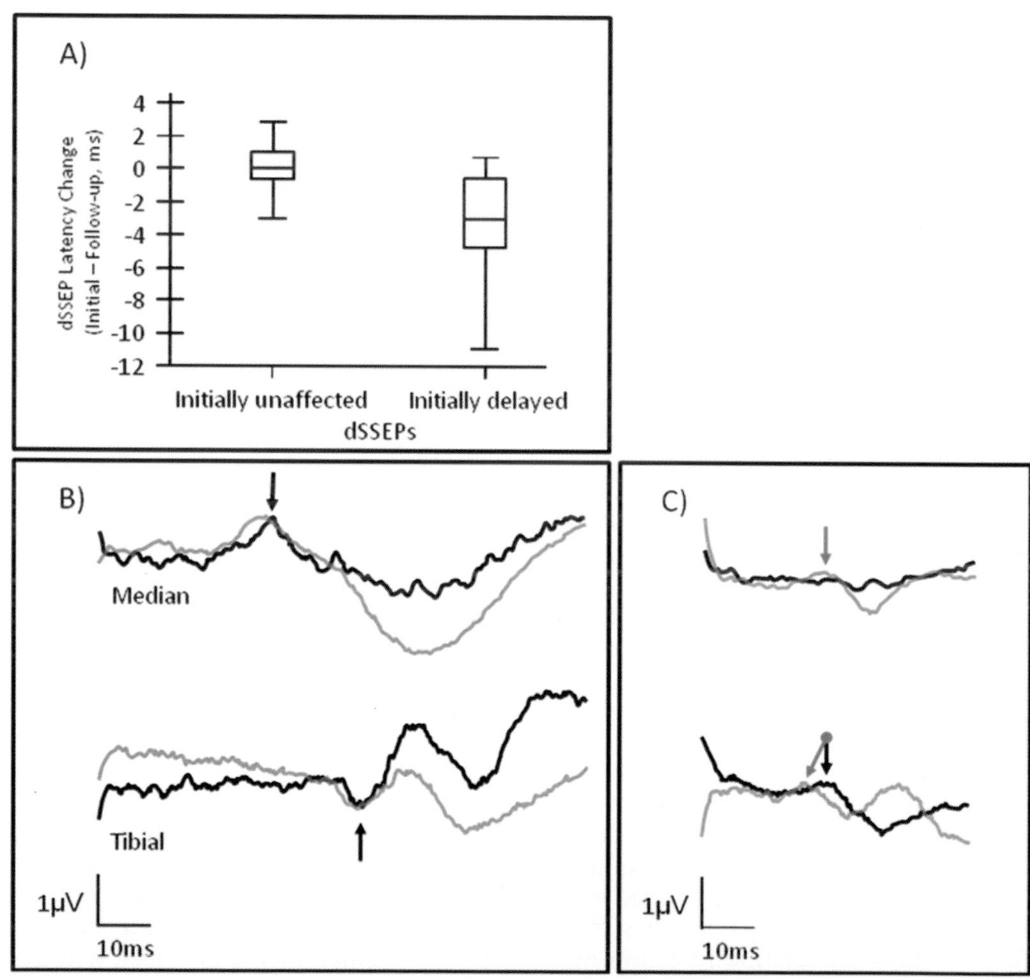

Fig. 46.3 **(A)** The aggregate change in cervical dermatomal somatosensory evoked potential (dSSEP) N1/onset latency in individuals with tetraplegia during spontaneous recovery. **(B)** Representative median and tibial nerve, and **(C)** dSSEPs recorded during the acute phase (<1 month after spinal cord injury; *black*), and on follow-up (*gray*) in the first year after SCI. (**[A]** Adapted from Kramer JK, Taylor P, Steeves JD, Curt A. Dermatomal somatosensory evoked potentials and electrical perception thresholds during recovery from cervical spinal cord injury. Neurorehabil Neural Repair 2010;24:309–317.)

in dermatomes initially (1) *unaffected* by the lesion remained stable on follow-up (*reliable*), (2) *delayed* remained stable or decreased toward more normal latencies on follow-up (*responsive*), and (3) *not recordable* could be interpreted at delayed latencies on follow-up (*responsive*).[25] The change in latency of initially delayed recordings appeared to be subthreshold for a functionally significant change in sensation according to EPT, though the emergence of abolished dSSEPs was related to the return of sensation. The key findings in this study were that the responsiveness of dSSEPs, observed in both individuals with complete and those with incomplete SCI, may otherwise have gone unnoticed by monitoring conventional SSEPs and S4-5 preservation.

The combined, segmental electrophysiological approach described herein has promising potential to measure important changes in spinal conduction in dissociated afferent spinal cord pathways near the lesion level affected by SCI, as well as to elucidate mechanisms related to functional sensory deficits and recovery. The additional information gained by acquiring unaffected dermatomes above the lesion level is useful as a within-subject control condition to account for variations in setup and recording during a longitudinally designed study, and to monitor and predict deleterious changes in sensation (i.e., safety). Technical requirements (i.e., training and expensive equipment) and practical concerns (i.e., time requirements), common to all EEG acquisition methods, are most frequently reported as limiting the clinical use of electrophysiology. The meaning of afferent electrophysiological changes is also not always so clear and requires consideration for multiple areas of change along the somatosensory axis. For example, decreased latency of evoked potentials may be attributable to mechanisms of repair at the lesion area (i.e., remyelination), though increasing amplitude may represent neuroplasticity in the somatosensory cortex.[34,35]

Conclusion

There are several limitations to assessing sensory function after SCI in addition to those described for AIS sensory outcomes (i.e., ordinal measurement scale, unresponsive to change) and advanced electrophysiological methods described in this chapter (i.e., expensive and time consuming). In clinical trials, electrophysiological outcomes cannot independently demonstrate the efficacy of treatment, but rather serve only as surrogate markers of improvements (i.e., proof of mechanism). Furthermore, the minimal clinically important difference (MCID) of changes in these outcomes remains largely unknown and warrants further study. A concern of using QST methods in the acute phase of SCI, during which time treatment for ongoing secondary complications (i.e., pain) may prevent adequate orientation of attention to the test stimulus, is the ability to establish a reliable baseline value to measure changes during recovery. Studies aimed at addressing the reliability of these outcome measures at different stages of SCI should be undertaken in the future.

The objective of sensory examination after SCI has been to measure the severity and level of spinal lesion for diagnosis and prognosis. With the advent of rehabilitation and cell-based therapies, and the need to judge preliminary safety, proof of mechanism, and efficacy during different stages of these clinical trials, an understanding of the initial sensory deficits and capacity to track changing sensation from early after injury (days to weeks) until chronic injury (months to years) are required. An important component of the sensory outcome tools will be to examine sensation within individual dermatomes that reflect different spinal segments above, at, and below the level of SCI. Although at present the clinical AIS sensory outcomes may be the most widely accepted method, the limitations of this method suggest that QST and electrophysiological methods may need to be applied in complement to gain a better understanding of somatosensory function and recovery following SCI.

Pearls

- The clinical sensory examination of light touch and pinprick is integral for diagnosis (i.e., injury level) and prognosis (i.e., injury severity) after SCI.
- QST and electrophysiology provide more detailed information regarding sensory impairments after SCI.
- Conduction in small (spinothalamic tract) and large diameter pathways (dorsal columns) can be assessed using similar electrophysiological approaches (CHEPs and SSEPs, respectively) to reveal the extent of damage in different areas of the spinal cord.
- Dermatomal electrophysiological approaches may be sensitive to subtle changes occurring in spinal segments close to the level of lesion during spontaneous recovery.

Pitfalls

- The clinical sensory exam is limited by an ordinal scale that is insensitive to differences in "impaired" sensation.
- SSEPs and CHEPs are more expensive and time-consuming to perform in comparison to standard clinical sensory examination techniques.
- Electrophysiological outcomes only serve as surrogate measures of function in clinical trials.

References

1. Cohen ME, Ditunno JF Jr, Donovan WH, Maynard FM Jr. A test of the 1992 International Standards for Neurological and Functional Classification of Spinal Cord Injury. Spinal Cord 1998;36(8):554–560
2. Marino RJ, Jones L, Kirshblum S, Tal J, Dasgupta A. Reliability and repeatability of the motor and sensory examination of the international standards for neurological classification of spinal cord injury. J Spinal Cord Med 2008;31(2):166–170
3. Mulcahey MJ, Gaughan J, Betz RR, Johansen KJ. The International Standards for Neurological Classification of Spinal Cord Injury: reliability of data when applied to children and youths. Spinal Cord 2007a;45(6):452–459
4. Mulcahey MJ, Gaughan J, Betz RR, Vogel LC. Rater agreement on the ISCSCI motor and sensory scores obtained before and after formal training in testing technique. J Spinal Cord Med 2007b; 30(Suppl 1):S146–S149
5. Mulcahey MJ, Gaughan J, Betz RR. Agreement of repeated motor and sensory scores at individual myotomes and dermatomes in young persons with complete spinal cord injury. Spinal Cord 2009; 47(1):56–61
6. Savic G, Bergström EM, Frankel HL, Jamous MA, Jones PW. Inter-rater reliability of motor and sensory examinations performed according to American Spinal Injury Association standards. Spinal Cord 2007;45(6):444–451
7. Curt A, Dietz V. Ambulatory capacity in spinal cord injury: significance of somatosensory evoked potentials and ASIA protocol in predicting outcome. Arch Phys Med Rehabil 1997a;78(1):39–43
8. Curt A, Rodic B, Schurch B, Dietz V. Recovery of bladder function in patients with acute spinal cord injury: significance of ASIA scores and somatosensory evoked potentials. Spinal Cord 1997b;35(6): 368–373
9. Curt A, Keck ME, Dietz V. Functional outcome following spinal cord injury: significance of motor-evoked potentials and ASIA scores. Arch Phys Med Rehabil 1998;79(1):81–86
10. Marino RJ, Graves DE. Metric properties of the ASIA motor score: subscales improve correlation with functional activities. Arch Phys Med Rehabil 2004;85(11):1804–1810
11. van Hedel HJ, Curt A. Fighting for each segment: estimating the clinical value of cervical and thoracic segments in SCI. J Neurotrauma 2006; 23(11):1621–1631
12. Bracken MB, Holford TR. Neurological and functional status 1 year after acute spinal cord injury: estimates of functional recovery in National Acute Spinal Cord Injury Study II from results modeled in National Acute Spinal Cord Injury Study III. J Neurosurg 2002;96(3, Suppl):259–266
13. Curt A, Van Hedel HJ, Klaus D, Dietz V; EM-SCI Study Group. Recovery from a spinal cord injury: significance of compensation, neural plasticity, and repair. J Neurotrauma 2008;25(6):677–685
14. Ditunno JF Jr, Cohen ME, Hauck WW, Jackson AB, Sipski ML. Recovery of upper-extremity strength in complete and incomplete tetraplegia: a multicenter study. Arch Phys Med Rehabil 2000;81(4): 389–393
15. Fawcett JW, Curt A, Steeves JD, et al. Guidelines for the conduct of clinical trials for spinal cord injury as developed by the ICCP panel: spontaneous recovery after spinal cord injury and statistical power needed for therapeutic clinical trials. Spinal Cord 2007;45(3):190–205
16. Marino RJ, Ditunno JF Jr, Donovan WH, Maynard F Jr. Neurologic recovery after traumatic spinal cord injury: data from the Model Spinal Cord Injury Systems. Arch Phys Med Rehabil 1999;80(11): 1391–1396
17. Spiess M, Schubert M, Kliesch U, Halder P; EM-SCI Study group. Evolution of tibial SSEP after traumat-

ic spinal cord injury: baseline for clinical trials. Clin Neurophysiol 2008;119(5):1051–1061

18. Furlan JC, Fehlings MG, Tator CH, Davis AM. Motor and sensory assessment of patients in clinical trials for pharmacological therapy of acute spinal cord injury: psychometric properties of the ASIA Standards. J Neurotrauma 2008;25(11):1273–1301

19. Steeves JD, Lammertse D, Curt A, et al; International Campaign for Cures of Spinal Cord Injury Paralysis. Guidelines for the conduct of clinical trials for spinal cord injury (SCI) as developed by the ICCP panel: clinical trial outcome measures. Spinal Cord 2007;45(3):206–221

20. Spiess MR, Müller RM, Rupp R, Schuld C, van Hedel HJ; EM-SCI Study Group. Conversion in ASIA impairment scale during the first year after traumatic spinal cord injury. J Neurotrauma 2009;26(11):2027–2036

21. Kirshblum S, Millis S, McKinley W, Tulsky D. Late neurologic recovery after traumatic spinal cord injury. Arch Phys Med Rehabil 2004;85(11):1811–1817

22. Felix ER, Widerström-Noga EG. Reliability and validity of quantitative sensory testing in persons with spinal cord injury and neuropathic pain. J Rehabil Res Dev 2009;46(1):69–83

23. Hayes KC, Wolfe DL, Hsieh JT, Potter PJ, Krassioukov A, Durham CE. Clinical and electrophysiologic correlates of quantitative sensory testing in patients with incomplete spinal cord injury. Arch Phys Med Rehabil 2002;83(11):1612–1619

24. King NK, Savic G, Frankel H, Jamous A, Ellaway PH. Reliability of cutaneous electrical perceptual threshold in the assessment of sensory perception in patients with spinal cord injury. J Neurotrauma 2009;26(7):1061–1068

25. Kramer JK, Taylor P, Steeves JD, Curt A. Dermatomal somatosensory evoked potentials and electrical perception thresholds during recovery from cervical spinal cord injury. Neurorehabil Neural Repair 2010;24(4):309–317

26. Krassioukov A, Wolfe DL, Hsieh JT, Hayes KC, Durham CE. Quantitative sensory testing in patients with incomplete spinal cord injury. Arch Phys Med Rehabil 1999;80(10):1258–1263

27. Nicotra A, Ellaway PH. Thermal perception thresholds: assessing the level of human spinal cord injury. Spinal Cord 2006;44(10):617–624

28. Savic G, Bergström EM, Frankel HL, Jamous MA, Ellaway PH, Davey NJ. Perceptual threshold to cutaneous electrical stimulation in patients with spinal cord injury. Spinal Cord 2006;44(9):560–566

29. Kramer JL, Moss AJ, Taylor P, Curt A. Assessment of posterior spinal cord function with electrical perception threshold in spinal cord injury. J Neurotrauma 2008;25(8):1019–1026

30. Curt A, Dietz V. Electrophysiological recordings in patients with spinal cord injury: significance for predicting outcome. Spinal Cord 1999;37(3):157–165

31. Treede RD, Lorenz J, Baumgärtner U. Clinical usefulness of laser-evoked potentials. Neurophysiol Clin 2003;33(6):303–314

32. Wydenkeller S, Wirz R, Halder P. Spinothalamic tract conduction velocity estimated using contact heat evoked potentials: what needs to be considered. Clin Neurophysiol 2008;119(4):812–821

33. Wydenkeller S, Maurizio S, Dietz V, Halder P. Neuropathic pain in spinal cord injury: significance of clinical and electrophysiological measures. Eur J Neurosci 2009;30(1):91–99

34. Jurkiewicz MT, Mikulis DJ, McIlroy WE, Fehlings MG, Verrier MC. Sensorimotor cortical plasticity during recovery following spinal cord injury: a longitudinal fMRI study. Neurorehabil Neural Repair 2007;21(6):527–538

35. Kaas JH, Qi HX, Burish MJ, Gharbawie OA, Onifer SM, Massey JM. Cortical and subcortical plasticity in the brains of humans, primates, and rats after damage to sensory afferents in the dorsal columns of the spinal cord. Exp Neurol 2008;209(2):407–416

47

Electrical Stimulation Following Spinal Cord Injury

Graham H. Creasey

Key Points

1. After spinal cord injury, surviving peripheral nerves can be activated safely for many years by electrical stimulation.
2. Stimulation of efferent nerves can produce muscle contraction and useful function of the diaphragm, bladder, bowel, and limbs, and seminal emission.
3. Stimulation of afferent nerves can modify reflex activity and pain.
4. Stimulation of muscles via the skin surface may be useful for exercise.
5. Implanted devices, like pacemakers, facilitate long-term restoration of function.

After injury to the spinal cord, the remaining intact nerves in the central or peripheral nervous system can be stimulated electrically for various purposes. These may be diagnostic, to estimate the extent of damage to upper or lower motor neurons. Therapeutic purposes may include providing exercise or modifying existing function by inhibiting or enhancing reflexes or inhibiting pain, a process sometimes known as neuromodulation.[1] It is also possible to restore some useful movement to paralyzed muscles by stimulation of their lower motor neurons, using devices known as neural prostheses, to provide functional electrical stimulation (FES).[2]

Muscles with intact lower motor neurons may undergo disuse atrophy but remain responsive to electrical stimulation applied directly to the muscle cell or to the motor nerve. Such stimulation can be effective many years after spinal cord injury (SCI) in producing contraction, reversing disuse atrophy, and restoring function. Denervated muscles undergo progressive atrophy that can probably not be prevented by electrical stimulation.

The main requirements have been to develop safe and effective patterns of stimulation that can be applied long term using commercially viable devices. These requirements have been met in several areas.

Techniques

The least invasive techniques of applying electrical stimulation use electrodes applied to the skin surface. These are suitable for diagnostic and therapeutic purposes but are not always sufficiently selective or reproducible for restoring useful function; managing the electrodes, wires, and stimulators can become inconvenient for long-term use.

Fine wire electrodes inserted with a hypodermic needle are widely used for diagnostic purposes, and some, such as percutaneous electrodes, can be left in place safely for months or years for research purposes. They allow specific reproducible stimulation patterns to be developed and evaluated using stimulators outside the body, although some care is needed for maintaining the skin exit sites and external leads.

For long-term functional use, it is most convenient to have stimulators fully implanted within the body. These may be powered by implanted batteries, in which case revision surgery is required every few years to replace the batteries, although implantable rechargeable batteries are being developed. Alternatively, the implant is powered by radio frequency transmission from a controller outside the body; such a controller can be reprogrammed or replaced conveniently.

All implanted components must be designed to cause no harm to the tissues, whether electrical, chemical, or mechanical, and to be resistant to damage by body fluids or movement. Ideally, the implant should have a lifetime longer than that of the user, but in case of faults or improvements, provision should be made for repair or replacement.

Therapeutic Effects

Exercise

Electrical stimulation can increase strength in paralyzed lower-limb muscles of people with SCI;[3] with prolonged aerobic exercise, it can also improve muscle endurance.[4,5] There are also cardiovascular benefits,[6] increased HDL level,[7] and improved insulin sensitivity.[8] Combining arm cycle ergometry (ACE) and electrical stimulation leg cycle ergometry (LCE)[9,10] may have enhanced cardiovascular benefits. Chronic electrical stimulation LCE may increase lower extremity bone mineral density, or at least slow the progression of lower extremity osteopenia,[11–13] but when FES training is discontinued, lower extremity bone mineral density reverts to its previous level.

Neuromodulation

There are variable reports of the effects on spasticity of electrical stimulation of the limbs, posterior columns, or sacral nerves,[14–17] and this is not widely used for spasticity control after SCI. Neuromodulation shows some promise for inhibition of the hyperreflexic bladder by stimulation of the dorsal genital nerves or the pudendal nerves, particularly if it can be applied specifically when a bladder contraction is detected.[18]

Electrical stimulation is sometimes effective for neuromodulation of neuropathic or nociceptive pain after SCI, a subject addressed in Chapter 17.

Restoration of Function

Respiratory Function

Inspiratory Muscle Pacing

In individuals with high tetraplegia but preserved bilateral phrenic nerve function, the phrenic nerves can be stimulated electrically to induce diaphragm contraction so that the patients no longer require mechanical ventilation. In conventional methods, the diaphragm is activated by electrodes implanted surgically on both phrenic nerves in the thorax and connected to an implantable receiver with an external power supply and transmitter. Such systems have been implanted in over a thousand patients over the last 3 decades, and there are now three commercially available devices.[19] This method requires a thoracotomy, in-patient hospital stay, and high cost. In addition, the procedure requires phrenic nerve dissection and placement of electrodes directly on the nerves and therefore carries some risk of phrenic nerve injury. These disadvantages have limited the number of individuals willing to undergo diaphragm pacing.

An alternative procedure, currently under investigation, involves placement of electrodes into the muscular portion of the diaphragm near the entrance points of the phrenic nerve into the diaphragm.[20] This procedure is performed laparoscopically and can be done on an out-patient basis. The advantages of intramuscular placement of phrenic nerve electrodes include less risk of phrenic nerve injury and a reduction in overall cost. When placed near the motor point, as determined by intraoperative testing, intramuscular diaphragm stimulation results in virtually the same inspired volume production as that resulting from direct phrenic nerve stimulation.

Expiratory Muscles and Coughing

Forced expiration and cough production involve lower intercostal and abdominal muscle activation. Electrical stimulation of abdominal muscles using electrodes on the skin has been found to produce cough comparable with that produced with the manual assistance of a therapist.[21] Electrical stimulation of the expiratory muscles has also been investigated with electrodes implanted on the lower thoracic spinal cord.[22]

Bladder, Bowel, and Sexual Function

In patients with preserved conus medullaris and sacral nerves, improved voiding, continence, and erection can be achieved by electrical stimulation of the sacral nerves or roots. An implantable stimulator capable of improving bladder, bowel, and erectile function has been available commercially in some countries since 1982 and has been implanted successfully in several thousand patients with SCI (**Fig. 47.1**).

Voiding

Electrical stimulation of the sacral motor roots causes contraction of the bladder and lower bowel but also contraction of the external sphincters, which might be expected to be counterproductive and even harmful. However, intermittent bursts of stimulation can produce sustained contraction of the smooth muscle of the bladder or bowel while allowing the sphincter to relax during the intervals and permit urine or stool to be passed safely. Urine is voided with low residual volumes, resulting in a significant reduction of urinary tract infection.[23,24]

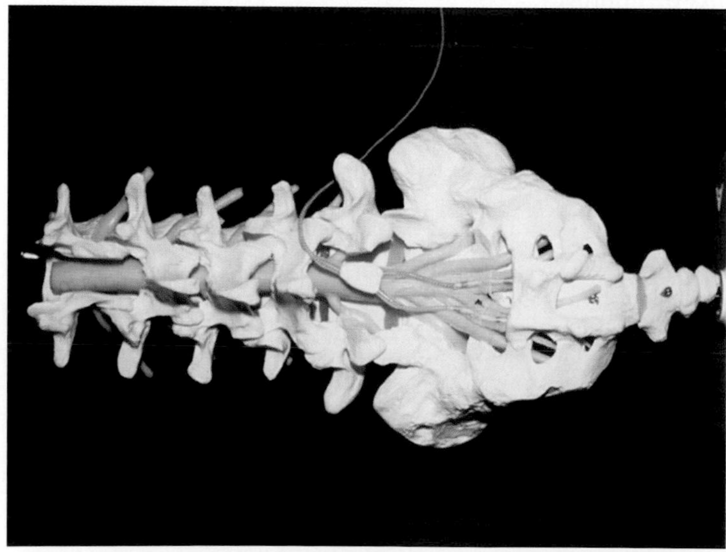

Fig. 47.1 Location of surgically implanted extradural electrodes on S3 and S4 nerves bilaterally, and one potential location for intradural posterior sacral rhizotomy at the level of L1.

Continence

Reflex incontinence can be reduced dramatically by surgical division of the sacral sensory roots, which is often performed when a sacral anterior nerve root stimulator is implanted, and this also reduces the risk of renal damage and autonomic dysreflexia. However, it also abolishes desirable functions, such as reflex erection and reflex ejaculation, and although there are alternative means of restoring these, its benefits must be weighed against its disadvantages.

Restoration of voiding and continence by the foregoing techniques reduces the need for antibiotic and anticholinergic medication, appliances, and hospital visits, resulting in reduced annual costs for bladder and bowel care; studies in Europe and the United States have indicated that within 5 to 8 years, these savings cover the cost of implanting and using the device.[25,26]

Current research is addressing alternatives to surgical rhizotomy for reducing hyperreflexia of the detrusor and sphincters, such as electrical block and inhibition of muscle contraction. Hyperreflexic contractions of the bladder can be inhibited by electrical stimulation of sacral afferent nerves by a variety of routes, including electrodes on sacral dermatomes, in the anus and vagina, in the ventral sacral foramina, on the dorsal genital nerves, and even on the posterior tibial nerves, but these techniques have not proved sufficiently effective in reducing reflex incontinence after SCI to be accepted into widespread clinical use.

Erection

Stimulation of intact parasympathetic efferent axons in S2 can produce erection for as long as stimulation is maintained. Electrodes are usually implanted at the same time as electrodes for restoring bladder and bowel function as already described.[27]

Ejaculation

Seminal emission can be obtained in most patients after SCI by applying stimulation via an electrode inserted temporarily into the rectum for "electroejaculation."[28]

Upper Limb Function

Restoration of useful function to patients with tetraplegia and preserved lower motor neurons to some upper limb muscles can be achieved by electrodes implanted in or on muscles in the forearm and hand and connected to an implanted stimulator. Implanted systems are usually enhanced by tendon transfers. Conversely, stimulation of paralyzed but innervated muscles can increase the number of potential tendon transfers.

Stimulation of flexors and extensors of the fingers and thumb, the adductor and opponens pollicis muscles, and sometimes wrist balancing muscles, can produce palmar grasp and release for large objects and key-pinch grasp for smaller items. Tendon transfers are used to stabilize the thumb, synchronize finger movement, and compensate for some denervated muscle groups.

A first-generation implant of this type using eight electrodes was implanted in over 200 patients with C5 or C6 tetraplegia by 35 centers in at least eight countries.[29] A user satisfaction survey at least 6 months after completing training with the device confirmed that users needed less adaptive equipment and less assistance from others; on average they used the device 5 days a week, and nearly half used it every day. The majority of patients were very satisfied with the system, and 80% said they would recommend it to others.[30]

Second-generation devices with 12 active stimulation channels and two myoelectric signal sensing channels are being investigated for improved control of the intrinsic muscles of the hand, wrist balance, pronation and supination, and elbow and shoulder position.[31] The triceps muscle is controlled to produce elbow extension and allow reaching above the head.

Research is also in progress on control of the paralyzed shoulder for people with high tetraplegia. Such control is complex because of its many potential movements, and there are limited voluntary movements available to a high tetraplegic to control a stimulator. Direct electrical connections with the cerebral cortex are being investigated as a control interface.[32]

Lower Limb Function

Surface and Percutaneous Electrode Systems

Electrical stimulation can provide individuals with thoracic or low cervical injuries with the ability to exercise, stand, transfer, and perform simple stepping. Standing can be achieved by activating both quadriceps, whereas a stride can be produced by activating the quadriceps of one leg while initiating a flexion withdrawal in the other. Selected individuals with neurologically incomplete SCI and some preserved motor and sensory function have been able to regain household or community mobility.[33]

Hybrid systems combining stimulation with orthoses have been fitted to patients with complete or incomplete thoracic or low-level cervical injuries. The energy required to operate these hybrid systems is less than that required for braces alone, but it increases rapidly with walking velocity due to an increased reliance on the arms and trunk muscles to move the body forward.[34]

Fully Implanted Electrode Systems

For long-term clinical application, implanted systems offer major advantages over surface and percutaneous stimulation, including improved convenience, cosmesis, and reliability. Exercise and standing have been reported with a cochlear implant modified to deliver 22 channels of stimulation,[35] and a 12-channel system for activation of the L2–S2 motor roots has been applied to a handful of volunteers.[36]

An eight-channel implanted stimulator with electrodes implanted in or on muscles has undergone clinical testing in a small number of subjects.[37] On average, subjects were able to stand for more than 10 minutes with 85% of their body weight on their legs. Some subjects were able to achieve short-distance mobility with a swing-to gait. Reciprocal stepping can be achieved with 16 channels of stimulation through the addition of a second implant to activate hip flexors and ankle dorsiflexors.[38]

All standing and walking neuroprostheses require assistive devices, such as crutches, walkers, or additional bracing, and this restricts the activities and environments in which the neuroprosthesis can be used. Current experimental lower extremity FES systems facilitate brief mobility-related tasks, allowing people with paraplegia to overcome physical obstacles, negotiate architectural barriers, and reach and manipulate objects that are otherwise inaccessible from the wheelchair.

Future Trends

Clinical

Electrically stimulated exercise of the lower limbs has been shown to enhance new neural cell birth and survival following chronic SCI in rats.[39] This demonstrates that FES can enhance cellular regeneration in the injured adult central nervous system and raises the possibility of controlled electrical activation of the nervous system for optimizing spontaneous regeneration and functional recovery in neurological injuries.

Technical

The trend in surgery to less invasive techniques affects the design and implantation of neural prostheses. Many electrodes and cables can be implanted percutaneously and tunneled under the skin to connect to a stimulator placed subcutaneously like a pacemaker.

Other developments include standards that will allow many components to be interconnected in wired and wireless networks within the body. This will allow systems to be assembled and upgraded as needed with minimal surgery; it also allows compatible components to be made by different manufacturers, permitting larger-scale production and reduced costs and increasing the flexibility with which systems can be assembled. This is likely to improve further the balance between function restored and the investment of time, energy, and money required.

Ultimately, the provision of improved care to SCI patients depends not primarily on development of new techniques but on their delivery by clinicians and funding agencies. This depends on collaboration to translate research into clinical application and on recognition by those responsible for health care funding of the return on investment achieved by restoring function to people with damage to the central nervous system.

Pearls

- Bladder, bowel, and sexual function after spinal cord injury can be substantially improved by an implanted stimulator of the sacral nerves or nerve roots.
- Hand grasp can be partly restored to tetraplegic subjects by electrical stimulation of peripheral nerves and muscles using an implant.
- Cough can be improved significantly in tetraplegic and high paraplegic patients by stimulation of the expiratory muscles, thereby reducing respiratory complications.

Pitfalls

- Electrical stimulation can only be applied to nerves remaining intact after SCI, such as lower motor neurons below the neurological level of the cord lesion.
- Spasticity and contractures may limit the function that can be restored by electrical stimulation.
- The relatively low incidence of SCI provides limited incentive for commercial development of electrical stimulation devices for this market alone.

References

1. Craggs M, McFarlane J. Neuromodulation of the lower urinary tract. Exp Physiol 1999;84(1):149–160
2. Creasey GH, Ho CH, Triolo RJ, et al. Clinical applications of electrical stimulation after spinal cord injury. J Spinal Cord Med 2004;27(4):365–375
3. Rodgers MM, Glaser RM, Figoni SF, et al. Musculoskeletal responses of spinal cord injured individuals to functional neuromuscular stimulation-induced knee extension exercise training. J Rehabil Res Dev 1991;28(4):19–26
4. Hooker SP, Figoni SF, Rodgers MM, et al. Physiologic effects of electrical stimulation leg cycle exercise training in spinal cord injured persons. Arch Phys Med Rehabil 1992b;73(5):470–476
5. Ragnarsson KT, Pollack S, O'Daniel W Jr, Edgar R, Petrofsky J, Nash MS. Clinical evaluation of computerized functional electrical stimulation after spinal cord injury: a multicenter pilot study. Arch Phys Med Rehabil 1988;69(9):672–677
6. Hooker SP, Figoni SF, Rodgers MM, et al. Physiologic effects of electrical stimulation leg cycle exercise training in spinal cord injured persons. Arch Phys Med Rehabil 1992b;73(5):470–476
7. Bauman WA, Alexander LR, Zhong Y-G, Spungen AM. Stimulated leg ergometry training improves body composition and HDL-cholesterol values. J Am Paraplegia Soc 1994a;17(4):201
8. Mohr T, Dela F, Handberg A, Biering-Sørensen F, Galbo H, Kjaer M. Insulin action and long-term electrically induced training in individuals with spinal cord injuries. Med Sci Sports Exerc 2001;33(8):1247–1252
9. Figoni SF. Exercise responses and quadriplegia. Med Sci Sports Exerc 1993;25(4):433–441
10. Glaser RM. Functional neuromuscular stimulation: exercise conditioning of spinal cord injured patients. Int J Sports Med 1994;15(3):142–148
11. Bloomfield SA, Mysiw WJ, Jackson RD. Bone mass and endocrine adaptations to training in spinal cord injured individuals. Bone 1996;19(1):61–68
12. Hangartner TN, Rodgers MM, Glaser RM, Barre PS. Tibial bone density loss in spinal cord injured patients: effects of FES exercise. J Rehabil Res Dev 1994;31(1):50–61
13. Mohr T, Podenphant J, Biering-Sorensen F, Galbo H, Thamsborg G, Kjaer M. Increased bone mineral density after prolonged electrically induced cycle training of paralyzed limbs in spinal cord injured man. Calcif Tissue Int 1997;61(1):22–25
14. Mirbagheri MM, Ladouceur M, Barbeau H, Kearney RE. The effects of long-term FES-assisted walking on intrinsic and reflex dynamic stiffness in spastic spinal-cord-injured subjects. IEEE Trans Neural Syst Rehabil Eng 2002;10(4):280–289
15. Seib TP, Price R, Reyes MR, Lehmann JF. The quantitative measurement of spasticity: effect of cutaneous electrical stimulation. Arch Phys Med Rehabil 1994;75(7):746–750
16. Pinter MM, Gerstenbrand F, Dimitrijevic MR. Epidural electrical stimulation of posterior structures of the human lumbosacral cord, III: Control Of spasticity. Spinal Cord 2000;38(9):524–531
17. Biering-Sørensen F, Laeessøe L, Sønksen J, Bagi P, Nielsen JB, Kristensen JK. The effect of penile vibratory stimulation on male fertility potential, spasticity and neurogenic detrusor overactivity in spinal cord lesioned individuals. Acta Neurochir Suppl (Wien) 2005;93:159–163
18. Kirkham AP, Shah NC, Knight SL, Shah PJ, Craggs MD. The acute effects of continuous and condi-

tional neuromodulation on the bladder in spinal cord injury. Spinal Cord 2001;39(8):420–428
19. Creasey G, Elefteriades J, DiMarco A, et al. Electrical stimulation to restore respiration. J Rehabil Res Dev 1996;33(2):123–132
20. DiMarco AF, Onders RP, Kowalski KE, Miller ME, Ferek S, Mortimer JT. Phrenic nerve pacing in a tetraplegic patient via intramuscular diaphragm electrodes. Am J Respir Crit Care Med 2002; 166(12 Pt 1):1604–1606
21. Jaeger RJ, Turba RM, Yarkony GM, Roth EJ. Cough in spinal cord injured patients: comparison of three methods to produce cough. Arch Phys Med Rehabil 1993;74(12):1358–1361
22. DiMarco AF, Romaniuk JR, Kowalski KE, Supinski G. Pattern of expiratory muscle activation during lower thoracic spinal cord stimulation. J Appl Physiol 1999;86(6):1881–1889
23. Schurch B, Rodic B, Jeanmonod D. Posterior sacral rhizotomy and intradural anterior sacral root stimulation for treatment of the spastic bladder in spinal cord injured patients. J Urol 1997;157(2): 610–614
24. van der Aa HE, Alleman E, Nene A, Snoek G. Sacral anterior root stimulation for bladder control: clinical results. Arch Physiol Biochem 1999;107(3):248–256
25. Wielink G, Essink-Bot ML, van Kerrebroeck PEV, Rutten FFH; Dutch Study Group on Sacral Anterior Root Stimulation. Sacral rhizotomies and electrical bladder stimulation in spinal cord injury, II: Cost-effectiveness and quality of life analysis. Eur Urol 1997;31(4):441–446
26. Creasey G, Dahlberg J. Economic consequences of an implanted neural prosthesis for bladder and bowel management. Arch Phys Med Rehab 2001;82:1520–1525
27. Brindley GS. Neuroprostheses used to restore male sexual or reproductive function. Baillieres Clin Neurol 1995;4(1):15–20
28. Kafetsoulis A, Brackett NL, Ibrahim E, Attia GR, Lynne CM. Current trends in the treatment of infertility in men with spinal cord injury. Fertil Steril 2006;86(4):781–789
29. Keith MW. Neuroprostheses for the upper extremity. Microsurgery 2001;21(6):256–263
30. Wuolle KS, Bryden AM, Peckham PH, Murray PK, Keith M. Satisfaction with upper-extremity surgery in individuals with tetraplegia. Arch Phys Med Rehabil 2003;84(8):1145–1149
31. Smith B, Tang Z, Johnson MW, et al. An externally powered, multichannel, implantable stimulator-telemeter for control of paralyzed muscle. IEEE Trans Biomed Eng 1998;45(4):463–475
32. Santhanam G, Ryu SI, Yu BM, Afshar A, Shenoy KV. A high-performance brain-computer interface. Nature 2006;442(7099):195–198
33. Graupe D, Cerrel-Bazo H, Kern H, Carraro U. Walking performance, medical outcomes and patient training in FES of innervated muscles for ambulation by thoracic-level complete paraplegics. Neurol Res 2008;30(2):123–130
34. Kobetic R, To CS, Schnellenberger JR, et al. Development of hybrid orthosis for standing, walking, and stair climbing after spinal cord injury. J Rehabil Res Dev 2009;46(3):447–462
35. Davis R, Eckhouse R, Patrick JF, Delehanty A. Computer-controlled 22-channel stimulator for limb movement. Acta Neurochir Suppl (Wien) 1987;39:117–120
36. Rushton DN, Perkins TA, Donaldson N, et al. LARSI: How to obtain favorable muscle contractions. In: Popovic D, ed. Proceedings of the Second Annual IFESS Conference (IFESS '97) and Neural Prosthesis: Motor Systems 5 (NP '97), Burnaby, British Columbia, Canada; The International Functional Electrical Stimulation Society. 16–21 August, 1997:163–164
37. Davis JA Jr, Triolo RJ, Uhlir JP, et al. Preliminary performance of a surgically implanted neuroprosthesis for standing and transfers—where do we stand? J Rehabil Res Dev 2001;38(6):609–617
38. Sharma M, Marsolais EB, Polando G, et al. Implantation of a 16-channel functional electrical stimulation walking system. Clin Orthop Relat Res 1998; (347):236–242
39. Becker D, Gary DS, Rosenzweig ES, Grill WM, McDonald JW. Functional electrical stimulation helps replenish progenitor cells in the injured spinal cord of adult rats. Exp Neurol 2010;222(2): 211–218

48

Operant Conditioning of Spinal Reflexes to Improve Motor Function after Spinal Cord Injury

Aiko K. Thompson and Jonathan R. Wolpaw

Key Points

1. Gradual activity-dependent plasticity shapes spinal cord function during early development and throughout life.
2. Spinal cord injury (SCI) often leads to abnormally functioning spinal reflexes that contribute to impaired movement control.
3. Thus a method that can induce and guide the plasticity in spinal cord pathways may offer a promising new therapeutic approach.
4. Operant conditioning of spinal reflexes induces central nervous system (CNS) multisite plasticity and can improve gait in animals with partial SCI.
5. Operant conditioning of spinal reflexes is possible in people and may improve gait in chronic incomplete SCI.

The spinal cord contains neural circuits that are capable of generating movement without direct input from the brain (i.e., reflexes and rhythmic movements) and are plastic throughout life.[1] Appropriate appreciation of the spinal cord's complex capacities for long-term activity-dependent plasticity has occurred only recently.[2,3] Methods for inducing and guiding this spinal cord plasticity could help to restore motor functions after spinal cord injuries (SCIs) or other chronic central nervous system (CNS) damage or disease.[3] Protocols for operant conditioning of spinal reflexes can be used to produce changes in specific spinal reflex pathways, and they might thereby contribute to the recovery of useful function.

Activity-Dependent Spinal Cord Plasticity

The spinal cord receives a continual barrage of descending and peripheral inputs throughout life. In the short term, these inputs produce appropriate movements (e.g., via voluntary muscle activation,[4,5] reflex modulation,[6–8] etc.). In addition, in the long term, they gradually establish and maintain spinal cord pathways in a state that supports the entire roster of motor behaviors.[9,10] Gradual activity-dependent plasticity, driven by descending and associated peripheral inputs, shapes spinal cord function during early development and throughout life.[11]

Developmental Plasticity of Spinal Cord

Both descending and peripheral inputs have crucial roles in the developmental plasticity that produces a normally functioning adult spinal cord that has characteristic adult reflex patterns and supports motor skills like posture, locomotion, dancing, and playing musical instruments. Disturbances to the descending activity early in life lead to an inappropriately functioning adult spinal cord. During early life, the corticospinal connections important for motor control and skill learning[12,13] develop their normal pattern of mainly contralateral innervation of limb muscles.[14] However, perinatal supraspinal damage (e.g., cerebral palsy) prevents the normal development of these pathways, and abnormal bilateral projections to the spinal cord may persist into adulthood. Perinatal disruption of descending activity also prevents proper development of the spinal proprioceptive reflexes[15,16] that contribute to normal motor behaviors[17,18] and results in motor disabilities in the adult. Similarly, properly functioning flexor withdrawal reflexes from noxious stimuli depend on appropriate descending and peripheral inputs during early development,[19,20] and descending activity is also crucial to the development of normal urinary function.[21]

Peripheral and descending inputs are both essential for shaping a properly functioning adult spinal cord. These inputs continue to modify spinal cord pathways throughout adult life. Because SCI disturbs both descending and peripheral activity, it produces motor dysfunction and spinal reflex abnormalities.

Abnormally Functioning Spinal Reflexes in Motor Dysfunction after Spinal Cord Injury

Normally, spinal reflexes are modulated in functionally appropriate ways that depend on the motor task. For instance, soleus Hoffmann reflex (H-reflex) gain is high during standing, much lower during walking, and even lower during running.[22] This task-dependent modulation of H-reflex gain prevents the saturation of motor output and the reflex feedback loop. Nonreciprocal inhibition, which arises largely from Golgi tendon organs and is present during standing, disappears or changes to excitation during some phases of walking.[23–25] In walking, the extensor muscles must remain active to support the body weight as long as the limb is loaded, and positive feedback from Golgi tendon organs serves to maintain extensor activity.[25–29] In general, reflex modulation across motor tasks appears to contribute to effective task execution.[25–27]

Injuries to the nervous system often lead to abnormally functioning spinal reflexes. Normal task-dependent modulation of the soleus H-reflex is greatly diminished or absent (or even reversed) in some subjects with incomplete SCI,[30,31] probably due to reduced presynaptic inhibition.[32] After SCI, normal nonreciprocal Ib inhibition of the soleus by medial gastrocnemius nerve stimulation is absent,[33] and recurrent inhibition of the soleus is exaggerated.[34] Such losses of appropriate reflex modulation contribute to motor dysfunction.

After SCI, altered spinal reflexes may interfere with the already weakened supraspinal control of gait.[30,31,35–37] Foot drop (drop and drag of the foot during the swing phase of the gait cycle), one of the most common problems after incomplete SCI, is probably due to changes in both spinal and supraspinal pathways. Ankle dorsiflexion is weakened after SCI due to disruption of the corticospinal connections that normally contribute to ankle dorsiflexion during the swing phase of walking.[4,5,38] The remaining dorsiflexion is often further reduced by exaggerated stretch reflex responses from extensor triceps surae muscles.[31,39] These reductions in dorsiflexion result in foot drop.

During walking in humans, reflexes normally change depending on the phase of the step cycle.[22,40,41] However, after SCI, not only task-dependent modulation (see earlier discussion)[37,42] but also phase-dependent modulation of the reflex is greatly diminished or absent.[30,31,39] In addition, abnormal reciprocal inhibition between the ankle plantar- and dorsiflexors may contribute to exaggerated stretch reflexes or foot drop.[35,37,42,43] (Other mechanisms may also contribute to such spastic movement disorders.[44]) **Figure 48.1** shows soleus H-reflexes, as well as soleus and tibialis anterior (TA) electromyography (EMG), during walking in a normal subject and in a subject with incomplete SCI. In the normal subject (**Fig. 48.1A**), H-reflex size is greatly modulated over the step cycle: it gradually increases from the beginning of stance, peaks at the end of stance (i.e., at about the same time as the peak soleus EMG activity), then rapidly decreases, and it stays low or is absent throughout the swing phase. In contrast, in **Fig. 48.1B**, the soleus H-reflex is suppressed after push-off (as it should be), but it recovers

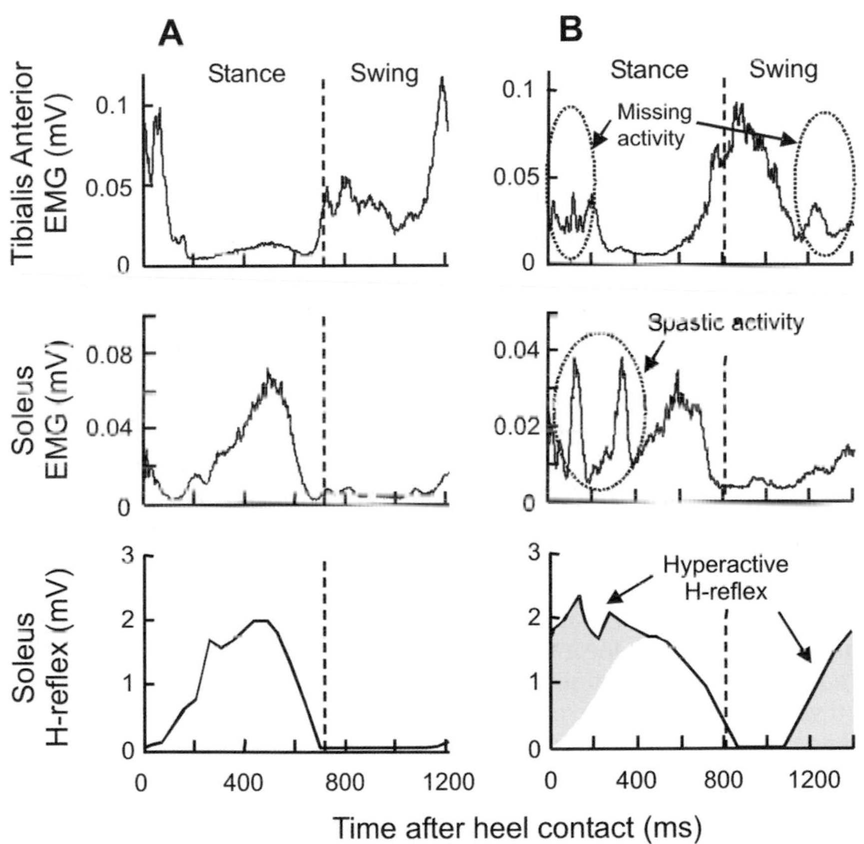

Fig. 48.1 Soleus and tibialis anterior (TA) electromyographic (EMG) activity and soleus H-reflex size during the step-cycle. The shaded areas in **(B)** indicate abnormally high reflex gain. **(A)** In a normal subject, two distinct bursts of TA EMG activity typically occur during the swing phase and the early stance phase: one from the end of stance to early swing and another during the swing-stance transition. Soleus EMG activity gradually increases from heel contact to push-off, then drops down to near zero, and remains low for the entire swing phase. The soleus H-reflex modulation pattern is similar to the soleus EMG pattern. **(B)** In a subject with chronic SCI, H-reflex modulation is impaired. The H-reflex is suppressed after push-off (i.e., at the end of stance), but it recovers in the middle of the swing phase and stays abnormally high through the midstance. This high soleus reflex gain probably contributes to the abnormally low TA activity during the late swing to early stance phase. In addition, in the presence of the abnormally high reflex gain during early stance, the foot dorsiflexion at heel contact, which stretches the soleus, triggers clonus (indicated by the dotted circle) and produces instability.

too soon (i.e., in the middle of the swing phase) and stays high through midstance. This probably contributes to the reduced second TA burst from the end of swing to early stance, which produces toe drop at the end of swing. In addition, the abnormally high H-reflex gain during early stance probably underlies the clonic soleus EMG activity seen in this subject (and many people with SCI) during early-middle stance. Such abnormal EMG activation produces instability during the stance-swing transition and in initial foot placement in early stance.[31,39] Another common locomotor reflex abnormality is a loss of reflex modulation throughout the step cycle (not shown).[30] It has been suggested that such loss of modulation reflects saturation of the reflex loop.[31]

Possible Therapeutic Benefits of Using Operant Conditioning to Induce and Guide Spinal Reflex Plasticity

H-reflex modulation is often impaired in subjects with chronic incomplete SCI, and this abnormality is likely to affect locomotor EMG activity.[30,45,46] As **Fig. 48.1B** illustrates, unsuppressed extensor reflex activity from swing to early stance may counteract ankle dorsiflexion and contribute to foot drop, and high reflex gain in the swing-stance transition may produce clonus that makes the ankle unstable. Thus decreasing extensor reflex gain or restoring its phase-dependent modulation might improve locomotion. In SCI-injured cats in which treadmill training had improved locomotion, the excitatory and inhibitory effects of group I pathways had also changed appropriately.[47] This provides evidence for the link between normalizing transmission in spinal reflex pathways and improving locomotion. Thus operant conditioning of spinal reflexes may offer a promising new approach to achieving therapeutic goals. The next sections review the reflex conditioning methodology, its results in normal animals and humans, and its initial applications to animals and humans with partial SCIs.

■ Operant Conditioning of Spinal Reflexes in Normal Animals and Humans

Operant Conditioning of Spinal Reflexes in Laboratory Animals

The standard protocol for operant conditioning of spinal reflexes was originally developed in monkeys,[48,49] adapted and used extensively in rats,[50] and recently tested in mice.[51] Although the protocol was first applied to the spinal stretch reflex,[49] subsequent work has focused on the H-reflex (and on reciprocal inhibition).[48,50,52,54] The rat H-reflex protocol is described here.[50,52] The monkey and mouse protocols are very similar.[48,51]

Rats are chronically implanted with fine-wire EMG electrodes in the soleus muscle and a stimulating cuff on the posterior tibial nerve. The implanted wires connect through a headmount and a flexible tether and commutator to EMG amplifiers and a nerve-cuff simulator. Soleus EMG is monitored continuously (24 h/d) in the freely moving animal. Whenever the absolute value of soleus EMG remains within a specified range for a random varying 2.3 to 2.7 second period, a stimulus through the nerve cuff that is kept just above M-wave threshold elicits the M-wave and the H-reflex. In the course of normal activity, the animal usually provides 2500 to 8000 of these H-reflex trials per day. For the first 10 days, the animal is exposed to the control mode, in which no reward occurs and the H-reflex is simply measured to determine its baseline (i.e., control) value. For the next 50 days, the rat is exposed to the up-conditioning (HRup) or down-conditioning (HRdown) mode, in which a food reward occurs if the H-reflex is above (HRup) or below (HRdown) a criterion value. Background EMG and M-wave amplitude remain constant throughout.

Figure 48.2 shows the results of the operant conditioning in rats, monkeys, and mice. In each species, chronic exposure to the up-(▲) or down-(▼) conditioning mode

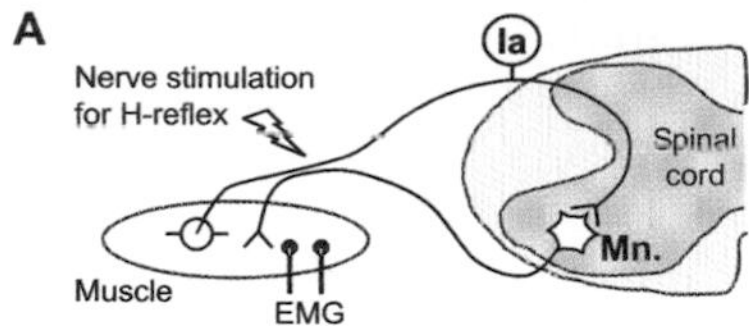

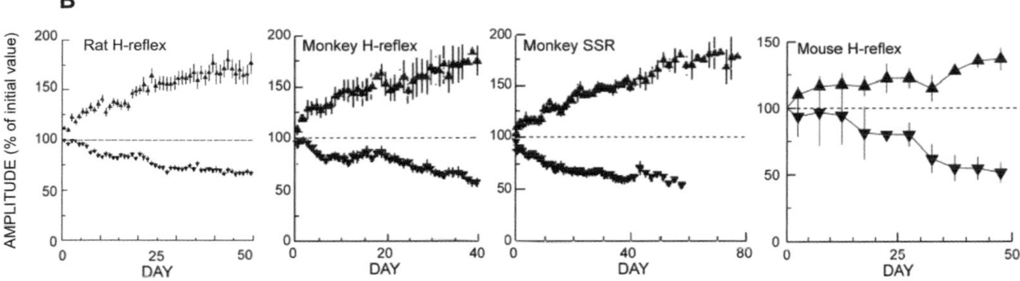

Fig. 48.2 **(A)** Main pathway of the spinal stretch reflex (SSR) and its electrical analog, the H-reflex. Excitation of the Ia spindle afferents (and possibly large group II afferents)[90,91] activates the motoneurons innervating the same muscle and its synergists. This activation is largely monosynaptic. If the afferents are excited by muscle stretch, the response is the SSR. If the afferents are excited by an electrical stimulus, the response is the H-reflex. Although the pathway is entirely spinal, it is strongly influenced by descending influence from the brain. **(B)** Operant up-conditioning and down-conditioning of a spinal reflex in different models. From left, soleus H-reflex in rats, triceps surae H-reflex in monkeys, biceps brachii SSR in monkeys, and triceps surae H-reflex in mice. In general, the time courses and magnitudes of change are similar across different species and muscles.[51–53] (Adapted from Wolpaw JR. The complex structure of a simple memory. Trends Neurosci 1997;20(12):588–594; Chen XY, et al. Reflex conditioning: a new strategy for improving motor function after spinal cord injury. Ann N Y Acad Sci 2010;1198(Suppl 1):E12–21; and Carp JS, Tennissen AM, Chen XY, Wolpaw JR. H-reflex operant conditioning in mice. J Neurophysiol 2006;96(4):1718–1727.)

gradually changes the size of the reflex in the correct direction. Successful conditioning, defined as a change of > 20% in the correct direction,[50,55] occurs in 75 to 80% of the animals. In the remainder, the reflex remains within 20% of its control value.

Operant Conditioning of the Soleus H-reflex in Normal Humans

Spinal reflex conditioning in humans uses a protocol comparable to that developed in animals. The protocol was first applied in humans to the biceps brachii stretch reflex[56,57] and more recently has been applied to the human soleus H-reflex.[58] The only significant difference from the animal protocol is that humans perform many fewer trials (i.e., only 2 to 5% as many), and these trials are confined to 1-hour sessions three times per week. Nevertheless, the human results are similar to the animal results in the gradual progression and final magnitude of reflex change. The newly developed soleus H-reflex protocol comprises six baseline sessions and 24 conditioning sessions at a pace of three sessions per week, and four follow-up sessions over the next 3 months. Sessions are always held at the same time of day to control for diurnal variation in the reflex.[59] In each session, the soleus H-reflex is elicited while the subject maintains a natural standing posture and a specified stable level of soleus background EMG. The size of the M-wave is kept constant within and across the sessions. In each baseline session, three blocks of 75 control H-reflexes (i.e., 225 H-reflexes) are elicited. In each conditioning or follow-up session, 20 control H-reflexes are elicited as in the baseline sessions, and then three blocks of 75 (i.e., 225) conditioned H-reflexes are elicited. In these conditioned H-reflex trials, the subject is asked to increase

(HRup mode) or decrease (HRdown mode) the H-reflex and is given visual feedback after each stimulus to indicate whether the resulting H-reflex was larger (HRup) or smaller (HRdown) than a criterion value. Good performance in changing the reflex size earns an additional monetary reward. Background EMG and M-wave size are kept stable throughout data collection.

Figure 48.3 summarizes the human soleus H-reflex conditioning results. Over the 24 conditioning sessions, H-reflex size gradually increased in six of eight HRup subjects and decreased in eight of nine HRdown subjects, resulting in final sizes of 140(± 12 standard error of mean [SEM])% and 69(± 6)% of baseline size, respectively. In these subjects, the final H-reflex change was the sum of within-session change (i.e., task-dependent adaptation) and across-session (i.e., long-term) change. Task-dependent adaptation appeared within four to six sessions and persisted thereafter, whereas long-term change began after 10 to 12 sessions and increased gradually thereafter. (Full presentation and discussion of task-dependent adaptation and long-term change can be found elsewhere.[58])

This study showed that people performing only 225 reflex conditioning trials a

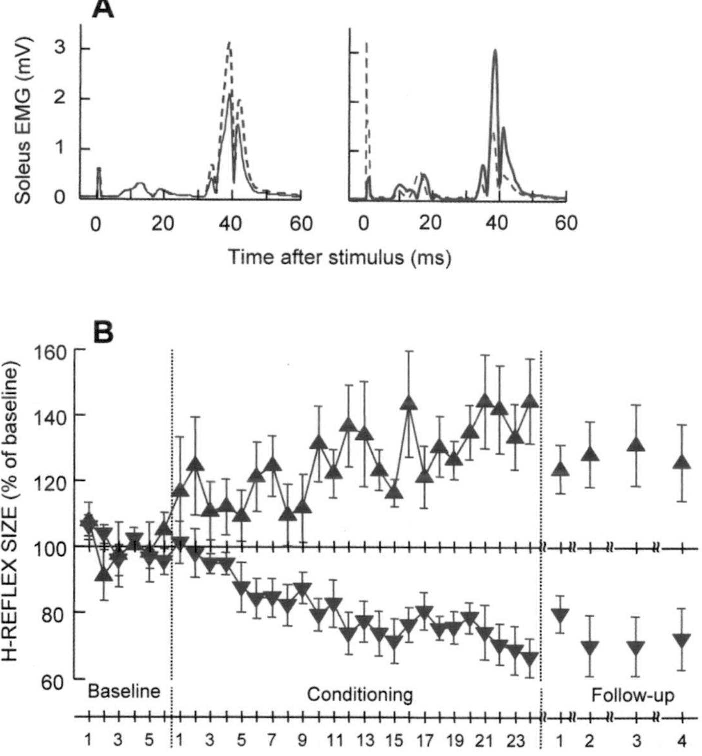

Fig. 48.3 Human subjects can learn to change H-reflex size in response to an operant conditioning protocol. **(A)** Average H-reflexes from two representative subjects for a baseline session (*solid*) and for the last conditioning session (*dashed*). After the 24 conditioning sessions, H-reflex size is larger in the up-conditioning (HRup) subject (*left*) and smaller in the down-conditioning (HRdown) subject (*right*). **(B)** Average H-reflexes (± SEM) for six successful HRup and eight successful HRdown subjects for baseline, conditioning, and follow-up (12, 30, 60, and 90 days after the end of conditioning) sessions. As in animals, H-reflex size gradually increases in the HRup group (*upward triangles*) and decreases in the HRdown group (*downward triangles*) over the course of the study. (With permission from Thompson AK, Chen XY, Wolpaw JR. Acquisition of a simple motor skill: task-dependent adaptation plus long-term change in the human soleus H-reflex. J Neurosci 2009;29(18):5784–5792.)

day, 3 days a week, displayed gradual reflex change similar in course and nearly equal in magnitude to that of animals that perform 20 to 50 times as many trials. This indicates that H-reflex conditioning is possible in humans and does not require the several thousand trials per day typically completed by animals. (Animals probably do not require that many trials either, but that remains to be determined.) The success rate of 82% (14 of 17 subjects changed H-reflex size significantly in the correct direction) was also comparable to that of animals.[48,50,52,58] In addition, this study showed that exposure to the reflex operant conditioning paradigm over several months induced both short-term adaptation and long-term plasticity in spinal reflex pathways. The long-term plasticity appeared to be a lasting change in the reflex pathway that persisted outside of the reflex conditioning paradigm and lasted for at least several months after cessation of reflex conditioning.[58] This suggests that it might be possible to use reflex conditioning protocols to guide such long-term plasticity so as to essentially reeducate abnormally functioning spinal reflex pathways and thereby alleviate motor disabilities associated with partial spinal cord injuries (**Fig. 48.1**). This possibility is supported by a recent study in rats with SCI.[60]

Current Understanding of the Spinal and Supraspinal Mechanisms of Reflex Conditioning

Spinal cord reflexes commonly function as parts of complex behaviors, such as locomotion.[6–8,41,61–64] At the same, these reflexes are themselves simple behaviors, and operantly conditioned changes in them are essentially simple skills (i.e., "adaptive behaviors acquired through practice" according to the *Compact Oxford English Dictionary*, 1993). Thus, operant conditioning of spinal reflexes can provide excellent models for studying the plasticity underlying motor skill learning.[11,12,52,65] An ongoing series of physiological and anatomical studies has begun to reveal the complex pattern of spinal and supraspinal plasticity underlying H-reflex conditioning.[11,12,52] A positive shift in motoneuron firing threshold (possibly due to a change in the activation voltage of Na^+ channels) can largely account for down-conditioning of the H-reflex.[52] Down-conditioning is also associated with marked increases in identifiable gamma aminobutyric acid (GABA)-ergic interneurons in the ventral horn and GABAergic terminals on the soleus motoneuron.[65] There is also evidence that changes occur in several other synaptic populations on the motoneuron, in motor unit properties, in other spinal interneurons, and even on the contralateral side of the spinal cord.[52] Up-conditioning and down-conditioning appear to have different mechanisms; they are not mirror images of each other. Up-conditioning may be due to plasticity in spinal interneurons.[65]

The corticospinal tract (CST) is the only major descending tract that is essential for H-reflex conditioning.[66–68] Thus it is presumably CST activity that changes the spinal cord. Furthermore, cerebellar–cortical connections appear to be essential for establishing and maintaining supraspinal plasticity that in turn establishes and maintains the spinal cord plasticity that is directly responsible for H-reflex change.[69,70] In sum, the data indicate that H-reflex conditioning depends on a hierarchy in which plasticity in the brain induces plasticity in the spinal cord.[58,67–71] Operant conditioning of a spinal reflex produces multisite plasticity that extends far beyond the reflex pathway conditioned and can therefore have complex effects on motor function.

Operant Conditioning of Spinal Reflexes after Spinal Cord Injuries

Operant conditioning is a powerful method for inducing changes in specific spinal pathways. Because abnormally functioning spinal reflexes contribute to movement disabilities (**Fig. 48.1**), methods for reducing reflex abnormalities may help to reduce motor disabilities. Segal and Wolf[57] showed that it is possible to operantly condition the biceps brachii stretch reflex in humans with incomplete SCI (**Fig. 48.4A**). In this initial study, they did not address the question of whether such conditioning can produce therapeutic benefits. Chen et al.[60] recently showed that up-conditioning of the soleus H-reflex can improve locomotion in rats with incomplete SCI (**Fig. 48.4B**). Midthoracic hemisection of the right lateral column shortens the right stance phase and thereby produces an asymmetry in locomotion. As **Fig. 48.4B** illustrates, H-reflex up-conditioning, which enhances the soleus burst during the stance phase, eliminates this asymmetry. This study suggests that reflex conditioning protocols might improve motor function in people with partial SCI.

Operant Conditioning of the Soleus H-reflex in Incomplete Spinal Cord Injury

The initial soleus H-reflex conditioning study in normal humans showed that exposure to the operant conditioning paradigm three times per week over several months induced both short-term adaptation and long-term plasticity in the reflex (see earlier discussion).[58] If such conditioning is possible in people with partial SCI, it could be used to guide long-term plasticity that reduces specific motor disabilities. To evaluate the therapeutic possibilities of this approach, we have begun to apply a soleus H-reflex down-conditioning protocol in people with spastic gait due to incomplete SCI.[72]

The initial subjects are adults with chronic (0.7 to 9 years postinjury) incomplete SCI who suffer from ankle extensor spasticity and foot drop. All are medically stable and ambulatory. The protocol is the same as the one used in normal subjects,[58] except for an increase in the number of conditioning sessions from 24 to 30. Six baseline and 30 down-conditioning sessions occur at the rate of three sessions per week for 12 weeks. Soleus and tibialis anterior background EMG and soleus M-wave size are maintained at constant levels throughout the study.

The initial results indicate that operant down-conditioning of the soleus H-reflex is possible in people after incomplete SCI. Three of the four subjects studied to date had significantly smaller H-reflexes after down-conditioning. **Fig. 48.4C** shows the before and after results for one of these subjects. Chen et al.[73,74] found that the success rate for reflex conditioning in rats with SCI was inversely correlated with the severity of the injury. In rats, the CST is essential for reflex conditioning,[67,68] and initial results from people with strokes suggest that the CST may also be important for conditioning in humans.[75] Thus incomplete SCIs that involve the CST may impair reflex conditioning. Nevertheless, the study of Segal and Wolf[57] and these new results indicate that conditioning is possible in many people with SCI, though it may take longer.

After successfully decreasing the soleus H-reflex, some of the subjects showed changes in locomotor EMG activity. **Figure 48.4D** shows soleus and TA locomotor EMG in a spastic subject before and after successful down-conditioning of the soleus H-reflex. Before conditioning, soleus EMG was comparable to that found in normal subjects (**Fig. 48.1**), but TA activity was much lower than normal, and this resulted in foot drop. After successful conditioning, the soleus burst was not noticeably different, whereas TA EMG had increased, especially during the swing-stance transition (i.e., the second burst of the swing-phase TA activity; compare with the normal subject in **Fig. 48.1A**). This increase in TA EMG served to reduce foot drop, although it was not enough to eliminate it completely. This subject also showed an increase in walking speed (i.e., reduction in 10 meter walk time from 54 to 24 seconds). The two other subjects in whom conditioning was successful also showed improvements in walking speed (15 to 55% reductions in 10 meter walking times). Whether such changes are specific to successful conditioning (and to the direction of conditioning), and how they are related to changes in gait kinematics, reflex modulation over the step-cycle, and other measures of spasticity remain to be determined.

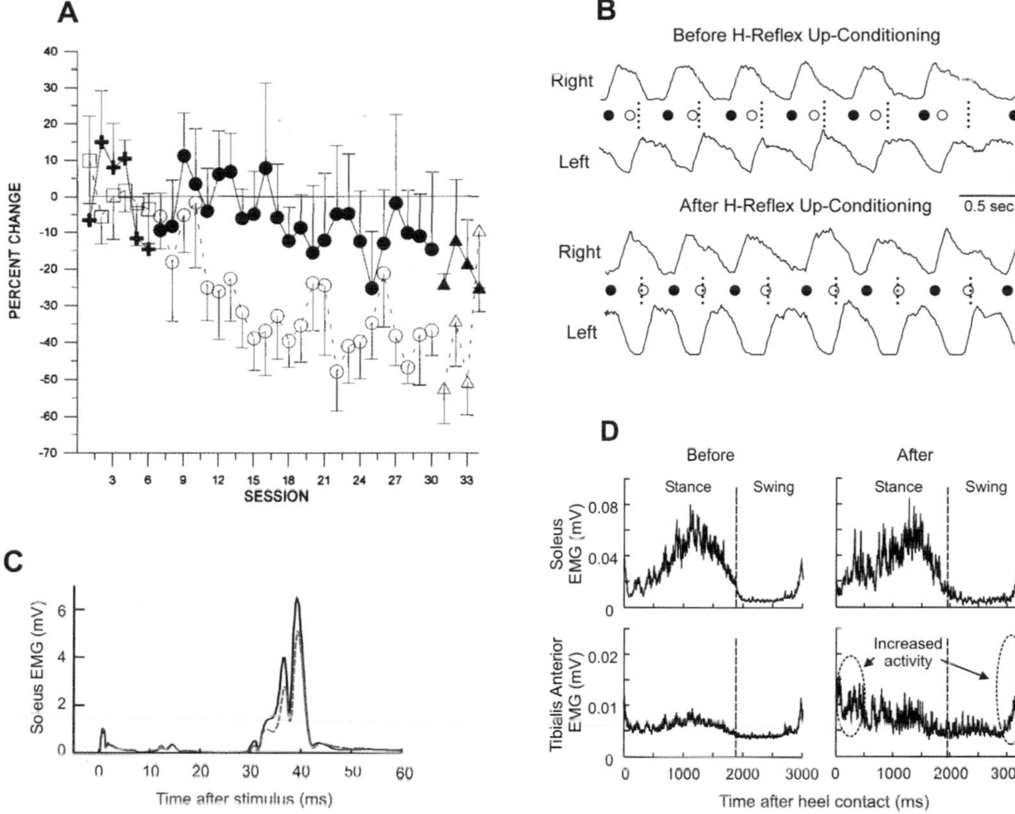

Fig. 48.4 **(A)** Average biceps brachii spinal stretch reflexes (± SEM) over 34 sessions (i.e., six baseline, 24 conditioning, and four follow-up sessions) in people with incomplete spinal cord injury (SCI) who were (□/○) or were not (+/●) exposed (i.e., the control group) to the down-conditioning protocol. In the down-conditioning group, spinal stretch reflex (SSR) size declines steadily over the conditioning sessions and remains low in the follow-up sessions. In contrast, SSR shows only a small insignificant decrease in the control group. **(B)** The effects of H-reflex up-conditioning on locomotion in a rat with midthoracic right lateral column transection. The traces show the electromyographic (EMG) bursts from right and left soleus muscles during treadmill locomotion before (*top*) and after (*bottom*) H-reflex up-conditioning has increased the size of the right soleus H-reflex. The presumed onsets of the right (●) and left (○) stance phases of locomotion are indicated in the middle. The short vertical dashed lines mark the midpoints between right burst onsets, where the left burst onsets should occur. Before H-reflex up-conditioning, the left burst onset occurs too early, and the gait is asymmetrical. H-reflex up-conditioning strengthens the right soleus EMG burst and corrects the left burst onset timing, and thereby reduces the gait asymmetry. Horizontal scale bar: 0.5 second vertical scale bar: 100 and 150 μV for the right and left EMG bursts, respectively. **(C)** Average H-reflexes in a representative subject with SCI for a baseline session (*solid*) and for the final conditioning session (*dashed*) (all 225 trials averaged for each trace). The final H-reflex is substantially smaller than the baseline H-reflex, whereas the background electromyographic (EMG) and M-wave size have not changed. **(D)** Soleus and tibialis anterior (TA) EMG activity during walking before and after soleus H-reflex down-conditioning in the same subject. Before H-reflex conditioning, there is almost no TA EMG activity throughout the step cycle. After down-conditioning, there is little change in soleus EMG, whereas TA EMG increases, especially in the late-swing to early-stance period. Increased TA activity in this period reduces foot-drop. (**[A]** from Segal RL, Wolf SL. Operant conditioning of spinal stretch reflexes in patients with spinal cord injuries. Exp Neurol 1994;130(2):202–213. **[B]** from Chen Y, Chen XY, Jakeman LB, Chen L, Stokes BT, Wolpaw JR. Operant conditioning of H-reflex can correct a locomotor abnormality after spinal cord injury in rats. J Neurosci 2006;26(48):12537–12543. Reprinted with permission.)

Therapeutic Applications of Reflex Conditioning

Spinal reflex conditioning protocols provide a unique new approach to rehabilitation. Because these protocols can target particular reflex pathways, they could be customized to address the particular motor deficits of each individual. It should be possible to design reflex conditioning protocols that complement existing therapeutic training methods, such as treadmill training[76–79] and constraint-induced movement therapy,[80–82] to maximize the recovery of useful motor function. Furthermore, when CNS regeneration becomes possible, methods such as spinal reflex conditioning could be essential for reeducating newly regenerated connections to support effective function.[80–82] Without the activity-dependent plasticity that could be induced and guided by appropriately targeted reflex conditioning protocols, regenerated connections are likely to display diffuse infantile-like responses and dysfunctional motor outputs. At the same time, these protocols clearly produce complex patterns of plasticity that extend well beyond the targeted reflex pathway.[2,12,54,65] Thus the principles critical for designing reflex conditioning protocols appropriate for individual patients will require careful study.

This new therapeutic approach has some limitations. At present, spinal reflex conditioning is successful in 75 to 80%, not 100%, of the subjects. This success rate could be lower, and the associated therapeutic effects may vary, among people with corticospinal tract damage (e.g., incomplete SCI) because studies to date indicate that the corticospinal tract is needed for successful reflex conditioning.[67,68] Furthermore, effective application of the current protocols requires a well-trained investigator or therapist with substantial knowledge of the relevant neurophysiology. However, this requirement may become less important in the future if a semiautomated hardware/software system for reflex conditioning becomes available.

Development of Other Operant Conditioning Protocols

Although the operant conditioning protocol described here has been applied mainly to the H-reflex and the spinal stretch reflex, comparable protocols might be applied to other reflexes. Indeed, operant conditioning of reciprocal inhibition has been described.[54] Extension to other reflex pathways (e.g., other proprioceptive or cutaneous reflexes, reflexes related to bladder or bowel function) could offer additional therapeutic possibilities. Furthermore, it may be possible to sharpen the focus of reflex conditioning by incorporating the conditioning protocol into complex motor skills, such as locomotion. Thus, for example, it should be possible to perform H-reflex conditioning trials during particular phases of the step-cycle. By focusing on the exact time when reflex gain is abnormal, such a protocol might help to restore functionally appropriate phase-dependent reflex modulation during walking.

Operant conditioning protocols that target corticospinal connections might also prove therapeutically valuable. The motor evoked potential (MEP) to transcranial magnetic stimulation (TMS) is reduced after SCI,[83] and recent studies suggest that functional recovery is accompanied by increased MEP size.[84] Our initial results suggest that operant up-conditioning of the TA MEP produced by TMS may strengthen CST connectivity after SCI[85] and may thereby improve control of ankle dorsiflexor muscles.[85,86] Finally, operant conditioning protocols might also focus on modifying EEG activity over the sensorimotor cortex so as to improve cortical control of motor function.[87]

Conclusion

SCI often produces abnormal spinal reflexes,[30,31,35–37] and abnormal reflexes can contribute to motor disabilities.[45,46,88,89] Therefore, methods for appropriately modifying reflex pathways might help to restore more effective motor function. Operant conditioning protocols can modify specific spinal reflexes in both normal people and people with partial SCIs.[56–58] Studies exploring the therapeutic potential of this new rehabilitation methodology in people with partial SCIs have recently begun. The initial results are encouraging. Furthermore, similar conditioning protocols could be developed to modify other spinal reflexes, corticospinal connections, or cortical activity, and might thereby also promote functional recovery.

Acknowledgments

Work in the authors' laboratories is supported by the National Institutes of Health (NS22189, HD36020, NS061823) and the New York State Spinal Cord Injury Research Trust (C023685).

References

1. Stein RB. The plasticity of the adult spinal cord continues to surprise. J Physiol 2008;586(Pt 12): 2823
2. Wolpaw JR, Carp JS. Plasticity from muscle to brain. Prog Neurobiol 2006;78(3-5):233–263
3. Wolpaw JR. The education and re-education of the spinal cord. Prog Brain Res 2006;157: 261–280
4. Capaday C, Lavoie BA, Barbeau H, Schneider C, Bonnard M. Studies on the corticospinal control of human walking, I: Responses to focal transcranial magnetic stimulation of the motor cortex. J Neurophysiol 1999;81(1):129–139
5. Schubert M, Curt A, Jensen L, Dietz V. Corticospinal input in human gait: modulation of magnetically evoked motor responses. Exp Brain Res 1997;115(2):234–246
6. Zehr EP, Stein RB. What functions do reflexes serve during human locomotion? Prog Neurobiol 1999;58(2):185–205
7. Stein RB. Presynaptic inhibition in humans. Prog Neurobiol 1995;47(6):533–544
8. Brooke JD, Cheng J, Collins DF, McIlroy WE, Misiaszek JE, Staines WR. Sensori-sensory afferent conditioning with leg movement: gain control in spinal reflex and ascending paths. Prog Neurobiol 1997;51(4):393–421
9. Nielsen J, Crone C, Hultborn H. H-reflexes are smaller in dancers from The Royal Danish Ballet than in well-trained athletes. Eur J Appl Physiol Occup Physiol 1993;66(2):116–121
10. Schneider C, Capaday C. Progressive adaptation of the soleus H-reflex with daily training at walking backward. J Neurophysiol 2003;89(2):648–656
11. Wolpaw JR, Tennissen AM. Activity-dependent spinal cord plasticity in health and disease. Annu Rev Neurosci 2001;24:807–843
12. Wolpaw JR. Spinal cord plasticity in acquisition and maintenance of motor skills. Acta Physiol (Oxf) 2007;189(2):155–169
13. Adkins DL, Boychuk J, Remple MS, Kleim JA. Motor training induces experience-specific patterns of plasticity across motor cortex and spinal cord. J Appl Physiol 2006;101(6):1776–1782
14. Eyre JA. Developmental plasticity of the corticospinal system. In: Boniface S, Ziemann U, eds. Plasticity in the Human Nervous System: Investigations with Transcranial Magnetic Stimulation. Cambridge: Cambridge University Press; 2003:62–89
15. Myklebust BM, Gottlieb GL, Agarwal GC. Stretch reflexes of the normal infant. Dev Med Child Neurol 1986;28(4):440–449
16. O'Sullivan MC, Miller S, Ramesh V, et al. Abnormal development of biceps brachii phasic stretch reflex and persistence of short latency heteronymous reflexes from biceps to triceps brachii in spastic cerebral palsy. Brain 1998;121(Pt 12): 2381–2395
17. Dietz V. Proprioception and locomotor disorders. Nat Rev Neurosci 2002;3(10):781–790
18. Dietz V, Müller R, Colombo G. Locomotor activity in spinal man: significance of afferent input from joint and load receptors. Brain 2002;125(Pt 12):2626–2634
19. Waldenstrom A, Thelin J, Thimansson E, Levinsson A, Schouenborg J. Developmental learning in a pain-related system: evidence for a cross-modality mechanism. J Neurosci 2003;23(20):7719–7725
20. Levinsson A, Luo XL, Holmberg H, Schouenborg J. Developmental tuning in a spinal nociceptive system: effects of neonatal spinalization. J Neurosci 1999;19(23):10397–10403
21. de Groat WC. Plasticity of bladder reflex pathways during postnatal development. Physiol Behav 2002;77(4-5):689–692
22. Stein RB, Capaday C. The modulation of human reflexes during functional motor tasks. Trends Neurosci 1988;11(7):328–332
23. Pearson KG, Collins DF. Reversal of the influence of group Ib afferents from plantaris on activity in medial gastrocnemius muscle during locomotor activity. J Neurophysiol 1993;70(3):1009–1017
24. Stephens MJ, Yang JF. Short latency, non-reciprocal group I inhibition is reduced during the stance phase of walking in humans. Brain Res 1996;743(1-2):24–31
25. Pearson KG. Proprioceptive regulation of locomotion. Curr Opin Neurobiol 1995;5(6):786–791
26. Dietz V, Duysens J. Significance of load receptor input during locomotion: a review. Gait Posture 2000;11(2):102–110
27. Duysens J, Clarac F, Cruse H. Load-regulating mechanisms in gait and posture: comparative aspects. Physiol Rev 2000;80(1):83–133
28. Hiebert GW, Whelan PJ, Prochazka A, Pearson KG. Contribution of hind limb flexor muscle afferents to

the timing of phase transitions in the cat step cycle. J Neurophysiol 1996;75(3):1126–1137
29. Whelan PJ, Hiebert GW, Pearson KG. Stimulation of the group I extensor afferents prolongs the stance phase in walking cats. Exp Brain Res 1995;103(1):20–30
30. Stein RB, Yang JF, Bélanger M, Pearson KG. Modification of reflexes in normal and abnormal movements. Prog Brain Res 1993;97:189–196
31. Yang JF, Fung J, Edamura M, Blunt R, Stein RB, Barbeau H. H-reflex modulation during walking in spastic paretic subjects. Can J Neurol Sci 1991;18(4): 443–452
32. Yang JF, Whelan PJ. Neural mechanisms that contribute to cyclical modulation of the soleus H-reflex in walking in humans. Exp Brain Res 1993;95(3): 547–556
33. Morita H, Shindo M, Momoi H, Yanagawa S, Ikeda S, Yanagisawa N. Lack of modulation of Ib inhibition during antagonist contraction in spasticity. Neurology 2006;67(1):52–56
34. Shefner JM, Berman SA, Sarkarati M, Young RR. Recurrent inhibition is increased in patients with spinal cord injury. Neurology 1992;42(11): 2162–2168
35. Crone C, Johnsen LL, Biering-Sørensen F, Nielsen JB. Appearance of reciprocal facilitation of ankle extensors from ankle flexors in patients with stroke or spinal cord injury. Brain 2003;126(Pt 2):495–507
36. Hiersemenzel LP, Curt A, Dietz V. From spinal shock to spasticity: neuronal adaptations to a spinal cord injury. Neurology 2000;54(8):1574–1582
37. Thompson AK, Estabrooks KL, Chong S, Stein RB. Spinal reflexes in ankle flexor and extensor muscles after chronic central nervous system lesions and functional electrical stimulation. Neurorehabil Neural Repair 2009;23(2):133–142
38. Petersen NT, Butler JE, Marchand-Pauvert V, et al. Suppression of EMG activity by transcranial magnetic stimulation in human subjects during walking. J Physiol 2001;537(Pt 2):651–656
39. Fung J, Barbeau H. Effects of conditioning cutaneomuscular stimulation on the soleus H-reflex in normal and spastic paretic subjects during walking and standing. J Neurophysiol 1994;72(5): 2090–2104
40. Schneider C, Lavoie BA, Capaday C. On the origin of the soleus H-reflex modulation pattern during human walking and its task-dependent differences. J Neurophysiol 2000;83(5):2881–2890
41. Sinkjaer T, Andersen JB, Larsen B. Soleus stretch reflex modulation during gait in humans. J Neurophysiol 1996;76(2):1112–1120
42. Boorman GI, Lee RG, Becker WJ, Windhorst UR. Impaired "natural reciprocal inhibition" in patients with spasticity due to incomplete spinal cord injury. Electroencephalogr Clin Neurophysiol 1996;101(2):84–92
43. Ashby P, Wiens M. Reciprocal inhibition following lesions of the spinal cord in man. J Physiol 1989;414:145–157
44. Aymard C, Katz R, Lafitte C, et al. Presynaptic inhibition and homosynaptic depression: a comparison between lower and upper limbs in normal human subjects and patients with hemiplegia. Brain 2000;123(Pt 8):1688–1702
45. Burne JA, Carleton VL, O'Dwyer NJ. The spasticity paradox: movement disorder or disorder of resting limbs? J Neurol Neurosurg Psychiatry 2005;76(1): 47–54
46. Dietz V, Sinkjaer T. Spastic movement disorder: impaired reflex function and altered muscle mechanics. Lancet Neurol 2007;6(8):725–733
47. Côté MP, Ménard A, Gossard JP. Spinal cats on the treadmill: changes in load pathways. J Neurosci 2003;23(7):2789–2796
48. Wolpaw JR. Operant conditioning of primate spinal reflexes: the H-reflex. J Neurophysiol 1987; 57(2):443–459
49. Wolpaw JR, O'Keefe JA. Adaptive plasticity in the primate spinal stretch reflex: evidence for a two-phase process. J Neurosci 1984;4(11):2718–2724
50. Chen XY, Wolpaw JR. Operant conditioning of H-reflex in freely moving rats. J Neurophysiol 1995;73(1):411–415
51. Carp JS, Tennissen AM, Chen XY, Wolpaw JR. H-reflex operant conditioning in mice. J Neurophysiol 2006;96(4):1718–1727
52. Chen XY, Chen Y, Wang Y, et al. Reflex conditioning: a new strategy for improving motor function after spinal cord injury. Ann NY Acad Sci 2010;1198(Suppl 1):E12–21
53. Wolpaw JR. The complex structure of a simple memory. Trends Neurosci 1997;20(12):588–594
54. Chen XY, Chen L, Chen Y, Wolpaw JR. Operant conditioning of reciprocal inhibition in rat soleus muscle. J Neurophysiol 2006;96(4):2144–2150
55. Wolpaw JR, Herchenroder PA, Carp JS. Operant conditioning of the primate H-reflex: factors affecting the magnitude of change. Exp Brain Res 1993;97(1):31–39
56. Wolf SL, Segal RL. Reducing human biceps brachii spinal stretch reflex magnitude. J Neurophysiol 1996;75(4):1637–1646
57. Segal RL, Wolf SL. Operant conditioning of spinal stretch reflexes in patients with spinal cord injuries. Exp Neurol 1994;130(2):202–213
58. Thompson AK, Chen XY, Wolpaw JR. Acquisition of a simple motor skill: task-dependent adaptation plus long-term change in the human soleus H-reflex. J Neurosci 2009;29(18):5784–5792
59. Lagerquist O, Zehr EP, Baldwin ER, Klakowicz PM, Collins DF. Diurnal changes in the amplitude of the Hoffmann reflex in the human soleus but not in the flexor carpi radialis muscle. Exp Brain Res 2006;170(1):1–6
60. Chen Y, Chen XY, Jakeman LB, Chen L, Stokes BT, Wolpaw JR. Operant conditioning of H-reflex can correct a locomotor abnormality after spinal cord injury in rats. J Neurosci 2006;26(48): 12537–12543
61. Yang JF, Stein RB. Phase-dependent reflex reversal in human leg muscles during walking. J Neurophysiol 1990;63(5):1109–1117
62. Mazzaro N, Grey MJ, Sinkjaer T. Contribution of afferent feedback to the soleus muscle activity during human locomotion. J Neurophysiol 2005;93(1): 167–177
63. Grey MJ, van Doornik J, Sinkjaer T. Plantar flexor stretch reflex responses to whole body loading/unloading during human walking. Eur J Neurosci 2002;16(10):2001–2007

64. Sinkjaer T, Andersen JB, Ladouceur M, Christensen LO, Nielsen JB. Major role for sensory feedback in soleus EMG activity in the stance phase of walking in man. J Physiol 2000;523(Pt 3):817–827
65. Wolpaw JR. What can the spinal cord teach us about learning and memory? Neuroscientist 2010;16(5):532–549
66. Chen XY, Chen Y, Chen L, Tennissen AM, Wolpaw JR. Corticospinal tract transection permanently abolishes H-reflex down-conditioning in rats. J Neurotrauma 2006;23(11):1705–1712
67. Chen XY, Carp JS, Chen L, Wolpaw JR. Corticospinal tract transection prevents operantly conditioned H-reflex increase in rats. Exp Brain Res 2002;144(1):88–94
68. Chen XY, Wolpaw JR. Probable corticospinal tract control of spinal cord plasticity in the rat. J Neurophysiol 2002;87(2):645–652
69. Wolpaw JR, Chen XY. The cerebellum in maintenance of a motor skill: a hierarchy of brain and spinal cord plasticity underlies H-reflex conditioning. Learn Mem 2006;13(2):208–215
70. Chen XY, Wolpaw JR. Ablation of cerebellar nuclei prevents H-reflex down-conditioning in rats. Learn Mem 2005;12(3):248–254
71. Chen XY, Carp JS, Chen L, Wolpaw JR. Sensorimotor cortex ablation prevents H-reflex up-conditioning and causes a paradoxical response to down-conditioning in rats. J Neurophysiol 2006;96(1):119–127
72. Pomerantz F, Wolpaw JR, Lichtman SW, DeFrancesco E, Thompson AK. Operant conditioning of the soleus H-reflex in spastic subjects after incomplete spinal cord injury. In: Society for Neuroscience 39th Annual Meeting 2009;79.9
73. Chen XY, Wolpaw JR, Jakeman LB, Stokes BT. Operant conditioning of H-reflex increase in spinal cord–injured rats. J Neurotrauma 1999;16(2):175–186
74. Chen XY, Wolpaw JR, Jakeman LB, Stokes BT. Operant conditioning of H-reflex in spinal cord-injured rats. J Neurotrauma 1996;13(12):755–766
75. Segal RL, Catlin PA, Cooke R, et al. Preliminary studies of modifications of hyperactive spinal stretch reflexes in stroke patients. In: Society for Neuroscience 1989;363.317
76. Edgerton VR, Courtine G, Gerasimenko YP, et al. Training locomotor networks. Brain Res Brain Res Rev 2008;57(1):241–254
77. Harkema SJ, Hurley SL, Patel UK, Requejo PS, Dobkin BH, Edgerton VR. Human lumbosacral spinal cord interprets loading during stepping. J Neurophysiol 1997;77(2):797–811
78. Maegele M, Müller S, Wernig A, Edgerton VR, Harkema SJ. Recruitment of spinal motor pools during voluntary movements versus stepping after human spinal cord injury. J Neurotrauma 2002;19(10):1217–1229
79. Wernig A, Nanassy A, Müller S. Laufband (LB) therapy in spinal cord lesioned persons. Prog Brain Res 2000;128:89–97
80. Wolf SL, Winstein CJ, Miller JP, et al; EXCITE Investigators. Effect of constraint-induced movement therapy on upper extremity function 3 to 9 months after stroke: the EXCITE randomized clinical trial. JAMA 2006;296(17):2095–2104
81. Taub E, Uswatte G. Constraint-induced movement therapy: bridging from the primate laboratory to the stroke rehabilitation laboratory. J Rehabil Med 2003 May;(41 Suppl):34–40
82. Taub E, Uswatte G, Pidikiti R. Constraint-Induced Movement Therapy: a new family of techniques with broad application to physical rehabilitation—a clinical review. J Rehabil Res Dev 1999;36(3):237–251
83. Davey NJ, Smith HC, Savic G, Maskill DW, Ellaway PH, Frankel HL. Comparison of input-output patterns in the corticospinal system of normal subjects and incomplete spinal cord injured patients. Exp Brain Res 1999;127(4): 382–390
84. Thomas SL, Gorassini MA. Increases in corticospinal tract function by treadmill training after incomplete spinal cord injury. J Neurophysiol 2005;94(4):2844–2855
85. Thompson AK, DeFrancesco E, Lichtman SW, Pomerantz F. Operant conditioning of motor evoked potentials to transcranial magnetic stimulation in people with chronic incomplete spinal cord injury. In: Society for Neuroscience 39th Annual Meeting 2009;79.10
86. Everaert DG, Thompson AK, Chong SL, Stein RB. Does functional electrical stimulation for foot drop strengthen corticospinal connections? Neurorehabil Neural Repair 2010;24(2):168–177
87. Daly JJ, Wolpaw JR. Brain-computer interfaces in neurological rehabilitation. Lancet Neurol 2008;7(11):1032–1043
88. Hultborn H. Changes in neuronal properties and spinal reflexes during development of spasticity following spinal cord lesions and stroke: studies in animal models and patients. J Rehabil Med 2003 May;(41 Suppl):46–55
89. Nielsen JB, Crone C, Hultborn H. The spinal pathophysiology of spasticity—from a basic science point of view. Acta Physiol (Oxf) 2007;189(2): 171–180
90. Zehr EP. Considerations for use of the Hoffmann reflex in exercise studies. Eur J Appl Physiol 2002;86(6):455–468
91. Magladery JW, Porter WE, Park AM, Teasdall RD. Electrophysiological studies of nerve and reflex activity in normal man, IV: The two-neurone reflex and identification of certain action potentials from spinal roots and cord. Bull Johns Hopkins Hosp 1951;88(6):499–519

49

Functional Restoration through Robotics

Martin Baggenstos, Geoffrey Ling, and James M. Ecklund

Key Points

1. Neuroprosthetic devices are helping to restore lost motor or sensory function as a result of aging, disease, or injury. They do so by acting as a bridge between functioning elements of the nervous system and dysfunctional limbs, prosthetic devices, damaged nerves, or receptor organs.
2. Functional electrical stimulation and brain–machine interfaces have helped promote the restoration of lost neural function and improve quality of life by interfacing with neuroprosthetic or robotic devices to allow the individual to regain some of the lost function.
3. Targeted reinnervation is a technique that can provide more natural control of prostheses than functional electrical stimulation and bypass brain–machine interface problems related to degradation from the body's natural immune response. This technique can provide both motor control and sensory feedback and can interface with new robotic prostheses or existing commercially available myoelectric prostheses, such as powered wrists or elbows.

Advances in robots and their control provide tremendous opportunities for restoring function to disabled patients. Over the past few decades, research in neuroscience and engineering and the merging of these two fields have enabled this. In engineering, remarkable end terminal devices, such as prosthetic hands, are the direct result of application of new materials, innovative designs, and on-board microprocessing. In neuroscience, there are new insights in how motor function and sensory perception are cortically controlled from innovations for extracting signals from both central and peripheral nervous system sources and algorithms for decoding these signals. Together, these achievements are enabling revolutionary ways of transforming user intent into user actions.

Disability is common. By far, the leading cause of disability is age-related frailty. The loss of either motor or sensory function can also be a result of traumatic brain and spinal cord injuries, amputations, and strokes. Currently, more than 200,000 patients in the United States have been involved in traumatic spinal cord injuries, with almost half of these patients being paralyzed below the neck. There are also more than 5,000,000 stroke survivors and 400,000 amputees living in the United States.[1] Emerging techniques using neural control, such as brain–machine interfaces (BMIs) with robotic devices, such as an exoskeleton or prosthetic limb, hold promise to more effectively restore a person's function than was previously thought possible.

The field of neuroprostheses focuses on technology to restore function through neural control. This is the critical feature of a neuroprosthesis and what clearly distinguishes it from a traditional prosthesis. The neuroprosthesis is controlled in ways that allow the patient to think naturally about an intended action and thereby to actuate the prosthesis to do that specific action (e.g., think about wiggling a finger and a robot finger wiggles, or think about moving a computer cursor left and the cursor moves left). This is distinct from how a traditional prosthesis (**Fig. 49.1**) is controlled using the myoelectric approach. Myoelectric control uses residual muscles to control artificial end terminal devices. To accomplish an intended action, a patient must think indirectly to actuate the device. For example, a prosthetic hook hand that is controlled by the biceps would require the patient to imagine flexing a forearm to open the hook hand such that a pencil could be grasped. This is clearly different than simply thinking about opening one's hand. Such indirect thinking makes even more complex actions, such as touch typing a keyboard, extremely difficult to achieve. So, by using the patient's natural intent, a neuroprosthesis can achieve levels of functionality far greater than that of a traditional prosthesis and likely to the same level of the native limb.

To use direct neural control, a neuroprosthesis must interact directly with the patient's nervous system. The site of interaction depends on where the lesion is and would need to be above the level of that disruption. Neuroprostheses can intercalate at any level of the nervous system from cortical gray to spinal anterior horn to peripheral nerve to neuromuscular junction to muscle. The approaches are varied and include peripheral ones, such as functional electrical stimulation (FES) and targeted reinnervation, and central ones, such as penetrating cerebral cortical electrodes and electrocorticography (ECoG). They also vary in terms of invasiveness. Surface electromyographic (EMG) and electroencephalographic (EEG) devices are virtually noninvasive, whereas cortical penetrating electrodes requiring craniotomy are invasive.

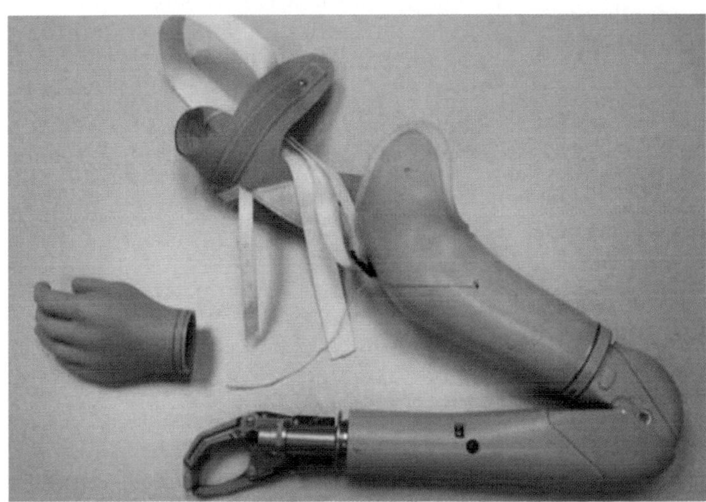

Fig. 49.1 Traditional upper extremity prosthesis that requires residual muscle actuation to provide basic control of the device, with limited pincer and elbow flexion function.

Recently, efforts to develop closed-loop systems (i.e., interactive motor efferent with sensory afferent components), have shown progress. True closed-loop controlled neuroprostheses will offer the highest level of natural function. Further advances in neuroprosthetic functional restoration will continue to require parallel work in engineering and neuroscience, as well as medical advances so that these extraordinary devices can be made clinically practical and acceptable to patients.

Types of Neuroprostheses

The development of neuroprostheses began with devices that electrically stimulated peripheral nerves or muscle. This was initially achieved using surface electrodes placed directly over muscles (surface EMG), or in close proximity to motor nerves (surface ENG). Eventually, development advanced to the level that some neuroprostheses functioned through direct cerebral cortical control.

It was originally proposed that direct interfaces between spared cortical or subcortical motor centers and artificial actuators could be employed to bypass spinal cord injury. This research resulted in the early development of BMI.[2] BMIs are devices that work in direct communication with the brain. The electrical signals used for actuation are derived from EEG, ECoG, or intracortical monitoring electrodes. Electrodes can be microwires placed individually or in arrays. The Utah Electrode Array (UEA) is a commonly used device, named by the researchers at the University of Utah and University of Michigan who developed it.[3] The UEA is silicon 4 mm × 4 mm platform with 100 1.5 mm long microelectrodes designed to be placed directly onto the surface of the brain with the microelectrodes penetrating into brain parenchyma. It can also be placed on a peripheral nerve. Initial research focused on motor prosthesis control, but continued advancements have led to the development of sensory prosthetic devices as well. Sensory prostheses record and process inputs from the environment and afferently transmit this information back to the appropriate cerebral sensory cortex. Notable examples of sensory prostheses include retinal implants for vision restoration and cochlear implants for hearing restoration.

Motor Prostheses

Implantable neuroprostheses for motor rehabilitation have been explored since the 1960s. Motor prostheses were devised that electrically directly stimulate muscles or motor nerves. Early technology was based almost exclusively on FES, an efferent approach. However, as robotic prosthetic limbs became more sophisticated (**Fig. 49.2**), other component technologies were developed that allowed for more complete integration. Afferent approaches are now included, such as biosensors to detect signals from the user's sensory nerves, muscles, or joints. Such information is relayed to a controller located inside the device, and together with feedback from the limb or actuator, action can be regulated more efficiently and precisely. Presently, intracortical BMIs are being developed to interface with the sensory cortex and thalamus with end terminal devices.

Because developing BMI systems is very complex and time consuming, beginning in 2000, the Brain–Computer Interface R&D Program at the Wadsworth Center of the New York State Department of Health began to develop a general purpose system for BMI research known as BCI2000.[4] The BCI2000 project facilitates research and development in the areas of data acquisition, stimulus presentation, and brain monitoring applications. The vision of the BCI2000 is that it will become a widely used software tool for diverse areas of real-time biosignal processing. It is currently free for nonprofit research and educational purposes and has been provided to over 400 laboratories worldwide.

Functional Electrical Stimulation

FES uses electrical stimulation to effect neuromuscular transmission peripherally by activating nerves that innervate paralyzed extremities. Initial studies of restoring movement to paralyzed limbs with

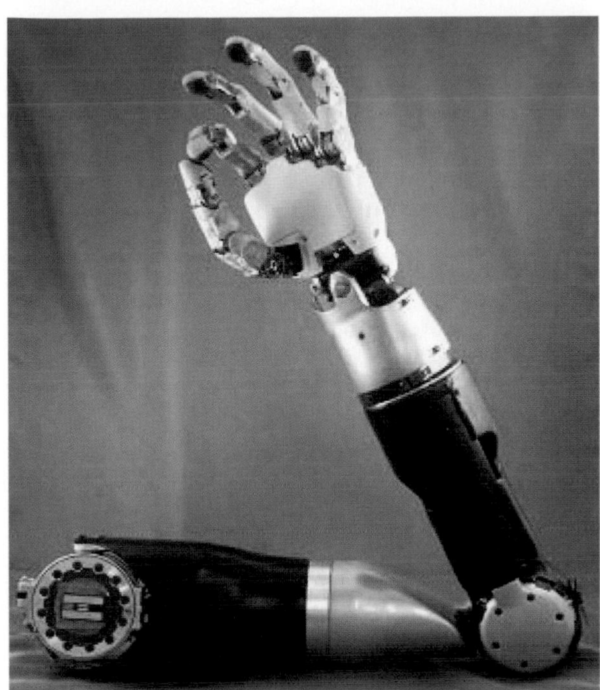

Fig. 49.2 New-generation robotic arm developed at Johns Hopkins Advanced Physics Laboratory. This arm can currently be used with external and indirect neural controls. Work is ongoing to develop brain–machine interface techniques for eventual direct neural control.

electrical stimulation date as far back as the mid-19th century.[5] The first truly modern FES device was developed in 1961. This early prototype used surface electrodes that activated the peroneal nerve to treat footdrop.[6] A decade later, implanted peroneal nerve stimulators to treat hemiplegic foot drop were introduced.[7,8] Also in the 1960s, radio frequency–controlled stimulators of the detrusor muscle in the bladder were implanted in a select number of incontinent patients.[9,10] In 1979, Brindley and colleagues implanted five paraplegic patients with sacral anterior root stimulators, all of whom were able to void when stimulated.[11] This led to larger human trials in the 1980s, in which similar devices controlled by an external transmitter were successfully implanted over the sacral ganglia. These devices would deliver intermittent stimulation, resulting in improved bladder emptying. They would also assist in defecation and restore the ability to sustain a full erection in male patients.

In 1991, BIOnic Neurons (BIONs) were developed. These are single-channel micromodule implants that are about the size of a grain of rice. Power and digital command signals are from inductive coils, which are positioned near or worn over the implant.[12] BIONs are used clinically for therapeutic muscle stimulation to electrically exercise paralyzed and weak muscles to prevent or reverse disuse atrophy. BIONs have gone through four generational iterations, all of which are designed to stimulate myelinated sensory or motor axons, typically in peripheral nerves. BION1 and BION2 require an external radio frequency–powered transmission coil for power and programming. An advantage of BION2 is that it allows for two-way signal transmission (stimulation and recording) through bidirectional telemetry. BION3 devices are focused on eliminating the continuous dependence of the implant on external coils for powering and control. A BION3 still requires an external transmission coil for programming and charging; however, downloaded stimulation paradigms can be implemented autonomously with power supplied through an on-board rechargeable battery. Finally, BION4 devices incorporate a rechargeable battery power similar to the BION3 but have a high-rate communication protocol that allows large numbers of implants to exchange information freely among themselves and with an external controller.[13]

In 1986, the Neurocontrol Freehand Stimulator (NFS), a surgically implanted FES device, was developed by the Cleveland FES Center at Case Western University. This is a radio frequency–powered motor neuroprosthesis that utilizes low levels of electrical current to stimulate peripheral nerves that innervate muscles in the forearm and hand to provide functional hand grasp patterns. The NFS involves implantation of up to eight electrodes in the muscles of the forearm and hand. Typically the NFS is implanted into the brachioradialis and extensor carpi radialis for voluntary wrist extension, and the posterior deltoid to triceps is used for elbow extension. The electrode wires are tunneled up the arm to a control box located under the skin in the pectoral region, and a movement detector is placed externally on the opposite shoulder. Opposite shoulder movement is then relayed to the control box, which is programmed to coordinate the activity in the electrodes and cause the hand to open and close. The device received US Food and Drug Administration (FDA) approval in 1997, and over 250 C5 and C6 quadriplegic patients have been successfully treated since that time.[14,15]

Design improvements in FES are under way to fine tune motor movement and to use implanted rechargeable power sources and wireless telemetry.[16] The limitations of FES devices are that they rely on indirect control because movement of underlying muscle activation from a nonparalyzed body part is used to trigger the coordinated electrical stimulation of muscles in the paralyzed limb.

Brain–Machine Interface

In the 1970s, early BMI work began at the University of California, Los Angeles (UCLA)[17] with support from the National Science Foundation and the Defense Advanced Research Projects Agency (DARPA). A BMI is simply a device that can decode human intent from brain cortical activity. By doing so, an alternate communication channel for people with severe motor impairments is created. Studies as early as the 1960s demonstrated that nonhuman primates could learn to voluntarily control the firing rate of primary motor cortex neurons using operant conditioning.[18–20] Algorithms were developed using motor cortex electrical signals. Such algorithms allow activity from motor cortex neurons to be made into intent. In the 1980s, Georgopoulos and his research team at Johns Hopkins University found a mathematical relationship between the electrical responses of single motor cortex neurons in rhesus macaque monkeys and the direction that the monkeys moved their arms. The research team also demonstrated that dispersed groups of neurons in different areas of the brain collectively controlled motor function. However, they were only able to record the firings of neurons in one area at a time because of the technical limitations imposed by their equipment.[21] Since then, rapid advances have occurred, with several groups being able to capture complex brain motor signals from groups of neurons to control external devices.[22]

Numerous studies and extensive research have been performed in regard to neural recording methods for BMI, such as microelectrodes, local field potentials, magnetic resonance imaging (MRI), and ECoG.[23–25] It has been shown that nonhuman primates can control robotic arms and hands using cortical control. Nicolelis at Duke University demonstrated cortical control of a computer cursor by monkeys with cortically implanted microwires. He then showed that these monkeys were able to control a robotic neuroprosthetic arm to move objects around a board.[26,27] Schwartz at the University of Pittsburgh then showed that nonhuman primates with cortically implanted UEAs can reach, grasp, and feed themselves food rewards using a cortically controlled neuroprosthetic upper extremity.[28] Hwang and Andersen at CalTech demonstrated that, by using signals from the posterior parietal cortex, neuroprosthetics can be controlled in near real time.[29] Schieber at the University of Rochester has shown monkeys can use cortical control to actuate individual fingers of a neuroprosthetic hand.[30] All of these investigators have shown what is possible with direct cortical control.

Noninvasive Brain–Machine Interfaces

Initially, studies on BMIs were based on scalp electroencephalograms (EEGs) due to their noninvasive nature and easy applications.[23] These EEG-based systems were developed as communication aids, such as moving a computer cursor or performing keyboard inputs, but were limited to these types of applications.[31,32] Scalp EEG recordings lack the spatial and temporal resolution that is required for dexterous control of a robot arm in real time due to reflecting electrical activity of millions of neurons in widespread areas of the cortex. Although these devices are easy to wear, the signals are suboptimal because of the skull dampening. To improve spatial resolution, MEG and functional magnetic resonance imaging (fMRI) were explored, but these applications required special equipment that is impractical for common everyday use.[25,33]

In the 1980s, an EEG-based BMI was developed that used the P300 brainwave response to allow the subject to communicate words, letters, and simple commands to a computer that converted the data through a speech synthesizer.[34] In the 1990s, Birbaumer from the University of Tübingen in Germany used EEG recordings of cortical potentials to give paralyzed patients limited control over a computer cursor. Ten patients were trained to move a computer cursor with these signals. The disadvantage was that the process was slow, training took many months, and, even after becoming expert with the system, patients required over an hour to assemble just 100 characters. In 1999, Peckham and his team at Case Western Reserve University used a 64-electrode EEG skullcap to provide limited hand movement to a quadriplegic patient. Mr. Jatich was instructed to concentrate on simple but opposite concepts like up and down, while his β-rhythm EEG output was analyzed. When a basic pattern was identified, it was used to control a switch, which later enabled the patient to control a computer cursor to drive nerve controllers embedded in his hands, restoring some movement. As before, the limited data that could be obtained by this method meant significant patient training to gain only rudimentary function. Because of the limitations associated with noninvasive BMIs, further research led to the development of semiinvasive BMIs.

Semiinvasive Brain–Machine Interfaces

To improve the shortcoming of EEGs, electrocorticograms (ECoGs) were investigated. ECoG grids were placed in the subdural space in the hope that signal attenuation from the skull would be attenuated. It was found that a neuronal electrical signal was indeed markedly enhanced. Sadly, in these early studies, in spite of this greater data stream, patients were still unable to perform dexterous robot control.[24] Nonetheless, ECoG devices produce signals with better resolution than do noninvasive BMIs, and they have a much lower risk of forming gliotic scar tissue than do fully invasive BMIs. In 2004, ECoG technology was first tried in adult human subjects by Leuthardt and Moran at Washington University in St. Louis. In 2006, a 14-year-old boy with epilepsy had an ECoG grid placed to localize his seizure focus. This ECoG grid was also linked to a computer running a BCI2000-based program that included the video game *Space Invaders*. The boy was then asked to perform various motor and speech tasks while the ECoG was acquired. The investigators were able to correlate the specific brain signals activated with certain movements and paired them with specific brain locations. The boy was then asked to play the simple two-dimensional *Space Invaders* game by moving his tongue and hand. The ECoG signals of his tongue and hand movements were correlated with the game cursor movement, which allowed him to play the game by simply moving his tongue and hand. His next task was to imagine the same movements, but not actually perform them with his hands or tongue. The result was the ability to play the video game by conscious thought. The results of this and similar studies along with advancements in fully invasive BMIs provide hope that conscious control of neuroprostheses can be achieved.

Invasive Brain–Machine Interfaces

Invasive BMI technology is the result of devices that are implanted directly into the gray matter of the brain. Deep brain stimulation is currently used in Parkinson disease, epilepsy, select pain conditions, and obsessive-compulsive disorder. Invasive devices produce the highest-quality signals of all BMI devices. The disadvantage is that they are prone to gliotic scar tissue formation, which can degrade the signals.[35] Using this approach, Wessberg and his team were among the first group of researchers to demonstrate that primates could control robots in one- and three-dimensional (1-D and 3-D) motion with cortical signals from chronically implanted electrodes.[36] In 1998, Kennedy and Bakay at Emory University implanted a cortical neuroprosthesis into Mr. Ray, a patient who was suffering from locked-in syndrome caused by a brain stem stroke in 1997. Using this neuroprosthesis, he acquired the ability to control a computer cursor and spell out words.[37] In 2003, Donohue at Brown University and Cyberkinetics developed a 96-electrode array called BrainGate. In 2005, Mr. Nagle, who suffered from a C3 spinal cord injury, was implanted with BrainGate and was subsequently able to control a computer mouse such that he could make words, draw pictures, and change the channel on a television. He was also able to open and close a prosthetic hand. The patient was also able to control a multijointed robot performing basic motions using cortical signals.[38] Currently, BrainGate2 is undergoing both safety and efficacy studies so as to obtain approval for a larger-cohort study with the intent of using the system to cortically control computers and other assistive devices. Although work continues to overcome the shortcoming of invasive BMIs' limitations, most notably gliosis, targeted muscle reinnervation has emerged as a practical, though more limited, alternative.

Targeted Muscle Reinnervation

Targeted muscle reinnervation (TMR) was developed by Kuiken and colleagues at Northwestern University to enable greater control of upper-extremity prosthetic limbs and to restore some sensory feedback for arm/hand amputee patients.[39–41] TMR is a method in which alternative muscle groups that are not biomechanically critical are deinnervated and then subsequently reinnervated with residual nerves from the amputated limb. This results in contractions in the targeted muscle responding to motor commands intended for the missing limb. EMG signals from these muscles are then used to actuate a prosthetic device. Traditionally, using myoelectric control, above-the-elbow amputees have to rely on body-powered technology, which uses bicycle cables to transfer the energy of chest and shoulder muscles to control a prosthetic limb. An improvement is using EMG signals from residual muscle groups to control the prosthesis. This strategy allows single-joint control and indirect control (e.g., residual biceps and triceps to control a prosthetic hook hand or wrist). TMR can overcome some of these limitations. TMR prosthetic control is intuitive to the patient because the EMG signal is generated by transferred residual limb nerves, unlike traditional myoelectric prosthetics, in which EMG signals have to be generated by muscles normally not involved in arm or wrist function. By transferring amputated upper-extremity nerves that had previously innervated the arm, to reinnervate nearby functionless muscle segments, the detection of the new EMG signals can be used to improve the control of a myoelectric prosthesis. For example, by transferring the median and distal radial nerve to other nerves innervating less functional muscle segments in the pectoralis region, the intact musculocutaneous (biceps) and proximal radial (triceps) signals are redirected. The EMG signals in the pectoralis region can then be captured to control elbow flexion and extension in a prosthetic device. The newly created EMG signals after successful multiple nerve transfers can also be used to control opening and closing of a prosthetic hand.[26] Chronic implants in BMI devices typically fail over time because the neuronal signals are degraded by tissue immune response to these foreign bodies.[35] TMR does not require implantation, so it does not have the issue of tissue foreign body response. With TMR, multiple yet independent EMG signals can be produced, leading to multiple simultaneous functions of the artificial limb.[42] Pragmatically, this technology allows all existing commercially available myoelectric prostheses, such as powered wrists or elbows, to be used, so patients do not have to incur additional expense acquiring new protheses.[40] Future research is being directed to provide improved thumb control as well as treatment for lower limb amputees. The hope is that nerves may be split further to provide even more independent signals, so that more functions can be controlled simultaneously with more degrees of freedom.

Sensory Prosthetics

Targeted Reinnervation

One challenge for full-natural-control artificial limbs is that prosthetic devices do not provide the user with any direct sensory feedback. In targeted sensory reinnervation, the skin near or over the targeted muscle is denervated, then reinnervated with afferent fibers of the remaining hand nerves.[39,43] This provides the amputee with a sense of the missing arm or hand being touched when the piece of skin that has been reinnervated is touched.[44,45] Sensory feedback in this manner has not been achieved by any other forms of prostheses. With further advancements in neuroprostheses, the goal is to achieve motor and sensory function similar to its original state prior to its loss from disease or injury.

Other Sensory Prosthetics

There has been significant research and development with prosthetic devices to enhance sensory modalities. These implants are beyond the scope of a text focusing on spinal cord injury, but they illustrate the potential for more direct sensory feedback to the nerves and brain itself. They include cochlear implants, auditory brain stem implants capable of stimulating the cochlear nucleus or inferior colliculus, and visual implants in the retina, optic nerves, medial geniculate ganglia, or visual cortex.

Future Technologies

Research for the future is being directed in several exciting directions. As this field matures it is very possible that patients with spinal cord injury could use their neural signals to control an exoskeleton enabling ambulation, or paralyzed limbs could be replaced with prosthetic, neurally controlled limbs. Exciting areas outside of spinal injury include using word-specific neural signals that occur before the speech is vocalized to communicate without the use of vocalized speech, and the use of neuroprostheses to bridge lesions in the hippocampus to restore memory.

Future-generation BMI electrode arrays are being designed with more biocompatible materials so as to evade the immunological response of the body in order for the implanted devices to function for decades.[46,47] Along with this is the development of wireless versions of neuroprosthetic devices, making the devices more convenient for the user.[48,49]

Disclaimer

The opinions expressed herein belong solely to the authors. They do not and should not be interpreted as belonging to or being endorsed by the Uniformed Services University of the Health Sciences, Defense Advanced Research Projects Agency, Walter Reed Army Medical Center, Department of the Army, or any branch of the US government.

Pearls

- Neuroprosthetic devices have dramatically helped improve the quality of life of disabled patients by reducing the physical and psychological impact of injury or disease.
- Functional restoration resulting from future advances in robotic prostheses combined with indirect and direct control mechanisms has the potential to outpace the functional expectations obtained with our standard biological repair techniques.
- Functional restoration through robotics has the potential to extend and enhance human capabilities.

Pitfalls

- The limitations of FES devices are that they rely on movement of underlying muscle activation from a nonparalyzed body part or an external device to trigger the coordinated electrical stimulation of muscles in the paralyzed limb or organ.
- Invasive BMI devices are prone to scar tissue buildup, which can cause the signal to become weaker or possibly lost as the body reacts to the foreign object.
- Current neuroprosthetic technology is limited to indirect control of limbs in upper extremity devices.

References

1. Kim HK, Park S, Srinivasan MA. Developments in brain-machine interfaces from the perspective of robotics. Hum Mov Sci 2009;28(2):191–203
2. Schmidt EM. Single neuron recording from motor cortex as a possible source of signals for control of external devices. Ann Biomed Eng 1980;8(4-6):339–349
3. Jones KE, Campbell PK, Normann RA. A glass/silicon composite intracortical electrode array. Ann Biomed Eng 1992;20(4):423–437
4. Krusienski DJ, Wolpaw JR. Brain-computer interface research at the Wadsworth Center developments in noninvasive communication and control. Int Rev Neurobiol 2009;86:147–157
5. Prochazka A, Mushahwar VK, McCreery DB. Neural prostheses. J Physiol 2001;533(Pt 1): 99–109
6. Liberson WT, Holmquest HJ, Scot D, Dow M. Functional electrotherapy: stimulation of the peroneal nerve synchronized with the swing phase of the gait of hemiplegic patients. Arch Phys Med Rehabil 1961;42:101–105
7. Waters RL, McNeal D, Perry J. Experimental correction of footdrop by electrical stimulation of the peroneal nerve. J Bone Joint Surg Am 1975;57(8):1047–1054
8. Strojnik P, Acimovic R, Vavken E, Simic V, Stanic U. Treatment of drop foot using an implantable peroneal underknee stimulator. Scand J Rehabil Med 1987;19(1):37–43
9. Bradley WE, Chou SN, French LA. Further experience with the radio transmitter receiver unit for the neurogenic bladder. J Neurosurg 1963;20:953–960
10. Stenberg CC, Burnette HW, Bunts RC. Electrical stimulation of human neurogenic bladders: experience with 4 patients. J Urol 1967;97(1):79–84
11. Brindley GS, Polkey CE, Rushton DN. Sacral anterior root stimulators for bladder control in paraplegia. Paraplegia 1982;20(6):365–381
12. Loeb GE, Zamin CJ, Schulman JH, Troyk PR. Injectable microstimulator for functional electrical stimulation. Med Biol Eng Comput 1991;29(6): NS13–NS19
13. Loeb GE, Richmond FJ, Baker LL. The BION devices: injectable interfaces with peripheral nerves and muscles. Neurosurg Focus 2006;20(5):E2
14. Hobby J, Taylor PN, Esnouf J. Restoration of tetraplegic hand function by use of the neurocontrol freehand system. J Hand Surg [Br] 2001;26(5): 459–464
15. Peckham PH, Keith MW, Kilgore KL, et al; Implantable Neuroprosthesis Research Group. Efficacy of an implanted neuroprosthesis for restoring hand grasp in tetraplegia: a multicenter study. Arch Phys Med Rehabil 2001;82(10):1380–1388
16. Pancrazio JJ, Peckham PH. Neuroprosthetic devices: how far are we from recovering movement in paralyzed patients? Expert Rev Neurother 2009;9(4):427–430
17. Vidal JJ. Toward direct brain-computer communication. Annu Rev Biophys Bioeng 1973;2: 157–180
18. Schmidt EM, McIntosh JS, Durelli L, Bak MJ. Fine control of operantly conditioned firing patterns of cortical neurons. Exp Neurol 1978;61(2): 349–369
19. Fetz EE. Operant conditioning of cortical unit activity. Science 1969;163(3870):955–958
20. Fetz EE, Baker MA. Operantly conditioned patterns on precentral unit activity and correlated responses in adjacent cells and contralateral muscles. J Neurophysiol 1973;36(2):179–204
21. Georgopoulos AP, Lurito JT, Petrides M, Schwartz AB, Massey JT. Mental rotation of the neuronal population vector. Science 1989;243(4888): 234–236
22. Lebedev MA, Nicolelis MA. Brain-machine interfaces: past, present and future. Trends Neurosci 2006;29(9):536–546
23. Wolpaw JR, McFarland DJ, Neat GW, Forneris CA. An EEG-based brain-computer interface for cur-

sor control. Electroencephalogr Clin Neurophysiol 1991;78(3):252–259
24. Leuthardt EC, Schalk G, Wolpaw JR, Ojemann JG, Moran DW. A brain-computer interface using electrocorticographic signals in humans. J Neural Eng 2004;1(2):63–71
25. Kamitani Y, Tong F. Decoding the visual and subjective contents of the human brain. Nat Neurosci 2005;8(5):679–685
26. Dumanian GA, Ko JH, O'Shaughnessy KD, Kim PS, Wilson CJ, Kuiken TA. Targeted reinnervation for transhumeral amputees: current surgical technique and update on results. Plast Reconstr Surg 2009;124(3):863–869
27. Brijesh R, Ravindran G. A spiking neural network of the CA3 of the hippocampus can be a neural prosthesis for lost cognitive functions. Conf Proc IEEE Eng Med Biol Soc 2007;2007:4755–4758
28. Velliste M, Perel S, Spalding MC, Whitford AS, Schwartz AB. Cortical control of a prosthetic arm for self-feeding. Nature 2008;453(7198):1098–1101
29. Hwang EJ, Andersen RA. Brain control of movement execution onset using local field potentials in posterior parietal cortex. J Neurosci 2009;29(45):14363–14370
30. Mollazadeh M, Aggarwal V, Singhal G, et al. Spectral modulation of LFP activity in M1 during dexterous finger movements. Conf Proc IEEE Eng Med Biol Soc 2008;2008:5314–5317
31. Wolpaw JR, Birbaumer N, McFarland DJ, Pfurtscheller G, Vaughan TM. Brain-computer interfaces for communication and control. Clin Neurophysiol 2002;113(6):767–791
32. Obermaier B, Müller GR, Pfurtscheller G. "Virtual keyboard" controlled by spontaneous EEG activity. IEEE Trans Neural Syst Rehabil Eng 2003;11(4):422–426
33. Mellinger J, Schalk G, Braun C, et al. An MEG-based brain-computer interface (BCI). Neuroimage 2007;36(3):581–593
34. Farwell LA, Donchin E. Talking off the top of your head: toward a mental prosthesis utilizing event-related brain potentials. Electroencephalogr Clin Neurophysiol 1988;70(6):510–523
35. Polikov VS, Tresco PA, Reichert WM. Response of brain tissue to chronically implanted neural electrodes. J Neurosci Methods 2005;148(1):1–18
36. Wessberg J, Stambaugh CR, Kralik JD, et al. Real-time prediction of hand trajectory by ensembles of cortical neurons in primates. Nature 2000;408(6810):361–365
37. Kennedy PR, Bakay RA. Restoration of neural output from a paralyzed patient by a direct brain connection. Neuroreport 1998;9(8):1707–1711
38. Hochberg LR, Serruya MD, Friehs GM, et al. Neuronal ensemble control of prosthetic devices by a human with tetraplegia. Nature 2006;442(7099):164–171
39. Kuiken TA, Miller LA, Lipschutz RD, et al. Targeted reinnervation for enhanced prosthetic arm function in a woman with a proximal amputation: a case study. Lancet 2007;369(9559):371–380
40. Kuiken T. Targeted reinnervation for improved prosthetic function. Phys Med Rehabil Clin N Am 2006;17(1):1–13
41. Kuiken TA, Li G, Lock BA, et al. Targeted muscle reinnervation for real-time myoelectric control of multifunction artificial arms. JAMA 2009;301(6):619–628
42. Kuiken T, Miller L, Lipschutz R, Stubblefield K, Dumanian G. Prosthetic command signals following targeted hyper-reinnervation nerve transfer surgery. Conf Proc IEEE Eng Med Biol Soc 2005;7:7652–7655
43. Marasco PD, Schultz AE, Kuiken TA. Sensory capacity of reinnervated skin after redirection of amputated upper limb nerves to the chest. Brain 2009;132(Pt 6):1441–1448
44. Kuiken TA, Marasco PD, Lock BA, Harden RN, Dewald JP. Redirection of cutaneous sensation from the hand to the chest skin of human amputees with targeted reinnervation. Proc Natl Acad Sci U S A 2007;104(50):20061–20066
45. Kuiken TA, Dumanian GA, Lipschutz RD, Miller LA, Stubblefield KA. The use of targeted muscle reinnervation for improved myoelectric prosthesis control in a bilateral shoulder disarticulation amputee. Prosthet Orthot Int 2004;28(3):245–253
46. He W, Bellamkonda RV. Nanoscale neuro-integrative coatings for neural implants. Biomaterials 2005;26(16):2983–2990
47. He W, McConnell GC, Bellamkonda RV. Nanoscale laminin coating modulates cortical scarring response around implanted silicon microelectrode arrays. J Neural Eng 2006;3(4):316–326
48. Harrison RR, Kier RJ, Chestek CA, et al. Wireless neural recording with single low-power integrated circuit. IEEE Trans Neural Syst Rehabil Eng 2009;17(4):322–329
49. Song YK, Borton DA, Park S, et al. Active microelectronic neurosensor arrays for implantable brain communication interfaces. IEEE Trans Neural Syst Rehabil Eng 2009;17(4):339–345

50

Peripheral Nerve Grafts and the Repair of Axonal Circuits Following Spinal Cord Injury

H. Francis Farhadi and Allan D. Levi

Key Points

1. Schwann cell or peripheral nerve grafting can partially counteract secondary injury mechanisms and promote ensheathment and myelination distal to the injury site.
2. Combinatorial strategies have yielded growth of certain critical brain stem tracts into Schwann cell or peripheral nerve grafts with associated improvements in gross locomotor recovery.
3. To date, the required combination of neuroprotective and regenerative strategies has yet to be identified that would promote functional restoration of corticospinal fibers required for fine motor control.

Trauma to the adult mammalian spinal cord results in progressive neuronal and glial cell death, axonal degeneration, and functional loss involving motor, sensory, and autonomic systems. Given the limited endogenous repair capacity of the spinal cord, functional recovery can occur either through (1) neuroprotective therapies to reduce secondary tissue loss and associated functional deficits or (2) molecular, cellular, and pharmacological treatments capable of replacing lost tissue or promoting axon regeneration and reconnection to restore lost function.

Transplantation of a variety of glial, immune, or undifferentiated stem cells to achieve repair following spinal cord injury (SCI) has resulted in reduced progressive tissue loss[1] and has retarded axonal dieback; has promoted sensory, proprio-, and supraspinal axon regeneration[2–5]; has facilitated myelination[3,6,7]; and has improved functional outcome.[3,4,8,9] Taken together, these studies have demonstrated the versatility of cellular implants in overcoming many key obstacles encountered following experimental SCI, making them ideal therapeutic candidates for repair.

Schwann cells (SCs), the myelinating cells of the peripheral nervous system that promote axonal regeneration following peripheral nerve (PN) injury, have also been shown to support central nervous system (CNS) axon growth either as PN grafts or as purified fluid grafts.[10–12] SCs provide multiple levels of support for growing axons in vivo; these range from physical guidance for axons by aligning into parallel arrays, to the synthesis of a variety of growth-promoting neurotrophic factors,[13,14] and both cell-adhesion molecules, such as N-CAM and L1,[15] and extracellular matrix components, including laminin, collagen, and heparan sulfate proteoglycan, which axons attach to and use as permissive substrates for growth and regeneration. Ultimately, SCs ensheathe and myelinate regenerating axons once a stable interrelationship is established.

This chapter provides a critical analysis of animal studies investigating the ability of transplanted SCs or PN grafts, alone or in combination, with known neuroprotective and regenerative strategies, to enhance axonal regeneration and functional recovery following experimentally induced contusive, crush, complete transection, or hemisection injuries of the spinal cord. To date, the vast majority of such studies have involved rodents, with assessment of functional recovery performed using standardized measures of simple cortically driven locomotive tasks.[16] Although such transplantation paradigms are promising, it remains to be determined whether such grafting will ultimately promote recovery of complex voluntary behaviors, such as reaching and grasping, as seen in humans.

Historical Perspective

In the early 1900s, Jorge Francisco Tello y Muñóz, a disciple of Santiago Ramón y Cajal, was the first investigator to test the ability of PN tissue to promote regeneration in the central nervous system. He placed slices of degenerating PN segments into lesioned rabbit cerebral cortex.[17] Histological examination revealed that nascent nerve fibers in the cortex appeared to converge onto the grafted pieces of PN. This finding led Ramón y Cajal to speculate that, given a suitable microenvironment, central neurons indeed could regenerate axons.

It was not until the 1980s and the seminal studies performed by Aguayo and colleagues that this initial discovery was ultimately substantiated.[10,18] This group showed that, following the removal of a segment of spinal cord and the placement of a piece of PN into the resulting gap, axonal projections were seen to project into the transplanted peripheral nerve. These projections were confirmed by neuroanatomical tracing to originate from the proximal stump central neurons, primarily from adjacent sensory and propriospinal neurons in the spinal cord itself as well as from a subset of brain stem spinal axons.[10,19] It thus became established that the PN environment is intrinsically conducive for CNS axon regeneration. Ultimately, this finding led to the observation that SCs are the essential component of this permissive environment,[20] which, in turn, laid the foundation for transplantation of SCs into the injured spinal cord.

Nevertheless, even at this early stage, Ramón y Cajal recognized that to effectively repair the CNS, a combination strategy involving both support for survival (growth factors) and specific guidance substances would be required.[17] Over the past 2 decades, the multiple secondary injury processes that result in progressive destruction of spinal cord tissue (primarily leading to apoptotic cell death of neurons and oligodendrocytes) have been progressively elucidated. In conjunction, research efforts have also progressively focused on combinatorial strategies aimed at counteracting these molecular and cellular obstacles.

Grafting in Animal Spinal Cord Injury Models

The development of standardized rodent injury models that recapitulate various aspects of human SCI, along with the established procedures that assess functional recovery, have enabled study of a multitude of potential therapeutic interventions. Human SCI is particularly well modeled by either graded contusion or compression injuries, which allow for varying degrees of sparing depending on the magnitude of the impact used.[21–24] For instance, following contusion injuries (which constitute the most common type of SCI reported clinically), both rats[25,26] and humans[27] form fluid-filled cystic cavities over the course of weeks, resulting in an absence of structural support and axonal growth within the lesion. At the lesion margins, injured axons terminate in dystrophic endings, indicating abortive axonal growth.

Complete Transection/Schwann Cell Bridge Models

In this model, an SC-filled polymer tube containing a viscous medium is placed at the rostral stump or between the completely severed stumps of the severed spinal cord.[5,12] Given the nature of the injury, the potential of confounding from spared and sprouted fibers is eliminated, allowing identification of regenerated axons with certainty. Axonal conduction across the transected cord has been demonstrated.[28,29] Yet, while the primarily sensory and propriospinal axons extending from both spinal cord stumps into the SC bridge are ensheathed and even myelinated (~10%) by SCs, the regenerative response is deficient in several aspects. As when using PN grafts alone,[30] these include scar formation at the interface with the spinal cord involving accumulation of chondroitin sulfate proteoglycans,[31] very minimal response of brain stem neurons, and the absence of axonal projections across the bridge to enter the spinal cord itself. Because brain stem axons can enter the distal spinal cord when the PN graft lies immediately adjacent to neuronal cell bodies[10] (but not when placed remotely within the thoracic spinal cord[30]), successful axonal regeneration appears to be dependent on the distance between the neuronal cell body and the graft, rather than an inability of brain stem axons to respond to SC cues.

Accordingly, several combinatorial paradigms have been evaluated using the complete transection model. These include SCs with methylprednisolone,[32] SCs with brain-derived neurotrophic factor (BDNF) and neurotrophin-3 (NT-3) infused around the SC bridge,[33] SCs transduced to secrete BDNF implanted into and caudal to the lesion site,[34] SCs plus olfactory-ensheathing cells,[35] and SCs plus olfactory-ensheathing cells plus chondroitinase.[36] As compared with implantation of SCs alone, each of these combination strategies showed a modest but statistically significant improvement in outcome measures, including increased numbers of myelinated axons on the bridge, increased numbers of regenerated axons from brain stem neurons, and increased numbers of regenerated axons extending beyond the bridge into the spinal cord. However, these findings have translated into only modestly improved locomotor function in a few paradigms.[36]

Alternatively, the use of PN grafts to bridge the interstump gap is associated with several relative potential advantages, including the provision of a suitable microenvironment for myelination of regenerating axons within the SC tubes, the ability to overcome relatively long distances with appropriately sized grafts, and the ability to target axonal growth toward specific target regions of interest. Cheng and colleagues first reported partial restoration of hindlimb function using a paradigm involving a T8–9 laminectomy, removal of a 5 mm spinal cord segment, and implantation of multiple intercostal nerve white matter to gray matter bridges with the engrafted area filled with an acidic fibroblast growth factor (aFGF)-containing fibrin glue[37,38] (**Fig. 50.1**). Detailed gait analysis at 3- and 4-month postinjury intervals revealed progressive improvements in coordinated hindlimb recruitment patterns, with 25 to 30% of movements ultimately involving some hindlimb use in rats treated with both the grafts and aFGF.[37]

Further investigations employing this approach have confirmed the presence of neurofilament positive axons extending across the grafted area, serotonin-labeled and anterogradely labeled corticospinal axons below the lesion site, as well as several retrogradely labeled supraspinal neuronal populations (including reticulospinal, vestibulospinal, raphe, and red nuclei) whose degree of activation is generally considered to be proportional to

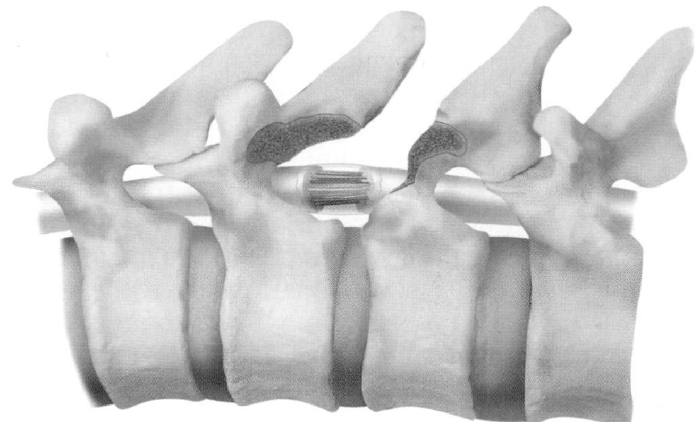

Fig. 50.1 Reproduction of an original figure by Cheng and colleagues describing their paradigm involving removal of a 5 mm spinal cord segment and implantation of multiple intercostal nerve white matter to gray matter bridges. (From Cheng H, Cao Y, Olson L. Spinal cord repair in adult paraplegic rats: partial restoration of hind limb function. Science 1996;273(5274):510–513. Reprinted with permission.

the extent of goal-directed locomotive recovery observed following complete spinal cord transection.[38–41] In particular, although serotonergic fibers tend to regenerate at a comparatively slower rate, they have been shown to directly activate the spinal locomotor circuit under physiological conditions.[42] The PN graft-mediated regeneration is also associated with electrophysiological evidence of both sensory and motor conduction across the transection site.[40] Finally, the combined treatment is associated with diminished astrocytic scar formation, activated macrophage migration, and inhibitory proteoglycan deposition,[43] all of which are conducive to enhanced CNS regeneration.

The original PN graft repair strategy reported by Cheng and colleagues[38] involved white to gray matter bridging to avoid the presumed inhibition of axonal regeneration by white matter. However, similar aFGF treatment but with direct apposition of the transected spinal cord stumps and placement of surrounding dorsal and ventral PN grafts has also been shown to result in a similar extent of supraspinal axonal regeneration, the presence of lumbar motor potentials, and partial recovery of locomotor function following complete transection.[44] Although the intricate bridging of white to gray matter thus does not appear absolutely necessary for functional locomotor recovery, it remains that only modest axonal regeneration is generally observed from supraspinal nuclei; in this study, for instance, functional recovery could only be correlated with corticospinal fiber density in caudal gray matter, which was at least partly due to the overall modest regenerative response achieved. Finally, it remains to be determined whether the observed long-tract regeneration improves functional recovery directly or rather through the stimulation of local neuronal circuitry. Given that regenerating fibers are primarily found within gray matter irrespective of the type of PN graft repair performed, it appears more likely that local interneurons or motoneurons are being stimulated directly to allow central pattern generator–mediated locomotion.[44]

Partial Transection/Schwann Cell Bridge Models

Following partial spinal cord transections, recovery of function has been associated with plasticity of the corticospinal and rubrospinal tracts rostral to the lesion.[45,46] The influence of SC or PN transplants in such injuries is of particular interest given that most human injuries are partial and thus leave spared tissue. As with complete transection, SC implantation also leads to enhanced sensory and propriospinal axon regeneration and myelination.[47,48] In fact, axons are observed to extend within the SC hemichannels in rats as early as 2 days postinjury; a few reach the caudal graft–

host interface, and, unlike with complete transections, some axons are even found within the caudal cord at 2 or 3 months following injury.[48] Although the presence of spared tissue clearly contributes to this enhanced axonal regeneration, as increased fibers are found within Matrigel-only bridges (BD Biosciences, Franklin Lakes, NJ) and some brain stem fibers (e.g., raphespinal, coeruleospinal, and rubrospinal) are even seen within the grafts following hemisection injuries,[48] the degree of contribution from sprouting of spared fibers remains an unresolved issue.

One of the most pressing and as yet unresolved problems in applying the data from these rodent studies to the human condition is to determine whether the observed regeneration is simply influencing the intrinsic and relatively simple central pattern generators in the rodent or whether there is an actual positive influence on more complex behavioral tasks. The testing of voluntary cortically driven tasks in the rodent is limited; thus testing in the nonhuman primate can establish whether grafting will promote recovery of complex voluntary behaviors such as reaching and grasping.

Importantly, whether the same regenerative potential as seen with rodents exists in the more complex primate CNS in response to PN grafts or their constituents is not well known. In a study by Levi and colleagues,[49] monkeys underwent T11 laminectomies and resection of a 1 cm length of hemispinal cord. In the experimental group, intercostal nerves were grafted along with fibrin glue containing acidic fibroblast growth factor. At 4 months postgrafting, regeneration of the CNS from proximal spinal axons into the PN grafts was observed. One of the basic tenets of regeneration previously established after rodent SCI was thus demonstrated in primates with this study, namely, that regeneration of CNS axons is possible when afforded a permissive environment. However, unlike in rodents, the grafts did not promote any regeneration beyond the lesion site even though an increase in regenerated myelinated axons was observed in the region of the hemisected cord itself. As such, although skilled hindlimb function was not recovered, some improvement in locomotion was noted (as measured by maximal treadmill velocities achieved), perhaps as a result of either trophic influences, local sprouting, or central pattern generator enhancement. The main challenge thus remains to induce the graft-derived regenerating fibers to reenter the injured spinal cord and to establish that the regenerating fibers have a positive influence on more complex (e.g., fine motor) behaviors.

Contusion/Graft Implantation Model

SC transplants have been used in numerous rodent studies following moderate to severe thoracic spinal cord contusion injuries. When compared with control rats injected with cell culture medium only, SC-implanted rats contained a ~2.4-fold increase in SC-myelinated axons,[11] indicating a contribution beyond that provided by endogenous SCs having migrated into the lesion site. Both transplanted and host SCs survive following contusional injuries, populate and fill the lesional area, and myelinate axons in ratios comparable to those observed following transections.[50–53]

SC transplants specifically reduce spinal cord cystic cavitation by enhancing neuronal survival and, in most studies, white matter sparing as well, thus accounting for the increased numbers of retrogradely labeled propriospinal and reticulospinal neurons.[11,50,53,54] Transplanted SCs also promote axonal growth into contused areas, and, as for transection models, these primarily arise from local propriospinal and sensory neurons with very little penetration from supraspinal axonal populations.[11,50,53,54]

As such, functional outcome measures, including the Basso, Beattie, and Bresnahan (BBB) rating scale or forelimb and grip strength measurements, have been shown to be only modestly improved in some studies, primarily when white matter sparing was also observed.[11,54] White matter preservation thus appears to be a key contribution, because those investigations that failed to demonstrate any improvement in functional outcomes[3,50] still demonstrated axonal extension into SC transplants.

PN grafts have also been used to promote recovery following acute or chronic spinal contusion injuries.[55] In a unilateral cervical contusion model, apposition of a predegenerated tibial nerve to the rostral cyst cavity wall, at 7 or 28 days postinjury, led to enhanced regeneration of brain stem and propriospinal neurons into the PN graft only and not beyond the graft–caudal spinal cord interface. Concomitant aspiration of cellular debris and clot from the cystic cavity reassuringly did not negatively impact on functional outcome measures, indicating that manipulation of the traumatic cyst prior to transplantation may also represent a viable therapeutic adjunct in clinical settings. Nevertheless, in the absence of any additional interventions, no difference in functional recovery is evident in this model beyond that which occurs spontaneously over time.[55]

Remaining Obstacles and Future Prospects

Taken together, SC and PN grafts undeniably show multiple beneficial effects following transplantation into the injured spinal cord. They promote white matter sparing and sensory and propriospinal axon growth into the transplanted area. They also myelinate ingrowing axons and help reestablish axonal conduction. However, by themselves they are not sufficient to promote either substantial supraspinal sensory, motor, or autonomic axon ingrowth or exiting from the graft area into the host spinal cord. As a result, functional restoration remains lacking, particularly in regard to locomotion.

This may be due, in part, to the restriction of SCs to the site of injury and the relative inability to enter and migrate within the astrocyte-rich environment caudal to the site of the lesion.[52,56] The ability to assess SC survival has been limited due to the lack of specific cellular labels for long-term in vivo tracking of transplanted cells. SCs acutely transplanted have nevertheless been shown to have lower survival rates than SCs transplanted 1 week following injury.[52] Moreover, SCs appear to fill large cystic cavities only when transplanted together with a synthetic matrix or with a PN graft.[36,57,58]

Although the degree of white matter preservation has often been assessed in animal studies, it appears that, more specifically, the integrity and identity of the tracts that remain intact (or are restored) are more closely related to functional outcomes.[59–61] As detailed later in the chapter, primarily combinatorial strategies to date have yielded growth into the SC grafts of critical brain stem tracts (including reticulospinal, coeruleospinal, and long-descending propriospinal) required for the initiation of stepping movements. In contrast, rubrospinal and especially corticospinal fibers, both of which are more involved with fine motor control, have proven to be poorly responsive to combinatorial strategies used to date.[62]

Alternative Sources of Schwann Cells

Traditionally, SCs have been isolated from PNs and induced to proliferate in vitro to obtain high numbers and pure cell populations. Importantly, similar procedures are available to harvest human SCs, including potentially from the peripheral nerve of a person with SCI. This process is associated with only minor morbidity risks and eliminates the need for the immunosuppression required following autologous transplantation.[63–65]

Recently, however, several reports have suggested that many of the limitations associated with adult PN-derived SCs may be overcome by obtaining SCs from alternative sources. Cells with an SC-like phenotype have been differentiated in vitro from bone marrow stromal cells (BMSCs) and from skin-derived precursors (SKPs) and examined following transplantation into the completely transected or contused spinal cord.[66,67] Both of these non PN-derived SCs were able to enhance the regeneration of descending brain stem axons and also yield modest functional improvements; whereas BMSC-SC bridges enhance non-weight-bearing hindlimb movement in completely transected SCs, SKP-SCs increased the number of animals achieving occasional forelimb–hindlimb coordination by ~46%. SKP-SCs in particular appear promising because, in addition to their ability to populate cystic lesions and myelinate central and peripheral axons, they appear to display improved integration and migration within the normally inhibitory host environment and also to possibly modify adjacent tissues by reducing reactive gliosis and altering growth factor expression.[66]

Cotransplantation of Different Cell Types

Combination treatments with other cell types have been pursued by some investigators to exploit potentially additive or synergistic effects. In particular, olfactory ensheathing cells (OECs) possess certain SC-like properties, but they are also uniquely able to intermingle with astrocytes in vivo and in vitro.[68,69] As such, cotransplanted OECs have been shown to enhance the exit of axons from the SC bridge into the caudal spinal cord[35] by likely making the SC–astrocyte interface more permissive for axonal crossing. Within the grafted area, OECs appear to play a primarily supportive role because they do not associate with myelinated axonal profiles themselves but rather appear to provide a structural framework for the SCs to, in turn, enhance myelination.[70,71] It nevertheless remains controversial to what degree OECs enhance axonal regeneration and functional recovery beyond SC implantation alone,[56] with different studies reaching contradictory conclusions with respect to the response of brain stem neuronal populations as well as in myelinated axon counts.[1,11] Among several potential confounders, further work will be required to delineate both the optimal source for these cells and the optimal postlesion time for implantation.

Neuroprotective and Regenerative Strategies

The majority of SCs undergo necrotic cell death following implantation into either the acute, subacute, or chronically injured spinal cord.[51,53] Several pharmacological agents have been shown to reduce post-SCI degeneration, including methylprednisolone, monosialoganglioside, and cyclic adenosine monophosphate (cAMP).[72] Interestingly, these agents, in particular cAMP, also appear to independently enhance axonal regeneration.[73] Following contusive SCI, immediate and prolonged administration of Rolipram (Sigma Chemicals Co., St. Louis, MO), a phosphodiesterase-4 inhibitor, significantly increases both white matter sparing and the number of SC-myelinated axons within the lesion, and also improves several functional outcome measures.[3] When coadministered with SCs and cAMP (triple combination), a significant improvement was noted in the overall BBB score. It remains to be determined whether cAMP directly enhances the survival and myelination capacity of the transplanted cells or whether the recruitment of endogenous SCs is also promoted. Taken together, these cAMP studies, as well as the wealth of data suggesting that methylprednisolone promotes transplant survival and brain stem/propriospinal/sensory axonal regeneration into SC bridges,[32,74] suggest that additional neuroprotective agents should be evaluated along with SC transplants.

Neurotrophic factors represent strong candidates for combination therapies given their well-recognized ability to promote neuronal survival as well as axonal regeneration/sprouting even on inhibitory substrates. Neurotrophic factor delivery following SCI can promote additional axonal regeneration into SC or PN implants,[33] although specific axonal populations respond differentially to specific factors either alone or in combination. Although propriospinal neurons extend projections into SC or PN grafts following glial-derived neurotrophic factor, NT-3, or BDNF factor treatment, sensory neurons appear to be more responsive specifically to nerve growth factor (NGF) and BDNF.[7,33,34,75,76] Acidic fibroblast growth factor has been shown to prevent the die back phenomenon of the corticospinal tract and to promote sprouting and regeneration across the zone of injury through either SC guidance channels or PN grafts following complete thoracic transection injuries.[77] Despite the long distances between the delivery site and brain stem neuronal cell bodies, several of these neuronal populations also become responsive when SC or PN grafting is combined with neurotrophic factor treatment.[33,34] Finally, neurotrophic factors appear to influence the survival and proliferation of the transplanted SCs themselves because grafts expressing D15A (a chimeric protein that mimics the activity of both BDNF and NT-3) or NGF[7,50] are enlarged as compared with controls, and this correlates with enhanced axonal ingrowth.

Promoting Entry and Extension into the Host Spinal Cord

A multitude of extracellular matrix molecules combine with reactive astroglia to form a dense scar in the zone of injury, which in turn acts as a barrier to regenerating axons.[78] Thus, additional interventions are necessary to enhance the reentry of regenerating axons into the host spinal cord. One promising approach involves the controlled administration of chondroitinase ABC (ChABC), which has shown efficacy in both SC implantation and PN grafting models.[36,79] Following a cervical hemisection injury, ChABC promoted axonal regrowth for ~1.2 mm into the caudal spinal cord, with regenerated fibers showing prominent branching and varicosities at their terminal ends and the extent of regeneration correlating well with functional assessments.[79] As expected, exiting axons from an SC-OEC-ChABC graft have been shown to primarily arise from local propriospinal neurons but, interestingly, also from more rostral levels, including raphe, vestibular, and reticular nuclei.[36]

Given the well-established inhibitory properties of CNS myelin and its constituent proteins for axonal elongation, combination strategies aimed at directly counteracting this effect within the host spinal cord appear particularly attractive[80] but have yet to be fully explored. In addition to promoting long-distance regeneration into SC grafts as discussed earlier, BDNF or NT-3 infusion caudal to the SC bridge independently also attracts propriospinal axons beyond the graft and into the host caudal cord tissue over several millimeters.[75] Although the underlying mechanisms of this action remain to be fully elucidated, it is possible that these neurotrophic factors support axonal growth over the inhibitory host environment via a cAMP-dependent mechanism.[3] Other options include either adjunctive myelin inhibitor blockade (e.g., as for Nogo-A)[81] or more general activation of the Rho pathway itself through the use of Rho kinase inhibitors.[82]

Conclusion

Although SC transplantation and PN grafting remain promising candidates for promoting functional repair following SCI, it is now apparent that they will need to be employed as part of optimized combination strategies. Using SCs from alternate sources or in combination with other cell types, such as OECs, and in conjunction with neurotrophic, glial scar-modifying, or myelin-inhibition blocking factors, may enhance the ingrowth of long-descending axons as well as the exit of fibers caudally into the host spinal cord. Similarly, PN grafts have yet to be assayed using combined strategies to promote regenerating axon graft entry, exit, and subsequent elongation toward synaptic targets. Future investigations will focus on these promising avenues to enhance transplant survival, host tissue sparing, and axonal growth across the implant–host interface.

Pearls

- A series of secondary injury processes following SCI combine to promote progressive cell death, degeneration, and functional loss of key fiber tracts. Cellular transplantation has been shown to counteract many of these sources of secondary injury.
- SC or peripheral nerve grafting alone results in ensheathment and even myelination distal to the injury site, but the regenerative response is deficient in several respects. This is attributable partly to a poor response of critical brain stem neuronal subpopulations as well as scar formation at the interface with the spinal cord.
- Several combinatorial strategies have been shown to further enhance the regenerative response and functional outcome in animal models. These include cotransplantation of different cell types and use of neurotrophic factors, as well as agents that modify the inhibitory extracellular environment.

Pitfalls

- Rodent SCI studies to date have used standardized measures of simple cortically driven locomotive tasks as outcome measures. It remains to be determined whether cellular grafting can ultimately promote recovery of complex voluntary behaviors, such as reaching and grasping, as seen in humans.
- Faithful in vivo identification and tracking of transplanted cells remain inadequate. As such, the precise mechanisms by which these cells promote recovery and thus the optimal combinatorial treatments remain incompletely defined.

References

1. Pearse DD, Marcillo AE, Oudega M, Lynch MP, Wood PM, Bunge MB. Transplantation of Schwann cells and olfactory ensheathing glia after spinal cord injury: does pretreatment with methylprednisolone and interleukin-10 enhance recovery? J Neurotrauma 2004;21(9):1223–1239
2. Li Y, Field PM, Raisman G. Repair of adult rat corticospinal tract by transplants of olfactory ensheathing cells. Science 1997;277(5334):2000–2002
3. Pearse DD, Pereira FC, Marcillo AE, et al. cAMP and Schwann cells promote axonal growth and functional recovery after spinal cord injury. Nat Med 2004;10(6):610–616
4. Ramón-Cueto A, Cordero MI, Santos-Benito FF, Avila J. Functional recovery of paraplegic rats and motor axon regeneration in their spinal cords by olfactory ensheathing glia. Neuron 2000;25(2):425–435
5. Xu XM, Chen A, Guénard V, Kleitman N, Bunge MB. Bridging Schwann cell transplants promote axonal regeneration from both the rostral and caudal stumps of transected adult rat spinal cord. J Neurocytol 1997;26(1):1–16
6. Lankford KL, Imaizumi T, Honmou O, Kocsis JD. A quantitative morphometric analysis of rat spinal cord remyelination following transplantation of allogenic Schwann cells. J Comp Neurol 2002;443(3):259–274
7. Weidner N, Blesch A, Grill RJ, Tuszynski MH. Nerve growth factor-hypersecreting Schwann cell grafts augment and guide spinal cord axonal growth and remyelinate central nervous system axons in a phenotypically appropriate manner that correlates with expression of L1. J Comp Neurol 1999;413(4):495–506
8. Li Y, Decherchi P, Raisman G. Transplantation of olfactory ensheathing cells into spinal cord lesions restores breathing and climbing. J Neurosci 2003;23(3):727–731
9. Rapalino O, Lazarov-Spiegler O, Agranov E, et al. Implantation of stimulated homologous macrophages results in partial recovery of paraplegic rats. Nat Med 1998;4(7):814–821
10. David S, Aguayo AJ. Axonal elongation into peripheral nervous system “bridges” after central nervous system injury in adult rats. Science 1981;214(4523):931–933
11. Takami T, Oudega M, Bates ML, Wood PM, Kleitman N, Bunge MB. Schwann cell but not olfactory ensheathing glia transplants improve hindlimb locomotor performance in the moderately contused adult rat thoracic spinal cord. J Neurosci 2002;22(15):6670–6681
12. Xu XM, Guénard V, Kleitman N, Bunge MB. Axonal regeneration into Schwann cell-seeded guidance channels grafted into transected adult rat spinal cord. J Comp Neurol 1995;351(1):145–160
13. Acheson A, Barker PA, Alderson RF, Miller FD, Murphy RA. Detection of brain-derived neurotrophic factor-like activity in fibroblasts and Schwann cells: inhibition by antibodies to NGF. Neuron 1991;7(2):265–275
14. Rende M, Muir D, Ruoslahti E, Hagg T, Varon S, Manthorpe M. Immunolocalization of ciliary neuronotrophic factor in adult rat sciatic nerve. Glia 1992;5(1):25–32
15. Chernousov MA, Yu WM, Chen ZL, Carey DJ, Strickland S. Regulation of Schwann cell function by the extracellular matrix. Glia 2008;56(14):1498–1507
16. Zörner B, Filli L, Starkey ML, et al. Profiling locomotor recovery: comprehensive quantification of

impairments after CNS damage in rodents. Nat Methods 2010;7(9):701–708

17. Ramon y Cajal S. Study of regenerative processes of the cerebrum. In: May RM De Felipe J, Jones EG, eds. Cajal's Degeneration and Regeneration of the Nervous System. New York: Oxford University Press; 1991:734–750
18. Richardson PM, McGuinness UM, Aguayo AJ. Axons from CNS neurons regenerate into PNS grafts. Nature 1980;284(5753):264–265
19. Richardson PM, McGuinness UM, Aguayo AJ. Peripheral nerve autografts to the rat spinal cord: studies with axonal tracing methods. Brain Res 1982;237(1):147–162
20. Enver MK, Hall SM. Are Schwann cells essential for axonal regeneration into muscle autografts? Neuropathol Appl Neurobiol 1994;20(6): 587–598
21. Basso DM, Beattie MS, Bresnahan JC. Graded histological and locomotor outcomes after spinal cord contusion using the NYU weight-drop device versus transection. Exp Neurol 1996;139(2): 244–256
22. Behrmann DL, Bresnahan JC, Beattie MS, Shah BR. Spinal cord injury produced by consistent mechanical displacement of the cord in rats: behavioral and histologic analysis. J Neurotrauma 1992;9(3):197–217
23. Fehlings MG, Tator CH. The relationships among the severity of spinal cord injury, residual neurological function, axon counts, and counts of retrogradely labeled neurons after experimental spinal cord injury. Exp Neurol 1995;132(2):220–228
24. Scheff SW, Rabchevsky AG, Fugaccia I, Main JA, Lumpp JE Jr. Experimental modeling of spinal cord injury: characterization of a force-defined injury device. J Neurotrauma 2003;20(2):179–193
25. Guizar-Sahagun G, Grijalva I, Madrazo I, et al. Development of post-traumatic cysts in the spinal cord of rats-subjected to severe spinal cord contusion. Surg Neurol 1994;41(3):241–249
26. Stokes BT, Jakeman LB. Experimental modelling of human spinal cord injury: a model that crosses the species barrier and mimics the spectrum of human cytopathology. Spinal Cord 2002;40(3): 101–109
27. Bunge RP, Puckett WR, Becerra JL, Marcillo A, Quencer RM. Observations on the pathology of human spinal cord injury: a review and classification of 22 new cases with details from a case of chronic cord compression with extensive focal demyelination. Adv Neurol 1993;59:75–89
28. Imaizumi T, Lankford KL, Kocsis JD. Transplantation of olfactory ensheathing cells or Schwann cells restores rapid and secure conduction across the transected spinal cord. Brain Res 2000;854(1-2):70–78
29. Pinzon A, Calancie B, Oudega M, Noga BR. Conduction of impulses by axons regenerated in a Schwann cell graft in the transected adult rat thoracic spinal cord. J Neurosci Res 2001;64(5):533–541
30. Richardson PM, Issa VM, Aguayo AJ. Regeneration of long spinal axons in the rat. J Neurocytol 1984;13(1):165–182
31. Plant GW, Bates ML, Bunge MB. Inhibitory proteoglycan immunoreactivity is higher at the caudal than the rostral Schwann cell graft-transected spinal cord interface. Mol Cell Neurosci 2001;17(3):471–487
32. Chen A, Xu XM, Kleitman N, Bunge MB. Methylprednisolone administration improves axonal regeneration into Schwann cell grafts in transected adult rat thoracic spinal cord. Exp Neurol 1996;138(2):261–276
33. Xu XM, Guénard V, Kleitman N, Aebischer P, Bunge MB. A combination of BDNF and NT-3 promotes supraspinal axonal regeneration into Schwann cell grafts in adult rat thoracic spinal cord. Exp Neurol 1995;134(2):261–272
34. Menei P, Montero-Menei C, Whittemore SR, Bunge RP, Bunge MB. Schwann cells genetically modified to secrete human BDNF promote enhanced axonal regrowth across transected adult rat spinal cord. Eur J Neurosci 1998;10(2):607–621
35. Ramón-Cueto A, Plant GW, Avila J, Bunge MB. Long-distance axonal regeneration in the transected adult rat spinal cord is promoted by olfactory ensheathing glia transplants. J Neurosci 1998;18(10):3803–3815
36. Fouad K, Schnell L, Bunge MB, Schwab ME, Liebscher T, Pearse DD. Combining Schwann cell bridges and olfactory-ensheathing glia grafts with chondroitinase promotes locomotor recovery after complete transection of the spinal cord. J Neurosci 2005;25(5):1169–1178
37. Cheng H, Almström S, Giménez-Llort L, et al. Gait analysis of adult paraplegic rats after spinal cord repair. Exp Neurol 1997;148(2):544–557
38. Cheng H, Cao Y, Olson L. Spinal cord repair in adult paraplegic rats: partial restoration of hind limb function. Science 1996;273(5274):510–513
39. Hase T, Kawaguchi S, Hayashi H, Nishio T, Mizoguchi A, Nakamura T. Spinal cord repair in neonatal rats: a correlation between axonal regeneration and functional recovery. Eur J Neurosci 2002;15(6):969–974
40. Lee YS, Hsiao I, Lin VW. Peripheral nerve grafts and aFGF restore partial hindlimb function in adult paraplegic rats. J Neurotrauma 2002;19(10): 1203–1216
41. Lee YS, Lin CY, Robertson RT, Hsiao I, Lin VW. Motor recovery and anatomical evidence of axonal regrowth in spinal cord-repaired adult rats. J Neuropathol Exp Neurol 2004;63(3):233–245
42. Ribotta MG, Provencher J, Feraboli-Lohnherr D, Rossignol S, Privat A, Orsal D. Activation of locomotion in adult chronic spinal rats is achieved by transplantation of embryonic raphe cells reinnervating a precise lumbar level. J Neurosci 2000;20(13):5144–5152
43. Lee MJ, Chen CJ, Cheng CH, et al. Combined treatment using peripheral nerve graft and FGF-1: changes to the glial environment and differential macrophage reaction in a complete transected spinal cord. Neurosci Lett 2008;433(3):163–169
44. Tsai EC, Krassioukov AV, Tator CH. Corticospinal regeneration into lumbar grey matter correlates with locomotor recovery after complete spinal cord transection and repair with peripheral nerve grafts, fibroblast growth factor 1, fibrin glue, and spinal fusion. J Neuropathol Exp Neurol 2005;64(3):230–244
45. Thallmair M, Metz GA, Z'Graggen WJ, Raineteau O, Kartje GL, Schwab ME. Neurite growth inhibi-

tors restrict plasticity and functional recovery following corticospinal tract lesions. Nat Neurosci 1998;1(2):124–131

46. Z'Graggen WJ, Metz GA, Kartje GL, Thallmair M, Schwab ME. Functional recovery and enhanced corticofugal plasticity after unilateral pyramidal tract lesion and blockade of myelin-associated neurite growth inhibitors in adult rats. J Neurosci 1998;18(12):4744–4757

47. Hsu JY, Xu XM. Early profiles of axonal growth and astroglial response after spinal cord hemisection and implantation of Schwann cell-seeded guidance channels in adult rats. J Neurosci Res 2005;82(4):472–483

48. Xu XM, Zhang SX, Li H, Aebischer P, Bunge MB. Regrowth of axons into the distal spinal cord through a Schwann-cell-seeded mini-channel implanted into hemisected adult rat spinal cord. Eur J Neurosci 1999;11(5):1723–1740

49. Levi AD, Dancausse H, Li X, Duncan S, Horkey L, Oliviera M. Peripheral nerve grafts promoting central nervous system regeneration after spinal cord injury in the primate. J Neurosurg 2002;96(2, Suppl):197–205

50. Golden KL, Pearse DD, Blits B, et al. Transduced Schwann cells promote axon growth and myelination after spinal cord injury. Exp Neurol 2007;207(2):203–217

51. Hill CE, Hurtado A, Blits B, et al. Early necrosis and apoptosis of Schwann cells transplanted into the injured rat spinal cord. Eur J Neurosci 2007;26(6):1433–1445

52. Hill CE, Moon LD, Wood PM, Bunge MB. Labeled Schwann cell transplantation: cell loss, host Schwann cell replacement, and strategies to enhance survival. Glia 2006;53(3):338–343

53. Pearse DD, Sanchez AR, Pereira FC, et al. Transplantation of Schwann cells and/or olfactory ensheathing glia into the contused spinal cord: survival, migration, axon association, and functional recovery. Glia 2007;55(9):976–1000

54. Schaal SM, Kitay BM, Cho KS, et al. Schwann cell transplantation improves reticulospinal axon growth and forelimb strength after severe cervical spinal cord contusion. Cell Transplant 2007;16(3): 207–228

55. Sandrow HR, Shumsky JS, Amin A, Houle JD. Aspiration of a cervical spinal contusion injury in preparation for delayed peripheral nerve grafting does not impair forelimb behavior or axon regeneration. Exp Neurol 2008;210(2):489–500

56. Raisman G, Li Y. Repair of neural pathways by olfactory ensheathing cells. Nat Rev Neurosci 2007;8(4):312–319

57. Martin D, Robe P, Franzen R, et al. Effects of Schwann cell transplantation in a contusion model of rat spinal cord injury. J Neurosci Res 1996;45(5):588–597

58. Nomura H, Tator CH, Shoichet MS. Bioengineered strategies for spinal cord repair. J Neurotrauma 2006;23(3-4):496–507

59. Arvanian VL, Schnell L, Lou L, et al. Chronic spinal hemisection in rats induces a progressive decline in transmission in uninjured fibers to motoneurons. Exp Neurol 2009;216(2):471–480

60. Takeoka A, Kubasak MD, Zhong H, Kaplan J, Roy RR, Phelps PE. Noradrenergic innervation of the rat spinal cord caudal to a complete spinal cord transection: effects of olfactory ensheathing glia. Exp Neurol 2010;222(1):59–69

61. Takeoka A, Kubasak MD, Zhong H, Roy RR, Phelps PE. Serotonergic innervation of the caudal spinal stump in rats after complete spinal transection: effect of olfactory ensheathing glia. J Comp Neurol 2009;515(6):664–676

62. Fortun J, Hill CE, Bunge MB. Combinatorial strategies with Schwann cell transplantation to improve repair of the injured spinal cord. Neurosci Lett 2009;456(3):124–132

63. Casella GT, Bunge RP, Wood PM. Improved method for harvesting human Schwann cells from mature peripheral nerve and expansion in vitro. Glia 1996;17(4):327–338

64. Levi AD, Bunge RP. Studies of myelin formation after transplantation of human Schwann cells into the severe combined immunodeficient mouse. Exp Neurol 1994;130(1):41–52

65. Morrissey TK, Kleitman N, Bunge RP. Isolation and functional characterization of Schwann cells derived from adult peripheral nerve. J Neurosci 1991;11(8):2433–2442

66. Biernaskie J, Sparling JS, Liu J, et al. Skin-derived precursors generate myelinating Schwann cells that promote remyelination and functional recovery after contusion spinal cord injury. J Neurosci 2007;27(36):9545–9559

67. Kamada T, Koda M, Dezawa M, et al. Transplantation of bone marrow stromal cell-derived Schwann cells promotes axonal regeneration and functional recovery after complete transection of adult rat spinal cord. J Neuropathol Exp Neurol 2005;64(1): 37–45

68. Lakatos A, Barnett SC, Franklin RJ. Olfactory ensheathing cells induce less host astrocyte response and chondroitin sulphate proteoglycan expression than Schwann cells following transplantation into adult CNS white matter. Exp Neurol 2003;184(1):237–246

69. Santos-Silva A, Fairless R, Frame MC, et al. FGF/heparin differentially regulates Schwann cell and olfactory ensheathing cell interactions with astrocytes: a role in astrocytosis. J Neurosci 2007; 27(27):7154–7167

70. Boyd JG, Jahed A, McDonald TG, et al. Proteomic evaluation reveals that olfactory ensheathing cells but not Schwann cells express calponin. Glia 2006;53(4):434–440

71. Boyd JG, Lee J, Skihar V, Doucette R, Kawaja MD. LacZ-expressing olfactory ensheathing cells do not associate with myelinated axons after implantation into the compressed spinal cord. Proc Natl Acad Sci USA 2004;101(7):2162–2166

72. Hall ED, Springer JE. Neuroprotection and acute spinal cord injury: a reappraisal. NeuroRx 2004; 1(1):80–100

73. Hannila SS, Filbin MT. The role of cyclic AMP signaling in promoting axonal regeneration after spinal cord injury. Exp Neurol 2008;209(2): 321–332

74. Guest JD, Rao A, Olson L, Bunge MB, Bunge RP. The ability of human Schwann cell grafts to promote regeneration in the transected nude rat spinal cord. Exp Neurol 1997;148(2):502–522

75. Bamber NI, Li H, Lu X, Oudega M, Aebischer P, Xu XM. Neurotrophins BDNF and NT-3 promote axonal re-entry into the distal host spinal cord through Schwann cell-seeded mini-channels. Eur J Neurosci 2001;13(2):257–268

76. Iannotti C, Li H, Yan P, Lu X, Wirthlin L, Xu XM. Glial cell line-derived neurotrophic factor-enriched bridging transplants promote propriospinal axonal regeneration and enhance myelination after spinal cord injury. Exp Neurol 2003;183(2):379–393

77. Bregman BS, Coumans JV, Dai HN, et al. Transplants and neurotrophic factors increase regeneration and recovery of function after spinal cord injury. Prog Brain Res 2002;137:257–273

78. Silver J, Miller JH. Regeneration beyond the glial scar. Nat Rev Neurosci 2004;5(2):146–156

79. Houle JD, Tom VJ, Mayes D, Wagoner G, Phillips N, Silver J. Combining an autologous peripheral nervous system "bridge" and matrix modification by chondroitinase allows robust, functional regeneration beyond a hemisection lesion of the adult rat spinal cord. J Neurosci 2006;26(28): 7405–7415

80. Brösamle C, Huber AB, Fiedler M, Skerra A, Schwab ME. Regeneration of lesioned corticospinal tract fibers in the adult rat induced by a recombinant, humanized IN-1 antibody fragment. J Neurosci 2000;20(21):8061–8068

81. Maier IC, Ichiyama RM, Courtine G, et al. Differential effects of anti-Nogo-A antibody treatment and treadmill training in rats with incomplete spinal cord injury. Brain 2009;132(Pt 6): 1426–1440

82. McKerracher L, Higuchi H. Targeting Rho to stimulate repair after spinal cord injury. J Neurotrauma 2006;23(3-4):309–317

VI

Resources

51

Population-Based Spinal Cord Injury Registries: Potential Impacts and Challenges

Marcel F. Dvorak, Catherine A. McGuinness, Michael G. Fehlings, and Vanessa K. Noonan

Key Points

1. Prospective data registries provide an effective way of tracking outcomes and epidemiology and can be useful in collecting valuable observational data that can inform clinical practice.
2. A registry should be focused on key data elements to be useful.
3. To ensure that the data collected remain focused, specific research questions should be formulated when setting up the registry.
4. Challenges in setting up such registries can include issues of privacy related to collecting data on patients, which is a further incentive to have focused research questions making the value and intended use of the data clear to those concerned.

As research funding becomes scarcer, the focus and practical impact of clinical research activities are coming under increased scrutiny by the agencies that provide funding for research.[1] Governmental funding agencies, industry, and nonprofit foundations are more cognizant of the outputs and outcomes of the research that they do support and are more likely to consider investing in research activities that are mission driven, focused on a clinical need, and strictly managed, as opposed to more exploratory endeavors. In this environment, it is more difficult to obtain financial and conceptual support for population-based observational studies that are often the outputs of patient registries. Patient registries, therefore, must be clear with respect to their outputs and deliverables.

Advances in the care of acute traumatic spinal cord injury (SCI) have meant that patients who experience SCI are now expected to survive and in many cases recover from their injuries.[2] The Rick Hansen Spinal Cord Injury Registry (RHSCIR) is a pan-Canadian patient registry that was initiated in 2002. This chapter describes why registries are important, what unique contributions the RHSCIR can make to improving patient care, and some of the challenges in establishing the RHSCIR, specifically, the impact of new privacy legislation on the registry, the influence this has had on the quality and quantity of data obtained, and how the RHSCIR has addressed these privacy issues. The RHSCIR will be used as an example of a population-based prospective data collection project; however, we acknowledge that other organizations, such as the North American Clinical Trials Network (NACTN) and the European Multicentre Study about Spinal Cord Injury (EMSCI), are establishing similar datasets.

Why Is It Important to Have a Spinal Cord Injury Registry?

A patient registry is defined as "an organized system that uses observational study methods to collect uniform data (clinical and other) to evaluate specified outcomes for a population defined by a particular disease, condition, or exposure, that serves predetermined scientific, clinical, or policy purpose(s)" and a "patient registry database describes a file (or files) derived from the registry."[2] The work of a registry is to identify and encourage the use of therapies and techniques that are effective, while minimizing reliance on those that are not. In the environment of cost containment and rapidly advancing technological capability, there is a strong need to determine which acute care, rehabilitation, and postdischarge community therapeutic interventions will lead to improved long-term patient outcomes, and to collect observational population-based data with long-term follow-up to allow this to be determined. Costs of acute surgical care and inpatient rehabilitation care, combined with restrictions on access to care, make this a critically important issue.

The collection and reporting of observational data, when combined with advances in medical and technological surgical care over the past half-century, have led to dramatic improvements in the care of patients with acute SCI.[3] The care improvements that affect patients include the advent of specialized centers of SCI care[4,5]; new techniques for anesthesia,[6] hemodynamic monitoring,[7] and improved thromboprophylaxis[8,9]; advances in surgical instrumentation; and technical advances that enable safe, early, and definitive surgical decompression and stabilization.[10,11]

Registries facilitate the collection of data for long-term observational studies, to determine evidence-based best practices for the treatment and care of those with SCI. Although randomized, controlled trials (RTCs) are considered the gold standard for evaluating new treatments, the RCT approach of creating an "ideal situation" by standardizing all aspects of the study may not always be necessary, appropriate, possible, nor adequate for evaluating treatments and therapies, particularly for SCI, where the numbers of patients are relatively small compared with other diseases and injury conditions.[12–15] In the clinical setting, it is difficult to establish control groups, particularly when invasive or surgical therapies are being examined. A well-designed observational study can assess interventions and practices commonly used in the clinical setting by controlling for known confounders.[16,17] If a registry collects a population-based sample (or one that represents the complete population at least in some geographic locations), then the relevance and generalizability of the data increase dramatically; the data in the registry then represent the circumstances in a day-to-day clinical situation.

One need only look at the impact of several large clinical trials on SCI to question whether they have had any positive influence on patient care or outcomes.[18–22] In fact, the multiple clinical trials on the use of methylprednisolone have, if anything, caused uncertainty among patients, physicians, and the legal community, while the question of effectiveness remains largely unanswered.[19,23,24] At the same time, large-scale observational studies have made substantial advances in answering questions related to therapeutic effectiveness in relation to thromboprophylaxis,[8,9] surgical timing for SCI,[25] and other spinal conditions.[26–28] One might argue that most of the substantial advances in patient care have come as the result of clinical and technological advances that have been reported initially as small case series and have slowly gained acceptance despite the low quality of the literature supporting these changes in practice.

What Unique Contributions to Patient Care Can the RHSCIR Make?

The RHSCIR was initiated with the goal of creating a national registry of individuals who sustain an acute traumatic SCI to enable translational research, to promote excellence in clinical practice, to facilitate the translation of therapeutic interventions for SCI, and to foster enhanced quality of life for people living with SCI. The RHSCIR leads and supports the collection and analysis of observational data for the purpose of conducting large-scale observational studies that facilitate the investigation of the potential links between the processes of care delivery and patient outcome. The RHSCIR model of translational research not only includes "the process of applying ideas, insights and discoveries generated through basic scientific inquiry to the treatment or prevention of disease or injury" but also takes into account the flow of information in the other direction, from the patient to inform the researchers. The registry populates economic and business case models, thus adding a dimension of transparent accountability to the researchers and influencing health care policy.

The integration of patient data from one phase of care to the next—prehospital to acute to rehab and then into community—allows health care providers to obtain information on the long-term outcomes of persons with SCI. Often it is the interventions applied or withheld in the first moments following injury (i.e., appropriate immobilization, timely imaging and decompression, etc.) that have a profound influence on eventual outcome. Reporting on a subacute rehabilitation intervention without controlling for and describing the acute interventions that might influence eventual outcome leaves one open to significant bias. Understanding how the patient was affected and influenced by various treatments encourages the validation of existing best practices, and will encourage surgeons and rehabilitation specialists to make best practice treatment decisions for other patients. Furthermore, it will be possible to evaluate the degree to which clinicians are following evidence-based guidelines, and this will provide a mechanism to improve the quality of care provided.

The existence of a national registry ensures that all data collected have standardized definitions and the patient registry database is linked to the primary data source, thereby streamlining data collection, eliminating duplicate data collection, and ensuring a consistent dataset is collected on all patients, which includes information from their first encounter with the medical system, through rehabilitation and community integration, through to periodic updates. From a health services provision perspective, this continuity of data flow is important.

Observational studies and RCTs have complementary roles in evaluating evidence for patient care and treatment, and a registry can enable both types of studies. The development of the RHSCIR has been a long-term project requiring considerable effort to create a national infrastructure. We are currently using the RHSCIR to conduct observational studies and are set to begin to use the RHSCIR program and technology infrastructure to manage the data collection for several clinical trials.

A national registry ensures the quality and consistency of research data. At present, research-minded health care professionals, lacking a centrally organized place to store data, often track treatment in stand-alone, personal databases. Many of these databases are not linked, so that the patient information is not continuous from one phase of treatment to another, patients may be entered multiple times in different datasets, patients are lost when they enter another phase of care or when they move to another community, and the data are collected in a nonstandardized format that makes comparisons between sites impossible. Furthermore, these individual physician- or site-based databases also use unique outcome tools that may not have been validated from a psychometric point of view. The use of nonstandard and unvalidated outcomes further complicates analysis between sites. A common terminology and standardized data collection processes, the use of unique patient identifiers to track patients from one geographical location or phase of treatment to the next, detailed procedures to ensure data quality, and the use of sophisticated technology to create a centralized place for data storage are all critical components of the RHSCIR. We have found that implementing standardized data collection protocols at certain sites, through a process of training and site visits and by mandating the use of standardized motor score assessment and recording, has resulted in substantial changes to the assessment and documentation of spinal cord impairment at these sites. Simply establishing a process for measuring and recording a neurological impairment can result in substantial improvements in the techniques used for neurological assessment at a given site.

The final benefit of a registry is the value that it can offer to patients. A registry allows patients, if they consent ahead of time, to be contacted for continuing care, innovative therapies, and the like. If a new therapy or treatment is developed, eligible patients can be rapidly identified and contacted with respect to the new study or treatment. The RHSCIR Web site will eventually provide information about new technologies and new service initiatives to interested patients. Because the registry acts as a single point of contact between the patients and researchers, the burden to the patient and health care provider is reduced. This single point of contact will aid the patient by answering questions or addressing concerns about the registry and can help to manage appropriate referrals to support services. The registry also informs and educates researchers/clinicians so that more data are collected as part of clinical practice instead of being obtained through separate interviews with patients; this also improves data consistency and promotes evidence-based practice. Finally, the RHSCIR, part of the Rick Hansen Institute (http://www.rickhanseninstitute.org), connects patients to a national network of people committed to reducing the incidence of permanent paralysis, reducing secondary complications related to SCI, and improving outcomes and quality of life. These benefits are listed in **Table 51.1**.

Functional Aspects of RHSCIR

The RHSCIR is a pan-Canadian initiative, collecting data through a network of 13 local member sites located in eight provinces to date (**Fig. 51.1** and **Table 51.2**). The data collected by the RHSCIR include detailed information on incident cases of traumatic SCI, American Spinal Injury Association (ASIA) Impairment Scale A, B, C, D, and cauda equina injuries, and are aligned with the International SCI Data Sets.[29] The data include sociodemographic data, medical history, diagnoses, interventions, procedures, and complications. Data are collected during the acute and rehabilitation phases through to community integration using patient-reported outcome measures at 1 and 2 years postinjury and at 5-year intervals until death. It is expected that the inclusion criteria will extend in the future to those with non-traumatic SCI, as the potential long-term impacts of the registry will benefit all persons with spinal cord impairment and will enroll individuals living with longstanding SCI.

A key challenge of acute traumatic SCI is obtaining consent from patients. Patients with minimal impairment are often discharged before engaging in the informed consent process required by the Personal Information Protection and Electronic Documents Act (PIPEDA) regarding their participation in a registry or research studies. For this reason, the RHSCIR has developed several strategies, including the collection of data from both responding and nonre-

Table 51.1 Benefits to Patients as a Result of Participating in a Registry

• Patients may have the opportunity to learn about new therapies or treatments. A Web site can eventually provide information about new technologies and new service initiatives.
• The burden to the patient and the health care provider is reduced by the registry's acting as the single point of contact between the patient and researchers.
• This single point of contact will aid the patient by answering questions or addressing concerns about the registry and can help to manage appropriate referrals to support services.
• Researchers/clinicians are informed and educated so that more data collected are part of clinical practice instead of obtained from patients. This also improves data consistency.
• All registry consents and information are provided in one package, so coordination and explanation of information is more streamlined.
• Through other activities associated with the Rick Hansen institute (RHI) , patients can be connected to people committed to reducing incidence of traumatic spinal cord injury and improving outcomes and quality of life.

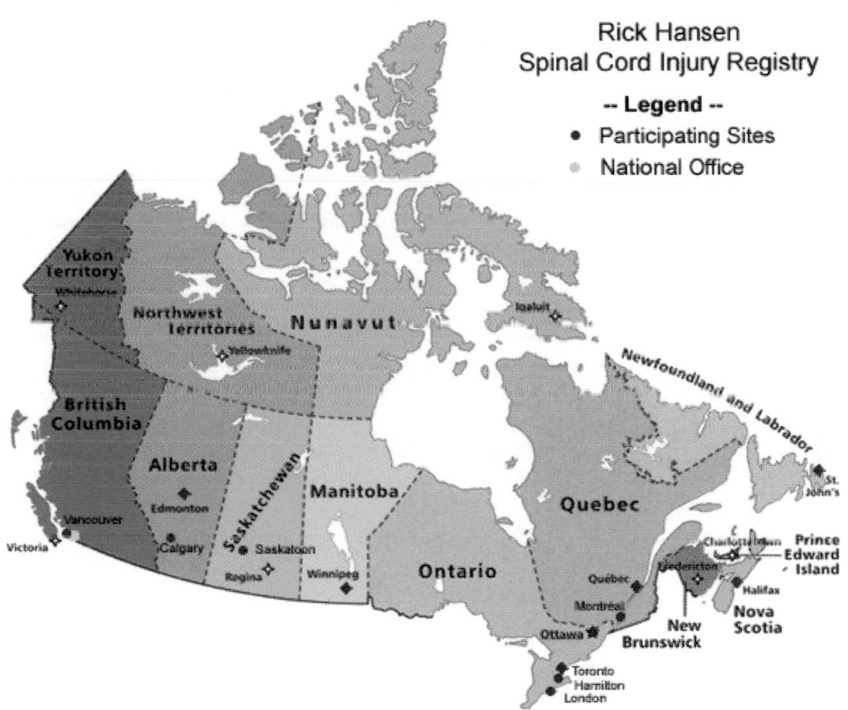

Fig. 51.1 Rick Hansen Spinal Cord Injury Registry member sites.

sponding patients. Patients are presented with consent packages, which contain the RHSCIR privacy policies, so that they have a full understanding of what will be done with the data. A coordinator is present to explain and obtain consents from the responding patients, a process that often requires repeated visits to ensure the patient has an opportunity to ask questions and is fully informed before consent is obtained. Patients who are nonresponders, either because they are discharged or chose not

Table 51.2 Registries at Time of Publication and Privacy Law Influencing the Registries

Province and numbers of registry sites	Estimated enrollment per year	Privacy law influencing the registries
British Columbia 2 sites	150	Freedom of Information and Protection of Privacy Act (FOIPPA) Personal Information Protection Act (PIPA) Bill 24
Alberta 5 sites	160	Health Information Act PIPA FOIPPA
Saskatchewan 2 sites	25	FOIPPA Personal Information Protection and Electronic Documents Act (PIPEDA) Health Information Act Local Authority Freedom of Information and Protection of Privacy Act
Manitoba 2 sites	50	FOIPPA PIPEDA Health Information Act
Ontario Anticipate 11 sites	440	FOIPPA PIPEDA Personal Health Information Protection Act Municipal Freedom on Information and Protection of Privacy Act
Quebec 5 sites	150	Act Respecting the Protection of Personal Information in the Private Sector Act Respecting Access to Documents Held by Government Bodies and the Protection of Personal Information
Prince Edward Island*		FOIPPA PIPEDA
Newfoundland 2 sites	20	FOIPPA PIPEDA
Nova Scotia 2 sites	30	FOIPPA PIPEDA
New Brunswick 2 sites		FOIPPA PIPEDA
Yukon*		FOIPPA PIPEDA
NWT*		FOIPPA PIPEDA
Nunavut*		FOIPPA PIPEDA
TOTAL SITES 33	1028	

*Asterisk indicates that there is no Rick Hansen Spinal Cord Injury Registry site in this province at the time of publication.

to participate, are included in the registry using an abstracted core dataset only; this contains minimal deidentified data about the type of injury to ensure that the registry is collecting population-based information with no selection bias. Participation in the registry at a core dataset level does not require direct personal contact between registry staff and the patient because the data are either collected as a part of the processes of care or abstracted from the medical record. Participation at this level requires no direct involvement of patients beyond their consent to participate. Participation in the full registry requires direct patient contact and consent to obtain accurate sociodemographic and socioeconomic data and to enable subsequent contact with the patient in the community to complete patient reported outcomes during scheduled follow-ups.

The data, once collected, will create a comprehensive picture of the care management process, including patient characteristics, all treatments and care processes, as well as patient outcomes. The data will undergo multivariate analysis to determine if specific patient interventions and differences in treatments result in different outcomes, which we hope will result in the development of evidence-based best practices. The registry data can also be used to identify the patients who may benefit from new therapies or innovative treatments, for potential inclusion in clinical trials. The registry data may also be used for quality improvement, to determine if best practices are being implemented at each site and to ensure that the same quality of care is being delivered across Canada.

Challenges and the Impact of Privacy Legislation

The implementation of new privacy legislation has led to significant challenges for setting up the registry. Recognizing ethical and legal obligations, RHSCIR decided to meet these challenges by opting for the highest possible standards of data collection, management, use and storage, privacy and security, operations management, quality assurance, and quality system management. The collection of information about procedures and outcomes needs to be mandated as an integral component of clinical care for patients with SCI.

In recent commentaries, new privacy legislation has imposed limitations on observational research, specifically leading to decreased participation and a selection bias in studies.[30–34] Canada's PIPEDA requires study participants to provide informed consent; although institutional review boards can waive this requirement in very select circumstances, this seems to occur only rarely.[32]

The RHSCIR was initiated in the same way as a multicenter clinical research study, which meant obtaining an institutional review board/research ethics board (IRB/REB) approval at each site; this allowed the RHSCIR to collect the data at each of the local member sites located across Canada. Since the inception of the registry, new privacy legislation has been introduced, both nationally and provincially. This includes the implementation of provincial privacy legislation, which varies from province to province and is described in **Table 51.2**. Not only is legislation different from one province to the next, but the interpretation of the legislation can differ between the privacy commissioners at a provincial level and the privacy officers at the institutional and health authority level. Similar variations are seen within the ethics boards regarding ownership, use, and transfer of locally collected data, accessed on a national basis, from one institution to the next. These differences in legislation and interpretation are creating challenges for the registry to standardize policies and procedures from one registry site to another. Furthermore, many of the provinces are still introducing new legislation, which means that the regulatory environment will continue to change and evolve, requiring the registry to accommodate these changes.

RHSCIR Provides a Solution: Privacy and Beyond

To respond to the challenges presented by privacy legislation, and the anticipated future changes to these privacy standards, RHSCIR is choosing to comply with the highest standards for privacy and quality management possible. The registry is setting up a Quality System for the collection and storage of data that is compliant with the International Conference on Harmonization of Technical Requirements for Registration of Pharmaceuticals for Human Use (ICH) standard. The ICH is an international body that makes recommendations for harmonization in the interpretation and application of technical guidelines and requirements, to allow more economical use of human, animal, and material resources, while maintaining safeguards on quality, safety and efficacy, and regulatory obligations to protect public health. This standard is expected to be used by Health Canada for oversight of patient registries in the future. By making the decision to operate under this standard, the RHSCIR is choosing to comply with an international standard for privacy and ethics, which will enable the registry to work in collaboration with other initiatives worldwide[35] to better benefit the SCI population.

The Quality System for the registry will be costly to implement, maintain, and monitor. The Quality System will include policies and standard operating procedures related to security, education and training, consent, data and record management and storage, document management, corrective and preventative action (CAPA), continuous quality improvement, internal and external audits and monitoring, vendor qualification, and system maintenance and change control. Although many of the expenses of setting up the Quality System will be incurred in the beginning, the Quality System will ensure that the registry operates efficiently and cost-effectively and conforms to the highest standards possible to meet all privacy legislations. So, while this system is costly, we anticipate that the improvements made possible in treatment and care for those with SCI will justify the costs in the long run.

Data stewardship for the RHSCIR is provided by the Rick Hansen Institute (RHI), which will govern and manage the collection, storage, and use of the data. An executive scientific committee, which includes clinicians, researchers, and people with SCI, will ensure data access in accordance with principles of academic integrity and ethics. The RHI aims to minimize disability and maximize the quality of life of people with SCI, and to enhance health, social, and economic outcomes through seamless coordination among the many organizations that provide services to people with SCI.

Although we have addressed many of the privacy and data challenges facing the registry, we anticipate that others will emerge as we move forward, for example, in negotiating data-sharing agreements and service agreement with local sites. We intend to address each of these challenges by carefully evaluating the privacy and patient impacts of each of our actions, and acting appropriately.

Conclusion

The benefits of developing a patient registry include developing infrastructure for clinical trials; providing a mechanism to identify, validate, and translate best practices to health care professionals, policy makers, and consumers; and facilitating research studies.[36] A key priority of the registry is to protect the privacy of the participants and the confidentiality of the data. The RHSCIR must ensure that there are privacy policies and many levels of security in place to satisfy privacy officers.

One issue that deserves mention is the issue of patient consent in a public health care system. Canada has a public health care system, where the care provided to all patients (including those with SCI) is provided by the government. In a publicly funded health care system like Canada's, we believe that through a social contract patients have an obligation to provide access to their health care information to facilitate the efficient and effective operations of the system. This raises the issue of where this "operational" data collection ends and where the collection of pure research data begins, or in other words, when is it necessary for patients to provide consent for their data to be recorded? The requirement for patient consent varies from province to province. No matter what the perceived obligation is for the patient to provide information, what is most important is that data collection, storage, and use are done properly, to ensure data are sound, with attention to quality, and that the privacy of patients is respected.

Although many challenges have been overcome during the implementation of the pilot phase of the registry, other issues are ongoing as a result of the changing legislative climate. The research community needs to be aware of the public's increased awareness of privacy issues and respond to the demands for being informed regarding the use of personal information. The future likely holds a balance by registries providing a privacy policy to their prospective registrants and collecting consent and abstracted datasets, or by adopting an "opt out" policy, whereby patients are enrolled in the registry unless they choose to "opt out."

Acknowledgment

Thanks to Sylvia Kingsmill from Anzen Consulting and Chrystal Palaty for their assistance with this manuscript.

Pearls

- Prospective data registries are an effective way to track outcomes and other key epidemiological data.
- It is strongly recommended that data collection be focused on key data elements.

Pitfalls

- The most common error in setting up a prospective dataset is to collect too much information. If the data fields are too numerous, then the quality of the data collected will suffer, and many of the elements that are collected will perhaps never actually be analyzed or utilized. This can be avoided by identifying data elements in a disciplined fashion and by basing the data collection on well formulated research questions that are identified a priori.

References

1. Campbell EG. The future of research funding in academic medicine. N Engl J Med 2009;360(15): 1482–1483
2. Gliklich RE, Dreyer NA, eds. Registries for evaluating patient outcomes: a user's guide. 2nd ed. Outcome DECIDE Center, contract no. HHSA-290200500351TO3. AHRQ publication no. 10-EHC049. Rockville, MD: Agency for Healthcare Research and Quality, September 2010
3. Fisher CG, Noonan VK, Dvorak MF. Changing face of spine trauma care in North America. Spine (Phila Pa 1976) 2006;31(11, Suppl):S2–S8, discussion S36
4. Bagnall AM, Jones L, Richardson G, Duffy S, Riemsma R. Effectiveness and cost-effectiveness of acute hospital-based spinal cord injuries services: systematic review. Health Technol Assess 2003;7(19):iii, 1–92
5. Jones L, Bagnall A. Spinal injuries centres (SICs) for acute traumatic spinal cord injury. Cochrane Database Syst Rev 2004;(4):CD004442
6. Babinski MF. Anesthetic considerations in the patient with acute spinal cord injury. Crit Care Clin 1987;3(3):619–636
7. Stene JK, Grande CM. General anesthesia: management considerations in the trauma patient. Crit Care Clin 1990;6(1):73–84
8. Deep K, Jigajinni MV, McLean AN, Fraser MH. Prophylaxis of thromboembolism in spinal injuries—results of enoxaparin used in 276 patients. Spinal Cord 2001;39(2):88–91
9. Jones T, Ugalde V, Franks P, Zhou H, White RH. Venous thromboembolism after spinal cord injury: incidence, time course, and associated risk factors in 16,240 adults and children. Arch Phys Med Rehabil 2005;86(12):2240–2247
10. Bagnall AM, Jones L, Duffy S, Riemsma RP. Spinal fixation surgery for acute traumatic spinal

cord injury. Cochrane Database Syst Rev 2008; (1):CD004725
11. Fehlings MG, Tator CH. An evidence-based review of decompressive surgery in acute spinal cord injury: rationale, indications, and timing based on experimental and clinical studies. J Neurosurg 1999;91(1, Suppl):1–11
12. Horn SD, DeJong G, Ryser DK, Veazie PJ, Teraoka J. Another look at observational studies in rehabilitation research: going beyond the holy grail of the randomized controlled trial. Arch Phys Med Rehabil 2005;86(12, Suppl 2):S8–S15
13. Leurs LJ, Buth J, Harris PL, Blankensteijn JD. Impact of study design on outcome after endovascular abdominal aortic aneurysm repair: a comparison between the randomized controlled DREAM-trial and the observational EUROSTAR-registry. Eur J Vasc Endovasc Surg 2007;33(2):172–176
14. Pibouleau L, Boutron I, Reeves BC, Nizard R, Ravaud P. Applicability and generalisability of published results of randomised controlled trials and non-randomised studies evaluating four orthopaedic procedures: methodological systematic review. BMJ 2009;339:b4538 10.1136/bmj.b4538.:b4538
15. Röder C, Müller U, Aebi M. The rationale for a spine registry. Eur Spine J 2006;15(Suppl 1): S52–S56
16. Black N. Why we need observational studies to evaluate the effectiveness of health care. BMJ 1996;312(7040):1215–1218
17. Black N. What observational studies can offer decision makers. Horm Res 1999;51(Suppl 1): 44–49
18. Bracken MB. Methylprednisolone and acute spinal cord injury: an update of the randomized evidence. Spine (Phila Pa 1976) 2001;26(24, Suppl):S47–S54
19. Bracken MB, Aldrich EF, Herr DL, et al. Clinical measurement, statistical analysis, and risk-benefit: controversies from trials of spinal injury. J Trauma 2000;48(3):558–561
20. Bracken MB, Shepard MJ, Collins WF, et al. A randomized, controlled trial of methylprednisolone or naloxone in the treatment of acute spinal-cord injury: results of the Second National Acute Spinal Cord Injury Study. N Engl J Med 1990;322(20):1405–1411
21. Geisler FH, Coleman WP, Grieco G, Poonian D; Sygen Study Group. The Sygen multicenter acute spinal cord injury study. Spine (Phila Pa 1976) 2001;26(24, Suppl):S87–S98
22. Geisler FH, Dorsey FC, Coleman WP. Recovery of motor function after spinal-cord injury—a randomized, placebo-controlled trial with GM-1 ganglioside. N Engl J Med 1991;324(26):1829–1838
23. Coleman WP, Benzel D, Cahill DW, et al. A critical appraisal of the reporting of the National Acute Spinal Cord Injury Studies (II and III) of methylprednisolone in acute spinal cord injury. J Spinal Disord 2000;13(3):185–199
24. Hurlbert RJ. Methylprednisolone for acute spinal cord injury: an inappropriate standard of care. J Neurosurg 2000;93(1, Suppl):1–7
25. Baptiste DC, Fehlings MG. Update on the treatment of spinal cord injury. Prog Brain Res 2007;161:217–233
26. Atlas SJ, Keller RB, Wu YA, Deyo RA, Singer DE. Long-term outcomes of surgical and nonsurgical management of lumbar spinal stenosis: 8 to 10 year results from the Maine lumbar spine study. Spine (Phila Pa 1976) 2005;30(8):936–943
27. Park DK, An HS, Lurie JD, et al. Does multilevel lumbar stenosis lead to poorer outcomes?: a subanalysis of the Spine Patient Outcomes Research Trial (SPORT) lumbar stenosis study. Spine (Phila Pa 1976) 2010;35(4):439–446
28. Weinstein JN, Lurie JD, Tosteson TD, et al. Surgical compared with nonoperative treatment for lumbar degenerative spondylolisthesis. four-year results in the Spine Patient Outcomes Research Trial (SPORT) randomized and observational cohorts. J Bone Joint Surg Am 2009;91(6):1295–1304
29. DeVivo M, Biering-Sørensen F, Charlifue S, et al; Executive Committee for the International SCI Data Sets Committees. International Spinal Cord Injury Core Data Set. Spinal Cord 2006;44(9): 535–540
30. Gershon AS, Tu JV. The effect of privacy legislation on observational research. CMAJ 2008; 178(7):871–873
31. Silver FL, Kapral MK, Lindsay MP, Tu JV, Richards JA; Registry of the Canadian Stroke Network. International experience in stroke registries: lessons learned in establishing the Registry of the Canadian Stroke Network. Am J Prev Med 2006;31(6, Suppl 2):S235–S237
32. Thompson J. Ethical challenges of informed consent in prehospital research. CJEM 2003; 5(2):108–114
33. Tu JV, Willison DJ, Silver FL, et al; Investigators in the Registry of the Canadian Stroke Network. Impracticability of informed consent in the Registry of the Canadian Stroke Network. N Engl J Med 2004;350(14):1414–1421
34. Willison D. Privacy and the secondary use of data for health research: experience in Canada and suggested directions forward. J Health Serv Res Policy 2003;8(Suppl 1):S1, 17–23
35. Melloh M, Staub L, Aghayev E, et al. The international spine registry SPINE TANGO: status quo and first results. Eur Spine J 2008;17(9):1201–1209
36. Wyndaele M, Wyndaele JJ. Incidence, prevalence and epidemiology of spinal cord injury: what learns a worldwide literature survey? Spinal Cord 2006;44(9):523–529

52

Resources to Empower and Expand the Opportunities of People with Spinal Cord Injury

Kay Harris Kreigsman, Sara Palmer, and Jeffrey B. Palmer

Key Points

1. People with SCI can continue to participate in meaningful social roles, with additional supports and assistance in place.
2. When health care providers are aware of the possibilities for people with SCI, they are better able to enhance their social participation and quality of life.
3. Health care providers who refer people with SCI and their families to appropriate resources empower them to engage in meaningful relationships, explore their interests, and realize their goals.

Spinal cord injury (SCI) is sometimes seen as narrowing the scope of activities and opportunities for the person who is injured. It may be assumed that, because individuals with SCI are physically unable to perform many activities of daily living, their participation in leisure, social, and vocational pursuits is over. Observers may perceive the injury as altering or destroying the person's predisability world and may be unable to imagine opportunities for a good quality of life in the future.

Some health care providers, including physicians, nurses, and other clinical health professionals, have a similar, erroneous view of life after SCI. This is unfortunate; if the health care team views SCI as the end of a person's ability to engage fully in life, the bias may be internalized by their patients and become reality. In fact, multiple avenues for engaging in productive and enjoyable activities are currently available for people with SCI and other disabilities. It is important that clinicians know about, and can direct their patients to, the resources that can enable people with SCI to live productive, satisfying, and creative lives.

Resources like those listed in this chapter empower medical professionals with referral recommendations to help their patients. This listing includes not only medical and rehabilitation resources but also those that address socialization, hobbies, employment, family, sports, equipment and technology, sexuality, and travel for those with SCI. When medical professionals share this information with their patients with SCI, the patients become empowered to use what they learn to achieve their own life goals.

The following lists of resources for people with SCI and their families have been selected because of their helpfulness and relevance as well as their general availability in print and their accessibility via computer Web sites. Some have greater public recognition than others. General information resources are listed first, followed by various types of resources grouped alphabetically by topic.

General Information

Selections include informative books and resource guides about SCI; memoirs and stories of people living with SCI; and magazines, periodicals, Internet sites, and organizations for people with SCI.

Books

- *An Introduction to Spinal Cord Injury: Understanding the Changes.* 4th ed. Washington, DC: Paralyzed Veterans of America; 2001. Available from Paralyzed Veterans of America, 801 Eighteenth Street NW, Washington, DC 20006. An electronic copy is available free at www.pva.org.
- Burns, SP, Hammond MC, eds. *Yes You Can! A Guide to Self-Care for Persons with Spinal Cord Injury.* 4th edition. Washington, DC: Paralyzed Veterans of America; 2009. Available from Paralyzed Veterans of America, 801 Eighteenth Street NW, Washington, DC 20006 or at www.pva.org. The book can be downloaded free at the PVA Web site.
- Karp G. *Life on Wheels: The ABC Guide for Living Fully with Mobility Issues.* 2nd ed. New York: Demos Medical Publishing; 2009.
- Maddox S. *Paralysis Resource Guide.* 2nd ed. Springfield, NJ: Christopher & Dana Reeve Paralysis Resource Center; 2007.
- *New Mobility Magazine's Spinal Network: The Total Wheelchair Resource Book.* 4th ed. Horsham: PA: No Limits Communications. Also available at www.spinalnetwork.net.
- Palmer S, Kriegsman KH, Palmer JB. *Spinal Cord Injury: A Guide for Living,* 2nd ed. Baltimore, MD: Johns Hopkins University Press; 2008.

Memoirs and Personal Stories of Living with Spinal Cord Injury

- Cole, J. *Still Lives: Narratives of Spinal Cord Injury.* Cambridge, MA: MIT Press; 2004.
- Hockenberry J. *Moving Violations: War Zones, Wheelchairs, and Declarations of Independence.* New York: Hyperion; 1995.
- Holicky R. *Roll Models: People Who Live Successfully following Spinal Cord Injury and How They Do It.* Victoria, BC: Trafford; 2004. Also available through the Paralyzed Veterans of America; see listing under organizations.
- Karp G, Klein SD, eds. *From There to Here.* Horsham, PA: No Limits Communications; 2004.
- Reeve C. *Still Me.* New York: Random House; 1998.

Magazines and Periodicals

- *Ability.* Published bimonthly. C. R. Cooper Publishing, 1682 Langley Avenue, Irvine, CA 2714. Covers a wide range of medical, social, and lifestyle topics of interest to people with various disabilities. Web site: www.abilitymagazinne.com.
- *Action.* United Spinal Association, 75–20 Astoria Boulevard, Jackson Heights, New York, NY 11370. Phone: 800-404-2898. Web site: www.unitedspinal.org. Available in audio format, by request.
- *Enabled Online.com.* An online magazine providing information and re-

sources for people with disabilities. Web site: www.enabledonline.com.

- *New Mobility: Disability Culture and Lifestyles.* Miramar Communications Inc., 23815 Stuart Ranch Road, PO Box 8987, Malibu, CA 90265. Web site: www.newmobility.com.
- *Paraplegia News.* Paralyzed Veterans of America, 2111 East Highland Street, Suite 180, Phoenix, AZ 85016–4702. Web site: www.pvamagazines.com/pnnews.
- *The Ragged Edge.* An online magazine published by the Avocado Press, Inc., Box 145, Louisville, KY 40201. Web site: www.ragged-edge-mag.com.
- *SCI Life Newspaper.* National Spinal Cord Injury Association, 6701 Democracy Boulevard, Suite 300–9, Bethesda, MD. Phone: 800-962-9629.

Videos

- Northwest Regional Spinal Cord Injury System Web site for both text and video resources. www.sci.washington.edu. Video resources include *Conversations About Living with Spinal Cord Injury*; *Personal Caregivers*; and *Getting Your Life Back after Spinal Cord Injury: Finding Meaning through Volunteering, School and Work.* Other videos focus on Social Security Insurance and Supplemental Security Income, osteoporosis in SCI, autonomic dysreflexia, and hypnosis for pain management, among other topics.

Internet Sites

- www.disaboom.com. A Web site with links to a wide variety of disability organizations
- www.mobilewomen.org. Addresses needs of women using wheelchairs.
- www.ninds.nih.gov/disorders/sci/sci.htm. This Web site is part of the National Institute of Neurological Disorders and Stroke, and provides information on spinal cord injury treatment, research and resources.
- www.spinalcordcentral.org A Web site of information for people living with SCI, operated jointly by United Spinal Association and National Spinal Cord Injury.

Organizations

- American Paralysis Association, 500 Morris Avenue, Springfield, NJ 07081. Phone: 800-225-0292. Web site: www.apacure.com.
- Christopher and Dana Reeve Paralysis Resource Center, 636 Morris Turnpike, Suite 3A, Short Hills, NJ 07078. Phone: 800-225-0292. Web site: www.paralysis.org.
- National Spinal Cord Injury Association, 6701 Democracy Boulevard, Suite 300–9, Bethesda, MD. Phone: 800-962-9629. Web site: www.spinalcord.org.
- Paralyzed Veterans of America, 801 Eighteenth Street, NW, Washington, DC 20006. Phone: 800-795-4327 TTD. Web site: www.pva.org.
- Spinal Cord Injury Network International, 3911 Princeton Drive, Santa Rosa, CA 95405. Phone: 800-548-CORD (548-2673). Web site: www.spinal@sonic.net.
- Spinal Cord Injury Information Network, UAB Model SCI System, Office of Research Services, 619 19th Street, Birmingham, AL 35249–7330. Phone: 205-934-3283 Web site: www.spinalcord.uab.edu.
- United Spinal Association, 75–20 Astoria Boulevard, Jackson Heights, New York, NY 11370 Phone: 718-803-3782. Web site: www.unitedspinal.org.

Accessible Design

- Accessible design, sometimes called universal design, refers to the design of homes and buildings that can be used by anyone, with or without a disability. Accessible designs are safe and barrier-free.

- *Accessible Home Design: Architectural Solutions for the Wheelchair User*. 2nd ed. Published by Paralyzed Veterans of America; see listing under Organizations.
- Amherst Homes, Inc., 7378 Charter Cup Lane, Westchester, OH 45069. Phone: 513-891-3303.
- The Center for Universal Design, North Carolina State University, Box 8613, Raleigh, NC 27695–8613. Phone: 800-647-6777. Web site: www.design ncsu.edu.
- Concrete Change, 600 Dancing Fox Road, Decatur, GA 30032. Phone: 404-378-7455. Mission is to make every home "visitable." Web site: http://concretechange.home.mindspring.com/.
- Lifease, Inc., 2451 Fifteenth Street, NW, New Brighton, MN 55112. Phone: 612-636-6869. Web site: www.lifease.com.

Internet Sites

- www.disabilityinfo.gov.
- www.universaldesignonline.com/index.html.

The Americans with Disabilities Act (ADA), Disability Rights, and Advocacy

ADA became law in 1990. It prohibits discrimination against people with disability in employment, transportation, public accommodation, communications, and governmental activities. Interpretations of the ADA continue to evolve through legal challenges. Familiarity with the most current applications of the ADA helps people with SCI to understand their legal rights. Other resources in this section address legal rights in the specific areas of housing and accessibility.

- Americans with Disabilities Act (ADA) Information. Phone: 800-466-4ADA. Web site: www.ada.gov.
- Disability Rights Education and Defense Fund (DREDF), 2212 Sixth Street, Berkeley, CA 94710. Phone: 415-644-2555. Provides information on disability rights laws and policy. Publishes a free newsletter, *Disability Rights News*.
- *Fair Housing: How to Make the Law Work for You*. Washington, DC. Available electronically from Paralyzed Veterans of America at www.pva.org.
- National Association of Governors' Committees on People with Disabilities. Phone: 916-654-1764. Web site: www.nagcpd.com. Promotes equal access to employment, programs, and services for people with disabilities. Provides monthly updates of information and resources on the following: grants, scholarships, internships and other funding opportunities; publications, media resources and releases; conferences, events, meetings and courses; Web sites on disability topics and issues, including accessible living, advocacy, laws, education, employment, funding, government, Internet disability job board, policy-related information, sports and recreation, statistics, transportation, travel, veterans, women, and youth; and resolving issues.
- United States Access Board. Web site: www.access-board.gov. An independent federal agency whose primary mission is technical assistance on accessibility for people with disabilities.
- US Department of Housing and Urban Development, Office of Fair Housing and Equal Opportunity, 451 Seventh Street, SW, Washington, DC 20410. Provides information on housing rights and resources for people with disabilities, and for those who encounter discrimination in housing. Phone: 202-708-1112. Web site: www.hud.gov.

Arts

Participation in a wide variety of visual and performance arts is available to people with disabilities. Appropriate technology or assistance may be needed to facilitate these experiences for people with severe SCI. Expressive arts are a source of pleasure, creativity, and mastery.

- Mouth and Foot Painting Artists, 2070 Peachtree Court, Suite 101, Atlanta, GA 30341 Phone: 770-986-7764. Web site: www.mfpusa.com.
- That Uppity Theater Company, 4466 West Pine Blvd., Suite 13C, St. Louis, MO 63108. Phone: 314-995-4600. Web site: www.uppityco.com. A theater company for actors with and without disabilities.
- VSA Arts, 818 Connecticut Avenue NW, Suite 600, Washington, DC 20006. Phone: 800-933-8721. Web site: www.vsarts.org. This nonprofit organization provides opportunities for people with disabilities to learn through, participate in, and enjoy visual and performing arts.

Driving

Transportation is a major issue for people with physical disabilities. Depending on the level of injury, many people with SCI can continue to drive a car or van that has been modified, for example, with hand controls, a wheelchair storage or locking device, or a built-in ramp. Many rehabilitation centers have driver training programs for people with disabilities. Some car manufacturers have discount programs for modifications required to enable a person to drive.

- *Adaptive Automotive Equipment: A Consumer's Guide*. A brochure published by the United Spinal Association, available on their Web site: www.unitedspinal.org/pdf/ahc.pdf.
- Association for Driver Rehabilitation Specialists (ADED), PO Box 49, Edgerton, WI 53534. Phone: 608-884-8833. Web sites: www.driver-ed.org; www.aded.net.
- National Highway Traffic Safety Administration. Adapting Motor Vehicles for People with Disabilities. Brochure available on their Web site: www.nhtsa.gov/cars/rules/adaptive/brochure/brochure.html.
- Family Village, adaptive driving and vehicle adaptation sources. Web site: www.familyvillage.wisc.edu/at/driving.htm.

Equipment and Technology

Technological equipment and assistive devices are important components in the lives of people with SCI. Consumers do not always know what is available and where to find what they need; the search can be time consuming and frustrating. Following are some resources to help make it easier.

- Abledata, 8455 Colesville Road, Suite 935, Silver Spring, MD 20910. Phone: 800-227-0216. Web site: www.abledata.com. Maintains a database with over 15,000 listings of adaptive devices for all disabilities.
- Assistive Technology News. Web site. www.atechnews.com. Featuring articles on new technologies.
- *The First Whole Rehab Catalog: A Comprehensive Guide to Products and Services for the Physically Disadvantaged.* Crozet, VA: Betterway Publications; 1990. Available from Betterway Publications, Box 219, Crozet, VA 22932.
- Karp G. *Choosing a Wheelchair: A Guide for Optimal Independence.* Sebastopol, CA: O'Reilly and Associates; 1998.
- Sammons Preston and Enrichments, PO Box 5071, Bolingbrook, IL 60440–5071. Phone: 800-323-5547; fax: 800-547-4333. A mail-order catalog for accessibility aids.

Family and Caregiver Resources

SCI affects not only the person who is injured but also the family. Family roles may change, even in the short term, during SCI treatment and rehabilitation. For people with SCI and their family members, *change* is the operative word as they trade responsibilities, independence, dependence, and caregiving, Appropriate supportive referrals may help families adjust and adapt to their new reality and be open to the learning that is necessary to be successful.

- Family Caregiver Alliance, 180 Montgomery Street, Suite 1100, San Francisco, CA 94104. Phone: 800-445-8106. Web site: www.caregiver.org.
- Holicky, Richard. *Taking Care of Yourself while Providing Care: A Guide for Those Who Assist and Care for Their Spouses, Children, Parents and Other Loved Ones Who Have Spinal Cord Injuries.* Englewood, CO: Craig Hospital; 2000.
- Kriegsman KH, Zaslow EL, and D'zmura-Rechsteiner J. *Taking Charge: Teenagers Talk about Life and Physical Disabilities.* Rockville, MD: Woodbine House; 1992.
- National Family Care Givers Association, 10605 Concord Street, Suite 501, Kensington, MD 20895–2504. Phone: 800-896-3650. Web site: www.nfcacares.org.
- Palmer S, Kriegsman KH, Palmer JB. *Spinal Cord Injury: A Guide for Living.* Baltimore, MD: Johns Hopkins University Press; 2008.
- Through the Looking Glass: National Resource Center for Parents with Disabilities, 2198 Sixth Street, #100, Berkeley, CA 94710–2204. Web site: www. lookingglass.org.

Insurance and Financial Information

Many individuals with SCI rely on private medical and disability insurance, Social Security Disability, or Medicare to cover their extraordinary medical expenses and provide income if they are not able to work. Yet these programs can be perplexing and complicated. Financial impacts of SCI on the individual and family are significant and ongoing; understanding how to obtain financial assistance and benefits is essential.

- Centers for Medicare and Medicaid Services (CMS), US Department of Health and Human Services. Web site: www.cms.hhs.gov.
- Information on Medicare and Medicaid benefits and programs, the Medicaid Waiver, and other programs and services provided by these government health insurance programs.
- *Mercer's 2010 Guide to Social Security*. 38th ed. Louisville, KY: Mercer; 2010. Available online from www .mercer.com.
- *Mercer's 2010 Medicare Booklet.* 27th ed. Louisville, KY: Mercer; 2010. Available online from www.mercer.com.
- Medicare information. Phone: 800-MEDICARE. Web site: www.medicare .gov.
- *On the Move: A Financial Guide for People with Spinal Cord Injury*. Available from the Paralyzed Veterans of America or the National Spinal Cord Injury Association; see listing under Organizations.
- Social Security Administration. Information on Social Security disability and retirement benefits, the application process and locating your local Social Security office. Web site: www.ssa.gov.
- *What You Should Know about Health Insurance: Guidelines for Persons Living with SCI.* Available from the National Spinal Cord Injury Association; see listing under Organizations.

Mental Health Services and Peer Support

Integrating an SCI into one's life and self-image can be daunting for some people, either at the onset of the SCI or later in life. There are supportive resources for those encountering depression, anger, and anxiety, among other feelings, that may derail the person's ability to progress physically, mentally, or psychologically. Appropriate referrals allow the person to get back on track.

- American Association of Marriage and Family Therapists, 112 South Alfred Street, Alexandria, VA 22314–3061. Phone: 703-838-9808. Provides a Therapist Locator service to help with find a qualified marriage counselor in your local area. Web site: www.therapistlocator.net.
- American Psychiatric Association, 1000 Wilson Boulevard, Suite 1825, Arlington, VA 22209. Phone: 800-35-PSYCH. Web site: www.psych.org.
- American Psychological Association, 750 First Street, NE, Washington, DC 20002. Phone: 800-374-2721. Web site: www.apa.org.
- Determined 2 Heal, 8112 River Falls Drive, Potomac, MD 20854. Phone: 703-795-5711. Web site: www.determined2heal.org. Provides information on, psychosocial recovery, support, research, and prevention.
- National Association of Social Workers, 750 First Street, NE, Suite 700, Washington, DC 20002. Telephone: 202-408-8600. Web site: www.socialworkers.org.
- United Spinal Association's Peer-Mentoring Program. Connects newly injured persons with people experienced in living with SCI, to provide role modeling and support. Contact: Jerome Kleckley, LMSW, Director of Social Services, United Spinal Association, 718-803-3782, ext. 267.

Research

Research on stem cells and nerve regeneration as well as new rehabilitation techniques and technologies for treating SCI are ongoing and include many promising approaches. Keeping abreast of the latest research helps patients learn about new treatments, discuss the risks and benefits with their physicians, and decide whether to participate in research trials.

- Christopher Reeve Paralysis Foundation, 636 Morris Turnpike, Suite 3A, Short Hills, NJ 07078. Phone: 800-225-0292. Web site: www.christopherreeve.org.
- The International Center for Spinal Cord Injury, Kennedy Krieger Institute, 707 N. Broadway, Baltimore, MD 21205. Phone: 888-923-9222. Web site: www.spinalcordrecovery.org.
- Miami Project to Cure Paralysis, University of Miami School of Medicine, 1600 NW Tenth Avenue, R-48, Miami, FL 33136. Phone: 800-782-6387. Web site: www.miamiproject.miami.edu.
- National Center for the Dissemination of Disability Research. Web site: www.neddr.org. Information developed for the public from National Institute of Disability and Rehabilitation Research (NIDRR) research. Topics include assistive technology, employment, and women with disabilities. Includes listings of Model Spinal Cord Injury Systems, disability statistics, links to other NIDRR sites.
- National Rehabilitation Information Center. Web site: www.naric.com/naric. Research results, audiovisuals, and publications about disability research. Publications available include a guide to the ADA and directory of national information resources.

Sexuality, Fertility, and Pregnancy

The first question a person usually asks after incurring SCI is "Will I live?" Often, the next question is "Can I still have sex?" People with SCI are interested in learning more about the impact of the injury on intimacy, including sexuality, fertility, and pregnancy. Following are resources and information to help people with SCI and their families in this area.

- American Association of Sexuality Educators, Counselors and Therapists, PO Box 1960, Ashland, VA 23005–1960. Phone: 804-752-0026. Web site: www.aasect.org.
- American Society of Reproductive Medicine, 1209 Montgomery Highway, Birmingham, AL 35216–2809. Phone: 205-978-5000. Website: www.asrm.org.
- Baer J. *Is Fred Dead: A Manual on Sexuality for Men with Spinal Cord Injuries.* Pittsburgh, PA: Dorrance Publishing; 2004.
- Ducharme SH, Gill KM. *Sexuality after Spinal Cord Injury: Answers to Your Questions.* Baltimore, MD: Paul Brookes; 1997.
- A Guide and Resource Directory to Male Fertility following SCI/C: A Miami Project Resource. Web site: www.themiamiproject.org.
- Guter B, Killacky JR. *Queer Crips: Disabled Gay Men and Their Stories.* New York: Harrington Park Press; 2004.
- Rogers J. *The Disabled Woman's Guide to Pregnancy and Birth.* 2nd ed. New York: Demos Medical Publishing; 2006.
- *Sexuality Reborn* (video, 48 minutes). Produced by Kessler Institute for Rehabilitation, 1199 Pleasant Valley Way, West Orange, NJ 07052. Phone: 800-248-3321, ext. 6977. This video explores the relationships and sexuality of four couples, in which at least one partner has a disability. They demonstrate and share their experiences on self-esteem, sexual functioning, and intercourse.
- www.sexualhealth.com. Web site with information about sexuality; has a Disability and Chronic Conditions section.

Sports, Fitness, and Outdoor Recreation

Many people with SCI have been active, athletic, and sports oriented before their injuries. These resources show them that those days are not over; in fact, there are assistive devices, adapted equipment, and modified games that will allow them to participate in team and individual sports and active outdoor recreation.

- American Canoe Association, 7432 Alban Station Blvd., Suite B-226, Springfield, VA 22159–2311.
- Buckmasters American Deer Foundation. Web site: www.badf.org/Disabled_Hunters/adaptiveEquip.html. Site for hunters with disabilities.
- *Easy Access to National Parks.* San Francisco: Sierra Club; 1998. A guide to accessible places in national parklands. Available from Sierra Club Books, 100 Bush Street, San Francisco, CA 94101.
- Handicapped Scuba Association International, 1104 El Prado, San Clemente, CA 92672–4637. Independent diver training and certifying agency. Offers Dive Buddy Program.
- *Murderball* (film, available on DVD and video). Codirected by Henry Alex Rubin and Dana Adam Shapiro. Produced by Jeffrey Mandell and Dana Alex Shapiro. This is a documentary about wheelchair rugby, and the journey of the American "quad" rugby team to the Olympics. For more information on this sport, including locating a team, contact the United States Quad Rugby Association at www.quadrugby.com.
- National Ability Center, Parks City, UT. Phone: 435-694-3991. Web site: www.nac1985.org. Specializes in accessible recreation, sports, and leisure activities.

- National Association of Handicapped Outdoor Sportsmen, Inc., RR 6, Box 25, Centralia, IL 62801.
- National Center on Physical Activity and Disability. Web site: www.ncpad.org. Phone: 800-900-8086.
- National Foundation of Wheelchair Tennis, 940 Calle Amanecer, Suite B, San Clemente, CA 92672.
- National Park Service, 1849 C Street NW, Mail stop 7253 MIB, Washington, DC 20240. Provides listings of national parks with accessible camping areas and a Golden Access Passport for individuals who have permanent visual or physical disabilities.
- National Wheelchair Basketball Association, 110 Seaton Building, University of Kentucky, Lexington, KY 40506. Web site: www.nwba.org.
- North American Riding for the Handicapped Association, Inc. (NARHA) (horse riding), PO Box 33150, Denver, CO 80238. Web site: www.narha.org.
- Shake-a-Leg, Inc., 76 Dorrance Street, Suite 300, Providence, RI 02903. Phone: 401-421-1111. Web site: www.shake@shakealeg.org. Offers therapy and recreational services to people with disabilities, with an emphasis on independent living and leisure/fitness; an Adaptive Sailing program; and a summer camp program for children with disabilities, ages 7 to 14.
- *Sports 'N' Spokes* magazine. Paralyzed Veterans of America, 2111 East Highland Street, Suite 180, Phoenix, AZ 85016–4702. Phone: 602-224-0500.
- United States Golf Association, PO Box 708, Far Hills, NJ 07931. Modified rules for golfers with disabilities.
- United States Handcycling Federation, PO Box 2245, Evergreen, CO 80437.
- United States Quad Rugby Association, 5821 White Cypress Drive, Lake Worth, FL 22467–6230.
- Wheelchair Sports USA, 10 Lake Circle, Suite G19, Colorado Springs, CO 80906. Information on archery, shooting, swimming, table tennis, weight lifting, track and field, in addition to specifics on local competition.
- Wilderness Inquiry, Inc., 1313 Fifth Street, PO Box 84, Minneapolis, MN 55414. Phone: 800-728-0719. Web site: www.wildernessinquiry.org. Wilderness (land and water) excursions for people with and without disabilities.
- Wilderness on Wheels Foundation, 7125 W Jefferson Ave., No. 155, Lakewood, CO 80235. Accessible camping, hiking, and fishing.

Transportation and Travel

Travel by train or airplane may be necessary for a person with SCI to conduct business or visit family. Traveling as a tourist to distant cities or natural environments is a source of enjoyment for many people. Although it requires planning and some advance homework, travel by car, air, train, or boat is popular among people with SCI and their families.

- Access-Able Travel Source, PO Box 1796, Wheat Ridge, CO 80034. Web site: www.access-able.com.
- Accessible Europe. Phone: 011-39-011-30-1888. Travel agencies in Italy, specializing in accessible tourism. Web site: www.accessibleeurope.com.
- Accessible Journeys. Phone: 800-846-4537. Web site: www.disabilitytravel.com. Organizes wheelchair travel for groups and individuals, including cruises.
- *The Air Carrier Access Act: Make It Work for You.* Washington, DC. Available from Paralyzed Veterans of America; see listing under Organizations.
- Emerging Horizons, PO Box 278, Ripon, CA 95366.
- International Association for Medical Assistance to Travelers. Phone: 716-754-4883. Web site: www.iamat.org. This organization provides access to English-speaking medical care providers for English-speakers traveling in foreign countries.
- Mersey River Chalets. Nova Scotia, Canada. Web site: www.merseyriverchallets.ns.ca. Accessible accommodations and nature activities.

- *New Horizons: Information for the Air Traveler with a Disability.* Washington, DC: US Department of Transportation. Available from US Department of Transportation, Aviation Consumer Protection Division, C-75, 400 Seventh Street, SW, Washington, DC 20590. Web site: www.gov/airconsumer/horizons.htm. The Web site has the full text of the document.
- Society for the Advancement of Travel for the Handicapped, 347 Fifth Avenue, Suite 610, New York, NY 10016.
- Travelin' Talk Network, 130 Hillcrest Plaza, Suite 102, PO Box 3534, Clarksville, TN 37043. Phone: 615-552-6670. Web site: www.travelintalk.net. A network of over 1000 people who offer help and services to travelers with disabilities. Membership benefits include discounts at various motels.

Education, Vocational Rehabilitation, and Employment

SCI can disrupt a person's educational and career trajectory. If it is not possible for the injured person to return to his or her previous job, retraining and employment in a different line of work may be possible. These resources provide information about how to get assistance with education, job training, and employment.

- State Vocational Rehabilitation. Under the provisions of the Rehabilitation Act, every state government offers vocational rehabilitation services to help people with disabilities obtain education and job training and return to gainful employment. A list of state Vocational Rehabilitation agencies can be found online. Web site: www.workworld.org/wwwebhelp/state_vocational_rehabilitation_vr_agencies.htm.
- *Working!* Published quarterly. Goodwill Industries International Inc., 9200 Rockville Pike, Bethesda, MD 20814. Available online. Website: www.goodwill.org.

Internet Sites

- www.dol.gov/odep. United States Department of Labor's Office of Disability Employment Policy's Web site provides technical assistance and information for individuals with disabilities.
- www.jobaccess.org. A Web site where people with disabilities can post their résumés and connect with employers to find jobs.

VII

Achieving Success

53

Neurogenomic and Neuroproteomic Approaches to Studying Neural Injury

Joy D. Guingab-Cagmat, Firas H. Kobeissy, Mary V. Ratliff, Peng Shi, Zhiqun Zhang, and Kevin K. W. Wang

Key Points

1. The fields of neurogenomics/neuroproteomics are still in the developing stage due to several factors. The full potential of these areas remains to be explored and will reveal integral signature molecules known as biomarkers that can be associated with injury severity, cellular mechanisms, and biological networks specific to the particular brain disorder in question.
2. The complexity of the central nervous system (CNS) and associated brain disorders necessitates the use and development of relevant animal models of experimental CNS injury that can mimic human spinal or brain injury.
3. Introducing various advanced analytical tools (multidimensional separation techniques, neuroproteomics, neurogenomics, and biochemical testing) would facilitate the identification of key biological hits (proteins and/or genes) that can highlight the underlying mechanisms involved in the area of neural injury.

Traumatic brain injury (TBI) is defined as neurotrauma caused by a mechanical force that is applied to the head.[1] Annually in the United States, there are ~2 million incidents that involve TBI. Of these, nearly 100,000 patients die, another 500,000 are hospitalized, and thousands of others suffer short- and long-term effects.[2] The medical costs associated with caring for TBI patients are extremely high, as are the costs of lost productivity from TBI victims. Although this is one of the leading health epidemics in the country, there are currently no US Food and Drug Administration–approved treatments. Spinal cord injury (SCI) is considered among the most frequent causes of mortality and morbidity in every medical care system around the world. The incidence of SCI in the United States alone is estimated to be 11,000 new cases each year, affecting a total of 183,000 to 230,000 individuals.[3] There are ~900 to 1000 cases per million in the general population.[4]

TBI and SCI often result in permanent neurological damage due to the fact that neurons lack regenerative ability. After the initial injury occurs, many destructive processes cause secondary injury, such as edema and intracranial hemorrhages, resulting in more cell death and spreading tissue loss. Many studies have sought to find a way to enhance neuroprotective devices and find a mechanism that allows for neuronal cell regeneration.[5,6] Studies have demonstrated the benefits of mild to moderate hypothermia in animal models of TBI and SCI.[7] Stem cell–based treatment has been applied to experimental SCI models and has shown promising results.[8]

Genomics and proteomics could be very helpful in identifying specific proteins that are involved in such regeneration for the benefit of patients of TBI and SCI. Genomics and proteomics are powerful, complementary tools that play an important role in the study of neural injury. Over the past few years advances in the fields of neuroproteomics and neurogenomics have led to the discovery of many candidate biomarkers to help identify the mechanism of TBI. Identification of these biomarkers could lead to a more cost-effective and more time-efficient way to diagnose brain injury than the current techniques, such as magnetic resonance imaging (MRI) and computed tomographic (CT) scans. The expanding field of neuroproteomics gives a broader view of protein dynamics in TBI and SCI. Several studies have demonstrated the role of proteomics[1,9] and genomics[10,11] in providing significant insight into changes, modifications, and functions in certain proteins post-TBI. Proteomic approaches have been applied to studying rat models to identify novel proteins following SCI.[11,12] A study by Kunz and colleagues used proteomics methods to identify novel proteins associated with chronic pain in SCI.[13] Understanding the mechanism behind cell regeneration after SCI has been the aim of several studies.[9,14] Genomics studies using microarray technologies include genome-based expression profiling in SCI rat models.[15] Different neuroproteomic methods and protocols have been described in a book coedited by Ottens and Wang,[16] including a two-dimensional (2-D) gel electrophoresis-based proteomic approach to study the proteome and phosphoproteome of the rat spinal cord lesion epicenter at 24 hours after spinal cord contusion.[17]

■ Gene Expression Profiling of Experimental Traumatic Spinal Cord Injury

SCI elicits complex sequelae of destructive and neuroprotective cellular cascades. The alteration in transcription of the molecular events occurring during the post-SCI period holds the key for these cascades. Recent technological developments provide the ability to analyze changes in gene expression across tens to thousands of transcripts on the same tissue sample. Thus it provides a unique opportunity to take gene expression pattern profiles out of the specific SCI system under study and relate them to general CNS neuronal injury.

There are several different technologies used for the simultaneous study of multiplex gene expression, including DNA microarrays, serial analysis of gene expression, Northern blot, nuclease protection assay (NPA), subtractive hybridization, and real-time reverse transcriptase-polymerase chain reaction (RT-PCR).[18]

Recently, mRNA differential profiles after SCI have been extensively performed to provide better understanding of the pathophysiology and formulation of a rational approach to treatment design after SCI.[19] However, due to the different SCI experimental designs, such as SCI injury paradigm, animal strains, and differing magnitude, injury site, and data analysis, direct comparisons of results across different groups are yet to be fully appreciated when one is trying to generate a global picture of transcriptional regulation following SCI.[20]

The most common animal model used for SCI study is contusive SCI. Studies have examined the transcription changes over extended periods of time, ranging from hours to months after injury (**Table 53.1**). Considering the life span differences between rodents and human beings, we summarized the data into three categories: acute, subacute, and chronic phase post-SCI.

Genes involved in inflammation, immune cell recruitment, and extravasation are highly upregulated during the acute phase postinjury. Transcriptional changes in inflammation-related molecules, such as cyclooxygenase 2 (COX2), levels of proinflammatory cytokines, such as interleukins (IL-1a, IL-1b, IL-4R, and IL-2Ra) and tumor necrosis factor (TNF)-α, are increased at early time points between 30 minutes and 6 hours post-SCI. This is followed by interstitial cell adhesion molecule (ICAM) and e- and p-selectin expression, which further recruit inflammatory cells to the injured sites, initiating secondary cytokine and inflammation signaling, such as IL-6, Fcg receptors (FcgRII and III) and classical complement (C1qb). Immediate early and cell cycle genes (cyclin D1, gadd45, krox24, NGF1-B); Scya2 or monocyte chemoattractant protein-1 (MCP-1); transcription factors, in particular those involved in cell damage and death, such as NF-κB, c-jun; suppressor of cytokine signaling 3 (SOCS-3), hsp70 and Bax, are upregulated in the epicenter samples post-SCI. Also, strong Janus kinase (JAK) and signal transducer and activator of transcription (STAT) activation might, however, represent an early attempt of the SCI repair and regeneration.[20–22]

Another common finding at early transcriptional changes after SCI is the downregulation of ion channels and transport involved in cell excitability, such as *N*-methyl-D-aspartate (NMDA) receptor, glutamate transporter, and potassium ion channel, which are followed by cytoskeletal protein loss, such as neurofilament L and H (NFL, NFH), tau, and microtubule associated protein 2 (MAP-2). The spectrum of these gene expression changes reflects the initial tissue loss after SCI.[23]

Table 53.1 Microarray Studies of Experimental Traumatic Spinal Cord Injury Indicating Injury Type and Level, Sex and Animal Model Used, Region Examined, and Time Point Analysis

Injury type	Injury level	Animal species	Sex of animals	Regions examined	Time points	Reference
OSU contusion	T8,	Rat (Fisher)	F	Epicenter, rostral, caudal	3 h, 24 h, 7 d, 35 d	Aimone et al., 2004[31]
Weight drop	T10-11	Rat (SD)	M	Epicenter, rostral, caudal	4 h, 24 h, 7 d	De Biase et al., 2005[20]
MASCIS	C4-5	Rat (SD)	F	Epicenter	1, 3, 10, 30, 90 d	Velardo et al., 2004[22]
MASCIS	T9	Rat	F	Epicenter	3 h, 24 h,	Song et al., 2001[18]
MASCIS	T9-10	Rat (Long-Evans)	F/M	Epicenter, caudal	6 h, 12 h, 24 h, 48 h	Carnel et al., 2001[57]
Weight drop	T8-9	Rat (SD)	M	epicenter	0.5 h, 4 h, 24 h, 7 d	Di Giovanni et al., 2003[58]

Abbreviations: MASCIS, Multicenter Animal Spinal Cord Injury Study; OSU, Ohio State University; SD, Sprague-Dawley.

After 24 hours postinjury, growth-associated molecules and growth factors start to be expressed, showing an attempt of the lesioned central nervous system (CNS) to regenerate and regrow. At 24 hours, a number of proteins have been shown to be upregulated, including nerve growth factor (NGF), brain-derived neurotrophic factor (BDNF), platelet-derived growth factor (PDGF), bone-morphogentic proteins (BMP), motor neuron-survival factor and fibroblast-growth-factor (FGF) receptor 1, insulin-like growth factor (IGF-I and II) and receptor, molecules possibly invovled in neuritogenesis (dynamin and attractin), and vascular adhesion molecules (VCAM).[24]

During the subacute period postinjury, the overall pattern of gene expression changes dramatically from damage-dominant transcriptional profile to one of active repair involving cellular proliferation and migration, which includes cell cycle genes (cyclin A2, cyclin G1, cell division cycle G25, oncogenes) and associated cytoskeletal and signal transcripts. These growth-promoting transcripts, such as c-myc, v-jun, and c-fos, are initiators of cell-cycle activity and protein synthesis and are followed at day 3 by large increase in transcripts coding for cellular division and the translational apparatus. A subset of growth factor gene families includes IGF, activin, follostatin, thyroid and steroid hormones, transforming growth factor b (TGFb), and those that moderate downstream growth factor signaling are substantially increased following SCI. Downregulation of neurotransmitter receptor, transporter, and synaptic molecules continues, such as NMDA receptor (NMDAR), glutamate receptor, rab3, and SNAP-25A, and contributes to secondary tissue damage.[22,24–26]

Several studies have investigated gene expression changes occurring in the chronic phase following SCI. The gene families expressed after 7 days postinjury are devoted to tissue repair and partial restoration of neural injury. Two categories are used according to the functional states of molecules after spinal injury. One group of genes is upregulated at chronic phase postinjury. These genes signify repair-directed transcript expression, which include matrix and blood vessel remodeling, antioxidant action, and blood–spinal cord barrier reestablishment. Gene families devoted to the regulation of angiogenesis and formation of tight junctions, including ICAM, P-selectin, VCAM-1, integrin ß-4, glypican-3, vitronectin, F-spondin, heparin sulfate proteoglycan core protein, tenasin-x, Apo-E, and angiopoietin-2, are upregulated following SCI. Other transcripts, such as angiopoietin and pleiotrophin, IGF, BMP4 and 6 are also detected upregulated.[22,27]

Glutathione S-transferase, a known blood–spinal cord barrier marker, and glial fibrillary acidic protein (GFAP) continue to increase as late as 42 days after injury, suggesting blood–spinal cord barrier reconstruction. The genes for the reactive oxygen species (ROS) scavengers metallothionein 1 and II (MTI and II) and genes associated with pathways that induce MTI and II were robustly upregulated in the epicenter samples at 3 hours, 7 days, and 35 days.[28,29] Structural protein vimentin, heme metabolism HO-1/HSP32, chaperon HSP27, transcriptor silencer factor-B, EGR1 (Krox-24), and osteopontin were observed to be upregulated in the acute phase and at 42 days.[30]

Expression of cathepsins B, C, D, K, and L was reported upregulated in the epicenter at 35 days and even longer at 42 days.[30,31] In contrast, it has been reported that cathepsin B and D are involved in the degradation of serum amyloid A, which causes amyloid plaque in Alzheimer disease. The long-term increased expression of genes coding for cathepsin proteases may coordinate with modulation of the neurodegeneration.[32]

The upregulation of transcripts associated with neurodegeneration, such as synucleins, prion protein, amyloid precursor protein binding protein-1, and neurodegeneration-associated protein-1, at 30 to 90 days postinjury strongly supports the neurodegeneration process during the chronic period after SCI.[22,32]

Another group of altered genes during the chronic phase belongs to a family that decreases in expression immediately after injury and slowly returns to normal transcript levels at a later time. This group of genes includes those encoding neurotransmitter receptors (NMDAR, glutamate receptor), transporters [glycine transporter 1, gamma aminobutyric acid (GABA) transport proteins], ion pumps (Ca^{2+}-ATPase, Na^{+}/K^{+}-ATPase), and synaptic proteins (synapsin I and II, syntaxin 2, synaptobrevin 2, synaptotagmin, synaptophysin, and SNAP25A).[31,32]

Rather than targeting transcription level, recent technology provides a powerful tool (microRNA array) to reveal the consequences after SCI at the gene regulation level.[33] MicroRNAs (miRNAs) are a recently discovered class of small RNA molecules implicated in a wide range of diverse gene regulation mechanisms. Liu et al. identified three groups of miRNA that correlated the temporal expression postcontusion SCI.[34]

In summary, the development of technology of genes on the chips, it provides tremendous information and unravels the mechanisms underlying SCI to limit secondary damage and promote regeneration and ultimately improve the functional outcome of patients.

Mass Spectrometry–Based Proteomics

Mass spectrometry (MS)-based proteomics workflow applicable to any type of biological sample, whether collected from human, animal, or cell culture models, can be organized into three stages: protein separation, protein identification and quantification, and bioinformatics analysis. Recent research articles describing the use of MS-based proteomics for studying protein expression changes in SCI have been published.[11,12,14,35]

Two-dimensional polyacrylamide gel electrophoresis (2-D-PAGE) has been the classical method of separation, visualization, and analysis of complex mixtures containing thousands of proteins. The first dimension involves isoelectric focusing, which separates proteins by their isoelectric point (pI) on a pH gradient strip. The second dimension resolves the proteins according to molecular weight, using a polyacrylamide gel. The spots are commonly visualized by Coomasie or silver staining methods. Despite the excellent resolving power of 2-D-PAGE, several limitations are present, including low sensitivity and poor reproducibility and the inability to resolve membrane proteins. This is due to their low abundance, high pI, and insolubility in aqueous buffers used in the isoelectric focusing step. Another separation technique relies on the separation by hydrophobicity or by charge where reproducible fractionation and eventually concentration of proteins of interest from the complex protein mixture is achieved. This method is referred to as cation anion exchange/polyacrylamide gel electrophoresis (CAX-PAGE), which is an approach developed in our laboratory that couples ion exchange chromatography for protein fractionation and 1D gel electrophoresis for protein separation, which is followed by MS analysis, as is discussed next.[36–38]

MS relies on the digestion of gel-separated proteins to peptides by sequence-specific proteases, such as trypsin. Tandem MS coupled to liquid chromatography (LC-MSMS) is among the major MS techniques used for proteomics analysis. The major advantage of tandem MS over other proteomics techniques is that it provides amino acid sequence information for the peptides that is more specific for identification of the protein. Tandem MS data are searched against a protein database using bioinformatics software. The peptides are matched to theoretical peptides in the database, and scores of how well the peptides match are generated. The database search output provides a list of identified proteins associated with the peptides. **Figure 53.1** shows an example of a database search report of an excised band from a TBI sample. This illustrates that a single gel band can contain multiple proteins even after protein separation using a multidimensional approach like CAX-PAGE. Correct identification of the proteins depends on correct peptide identification. Another proteomics approach is quantitative pro-

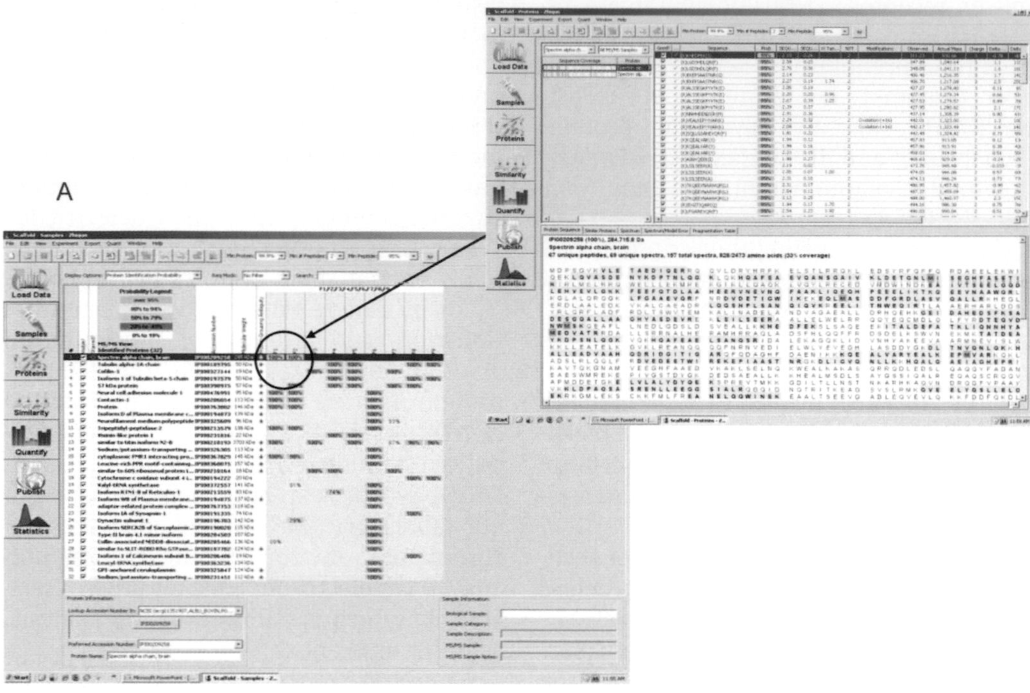

Fig. 53.1 An example of the bioinformatic output of processed tandem mass spectrometry (MSMS) spectra collected from tryptic digests of excised gel bands. **(A)** At the set criteria (protein probability > 99.9% and peptide probability > 95%), several proteins were identified in each sample (band). **(B)** Peptide tandem mass spectra indicated presence of α-spectrin in sample F1.

teomics. Quantitative proteomics provides an accurate picture of the dynamics of protein. Different strategies for quantifying proteins use sample labeling with stable isotopes as well as label-free methods. Label-free quantitative proteomics is an approach of growing interest among researchers. The stable isotope labeling method has been the gold standard in quantitative proteomics. It creates a mass shift to distinguish identical peptides from different samples with a single analysis. Alternative ways of introducing the stable isotopes into the peptides or proteins have been developed. One major labeling approach involves introduction of metabolic precursors with isotope labels in growth media of living cells. The multiplexing introduction of these proteomics techniques in assessing biomarker identification is an ideal approach for high throughput quantitative analysis of complex samples.

Neuroproteomic Analysis of Spinal Cord and Brain Injury

Several neuroproteomic studies have been initiated in the field of neurotrauma with an aim of elucidating CNS injury–specific and sensitive putative biomarkers, as will be described later. In the area of SCI, most studies have utilized spinal cord tissue to assess globally altered proteins in the area of injury due to the nature of injury that is more localized and focused compared with TBI.[12,14,35,39] Kang et al. employed a rat model of SCI that used a microscissor incision surgical procedure to cut the spinal cord between T9 and T10.[12] Tissue from the injured spinal cord was collected after 24 hours for global protein changes by using 2-DE and matrix-assisted laser desorption/ionization-time of flight MS (MALDI-TOF MS). Differential protein expression between normal and traumatic injured spinal cord tissues was compared. Injured spinal cord tissue showed 39 upregulated proteins, which included neurofilament light chain, annexin 5, heat shock protein, tubulin b, peripherin, glial fibrillary acidic protein delta, peroxiredoxin 2, and apolipoprotein A. On the other hand, 21 proteins showed downregulation. Protein alterations were validated using immunohistochemistry and Western blotting techniques. The majority of the modulated proteins in the injured spinal cord tissue belonged to the following major categories: transporters, signal transduction, protein synthesis and processing, metabolism, angiogenesis/circulatory system, apoptosis, cell adhesion and migration, cell cycle, neural function, carcinogenic specific, and DNA-binding protein. Injured spinal cord tissues upregulated neural-specific proteins, including neurofilament, glial fibrillary acidic protein, tubulin a, neurofilament 3, tubulin b, and peripherin. Altered neural-specific proteins were considered most likely to be involved in a wound-healing response coupled with neurogenesis and gliogenesis. With their important findings, the authors did not propose any candidates among the identified proteins to serve as potential SCI markers.

Similarly, in another study, Ding et al. compared a rat thoracic spinal cord transection model with thoracic laminectomy (as a sham control) for global protein changes after 5 days post–spinal injury.[11] In this study, the authors dissolved the analyzed tissue in a sequential-extraction strategy using two different buffers (water soluble and water insoluble); such fractionation facilitates the isolation of insoluble and low-abundance proteins for the 2-D pattern comparative analysis. Comparative analysis utilized 2-DE-MALDI-TOF MS/nano-ESI-MS/MS. Interestingly, the proteins identified were shown to be upregulated, with a total of 30 protein spots. However, the cutoff value for the identified spots was set at 1.5-fold change. Identified proteins were functionally categorized in different groups, such as stress-responsive and metabolic changes, lipid and protein degeneration, neural survival and regeneration. In a recent study by Singh et al., a peripheral nerve injury rat model was performed to study the global expression changes of synaptosome-associated proteins in spinal cord dorsal horn, which can reflect the underlying mechanisms involved in neuropathic pain occurring after SCI.[35] Similar to other studies, 2DE-MALDI-TOF MS was utilized to investigate protein changes. Samples were collected 14 days post–spinal injury and were subjected to proteomic analysis. The 2-DE-MS analysis revealed 27 proteins with differential expression between control and injured samples. These included proteins involved in transmission, cellular metabolism, membrane receptor trafficking, oxidative stress, apoptosis, and degeneration. Interestingly, Western blotting validation reflected differential protein subcellular distribution in dorsal horn cells, which can reflect the dynamics occurring within the different compartments in the injured neurons. Finally, an elegant study by Tsai et al. evaluated the role of acidic fibroblast growth factor (aFGF), a potent neurotrophic factor, after a rat model of SCI.[14] Proteomics and bioinformatics approaches were adapted to investigate changes in the global protein changes of the damaged spinal cord tissue when experimental rats were treated with or without aFGF at 24 hours after injury. It is of note that, after aFGF treatment, injured rats showed significant functional/behavioral recovery accompanied by the downregulation of proteins involved in the process of secondary injury, such as astrocyte activation (glial fibrillary acidic protein), inflammation (S100B), and scar formation (keratan sulfate proteoglycan lumican), which led to the blocking of spinal cord regeneration. These data were validated using reverse transcriptase polymerase chain reaction (RT-PCR), which gives high credibility to the proteomic changes observed after spinal injury. Taken together, these proteomic studies evaluated protein changes in the area of the injury site. Protein analysis was performed at different time points (24 hours, 5 days, 14 days, and 28 days) along with different models of spinal cord injury techniques (spinal transection vs a weight drop method), which makes comparative proteomics analysis between the studies hard to achieve.

On the other hand, TBI studies have utilized body fluids like blood/serum in addition to injured tissue to identify clinical markers that may correlate with the severity of the injury. One of the studies by Burgess et al. evaluated altered differential proteins in normal human postmortem cerebrospinal fluid (CSF) via a modified proteomic approach that combined immunoaffinity depletion of abundant CSF proteins, off-gel electrophoresis, SDS-PAGE and protein identification by LC-MSMS.[40] Postmortem samples were used to mimic the proteolytic damage occurring after brain trauma or neurodegeneration. Of the 229 proteins identified, a total of 172 were not previously described. The findings of this study showed that the use of postmortem CSF (non-TBI samples) to evaluate altered protein levels mimicked the changes occurring in the brain following a traumatic insult. Furthermore, the identification of differential proteins of intracellular origin in the CSF corroborates the suggestion that there is protein leakage into the CSF following brain injury.[41,42] Thus, this method of protein detection might be ideal to identify biomarkers in body fluids to determine the extent and severity of brain injury.

In another study, Siman et al. evaluated CSF for proteins in a rat model of mild/moderate experimental TBI. In their experiments, tau protein fragments of 17 kDa, aII-spectrin breakdown product of 150 kDa (SBDP150), and collapsing response-mediated protein-4 were found to be released as a general response to the brain insult. Other proteins, such as growth associate protein-43 (GAP-43) and 14–3-3z, were suggestive of necrotic neurodegeneration, whereas proteins like aII-spectrin breakdown product of 120 kDa (SBDP120) were suggestive of apoptotic cell death. The presence of the aforementioned proteins in the CSF of mild/moderate experimental brain injury was identified by employing 2-D-PAGE with MALDI-TOF MS analysis. The identified proteins released into the CSF following brain trauma have the potential to be considered surrogate biomarkers and may have the potential for increasing our understanding of brain injury severity.[43]

Finally, in one of the TBI studies from our laboratory, we utilized one-dimensional (1-D)-difference in gel electrophoresis (DIGE) protein separation in series with reversed-phase chromatography tandem MS peptide analysis to discover putative TBI biomarkers in the rat model.[36] Although our protein hits were far-reaching (57 downregulated and 74 upregulated in TBI), limited protein separation confounded the results. For this purpose, our laboratory introduced an offline multidimensional separation platform termed cation-anion exchange chromatography-polyacrylamide gel electrophoresis/reversed phase-tandem mass spectrometry (CAX-PAGE/RPLC-MSMS), which is composed of tandem ion exchange fractionation followed by 1-D-PAGE separation as a novel approach for identifying biomarkers and protein breakdown products (degradomes) (**Fig. 53.2**).[44,45] Our platform, comprising nine sequential steps, is based on the theory that offline separation will enhance the discovery of differential sets of protein markers and avoid some of the limitations encountered in traditional 2-D-PAGE, including limited resolution, mass range, and reproducibility.[44,45] As an application, we employed our CAX/neuroproteomic analysis on cortical samples of rats subjected to controlled cortical impact

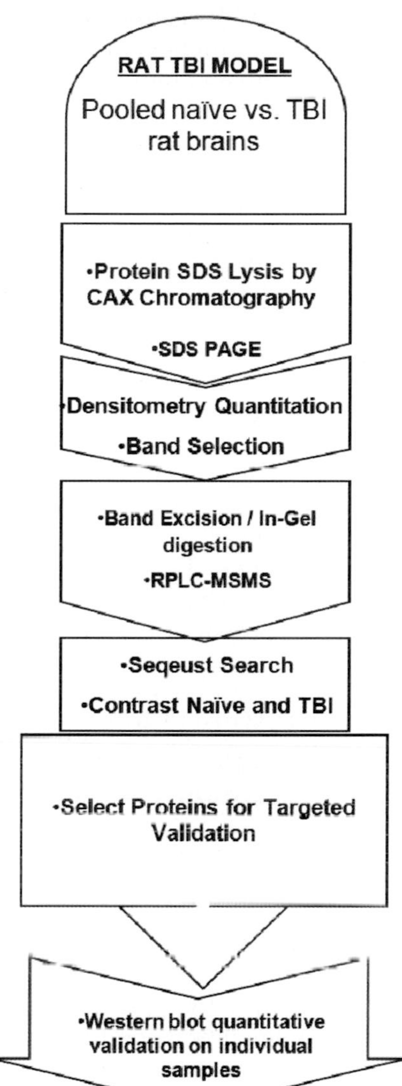

Fig. 53.2 Cation–anion exchange chromatography coupled to one-dimensional chromatography (CAX-PAGE) platform as a novel multidimensional protein separation technique, followed by reversed-phase tandem mass spectrometry coupled to liquid chromatography (LC-MSMS). **(A)** The sequential steps of the CAX-PAGE platform applied to traumatic brain injury samples. **(B)** One dimensional PAGE (ID-PAGE) showing side-by-side runs of naive and injured samples. **(C)** Immunoblotting validation of selected proteins.

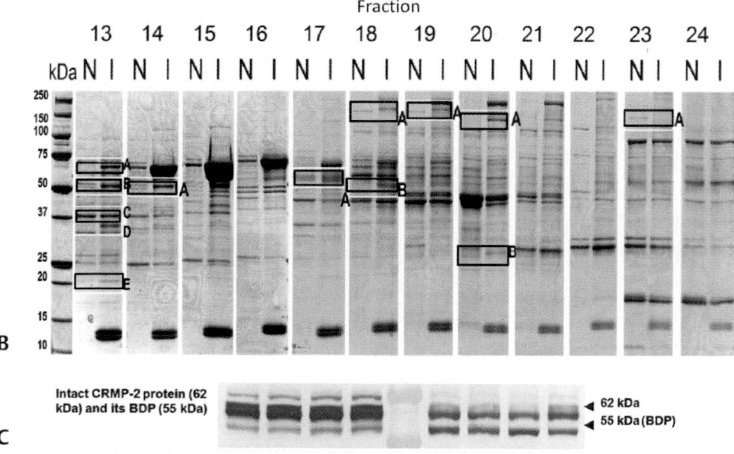

(CCI) experimental TBI (48 hours postinjury). Of interest, our neuroproteomic analysis identified 59 differential protein components, of which 21 decreased and 38 increased in levels after TBI. Among the downregulated proteins are CRMP-2, GAPDH, MAP-2A/2B, and hexokinase. Conversely, C-reactive protein and transferrin were found upregulated. One main advantage of this technique is its ability to elucidate degradomic substrates of different protease systems; thus our data identified the elevated levels of the breakdown products of several proteins, including CRMP-2, synaptotagmin, and aII-spectrin after TBI, as shown in **Fig. 53.2**. Results from this work identified novel protease substrates, such as CRMP-2, synaptotagmin, and aII-spectrin, which provided insight into TBI proteolytic pathways.[45]

■ Antibody-Based Proteomics in Brain Injury

Complementary to mass spectrometry-based proteomic methods, novel proteomic techniques utilizing antibody-based methods have been recently introduced. These techniques have several advantages: probes can provide (1) high specificity and selectivity, (2) better compatibility with complex high-protein-content samples (such as plasma), and (3) rapid confirmation of identified hits. On the other hand, one major disadvantage of an antibody-based method is its inability to identify novel biomarkers not included on the array. One application is the use of high-throughput immunoblotting technology and the antibody panel/arrays, which have been applied in TBI studies. High-throughput immunoblotting (HTPI) technology is a manifold immunoblotting system with 40 useable channels that allows nonlabeled samples to be PAGE-resolved in each lane.[46] In one study from our laboratory, we utilized HTPI to identify a comprehensive set of protease substrates (degradomes) for calpains and caspase-3, which were compared with experimental TBI.[39] In our experiment, we employed 1000 monoclonal antibodies targeting human and rat proteins to compare rat hippocampal lysates from four different treatment groups, namely (1) naive, (2) TBI (48 hours after controlled cortical impact), (3) in vitro calpain digestion, and (4) in vitro caspase-3 digestion. We identified 92 proteins of interest, of which 54 were substrates sensitive to calpain-2 digestion and 38 were sensitive to caspase-3 proteolysis. In addition, 48 protein hits were downregulated, whereas only nine proteins were shown to be upregulated following TBI. The study also revealed an array of novel proteins, such as b-spectrin, synaptotagmin-1, striatin, and synaptojanin-1, as substrates vulnerable to proteolysis following TBI. These findings indicate that these proteins can be studied as potential TBI biomarkers.

■ Neurosystems Biology Analysis and the Field of Central Nervous System Injury

Neurosystems biology, application of systems biology to neuroscience, has been well documented. Neurosystems biology represents a mathematical model capable of predicting the altered processes or functions of a complex system under normal and perturbed conditions. In this regard, neuroproteomics constitutes one key component of neurosystems biology. It discusses the global changes involved in neurological perturbations, integrating the final outcomes into a global functional network map.[47,48] According to Choudhary and Grant, neurosystems biology includes the genome, transcriptome, proteome, organelle and subcellular structures, synapse, cells, circuits, brain, and behavior, as shown in **Fig. 53.3**.[49] The application of neurosystems biology in the field of CNS injury is still in its infancy. Currently, studies have been initiated to decipher the dynamics of proteins and peptides in certain brain regions and quantitatively detect their changes at a subcellular level.

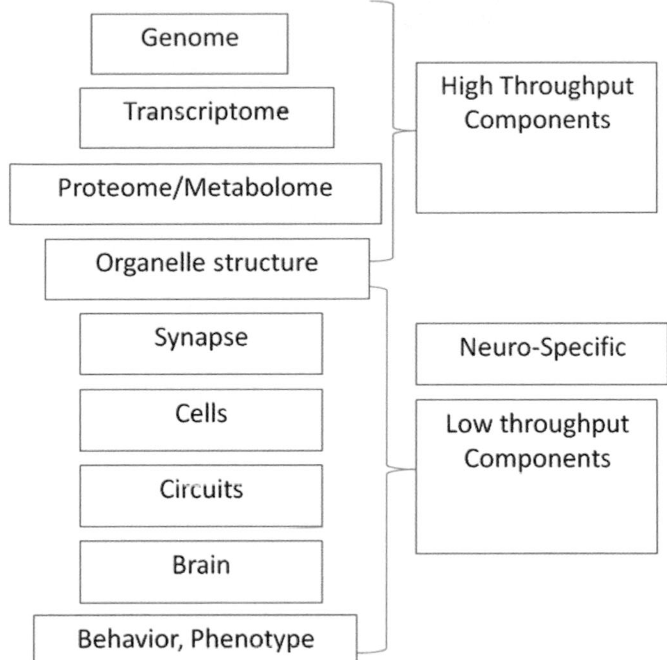

Fig. 53.3 Components of the neurosystems biology. The eight components of neurosystems biology illustrating the available analysis techniques; the first four components are common among other systems biology, the last five are specific to the neuronal system. (Modified from Choudhary and Grant, 2004)[49]

In one study, using nanoLC ESI-Q-TOF MS, peptide expression was characterized with its unique distribution in different brain regions to achieve standardized spatial distribution of these peptides.[50,51] Several synapse studies (synaptosome, synaptic plasma membrane, synaptic vesicles and postsynaptic densities) led to the identification of distinct functional classes of proteins known to be involved with synaptic physiology. Some of these proteins indicate they may have novel functions, and some were found to be without a known function. These types of studies will enable researchers to assess biomarkers related to synaptic pathology, specifically in neuronal injury to elements of the presynaptic terminal and postsynaptic density. In the context of biomarker identification, several studies have looked at genomics and neuroproteomics as a means of achieving a global understanding of how the neural system operates at the normal versus diseased condition.[52–56]

Conclusion

Neural injury, including SCI and brain injury, represents a major national health problem without a US Food and Drug Administration–approved therapy. Recently, the emerging fields of neuroproteomics and neurogenomics have made major advances in the area of neurotrauma research, where several candidate markers have been identified and are being evaluated for their efficacy as biological biomarkers and as tools to identify the underlying mechanism of neuronal injury. The application of neuroproteomics/neurogenomics has revolutionized the characterization of protein/gene dynamics, leading to a greater understanding of postinjury biochemistry. Genomics and proteomics are complementary approaches, and the integration of the datasets from genomic and proteomic experiments through bioinformatics enables generation of useful databases to aid researchers in understanding the mechanism of neural injury.

Pearls

- Designing relevant animal models of experimental neural injury that mimics human (spinal or brain injury) remains a major step toward major advancements in the area of neuroproteomics.
- The level of brain proteome complexity and the potential limitations of neuroproteomic-brain injury–related research necessitate the use of more advanced analytical tools (multidimensional separation techniques, proteomics, genomics, and biochemical testing) for significant breakthroughs in the area of neural injury.
- Recognizing that the field of neurogenomics is still in the developing stage, the full potential of this field remains to be explored and will reveal integral molecular and cellular mechanisms of gene dynamics involved in various nervous system disorders.

Pitfalls

- The current lack of a sensitive tool to assess the severity of SCI can be addressed by the utility of neuroproteomics and neurogenomics through identification of a panel of biomarkers for accurate SCI diagnosis and prognosis.
- The use of neuroproteomics/neurogenomics approach alone is sufficient to elucidate markers of neural injury. The application of neurosystems biology would assist in integrating proteomics and genomics data to generate a global understanding of certain neural biological entities, such as receptors, synapses, or organelle structures.
- The field of neural injury is not limited to brain-related science, but includes other fields, such as bioinformatics, mathematics, and other basic sciences; these are needed to establish comprehensive functional interaction maps on various high-throughput (proteomics and genomics) data, which would be considered the first step toward establishing neurosystems biology.

References

1. Denslow N, Michel ME, Temple MD, Hsu CY, Saatman K, Hayes RL. Application of proteomics technology to the field of neurotrauma. J Neurotrauma 2003;20(5):401–407
2. Pineda JA, Wang KK, Hayes RL. Biomarkers of proteolytic damage following traumatic brain injury. Brain Pathol 2004;14(2):202–209
3. Ehde DM, Gibbons LE, Chwastiak L, Bombardier CH, Sullivan MD, Kraft GH. Chronic pain in a large community sample of persons with multiple sclerosis. Mult Scler 2003;9(6):605–611
4. Ravenscroft A, Ahmed YS, Burnside IG. Chronic pain after SCI. A patient survey. Spinal Cord 2000; 38(10):611–614
5. Tederko P, Krasuski M, Kiwerski J, Nyka I, Białoszewski D. Repair therapies in spinal cord injuries. Ortop Traumatol Rehabil 2009;11(3): 199–208
6. Tederko P, Krasuski M, Kiwerski J, Nyka I, Białoszewski D. Strategies for neuroprotection following spinal cord injury. Ortop Traumatol Rehabil 2009;11(2):103–110
7. Dietrich WD, Bullock MR, Kochanek PM. Hypothermic therapies targeting brain and spinal cord injury. Introduction. J Neurotrauma 2009; 26(3):297–298
8. Ao Q, Wang AJ, Chen GQ, Wang SJ, Zuo HC, Zhang XF. Combined transplantation of neural stem cells and olfactory ensheathing cells for the repair of spinal cord injuries. Med Hypotheses 2007; 69(6):1234–1237
9. Katano T, Mabuchi T, Okuda-Ashitaka E, Inagaki N, Kinumi T, Ito S. Proteomic identification of a novel isoform of collapsin response mediator protein-2 in spinal nerves peripheral to dorsal root ganglia. Proteomics 2006;6(22):6085–6094
10. Redell JB, Liu Y, Dash PK. Traumatic brain injury alters expression of hippocampal microRNAs: potential regulators of multiple pathophysiological processes. J Neurosci Res 2009;87(6): 1435–1448
11. Ding Q, Wu Z, Guo Y, et al. Proteome analysis of up-regulated proteins in the rat spinal cord induced by transection injury. Proteomics 2006;6(2):505–518
12. Kang SK, So HH, Moon YS, Kim CH. Proteomic analysis of injured spinal cord tissue proteins using 2-DE and MALDI-TOF MS. Proteomics 2006;6(9):2797–2812
13. Kunz S, Tegeder I, Coste O, et al. Comparative proteomic analysis of the rat spinal cord in inflammatory and neuropathic pain models. Neurosci Lett 2005;381(3):289–293

14. Tsai MC, Shen LF, Kuo HS, Cheng H, Chak KF. Involvement of acidic fibroblast growth factor in spinal cord injury repair processes revealed by a proteomics approach. Mol Cell Proteomics 2008;7(9):1668–1687
15. Malaspina A, Jokic N, Huang WL, Priestley JV. Comparative analysis of the time-dependent functional and molecular changes in spinal cord degeneration induced by the G93A SOD1 gene mutation and by mechanical compression. BMC Genomics 2008;9:500
16. Ottens AW, Wang KW, eds. Neuroproteomic Methods and Protocols. Methods in Molecular Biology, Vol 566. Dordrecht: Humana Press; 2009
17. Chen A, Springer JE. Neuroproteomic methods in spinal cord injury. Methods Mol Biol 2009; 566:57–67
18. Song G, Cechvala C, Resnick DK, Dempsey RJ, Rao VL. GeneChip analysis after acute spinal cord injury in rat. J Neurochem 2001;79(4):804–815
19. Bauchet L, Lonjon N, Perrin FE, Gilbert C, Privat A, Fattal C. Strategies for spinal cord repair after injury: a review of the literature and information. Ann Phys Rehabil Med 2009;52(4):330–351
20. De Biase A, Knoblach SM, Di Giovanni S, et al. Gene expression profiling of experimental traumatic spinal cord injury as a function of distance from impact site and injury severity. Physiol Genomics 2005;22(3):368–381
21. Tseng LH, Chen I, Lin YH, Liang CC, Lloyd LK. Genome-based expression profiling study following spinal cord injury in the rat: An array of 48-gene model. Neurourol Urodyn 2010;29(8): 1439–1443
22. Velardo MJ, Burger C, Williams PR, et al. Patterns of gene expression reveal a temporally orchestrated wound healing response in the injured spinal cord. J Neurosci 2004;24(39):8562–8576
23. Zhang SX, Underwood M, Landfield A, Huang FF, Gison S, Geddes JW. Cytoskeletal disruption following contusion injury to the rat spinal cord. J Neuropathol Exp Neurol 2000;59(4):287–296
24. Lacroix-Fralish ML, Tawfik VL, Tanga FY, Spratt KF, DeLeo JA. Differential spinal cord gene expression in rodent models of radicular and neuropathic pain. Anesthesiology 2006;104(6):1283–1292
25. Nesic O, Svrakic NM, Xu GY, et al. DNA microarray analysis of the contused spinal cord: effect of NMDA receptor inhibition. J Neurosci Res 2002;68(4):406–423
26. Yang Y, Xie Y, Chai H, et al. Microarray analysis of gene expression patterns in adult spinal motoneurons after different types of axonal injuries. Brain Res 2006;1075(1):1–12
27. Benton MG, Glasser NR, Palecek SP. Deletion of MAG1 and MRE11 enhances the sensitivity of the Saccharomyces cerevisiae HUG1P-GFP promoter-reporter construct to genotoxicity. Biosens Bioelectron 2008;24(4):736–741
28. Urso ML, Chen YW, Scrimgeour AG, Lee PC, Lee KF, Clarkson PM. Alterations in mRNA expression and protein products following spinal cord injury in humans. J Physiol 2007;579(Pt 3):877–892
29. Hashimoto M, Koda M, Ino H, et al. Gene expression profiling of cathepsin D, metallothioneins-1 and -2, osteopontin, and tenascin-C in a mouse spinal cord injury model by cDNA microarray analysis. Acta Neuropathol 2005;109(2):165–180
30. Resnick DK, Schmitt C, Miranpuri GS, Dhodda VK, Isaacson J, Vemuganti R. Molecular evidence of repair and plasticity following spinal cord injury. Neuroreport 2004;15(5):837–839
31. Aimone JB, Leasure JL, Perreau VM, Thallmair M; Christopher Reeve Paralysis Foundation Research Consortium. Spatial and temporal gene expression profiling of the contused rat spinal cord. Exp Neurol 2004;189(2):204–221
32. Bareyre FM, Schwab ME. Inflammation, degeneration and regeneration in the injured spinal cord: insights from DNA microarrays. Trends Neurosci 2003;26(10):555–563
33. Nakanishi K, Nakasa T, Tanaka N, et al. Responses of microRNAs 124a and 223 following spinal cord injury in mice. Spinal Cord 2010;48(3): 192–196
34. Liu NK, Wang XF, Lu QB, Xu XM. Altered microRNA expression following traumatic spinal cord injury. Exp Neurol 2009;219(2):424–429
35. Singh OV, Yaster M, Xu JT, et al. Proteome of synaptosome-associated proteins in spinal cord dorsal horn after peripheral nerve injury. Proteomics 2009;9(5):1241–1253
36. Haskins WE, Kobeissy FH, Wolper RA, et al. Rapid discovery of putative protein biomarkers of traumatic brain injury by SDS-PAGE-capillary liquid chromatography-tandem mass spectrometry. J Neurotrauma 2005;22(6):629–644
37. Ottens AK, Kobeissy FH, Wolper RA, et al. A multidimensional differential proteomic platform using dual-phase ion-exchange chromatography-polyacrylamide gel electrophoresis/reversed-phase liquid chromatography tandem mass spectrometry. Anal Chem 2005;77(15):4836–4845
38. Wang KK, Ottens A, Haskins W, et al. Proteomics studies of traumatic brain injury. Int Rev Neurobiol 2004;61:215–240
39. Abdi F, Quinn JF, Jankovic J, et al. Detection of biomarkers with a multiplex quantitative proteomic platform in cerebrospinal fluid of patients with neurodegenerative disorders. J Alzheimers Dis 2006;9(3):293–348
40. Burgess JA, Lescuyer P, Hainard A, et al. Identification of brain cell death associated proteins in human post-mortem cerebrospinal fluid. J Proteome Res 2006;5(7):1674–1681
41. Dumont D, Noben JP, Raus J, Stinissen P, Robben J. Proteomic analysis of cerebrospinal fluid from multiple sclerosis patients. Proteomics 2004;4(7):2117–2124
42. Hammack BN, Fung KY, Hunsucker SW, et al. Proteomic analysis of multiple sclerosis cerebrospinal fluid. Mult Scler 2004;10(3):245–260
43. Siman R, McIntosh TK, Soltesz KM, Chen Z, Neumar RW, Roberts VL. Proteins released from degenerating neurons are surrogate markers for acute brain damage. Neurobiol Dis 2004;16(2): 311–320
44. Svetlov SI, Xiang Y, Oli MW, et al. Identification and preliminary validation of novel biomarkers of acute hepatic ischaemia/reperfusion injury using dual-platform proteomic/degradomic approaches. Biomarkers 2006;11(4):355–369

45. Kobeissy FH, Ottens AK, Zhang Z, et al. Novel differential neuroproteomics analysis of traumatic brain injury in rats. Mol Cell Proteomics 2006;5(10):1887–1898
46. Ananiadou S, Kell DB, Tsujii J. Text mining and its potential applications in systems biology. Trends Biotechnol 2006;24(12):571–579
47. Grant SG. Systems biology in neuroscience: bridging genes to cognition. Curr Opin Neurobiol 2003;13(5):577–582
48. Grant SG, Blackstock WP. Proteomics in neuroscience: from protein to network. J Neurosci 2001;21(21):8315–8318
49. Choudhary J, Grant SG. Proteomics in postgenomic neuroscience: the end of the beginning. Nat Neurosci 2004;7(5):440–445
50. Svensson M, Sköld K, Svenningsson P, Andren PE. Peptidomics-based discovery of novel neuropeptides. J Proteome Res 2003;2(2):213–219
51. Sköld K, Svensson M, Kaplan A, Björkesten L, Aström J, Andren PE. A neuroproteomic approach to targeting neuropeptides in the brain. Proteomics 2002;2(4):447–454
52. Fornage M, Swank MW, Boerwinkle E, Doris PA. Gene expression profiling and functional proteomic analysis reveal perturbed kinase-mediated signaling in genetic stroke susceptibility. Physiol Genomics 2003;15(1):75–83
53. Lipsky RH, Goldman D. Genomics and variation of ionotropic glutamate receptors. Ann N Y Acad Sci 2003;1003:22–35
54. Lipsky RH, Jiang X, Xu K, et al. Genomics and variation of ionotropic glutamate receptors: implications for neuroplasticity. Amino Acids 2005; 28(2):169–175
55. Rosen MR, Binah O, Marom S. Cardiac memory and cortical memory: do learning patterns in neural networks impact on cardiac arrhythmias? Circulation 2003;108(15):1784–1789
56. Ruff S, Marie N, Celsis P, Cardebat D, Démonet JF. Neural substrates of impaired categorical perception of phonemes in adult dyslexics: an fMRI study. Brain Cogn 2003;53(2):331–334
57. Carmel JB, Galante A, Soteropoulos P, Tolias P, Reece M, Young W, et al. Gene expression profiling of acute spinal cord injury reveals spreading inflammatory signals and neuron loss. Physiol Genomics 2001;7(2):201–213
58. Di Giovanni S, Knoblach SM, Brandoli C, Aden SA, Hoffman EP, Faden AI. Gene profiling in spinal cord injury shows role of cell cycle in neuron death. Ann Neurol 2003;53(4):454–468

54

Breakthroughs of the Last Twenty Years

Kevin Chao, Terry C. Burns, Maxwell Boakye, and Michael G. Fehlings

Over the last 20 years there have been numerous breakthroughs in the evaluation and management of spinal cord injury (SCI). This chapter discusses ten of the most significant breakthroughs of the last 20 years (**Fig. 54.1**). The ten advances span seven key areas, with stem cells currently being the most heavily investigated (**Fig. 54.2**). The ten areas may also be classified into four major themes: repair, neurorestoration, medical management, and surgical management (**Fig. 54.3**). The ten breakthroughs are not presented in order of importance. Most of the breakthroughs are covered in detail in several chapters in the book, but they are presented here to highlight their importance and to present an overview in a single chapter. The reader is referred to appropriate sections of the book for further details.

■ Neuroprotection

On average, each mammalian neuron is synaptically connected to 5000 other neurons. Although much attention in recent years has been given to neuroregeneration, including cell replacement and axonal regeneration, the challenges associated with such attempted "rewiring" must not be underestimated. The critical first task in maximizing functional outcome after SCI is preservation of existing circuitry. Fortunately, most SCIs represent contusion rather than transection, and much of the damage is due to secondary cell death, presenting opportunities for meaningful intervention. To this end, enormous gains have been made in the past 20 years in understanding inflammation, excitotoxicity, and free radical effects, as well as apoptotic and neurotrophic pathways (see Chapter 4 for further discussion of pathophysiology).

Minocycline is a tetracycline analogue that has been found to mitigate injury in animal models of SCI. Its efficacy is likely due in part to simultaneous disruption of apoptotic pathways via inhibition of mitochondrial cytochrome c, as well as downregulation of multiple inflammatory mediators and microglial activation.[1,2] Findings of improved functional outcomes obtained from preclinical studies of SCI in multiple laboratories and multiple species[1,3] prompted initiation (in 2004) of a prospective randomized phase 1/2 trial in Calgary (scheduled for completion in 2010). A separate trial employing minocycline in combination with the immunosuppressant tacrolimus is reportedly in progress in Saudi Arabia.[3]

Riluzole is a sodium channel blocker that additionally inhibits presynaptic calcium channels, thereby blocking glutamate-mediated excitotoxicity after central nervous system (CNS) injury. It has been in use for amyotrophic lateral sclerosis (ALS) since 1997 and was shown in a recent Cochrane meta-analysis to prolong survival by 2 to 3 months.[4] Improved recovery of function with riluzole has been observed in animal

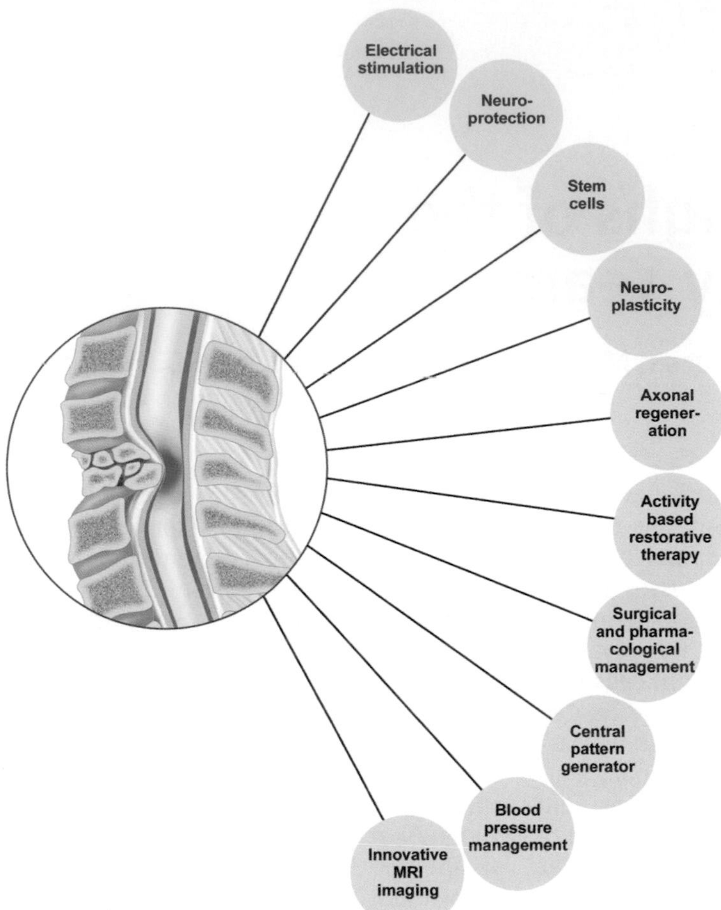

Fig. 54.1 Ten major breakthroughs in spinal cord Injury research and management in the last 20 years.

models of SCI since 1996.[3] A phase 1 clinical trial for acute SCI is being undertaken by the North American Clinical Trials Network (NACTN). Plans are under way, based on the outcomes of this study, to undertake a phase 2/3 randomized, controlled trial with riluzole.

Clinical trials have also been undertaken with other putative neuroprotective agents, including GM-1, TRH, gacyclidine, nimodipine, and naloxone. However, due to failure to meet primary end points in admittedly often-underpowered clinical studies, these drugs are no longer under active clinical development for SCI.[3] Lessons from these trials, including the importance of adequate power and selection of appropriate outcome measures, among other details of trial design, will help to improve the quality of ongoing and upcoming trials. At this time, a surplus of candidate neuroprotective agents, including a variety of multifunctional cytokines, such as VEGF, GDNF, nerve growth factor (NGF), EPO, brain-derived neurotrophic factor (BDNF), and neurotrophin-3 (NT-3), have each shown benefit in animal models of SCI and, together with strategies to promote remyelination, neurite outgrowth, and synaptic plasticity, offer significant hope for the future ability to ameliorate SCI-associated deficits.[5–7] As noted elsewhere, multimodal interventions targeting several pathways in the degenerative and regenerative processes may offer

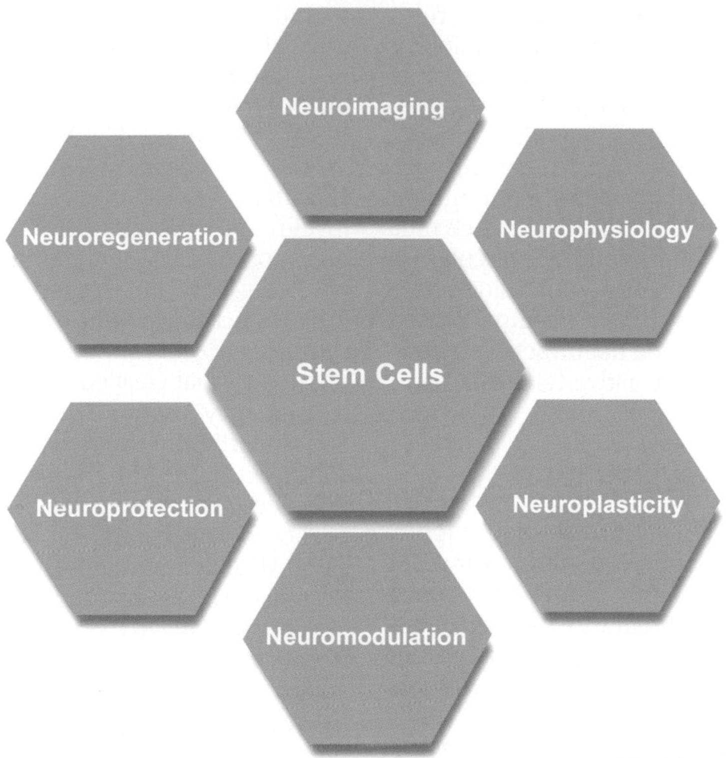

Fig. 54.2 These breakthroughs span seven main research areas: neuroimaging, neurophysiology, neuromodulation, neuroplasticity, neuroregeneration, neuroprotection, and stem cells, which are currently the center of attention.

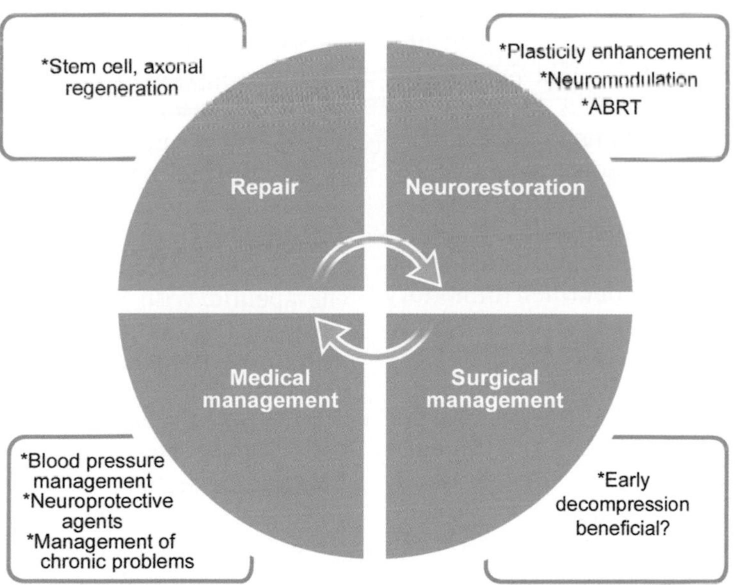

Fig. 54.3 Ten major breakthroughts, spanning seven main research areas (neuroimaging, neurophysiology, neuromodulation, neuroplasticity, neuroregeneration, neuroprotection, and stem cells, which are the center of attention now) have occurred in SCI research and management in the last twenty years. The breakthroughs can be classified into four thematic areas: repair, neurorestoration, medical management, and surgical management.

the greatest likelihood of achieving functional recovery. Pharmacological inhibition of a single apoptotic pathway, for example, may leave cells vulnerable to death via alternate apoptotic or nonapoptotic pathways. By contrast, interventions to concurrently modulate the inflammatory environment, provide trophic support, enhance free radical scavenging, and promote revascularization may, in combination with a blockade of cell death pathways, yield maximal preservation of neurons and fiber tracts for subsequent remyelination and outgrowth.

■ Axonal Regeneration

CNS neurons of certain fish and amphibians are capable of regeneration. However, regeneration of adult mammalian axons is restricted essentially to the peripheral nervous system. Although some limited sprouting of rodent CNS axons was observed by Ramon y Cajal in the 1920s, facilitated by transplants of peripheral nerve,[8] it was not until Richardson et al. demonstrated projection of labeled spinal axons across a 10 mm sciatic nerve graft in 1980[9] that the regenerative capacity of at least some CNS axons was given serious consideration. Thus began a fruitful search for factors that might explain the reluctance of CNS neurons to regenerate in their native environment. Caroni et al. in the late 1980s demonstrated that the myelin membrane of oligodendrocytes is inhibitory to axonal growth.[10,11] A monoclonal antibody was developed that could block the action of identified inhibitory fractions from myelin in vitro.[12] Administered in vivo, this antibody led to improved functional performance in spinal cord–lesioned rodents.[13] Ultimately, the antibody was used to isolate and sequence its target antigen, which was subsequently termed Nogo-A.[14] Interestingly, Nogo-A knockout animals showed less consistent regeneration than did wild-type animals treated with Nogo antibodies, suggesting increased inhibition via compensatory pathways.[15] A growing list of other myelin-associated factors, components of the glial scar that forms after injury, now exists, each of which has been shown to inhibit neuronal growth cones in vitro. Examples include chondroitin sulfate proteoglycans (CSPGs), a family of inhibitory molecules in the glial scar, myelin-associated glycoprotein (MAG), and oligodendrocyte myelin glycoprotein (OMG).[16] Enzymatic digestion of CSPG via chondroitinase ABC has been shown to ameliorate growth cone inhibition, though failure of impaired CSPG synthesis to yield similar results raises the possibility that cleaved glycoaminoglycans (GAGs) may promote neurite outgrowth and underlie the improvements seen with chondroitinase ABC.[15] In 2006, Novartis initiated a multicenter open-label phase 1 trial of intrathecal infusion of various doses of ATI355, a humanized Nogo antibody. Results of the anticipated 51 patients were expected in late 2010, but as of this writing they have not been published.

Analysis of the signal transduction pathways of growth-cone inhibitory compounds has revealed that all such identified compounds act via activation of the guanosine triphosphatase Rho, which in turn is activated by, and binds to, Rho kinase (ROCK).[16] ROCK regulates actin cytoskeleton, and, thereby, growth cone dynamics. McKerracher and Higuchi identified a specific inhibitor of Rho called C3 transferase, produced by *Clostridium botulinum*, which acts at the final common pathway of growth cone regulation[17] and has been shown to promote axonal regeneration and functional recovery in murine SCI.[18] Clinical trials have been initiated by BioAxone Therapeutic, with BA-210, a recombinant version of the C3 transferase with improved membrane permeability. This compound (Cethrin, Alseres Pharmaceuticals, Inc., Hopkinton, MA) was administered epidurally within 7 days of injury during spinal stabilization surgery, in combination with fibrin sealant as a delivery vehicle. Results of the open-label phase 1/2a trial, wherein 27% conversion was observed from American Spinal Injury Association (ASIA) grade A to grade B, C, or D, have prompted efforts to translate this into a phase 2/3 randomized, controlled trial.[3]

The low endogenous levels of adult neurite outgrowth likely represent a mechanism to preserve complex circuitry in higher organisms, thus therapeutic reversal of this stability may open the door for certain unintended effects on sensorimotor function. Moreover, much remains to be learned regarding optimal timing of growth-cone-promoting therapies, as well as the functionality, activity-dependence, and consolidation of any new synaptic connections.[19] Nevertheless, ample proof of principle suggests axonal regeneration is likely to be a fundamental contributor to functional regeneration following SCI and may ideally provide critical substrate for neural plasticity, including regulation of central pattern generators (CPGs).

■ Stem Cell Therapy and Cellular Transplantation

Although stem cells have been subject to extraordinarily high expectations, founded more on media hype than on scientific data points, they remain among the most versatile and promising potential therapies for SCI. While neurons from both embryonic and neural stem cells (NSCs) have been shown to survive and form synaptic connections in vivo,[20,21] functional benefits in SCI after transplantation of NSCs, MSCs, and other stem or progenitor cells are likely to be attributable in large part to their supportive properties. CNS and bone-marrow-derived stem cells may migrate to the region of injury, modulate inflammation, promote angiogenesis, promote neurite outgrowth, and enhance synaptic plasticity.[22] Mechanisms underlying these actions remain incompletely elucidated; however, secretion of a diverse array of neuroprotective compounds has been observed.

NSCs are known to exist in the hippocampus and forebrain subventricular zone throughout life. However, numerous groups have additionally reported isolation of NSCs from spinal cord. The exact etiology of such cells is controversial; whereas some argue a latent subventricular zone NSC population exists throughout the neuraxis,[23] findings that oligodendrocyte progenitor cells may dedifferentiate into NSCs under in vitro conditions challenge the assumption that NSCs necessarily exist as such in the spinal cord.[24] Several attempts have been made to mobilize endogenous stem or progenitor cells via genetic manipulation and infusion of cytokines[25]; however, a neurogenic response has largely been minimal, and functional consequences may likely be attributable to the treatment itself rather than any new neurons that might be generated as a result.[26] Endogenous bone marrow mononuclear cells, including macrophages, are mobilized to the site of CNS injury and have been found to be responsible for significant spontaneous recovery.[27] Amplification of this response via administration of GCSF[28] or even direct transplantation of autologous macrophages has also been shown to yield marked benefit. Transplantation of autologous macrophages at the time of spinal stabilization surgery has been investigated in an open-label phase 1 clinical trial by Procord.[29] ASIA score improvement was noted in five of 16 enrolled patients and a phase 2 study was initiated. Benefits from macrophages may be attributable to secretion of prosurvival cytokines and enhanced phagocytosis of potentially harmful injury-associated debris. T cell-based vaccination is based similarly on the principle of timely removal of harmful degradation products as well as provision of growth factors.[30] The phase 2 Procord study was halted prematurely due to financial challenges experienced by the sponsoring company.

Secondary neuronal death after SCI may be due in part to demyelination. Oligodendrocyte precursor cells (OPCs) from hESCs have been shown to spontaneously remyelinate congenitally myelin-deficient mice. Functional recovery in rats with SCI after hESC-derived OPC transplantation has been robust, and Geron was granted US Food and Drug Administration (FDA) approval for a clinical trial in early 2009.[31] The first patients have now been enrolled in the trial. Given the capacity of hESCs to form teratomas, careful attention is appropriately being paid to preclinical safety studies; the trial is currently on hold during investigation of small cysts observed in transplanted animals at later time points. Used in appropriate combinations with other trials, stem cells may have the capacity to mediate significant functional benefits. A recent open-label trial for chronic SCI by Moviglia employed a sequential combination of intraarterial bone marrow mononuclear cells to improve angiogenesis followed by T cell therapy and finally by infusion of autologous NSCs. Although results remain to be replicated by other groups or validated via a randomized double-blind placebo-controlled trial, five of eight treated patients evolved from ASIA A to ASIA D, regaining at least some capacity for ambulation.[31]

Plasticity

The breakthrough here is the realization that significant plasticity and reorganization occur in the neuraxis after SCI. Transcranial magnetic stimulation and functional magnetic resonance imaging studies have provided evidence of significant plasticity in the sensorimotor cortex after SCI (see Chapter 46 for review). This involves activation of new areas and displacements of activation maxima. This plasticity is dynamic and evolves with time. There is also evidence that significant plasticity accompanies training and rehabilitation.[32,33] Clinical implications are unclear at the present time, but the extent and pattern of plasticity may be used as potential markers of recovery. There is significant rewiring of circuits after partial lesions. There is a modest regrowth of axons and a rewiring of circuits so that the cortex can reach the spinal cord through different circuits (via reticulospinal or propriospinal circuits). In that context, the implication of propriospinal pathways has become important.[34–36]

An area of plasticity research involves attempts to modulate spinal cord plasticity to improve recovery. This area of research is in its infancy and involves modulation of the Hoffmann reflex (H-reflex) and other spinal reflexes, such as reciprocal inhibition, to improve recovery.[37–39]

Techniques for understanding plasticity and development of new plasticity-enhancing techniques, such as paired association stimulation, prolonged somatosensory stimulation, theta burst stimulation, transcranial direct current stimulation and repetitive transcranial stimulation, represent breakthroughs that are likely to lead to greater enhancement of plasticity and a greater understanding of the relationship between plasticity and recovery.[40–48]

Central Pattern Generator

The breakthrough here was the establishment of the role of the CPG in neurological recovery after SCI. The notion of the CPG is unique and refers to the ability of spinal circuitry to generate an organized rhythmic activity all by itself (of course normally under the control of descending commands and afferents).[49] The activity of the CPG is rhythmic, automatic, activated by neurotransmitter or proprioceptive information (e.g., from activity-based training). It can also be activated by pharmacology or electrical stimulation. It is under supraspinal control and can undergo plasticity during training. Significant evidence now exists implicating the CPG in the recovery of locomotion after partial spinal lesions.[50,51] There is increasing evidence for a human CPG.[52–56] The role of the human CPG in SCI is discussed in detail in Chapter 49.

Activity-Based Restorative Therapy

The breakthrough here is the increasing evidence that recovery can be achieved by specific activity-based therapies and the notion that plasticity of spinal circuits is activity dependent. This represents a significant departure from previous rehabilitation philosophies that focused more on development of compensatory strategies. Repetitive practice using task-specific sensory input can engage key spinal locomotor networks and improve recovery.[57] Potential mechanisms include increased gene expression, synaptogenesis, increased reorganization, and repair along the neural axis and engagement of the CPG. Physiological benefits include optimization of cardiovascular functioning and musculoskeletal restoration, including increase in bone mineral density, muscle strength, and tone.[58] Locomotor training is probably the most well known activity-based therapy and has been shown to increase supraspinal plasticity.[32,33] Great interest in human locomotor studies followed the observation that cats with complete transections of the spinal cord recovered locomotor stepping response after intense treadmill training involving partial body weight support and optimization of assistance during stance cycle. Subsequently, several locomotor training regimens have been investigated, including manual and robotic body weight support treadmill training (BWSTT) and functional electrical stimulation augmented ergometry and training methods. The roles in rehabilitation are discussed in detail in the sections on plasticity and rehabilitation (see Chapters 48, 49, and 50).

Management of Blood Pressure

The significant breakthrough here was the realization of the importance of vascular changes in the injured spinal cord with resultant loss of autoregulation and ischemia.[59] This basic science knowledge has been translated into the clinical recognition of the importance of blood pressure management in the prevention of secondary injury after acute SCI. Significant evidence has accumulated regarding benefits of close monitoring and aggressive maintenance of blood pressure after significant injury.[60–62] An extensive evidence-based guideline recommends avoidance of systolic blood pressure < 90 mmHg or corrected as soon as possible and maintenance of mean arterial pressure at 85 to 90 mmHg during the first 7 days after SCI.[63,64] The lack of clinically relevant methods to directly measure spinal cord blood flow remains an ongoing challenge and represents an opportunity for innovation. These are discussed in more detail in Chapter 9.

Development of Diffusion Tensor Imaging

The breakthrough here is the development of imaging technology with the potential to visualize preserved white matter pathways in SCI. This will likely revolutionalize the classification of SCIs based on direct visualization of anatomical tracts. The ASIA scale and motor scores, as well as magnetic resonance imaging (MRI) parameters like the presence of hematoma, have proven valuable in predicting recovery. However, both the ASIA scale and MRI are unable to identify potentially salvageable white matter tracts. This disadvantage will be overcome by diffusion tensor imaging (DTI). DTI also provides quantitative markers of injury, such as the fractional anisotropy and apparent diffusion coefficient, that may become important surrogate markers of recovery (see Chapter 46 for further discussion).

Functional Electrical Stimulation

Despite major advances in our understanding of neuroregenerative processes, effective regeneration therapy for people with SCI remains elusive. In fact, the improved quality of life, function, and life expectancy after SCI have risen largely from work in specialized SCI medical care and comprehensive rehabilitation. Many medical complications associated with SCI are now preventable or managed more efficiently—thromboembolic disease, pressure ulcers, respiratory insufficiency, male sexual dysfunction, constipation, and renal failure, to name a few. In the absence of a cure for the site of injury, we have sought ways to overcome specific deficits created by SCI—functional electrical stimulation (FES) is the epitome of such endeavors.

FES, once merely a sci-fi fantasy, has been enabled by achievements in electronics, microprocessing, neuroscience, and rehabilitation. FES systems now allow certain people with SCI to reclaim meaningful use of their hands, to stand, or to take steps. Some have regained some control of bladder and bowel evacuation,[65] others the ability to overcome male sexual dysfunction. Beyond enabling specific motor functions, FES has been shown to increase muscle bulk, improve cardiovascular performance, prevent pressure ulcers, treat osteoporosis and contractures, control spasticity, and improve depression.[66,67]

The majority of FES systems work by direction stimulation of a peripheral nerve. The energy required to activate muscle contraction via direct muscle fiber stimulation is roughly 100 times that of nerve stimulation—too unsafe to be applied multiple times. The main components of FES systems are basically the same—a power source, command processor, stimulator, lead wires, electrodes, and sensors. Delivery of the stimulation is through a variable number of lead wires to either surface, percutaneous, or implanted electrodes. An external control unit typically houses the power source (batteries), receives information from the user and sensors, and transforms this information into commands that are sent to the stimulator for a specific motor end effect. In open loop control programs, a stimulation results in a specific function (e.g., knee extension) without autocorrection through processing of feedback sensor information. Closed loop programs incorporate information on muscle force and joint motion from sensors and modify the output stimulation accordingly for more complex functions (e.g., taking a step).

Surface systems are inexpensive and can be safely placed in the clinic, but accurate placement is difficult, and stimulation often lacks specificity, can be painful, and can be cosmetically unacceptable. Surface systems are best for diagnostics and short-term therapeutic use. Percutaneous leads are often used temporarily for muscle conditioning. They are easier to place accurately than surface electrodes, but long-term use carries the risk of infection and granuloma formation. In implanted FES systems, the electrodes, lead wires, and stimulators are internalized while the control unit and battery are external—they communicate through radio frequency telemetry. Unfortunately, no implantable battery today can meet the energy demand of a multichannel FES system.

Naturally, the lower motor neuron (LMN) must be intact for an FES system to work. Other criteria for effective application of FES include the following: (1) the strength of muscle contraction must be forceful, controllable, and repeatable; (2) neural structures must not be damaged by the stimulus; and (3) the method of stimulus delivery must be acceptable to the patient and not be unbearably painful. Several FES systems have been approved by the FDA; a select few are available only in Europe or Japan.

Cervical SCI patients with preserved C7 and C8 segments or higher benefit most from upper limb FES systems, given that hand grasp, hold, and release may be restored. Significant spasticity or joint contractures make meaningful use of the hand or arm difficult. Current systems provide some patients the ability to hold and release larger objects like bottles and cans, or even to use finer items like keys.

For lower limb function, FES currently enables SCI patients to stand and perform limited transfers, but no system allows for functional walking. In many ways, locomotion is far more complex than it may seem—beyond the loss of large muscles in the lower extremities, most patients with SCI lose proprioceptive feedback as well as control of trunk muscles for maintaining erect posture and balance. Technology limitations include high energy expenditure (due to inadequate efficient coordination of muscle activation), heavy batteries, unreliable hardware, and reliance on visual feedback, among others. FES systems will not replace wheelchairs as the main means of mobility for SCI patients in the foreseeable future.

Direct stimulation of the phrenic nerve (i.e., electrophrenic respiration or EPR) either in the cervical or thoracic region allows for some high cervical SCI patients to become independent of ventilatory support.[68] Because spontaneous recovery of diaphragm function sometimes occurs even a year after initial injury, people generally wait 4 to 6 months before EPR is considered. The diaphragm often suffers from disuse atrophy, thus commonly 2 to 3 months of diaphragm reconditioning must occur after implantation for complete independence from a ventilator. With adequate teaching, reconditioning, and support, respiratory complications from EPR are equivalent to the current standard and afford patients dramatically improved quality of life.

Regular bladder catheterization has dramatically reduced morbidity and mortality from urinary retention in SCI patients. Sacral anterior root stimulation for bladder control has been reported since the 1970s. Refinement of this approach led to development of the Finetech-Brindley bladder system (formerly marketed as "Vocare" in the United States), which has been shown to produce bladder emptying and continence in select SCI patients. The biggest drawback of this technique is the need to perform a dorsal S2-4 rhizotomy, which leads to irreversible loss of reflex erection and ejaculation, to secure continence between stimulation and decrease detrusor and sphincter dyssynergy. Studies show that 80 to 90% of users can urinate on demand, with postvoid residuals of less than 50 mL; between-stimulus continence is preserved in more than 85%. Similar but less well-documented achievements have been made with regard to bowel evacuation. As for male sexual dysfunction, FES of intact anterior sacral nerve roots, especially S2, produces sustained penile erection for the duration of stimulation. Likewise, ejaculation can be generated by stimulation of the presacral sympathetic plexus. However, because other methods of achieving erection and ejaculation exist, FES systems are not typically implanted solely for treatment of male sexual dysfunction.

Advances in microelectronics, computer technologies, and neurophysiology have helped create decent FES systems. As components are miniaturized and our understanding of the physiology of myoelectric systems improves, FES systems will surely boast improved functionality and accessibility. With recent research in brain–machine interfaces showing the promise of enabling tetraplegic patients to perform motor tasks by thought, we can be optimistic about the future for SCI patients[69] (see Chapters 52 and 54 for further discussion).

■ Early Interventions after Spinal Cord Injury: Steroids and Surgical Decompression in Acute Spinal Cord Injury

For decades, the prevailing attitude about SCI was that all the damage to the CNS occurs at the time of injury and that the damage is irreversible. Hemodynamic stabilization of the trauma patient claimed top priority. Because outcomes were thought to be totally determined by the extent of initial injury, little attention was paid to examining the effect of prompt interventions, such as drugs or decompressive surgery, on the "natural course" of SCI. It is now recognized that much of the degeneration of the spinal cord after SCI is due to a multifactorial secondary injury process that occurs over minutes, to hours, to days. For instance, production of reactive oxygen-induced lipid peroxidation (LP) has been found to play a key role in this process. Demonstration of LP inhibition by the glucocortico steroid methylprednisolone (MP) in animal SCI models led to important clinical trials in humans, the results of which have been the focus of intense debate for nearly 20 years.[70–74] However, due to concerns regarding the relatively small effect sizes seen in the National Acute Spinal Cord Injury Study 2 (NASCIS-2) and NASCIS-3 trials, coupled with potential adverse effects of immunosuppression on wound healing and resistance to infection, many clinicians have questioned whether steroids should be routinely used in acute traumatic SCI. Currently, the use of steroids is not considered standard of care by several evidence-based guidelines.[70,75–78] To clarify, the guidelines committee of the AANS/CNS Joint Section on Disorders of the Spine and Peripheral Nerves concluded that use of methylprednisolone in treatment of acute SCI in adults can only be supported as a "treatment option" and not a standard of care.[75] The controversy surrounding the use of steroids is discussed in detail in Chapter 11.

Early surgical decompression for acute SCI is another area of controversy where recent research seems to be pushing practice paradigms in a new direction. Decompression of the injured spinal cord is thought to prevent or attenuate secondary injury mechanisms. This theory is supported by work done in purebred dogs,[79,80] where a time-dependent benefit in hindleg motor function from early surgical decompression done within 6 hours of injury was observed. Rabinowitz et al.[79] further showed that this effect was independent of administration of methylprednisolone.

Despite the widespread use of surgery in patients with SCI, its application varies widely. The presence and duration of a therapeutic window were merely suggested by numerous Class III and limited Class II studies.[81–83] The Surgical Treatment for Acute Spinal Cord Injury Study (STASCIS) group was formed in 1992 by the Spinal Cord Injury Committee of the Joint Section on Neurotrauma and Critical Care of the AANS and CNS, with the goal of conducting prospective, controlled trials to determine the role and timing of decompressive surgery after acute SCI.[74,84] Of the 222 patients with follow-up available at 6 months postinjury, 19.8% of patients undergoing early surgery showed a 2 grade improvement in AIS, compared to 8.8% in the late decompression group (OR = 2.57, 95% Cl:1.11,5.97). In the multivariate analysis, adjusted for preoperative neurological status and steroid administration, the odds of at least a 2 grade AIS improvement were 2.8 times higher amongst those who underwent early surgery as compared to those who underwent late surgery (OR = 2.83, 95% Cl:1.10,7.28). They concluded that "Decompression prior to 24 hours after SCI can be performed safely and is associated with improved neurologic outcome, defined as at least a 2 grade AIS improvement at 6 months follow-up."[85]

It is important to note that the STASCIS study enrolled only patients with subaxial cervical spine injury. Upon conclusion of the study and publication of the results, careful analysis must be done before any new treatment guidelines are made, but positive results may shift current practice paradigms toward more urgent management of spinal cord compression (see Chapter 27 for further discussion). It is noteworthy that a consensus panel of the Spine Trauma Study Group has recommended early intervention for patients with traumatic SCI and that this approach is favored by the vast majority of clinicians, as determined by a recently published international survey.[86,87]

References

1. Teng YD, Choi H, Onario RC, et al. Minocycline inhibits contusion-triggered mitochondrial cytochrome c release and mitigates functional deficits after spinal cord injury. Proc Natl Acad Sci USA 2004;101(9):3071–3076
2. Wells JE, Hurlbert RJ, Fehlings MG, Yong VW. Neuroprotection by minocycline facilitates significant recovery from spinal cord injury in mice. Brain 2003;126(Pt 7):1628–1637
3. Hawryluk GW, Rowland J, Kwon BK, Fehlings MG. Protection and repair of the injured spinal cord: a review of completed, ongoing, and planned clinical trials for acute spinal cord injury. Neurosurg Focus 2008;25(5):E14
4. Miller RG, Mitchell JD, Lyon M, Moore DH. Riluzole for amyotrophic lateral sclerosis (ALS)/motor neuron disease (MND). Cochrane Database Syst Rev 2007;(1):CD001447
5. Lu P, Tuszynski MH. Growth factors and combinatorial therapies for CNS regeneration. Exp Neurol 2008;209(2):313–320
6. Onose G, Anghelescu A, Muresanu DF, et al. A review of published reports on neuroprotection in spinal cord injury. Spinal Cord 2009;47(10): 716–726
7. White RE, Jakeman LB. Don't fence me in: harnessing the beneficial roles of astrocytes for spinal cord repair. Restor Neurol Neurosci 2008;26(2-3): 197–214

8. Ramon y Cajal S. Degeneration and Regeneration of the Nervous System. Vol 2. Haffner Publishing; 1928
9. Richardson PM, McGuinness UM, Aguayo AJ. Axons from CNS neurons regenerate into PNS grafts. Nature 1980;284(5753):264–265
10. Caroni P, Savio T, Schwab ME. Central nervous system regeneration: oligodendrocytes and myelin as non-permissive substrates for neurite growth. Prog Brain Res 1988;78:363–370
11. Caroni P, Schwab ME. Two membrane protein fractions from rat central myelin with inhibitory properties for neurite growth and fibroblast spreading. J Cell Biol 1988;106(4):1281–1288
12. Caroni P, Schwab ME. Antibody against myelin-associated inhibitor of neurite growth neutralizes nonpermissive substrate properties of CNS white matter. Neuron 1988;1(1):85–96
13. Bregman BS, Kunkel Bagden E, Schnell L, Dai HN, Gao D, Schwab ME. Recovery from spinal cord injury mediated by antibodies to neurite growth inhibitors. Nature 1995;378(6556): 498–501
14. Chen MS, Huber AB, van der Haar ME, et al. Nogo-A is a myelin-associated neurite outgrowth inhibitor and an antigen for monoclonal antibody IN-1. Nature 2000;403(6768):434–439
15. Rolls A, Shechter R, Schwartz M. The bright side of the glial scar in CNS repair. Nat Rev Neurosci 2009;10(3):235–241
16. Yiu G, He Z. Glial inhibition of CNS axon regeneration. Nat Rev Neurosci 2006;7(8):617–627
17. McKerracher L, Higuchi H. Targeting Rho to stimulate repair after spinal cord injury. J Neurotrauma 2006;23(3-4):309–317
18. Dergham P, Ellezam B, Essagian C, Avedissian H, Lubell WD, McKerracher L. Rho signaling pathway targeted to promote spinal cord repair. J Neurosci 2002;22(15):6570–6577
19. Maier IC, Ichiyama RM, Courtine G, et al. Differential effects of anti-Nogo-A antibody treatment and treadmill training in rats with incomplete spinal cord injury. Brain 2009;132(Pt 6): 1426–1440
20. Cizkova D, Kakinohana O, Kucharova K, et al. Functional recovery in rats with ischemic paraplegia after spinal grafting of human spinal stem cells. Neuroscience 2007;147(2):546–560
21. Yan J, Xu L, Welsh AM, et al. Extensive neuronal differentiation of human neural stem cell grafts in adult rat spinal cord. PLoS Med 2007;4(2): e39
22. Xu XM, Onifer SM. Transplantation-mediated strategies to promote axonal regeneration following spinal cord injury. Respir Physiol Neurobiol 2009;169(2):171–182
23. Horner PJ, Power AE, Kempermann G, et al. Proliferation and differentiation of progenitor cells throughout the intact adult rat spinal cord. J Neurosci 2000;20(6):2218–2228
24. Kondo T, Raff M. Chromatin remodeling and histone modification in the conversion of oligodendrocyte precursors to neural stem cells. Genes Dev 2004;18(23):2963–2972
25. Carlén M, Meletis K, Barnabé-Heider F, Frisén J. Genetic visualization of neurogenesis. Exp Cell Res 2006;312(15):2851–2859
26. Ohori Y, Yamamoto S, Nagao M, et al. Growth factor treatment and genetic manipulation stimulate neurogenesis and oligodendrogenesis by endogenous neural progenitors in the injured adult spinal cord. J Neurosci 2006;26(46):11948–11960
27. Shechter R, London A, Varol C, et al. Infiltrating blood-derived macrophages are vital cells playing an anti-inflammatory role in recovery from spinal cord injury in mice. PLoS Med 2009;6(7):e1000113
28. Luo J, Zhang HT, Jiang XD, Xue S, Ke YQ. Combination of bone marrow stromal cell transplantation with mobilization by granulocyte-colony stimulating factor promotes functional recovery after spinal cord transection. Acta Neurochir (Wien) 2009;151(11):1483–1492
29. Knoller N, Auerbach G, Fulga V, et al. Clinical experience using incubated autologous macrophages as a treatment for complete spinal cord injury: phase I study results. J Neurosurg Spine 2005;3(3):173–181
30. Ziv Y, Avidan H, Pluchino S, Martino G, Schwartz M. Synergy between immune cells and adult neural stem/progenitor cells promotes functional recovery from spinal cord injury. Proc Natl Acad Sci U S A 2006;103(35):13174–13179
31. Moviglia GA, Varela G, Brizuela JA, et al. Case report on the clinical results of a combined cellular therapy for chronic spinal cord injured patients. Spinal Cord 2009;47(6):499–503
32. Thomas SL, Gorassini MA. Increases in corticospinal tract function by treadmill training after incomplete spinal cord injury. J Neurophysiol 2005;94(4):2844–2855
33. Winchester P, McColl R, Querry R, et al. Changes in supraspinal activation patterns following robotic locomotor therapy in motor-incomplete spinal cord injury. Neurorehabil Neural Repair 2005;19(4):313–324
34. Zaporozhets E, Cowley KC, Schmidt BJ. Propriospinal neurons contribute to bulbospinal transmission of the locomotor command signal in the neonatal rat spinal cord. J Physiol 2006;572(Pt 2):443–458
35. Courtine G, Song B, Roy RR, et al. Recovery of supraspinal control of stepping via indirect propriospinal relay connections after spinal cord injury. Nat Med 2008;14(1):69–74
36. Cowley KC, Zaporozhets E, Schmidt BJ. Propriospinal neurons are sufficient for bulbospinal transmission of the locomotor command signal in the neonatal rat spinal cord. J Physiol 2008;586(6): 1623–1635
37. Perez MA, Field-Fote EC, Floeter MK. Patterned sensory stimulation induces plasticity in reciprocal Ia inhibition in humans. J Neurosci 2003;23(6):2014–2018
38. Thompson AK, Chen XY, Wolpaw JR. Acquisition of a simple motor skill: task-dependent adaptation plus long-term change in the human soleus H-reflex. J Neurosci 2009;29(18):5784–5792

39. Wolpaw JR. Spinal cord plasticity in acquisition and maintenance of motor skills. Acta Physiol (Oxf) 2007;189(2):155–169
40. Beekhuizen KS, Field-Fote EC. Massed practice versus massed practice with stimulation: effects on upper extremity function and cortical plasticity in individuals with incomplete cervical spinal cord injury. Neurorehabil Neural Repair 2005;19(1):33–45
41. Belci M, Catley M, Husain M, Frankel HL, Davey NJ. Magnetic brain stimulation can improve clinical outcome in incomplete spinal cord injured patients. Spinal Cord 2004;42(7):417–419
42. Fregni F, Boggio PS, Lima MC, et al. A sham-controlled, phase II trial of transcranial direct current stimulation for the treatment of central pain in traumatic spinal cord injury. Pain 2006;122(1-2):197–209
43. Fregni F, Pascual-Leone A. Technology insight: noninvasive brain stimulation in neurology-perspectives on the therapeutic potential of rTMS and tDCS. Nat Clin Pract Neurol 2007;3(7):383–393
44. Huang YZ, Edwards MJ, Rounis E, Bhatia KP, Rothwell JC. Theta burst stimulation of the human motor cortex. Neuron 2005;45(2):201–206
45. Stefan K, Kunesch E, Cohen LG, Benecke R, Classen J. Induction of plasticity in the human motor cortex by paired associative stimulation. Brain 2000;123(Pt 3):572–584
46. Talelli P, Greenwood RJ, Rothwell JC. Exploring Theta Burst Stimulation as an intervention to improve motor recovery in chronic stroke. Clin Neurophysiol 2007;118(2):333–342
47. Valero-Cabré A, Pascual-Leone A. Impact of TMS on the primary motor cortex and associated spinal systems. IEEE Eng Med Biol Mag 2005;24(1):29–35
48. Valle AC, Dionisio K, Pitskel NB, et al. Low and high frequency repetitive transcranial magnetic stimulation for the treatment of spasticity. Dev Med Child Neurol 2007;49(7):534–538
49. Grillner S, McClellan A, Sigvardt K, Wallén P. On the spinal generation of locomotion, with particular reference to a simple vertebrate: the lamprey. Birth Defects Orig Artic Ser 1983;19(4):347–356
50. Barrière G, Leblond H, Provencher J, Rossignol S. Prominent role of the spinal central pattern generator in the recovery of locomotion after partial spinal cord injuries. J Neurosci 2008;28(15): 3976–3987
51. Rossignol S, Barrière G, Alluin O, Frigon A. Reexpression of locomotor function after partial spinal cord injury. Physiology (Bethesda) 2009; 24:127–139
52. Nadeau S, Jacquemin G, Fournier C, Lamarre Y, Rossignol S. Spontaneous motor rhythms of the back and legs in a patient with a complete spinal cord transection. Neurorehabil Neural Repair 2010;24(4):377–383
53. Minassian K, Persy I, Rattay F, Pinter MM, Kern H, Dimitrijevic MR. Human lumbar cord circuitries can be activated by extrinsic tonic input to generate locomotor-like activity. Hum Mov Sci 2007;26(2):275–295
54. Dietz V. Spinal cord pattern generators for locomotion. Clin Neurophysiol 2003;114(8): 1379–1389
55. Dimitrijevic MR, Gerasimenko Y, Pinter MM. Evidence for a spinal central pattern generator in humans. Ann N Y Acad Sci 1998;860:360–376
56. Calancie B. Spinal myoclonus after spinal cord injury. J Spinal Cord Med 2006;29(4):413–424
57. Behrman AL, Nair PM, Bowden MG, et al. Locomotor training restores walking in a nonambulatory child with chronic, severe, incomplete cervical spinal cord injury. Phys Ther 2008;88(5):580–590
58. Sadowsky CL, McDonald JW. Activity-based restorative therapies: concepts and applications in spinal cord injury-related neurorehabilitation. Dev Disabil Res Rev 2009;15(2):112–116
59. Tator CH, Fehlings MG. Review of the secondary injury theory of acute spinal cord trauma with emphasis on vascular mechanisms. J Neurosurg 1991;75(1):15–26
60. Vale FL, Burns J, Jackson AB, Hadley MN. Combined medical and surgical treatment after acute spinal cord injury: results of a prospective pilot study to assess the merits of aggressive medical resuscitation and blood pressure management. J Neurosurg 1997;87(2):239–246
61. Ploumis A, Yadlapalli N, Fehlings MG, Kwon BK, Vaccaro AR. A systematic review of the evidence supporting a role for vasopressor support in acute SCI. Spinal Cord 2010;48(5):356–362
62. Ahn H, Fehlings MG. Prevention, identification, and treatment of perioperative spinal cord injury. Neurosurg Focus 2008;25(5):E15
63. Management of acute central cervical spinal cord injuries. Neurosurgery 2002;50(3, Suppl): S166–S172
64. Blood pressure management after acute spinal cord injury. Neurosurgery 2002;50(3, Suppl): S58–S62
65. Creasey GH, Grill JH, Korsten M, et al; Implanted Neuroprosthesis Research Group. An implantable neuroprosthesis for restoring bladder and bowel control to patients with spinal cord injuries: a multicenter trial. Arch Phys Med Rehabil 2001;82(11):1512–1519
66. Hamid S, Hayek R. Role of electrical stimulation for rehabilitation and regeneration after spinal cord injury: an overview. Eur Spine J 2008;17(9):1256–1269
67. Ragnarsson KT. Functional electrical stimulation after spinal cord injury: current use, therapeutic effects and future directions. Spinal Cord 2008;46(4):255–274
68. Glenn WW, Brouillette RT, Dentz B, et al. Fundamental considerations in pacing of the diaphragm for chronic ventilatory insufficiency: a multi-center study. Pacing Clin Electrophysiol 1988;11(11 Pt 2):2121–2127
69. Hochberg LR, Serruya MD, Friehs GM, et al. Neuronal ensemble control of prosthetic devices by a human with tetraplegia. Nature 2006;442(7099):164–171
70. Fehlings MG; Spine Focus Panel. Summary statement: the use of methylprednisolone in acute spinal cord injury. Spine (Phila Pa 1976) 2001;26(24, Suppl):S55
71. Bracken MB, Holford TR. Neurological and functional status 1 year after acute spinal cord injury: estimates of functional recovery in National Acute Spinal Cord Injury Study II from results modeled

in National Acute Spinal Cord Injury Study III. J Neurosurg 2002; 96(3, Suppl)259–266
72. Bracken MB, Shepard MJ, Collins WF Jr, et al. Methylprednisolone or naloxone treatment after acute spinal cord injury: 1-year follow-up data: results of the Second National Acute Spinal Cord Injury Study. J Neurosurg 1992;76(1):23–31
73. Bracken MB, Shepard MJ, Collins WF, et al. A randomized, controlled trial of methylprednisolone or naloxone in the treatment of acute spinal-cord injury: results of the Second National Acute Spinal Cord Injury Study. N Engl J Med 1990;322(20):1405–1411
74. Baptiste DC, Fehlings MG. Update on the treatment of spinal cord injury. Prog Brain Res 2007;161:217–233
75. Pharmacological therapy after acute cervical spinal cord injury. Neurosurgery 2002;50(3, Suppl):S63–S72
76. Hugenholtz H. Methylprednisolone for acute spinal cord injury: not a standard of care. CMAJ 2003;168(9):1145–1146
77. Hurlbert RJ. Methylprednisolone for acute spinal cord injury: an inappropriate standard of care. J Neurosurg 2000;93(1, Suppl):1–7
78. Sayer FT, Kronvall E, Nilsson OG. Methylprednisolone treatment in acute spinal cord injury: the myth challenged through a structured analysis of published literature. Spine J 2006;6(3):335–343
79. Rabinowitz RS, Eck JC, Harper CM Jr, et al. Urgent surgical decompression compared to methylprednisolone for the treatment of acute spinal cord injury: a randomized prospective study in beagle dogs. Spine (Phila Pa 1976) 2008;33(21): 2260–2268
80. Delamarter RB, Sherman J, Carr JB. Pathophysiology of spinal cord injury: recovery after immediate and delayed decompression. J Bone Joint Surg Am 1995;77(7):1042–1049
81. Fehlings MG, Perrin RG. The role and timing of early decompression for cervical spinal cord injury: update with a review of recent clinical evidence. Injury 2005;36(Suppl 2):B13–B26
82. Fehlings MG, Perrin RG. The timing of surgical intervention in the treatment of spinal cord injury: a systematic review of recent clinical evidence. Spine (Phila Pa 1976) 2006;31(11, Suppl):S28–S35, discussion S36
83. Fehlings MG, Tator CH. An evidence-based review of decompressive surgery in acute spinal cord injury: rationale, indications, and timing based on experimental and clinical studies. J Neurosurg 1999;91(1, Suppl):1–11
84. Ng WP, Fehlings MG, Cuddy B, et al. Surgical Treatment for Acute Spinal Cord Injury Study pilot study #2: evaluation of protocol for decompressive surgery within 8 hours of injury. Neurosurg Focus 1999;6(1):e3
85. Fehlings MG, Vacarro A, Wilson JR, Singh A, Cadotte D, Harrop JS, et al. Early versus delayed decompression for traumatic cervical spinal cord injury: results of the Surgical Timing in Acute Spinal Cord Injury Study (STASCIS). PLoS ONE 2012;7(2):e32037
86. Fehlings MG, Wilson JR. Timing of surgical intervention in spinal trauma: what does the evidence indicate? Spine (Phila Pa 1976) 2010;35(21, Suppl):S159–S160
87. Fehlings MG, Rabin D, Sears W, Cadotte DW, Aarabi B. Current practice in the timing of surgical intervention in spinal cord injury. Spine (Phila Pa 1976) 2010;35(21, Suppl):S166–S173

Index

Note: Page numbers followed by *f* and *t* indicate figures and tables, respectively.

B

C

Index

D

E

F

G

H

I

M

S

T

V

W

Y

Z